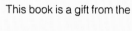

INFECTIOUS DISEASES and ANTIMICROBIAL THERAPY of the EARS, NOSE and THROAT

INFECTIOUS DISEASES and ANTIMICROBIAL THERAPY of the EARS, NOSE and THROAT

Jonas T. Johnson, M.D., F.A.C.S.

Professor
Departments of Otolaryngology and Radiation Oncology
The University of Pittsburgh School of Medicine
Pittsburgh, Pennsylvania

Victor L. Yu, M.D.

Professor
Department of Medicine
The University of Pittsburgh School of Medicine
Chief, Infectious Disease Section
Veterans Affairs Medical Center
Pittsburgh, Pennsylvania

W.B. SAUNDERS COMPANY
A Division of Harcourt Brace & Company
Philadelphia London Toronto Montreal Sydney Tokyo

W.B. SAUNDERS COMPANY
A Division of Harcourt Brace & Company

The Curtis Center
Independence Square West
Philadelphia, Pennsylvania 19106

Library of Congress Cataloging-in-Publication Data

Infectious diseases and antimicrobial therapy of the ears, nose and throat / [edited by] Jonas T. Johnson, Victor L. Yu.—1st ed.

    p.   cm.

ISBN 0–7216–6154–8

1. Communicable diseases.   2. Ear—Diseases.   3. Nose—Diseases.
4. Throat—Diseases.   5. Anti-infective agents.   I. Johnson, Jonas T.
II. Yu, Victor L.
[DNLM: 1. Otorhinolaryngologic Diseases—drug therapy.
2. Communicable Diseases—drug therapy   3. Antibiotics—therapeutic use.
WV 140 I43 1997]

RF49.I53I55 1997   617.5′ 1061—dc20

DNLM/DLC   96–7414

INFECTIOUS DISEASES AND ANTIMICROBIAL THERAPY OF
THE EARS, NOSE AND THROAT   ISBN 0–7216–6154–8

Printed in the United States of America.

Last digit is the print number: 9   8   7   6   5   4   3   2   1

This textbook is dedicated to our families,
who have provided the
continuing support to make this book a successful project.

Janis C. Johnson
Olin, Rurik, and Ivar Johnson

Deborah Yu
Chen and Ting Yu

Contributors

JACK ANON, M.D.
Assistant Clinical Professor, Department of Otolaryngology, The University of Pittsburgh School of Medicine, Pittsburgh, Pennsylvania
Prophylaxis for Sinonasal Surgery

ROBERT D. ARBEIT, M.D.
Professor of Medicine, Boston University School of Medicine, Boston, Massachusetts; Associate Chief of Staff for Research, Veterans Administration Medical Center, Boston, Massachusetts
Staphylococcus aureus

EURICO ARRUDA, Ph.D., M.D.
Research Assistant Professor, Department of Internal Medicine, University of Virginia School of Medicine, Charlottesville, Virginia
Antiviral Agents

MICHAEL C. BACH, M.D.
Clinical Professor of Medicine, University of South Florida School of Medicine, Tampa, Florida; Hospital Epidemiologist, Manatee Memorial Hospital, Bradenton, Florida; Attending Physician, Infectious Disease, Sarasota Memorial Hospital and Doctors Hospital of Sarasota, Sarasota, Florida; L.W. Blake Hospital, Bradenton, Florida
Nocardia

ALDONA L. BALTCH, M.D.
Professor of Medicine, Professor of Pharmacology, Albany Medical College, Albany, New York; Chief, Infectious Disease Section, Stratton Veterans Administration Medical Center, Albany, New York
Pseudomonas aeruginosa and Aerobic Gram-Negative Bacilli

IRMGARD BEHLAU, M.D.
Research Associate, Department of Molecular Biology and Microbiology, Tufts University School of Medicine, Boston, Massachusetts
Antimycobacterial Agents; Mycobacterial Diseases: Tuberculosis, Leprosy, and Other Mycobacterial Infections

SUZANNE BELFIGLIO, Pharm.D.
Clinical Pharmacist, The University of Pittsburgh School of Medicine, Pittsburgh, Pennsylvania
Quinolones

DAVID F. BENNHOFF, M.D.
Assistant Clinical Professor, Otolaryngology, Case Western Reserve University, Cleveland, Ohio; Chief of Otolaryngology, Lakewood Hospital, Cleveland, Ohio
Actinomycosis

STEPHEN A. BERGER, M.D.
Associate Professor of Medicine, Tel Aviv University, Sackler School of Medicine, Tel Aviv, Israel; Director of Microbiology and Geographic Medicine, Tel Aviv Medical Center, Tel Aviv, Israel
Thyroid Infections

JOEL BERNSTEIN, Ph.D., M.D.
Associate Clinical Professor of Otolaryngology and Pediatrics, State University of New York School of Medicine and Biomedical Sciences, New York
Prophylaxis for Sinonasal Surgery

ANDREW BLITZER, M.D., D.D.S.
Professor of Clinical Otolaryngology, Director, Division of Head and Neck Surgery, College of Physicians and Surgeons of Columbia University, New York, New York; Senior Attending Otolaryngologist and Director, New York Center for Voice and Swallowing Disorders, St. Luke's/Roosevelt Hospital Center, New York, New York
Fungal Sinusitis; Sialadenitis

CHARLES D. BLUESTONE, M.D.
Professor, Department of Otolaryngology, The University of Pittsburgh School of Medicine, Pittsburgh, Pennsylvania; Director, Department of Pediatric Otolaryngology, Children's Hospital of Pittsburgh, Pittsburgh, Pennsylvania
Otitis Media

DENNIS I. BOJRAB, M.D.
Clinical Professor, Department of Otolaryngology, Wayne State University, Detroit, Michigan; Chief, Department of Otolaryngology, William Beaumont Hospital, Royal Oak, Michigan; Director, Skull Base Surgery and Resident Education, Providence Hospital, Southfield, Michigan
External Otitis

ITZHAK BROOK, M.D., M.Sc.
Professor of Pediatrics, Georgetown University School of Medicine, Washington, D.C.; Staff Physician and Consultant Infectious Diseases, Naval Medical Center, Bethesda, Maryland; Hospital for Sick Children, Washington, D.C.
Miscellaneous Antibacterial: Chloramphenicol, Clindamycin, Metronidazole; Oropharyngeal Anaerobes

THOMAS E. BRUDERLY, D.O.
Chief Resident Otolaryngology, Flint Osteopathic Hospital, Flint, Michigan
External Otitis

DIANE M. CAPPELLETTY, Pharm.D.
Assistant Professor, College of Pharmacy and Allied Health Professions, Wayne State University, Detroit, Michigan
Aminoglycosides

VINCENT N. CARRASCO, M.D.
Assistant Professor of Surgery, University of North Carolina School of Medicine, Chapel Hill, North Carolina; Chief, Section of Otology, Neurotology, and Skull Base Surgery, University of North Carolina at Chapel Hill, North Carolina
Mastoiditis

JAMES D. CHERRY, M.D., M.Sc.
Professor of Pediatrics, UCLA School of Medicine, Los Angeles, California; Attending Physician, UCLA Children's Hospital and UCLA Medical Center, Los Angeles, California
Whooping Cough (Pertussis)

CHEN-CHIA CHIOU, M.D.
Lecturer, School of Medicine, National Yang-Ming University, Taipei, Taiwan; Attending Physician, Department of Pediatrics, Veterans General Hospital—Kaohsiung, Kaohsiung, Taiwan
Diphtheria

RICHARD A. CHOLE, Ph.D., M.D.
Professor and Chair, Department of Otolaryngology, University of California at Davis, School of Medicine, Davis, California; Director of Ear, Nose, Throat and Head and Head and Neck Surgery, University of California at Davis, Medical Center, Sacramento, California
Prophylaxis for Oral Surgery and Fractures of the Facial Skeleton

ANTHONY W. CHOW, M.D.
Professor of Medicine, Division of Infectious Diseases, Department of Medicine, University of British Columbia, Vancouver, British Columbia, Canada; Consultant, Division of Infectious Diseases, Department of Medicine, Vancouver Hospital Health Sciences Center, Vancouver, British Columbia, Canada
Orofacial Infections; Odontogenic Infections

MARTHA E. CORCORAN, M.D.
Assistant Professor of Clinical Otolaryngology, University of California at Davis, School of Medicine, Davis, California; Chief, Division of Otolaryngology, Veterans Administration System Clinics and Merrithew Memorial Hospital, Martinez, California
Prophylaxis for Oral Surgery and Fractures of the Facial Skeleton

ROBIN T. COTTON, M.D.
Professor of Otolaryngology–Head and Neck Surgery, University of Cincinnati College of Medicine, Cincinnati, Ohio; Director, Pediatric Otolaryngology and Maxillofacial Surgery, Children's Hospital Medical Center, Cincinnati, Ohio
Supraglottitis

THOMAS M. DANIEL, M.D.
Professor Emeritus, Case Western Reserve University School of Medicine, Cleveland, Ohio
Antimycobacterial Agents; Mycobacterial Diseases: Tuberculosis, Leprosy, and Other Mycobacterial Infections

ANNE DAVIS, M.B. Cl.B.
Honorary Clinical Tutor, Faculty of Medicine, Southampton University, Southampton, England; Consultant Otolaryngologist/Head and Neck Surgeon, Associate Clinical Director, Portsmouth Hospitals Trust, Portsmouth, England
Postoperative Meningitis

GARY V. DOERN, Ph.D.
Professor of Medicine, Pathology, and Molecular Genetics and Microbiology, University of Massachusetts Medical Center, Worcester, Massachusetts; Director, Clinical Microbiology Laboratories, University of Massachusetts Medical Center, Worcester, Massachusetts
Laboratory Diagnosis of Infectious Diseases

GEORGE M. ELIOPOULOS, M.D.
Associate Professor of Medicine, Harvard Medical School, Boston, Massachusetts; Assistant Chairman, Department of Medicine, Deaconess Hospital, Boston, Massachusetts
Vancomycin

ANN R. FALSEY, M.D.
Assistant Professor of Medicine, University of Rochester School of Medicine and Dentistry, Rochester, New York; Attending Physician, Rochester General Hospital, Rochester, New York
Viruses

JOACHIM FORSGREN, Ph.D., M.D.
Karolinska Institute, Division of Otorhinolaryngology, Huddinge Hospital, Stockholm, Sweden; Consultant, Ear, Nose, and Throat Surgeon, ENT Clinic, Huddinge Hospital, Stockholm, Sweden
The Microbe

IAN R. FRIEDLAND, M.D.
Director, Pediatric Infectious Diseases, Department of Pediatrics, Bragwanath Hospital and the University of Witwatersrand, Johannesburg, South Africa
Streptococci Including S. pneumoniae

DALE N. GERDING, M.D.
Professor and Associate Chair, Department of Medicine, Northwestern University Medical School, Chicago, Illinois; Chief, Medical Service, Veterans Administration Lakeside Medical Center, Chicago, Illinois
Nosocomial Diarrhea

PAUL W. GIDLEY, M.D.
Assistant Professor, Department of Otolaryngology—Head and Neck Surgery, University of Texas Medical School at Houston, Houston, Texas
Deep Neck Space Infections

STEVEN GOLD, M.D.
Resident, Department of Otolaryngology—Head and Neck Surgery, University of Cincinnati College of Medicine, Cincinnati, Ohio
AIDS in Otolaryngology

LUCIANO Z. GOLDANI, M.D., Ph.D.
Assistant Professor of Medicine, Infectious Diseases, Faculty of Medicine, Universidade Federal do Rio Grande do Sul, Porto Alegre, Brazil; Research Associate, Conselho, Brazil
Dimorphic and Miscellaneous Fungi

JENNIFER RUBIN GRANDIS, M.D.
Assistant Professor, Department of Otolaryngology, The University of Pittsburgh School of Medicine, Pittsburgh, Pennsylvania
Quinolones; Necrotizing (Malignant) External Otitis

KENNETH M. GRUNDFAST, M.D.
Professor, George Washington University School of Medicine, Department of Surgery and Department of Pediatrics, Washington, D.C.; Senior Attending Physician, Vice Chairman, Otolaryngology Department, Director, Hearing Disorders Clinic, Children's National Medical Center, Washington, D.C.
Tonsillitis

JACK M. GWALTNEY, M.D.
Professor of Medicine, Head, Division of Epidemiology and Virology, Wade Hampton Frost Professor of Epidemiology, University of Virginia Health Sciences Center, Charlottesville, Virginia
Management of Acute Sinusitis in Adults

CAROLINE BREESE HALL, M.D.
Professor of Pediatrics and Medicine in Infectious Diseases, University of Rochester School of Medicine and Dentistry, Rochester, New York
Viruses

MARGARET R. HAMMERSCHLAG, M.D.
Professor of Pediatrics and Medicine, Codirector, Pediatric Infectious Diseases, State University of New York Health Science Center at Brooklyn, Brooklyn, New York; Active Attending Physician, Kings County Hospital Center, Brooklyn, New York
Chlamydia

ULRICH HEININGER, M.D.
Assistant Professor, University of Erlangen-Nürnberg Medical School, Erlangen, Germany; Attending Physician, University Hospital for Children and Adolescents, Erlangen, Germany
Whooping Cough (Pertussis)

LINDEN T. HU, M.D.
Instructor in Medicine, Tufts University School of Medicine, Boston, Massachusetts; New England Medical Center, Boston, Massachusetts
Lyme Disease

C. GARY JACKSON, M.D.
Clinical Professor, Department of Surgery, Division of Otolaryngology—Head and Neck Surgery, University of North Carolina School of Medicine, Chapel Hill, North Carolina; Clinical Professor, Department of Otolaryngology—Head and Neck Surgery; Clinical Professor of Hearing and Speech Sciences, Vanderbilt University School of Medicine, Nashville, Tennessee
Antibiotic Prophylaxis in Otology and Neurotology

ALAN P. JOHNSON, Ph.D.
Clinical Scientist, Antibiotic Reference Unit, Central Public Health Laboratory, London, England
Enterococci

JONAS T. JOHNSON, M.D.
Professor, Departments of Otolaryngology and Radiation Oncology, The University of Pittsburgh School of Medicine, Pittsburgh, Pennsylvania
Special Problems in Sinusitis; Management of Postoperative Head and Neck Wound Infections; Principles of Antibiotic Prophylaxis; Prophylaxis for Contaminated Head and Neck Cranial Base Surgery

STUART JOHNSON, M.D., D.T.M. & H.
Assistant Professor, Department of Medicine, Northwestern University Medical School, Chicago, Illinois; Staff Physician, Infectious Disease Section, Veterans Administration Lakeside Medical Center, Chicago, Illinois
Nosocomial Diarrhea

CAROL A. KAUFFMAN, M.D.
Professor of Internal Medicine, University of Michigan Medical School, Ann Arbor, Michigan; Chief, Infectious Diseases Section, Veterans Administration Medical Center, Ann Arbor, Michigan
Antifungal Agents

JAMES D. KELLNER, M.D.
Assistant Professor of Pediatrics, University of Calgary, Calgary, Alberta, Canada; Staff Physician, Division of Infectious Diseases, Department of Pediatrics, Alberta Children's Hospital, Calgary, Alberta, Canada
Cervical Lymphadenitis

MARGARET A. KENNA, M.D.
Associate Professor of Otology and Laryngology, Harvard Medical School, Boston, Massachusetts; Associate in Otolaryngology, Department of Otolaryngology, Children's Hospital, Boston, Massachusetts
Laryngotracheobronchitis

JEROME O. KLEIN, M.D.
Professor of Pediatrics, Boston University School of Medicine, Boston, Massachusetts; Director, Division of Pediatric Infectious Diseases, Maxwell Finland Laboratory for Infectious Diseases, Department of Pediatrics, Boston City Hospital, Boston, Massachusetts
Haemophilus influenzae

MARK S. KLEMPNER, M.D.
Professor of Medicine, Tufts University School of Medicine, Boston, Massachusetts; Vice Chairman, Department of Medicine, New England Medical Center, Boston, Massachusetts
Lyme Disease

WILLIAM LAWSON, M.D., D.D.S.
Professor of Otolaryngology, Mt. Sinai School of Medicine, New York, New York; Attending Otolaryngologist, Mt. Sinai Medical Center, New York, New York; Director, Otolaryngology Service, Bronx Veterans Administration Hospital, Bronx, New York
Fungal Sinusitis; Sialadenitis

NORRIS K. LEE, M.D.
Assistant Professor, Department of Otorhinolaryngology—Head and Neck Surgery, Cornell University Medical Center, New York, New York
Complications of Sinusitis

PETER LEES, M.B., Ch.B., M.S.
Senior Lecturer in Neurosurgery, Faculty of Medicine, Southampton University, Southampton, England; Director of Research and Development, Honorary Consultant Neurosurgeon, Southampton University Hospitals NHS Trust, Southampton, England
Postoperative Meningitis

STEPHEN A. LERNER, M.D.
Professor of Medicine, Wayne State University School of Medicine, Detroit, Michigan
Aminoglycosides

MATTHEW E. LEVISON, M.D.
Professor of Medicine, Chief, Division of Infectious Diseases, Medical College of Pennsylvania and Hahnemann University, Philadelphia, Pennsylvania
Prophylaxis for Bacterial Endocarditis

JOHN Y. LIM, M.D.
Resident, Department of Otolaryngology, University of California at Davis
Prophylaxis for Oral Surgery and Fractures of the Facial Skeleton

CHIEN LIU, M.D.
Professor Emeritus of Medicine and Pediatrics, University of Kansas Medical Center, Kansas City, Kansas
Mycoplasma pneumoniae

JOSEPH P. LYNCH, III, M.D.
Professor of Internal Medicine, University of Michigan Medical Center, Ann Arbor, Michigan; Professor of Internal Medicine, Division of Pulmonary and Critical Care Medicine, University of Michigan Medical Center, Ann Arbor, Michigan
Nosocomial Pneumonia

RICHARD L. MABRY, M.D.
Professor, Department of Otolaryngology—Head and Neck Surgery, University of Texas Southwestern Medical Center, Dallas, Texas
Complications of Sinusitis

GERALD L. MANDELL, M.D.
Owen R. Cheatham Professor of the Sciences, Professor of Medicine, and Chief, Division of Infectious Diseases, University of Virginia School of Medicine, Charlottesville, Virginia; Attending Physician, University of Virginia Hospital, Charlottesville, Virginia
Beta-Lactam Antibiotics: Penicillins and Cephalosporins

GEORGE H. McCRACKEN, M.D.
Professor of Pediatrics, The Sarah M. and Charles E. Seay Chair in Pediatric Infectious Diseases, University of Texas Southwestern Medical Center, Dallas, Texas; Attending Physician, Children's Medical Center, Dallas, Texas
Streptococci Including S. pneumoniae

LUTFIYE MULAZIMOGLU, M.D.
Instructor in Infectious Disease, Marmara University School of Medicine, Department of Medicine, Section of Infectious Diseases, Istanbul, Turkey
Macrolides

M. HONG NGUYEN, M.D.
Assistant Professor of Medicine, University of Florida College of Medicine; Gainesville Veterans Administration Medical Center, Gainesville, Florida
Aspergillus; Candida

DAVID P. NICOLAU, Pharm.D.
Associate Clinical Professor, University of Connecticut School of Pharmacy, Storrs, Connecticut; Coordinator for Research, Department of Medicine, Division of Infectious Diseases and Pharmacy, Hartford Hospital, Hartford, Connecticut
Pharmacokinetic and Pharmacodynamic Principles in Antibiotic Usage

CHARLES H. NIGHTINGALE, Ph.D.
Research Professor, University of Connecticut School of Pharmacy, Storrs, Connecticut; Vice-President for Research, Hartford Hospital, Hartford, Connecticut
Pharmacokinetic and Pharmacodynamic Principles in Antibiotic Usage

LISBETH K. NORDSTROM-LERNER, M.D.
Infection Control Department, Sinai Hospital, Detroit, Michigan
Aminoglycosides

S. RAGNAR NORRBY, M.D., Ph.D.
Professor and Chairman, Department of Infectious Diseases, University Hospital of Lund, Lund, Sweden
Beta-Lactam Antibiotics: Monobactams, Carbapenems

PEARAY L. OGRA, M.D.
Professor, University of Texas Medical Branch, Galveston, Texas; Chairman of Pediatrics, John Sealy Distinguished Chair in Pediatrics, Children's Hospital, Galveston, Texas
Host Defense

JANAK A. PATEL, M.D.
Associate Professor, University of Texas Medical Branch, Galveston, Texas; Consultant, Pediatric Infectious Diseases, Children's Hospital, Galveston, Texas
Host Defense

WILLIAM A. PETRI, JR., Ph.D., M.D.
Professor, Internal Medicine, Microbiology, and Pathology, University of Virginia School of Medicine, Charlottesville, Virginia; Attending Physician and Associate Director of Clinical Microbiology, University of Virginia Hospital, Charlottesville, Virginia
Beta-Lactam Antibiotics: Penicillins and Cephalosporins

MICHAEL E. PICHICHERO, M.D.
Professor of Microbiology and Immunology, Professor of Pediatrics, and Professor of Medicine, University of Rochester, Rochester, New York
Group A Beta-Hemolytic Streptococcal Tonsillopharyngitis

HAROLD C. PILLSBURY, M.D.
Professor and Chief, Thomas J. Dark Distinguished Professor of Surgery; Division of Otolaryngology and Head and Neck Surgery, University of North Carolina School of Medicine, Chapel Hill, North Carolina; Attending Physician and Surgeon, University of North Carolina Hospitals, Chapel Hill, North Carolina
Mastoiditis

RICHARD QUINTILIANI, M.D., Ph.D.
Professor of Medicine, University of Connecticut School of Medicine, Farmington, Connecticut; Director, Anti-Infective Research and Pharmacoeconomic Studies, Hartford Hospital, Hartford, Connecticut
Pharmacokinetic and Pharmacodynamic Principles in Antibiotic Usage

J. MARK REED, M.D.
Clinical Assistant Professor of Surgery (Otolaryngology), University of Mississippi Medical Center, Jackson, Mississippi
Supraglottitis

ANTHONY REINO, M.D.

Assistant Professor of Clinical Otolaryngology, Department of Otolaryngology—Head and Neck Surgery, Mt. Sinai School of Medicine, New York, New York; Staff Physician, Veterans Affairs Medical Center, Bronx, New York; Assistant Attending Physician, Mt. Sinai Medical Center, New York, New York; Attending Physician, Veterans Affairs Medical Center, Bronx, New York; Assistant Attending Physician, City Hospital Center, Elmhurst, New York
Sialadenitis

HEIDI D. REMULLA, M.D.

Fellow, Ophthalmic Plastics and Orbital Surgery, Massachusetts Eye and Ear Infirmary, Boston, Massachusetts
Dacryocystitis

MICHAEL RONTAL, M.D.

Associate Clinical Professor, Department of Otolaryngology—Head and Neck Surgery, University of Michigan Medical School, Ann Arbor, Michigan
Prophylaxis for Sinonasal Surgery

PETER A.D. RUBIN, M.D.

Director, Eye Plastics and Orbit Center, Massachusetts Eye and Ear Infirmary, Boston, Massachusetts
Dacryocystitis

BRITTA RYNNEL-DAGÖÖ, Ph.D., M.D.

Associate Professor, Karolinska Institute, ENT Clinic, Huddinge Hospital, Stockholm, Sweden
The Microbe

ANDERS SAMUELSON, Ph.D., M.D.

Karolinska Institute, Division of Clinical Bacteriology, Huddinge Hospital, Stockholm, Sweden
The Microbe

MOSELIO SCHAECHTER, Ph.D.

Distinguished Professor Emeritus, Tufts University School of Medicine, Boston, Massachusetts; Adjunct Professor, San Diego State University, San Diego, California
Establishment of Infectious Diseases

NINA SINGH, M.D.

Director, HIV Clinic, and Chief, Transplant Infectious Diseases, Veterans Administration Medical Center, Pittsburgh, Pennsylvania
AIDS in Otolaryngology

RAYMOND P. SMITH, M.D.

Associate Professor of Medicine, Albany Medical College, Albany, New York; Assistant Chief, Infectious Disease Section, Stratton Veterans Administration Medical Center, Albany, New York
Pseudomonas aeruginosa and Aerobic Gram-Negative Bacilli

JAMES STANKIEWICZ, M.D.

Professor and Vice-Chairman, Department of Otolaryngology—Head and Neck Surgery, Loyola University Medical Center, Chicago, Illinois; Staff Attending Physician, Loyola University Medical Center, Chicago, Illinois; Courtesy Staff, Children's Memorial Hospital, Chicago, Illinois
Chronic Sinusitis

DENNIS L. STEVENS, Ph.D., M.D.

Professor of Medicine, University of Washington School of Medicine, Seattle, Washington; Chief, Infectious Diseases, Veterans Affairs Medical Center, Boise, Idaho
Streptococcus pyogenes

CHARLES M. STIERNBERG, M.D.

Professor and Chairman, Department of Otolaryngology—Head and Neck Surgery, Assistant Dean for Continuing Medical Education, University of Texas Medical School at Houston, Houston, Texas; Chief of Otolaryngology Service, Hermann Hospital, Chief of Otolaryngology Service, LBJ General Hospital, Houston, Texas
Deep Neck Space Infections

IAN S. STORPER, M.D.

Assistant Professor of Otolaryngology, Director of Neurotology, Columbia University College of Physicians and Surgeons, New York, New York; Assistant Attending Physician, Columbia-Presbyterian Medical Center, New York, New York
Antibiotic Prophylaxis in Otology and Neurotology

SCOTT P. STRINGER, M.D.

Associate Professor and Vice-Chair, University of Florida College of Medicine, Gainesville, Florida
Peritonsillar Abscess

ALAN M. SUGAR, M.D.

Associate Professor, Department of Medicine, Boston University School of Medicine, Boston, Massachusetts; Assistant Visiting Physician, Boston University Medical Center Hospital
Aspergillus; Mucormycosis; Candida; Dimorphic and Miscellaneous Fungi

THOMAS A. TAMI, M.D.

Associate Professor, Department of Otolaryngology—Head and Neck Surgery, University of Cincinnati College of Medicine, Cincinnati, Ohio
AIDS in Otolaryngology

STEPHEN C. THRELKELD, M.D.

Clinical and Research Fellow, Harvard Medical School, Boston, Massachusetts; Fellow, Infectious Disease Unit, Massachusetts General Hospital, Boston, Massachusetts
Miscellaneous Antibacterial: Trimethoprim-Sulfamethoxazole; The Tetracyclines

MAUREEN R. TIERNEY, M.D.

Assistant Professor of Medicine, Harvard Medical School, Boston, Massachusetts; Chief, Division of Infectious Diseases, West Roxbury Medical Center, Veterans Administration, Boston, Massachusetts
Miscellaneous Antibacterial: Trimethoprim-Sulfamethoxazole; The Tetracyclines

RONALD B. TURNER, M.D.

Associate Professor, Pediatrics and Laboratory Medicine, Department of Pediatrics, Medical University of South Carolina, Charleston, South Carolina
The Common Cold

ABRAHAM VERGHESE, M.D.

Professor of Medicine, Texas Tech Health Sciences Center, El Paso, Texas
Moraxella (Branhamella) catarrhalis

ELLEN R. WALD, M.D.

Professor of Pediatrics and Otolaryngology, The University of Pittsburgh School of Medicine, Pittsburgh, Pennsylvania; Division Chief, Allergy, Immunology and Infectious Disease, Children's Hospital of Pittsburgh, Pittsburgh, Pennsylvania
Management of Acute Bacterial Sinusitis in Children

ELAINE E.L. WANG, M.D.C.M., M.Sc.
Associate Professor, Department of Pediatrics, Faculty of Medicine, University of Toronto, Toronto, Ontario, Canada; Director, Clinical Epidemiology Unit; Staff, Division of Infectious Diseases, The Hospital for Sick Children, Toronto, Ontario, Canada
Cervical Lymphadenitis

RANDAL S. WEBER, M.D.
Gabriel Tucker Professor and Vice-Chair, Department of Otorhinolaryngology—Head and Neck Surgery, University of Pennsylvania Health System, Philadelphia, Pennsylvania
Management of Postoperative Head and Neck Wound Infections; Prophylaxis for Contaminated Head and Neck and Cranial Base Surgery

JANE L. WEISSMAN, M.D.
Departments of Radiology and Otolaryngology, The University of Pittsburgh School of Medicine, Pittsburgh, Pennsylvania; Director, Head and Neck Imaging, The University of Pittsburgh Medical Center, Pittsburgh, Pennsylvania
Imaging the Paranasal Sinuses

PAUL L. WILLIAMS, M.D., M.Sc.
Department of Medicine, Visalia Medical Clinic, Visalia, California
Coccidioidomycosis

AYAL WILLNER, M.D.
Assistant Professor, George Washington University School of Medicine; Attending Physician, Children's National Medical Center, Department of Otolaryngology, Washington, D.C.
Tonsillitis

JONATHAN R. WORKMAN, M.D.
Resident, Division of Otolaryngology and Head and Neck Surgery, University of North Carolina School of Medicine, Chapel Hill, North Carolina
Mastoiditis

LOWELL S. YOUNG, M.D.
Clinical Professor of Medicine, University of California, San Francisco, California; Chief, Division of Infectious Diseases, California Pacific Medical Center, San Francisco, California; Director, Kuzell Institute for Arthritis and Infectious Diseases, California Pacific Medical Center, San Francisco, California
Macrolides

VICTOR L. YU, M.D.
Professor, Department of Medicine, The University of Pittsburgh School of Medicine, Chief, Infectious Disease Section, Veterans Affairs Medical Center, Pittsburgh, Pennsylvania
Quinolones; Necrotizing (Malignant) External Otitis

Preface

▼

Five decades after the introduction of the modern antimicrobial era, the physician is faced by an increasingly complex world as evidenced by a broad spectrum of microbes that have changing patterns of drug susceptibility producing a wide range of disease. It is estimated that 25%–40% of patients who present to the primary care physician have complaints referable to the ears, nose, and throat. The majority of these diseases are infectious in nature.

Infectious Diseases and Antimicrobial Therapy of the Ears, Nose and Throat has been developed based upon the foundation of our understanding of infectious disease, including the disciplines of anatomy, microbiology, immunology, and pharmacology.

This text was prepared by a multidisciplinary faculty of authorities whose clearly defined goal was to produce a comprehensive but practical text aimed at facilitating the diagnosis and management of patients with infectious diseases of the ears, nose, and throat. The text has been organized to facilitate understanding of the microbes important to infections of the ears, nose, and throat and of the antimicrobials used to treat these infectious agents and to provide an overview of the syndromes most commonly encountered. In an effort to make each chapter comprehensive, some duplication of material is required. We hope you find this text to be an indispensable addition to your medical library.

JONAS T. JOHNSON
VICTOR L. YU

Acknowledgments

▼

We gratefully acknowledge the intellectual assistance and hard work of many individuals who have facilitated completion of this textbook. We are indebted to Lawrence McGrew of the W.B. Saunders Company, whose editorial assistance has been invaluable. We are grateful to Loni Zienkiewicz, Scott Filderman, and Linda R. Garber, also of Saunders, for their assistance in the publishing process. We thank Drs. Raymond Karasic and Melinda Wharton for review of selected chapters. Finally, we are especially appreciative of the efforts made on our behalf by Sharon Coutch, Shirley Brinker, and Linda Szalla, without whose assistance this text would have never come to completion.

JONAS T. JOHNSON
VICTOR L. YU

Contents

SECTION I
GENERAL PRINCIPLES

Moselio Schaechter

Establishment of Infectious Diseases

▼

Physicians come upon an enormous number of facts about infectious agents and the diseases they cause. In order to deal with this avalanche of information, it is desirable to develop a conceptual framework on which to hang such a multitude of facts. This framework is based on the features that characterize all forms of parasitism. It comprises two generalizations, as follows:

1. The following events take place in all infectious diseases:
   Encounter: the agent meets the host.
   Entry: the agent enters the host.
   Spread: the agent spreads from the site of entry.
   Multiplication: the agent multiplies in the host.
   Damage: the agent, the host response, or both cause tissue damage.
   Outcome: the agent or the host wins out, or they learn to coexist.
2. All these steps require the breaching of host defenses. What distinguishes one parasite from another is the manner in which each elicits and combats these host defenses.

ENCOUNTER

Microbiologically, humans have a sterile existence in the mother's womb and usually encounter microorganisms at birth. This is true for two reasons: first, the fetus is well shielded from the microorganisms in the exterior environment by the fetal membranes; second, the mother is not a likely source of microorganisms. The mother's blood carries infectious agents only sporadically and in small numbers, and the placenta is a formidable obstacle to the passage of microorganisms into the fetus. Still, passage is possible, and congenital infections are acquired in this way. Some examples of microbe-host encounters are listed in Table 1–1.

First Encounters

During parturition, the newborn comes in contact with microorganisms present on the mother's vaginal canal and skin. Not only do these microorganisms colonize the newborn, but with relative frequency they cause disease. The ear, nose, and throat seem particularly vulnerable, leading to such early-onset diseases as gonococcal ophthalmia and herpes simplex. The child is born with considerable defenses acquired from the mother, such as circulating antibodies, but in time, these defenses wane and the infant must cope on its own.

Exogenously Acquired Disease

Exogenously acquired diseases are those that result from the encounter with agents in the environment. Thus, people "catch" a cold from other people or become infected with such environmental organisms as *Pseudomonas* during or after surgery. With the exception of infections of the upper respiratory tract, exogenously acquired diseases are not the most common diseases encountered in otolaryngologic practice.

Endogenously Acquired Diseases

Endogenously acquired diseases are those that result from encounters with agents in or on the body. The ears, nose, and throat are especially vulnerable to infections of this kind because they are so densely colonized. In addition, the integuments of these and adjacent areas are frequently interrupted by trauma or surgery; thus, there is the possibility of infections. Members of the microbial biota that are normally present on the mucous membranes or skin may cause disease when they penetrate into deeper tissues. For example,

Table 1–1. EXAMPLES OF ENCOUNTERS AND DISEASE PREVENTION

Type of Contact	Example	Type of Agent	Source	Strategy for Prevention
Inhalation	Common cold	Virus	Aerosol from infected persons	None
	Coccidioidomycosis	Fungus	Soil	None
Ingestion	Typhoid fever	Bacterium	Water, food	Sanitation
	Salmonella food poisoning	Bacterium	Food	Sanitation
Sexual contact	Gonorrhea	Bacterium	Person	Social behavior
Wound	Surgical infections	Bacteria	Normal flora, surroundings	Aseptic techniques
Insect bite	Malaria	Protozoan	Mosquito	Insect control

a cut invaded by the staphylococci that inhabit the healthy skin may lead to pus formation. The encounter with the agent took place long before the disease, namely, at the time of colonization of the skin by the staphylococci. The distinction must be made therefore between colonization and disease. Colonization denotes the presence of microorganisms in a site of the body and does not necessarily imply that their presence leads to tissue damage and signs and symptoms of disease. Colonization does suggest, however, that the microorganisms can multiply at the site.

The difference between endogenous and exogenous disease is sometimes quite sharp, as in the common cold, influenza, or diphtheria. However, in many other instances, the demarcation becomes less clear because it may be difficult to define what constitutes the normal biota. For example, certain strains of virulent streptococci may be harbored in the throat for a considerable time but only rarely cause pharyngitis. To the question "Was the streptococcus a member of the normal biota?" the answer is yes if "normal biota" means organisms in or on the body that are not in the process of causing disease; the answer is no upon considering that this kind of streptococcus is found in the throat of only about 5% of all healthy people. There is no easy way out of this ambiguity, and the term "normal biota" must be used in an operational sense.

The clinical manifestations of infection in the ear, nose, and throat depend, of course, on the causative agent. Thus, viruses are particularly important in the upper respiratory tract and account for most of the cases of pharyngitis. Bacteria are the most important causes of otitis media, sinusitis, epiglottitis, bronchitis, and pneumonia. Fungi and protozoa rarely cause serious infections at these sites in normal individuals but may be of importance in the compromised host.

ENTRY

Much of what is normally considered as being inside the body is connected topologically with the outside. For instance, the epithelia of the nose, the oropharynx, the larynx, the middle ear, and the sinuses are in direct connection with the exterior. The term "entry," then, denotes either the ingress of microorganisms into body cavities that are contiguous with the outside or their penetration into deeper tissue after crossing an epithelial barrier.

Ingress: Entry Without Crossing Epithelial Barriers

Inhalation

Infections of the upper reaches of the respiratory tract are usually acquired by inhalation of airborne droplets or aerosols. For a number of infections of these sites, little is known about the actual epithelial layer that is first colonized by the invading microorganisms. Thus, it is assumed that the viruses that cause the common cold first land on the nasal epithelium, although there is little evidence to prove it.

To enter the respiratory system, microorganisms face a series of aerodynamic and hydrodynamic obstacles. Microor-

ganisms are inhaled from aerosol droplets or dust particles in the air. The air column is not uniform; it is affected by complex anatomic structures (nasal turbinates, oropharynx, larynx). As a result, the surgical removal of the larynx predisposes to diseases of the lower respiratory tract. Once microorganisms arrive at the lower reaches of the respiratory tree, they face the upward-sweeping action of the ciliary epithelium. Persons in whom this action is impaired (e.g., heavy smokers) are more likely to get sick with pneumonia.

Ingestion

Virtually all the pathogens of the alimentary tract enter through the mouth; some cause disease there and in the pharynx. The mouth is the portal that allows microorganisms to enter the body on food, fluids, or fingers. The defenses of the mouth are as follows:

- The mechanical action of saliva and the tongue. More than 1 L of saliva daily is produced, which mechanically dislodges and flushes microorganisms from mucosal surfaces with assistance from the tongue. Should salivary flow be reduced, as with dehydration or during fasting, the bacterial content of saliva increases markedly.

- The nonpathogenic resident biota, especially bacteria, but also fungi (e.g., *Candida*) and protozoa (e.g., the ameba *Entamoeba gingivalis*). These organisms resist the establishment of newcomers both by the occupancy of suitable sites and by the production of acids and other metabolic inhibitors.

- Antimicrobial constituents of saliva, notably lysozyme and secreted antibodies. Lysozyme is effective mainly against gram-positive bacteria. Secretory immunoglobulin A (IgA) selectively inhibits the adherence of certain bacteria to mucosal cells.

Bacteria evade these host defenses in part by being able to stick to teeth or mucosal surfaces. Attachment to teeth is indirect, on a coating of sticky macromolecules, mainly proteins, called the dental pellicle. The bacteria produce polysaccharides that aid adherence. For example, *Streptococcus mutans* transforms sucrose into polysaccharides, dextrans and levans, that are particularly sticky. The substances are layered on the pellicle to form a matrix that allows further adherence of other organisms. The result is dental plaque, one of the densest collections of bacteria in the body. Microbial metabolism in plaque transforms dietary sugar into acids, mainly lactic acid, that are responsible for dental caries. Other bacteria, especially strict anaerobes, reside in the gingival crevices between the tooth and gum and escape the washing effects of the saliva and of normal tooth-brushing.

An example of other factors involved in colonization is the adhesive protein fibronectin. This protein coats the mucosal surfaces of epithelial cells and attaches preferentially to gram-positive organisms. Fibronectin is probably important in establishing the nature of the bacterial biota in the mouth and pharynx, as suggested by the following findings. The oropharynx of individuals in poor general health, including many hospitalized patients, is deficient in fibronectin. With low levels of this protein, gram-negative organisms tend to displace gram-positive organisms, in part because the fibronectin-denuded mucosal cells reveal on their surface receptors for components of bacterial pili or fimbriae, adhesive organelles found on gram-negative but not on gram-positive bacteria.

Penetration: Entry After Crossing Epithelial Barriers

Direct Penetration

Penetration into tissues takes many forms. Some microorganisms can pass directly through epithelia, especially mucous membranes that consist of a single cell layer. To penetrate the skin, which is tough and multilayered, most infecting agents must be carried across by insect bites or must await breaks in the skin. To penetrate into mucosal epithelial cells, many agents first interact with specific receptors on the surface of the host cell. This phenomenon has been studied with viruses, some of which have a complex mechanism for attachment and internalization. For instance, influenza viruses have surface components that bind to receptors on the surface of sensitive host cells. Binding is soon followed by the uptake of the virus particles by the cells. In the case of bacteria, these two functions, attachment and internalization, are also being studied. One strategy for such studies is to clone bacterial genes that confer the ability to enter cells into strains that are normally noninvasive. This strategy has resulted in identification of a number of adhesins, bacterial components that are involved in adherence to host cells.

Penetration Aided by White Blood Cells

Microorganisms may also be carried actively into tissue by white blood cells or by the macrophages that lie on the outside of the body. For example, the macrophages that reside in the alveoli of the lungs, known as dust cells, can pick up infectious agents by phagocytosis. Most of the time these cells carry bacteria upward on the ciliary epithelium, but occasionally these macrophages can reenter the body and carry their load of microorganisms into deeper locations. Such a mechanism of cell-mediated entry may function at the mucous membranes of the upper respiratory and digestive tracts as well, but this has not yet been well documented.

Cuts and Wounds

Penetration from cuts and wounds is a common occurrence that is usually unnoticed because it does not normally lead to symptoms of disease. For example, brushing one's teeth or defecating vigorously causes minute abrasions of epithelial membranes. Bacteria can then penetrate in small numbers into the blood, but they are rapidly removed by the filtering mechanisms of the reticuloendothelial system. However, if internal tissues are damaged or the defense mechanisms are disrupted, circulating bacteria may gain a foothold and cause serious diseases. An example is subacute bacterial endocarditis, a disease that was devastating before antibiotics. This disease was usually caused by oral streptococci that became implanted on heart valves damaged by a previous disease, most commonly rheumatic fever.

Organ Transplants and Blood Transfusion

Organisms can penetrate into deeper tissue as the result of organ transplants or blood transfusions. For instance, transplants of corneas have been known to result in the infection of recipients with a virus that causes a slow degenerative disease of the central nervous system (Creutzfeldt-Jakob disease). A transplanted organ is not necessarily the source of infection, since the immune response of transplant recipients must be suppressed in order to avoid graft rejection. In such a patient, an endogenous virus may now be able to multiply.

Of the infectious agents that may be acquired via blood transfusions, none causes greater concern than the virus of acquired immunodeficiency syndrome (AIDS). Many others, such as hepatitis B virus, can also be transmitted in this manner. Screening of blood in blood banks has become imperative.

The Importance of Inoculum Size

The likelihood that organisms from the biota of the skin or mucous membranes might cause disease depends on many factors. Among them is the size of the inoculum, meaning that a few organisms are unlikely to result in an infection; it usually takes many infecting agents to overcome the local defenses. The effect of the inoculum size can be readily demonstrated in experimental infections. A spontaneous example is what happens when people take baths in contaminated hot tubs. At times, the water can become a culture broth, with as many as 100 million *Pseudomonas* per milliliter. In such numbers, bacteria that are normally harmless can overcome the normal defenses of the skin and cause skin infection all over the body. Clearly, what a surgeon tries to achieve in preparing an area before making an incision is to reduce the number of bacteria that may invade a surgical wound. Infections are almost inevitable if high numbers of microorganisms are deposited in deeper tissues, either from dirty skin or from contamination by soil or other microberich material. This requires a great deal of attention in the treatment of patients with open wounds, even in the modern era of powerful antimicrobial drugs.

SPREAD

The term "spread" suggests direct, lateral propagation of organisms from the original site of entry to contiguous tissues and also refers to dissemination to distant sites. Either way, microorganisms spread and multiply only if they overcome host defenses. Spread sometimes precedes and sometimes follows microbial multiplication in the body. For instance, the parasite that causes malaria enters the body through a mosquito bite and is distributed throughout the blood stream before it has a chance to increase in numbers; on the other hand, staphylococci that infect a cut multiply locally before spreading to distant sites.

Appreciating the role of host defenses in impeding the

spread of microorganisms requires a fair understanding of the immune response and of the innate defense mechanisms. Owing to the dynamic nature of host-parasite interactions, for every defense mechanism microbes develop strategies to try to overcome it. The host, in turn, adapts to such new challenges, and the adaptation elicits yet different responses from the agents. This intricate counterpoint is played out, sometimes over extended periods, until one of three things happens: (1) the host wins, (2) the parasite overcomes the host, or (3) they learn to live with each other in an uneasy truce. Some examples of issues of bacterial colonization are presented in Table 1–2.

Anatomic Factors

The pattern of spread of microorganisms from a given site is often dictated by anatomic considerations, so a knowledge of human anatomy often aids understanding of infectious diseases. An example is orbital cellulitis, inflammation of the submucosal connective tissue of the eye socket, which is a complication of acute sinusitis. The anterior and lateral border of the ethmoid sinuses forms the medial and superior border of the orbit. The orbit is then separated from the ethmoid sinus by the lamina papyracea, literally a paper-thin piece of bone. Infection in the ethmoid sinus may break through this thin piece of bone and enter the orbit. If the infection is localized, it becomes an intraorbital but extraocular abscess. Another example is infection of the middle ear, a condition more common in children than in adults. This age difference is explained in part by developmental changes that take place in the eustachian tube with growth. These conduits are nearly horizontal in children and become more steeply inclined with age. For this and other reasons, the eustachian tubes of children do not drain as well as those of adults.

A speculative but intriguing notion is that viruses and other infectious agents may penetrate the body via the olfactory nerve endings, the only elements of the nervous system in direct contact with the exterior. In experimental studies, it has been shown that herpes viruses can reach the brain by this route. The ameba *Naegleria,* which causes a rare but lethal meningoencephalitis, is also thought to penetrate the central nervous system by trauma to the cribriform plate, as might happen when a person dives into water containing these amebae.

Spread of microorganisms is greatly influenced by fluid dynamics. Thus, infected fluids in the interior of the body tend to flow along fascial planes. For example, infection of one site in the meninges usually results in generalized meningitis because there are no barriers to impede the spread of the infected cerebrospinal fluid. The same is true for the pleura, the pericardium, and the synovial cavities. Of course, the most extensive liquid system of the body, the blood, is replete with defense mechanisms. All the liquids of the body contain different antimicrobial defense factors, which, if overcome, result in disease.

Active Participation by Microorganisms

Infectious agents are not always silent partners in the process of spreading. Some contribute to it by moving actively. Some of these movements appear random; others probably occur in response to chemotactic signals. Spreading can also be facilitated by chemical rather than mechanical action. For instance, streptococci manufacture a variety of extracellular hydrolases that let them break out of the walling-in force of the inflammatory response. They make a protease that breaks up fibrin, a hyaluronidase that hydrolyzes hyaluronic acid of connective tissue, and a deoxyribonuclease that reduces the viscosity of pus caused by the release of deoxyribonucleic acid from lysed white blood cells. Other bacteria make elastases, collagenases, or other powerful proteases. Such organisms can break through some of the natural surface barriers or can penetrate through thick, viscous pus that would otherwise impede their spread.

DAMAGE

In the ears, nose, and throat, there are nearly as many kinds of damage as there are infectious diseases. The type and intensity of the damage depend on the tissues and organs affected, making generalizations difficult. Damage in infectious processes may be loosely categorized as due to (1) mechanical causes, (2) cell death, (3) pharmacologic alterations of metabolism, and (4) vehement host responses. These manifestations are interrelated, and several are usually seen at one time.

Mechanical Causes

Mechanical obstruction usually results not from the infectious agents alone but from the inflammatory response of the host elicited by their presence. Almost any duct or tubelike organ, thick or thin, may be obstructed by infections, sometimes with life-threatening consequences. An example is epiglottitis, a distinct clinical syndrome that can be rapidly fatal because the airway may become completely obstructed from swelling of the epiglottis and surrounding

Table 1–2. SOME ISSUES IN BACTERIAL COLONIZATION

Anticolonizing Powers of the Host	Examples of How Bacteria Overcome Them
Sweeping microbes away by liquid currents	Adhering to epithelial cells (e.g., streptococci adhering to the mucous membranes of the oropharynx)
Killing microbes by the host's phagocytes	Avoiding being taken up (e.g., the meningococcus is surrounded by a slimy capsule that impairs uptake by neutrophils)
	Killing the phagocytes (e.g., certain streptococci produce toxins that make holes in neutrophil membranes)
Starving bacteria for lack of needed nutrient	Obtaining nutrients from host cells (e.g., certain staphylococci lyse blood cells and use their hemoglobin as a source of iron)

structures. This condition is more serious in children, because their proportionally smaller airways are more readily compromised by a swollen epiglottis.

In the case of croup, the characteristic obstruction of the upper airway results from swelling of the tracheal mucous membrane. Because the cartilage rings in the tracheal wall are nonexpandable, swelling of the mucous membrane results in narrowing of the tracheal lumen, which worsens during inspiration, resulting in inspiratory stridor. Histamine and IgE antibody specific for parainfluenza viruses, the most common agents of this disease, have been detected in nasopharyngeal secretions of children with croup, suggesting that immunologic mechanisms involving inflammatory mediators may be involved in pathogenesis.

Bacteria-induced hyperplasia of the tissues surrounding the nose and throat is seen in a rare disease, rhinoscleroma, in which the production of granulomatous tissue is so copious as to threaten to occlude the upper air passages.

Cell Death

The effect of cell death depends on (1) which cells are involved, (2) how many cells are infected, and (3) how quickly the infection proceeds. If the cells belong to an essential organ, such as the heart or the brain, the outcome is likely to be serious and could even be fatal. Sometimes the effects of cell death are easily seen. For instance, in patients with necrotizing myositis, lysis of red blood cells and the outpouring of hemoglobin may result in a reddish or burgundy appearance of serum and urine.

Some bacteria kill cells by poisoning them with toxins. Sometimes toxins function in the immediate surroundings of the bacteria that produce them. Other bacteria produce toxins that act at great distances. An example is diphtheria, in which bacteria in the throat produce a toxin that affects the heart and the nervous system. Toxins produced by bacteria are among the most powerful cell poisons known, and they work at extraordinarily low concentrations. It has been estimated that a single molecule of diphtheria toxin is sufficient to kill a sensitive cell.

Pharmacologic Alterations of Metabolism

Certain infectious diseases do not involve the direct killing of cells. Among these are some of the most severe, such as tetanus, botulism, and cholera. They are caused by bacterial toxins that alter important aspects of metabolism in ways that resemble the action of hormones or other pharmacologic effectors. Tetanus toxin works on motor cells, leading to a spastic paralysis. Botulism toxin interferes with the release of acetylcholine at cholinergic synapses and neuromuscular junctions, resulting in a flaccid paralysis. Cholera toxin increases the level of cyclic adenosine monophosphate in intestinal cells, leading to massive diarrhea because of loss of water and electrolytes. In all these cases, the affected cells remain intact.

Vehement Host Responses

The symptoms of infectious diseases are most often produced not by the microorganisms alone but by the response of the host to their presence. Rarely is the host response so finely tuned that the response does just what is desired of it. Its overemphatic expression may well help the host survive in the long run, but it contributes greatly to the immediate signs and symptoms. Two manifestations of overemphatic host response are damage due to inflammation and damage from the immune response.

Inflammation

The ears, nose, and throat, being densely colonized and open to the environment, are among the sites of the body most prone to inflammatory infections. Many of these diseases are caused by members of the normal microbial biota. Thus, the bacteria of the indigenous oral biota are not highly virulent, but when there is a break in the mucosal barrier, such as with advanced gingivitis (periodontal disease), they may invade surrounding healthy tissue.

The most familiar example of inflammation is pus, which consists of a mixture of dead and live white blood cells, bacteria, and exudate. Pus results from the rapid migration of neutrophils to a site where bacteria are present. Neutrophils are called up by chemotactic substances produced by the bacteria as well as by tissue and serum components. When neutrophils die, they release powerful hydrolases from their lysosomal granules. These enzymes damage surrounding tissues, extending the lesion to adjacent areas.

When pus is walled off, the lesion is called an abscess. An example is a peritonsillar abscess, caused in about half the cases by β-hemolytic streptococci. Despite their relatively sequestered location, microorganisms advertise their presence by producing chemotaxins, and neutrophils arrive at the scene to join the battle. It should be noted that the anatomic location of this battlefield is all-important. An abscess in the skin may be painful, but one in the brain could be fatal. Pus may be damaging locally, but such damage is a small price to pay for containing the infection. Patients with genetic defects in neutrophil function suffer from severe recurrent infections. Despite antibiotic treatment, many such patients do not survive into adolescence.

In the soft tissues about the oral cavity, a synergistic cooperation among several different types of bacteria, both aerobic and strictly anaerobic, can lead to a severe and rapidly advancing mixed infection. Ludwig's angina, a polymicrobial infection of the sublingual and submandibular spaces that arises from a tooth (often the 2nd and 3rd mandibular molars), is a cellulitis that may at times progress rapidly, compromise the airway, and threaten the patient with asphyxiation.

Although the posterior nasopharynx merges with the oropharynx, there are important differences between infections of the nose and throat. Most infections of the nasopharynx are caused by viruses and give rise to the signs and symptoms that are known collectively as the common cold. Approximately 40%–50% of colds are caused by the rhinovirus group. Coronaviruses are the next most common group of agents, accounting for approximately 10% of colds. The remainder are caused by a variety of other respiratory viruses. Although a person with a cold may experience a scratchy feeling in the throat, nasal symptoms are usually more prominent. Bacterial infection of the nose occurs occasionally but is not a common clinical problem.

Viruses and bacteria are the most common etiologic agents of pharyngitis. It is difficult to differentiate between a viral and a bacterial cause on the basis of clinical findings; in practice, the distinction is made by performing a throat culture or a rapid diagnostic test to detect group A streptococci, which are by far the most important bacterial cause of pharyngitis. Other streptococci account for a small proportion of cases, as do gonococci in sexually active individuals. In the past, oropharyngeal diphtheria caused an important form of pharyngitis, but this disease is rarely seen in developed countries today. Among the viruses, the adenovirus group is particularly prominent and may be suspected if conjunctivitis is also present (pharyngoconjunctival fever). In adolescents and young adults, Epstein-Barr virus is a common cause of pharyngitis, which is one of the manifestations of infectious mononucleosis. The enteroviruses, especially the group A coxsackieviruses, sometimes produce small vesicles on the mucous membrane of the throat, a clinical condition called herpangina.

The presence of bacteria in tissues also elicits a generalized reaction known as the acute-phase response. Bacteria set off the outpouring of a powerful protein called interleukin-1, which acts on the fever centers to raise body temperature. Interleukin-1 stimulates the synthesis of substances called prostaglandins, which work on the thermoregulatory center of the brain. Prostaglandins are also responsible for the feeling of malaise, the well-known sensation of "feeling sick" that accompanies the common cold. Aspirin and acetaminophen interfere with the production of prostaglandins, thereby reducing fever and malaise.

With many gram-negative bacteria, the acute-phase response is elicited by a major component of their surface, a lipopolysaccharide known as endotoxin. In small amounts, endotoxin elicits fever and mobilizes certain defense mechanisms. In large amounts, it causes shock and intravascular coagulation. Thus, the body response to the presence of these bacteria depends on the amount of endotoxin present.

The Immune Response

The immune response is complex and has multiple manifestations. There are many ways in which it may go awry and cause damage. Immune responses are usually classified as "humoral," related to circulating antibodies, and "cellular," elicited by special cells of the immune system. Both may cause damage.

Although the immune responses may cause tissue damage, in most instances there is a benefit. The point is illustrated in people who have genetic or acquired defects in their immune system. The advent and spread of AIDS have placed hundreds of thousands of persons in this category. Such patients are ravaged and later killed by microorganisms that cause little or no disease in healthy persons. In the immunocompetent person, for example, active tuberculosis causes much damage; if this damage leads to death, it does so usually only after many years. In the immunocompromised patient, the disease can become rampant in a much shorter period.

Humoral Immunity. Infecting agents elicit the formation of specific antibodies. In the circulation and in tissues, antibodies combine with the infecting agents or with some of their soluble products. These antigen-antibody complexes evoke an inflammatory response. In the presence of antigen-antibody complexes, the complement system becomes activated by a series of proteolytic reactions known as the classic pathway of activation. Complement can also be activated by the presence of microorganisms alone, resulting in the alternative pathway. The products of these proteolytic cleavages are pharmacologically active. Some work on platelets and white blood cells to produce substances that increase vascular permeability and vasodilation. The result is edema, the outpouring of fluids into tissues. Other complement factors act on white blood cells, some as chemotaxins, others to make bacteria more easily phagocytized. The result of these activities is, on the one hand, the mobilization of powerful defenses against invading microorganisms and, on the other hand, inflammation.

Antigen-antibody complexes sometimes are deposited on the membrane of the glomeruli of the kidneys, resulting in impairment of kidney function, a condition called glomerulonephritis. This condition is seen as the aftermath of certain streptococcal and viral infections. Similar effects also take place in blood vessels, leading to visible skin rashes.

Cellular Immunity. A different type of response is expressed by special cells of the immune system and is called cell-mediated immunity (CMI). This complex phenomenon leads to the activation and mobilization of macrophages, the powerful phagocytic cells that participate in the later stages of inflammation, to clean up debris and remaining microorganisms.

CMI is associated with chronic inflammation, the histologic changes that limit the spread of infections but also cause lesions in tissues. These damaging activities are characteristic of chronic infections, which are often caused by intracellular microorganisms and viruses. An example is chronic tuberculosis, in which the main damage to tissue is due to CMI. It is elicited by the tubercle bacilli, which have the ability to persist in cells for a long time. As a result, pathologic changes associated with CMI lead to the production of tubercles or granulomas and eventually to destruction of tissue cells.

OUTCOME

There is nothing simple about infectious diseases, either mild or life-threatening. A high number of properties of the invading agent and the host lead to an intricate and ever-changing interplay. It is not always possible to figure out the relative role of the known properties, let alone those that await discovery. To complicate matters, humans are beset by a huge number of possible invaders. New ones emerge apparently under our very eyes, to be added to the long list.

Joachim Forsgren
Britta Rynnel-Dagöö
Anders Samuelson

CHAPTER TWO

The Microbe

▼

In this chapter, a number of surface-exposed bacterial cell components and other factors of importance for pathogenicity are discussed. The cell envelope of gram-negative bacteria is a complex structure with inner and outer membranes separated by the periplasm, containing a murein sac consisting of peptidoglycan. The outer membrane is a bilayer of phospholipids in which the lipopolysaccharides (LPSs) and outer membrane proteins (OMPs) are anchored. Fimbriae or pili may also be present on the bacterial surface. The gram-positive cell wall contains two major components, peptidoglycans and teichoic acids. A variety of different carbohydrates and proteins, depending on the species, are also present. Examples are the M proteins of group A streptococci and the immunoglobulin-binding protein of *Staphylococcus aureus.* Gram-negative as well as gram-positive bacteria may be surrounded by a polysaccharide capsule. For a detailed insight into these issues concerning the respective pathogens, see Chapter 6.

All measures developed by pathogenic microbes to promote disease and persistence could be regarded as virulence factors. With a working principle of genetic trial and error and rapid replication, and under favorable circumstances, microbes posses a tremendous potential for rapid adaptive changes relative to their environment by mass action.

The interaction between microbe and host eventually leading to infection is a process that can be divided schematically into four steps: entry, colonization, invasion, and persistence. The various countermeasures microbes use to combat the immune mechanisms of the host are given in Table 2–1. The initial events in this process on mucosal surfaces and in tissues are highly specific and display a marked species and tissue tropism highlighting differences at the cellular and molecular levels of the mechanisms involved. Microbes have developed different strategies, displayed in the various steps of the pathogenesis. A successful outcome for the microbe is when it can grow and multiply, whether in the mucus blanket on top of a mucous membrane or in the cytoplasm of an invaded host cell. An example of the first situation is the nasopharyngeal colonization by a potential pathogen like nontypable, nonencapsulated *Haemophilus influenzae,* which most of the time is not harmful to the host. An example of the second situation is microbial persistence, which manifests clinically as a chronic infection with ulterior tissue damage due to unsuccessful immunologic clearance by the host. The consequences are thus equally dependent on the immune status of the host.

In the unprimed individual, nonspecific and innate defense mechanisms—such as mucociliary clearance, the action of microbicidal substances, and phagocytosis—are first engaged. In a later phase, an immune response is mounted, comprising the synthesis of specific antibodies and the targeting of cytotoxic cells.

Because the following discussion deals in particular with various virulence factors and microbial strategies for evasion of innate and adaptive host defenses, the reader in need of a review of these functions should see Chapter 3.

COLONIZATION

Affinity for Mucus and Cilia; Ciliostasis

The mucus blanket covering large areas of the respiratory tract epithelium is a complex mixture of secreted molecules, cells, and debris. Mucus glycoproteins, called mucins, represent the main components of mucus in the respiratory tract. They are secreted by the goblet cells of the epithelium and the mucous glands of the respiratory mucosa. Mucins are large, highly glucosylated glycoproteins with a molecular mass of up to one million daltons. The mucin molecules are covered with carbohydrate chains, oligosaccharides with 1–20 sugars, which represent a mosaic of potential sites for the attachment of microorganisms. Once trapped on the mucus blanket, the bacteria are likely to be eliminated from the respiratory tract by mucociliary clearance. Under favorable circumstances for the bacteria, trapping by mucus may also be the first step of colonization and further multiplication within the host. Several bacterial species with relevance

Table 2–1. PRINCIPAL MICROBIAL COUNTERMEASURES TO HOST DEFENSE MECHANISMS

Colonization

Affinity for mucus and cilia; ciliostasis
Attachment to mucosal surfaces: adherence
Evasion of host innate microbicidal agents
Proteolysis of secretory antibodies

Infection/Invasion

Defense against complement
Defense against phagocytosis
    Inhibition of phagocyte recruitment
    Antiphagocytic mechanisms
    Killing of phagocytes
Subversion of immune responses
    Alteration of lymphocyte function
    Depletion of lymphocytes
    Alteration of cytokine expression

Persistence

Antigenic variations
Intracellular survival
Viral latency

for respiratory tract disease, including *H. influenzae, Streptococcus pneumoniae,* and *Pseudomonas aeruginosa,* attach to mucus or mucins.[1]

To enable bacterial attachment to epithelial cells and the establishment of a clinical infection, the bacterium must overcome the defense mechanism of mucociliary clearance. This can be achieved by toxic substances present in the bacterial cell wall like lipopolysaccharides (e.g., *H. influenzae*) or glucopeptides derived from peptidoglycan (e.g., *Bordetella pertussis* and *Neisseria gonorrhoeae*). These substances have cytotoxic effects on ciliated epithelial cells that lead to sloughing of cells and paralysis of cilia—ciliostasis.[2]

Attachment to Mucosal Surfaces: Adherence

Adherence is the initial interaction of a microorganism with its host and a prerequisite for colonization. A distinction must, however, be made between colonization and disease. Colonization denotes the presence of microorganisms at a site of the body and does not necessarily imply tissue damage or signs and symptoms of disease. It does suggest, however, that the microorganisms have invaded that site of the body and can multiply there.

S. pneumoniae is a true pathogen causing pneumonia and otitis media. Still, it is a member of the normal flora in most children. Thus, it is sometimes hard to distinguish between endogenous and exogenous infections because the normal flora cannot always be defined precisely.

Some parts of the respiratory tract, such as the eustachian tube, the nasal cavities, the sinuses, and the trachea, are outlined by a ciliated respiratory epithelium, which prevents stable attachment of microbes. These domains are, in fact, virtually sterile. In other regions, such as the nasopharynx, the oropharynx, and the oral cavity, the mucosa also includes patches of squamous epithelium. These areas are colonized by a high number of microbes, the majority being members of the normal flora but some being potentially pathogenic.

Adhesion Mechanisms

Microorganisms have surface-exposed molecules, called adhesins, that promote adherence to surface receptors on the host cell. These ligands are often species- and tissue-specific. Species specificity of adherence of microbial pathogens has been demonstrated for poliovirus and the major group of rhinoviruses, in which viral receptors are present on human but not on murine cells. Tissue tropism often relies on the existence of specific receptors on the surface of certain cells. An adhesin may have more than one receptor, and a single receptor may be recognized by many adhesins. Species or tissue specificity for receptors of microbial adhesins has suggested an approach to their identification: transfection of DNA from a receptor-positive to a receptor-negative cell line, followed by identification of the receptor DNA. This procedure has been used to identify the intercellular adhesion molecule 1 (ICAM-1) as the receptor for the major group of rhinoviruses and to identify the poliovirus receptor, a member of the immunglobulin gene superfamily.

The interaction between adhesin and receptor may be affected or even improved by host mechanisms. Thus, many adhesins require proteolytic fragmentation to manifest full biologic activity. For example, the membrane fusion activity, that is needed for full viral activity requires processing by a host protease. This concept of posttranslational processing may also to some extent explain tissue tropism, as the specific proteases may be present only in certain tissues.

Rhinoviruses display considerable antigenic diversity—nearly 100 different serotypes have been recognized. Infected humans, particularly children, are the only known reservoir for these viruses. It has been found that most of the various rhinovirus serotypes bind to the same host cell receptor, notably the ICAM-1, known to play an important role in cell-to-cell adhesion processes. The expression of ICAM-1 is, furthermore, increased by certain inflammatory mediators, and the infection itself may thus contribute to spread of the disease. It has been hypothesized that one strategy used by viruses to escape the immune surveillance of the host is to protect the receptor attachment site in a narrow surface depression so that it is not available to neutralize antibodies, the so-called canyon hypothesis.[3]

The number of studies that identify the attachment site on a viral surface is still limited. The binding site has been described for influenza virus and human rhinovirus (HRV). The three-dimensional structure of HRV14 is known. The surface has deep depressions, or "canyons," surrounded by hypervariable regions that can bind neutralizing antibodies. The narrow canyon is outlined by conserved molecular residues, which are inaccessible to the broad antigen-binding region of antibodies but can bind very small molecules. The strategy employed by HRV14 to protect the virus receptor attachment site may also be used by many other types of viruses.

Structures Mediating Attachment

Many microbial adhesins are lectins and recognize carbohydrate structures that can be investigated in inhibition assays, by which different oligosaccharides can be tested for inhibition of adherence. Some bacteria have specific structures, called fimbriae or pili, that mediate attachment to host tissues. Fimbriae are proteinaceous, rodlike structures 2–7 nm in length, that cover the bacterial surface in numbers varying from 100–1000 per cell. Some *Escherichia coli* strains expressing so-called P fimbriae are found to be uropathogenic ("P" for pyelonephritis) and bind specifically to uroepithelial cells via glycolipid receptors. P fimbriae undergo a type of phase variation in which individual bacteria can turn on and off the expression of fimbrial genes. This feature might help the bacterium avoid recognition by the immune system.

Binding of group A streptococci to buccal cells has been well studied. A candidate streptococcal adhesin involved in colonization is lipoteichoic acid, which is a cell-wall component of many gram-positive bacteria. Streptococci with large amounts of lipoteichoic acid are very sticky and also bind specifically to fibronectin, a protein coating the epithelial cells of the oropharynx.

Fibronectin is an adhesive protein found in large amounts on mucosal surfaces of the respiratory tract and may hide surface receptors for fimbriae. It has a strong affinity for gram-positive organisms. Fibronectin may be important in establishing the nature of the bacterial flora in the mouth and pharynx. With low levels of this protein, fimbriae become available for binding, perhaps explaining why gram-negative organisms may displace gram-positive organisms. Individuals in poor health have low mucosal levels of fibronectin, which may result in a higher frequency of gram-negative infections in hospitalized patients.

S. pneumoniae and typable (capsulated) as well as nontypable (nonencapsulated) *H. influenzae* attach to epithelial—mainly nasopharyngeal—cells. Pneumococci bind via glycoconjugates containing the disaccharide GlcNaAcβ1-4Gal. Pili and fimbriae are well-characterized mediators of adhesion and colonization for *H. influenzae*. Nonpilus mediators of adherence have also been identified. Of special interest are the so-called high-molecular-weight proteins that mediate attachment to human epithelial cells and macrophages. Notably, the high-molecular-weight proteins have structural and probably functional similarities with the filamentous hemagglutinin found on *B. pertussis* (discussed later).

Microflora of the Respiratory Tract

The nasopharyngeal microflora is established early in childhood, and its composition of nonpathogenic commensals and potentially pathogenic bacteria may be influenced by a variety of factors, such as genetic differences in the host, the number of household contacts, diet (especially breast-feeding versus formula feeding), and age. This complex situation contributes to a considerable variation in the reported frequencies of nasopharyngeal bacterial carriage. Longitudinal studies with repeated upper respiratory tract cultures from the same population over several years have contributed to the understanding of the dynamics and turnover of bacteria in these regions.

The nasopharyngeal commensal bacterial flora comprises a great number of nonpathogenic species, aerobes as well as anaerobes. Potentially pathogenic bacteria such as *S. pneumoniae*, *H. influenzae* (the majority being nontypable), *Moraxella (Branhamella) catarrhalis* and, to some extent, *Streptococcus pyogenes* are frequently isolated, especially in the younger age groups.

Close to 100% of children studied have been found to be colonized with pneumococci at least once during the first 2 years of life. The age of the first encounter with a pneumococcal strain ranged from 4 days to 8 months, and the same capsular type could be carried for as long as 17 months. The acquisition of *H. influenzae* strains has been monitored in children from birth to 2 years of age; the colonization rate increases with age and reaches about 30% at 2 years of age. Surveys have indicated that up to 80% of persons are carriers.

One common feature of these potentially pathogenic bacteria is that the colonization rate declines with age and that less than 10% of adults carry bacteria in the nasopharynx. It has been posited that local immune mechanisms, mainly secretory immunoglobulin A (IgA) antibodies, could protect against colonization. An interesting finding is that, in adults with antibody deficiencies, colonization with *H. influenzae* is far more common than in healthy adults. This finding is in accordance with the relatively high colonization rate in young children with immature immune systems as reflected by specific serum antibody activity. Development of immu-

nity against, for example, nontypable *H. influenzae* is hampered and perhaps delayed by the considerable antigenic heterogeneity of bacterial cell-wall components, fimbriae, proteases, and so on.

Whether the pattern of nasopharyngeal colonization in clinically infection-free intervals is different in infection-prone versus healthy individuals is still a matter of controversy. In one study using nasopharyngeal swab cultures, *H. influenzae* was obtained twice as often in otitis-prone children compared with non–otitis-prone children, regardless of the otologic status.[4] In a later study, all three middle ear pathogens in the nasopharynx were compared in otitis-prone and healthy children.[5] Nontypable *H. influenzae* was carried more than seven times as often in otitis-prone children as in non–otitis-prone children, although in other studies, no such differences could be found.

Oropharynx

Group A streptococci frequently colonize the throats of asymptomatic individuals. Pharyngeal carriage rates among normal schoolchildren vary with geographic location and season. Carriage rates of 15%–20% have been noted in several studies. The carriage rate in adults is considerably lower.

Oral Cavity

There is a massive colonization of the mouth, with a high number of different bacterial species, of which the majority are nonpathogenic. In fact, the gingival pockets surrounding the teeth are filled with bacteria. However, these microbes only occasionally cause infection, as, for example, in periodontitis, which results when overgrowth with particular bacterial strains occurs in the gingival crevices (see Chapter 55). Viridans streptococci, or "alpha-hemolytic *Streptococcus* species," comprise a number of bacteria inhabiting the normal oral cavity, where they make up 30%–60% of the flora. They include the mutans group, consisting of *Streptococcus mutans* and other related species, which are responsible for the development of dental caries. These organisms have surface proteins that bind to salivary glycoproteins deposited on teeth, forming sticky masses of bacteria called plaque.

Colonization and Disease

Colonization is a common phenomenon, particularly in early childhood, that rarely leads to infection. Still, bacterial colonization is a factor for pathogenicity and an essential step in disease production. Microorganisms may find their way into the eustachian tubes, sinuses, and bronchi where they may replicate. Under normal circumstances, defense mechanisms rapidly clear the threatening microorganisms. A defective tubal opening function (which is common in young children) or a viral infection with edema of the mucosal lining can obstruct the eustachian tube and give the organisms in the middle ear a chance to replicate and cause disease. A synergistic action between virus and bacteria-promoting disease has also been demonstrated for several viruses that can up-regulate the expression of receptors for bacteria on epithelial cells.

Mucosa-Associated Lymphatic Tissue and Nasopharyngeal Colonization

The adenoid, or pharyngeal tonsil, and the palatine and lingual tonsils form Waldeyer's ring at the entrance of the respiratory and gastrointestinal tracts. These lymphoid organs belong to the mucosa-associated lymphatic tissue (MALT) or, more particularly, to the nasopharyngeal mucosa-associated lymphatic tissue, as has been suggested. Experimental data support the view of this tissue as a gatekeeper of mucosal immunity, and the concept of compartmentalization of this secondary lymphoid organ is now fairly well established. Colonizing bacteria in the nasopharynx are taken up by a specialized crypt epithelium: bacterial antigens are transported within the highly organized lymphoid tissue and are presented to various cell populations, with important immunologic inductor and effector functions as a consequence.

Adenoids and tonsils have been suggested as sites of chronic infection owing to an increase of bacterial load in the tissue and/or a breakdown of immunologic defense mechanisms. This theory is likely regarding tonsils but more questionable for adenoids. Conflicting results on the effect of adenoidectomy on otitis media have been reported through the years. Adenoidectomy is by tradition not often performed before 3 years of age. Studies on the effect of the operation on recurrent episodes of acute otitis media, which is a disease of early childhood, have not been performed. On the other hand, a beneficial effect of adenoidectomy on the resolution of secretory otitis media (SOM) has been demonstrated in randomized, well-planned, and controlled studies. The role of the adenoid in the pathogenesis of SOM is, however, still unclear. The number of tonsillectomies and adenoidectomies has decreased dramatically in recent decades, although sleep apnea and nasal obstruction with hypertrophy of the lymphoid tissue are still indications for these operations (see Chapter 47). The operations are therefore sometimes performed in very young children. However, it is still a matter of debate whether these operations compromise the development and/or persistence of mucosal immunity in the region.

Evasion of Host Innate Microbicidal Agents

Lysozyme is an enzyme present in secretions such as tears and saliva. Its hydrolytic actions break up the murein in bacterial cell walls as well as the chitin in fungi. The entry of water into a bacterial cell causes lysis of the organism under hypo-osmotic conditions. Gram-positive bacteria are the main target for the antimicrobial action of lysozyme, as the outer membrane protects the cell wall of gram-negative bacteria.

Proteolysis of Secretory Antibodies

Several members of the oral microflora, such as *H. influenzae,* produce extracellular proteases that specifically inacti-

vate secretory IgA1. All proteases cleave the heavy chain of IgA1 in the hinge region. The products are monomeric fragment, antigen-binding (Fab) fragments with retained antigenic binding capacity and the fragment, crystallizable (Fc) portion associated with the secretory component. There are some indirect proofs of a pathogenetic role of these proteases. One example is the presence of enzyme-neutralizing antibodies in patient-convalescent sera and secretions.

Studies have shown considerable antigenic polymorphism of proteases, in particular among nontypable *H. influenzae* strains. Furthermore, a frequent exchange of clones expressing antigenically different IgA1 proteases has been observed in the upper respiratory tract in healthy children.[6] This may be a (principal) mechanism whereby *H. influenzae* evades the host immune response against IgA1 proteases. It may indirectly support the concept that protease activity is important for the colonization of *H. influenzae* on the respiratory epithelium.

INFECTION/INVASION

Defense Against Complement

When a microbe enters the blood stream of a nonimmune host, activation of the complement cascade through the binding of complement component 3b (C3b) to the surface of the microbe is followed by the formation of C3 convertase. This is the initial crucial step in the so-called alternative pathway of activation of complement. In the immune host, the binding of antibodies to target molecules on the invader triggers complement activation via the classic pathway, starting with the binding of complement fragment C1q to the immune complex. However, microorganisms display an array of countermeasures against the actions of complement[7] (Table 2–2).

If no suitable structure for the binding of C3b is presented on the surface of the pathogen, complement is not activated. This is the case for the gram-negative upper respiratory tract pathogen *H. influenzae.* In contrast, C3b binds well to the murein of *Staphylococcus aureus.* By coating the cell wall

Table 2–2. SOME ANTICOMPLEMENT DEFENSES OF MICROBES

Prevention of activation
  No suitable surface acceptor structure (e.g., *Haemophilus influenzae*)
  Covering of activator sites (e.g., capsule of *Staphylococcus aureus*)

"Molecular mimicry," or masquerading in host molecules
  Sialic acid–rich capsules, factor H binding (e.g., *Escherichia coli,* group B streptococci)
  Coating with circulating IgA antibodies (e.g., *Neisseria meningitidis*)
  Incorporation of decay-accelerating factor (e.g., *Schistosoma mansoni*)
  Complement receptor 1 homologue (herpes simplex virus)
  Virus-encoded secretion of C4-binding protein analogue (vaccinia virus)

Inactivation of complement components
  Complement component C3b (e.g., *Streptococcus pneumoniae*)
  Complement component C5a (e.g., *Pseudomonas aeruginosa,* group A streptococci)

Decoy of complement action
  Placement of target distant from outer membrane (e.g., *Salmonella enteritidis, E. coli*)
  Release of decoy molecules (e.g., *S. aureus, P. aeruginosa*)

with a capsule, the bacterium prevents the activation of complement through the alternative pathway.

The capsule of strains of *E. coli* and that of group B streptococci are rich in sialic acid, which is also bound to the lipopolysaccharide (LPS) of serum-resistant strains of *N. gonorrhoeae*. Because sialic acid is also present as a surface component of erythrocytes, immune recognition is probably disfavored in organisms with surface-exposed sialic acid. Moreover, sialic acid favors the binding of the complement system regulatory factor H, thereby constituting a nonactivator surface and enhancing the decay of alternative pathway C3 convertase.

Meningococci, having entered the blood stream, become coated with serum IgA antibodies. The immune complex thus formed does not activate complement through the classic pathway, because the Fc region of IgA has no binding site for C1q. Instead, the organisms become protected not only against complement but also against the further binding of antibodies of the IgG and IgM classes capable of complement activation through C1q binding.

Schistosoma mansoni larvae passing into the blood stream have developed an ingenious way of escaping from complement action. Their trick is to incorporate host decay-accelerating factor (DAF) into their membranes. With this masquerade, the schistosomes make use of a mechanism of protection against complement employed by the host cells themselves. DAF is a protein present in the membrane of host cells, and its physiologic function is to accelerate dissociation of C3 convertase formed by either the classic or the alternative pathway.

Another example of how an organism decoys the immune defense by making use of structures similar to those of the immune system is provided by the herpes simplex virus (HSV). One physiologic action of complement receptor 1 (CR1) is to downregulate complement activation by accelerating the dissociation of both C3 convertases. The HSV produces a surface glycoprotein, glycoprotein C, that mimicks parts of the CR1. The amino acid sequence of glycoprotein C and that of the CR1 are sufficiently homologous to allow the binding of C3b and thus promote the breakdown of formed C3 convertase. Yet another example in this context is the secretion by vaccinia-infected cells of a protein resembling the host's own regulatory C4-binding protein (C4bp). The virus-encoded C4bp binds to the C4b fragment of the classic pathway and thus both hinders the formation of C3 convertase and accelerates its decay.

Both *S. pneumoniae* and *Yersinia enterocolitica* possess surface enzymes that can degrade bound C3b and block further complement activation via the alternative pathway. The carboxypeptidase released by group A streptococci acts as a specific C5a (chemotaxin) inactivator, an effect shared with *P. aeruginosa* elastase, which in addition cleaves a number of other complement components.

In order for the complement system to exert its lytic effects on bacteria, the membrane attack complex (MAC) needs to be inserted into the bacterial cell membrane. Gram-positive bacteria, which lack an outer membrane but have a thick murein cell wall, generally resist the MAC. Examples of gram-negative bacteria not sensitive to the MAC are certain strains of *Salmonella enteritidis* and *E. coli*. It has been demonstrated that smooth strains with long O chains in the LPS molecules are virulent, whereas rough strains with shorter O chains are not, although both forms bind comparable amounts of C3b and consume equal amounts of the MAC components. The explanation is that the LPS molecules with long O antigen side chains act as decoys for the deposition of the MAC to sites distant from the outer membrane where it cannot harm the bacterium. A similar strategy of diversion using soluble substances has been developed by *S. aureus* and *P. aeruginosa*: teichoic acid is released by *S. aureus*, and mucoexopolysaccharide is released by *P. aeruginosa*. Both these substances are powerful activators of complement via the alternative pathway. Shedding of capsular polysaccharides and chunks of outer membranes serves the same purpose in other organisms. Again, the complement activation takes place at a site away from the bacterium so that it has no lytic effect.

Defense Against Phagocytosis

In the battle between invading microbes and the host, the phagocytic function of granulocytes and monocytes is the most powerful of the constitutive host defenses. It is therefore not surprising that microorganisms that are successful human pathogens have developed a wide array of mechanisms by which to escape the lethal action of phagocytosis.[8] In the in vivo situation, the actions of complement and phagocytosis work together. Thus, all microbial measures that abrogate the activation of complement also affect the process of phagocytosis.

Inhibition of Phagocyte Recruitment

C5a, the soluble cleavage product of complement factor 5, is the chief chemoattractant for neutrophils. As mentioned previously, certain bacteria possess proteins that can cleave C5a enzymatically. An example is the C5a peptidase of *S. pneumoniae*, which splits C5a at the carboxy terminal end, leaving a molecule that has lost its chemotactic capacity.

Another way of obstructing phagocyte recruitment is directed at phagocyte motility. *B. pertussis*, the agent of whooping cough, produces pertussis toxin that resembles cholera toxin in that it affects the cyclic adenosine monophosphate (cAMP) metabolism of the human host cells. Its enzymatic function is that of an adenosine diphosphate (ADP)–ribosyltransferase that catalyzes the transfer of the ADP group from coenzyme nicotinamide adenine dinucleotide to different target proteins. This is also the mechanism of diphtheria toxin, cholera toxin, and exotoxin A of *P. aeruginosa*. The target for ADP-ribosylation of the pertussis toxin is an adenylate cyclase regulatory G protein. Its ADP-ribosylation results in an increase of cAMP, which paralyzes the neutrophil and inhibits its oxidative burst. An extracellular adenylate cyclase also secreted by *B. pertussis* further adds to this action when taken up intracellularly.

Antiphagocytic Mechanisms

In order for microbes to become engulfed by the neutrophil, structures on the respective antagonists need to come into close physical contact. This interaction is mediated through phagocyte surface receptors directed at naturally occurring molecules on the microbe or via opsonins. Bacteria can severely frustrate this contact by wrapping up in a capsule and thus becoming almost impossible for the nonimmune host to phagocytize. A great number of species are capable of this strategy, such as pneumococci, group A streptococci, *H. influenzae,* and salmonellae. Classic in vitro experiments have demonstrated the striking difference between strains with rough (unencapsulated) and smooth (capsulated) colony morphology in how organisms are taken up and killed by phagocytes.

The group A streptococci have a more efficient shield against opsonization than their hyaluronate-containing capsules: the M protein. Under the microscope, M protein–bearing organisms are seen to have a woolly layer on their surface, owing to the protrusion of M protein molecules from the bacterial cell wall. The antiphagocytic effect of the M protein is caused by its binding of the plasma-clotting factor fibrinogen and its degradation products. The dense coating thus formed around the organism blocks the deposition of C3b. The importance of the M protein for virulence of *S. pyogenes* is demonstrated by the fact that strains devoid of M protein are readily killed by phagocytosis after being opsonized through C3b binding.

M protein molecules exposed to the host's immune system in spite of the fibrinogen coat induce the production of specific antibody. These antibodies effectively opsonize the bacteria and confer immunity. How, then, can the bacteria stay among humans as progressively more and more individuals become immune to the M protein? Through DNA recombination, the streptococci can change the genes encoding the opsonic epitopes of the M protein, giving rise to different serotypes. Because the antibodies are highly specific for the serotype against which they are mounted, they do not protect against any of the other approximately 80 existing serotypes. This is an example of antigenic variation as a means of persistence in the population as a whole.

Another way of interfering with the opsonization is the binding of antibodies to protein A. A cell-wall component of streptococci and staphylococci, protein A attaches unspecifically to the Fc portion of IgG. The Fc end of the antibody molecule then becomes inaccessible to the Fc receptors on phagocytes. Moreover, the specific antigen-binding domains of the Fab fragment are turned away from the target on the bacterial surface.

Killing of Phagocytes

A lethal weapon aiming to kill neutrophils and macrophages is a group of toxins called the leukocidins. They are elaborated by several pathogenic bacteria and can either work at distance, before the phagocyte-microbe contact is made, or function like a Trojan horse, taking their deadly action only after the organism has been ingested. Leukocidins form pores in the cell membrane in a fashion similar to the MAC of the complement system. Much the same as the consequence of MAC insertion into the membrane, channels are formed by leukocidin proteins, and water is allowed to enter the cell. When the cell membrane can no longer resist the intracellular pressure, the cell bursts, causing lysis. Even if this final point is not reached, low concentrations of the toxin can severely disturb the cellular functions of the phagocyte.

The alpha toxin of *S. aureus* consists of hexamers, has a molecular weight (MW) of 34 kD and forms pores with an internal diameter of 2–3 nm, which permits the transit of water and most small metabolites. Streptolysin O is an 89-kD protein monomer that binds to cholesterol in the cell membrane, creating pores with an inner diameter up to 30 nm. Streptolysin O acts on the lysosome membrane, causing hydrolytic enzymes to be discharged into the cytoplasm of the phagocyte. The cell is not primarily lysed by this mechanism but dies from intoxication by its own poisons. Eventually, however, the lysosomal enzymes pour out from the killed neutrophils and cause tissue damage. In delayed revenge, certain streptococci bear streptolysin S on their surface, which slays the phagocyte that ingested the bacteria after they have been killed intracellularly. Interestingly, it has been shown that *Shigella flexneri* is capable of inducing programmed cell death, or apoptosis, in human macrophages in vitro. In vivo, this mechanism could promote persistence of bacteria within host tissues. Alternately, virus persistence is favored if apoptosis of the infected cell is inhibited, as discussed later.

Subversion of Immune Responses

Alteration of Lymphocyte Function

Measles is immunosuppressive. T lymphocytes infected with measles virus do not die, but they lose certain functions, and B lymphocytes stop the production of immunoglobulins. After infection with measles, people have an increased risk of reactivation of herpes simplex infections and tuberculosis. Patients with cellular immune deficits, such as patients with acute leukemia, may get severe or fatal infections. The measles vaccine has reduced the incidence of the disease in developed countries, but measles remains a major killer of children in underdeveloped countries.

Depletion of Lymphocytes

Human immunodeficiency virus (HIV), the agent of acquired immunodeficiency syndrome (AIDS), preferentially infects helper T cells through interaction with the CD4 surface antigen. Many of the infected cells are killed by the replication of the virus. Depletion of helper T cells results in a reduction of the total number of circulating lymphocytes (lymphopenia) and a relative increase in the number of cytotoxic, CD8-positive lymphocytes. Subpopulations of other cell types, including monocytes, macrophages, natural killer (Nk) cells, and B lymphocytes, have been found to express the CD4 surface antigen. The loss of mainly helper T cells impairs the ability to produce specific antibodies. Even if patients with AIDS have elevated immunoglobulin levels in serum, children with HIV infections cannot respond with antibody production to the capsular polysaccharide antigens of, for example, the pneumococci and *H. influenzae* type B.

Alteration of Cytokine Expression

Cytokines are soluble proteins with widespread and diversified actions in cellular communications throughout all organs. By acting at any level of expression of these signal substances, immune responses can be modified in a manner favorable for the microbe.[9]

The action can be direct, as is the case with leishmaniasis, a disease associated with T cell unresponsiveness. Thus, it has been demonstrated that the protozoan leishmania, when grown in macrophages, suppress as the synthesis of interleukin-1 (IL-1). IL-1, interleukin-6 (IL-6), and tumor necrosis factor alpha (TNF-α) constitute the major proinflammatory cytokines. The action of IL-1 is crucial for the activation of both humoral and cellular immune defenses, which eventually eliminate the infection.

An example of a more complex and indirect effect comes from studies on the activities of interleukin-10 (IL-10). IL-10 is a pleiotropic growth and differentiation factor produced by monocytes, T cells, and B cells. It is a potent stimulator of antibody production and suppresses functions of macrophages, T cells, and NK cells. In fact, IL-10 inhibits all functions of interferon-γ (IFN-γ), promoting the killing of intracellular parasites, i.e., enhancing the expression of major histocompatibility complex (MHC) class II antigens necessary for antigen presentation to T cells, activation of intracellular killing of macrophages, and production of reactive oxygen intermediates.

Mycobacterium leprae, the causative agent in leprosy and a facultative intracellular bacterium, has been shown to stimulate the release of similar amounts of IL-10 from peripheral blood mononuclear cells of both healthy donors and leprosy patients, the major source of the IL-10 being macrophages. In vivo, the expression of messenger RNA (mRNA) encoding IL-10 is high in lepromatous lesions, whereas the T cell clones from the lesions produce small quantities of IL-10 protein in vitro. Taken together, the data indicate that *M. leprae* induces IL-10 production. In contrast, in the tuberculoid form of leprosy, in which the host's immune system has succeeded in limiting the disease, the expression of IL-10 mRNA is low, whereas that of IFN-γ mRNA is high.

It has been reported that patients with infectious mononucleosis induced by Epstein-Barr virus (EBV) transiently have high serum levels of IL-10 compared with healthy control subjects (in whom IL-10 was practically undetectable).[10] Using Burkitt's lymphoma cell lines, another group of investigators has suggested that the EBV latent membrane protein 1 (LMP-1) has an important role for the induction of human IL-10 (hIL-10).[11] Interestingly, the EBV genome contains an open reading frame with strong DNA and amino acid sequence homology to hIL-10. The translation product, viral IL-10 (vIL-10), appears to have extensive functional similarity to hIL-10. Furthermore, vIL-10 is expressed during the lytic phase of EBV infection but not during latency. Viral IL-10 could thus enhance the persistence of B cells infected at the site of virus replication. Moreover, both hIL-10 and vIL-10 have been shown to inhibit apoptotic cell death in T cells from patients with EBV-induced infectious mononucleosis.

In summary, microbes have developed different strategies for subverting the host's immune response by acting on the cytokine-signaling pathways, thus favoring infection.

PERSISTENCE

Antigenic Variations

A genetic diversity within different species of viruses, bacteria, and parasites is obviously important to the capability of the microorganisms to survive as a population. Such diversity makes possible the expression of different surface antigens with subsequent variation of other microbial pathogenicity factors. Specific strains among numerous bacterial subspecies express different virulence factors, such as pili, polysaccharide capsules, outer membrane proteins (OMP), LPSs, production of toxins, and proteases.[12]

Antigenic variation of a microbe is a mechanism for evasion of host defense mechanisms. An illustration of this is the protozoan *Trypanosoma brucei,* which causes sleeping sickness. To avoid eradication through antibody-dependent immunity, trypanosomes periodically change their surface glycoprotein. Within a single strain, several bacteria have the capability to change their surface antigens. This phenomenon, called phase variation, has been described for several bacterial genera, such as *Haemophilus* and *Neisseria.*[8]

As a relevant respiratory tract pathogen, *H. influenzae* is used here to exemplify this intrastrain variation. *H. influenzae* type B expresses fimbriae that are subject to phase variation.[13] Fimbriation is beneficial for the bacterium during the initial steps of colonization but disadvantageous in establishing systemic disease (e.g., septicemia, meningitis). Blood isolates are as a rule nonfimbriated but can, under laboratory conditions, be induced to produce fimbriae.

The LPS molecule is unique for gram-negative bacteria. It can be divided into three major parts: lipid A, the core, and the O-specific chain. Lipid A is to a great extent responsible for the systemic endotoxic effects of LPS (septic shock). The O-specific chain of *H. influenzae* is very different from that in species within the Enterobacteriaceae family. *Haemophilus* species lack the repeating units; instead, there are a low number of sugars. Such LPS is often referred to as lipo-oligosaccharide (LOS). LPSs from *Haemophilus* species as well as from *Neisseria* species have special features important for the pathogenicity of these bacteria. They include (1) short oligosaccharide parts with complicated, often branched, structures and a variable number of sialic acid residues; (2) variable phosphorylation of the KDO (3-deoxy-*manno*-octulosonic-acid) regions; (3) molecular mimicry between LPS structures and carbohydrate structures found on human cells; and (4) intrastrain phase variation of the LPS epitopes. Both capsulated and noncapsulated forms of *H. influenzae* are subject to phase variation, giving the bacterium the opportunity to adapt the expression of different structures of its LPS. The molecular basis for this capability has been described for *H. influenzae* type B (Hib). Three loci in the Hib genome, named *lic*1, *lic*2, and *lic*3, are partly responsible for the synthesis of LPS. The regulation of these loci involves the repeating tetramer (5′-CAAT-3′). Twenty to 30 repeats of this sequence are found heading the transcribed part of each locus. Presumably because of slipped-strand mispairing mutations, the reading frame can be altered, and different translation products (LPS molecules) occur. This sophisticated masquerade enables the bacterium to escape the antibody-dependent immune defense.[14]

Antigenic variations of the major OMPs of nontypable *H. influenzae* have been demonstrated on isolates from patients with chronic obstructive pulmonary disease. Genetically identical strains changed their OMP composition during persistent infection. Such OMPs are immunogenic, and a change in OMP structure may possibly impair binding of antibodies and subsequent phagocytosis by alveolar macrophages.[15]

Intracellular Survival

Several bacterial species are known as facultative intracellular parasites.[16] Some of these bacteria can elicit phagocytosis and thus enter cells not normally considered phagocytic, for instance, epithelial cells. Others can survive and multiply in the hostile environment inside "professional" phagocytes. Once the bacterium is inside, the intracellular environment offers protection against host defense mechanisms like complement and antibodies, which do not penetrate intracellularly. A number of commonly used antibiotics also have poor intracellular penetration. An often repeated theme is the abuse done to physiologic receptors by the invading microbes and the involvement of the cytoskeleton in the process of internalization.[17]

Enteropathogenic *E. coli* has been shown to induce tyrosine phosphorylation in epithelial cells and thereby initiates rearrangements of the cytoskeleton mediating uptake. *Salmonella typhimurium* invades epithelial cells by secretion of an invasion gene (*invA*)–encoded product that directly interacts with the epidermal growth factor receptor. The protein invasion expressed in *Yersinia pseudotuberculosis* promotes penetration of the host cell by binding to the cell adhesion molecules of the β_1 integrin superfamily. Uptake of *B. pertussis* is promoted by filamentous hemagglutinin containing an Arg-Gly-Asp sequence that interacts with the complement receptor 3 (CR3) on the macrophage surface. In a study using a rabbit model, it was shown that inhibition of the CR3 interaction disrupted the accumulation of viable intracellular bacteria but did not prevent pathologic changes in the lung.[18] In contrast, inhibition of bacterial recognition of carbohydrates on cilia and macrophages prevented pulmonary edema. It was therefore proposed that the intracellular localization within macrophages could promote persistence of *B. pertussis* in the lung without causing injury and that the extracellular presence of bacteria is responsible for disease. Long-term intracellular filamentous hemagglutinin–dependent entry and survival of *B. pertussis* in human macrophages have been reported.[19] This could perhaps be one explanation of the protracted clinical course of whooping cough.

Surface-exposed high-molecular-weight proteins of non-encapsulated *H. influenzae* have been characterized and shown to be related to the filamentous hemagglutinin of *B. pertussis* and to mediate attachment to human epithelial cells and to monocytes and macrophages. *H. influenzae* entry into epithelial cells, as a mechanism for evasion of host defenses and persistence, has been proposed as a result of in vitro invasion assays using cultured human conjunctival cells.[20] The addition of cytochalasin D, an inhibitor of microfilament formation, markedly decreased invasion. The intracellular presence of nonencapsulated *H. influenzae* in in vivo human adenoid tissue, in subepithelially located macrophage-like cells, has been described. This finding suggests that intracellular sequestration could be a way for this species to become resident in the nasopharynx.

Within the host cell, bacteria have evolved different strategies for evading intracellular killing. By inhibiting phagolysosomal fusion, a function mapped to a 4-kilobase DNA fragment of the *icm* locus, *Legionella pneumophila* survives in macrophages. *Listeria monocytogenes* and *S. flexneri* are capable of escape from the phagocytic vacuole into the cytoplasm, where a rich nutritional environment is offered. Both species can move in the cytosol, as a function of the *actA* gene product, a bacterial surface protein that interacts with actin filaments. In the case of *L. monocytogenes,* an actin polymer tail is formed that pushes the organism to the cell membrane, where exocytosis is induced. The vacuole formed is then phagocytized by the neighboring cell. It is thus possible for the bacterium to spread from cell to cell without having to leave the intracellular compartment.

Viral Latency

A number of viruses have developed coexistence with the host—viral latency—which differs from chronic infection and implies a long-term presence of virus in nonreplicating form. Latency is a feature of several infections but is best understood for the herpesvirus group, including herpes simplex virus as well as Epstein-Barr virus, cytomegalovirus, and varicella zoster virus.

Herpesvirus passes from cell to cell and does not enter the extracellular fluid. This behavior renders the virus invisible to host immune mechanisms such as circulating antibodies, cell-mediated responses, and interferons. The virus has found a privileged site. When virus is reactivated, and immune mechanisms are intact, the spread of virus is limited. If defenses are reduced, however, as in old age, during immunosuppressive treatment, or from immunodeficiency diseases, the virus can replicate and again cause disease.

References

1. Davies J, Carlstedt I, Nilsson AK, et al.: Binding of *Haemophilus influenzae* to purified mucins from the human respiratory tract. Infect Immun 1995; 63: 2485.
2. St. Gene III JW: Nontypeable *Haemophilus influenzae* disease: Epidemiology, pathogenesis, and prospects for prevention. Infect Agents Dis 1993; 2: 1.
3. Rossmann MG: The canyon hypothesis. J Biol Chem 1989; 264: 14587.
4. Freijd A, Bygdeman S, Rynnel-Dagöö B: The nasopharyngeal microflora of otitis-prone children, with emphasis on *H. influenzae.* Acta Otolaryngol (Stockh) 1984; 97:117.
5. Faden H, Brodsky L, Waz MJ, et al.: Nasopharyngeal flora in the first three years of life in normal and otitis-prone children. Ann Otol Rhinol Laryngol 1991; 100: 612.
6. Lomholt H, van Alphen L, Kilian M: Antigenic variation of immunoglobulin A_1 proteases among sequential isolates of *Haemophilus influenzae* from healthy children and patients with chronic obstructive pulmonary disease. Infect Immun 1993; 61: 4575.
7. Male D, Champion B, Cooke A, et al.: Complement. In: Advanced Immunology, 2nd ed. London: Gower Medical Publishing, 1991, p 151.
8. Plaut A: Microbial subversion of host defenses. In: Schaechter M, Medoff G, Eisenstein BI (eds): Mechanisms of Microbial Disease, 2nd ed. Baltimore: Williams & Wilkins, 1992, p 154.

9. Modlin RL, Nutman TB: Type 2 cytokines and negative immune regulation in human infections. Curr Opin Immunol 1993; 5: 511.

10. Taga H, Taga K, Wang F, et al.: Human and viral interleukin-10 in acute Epstein-Barr virus–induced infectious mononcleosis. J Infect Dis 1995; 171: 1347.

11. Nakagomi H, Dolcetti R, Bejarano MT, et al.: The Epstein-Barr virus latent membrane protein-1 (LMP1) induces interleukin-10 production in Burkitt lymphoma lines. Int J Cancer 1994; 57: 240.

12. Relman DA, Falkow S: A molecular perspective of microbial pathogenicity. In: Mandell GL (ed): Principles and Practice in Infectious Diseases, 4th ed. New York: Churchill Livingstone, 1995, p 19.

13. van Ham SM, van Alphen L, Mooi FR, van Putten JP: Phase variation of H. influenzae fimbriae: Transcriptional control of two divergent genes through a variable combined promotor region. Cell 1993; 73: 1187.

14. Weiser JN, Maskell DJ, Butler PD, et al.: Characterization of repetitive sequences controlling phase variation of Haemophilus influenzae lipopolysaccharide. J Bacteriol 1990; 172: 3304.

15. Groenveld K, van Alphen L, Eijk PP, et al.: Endogenous and exogenous reinfections by Haemophilus influenzae in patients with chronic obstructive pulmonary disease: The effect of antibiotic treatment on persistence. J Infect Dis 1990; 161: 512.

16. Pamer EG: Cellular immunity to intracellular bacteria. Curr Opin Immunol 1993; 5: 492.

17. Wick MJ, Madara JL, Fields BN, et al.: Molecular cross talk between epithelial cells and pathogenic microorganisms. Cell 1991; 67: 651.

18. Saukkonen K, Cabellos C, Burroughs M, et al.: Integrin-mediated localization of Bordetella pertussis within macrophages: Role in pulmonary colonization. J Exp Med 1991; 173: 1143.

19. Friedman RL, Nordensson L, Wilson L, et al.: Uptake and intracellular survival of Bordetella pertussis in human macrophages. Infect Immun 1992; 60: 4578

20. St. Gene III JW, Falkow S: Haemophilus influenzae adheres to and enters cultured human epithelial cells. Infect Immmun 1990; 58: 4036.

CHAPTER THREE

Janak A. Patel
Pearay L. Ogra

Host Defense

▼

The nasopharynx and oropharynx are important sites of entry by microorganisms and other particulate and gaseous matter into contiguous tissues such as sinuses, middle ear bullae, lower respiratory tract, and gastrointestinal tract. Microorganisms also invade distant organs by entry into the submucosal tissues and subsequently into the blood or lymph stream. The host defenses of the nasopharynx and oropharynx are, therefore, critical for maintenance of health. Advances in research have significantly improved understanding of the mucosal and systemic immune responses at these sites. However, a significant gap exists in the understanding of the role of immune defenses in the pathogenesis of recurrent infections of the sinuses, pharynx, and middle ear, which account for the frequent use of antimicrobial therapy. Additional studies of immune defenses may facilitate better approaches for immunomodulatory therapies.

The mechanisms of host defense can be divided into two functional divisions: the innate and the adaptive or acquired (Fig. 3–1). Innate immunity attempts to check pathogens before they cause overt infection. The mucus blanket, ciliary activity, cytokines, neutrophils, monocytes, and macrophages contribute to this system. If this first line of defense is penetrated, the adaptive immune system, controlled by lymphocytes, mounts a specific response to the pathogen in an attempt to eradicate it. The adaptive system remembers prior pathogens, so future responses occur more rapidly. Table 3–1 summarizes the immunologic characteristics in the tissues of head and neck during infection relative to those in the gastrointestinal and lower respiratory tracts. These characteristics are discussed further in this chapter.

INNATE IMMUNITY

The Mucus Blanket

The mucosal epithelial cells are the most effective first line of defense in the innate immune system. Most infectious organisms cannot penetrate the intact secretory blanket of the epithelial cells. The secretory blanket consists of two separate layers, the surface mucous (or gel) layer and a deeper aqueous (or serous, periciliary) layer, in which the base of the cilia is located. In the nose, particles trapped in the surface mucous layer are transported by mucociliary action to the posterior pharynx at the rate of 1 cm/min.[1] The surface mucus blanket is then swallowed and is constantly replaced about every 10 to 20 minutes under resting conditions. The mucus blanket is thus secreted constantly and is constantly removed and replaced. This rapid turnover contributes to the barrier function of the mucus blanket.

Microorganisms and other particulate matter are trapped in the mucus and are passively removed by these processes. The blanket is a selective sieve because large particles never reach the mucous membrane, whereas smaller molecules do so and are readily absorbed.

Mucus glycoproteins are a major constituent of the mucous layer. They constitute 15% of the total protein of nasal lavage, although the composition is at least 80% carbohydrate.[2] These glycoproteins provide a flexible, replaceable coat that absorbs water for hydration. A selective function of the mucus glycoprotein is to serve as a specific binding receptor for bacteria such as nontypable *Haemophilus influenzae*.[3]

The deeper periciliary or serous layer follows different kinetics from the surface mucous layer. The periciliary fluid contains most of the aqueous proteins listed in Table 3–2, many of which are derived from the serous cells of the submucosal glands. Unlike the surface mucous layer, which traps and exports foreign material away from the mucous membrane, the deeper periciliary fluid contains molecules such as lysozymes and lactoferrin, providing important host defense functions.[1] The proteins of the periciliary fluid reconstitute themselves within 10 to 20 minutes after repeated lavages and may require 4 to 24 hours to achieve resting concentrations.[4] The periciliary fluid does not turn over quickly, and the stability of this layer of fluid may provide many of the protective functions of secretions in host defense.

Regulation of Nasal Secretions

The production of nasal secretions containing mucus and other constituents is regulated by parasympathetic nerves.[5, 6] The resultant secretion is enriched for glandular proteins, although plasma proteins are also included. Adrenergic stimulation of the mucosa either has no effect on secretions or only mildly stimulates glandular secretion (β-adrenergic stimulation).[7] The mucosal lining of the nasopharynx and middle ear exhibits a number of sensory nerves containing the neuropeptides substance P, calcitonin gene–related peptide, (CGRP), vasoactive intestinal peptide, and gastrin-releasing peptide (GRP).[8–11] All of the sensory nerves have some fibers that apparently innervate submucosal glands. These neuropeptides, therefore, have the capacity to induce mucus and serous cell secretion. The mucosa is not only rich in nerves and blood vessels but also contains numerous mast cells. It is possible that interactions between histamine-containing mast cells and substance P–containing and CGRP-containing nerves—i.e., neurogenic inflammation—are one of the mechanisms involved in vessel permeability

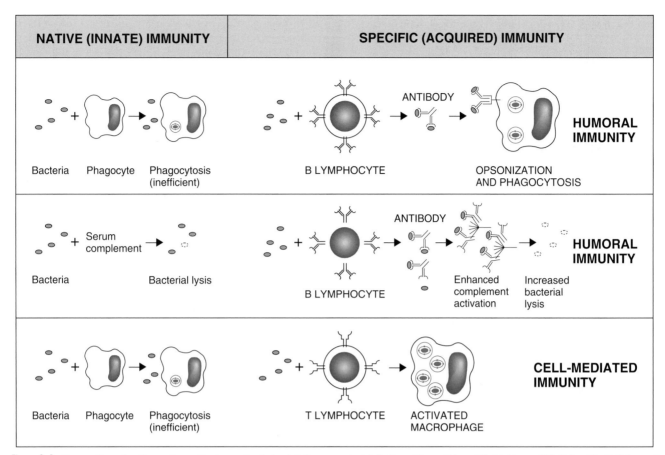

Figure 3–1. Cooperation of native and specific immunity in host defenses against infection. (From Abbas AK, Lichtman AH, Pober JS: Cellular and Molecular Immunology, 2nd ed. Philadelphia: WB Saunders Co., 1994, p 11.)

changes in otitis media with effusion, chronic sinusitis, and allergic rhinitis.[12] Several enzymes, including neutral endopeptidase, important in metabolizing neuropeptides, have also been localized to serous cells and endothelium of small blood vessels.[13]

The nasal secretions during upper respiratory tract infections are also under the control of inflammatory mediators such as histamine, leukotrienes, and prostaglandins, which are released by leukocytes and tissue cells involved in the inflammatory response. During the early stage of infection, the secretions are rich in plasma proteins, including immunoglobulin G (IgG) and albumin, whereas during the later stage, glandular proteins predominate.[1, 14] It has been suggested that the outpouring of plasma proteins might represent an important first line of defense at mucosal surfaces.

Ciliary System

The mucociliary system is composed of motile epithelial cilia and the mucus blanket. In the tissues of the head and neck, the ciliated epithelial cells line the nasopharynx, si-

Table 3–1. COMPARISON OF IMMUNOLOGIC CHARACTERISTICS

Feature	Intestinal Tract	Respiratory Tract	Middle Ear	Paranasal Sinuses	Nasopharynx
Ciliated epithelium	−	+ +	+	+ +	+
Mucus blanket	+ + +	+ + +	+ +	+ +	+ +
Production of IgA	+ + +	+	+	+	+ + +
IgG:IgA ratio	0.5–1.0	3–4	3–4	?	0.5–3
T-cell distribution					
Th1 cells	+ +	+ +	?	?	+ +
Th2 cells	+ +	+ +	?	?	+ +
Cytotoxic T lymphocytes	+ +	+ +	+ +	?	+ +
Cytokine production					
Proinflammatory	+ +	+ +	+ +	+ +	+ + +
Immnunoregulatory	+ +	+ +	+ +	+ +	+ +

*Grading from − (none) to + + + (strong); ? unknown.

Table 3–2. MAJOR CONSTITUENTS OF HUMAN NASAL SECRETIONS

Source	Products
Mucous cell products	Mucus glycoproteins
Serous cell products	Lactoferrin, lysozyme, s-IgA (dimeric) and secretory component, peroxidase, secretory leukoprotease inhibitor
Plasma proteins	Albumin, immunoglobulins (IgG, monomeric IgA, IgM, IgE), kallikrein, complements
Sensory nerves	Calcitonin gene–related peptide, substance P
Leukocytes and other cells	Interleukins 1–12, tumor necrosis factor α, interferons α, β, and γ, transforming growth factor β, macrophage inflammatory protein 1, monocyte chemotactic peptide 1, histamine, leukotrienes, tryptase, major basic protein, prostaglandins

nuses, and eustachian tube. The ciliary motion requires sequential coordination of the adjacent cilia. This coordination occurs because when a cilium begins to move among a group of stationary cilia, the clockwise swing of its recovery stroke brings it into contact with adjacent cilia, thereby stimulating the cilia on that side to commence their recovery strokes and causing them to excite their neighboring cilia. Such coordinated activity disappears, only to be followed by further waves propagated over the same group of cells. Calcium ion flux is associated with a change in the frequency of the ciliary beat.[15]

Cytokines

The nasopharyngeal epithelium can function as an immunologic organ by its ability to produce immunoregulatory cytokines. The mucosal tissues of the nasopharynx and oropharynx are capable of producing all the cytokines discovered to date, including interleukins 1 through 12 (IL-1 through IL-12), tumor necrosis factor α (TNF-α), interferons (IFNs), and transforming growth factor β (TGF-β). The sources and functions of various cytokines are summarized in Table 3–3. The cytokines produced by helper T cell subsets (Th1 and Th2) are divided into two distinct classes. Characteristically, Th1 cells secrete IL-2, IFN-γ, and lymphotoxin (TNF-β); Th2 cells secrete IL-4, IL-5, IL-6, and IL-10. A dichotomy of function between the two predominant helper subsets has been suggested. Th1 cells are associated with delayed-type hypersensitivity, whereas Th2 cells are associated with antibody responses and allergic responses. However, only the antiviral activity of interferons, the phagocyte recruitment property, and the natural killer (NK) cell–enhancing activity of certain cytokines contribute to innate host defenses.

Antiviral Role

Viral infection directly stimulates the production of type I IFN (i.e., IFN-α and IFN-β) by infected cells.[16] IFN-α and IFN-β show little structural similarity. Nevertheless, all type I IFN molecules bind to the same cell surface receptor and appear to induce a similar series of cellular responses. Type

I IFN inhibits viral replication by its effect on cells to synthesize a number of enzymes, such as 2′-5′ oligoadenylate synthetase, that collectively interfere with replication of viral RNA and DNA. The antiviral action of type I IFN is primarily paracrine in that a virally infected cell secretes IFN to protect neighboring cells not yet infected. A cell that has responded to IFN and is resistant to viral infection is said to be in an antiviral state.

Recruitment of Phagocytes

IL-8 is the most potent cytokine with chemoattractant property for neutrophils. It can be produced by local epithelial cells, endothelial cells, fibroblasts, and tissue macrophages.[17] IL-1α, IL-1β, and TNF-α, which are also produced by similar cells, increase the expression of adhesion molecules, such as intercellular adhesion molecule 1 (ICAM-1), on endothelial cells as well as the expression of its adhesion receptors—leukocyte function–associated antigen 1 (LFA-1) (CD11a/CD18 heterodimer complex) and glycoprotein Mac-1 (CD11b/CD18)—on surface membranes of neutrophils and blood monocytes/macrophages involved in innate defense.[18] The interactions between these as well as many other adhesion molecules and receptors contribute to the adhesion-dependent pathway used by leukocytes to bind to the endothelium and subsequently egress into the extravascular tissues at the site of infection. C5a (a complement product), leukotrienes, and prostaglandins are also potent chemotactic agents for phagocytes.

Phagocytes

As in most tissues of the body, the neutrophil is the predominant phagocyte accumulating in the tissues of the head and neck during the early stage of infection with either bacterial or viral pathogens. For example, middle ear fluids and nasal secretions from hosts with acute infection due to viral and bacterial pathogens contain predominantly neutrophils.[19–22] The role of the neutrophil is to contain bacterial infection by phagocytosis and extracellular release of antibacterial products. However, its role in viral infection is unknown. It is likely that during viral and bacterial infection, neutrophils also play a deleterious role by releasing mediators that produce tissue injury. For example, animals inoculated with nontypable *H. influenzae* have minimal tissue injury when the neutrophil migration is blocked by use of an antiadhesion molecule (anti-CD11b/CD18) antibody.[23]

Other leukocytes with phagocytic capability are eosinophils, monocytes, and macrophages. In innate immunity of the upper airway, however, the phagocytic role of these cells is considerably smaller. This is in contrast to the important phagocytic role of alveolar macrophages in the lower airway. Eosinophils are more specifically directed toward parasites rather than bacteria.

Lysozymes

Several nonspecific proteins in nasal secretions have broad-spectrum antimicrobial actions. Lysozymes are relatively

Table 3–3. SELECTED CHARACTERISTICS OF CYTOKINES

Cytokine	Cell Sources	Biologic Activities
IL-1	Macrophages, endothelial cells, fibroblasts, epithelial cells, T and B cells, and other cells	Acts on a large variety of cell targets Proliferation of B and T lymphocytes and fibroblasts Release of PGE_2 from fibroblasts, macrophages, and endothelial cells Release of TNF-α from macrophages Mediator of acute-phase response Mediator of neutrophilic exudate, edema, and mononuclear exudate at site of injury Mediator of angiogenesis Fever, sleep, anorexia, bone resorption
IL-2	T (Th1) and B cells	Acts on activated T and B lymphocytes and monocytes, generation of cytolytic T cells, and enhancement of cytolytic T cell responses Induction of IFN-γ secretion by T lymphocytes and, secondarily, activation of natural killer cell activity Induction of antibody synthesis and secretion by B lymphocytes Adoptive immunotherapy (LAK cells) against various tumors, particularly renal cell carcinoma and malignant melanoma Damage of endothelium at high doses
IL-3	T (Th1 and Th2) cells	Acts on myelomonocytic cells and other precursors of hematopoiesis Proliferation of colony-forming units Generation of monocytes, granulocytes, megakaryocytes, basophils, and eosinophils from bone marrow precursors Generation of normoblasts in conjunction with erythropoietin Enhancement of hematopoiesis during the immune response
IL-4	T (Th2) cells and mast cells	Acts on many lineages Induction of expression of HLA-DR on mast cells, resting B cells, and macrophages Causes immunoglobulin isotype switching on B cells from IgG to IgE Induces expression of CD23 (Fc receptor) on B cells Induces cytolytic T-cell reactivity and mitogenesis in helper T and cytotoxic T cells Induces production of IL-2 and IL-2 receptor Induces fusion of monocytes to form multinucleated giant cells Required for maturation of progenitor CD4 cells to the Th2 pattern of cytokine secretion
IL-5	T (Th2) cells	Limits B cell proliferation Generates eosinophils from bone marrow precursors Enhances IgA production Induces IL-2 receptor in T cells Enhances cytotoxic T-lymphocyte production Induces expression of CD23 on B cells
IL-6	T (Th2) and B cells, macrophages, fibroblasts, endothelial cells, myeloma cells, and others	Production in response to other cytokines (IL-1, TNF-α) Mediator of the acute-phase response by acting on liver Proliferation of cytotoxic T cells in conjunction with IL-1, IL-2, and TNF-α
IL-7	Thymic and bone marrow cells, splenic stromal cells	Generation of immature T and B cells No activity on mature T or B cells
IL-8	Macrophages, endothelial cells, fibroblasts, keratinocytes, alveolar epithelium, and others	Chemoattractant for polymorphonuclear leukocytes (PMNs) Induces degranulation and expression of receptors Promotes migration through endothelium of PMNs
IL-9	T lymphocytes (Th2 cells)	Growth of helper T cells independent of IL-2 and IL-4 Enhances responses of mast cells to IL-3 Stimulates erythropoiesis and megakaryopoiesis
IL-10	T (Th2) and B cells	Markedly reduces IFN-γ production by macrophages Promotes lymphocyte growth in combination with IL-3 and IL-4 Promotes cytotoxic T-cell growth and differentiation of antigen-specific CD8 + T cells in combination with IL-2
IL-11	Bone marrow stromal cells	Stimulates development of IgG B cells With IL-3, induces megakaryocyte development Shortens the G_0 period of early hematopoietic precursors and acts in conjunction with IL-3 in hematopoiesis like IL-6
IL-12	B lymphoblastoid cell line	Activates T-cell and NK-cell growth and differentiation

Modified from Beckman E: Cytokines in infectious diseases. Clin Microbiol Newsletter 1992; 14: 73–77 by Elsevier Science Inc.

small proteins (14,000 D) found in all body secretions. They represent 15%–30% of the protein normally found in nasal secretions and effectively prevent mucosal infections from most airborne bacteria.[1] Lysozymes are synthesized and secreted by the serous cells of submucosal glands and by neutrophils and macrophages. Lysozymes cleave murein, a complex polymer of amino acids and sugars or peptidoglycan, in the cell walls of bacteria and in the chitin found in fungi.[24] Lysozymes are not effective against intact gram-negative organisms, because the murein complex is hidden by the lipopolysaccharide outer membrane. The ability of the complement membrane attack complex (MAC) to break up the outer membrane allows cleavage of the exposed murein by lysozyme.

Lactoferrin

Lactoferrin is an antimicrobial protein made by serous glands that is both bacteriostatic and bactericidal to susceptible bacteria. Lactoferrin binds iron, thereby interfering with microbial iron metabolism, and presumably this action kills bacteria.[25] In general, dose-dependent killing or inhibition of microorganisms is caused by apolactoferrin but not by iron-saturated lactoferrin. Lactoferrin constitutes about 2%–4% of nasal proteins. It is suggested that lactoferrin acts in synergy with secretory IgA (s-IgA) for enhanced killing of pathogens.[26]

Acute-Phase Proteins

Acute-phase proteins, such as C-reactive protein, lipopolysaccharide-binding proteins, serum amyloid A protein, transferrin, complement factor B, and α_1-antitrypsin, are released from the liver as part of the inflammatory response. Their role may be stimulatory or inhibitory in the acute-phase response.[27] For example, α_1-antitrypsin inhibits the proteases that stimulate the production of kinins. Transferrin binds iron, thereby inhibiting bacterial growth by reducing the availability of iron necessary for growth. Lipopolysaccharide-binding proteins inactivate gram-negative bacterial endotoxins. C-reactive protein can bind serum lipids and opsonize *Streptococcus pneumoniae*.

The Complement System

The main functions of the complement system are to limit the spread of infectious agents and to facilitate the destruction of infectious agents by phagocytosis and/or lysis. The complement proteins interact with one another, with antibodies, and with cell-wall membranes. These interactions mediate such functions as immune adherence, phagocytosis, chemotaxis, and cytolysis. C5a facilitates the adherence of neutrophils and induces increased metabolic activity within the cells.[28] In the nonspecific early response to invasion with microorganisms, the alternative complement pathway can be activated in the absence of specific antigen-antibody complexes. Complement components C5a and C3b enhance the phagocytosis of invading organisms by inducing chemotaxis and opsonization. The complement components that make up the membrane attack complex (C5, C6, C7, C8, C9) are responsible for lysis of bacteria, viruses, fungi, protozoa, and virus-infected host cells.[27, 29] Complement-mediated killing of the organisms occurs by insertion of the MAC into the cell membrane, making it leaky and permeable to ions and water, and eventually leading to cell death. Along with this protective role, activation of the complement system also results in the formation of biologically active compounds capable of contributing to tissue damage.

During bacterial and viral infections of the tissues of the head and neck, complement products are readily detected in inflammatory fluids.[30–32] However, most investigations to date have been unable to correlate the levels of complement proteins with the presence or severity of disease.

Natural Killer (NK) Cells

NK cells are a subset of lymphocytes that lack the specific T-cell receptor for antigen recognition; therefore, they do

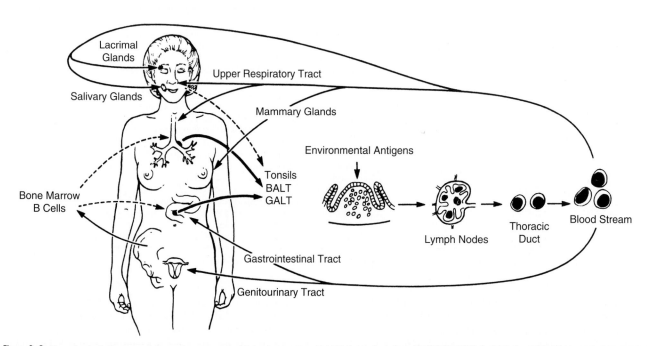

Figure 3–2. Hypothetical diagram of the common mucosal immune system (BALT [bronchus-associated lymphoid tissue]; GALT [gut-associated lymphoid tissue]). (From Mestecky J, Abraham R, Ogra PL: Common mucosal immune system and strategies for the development of vaccines effective at the mucosal sites. In: Ogra PL, Strober W, Mestecky J, et al. [eds]: Handbook of Mucosal Immunology. San Diego: Academic Press, 1994.)

not exhibit virus-specific activity. However, NK cells play an important early role in limiting the extent of certain mucosal viral infections.[33] NK cells can be activated to increase their ability to lyse target cells by treatment with type I IFN, IFN-γ, IL-12, TNF, or IL-2. These cells can acquire additional specificities by virtue of CD16-mediated recognition of targets coated with IgG antibodies. This form of cytolysis is called antibody-dependent cell-mediated cytotoxicity, and NK cells are its principal mediator. NK cells kill the target cells by granule exocytosis and induction of target cell DNA fragmentation and apoptosis.

ADAPTIVE IMMUNITY

Lymphoid Tissues of the Head and Neck and the Common Mucosal System

In the head and neck, the T and B lymphocytes reside both in the mucosa of the nasopharynx and oropharynx and in the lymph nodes. In the mucosa, the aggregation of lymphoid tissue referred to as Waldeyer's ring comprises palatine, lingual, adenoidal, and tonsillar lymphoid tissues.[34] These lymphoid tissues show a characteristic architecture that includes a reticular epithelium, a follicular region (or primary and secondary germinal centers that are covered with mantle zones), and extrafollicular regions. These nasopharynx-associated lymphoid tissues resemble other lymphoepithelial structures, such as bronchus-associated and gut-associated lymphoid tissues.[35] Indeed, the cells from palatine and nasopharyngeal tonsils have been proposed to contribute to the population of lymphoid cells at adjacent sites, such as sinuses and middle ear bullae and parotid gland, as well as at distant mucosal sites, such as the lower respiratory and digestive tracts.[36–38] This phenomenon has led to the development of the concept of a common mucosal immune system[35] (Fig. 3–2). For the middle ear, however, this concept is disputed by others.[39] Furthermore, it is not known whether infection restricted to the nasopharyngeal site alone generates antibodies at other mucosal sites.

The major regional lymph nodes of the head and neck are illustrated in Figure 3–3.[40] The superficial cervical lymph nodes lie on top of the sternomastoid muscle along the course of the external jugular vein. They receive afferents from the superficial tissues of the neck, mastoid, parotid nodes, and submaxillary glands. The mastoid lymph nodes receive drainage from the parietal scalp and inner surface of the pinna. The occipital lymph nodes receive drainage from the occipital scalp and upper posterior neck. The efferents terminate in the deep cervical glands. The deep cervical lymph nodes lie deep to the sternocleidomastoid muscle. The jugulodigastric lymph nodes lie at the angle of the jaw and drain the palatine tonsils. These lymph nodes frequently become enlarged in patients with tonsillitis or with tuberculous infection originating from the tonsils. The larynx, trachea, thyroid gland, and esophagus drain into the lower deep cervical glands. The submental lymph nodes receive superficial and deep drainage from the anterior tongue, lower lip, and chin on both sides of the midline. They send efferents to the submandibular and upper deep cervical glands. The submandibular lymph nodes lie adjacent to the subman-

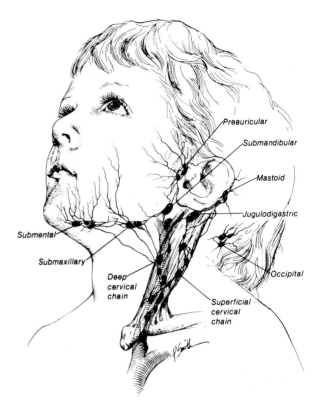

Figure 3–3. The lymphatic drainage and lymph nodes involved in infants and children with cervical lymphadenitis. (From Butler KM, Baker CJ: Cervical lymphadenitis. In: Feigin RD, Cherry JD [eds]: Textbook of Pediatric Infectious Diseases, 3rd ed., vol 1. Philadelphia: WB Saunders Co., 1992, p 221.)

dibular salivary gland and receive rather wide, superficial drainage from the lateral aspect of the lower lip, the vestibule of the nose, the cheeks, the medial portions of the eyelids, and the forehead. Deep drainage to these nodes arises from the posterior part of the mouth, gums, teeth, and tongue as well as from superficial and submental lymph nodes.

Because the majority of the lymphatic drainage of the head and neck goes to the submandibular and deep cervical nodes, it is not surprising that these glands are involved in more than 80% of young children with cervical adenitis. Submental and superficial cervical lymph node infection is seen less frequently. The lymphocytes of the lymphoid tissues of the head and neck and those derived from the circulation participate actively in humoral and cell-mediated immunity (Fig. 3–4).

Antigen Processing

Much of the processing of microbial antigens occurs in the tonsillar and adenoidal tissues[35, 41] (Fig. 3–5). The principal route of antigen uptake occurs in the crypts or furrows. Microfold cells (commonly referred to as M cells), which are important in antigen uptake, are present in the epithelium.[42] Other human leukocyte antigen (HLA)-DR–positive cells that exist deep in the crypt are also important in antigen uptake. Further antigen transport into follicles occurs via macrophages, interdigitating cells that are present in the extrafollicular areas, and follicular dendritic cells that are primarily present in the germinal centers.[43]

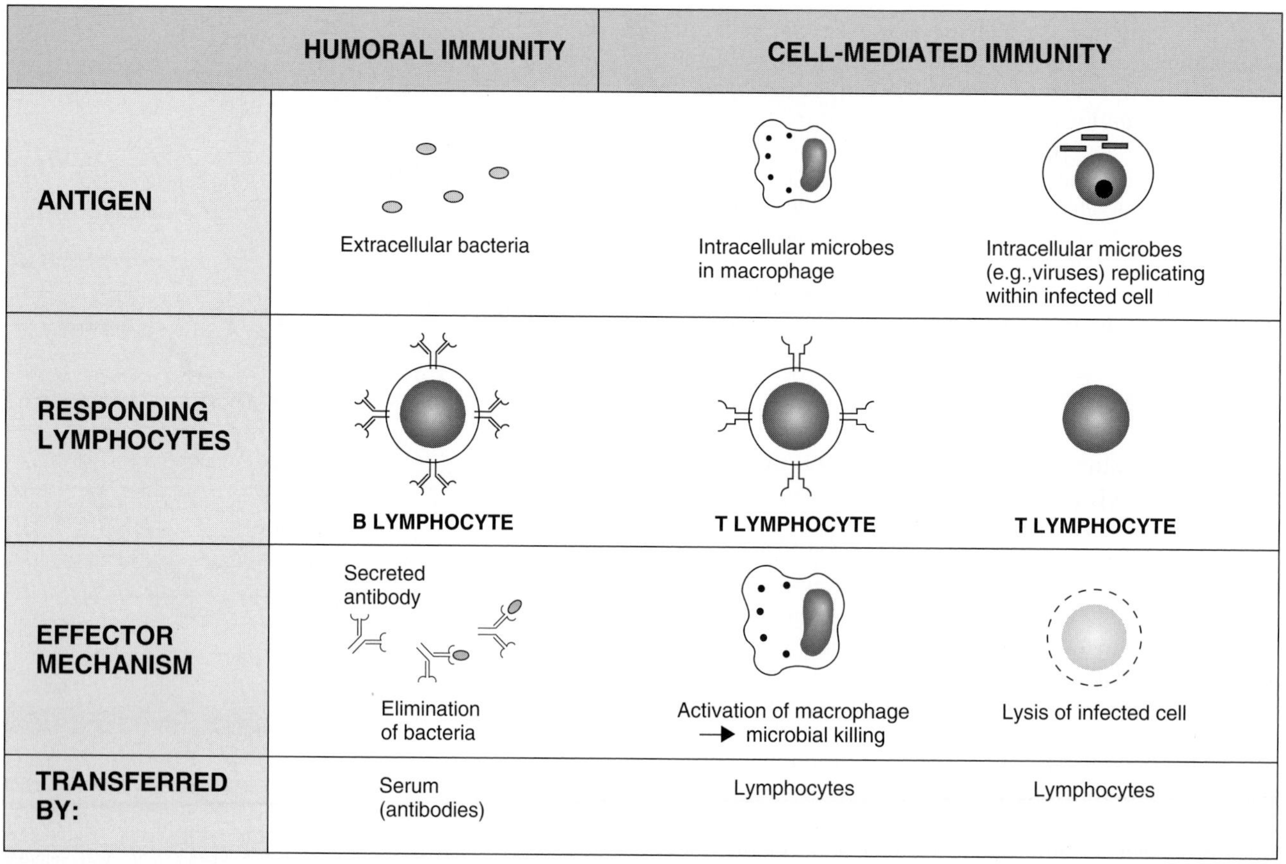

	HUMORAL IMMUNITY	CELL-MEDIATED IMMUNITY	
ANTIGEN	Extracellular bacteria	Intracellular microbes in macrophage	Intracellular microbes (e.g.,viruses) replicating within infected cell
RESPONDING LYMPHOCYTES	**B LYMPHOCYTE**	**T LYMPHOCYTE**	**T LYMPHOCYTE**
EFFECTOR MECHANISM	Secreted antibody / Elimination of bacteria	Activation of macrophage → microbial killing	Lysis of infected cell
TRANSFERRED BY:	Serum (antibodies)	Lymphocytes	Lymphocytes

Figure 3–4. Forms of specific immunity. (From Abbas AK, Lichtman AH, Pober JS: Cellular and Molecular Immunology, 2nd ed. Philadelphia: WB Saunders Co., 1994, p 7.)

T cells characteristically occupy the extrafollicular zones of the lymphoid tissues, but the helper T cells are also present in the germinal centers.[44] B cells are primarily present in the germinal center and the mantle zone but may also be found in the reticular epithelium. The average percentages of T and B cells in the lymphoid tissues are 42% and 52%, respectively. The majority of T cells are helper T cells.[45]

Immunoglobulins

The major source of local antibody production in the nasopharynx and oropharynx are the tonsils and adenoids. Actively Ig-secreting cells constitute no more than 2% of total cells of the lymphoid tissues.[46] IgG is the predominant immunogloblin. The numbers of B cells that produce IgA and IgM are about equal. IgA secretion is significantly greater in the palatine tonsils than in the regional lymph nodes.[47] IgG- and IgM-producing cells are found in the germinal centers, whereas IgG- and IgA-producing cells are found primarily in the extrafollicular zones and in the crypt of the epithelium. The production of immunoglobulins is under the influence of cytokines that exist in the microenvironment of the lymphoid tissues.

IgA

IgA is produced locally by plasma cells located within 50 μm of submucous glands (Fig. 3–6). The locally produced IgA is dimeric and is joined by the J-chain before secretion. Dimeric IgA binds to the secretory component produced by serous cells and forms s-IgA. s-IgA is transported transcellularly through the serous cells into glandular secretions and becomes a glandular secretory product. s-IgA constitutes about 15% of total protein in baseline secretions.[1, 48] It acts primarily by binding microorganisms in the airway lumen and by preventing attachment of these potential pathogens to the mucosa. During diseases such as recurrent tonsillitis, a significant reduction in IgA cells is seen in the follicle and in the extrafollicular area of the tonsils. Two IgA isotypes have been described in humans, IgA1 and IgA2.[49] These two isotypes are very similar in structure. IgA1 is the predominant type in serum (~85%) and tonsils, whereas in salivary secretions, it constitutes 55% of the immunoglobulins.[49–51]

Under certain conditions, some of the microorganisms are capable of subverting the activity of IgA1 by cleaving IgA1 into fragment, antigen-binding (Fab) and fragment, crystallizable fragments. This cleavage is caused by IgA1 proteases excreted from bacteria such as *H. influenzae, S. pneumoniae, Neisseria gonorrhoeae, Neisseria meningitidis,* some strains of *Streptococcus sanguis,* and *Streptococcus mitis.*[52–55] IgA2, on the other hand, is resistant to the activity of bacterial proteases.

IgG

IgG acts primarily in the mucosa itself to limit invasion by microorganisms that reach the epithelium. Although IgG is

Figure 3–5. Schematic representation of various tissue elements that are important for the immunologic functions of the human palatine tonsil (crypt in the center). (From Brandtzaeg P: Immune functions and immunopathology of palatine and nasopharyngeal tonsils. In: Bernstein JM, Ogra PL [eds]: Immunology of the Ear. New York: Raven Press, 1987.)

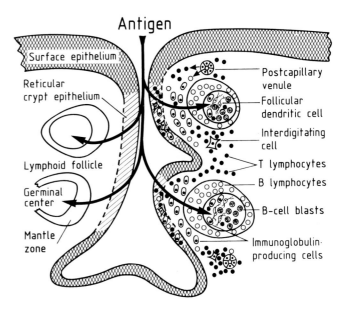

present in secretions (about 2%–4% of total protein in baseline secretions), it is found in a much higher concentration in the tissue fluid itself.[1, 48] IgG levels in secretions are increased up to 125 times by the process of vascular permeability.[1, 4] Thus, it is likely that one purpose of acute inflammation is to bathe the mucosa in an IgG-rich secretion. The nonspecific antimicrobial properties of mucus and the presence of normal amounts of IgG must compensate adequately for the functions of s-IgA because most IgA-deficient patients have a normal incidence of infections. In contrast, patients with IgG deficiency usually require treatment for recurrent respiratory infections. Thus, it appears that the protective functions served in the mucosa by IgG are of greater importance in preventing the development of respiratory infections than is s-IgA.

IgE

Among mucosal pathogens of the nasopharynx and oropharynx, only respiratory syncytial virus (RSV) has been well studied for its ability to induce production of virus-specific IgE antibodies.[56, 57] As with secretory IgA, IgE appears first bound to the surface of RSV-infected cells and later free in secretions. The significance of these antibodies in the host defenses of nasopharyngeal and oropharyngeal tissues is unknown, although the concentrations of IgE correlate with the release of histamine in nasopharyngeal secretions and the severity of lower airway disease.[56, 57]

Role of Cytokines in Mucosal Immunoglobulin Production

At the mucosal site, the expression of a specific isotype of immunoglobulin is regulated by cytokines that act either to mediate heavy-chain class switching or to stimulate the maturation of B lymphocytes expressing particular isotypes. The mucosal immune system is distinguished from other secondary lymphoid organs by the predominance of IgA in mucosal secretions. IL-4 and IL-5 increase the production of IgA in secretions. Both of these cytokines are produced by Th2 cells.[58] IL-2, a cytokine secreted by Th1 cells, can act to cause maturation to IgA secretion.[59] IL-6 is associated with growth and differentiation of B-lineage cells.[60] TGF-β inhibits both human T-cell proliferation and immunoglobulin secretion. However, TGF-β can synergize with IL-2 and IL-5 to enhance IgA secretion.[61, 62] TGF-β is particularly im-

Figure 3–6. Mechanism of immunoglobulin A transport and secretion in mucosal epithelia. (From Abbas AK, Lichtman AH, Pober JS: Cellular and Molecular Immunology, 2nd ed. Philadelphia: WB Saunders Co., 1994, p 234.)

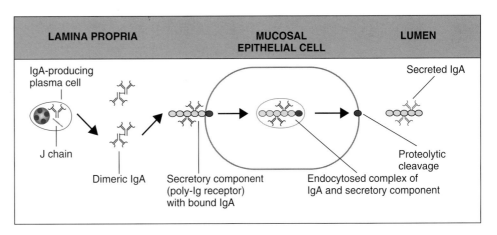

portant in switching of s-IgA–negative to s-IgA–positive cells.[63]

The combination of IL-2 and IL-4 causes a substantial increase in IgM secretion, whereas IFN-γ and IL-4 increase IgG secretion.[64] Th1 cells are relatively more efficient in stimulating IgG2a responses, whereas Th2 cells are more efficient in stimulating IgE responses.[65, 66] IL-10, which is produced by Th2 cells, inhibits cytokine production by Th1 cells.[67]

INFLAMMATORY MEDIATORS IN HOST DEFENSE

Inflammatory mediators at the site of infection may arise primarily from at least two different sources, (1) transudation of serum proteins (e.g., fibrinogen, the complements, the clotting factors, and plasminogen) and (2) release of inflammatory mediators by leukocytes and other local cells. The beneficial roles of complements and lysozymes were discussed earlier. The following discussion deals with other important mediators that are more frequently associated with inflammation and tissue injury than with recovery from infection.

Histamine

Histamine is a potent pharmacologic mediator of inflammation that influences smooth muscle activity, thus increasing the permeability of blood vessels. Its other functions are chemotaxis for eosinophils, blocking of T-lymphocyte function, and induction of mucociliary dysfunction.[68, 69] Histamine is stored in mast cells and basophils largely complexed to mucopolysaccharides such as heparin. During acute and chronic otitis media and sinusitis, significant quantities of histamine are detected in secreted fluids.[70–73] Indeed, combined viral and bacterial infections of the middle ear have been shown to have an additive effect on histamine content.[70] During chronic otitis media, the levels of histamine in tonsillar and adenoidal tissue are even higher than those in middle ear mucosa.[71] There is evidence that children with higher histamine levels in nasal mucosa may have underlying allergic disease.[74] Additional studies show that histamine induces mucociliary dysfunction.[75]

Histamine release during infection may also be mediated by chemokines such as macrophage inflammatory protein 1-α (MIP-1-α) and monocyte chemotactic peptide 1 (MCP-1), which have extremely potent effects on chemotaxis and degranulation of mast cells and basophils. One study has shown that MIP-1-α and MCP-1 are induced by both viral infection and bacterial infection of the middle ear.[76] There is an additive effect on levels of these chemokines when both viral and bacterial infections are present together. The levels of MCP-1 also correlate well with levels of histamine in middle ear fluids.

Lipid Mediators

Cellular phospholipases present in leukocytes and platelets and other cells are activated during inflammation and de-grade phospholipids to arachidonic acid.[28] Arachidonic acid can be metabolized by the enzyme cyclooxygenase to prostaglandins and by the enzyme lipoxygenase hydroxyeicosatetraenoic acid (HETE) as well as derivatives of 5-hydroperoxyeicosatetraenoic acid called leukotrienes. Subsequent enzymatic degradation by cyclooxygenase results in formation of prostaglandins, thromboxanes, or prostacyclins. The neutrophils, macrophages, and basophils are rich sources for 5,12-HETE, also called leukotriene B_4 (LTB_4). The leukotrienes, prostaglandins, thromboxanes, and prostacyclins participate in a variety of inflammatory processes that result in enhanced vascular permeability, tissue edema, and increased accumulation of inflammatory leukocytes.

The platelets and other leukocytes, such as basophils, produce a variety of analogues of phosphatidylcholine called platelet-activating factors (PAFs).[77] PAFs cause platelet aggregation and phagocyte chemoattraction, and they stimulate lysozomal enzyme release and reactive oxygen product formation by neutrophils, eosinophils, and macrophages. In addition, PAFs increase the stickiness of endothelial cells, thereby promoting leukocyte and platelet aggregation. The role of the lipid mediators in infections of the head and neck is highlighted by several studies. LTB_4, a product primarily of neutrophils, and other HETE metabolites have been detected in middle ear effusions in children with acute and chronic bacterial or viral otitis media.[78–80] In another study, it was shown that the levels of LTB_4 correlate with duration and severity of inflammation.[81] Additional studies have shown that LTC_4 and LTD_4 and PAF increase the resistance of the eustachian tube, thereby affecting its patency.[82]

Kinins

In addition to histamine, a group of small polypeptides of the kallikrein-kinin system have potent pharmacologic actions that dilate blood vessels and may also enhance leukocyte migration.[69] The kallikrein-kinin system is activated by the proteolytic activity of a variety of enzymes, including plasmin and trypsin, and activation of Hageman's factor and by acidification and dilution. The products of the kallikrein-kinin system have been shown to be involved in inflammation of the human nasopharynx and middle ear. In otitis media, the concentrations of kininogen appear to be greatest in the serous and seromucinous effusions and lowest in mucoid effusions.[83] Because kinins appear in the early phase of acute inflammation, it can be suggested that serous and seromucinous effusions may precede the mucoid type of middle ear effusions. Bradykinin has also been found in nasal secretions.[84] Topical application of bradykinin to nasal mucosa results in secretions rich in vascular proteins and is associated with increased nasal blood flow.[85]

HOST DEFENSES AGAINST BACTERIAL, VIRAL, AND FUNGAL INFECTIONS

Bacterial Infection

Nonspecific mechanisms such as neutrophil-mediated phagocytosis, lysozymes, defensins, and lactoferrin are the most important early host defense responses to bacterial pathogens. The mechanisms of activity of these innate defenses were discussed earlier. Among the adaptive responses, immunoglobulins provide the most important defense against bacterial infection in the soft tissues of the head and neck.

Defense Against Extracellular Bacteria

Humoral immunity is the principal response against extracellular bacteria.[33] The most important immunogenic components are cell-wall and capsular polysaccharide antigens, which directly stimulate B cells to produce antibodies. The best example of this type of T-cell–independent response is generated by pneumococcal capsular polysaccharide, which leads to production of IgG2 antibodies.

For protein antigens, $CD4^+$ T cells are involved in association with major histocompatibility (MHC) class II molecules, which present the antigen. These antigen-presenting cells could be macrophages, B cells, or other cell types. The IgG and IgM antibodies provide protective function by (1) opsonizing bacteria and enhancing phagocytosis by binding to Fcγ receptors on monocytes, macrophages, and neutrophils; (2) neutralizing bacterial toxins and preventing their binding to target receptors, a function also performed by IgA in secretions; and (3) activation of the complement system by IgG and IgM antibodies, which leads to production of a microbicidal membrane attack complex.

Defense Against Intracellular Bacteria

The major protective immune response against intracellular bacteria such as mycobacteria is cell-mediated immunity.[33] The macrophages that have ingested bacteria are activated to kill the bacteria by T-cell–derived cytokines, particularly IFN-γ. These T cells are of the $CD4^+$ class, which have presumably responded to extracellular release of antigen. For bacteria that release their antigens intracellularly into the cytoplasm, a cytotoxic T lymphocyte (CTL) response comprising $CD8^+$ T cells is elicited. CTLs produce IFN-γ and are also capable of lysing infected cells. The effectors of cell-mediated immunity, namely activated macrophages and CTLs, act in concert and may complement each other.

In contrast to viral infections, the role of NK cells in control of bacterial infection is not well understood.

Viral Infection

Cytotoxic T Lymphocytes

$CD8^+$ CTLs appear to be the major T-cell effectors with antiviral activity.[33] The CTL receptor recognizes a short peptide derived from an endogenously produced viral protein in the context of an MHC class I beta₂-microglobulin heterodimer expressed on the surface of an infected cell. Because MHC class I restriction elements are present on almost all cells except neurons, CTLs can exert their antiviral effect against almost all infected cells of mucosal surfaces. As viral infection of a cell is required for antigen presentation to a CTL receptor, CTLs cannot function to prevent viral infection; they must function to eliminate cells already in-

fected or, alternatively, restrict virus replication in cells already infected. The net effect of CTL activity is preventing further spread of virus and terminating infection in cells already infected.

The time of CTL activation during viral infection is consistent with this predominant role in the clearance of virus infection. For example, primary CTL activity peaks during RSV and influenza virus infections at days 5–7.[86, 87] This peaking occurs just before the viral replication is reduced. CTLs destroy virus-infected cells by inducing apoptosis and activating cellular enzymes that degrade viral genome. CTLs also produce IFN-γ, which stimulates the microbicidal activities of macrophages that have phagocytosed viruses.[88]

Helper T Cells

Although helper T (Th) cells are known to provide help to B cells, thereby augmenting antibody response, Th cells themselves have been shown to have direct antiviral activities in vivo. The contribution made by the direct antiviral activity of the Th response to the overall immunity that is induced appears to be of lower magnitude than that of the CTLs, consistent with the more limited distribution of its restricting element, the MHC class II α, β heterodimer, which is predominantly on B lymphocytes and antigen-presenting cells such as macrophages and dendritic cells.

IgG Antibodies

IgG antibodies present in blood can gain access to mucosal surfaces by passive diffusion and can exert antiviral activity. Much of the IgG antibody present at mucosal surfaces is derived from serum.[89] However, in the case of respiratory viruses, serum IgG antibodies restrict virus replication in the lung more effectively than in the trachea or nose.[90] One possible explanation is that serum antibodies can diffuse more readily across alveolar walls than across the mucosa of the upper respiratory tract. Virus-specific IgG antibodies produced by the local mucosa also can contribute to total antiviral activity in mucosal secretions.[91]

The mechanisms of the antiviral activity of IgG antibodies in vivo are related to direct neutralization of virus infectivity, as evidenced by the restriction of RSV replication in the nasopharynx of passively immunized subjects.[92] Indeed, there is evidence that complement-dependent immune cytolysis, antibody-dependent immune cytolysis, and antibody-dependent cell cytotoxicity are not required for the activity of IgG antibodies.[92]

IgA Antibodies

The major mediator of resistance to viral infection on mucosal surfaces are IgA antibodies. IgA antiviral antibodies are likely to play a major role in clearance of viral infection, modification of the severity of disease on reinfection, and prevention of infection on reexposure to virus. The major viral antigens that induce a protective antibody response are the surface glycoproteins of viruses that contain lipid envelopes and the proteins present on the surface of viruses. IgA antibodies recognize the same viral antigens as IgG antibodies. For instance, polyclonal IgA antibodies, like polyclonal IgG antibodies, recognize the hemagglutinin of influenza virus, the F and G glycoproteins (gps) of RSV, and gp340 of Epstein-Barr virus (EBV).[93–95]

The mucosal IgA response to viral infection is rapid after first infection and can be detected as early as day 3 following infection. The primary response peaks within the first 6 weeks and can decrease to a low level by 3 months.[96] This short duration of the primary mucosal antibody response is compatible with the susceptibility to reinfection that is common for viruses that infect mucosal surfaces. Reinfection results in a secondary antibody response, indicating immunologic memory characterized by a rapid rise in IgA antibody titer, a rise to a higher peak titer, and maintenance of detectable levels of antibody over a longer time.[97]

A variety of mechanisms contribute to loss of viral infectivity.[98] Aggregation of virus by IgA antibodies is associated with a decrease in viral activity. Because they are able to block virus particles from attaching to cell receptors, IgA antibodies to influenza may be more efficient than IgG antibodies in preventing attachment of virus to infected cells.[99] The polymeric nature of the IgA molecule is thought to contribute in part to this difference. IgA antibodies prevent the penetration of attached virus into the infected cell.[99] IgA antibodies, like IgG antibodies, also act to neutralize viruses after penetration of the host cell.[99] Furthermore, IgA antibodies can have other effects on the immune system, such as promoting uptake of viral antigens via immunoglobin receptors present on the specialized absorptive epithelial cells called M cells, which are in proximity to subepithelial macrophages.[100]

In addition to a mucosal IgA response, a serum IgA response occurs after mucosal viral infection.[101] The latter appears to be more sustained than the mucosal response. Some of the serum IgA antibodies are a spillover from mucosal sites, but some IgA cells of mucosal origin might seed systemic and other mucosal sites after infection. Although trafficking of B cells between mucosal sites occurs, the level of antiviral antibody and resistance to infection achieved at distant sites appear to be much less than at sites of direct antigenic stimulation.

Complement

Although it has not been established in vivo that complement-mediated neutralization might constitute a defense mechanism, there is in vitro evidence that antibody-mediated neutralization of viruses with lipid envelopes, such as RSV, is enhanced by complements.[102] Some viruses, such as EBV, use complement receptor as entry for infection.[103]

Host Defense Against Fungal Infections

Candidiasis

Candida is the prototypic opportunistic fungal pathogen of the oropharynx. It is normally held in check by as yet incompletely defined local factors, including competition with the resident bacterial flora and innate effectors of nonspecific mucosal resistance. Lymphocytes play a major role in the cell-mediated immunity in defense against mucocuta-

neous disease.[104] The importance of this arm of host defense is highlighted by the observations that (1) patients with chronic mucocutaneous candidiasis have dysfunction of their lymphocyte system and (2) patients with AIDS are highly susceptible to mucocutaneous *Candida* infection. Experimental evidence indicates that mannan is the important antigen influencing lymphocyte responses.

The phagocytic role of neutrophils is the most important arm of host defense that prevents systemic invasion by *Candida*. This is evident by the fact that patients with quantitative and qualitative neutrophil defects are at risk for systemic candidiasis. The role of complements and antibodies in opsonophagocytosis is unknown. IgA, IgM, and IgG classes of *Candida*-specific antibodies can be detected in salivary secretions and serum.[104, 105] There is in vitro evidence that both serum complement proteins and antibodies enhance phagocytosis.[106] However, there is consensus that complement and antibodies are not critical for phagocytosis and intracellular killing. On the contrary, there is evidence that high serum antibodies impair candidacidal activity of normal neutrophils.[107] The ingested *Candida* are killed by oxidative and nonoxidative means.[104]

In contrast to the strong evidence that identifies the neutrophil as the key cell in innate defenses against systemic *Candida* infections, the role of monocytes and macrophages is not as well defined.[104] Most of the in vitro data suggest that activated macrophages are more candidacidal than resident cells. However, the level of killing is modest, suggesting that many *Candida* may survive the initial encounter. Nonetheless, alveolar macrophages may play an important role in protection of the lower airway.

Aspergillosis

Aspergillosis is the most common fungal infection of the nose and paranasal sinuses. Host defense against invasive aspergillosis is virtually exclusively the province of innate mechanisms. Phagocytic response by neutrophils and monocytes, rather than antibody or T-cell response, provides the primary host defense.[108] The predisposition to aspergillosis seen in patients who have chronic granulomatous disease or selective defects in phagocyte killing or who are on corticosteroid therapy underscores the importance of oxidative killing in the human host defenses against aspergillosis. In normal hosts with indolent sinonasal aspergillosis, it is likely that previous chronic, recurrent sinus inflammation causes poor mucociliary clearance with the production of lactic acid and other organic acids, which in turn impairs the phagocytic and intracellular killing response of neutrophils and macrophages, thereby allowing infection with *Aspergillus*.

Zygomycosis

A less common but more lethal fungal infection is zygomycosis, including infections with *Mucor* species and *Rhizopus* species. These fungi colonize the sinuses and nasopharynx of some individuals. The neutrophil appears to be the primary component of the immune response against these organisms and may serve to prevent germination of inhaled spores.[109] Diabetes mellitus, in particular diabetic ketoacidosis, is the most common underlying disease in patients with mucormycosis. It is not known whether it is the ketoacidosis that affects the killing ability of neutrophils against these fungi. Iron may play a key role in lowering host defenses, as demonstrated by the tendency for deferoxamine therapy and hemodialysis to result in progression of both natural and experimental mucormycosis.[110, 111]

SPECIFIC HOST DEFENSES IN OTITIS MEDIA, SINUSITIS, PHARYNGITIS, AND TONSILLITIS

Otitis Media

The middle ear consists of the eustachian tube, tympanic cavity, antrum, and mastoid air cells. The mucosa of the middle ear is basically a respiratory type, although the tympanic cavity, antrum, and air cells are covered mostly by cuboidal and squamous cells with few secretory and ciliated cells.[112] Secretory glands of mixed type exist only in the cartilaginous portion of the eustachian tube. Although many lymphocytes, plasma cells, macrophages, neutrophils, and other inflammatory cells accumulate in inflamed mucosa, only a few immunocompetent cells (without organized follicles) are found in the normal middle ear mucosa.

During acute infection of the middle ear with bacteria and viruses, a variety of chemotactic cytokines have been detected in the middle ear effusions which are most likely produced locally in the middle ear. They include IL-1, IL-2, IL-6, IL-8, TNF-α, IFN-γ, MIP-1-α, and MCP-1.[76, 113–116] The initial source of these cytokines is probably local epithelial cells, fibroblasts, and macrophages. Adhesion molecules such as ICAM-1, vascular cell adhesion molecule, and E-selectin, which enhance leukocyte migration and leukocyte-leukocyte interactions, are also enhanced during the acute phase of infection.[116] Furthermore, complement products and inflammatory mediators such as histamine, leukotrienes, and prostaglandins are enhanced in the middle ear infection.[70, 78, 81] All of these substances induce the migration of and further enhance the release of mediators from neutrophils, lymphocytes, eosinophils, macrophages, basophils, and mast cells. These cells subsequently take part in elimination of pathogens by phagocytosis, cell cytotoxicity, and antibody-mediated neutralization.

Local antibodies produced are of the IgA, IgG, and IgM classes.[117] There is evidence that gut-associated and bronchus-associated lymphatic lymphoid tissues are two of the sources of IgA precursors for inflamed tubotympanic mucosa. Whereas specific antibodies in middle ear effusions against certain viruses are restricted to mainly IgA class antibodies, those against bacterial antigens belong to IgG, IgA, and IgM classes.[118, 119] The bacteria recovery rate in the middle ear fluids is inversely related to the dramatic increase in age of IgA and IgG levels in effusions. Studies by Faden and colleagues[120–122] shed light on the need for cooperation between systemic immunity and local immunity: in children with recurrent otitis media, the titer of strain-specific nontypable *H. influenzae* is much higher for the IgG class than for the IgM and IGA classes. Although antibody titers in middle ear fluids decline over time, serum antibody levels remain stable.[120] On the other hand, children develop a local anti-

body response to *Moraxella (Branhamella) catarrhalis* in the middle ear consisting of strain-specific IgG, IgM, and IgA but fail to develop a systemic antibody response in a uniform manner.[121, 122]

Sinusitis

The sinuses have not been studied well with respect to local and systemic immune responses during infections. Much of the information is derived from the study of immunity of the nasopharynx and nasal turbinates. Investigations have shown that cytokines such as IL-1, IL-6, IL-8, and IFN-γ are produced in the mucosa of the sinuses.[123, 124] The expression of vascular and epithelial adhesion molecules is also increased, facilitating migration of leukocytes to the sinus mucosa.[123, 124]

During acute sinusitis, the higher number of leukocytes seen in secretions is associated with infection with *S. pneumoniae* rather than nontypable *H. influenzae*.[125] During acute sinusitis, the sinus mucosa produces micoorganism-specific IgA, IgG, and IgM as well as lysozyme.[126, 127]

The single most important factor leading to purulent, acute sinusitis is upper respiratory tract viral infection. Viruses induce severe mucosal injury with deranged mucociliary activity. The host defense response is typical of that seen following rhinovirus infection. Studies with experimental rhinovirus of the nasopharynx show that the initial response consists almost exclusively of increased vascular permeability that lasts 2 days into infection. This response is probably driven by the generation of vasoactive amines such as bradykinin.[14] Secretions thereafter become enriched with glandular proteins as the infection resolves. This response is probably stimulated by either cholinergic or peptidergic mechanisms.[1]

In chronic sinusitis, the secretions contain high concentrations of the glandular proteins lysozyme and lactoferrin, suggesting that glands are driven to secrete excessively in patients with chronic inflammation.[1] Data also suggest that abnormal cholinergic responses result in limited capacity to secrete mucus and the antimicrobial factors necessary to combat new or recurrent infections.[1] Ineffective IgA response has also been implicated in the development of otitis media. In a study of patients with chronic sinusitis, nasal secretions were shown to contain high levels of IgA, but its specific activity against the M protein of *S. pneumoniae* was lower than that in nasal secretions from normal subjects.[128]

Another underlying clinical condition associated with the development of chronic sinusitis is asthma. In one study, about half of the nasopharyngeal secretions showed the presence of major basic protein, a proinflammatory product of eosinophils, which was most marked in patients with asthma.[129] These findings suggest that chronic sinusitis shares some of the findings seen in the airways of asthmatic patients and that the eosinophil might play a role in the pathogenesis of chronic sinusitis.

Host Defenses in Pharyngitis/Tonsillitis

Group A Streptococci

The factors responsible for the early host defense against group A streptococci in the pharynx and tonsils are poorly understood. Type-specific antibody against M protein, which greatly enhances phagocytosis, usually is not detectable until 6 to 8 weeks after initiation of infection; therefore, its primary role is probably not in the limitation or termination of active infection, but rather in the prevention of reinfection by the same serotype. Surface phagocytosis, first by monocytes and later by neutrophils, may be the primary mechanism of defense in the early stage of infection.[130] The rash and other toxic manifestations of scarlet fever have been attributed to the development of hypersensitivity to the erythrogenic (pyrogenic) toxins.[131] Toxic manifestations of the streptococcal toxic shock–like syndrome may also result from a direct influence of the pyrogenic exotoxins on cytokines such as TNF. Most of the processes involved in the development of poststreptococcal glomerulonephritis and acute rheumatic fever invoke immunologic responses in one way or another.

Epstein-Barr Virus

EBV infects the oropharyngeal epithelial cells and susceptible B lymphocytes within the lymphoid tissues of the pharynx. The immune response to EBV-infected transformed lymphocytes is complex and involves both humoral and cell-mediated immune responses. The antibodies are directed against viral antigens as well as unrelated antigens (heterophile antibodies).[132] The role of the heterophile antibodies in the pathogenesis or recovery from infection is unclear. The role of specific antibodies to EBV capsid antigen and other antigens is also not clear. The cellular immunity includes T lymphocytes and NK cells with cytotoxic properties. The mononuclear response seen in circulation is due to increased numbers of T lymphocytes. Despite this immune response and clinical recovery, the virus is not eliminated from the host. Thus, EBV shares the property of latency or persistence with other members of the herpesvirus group.

Mycoplasma Infection

Mycoplasma pneumoniae is a common cause of pharyngitis and is infrequently associated with otitis media and sinusitis. During the process of infection, neutralizing antibodies as well as autoantibodies are produced.[133] The IgG and IgA classes of antibodies have a clear role in recovery from disease. Neutrophils and macrophages appear to have relative difficulty in clearing this pathogen.

HOST DEFENSES IN ABNORMAL HOSTS

Immune Defense Disorders

The critical roles of the various arms of the immune responses in the nasopharynx and oropharynx, as discussed previously, are best realized in clinical situations in which the host demonstrates defects in immune responses. Table 3–4 summarizes the various types of host defense disorders that increase the susceptibility to specific infections. Table 3–5 summarizes the broad categories of microbial pathogens that are encountered in susceptible hosts.[134]

Selective IgA Deficiency

A special discussion on IgA deficiency (i.e., <10 mg/dL) of serum and secretory IgA deserves merit, because it is the most common well-defined immunodeficiency disorder. Its frequency in adults is 1:333. The mode of inheritance seems to be an autosomal dominant pattern with variable expressiv-

Table 3–4. HOST DEFENSE DISORDERS AND TYPICAL INFECTIOUS COMPLICATIONS IN THE NASOPHARYNX AND OROPHARYNX

Host Defense	Defective in	Infections
Nasal turbinates	Intubation	Sinusitis
Mucociliary clearance		
Cilia	Ciliary dyskinesia syndrome	Otitis media, sinusitis
	Infections (viral)	
Mucus blanket	Cystic fibrosis	Sinusitis
Immunoglobulins (Ig)		
Secretory IgA, IgA	IgA deficiency	Otitis media, sinusitis
IgG (including subclasses)	IgG subclass deficiency	Otitis media, sinusitis, mastoiditis
	Agammaglobulinemia	
	Hypogammaglobulinemia	
IgE	Hyper-IgE syndrome (Job's)	Otitis media, sinusitis
Cellular		
Neutrophils		
Number	Chemotherapy	Otitis media, sinusitis, mastoiditis, dental infections
	Congenital neutropenia	
Motility	Motility disorders	Otitis media, sinusitis, pharyngitis, gingivitis
Function	Chronic granulomatous disease	Ulcerative stomatitis
Lymphocytes		
Number	AIDS	Oral candidiasis, otitis media, sinusitis
Function	Chronic mucocutaneous candidiasis	Oral candidiasis
	Severe combined immunodeficiency	Oral candidiasis, sinusitis
	Wiskott-Aldrich syndrome	Otitis media, sinusitis
Complement	C3, C5 deficiency	Otitis media, sinusitis

Table 3–5. EFFECT OF HOST DEFENSE ABNORMALITIES ON SUSCEPTIBILITY TO INFECTION

Defect	Effect on Susceptibility to			
	Bacteria	Viruses	Fungi	Parasites
Phagocytes	Yes	No	Some (invasive *Candida*)	Yes
Cell-mediated	Some	Yes	Some (mucosal *Candida*)	Yes
Antibody	Yes	Yes	No	No
Complement	Yes	Yes	No	Some

Modified from Keutsch GT: Immunologic responses to infection. In: Feigin RD, Cherry JD (eds): Textbook of Pediatric Infectious Diseases, 3rd ed, vol 1. Philadelphia, WB Saunders Co., 1992.

ity. The basic defect leading to IgA deficiency is unknown, but it appears that the susceptibility gene may reside in the rare alleles and deletions in the MHC class III region on chromosome 6.[135] IgA deficiency can also be induced by environmental factors such as drugs. For example, IgA deficiency is known to remit either following discontinuation of Dilantin therapy or spontaneously.[136] Most patients with IgA deficiency have normal levels of other immunoglobulins, although IgG4 and IgG2 subclass deficiencies have been reported.

Persons with IgA deficiency have an increased incidence of infections of the mucosal sites, such as the respiratory, gastrointestinal, and urogenital tracts. In the upper respiratory tract, the presenting illnesses are chronic and recurrent sinusitis and otitis media. Nonetheless, many persons with IgA deficiency have apparently normal health. Indeed, studies suggest that the susceptibility to infection is related not to the degree of IgA deficiency but instead to the concomitant deficiencies of IgG4 and, to a lesser extent, IgG2.[137]

IgG Subclass Deficiencies

IgG subclass deficiencies have been described in both normal and abnormal hosts. The most common presenting illness is frequent upper and lower respiratory tract infections.[138] IgG2 subclass deficiency is frequently associated with selective IgA deficiency, as well as with IgA deficiency in ataxia-telangiectasia. IgG2 subclass deficiency may also occur as part of an evolving pattern of immunodeficiency, such as common variable immunodeficiency, suggesting that the presence of IgG subclass deficiency may be a marker for more general immune dysfunction.

The difficulties in the diagnosis of IgG subclass deficiencies are that the normal serum values are widely scattered and that commercial laboratory measurement is not well standardized. The more important issue is the identification of a patient who mounts a suboptimal specific and protective antibody response to protein and polysaccharide antigens. Typically, response to protein antigen occurs in the IgG1 and IgG3 subclasses, whereas response to polysaccharide antigen occurs in the IgG2 subclass.[139–140]

Host Defenses in the Malnourished Host

The mucosa of the nasopharynx and oropharynx is often the primary site of clinical symptoms due to malnutrition. Diminished secretory IgA has been noted in malnourished children.[141] Deficiencies in protein, vitamins A and B complex, ascorbic acid, and zinc are frequently associated with tissue changes that contribute to diminution of host resistance to infection. Illnesses due to respiratory infections have a higher morbidity in children deficient in vitamin A.[142] Specifically, mortality due to measles is substantially increased. Vitamin A supplementation during measles has been shown to be life-saving.

Severe protein malnutrition and xerophthalmia have been shown to suppress significantly the secretion of lysozymes into the tears of children, thereby impairing host defense against bacteria.[143] Large visible epithelial lesions may be caused by dietary deficiencies. Examples are cheilitis and angular stomatitis from riboflavin and pyridoxine deficiency, and the spongy gums of scurvy. Patients with protein-calorie malnutrition have decreased complement level as well as diminished antibody responses and phagocytosis.

References

1. Kaliner MA: Human nasal host defense and sinusitis. J Allergy Clin Immunol 1992; 90: 424–430.
2. Patow CA, Shelhamer J, Marom Z, et al.: Analysis of human nasal mucous glycoproteins. Am J Otolaryngol 1984; 5: 334–343.
3. Reddy MS, Murphy TF, Faden HS, Bernstein JM: Middle ear mucin glycoprotein: Purification and interaction with nontypeable *Haemophilus influenzae* and *Moraxella catarrhalis*. Presented at the Sixth International Symposium on Recent Advances in Otitis Media; June 4–8, 1995; Ft Lauderdale, Florida.
4. Kaulbach HC, White MV, Igarashi Y, et al.: Estimation of nasal epithelial lining fluid using urea as a marker. J Allergy Clin Immunol 1993; 92: 457–465.
5. Raphael GD, Meredith SD, Baraniuk JN, Kaliner MA: Nasal reflexes. Am J Rhinol 1988; 2: 109–116.
6. Raphael GD, Druce, HM, Baraniuk JN, Kaliner MA: Pathophysiology of rhinitis. I: Assessment of the sources of protein in methacholine-induced nasal secretions. Am Rev Respir Dis 1989; 138: 413–420.
7. Mullol J, Raphael GD, Lundgren JD, et al.: Comparison of human nasal mucosal secretion *in vivo* and *in vitro*. J Appl Physiol 1992; 89: 684–693.
8. Hellstrom S, Goldie P: Mechanisms of otitis media development: Neurogenic inflammation involved? Otolaryngol Clin North Am 1991; 24: 829–834.
9. Baraniuk JN, Lundgren, JD, Goff J, et al.: Calcitonin gene-related peptide in human nasal mucosa. J Appl Physiol 1990; 258: 81–88.
10. Baraniuk JN, Lundgren JD, Goff J, et al.: Gastrin releasing peptide (GRP) in human nasal mucosa. J Clin Invest 1990; 85: 998–1005.
11. Baraniuk JN, Lundgren JD, Okayama M, et al.: Vasoactive intestinal peptide (VIP) in human nasal mucosa. J Clin Invest 1990; 86: 825–831.
12. Okamoto Y, Shirotori K, Kudo K, et al.: Cytokine expression following the topical administration of substance P to human nasal mucosa: The role of substance P in nasal allergy. J Immunol 1993; 151: 4391–4398.

13. Ohkubo K, Baraniuk JN, Hohman RJ, et al.: Human nasal mucosal neutral endopeptidase (NEP): Location, quantitation, and secretion. Am J Respir Cell Mol Biol 1993; 9: 557–567.

14. Igarashi Y, Skoner D, Fireman P, et al.: Phases of nasal secretions during upper respiratory viral infections. Am Rev Respir Dis 1991; 143:A757.

15. Verdugo P: Ca^{2+}-dependent hormonal stimulation of ciliary activity. Nature (London) 1982; 283: 764–765.

16. Arruda E, Hayen FG: Role of cytokines in viral infections. In: Oppenheim J, Rossio J, Gearing A (eds): Clinical Applications of Cytokines. New York: Oxford University Press, 1993.

17. Durum SK, Oppenheim JJ: Proinflammatory cytokines and immunity. In: Paul WE (ed): Fundamental Immunology. New York: Raven Press, 1993.

18. Springer TA: Adhesion receptors of the immune system. Nature 1990; 346: 425.

19. Giebink GS, Juhn SK, Weber ML, Le CT: The bacteriology and cytology of chronic otitis media with effusion. Pediatr Infect Dis J 1982; 1: 98–103.

20. Westrin KM, Steirna P, Soderlund K: Microorganisms and leukocytes in purulent sinusitis: A symbiotic relationship in metabolism. Acta Otolaryngol Suppl (Stockh) 1994; 515: 18–21.

21. Berglund B, Kortekangas AE, Lauren P: Experimental inoculation of guinea pigs middle ear with respiratory syncytial virus. Acta Otolaryngol Suppl (Stockh) 1966; 224: 268–271.

22. Faden H, Ogra P: Neutrophils and antiviral defense. Pediatr Infect Dis J 1986; 5: 86–92.

23. Patel JA, Chonmaitre T, Schmalstieg F: Effect of modulation of polymorphonuclear leukocyte migration with anti-CD18 antibody on pathogenesis of experimental otitis media in guinea pigs. Infect Immun 1993; 61: 1132–1135.

24. Lim DJ, Liu YS, Birck H: Secretory lysozyme of the human middle ear mucosa: Immunocytochemical localization. Ann Otol Rhinol Laryngol Suppl 1976; 85: 50.

25. Arnold RR, Russell JE, Champion WJ, et al.: Bactericidal activity of human lactoferrin: Differentiation from the stasis of iron deprivation. Infect Immun 1982; 35: 792–799.

26. Watanabe T, Nagura H, Watanabe K, Brown WR: The binding of human lactoferrin to immunoglobulin A. FEBS Lett 1984; 168: 203–207.

27. Saez-Llorens X, Lagrutta F: The acute phase host reaction during bacterial infection and its clinical impact in children. Pediatr Infect Dis J 1993; 12: 83–87.

28. Gallin JI: Inflammation. In: Paul WE (ed): Fundamental Immunology. New York: Raven Press, 1993.

29. Joiner KA: Complement evasion by bacteria and parasites. Ann Rev Microbiol 1988; 42: 201–230.

30. Prellner K: Complements and other amplification mechanisms in otitis media. In: Bernstein JM, Ogra PL (eds): Immunology of the Ear. New York: Raven Press, 1987.

31. Su H, Boackle RJ: Interaction of the envelope glycoprotein of human immunodeficiency virus with C1q and fibronectin under conditions present in human saliva. Mol Immunol 1991; 28: 811–817.

32. Kaul TN, Welliver RC, Ogra PL: Appearance of complement components and immunoglobulins on nasopharyngeal epithelial cells following naturally acquired infection with respiratory syncytial virus. J Med Virol 1982; 9: 149.

33. Abbas AK, Lichtman AH, Pober JS: Cellular and Molecular Immunology, 2nd ed. Philadelphia: WB Saunders Co., 1994.

34. Brandtzaeg P: Immune functions and immunopathology of palatine and nasopharyngeal tonsils. In: Bernstein JM, Ogra PL (eds): Immunology of the Ear. New York: Raven Press, 1987.

35. Croitoru K, Bienenstock J: Characteristics and functions of mucosa-associated lymphoid tissue. In: Ogra PL, Strober W, Mestecky J, et al. (eds): Handbook of Mucosal Immunology. San Diego: Academic Press, 1994.

36. Quiding-Jarbrink M, Granstrom G, Nordstrom I, et al.: Induction of compartmentalized B-cell responses in human tonsils. Infect Immun 1995; 63: 853–857.

37. Watanabe N, Kato H, Mogi G: Induction of antigen-specific IgA-forming cells in the upper respiratory mucosa. Ann Otol Rhinol Laryngol 1989; 98: 523–529.

38. Kurono Y, Shimamura R, Mogi G: Inhibition of nasopharyngeal colonization of *Haemophilus influenzae* by oral immunization. Ann Otol Rhinol Laryngol 1992; 101: 11–15.

39. Ryan AF, Sharpe TA, Harris JP: Lymphocyte circulation of middle ear. Acta Otolaryngol (Stockh) 1990; 109: 278–287.

40. Butler KM, Baker CJ: Cervical lymphadenitis. In: Feigin RD, Cherry JD (eds): Textbook of Pediatric Infectious Diseases, 3rd ed. Philadelphia: WB Saunders Co., 1992.

41. Ogra PL: Effect of tonsillectomy and adenoidectomy on nasopharyngeal antibody response to polio virus. N Engl J Med 1971; 284: 59–64.

42. Owen R, Nemanic P: Antigen processing structures of the mammalian intestinal tract: An SEM study of lymphoepithelial organs. In: Becker R, Johari O (eds): Scanning Electron Microscopy. O'Hare, Illinois, AMF, 1978, pp 367–378.

43. Tew J, Thornbacke J, Steinman RM: Dendritic cells in the immune response. J Reticuloendothel Soc 1982; 31: 371–380.

44. Yamanaka N, Sambe S, Harabuchi Y, Kataura A: Immunological study of tonsils. Distribution of T cell subsets. Acta Otolaryngol (Stockh) 1983; 96: 509–516.

45. Bernstein JM, Yamanaka N, Nadal D: Immunobiology of the tonsils and adenoids. In: Ogra PL, Strober W, Mestecky J, et al. (eds): Handbook of Mucosal Immunology. San Diego: Academic Press, 1994.

46. Nadal D, Albini B, Schlapfer E, et al.: Role of Epstein-Barr virus and interleukin-6 in the development of lymphomas of human origin in SCID mice engrafted with human tonsillar mononuclear cells. J Gen Virol 1992; 73: 113–121.

47. Woloschak G, Liarakos C, Tomasi T: Identification of the major immunoglobulin heavy chain poly A RNA in murine lymphoid tissues. Mol Immunol 1986; 23: 645–653.

48. Raphael GD, Baraniuk JN, Kaliner MA: How the nose runs and why. J Allergy Clin Immunol 1991; 87: 457–467.

49. Underdown BJ, Mestecky J: Mucosal immunoglobulins. In: Ogra PL, Strober W, Mestecky J, et al. (eds): Handbook of Mucosal Immunology. San Diego: Academic Press, 1994.

50. Challacombe SJ, Shirlaw PJ: Immunology of Diseases of the Oral Cavity. II: Oral mucosal diseases. In: Ogra PL, Strober W, Mestecky J, et al. (eds): Handbook of Mucosal Immunology. San Diego: Academic Press, 1994.

51. Kett L, Brandtzaeg P, Radl J, Haaijman J: Different subclass distribution of IgA-producing cells in human lymphoid organs and various secretory tissues. J Immunol 1986; 136: 3631–3635.

52. Kilian M, Holmgren K: Ecology and nature of immunoglobulin A1 protease–producing streptococci in the human oral cavity and pharynx. Infect Immun 1981; 31: 868–873.

53. Kilian M, Mestecky J, Schrohenloher RE: Pathogenic species of the genus *Haemophilus* and *Streptococcus pneumoniae* produce immunoglobulin A1 protease. Infect Immun 1979; 26: 143–149.

54. Plaut AG, Genco RJ, Tomasi T: Isolation of an enzyme from *Streptococcus sanguis* which specifically cleaves IgA. J Immunol 1974; 113: 289–291.

55. Plaut AG, Gilbert JV, Artenstein MS, Capra JD: *Neisseria gonorrhoeae* and *Neisseria meningitidis*: Extracellular enzyme cleaves human immunoglobulin A. Science 1975; 190: 1103–1105.

56. Welliver RC, Kaul TN, Ogra PL: The appearance of cell-bound IgE in respiratory tract epithelium after respiratory syncytial virus infection. N Engl J Med 1980; 303: 1198–1202.

57. Welliver RC, Wong DT, Sun M, et al.: The development of respiratory syncytial virus–specific IgE on the release of histamine in nasopharyngeal secretions after infection. N Engl J Med 1981; 305: 841–846.

58. Mosmann TR, Coffman RL: Th1 and Th2 cells: Different patterns of lymphokine secretion lead to different functional properties. Annu Rev Immunol 1989; 7: 145–173.

59. Coffman RL, Shrader B, Carty J, et al.: A mouse T cell product that preferentially enhances IgA production. I: Biologic characterization. J Immunol 1987; 139: 3685–3690.

60. Van Snick J: Interleukin-6: An overview. Annu Rev Immunol 1990; 8: 253–278.

61. Kim P-H, Kagnoff MF: Transforming growth factor β1 is a costimulator for IgA production. J Immunol 1990; 144: 3411–3416.

62. Sonada E, Matsumoto R, Hitoshi E, et al.: Transforming growth factor β induces IgA production and acts additively with interleukin 5 for IgA production. J Exp Med 1989; 170: 1415–1420.

63. Lebman DA, Lee FD, Coffman RL: Mechanism for transforming growth factor β and IL-2 enhancement of IgA expression in lipopolysaccharide-stimulated B cell cultures. J Immunol 1990; 144: 952–959.

64. Lebman DA, Coffman RL: Cytokines in the mucosal immune system.

In: Ogra PL, Strober W, Mestecky J, et al. (eds): Handbook of Mucosal Immunology. San Diego: Academic Press, 1994.

65. Snapper CM, Peschel C, Paul WE: IFN-γ stimulates IgG2a secretion by murine B lymphocytes stimulated with bacterial lipopolysaccharide. J Immunol 1988; 140: 2121–2127.

66. Lebman DA, Coffman RL: Interleukin 4 causes isotype switching to IgE in T cell–stimulated clonal B cell cultures. J Exp Med 1988; 168: 853–862.

67. Chen WF, Zlotnik A. IL-10, a novel cytotoxic T cell differentiation factor. J Immunol 1991; 147: 528–534.

68. Tillinghast JP, Metcalf DD: Pharmacologic mediators of inflammation. In: Bernstein JM, Ogra PL (eds): New York: Raven Press, 1987.

69. Schwartz LB, Austen KF: The mast cell and mediators of immediate hypersensitivity. In: Samter M, Talmage DW, Frank MM, et al. (eds): Immunological Diseases. Boston: Little, Brown, 1988.

70. Chonmaitre T, Patel JA, Lett-Brown MA, et al.: Virus and bacteria enhance histamine production in middle ear fluids of children with acute otitis media. J Infect Dis 1994; 169: 1265–1270.

71. Palva T, Taskinen E, Lehtinen T, et al.: Mast cells and histamine in adenoid tissue and middle ear. Acta Otolaryngol 1991; 111: 349–353.

72. Berger G, Ophir D: Possible role of adenoid mast cells in the pathogenesis of secretory otitis media. Ann Otol Rhinol Laryngol 1994; 103: 632–635.

73. Raphael GD, Meredith SD, Baraniuk JN, et al.: The pathophysiology of rhinitis. II: Assessment of the sources of protein in histamine-induced nasal secretions. Am Rev Respir Dis 1989; 139: 791–800.

74. Meltzer EO, Orgel HA, Jalowayski AA: Histamine levels and nasal cytology in children with chronic otitis media and rhinitis. Ann Allergy Asthma Immunol 1995; 74: 406–410.

75. Esaki Y, Ohashi Y, Furuya H, et al.: Histamine-induced mucociliary dysfunction and otitis media with effusion. Acta Otolaryngol (Suppl) 1991; 486: 116–134.

76. Patel JA, Sim T, Owen M, et al.: Influence of viral infection on middle ear chemokine response in acute otitis media. Presented at the Sixth International Symposium on Recent Advances in Otitis Media; June 4–8, 1995; Ft Lauderdale, Florida.

77. Camussi G, Brentjens J, Bussolino F, Tetta C: Role of platelet activating factor in immunopathological reactions. In: Otterness I (ed): Advances in Inflammation Research, vol 2. New York: Raven Press, 1986.

78. Nonomura N, Giebink GS, Zelterman D, et al.: Early biochemical events in pneumococcal otitis media: Arachidonic acid metabolites in middle ear fluids. Ann Otol Rhinol Laryngol 1991; 100: 385–388.

79. Jung TTK, Linda L: Prostaglandins, leukotrienes and other arachidonic acid metabolites in the pathogenesis of otitis media. Laryngoscope 1988; 98: 980–993.

80. Jung TTK, Park YM, Schlund D, et al.: Effect of prostaglandin, leukotriene and arachidonic acid on experimental otitis media with effusion in chinchillas. Ann Otol Rhinol Laryngol 1990; 99: 28–32.

81. Chonmaitre T, Patel JA, Garofalo R, et al.: Role of leukotriene B4 and interleukin-8 in acute viral and bacterial otitis media. Ann Otol Rhinol Laryngol (accepted for publication).

82. Minami T, Kubo N, Tomoda K, Kumazawa T: Effects of various inflammatory mediators on eustachian tube patency. Acta Otolaryngol 1992; 112: 680–685.

83. Bernstein JM, Steger R, Back N: The kallikrein-kinin system in otitis media with effusion. Trans Am Acad Ophthalmol Otolaryngol 1979; 86: 249.

84. Proud D, Baumgartin CR, Naclerio RM, Ward PE: Kinin metabolism in human nasal secretions during experimentally induced allergic rhinitis. J Immunol 1987; 138: 428–434.

85. Holmberg K, Bake B, Pipkorn U: Vascular effects of topically applied bradykinin on the human nasal mucosa. Eur J Pharmacol 1990; 175: 35–41.

86. Chiba Y, Higashidate Y, Suga K, et al.: Development of cell-mediated cytotoxic immunity to respiratory syncytial virus in human infants following naturally acquired infection. J Med Virol 1989; 28: 133–139.

87. Dolin R, Murphy BR, Caplan EA: Lymphocyte blastogenic responses to influenza virus antigens after influenza infection and vaccination in humans. Infect Immun 1978; 19: 867–874.

88. Morris AG, Lin Y-L, Askonas BA: Immune interferon release when cloned cytotoxic T-cell line meets its correct influenza-infected target cells. Nature 1982; 295: 150–152.

89. Wagner DK, Clements ML, Reimer CB, et al.: Analysis of IgG antibody responses after live and inactivated influenza A vaccine indicate that nasal wash is a transudate from serum. J Clin Microbiol 1987; 25: 559–562.

90. Kris RM, Yetter RA, Cogliano R, et al.: Passive serum antibody causes temporary recovery from influenza infection of the nose, trachea, and lung of nude mice. Immunology 1988; 63: 349–353.

91. Ogra PL, Coppola PR, MacGillivray MH, Dzierba JL: Mechanism of mucosal immunity to viral infections in γA immunoglobulin-deficiency syndromes. Proc Soc Exp Biol Med 1974; 145: 811–816.

92. Prince GA, Hemming VG, Horswood RL, et al.: Mechanism of antibody-mediated viral clearance in immunotherapy of respiratory syncytial virus infection in cotton rats. J Virol 1990; 64: 3091–3092.

93. Clements ML, Betts RF, Tierney EL, Murphy BR: Serum and nasal wash antibodies associated with resistance to experimental challenge with influenza A wild-type virus. J Clin Microbiol 1986; 24: 157–160.

94. Murphy BR, Graham BS, Prince GA, et al.: Serum and nasal-wash immunoglobulin G and A antibody response of infants and children to respiratory syncytial virus F and G glycoproteins following primary infection. J Clin Microbiol 1986; 23: 1009–1014.

95. Yao QY, Rowe M, Morgan AJ, et al.: Salivary and serum IgA antibodies to the Epstein-Barr virus glycoprotein gp340: Incidence and potential for virus neutralization. Int J Cancer 1991; 48: 45–50.

96. Blandford G, Heath RB: Studies on the immune response and pathogenesis of Sendai virus infection of mice. I: The fate of viral antigens. Immunology 1972; 22: 637–649.

97. Wright PF, Murphy BR, Kervina M, et al.: Secretory immunological response after intranasal inactivated influenza A virus vaccinations: Evidence for immunoglobulin A memory. Infect Immun 1983; 40: 1092–1095.

98. Outlaw MC, Dimmock NJ: Mechanisms of neutralization of influenza virus on mouse tracheal epithelial cells by mouse monoclonal polymeric IgA and polyclonal IgM directed against the viral haemagglutinin. J Gen Virol 1990; 71: 69–76.

99. Outlaw MC, Dimmock NJ: Insights into neutralization of animal viruses gained from study of influenza virus. Epidemiol Infect 1991; 106: 205–220.

100. Weltzin R, Lucia-Jandris P, Michetti P, et al.: Binding and transepithelial transport of immunoglobulins by intestinal M cells: Demonstration using monoclonal IgA antibodies against enteric viral proteins. J Cell Biol 1989; 108: 1673–1685.

101. Friedman MG, Phillip M, Dagan R: Virus-specific IgA in serum, saliva, and tears of children with measles. Clin Exp Immunol 1989; 75: 58–63.

102. Kaul TN, Welliver RC, Ogra PL: Comparison of fluorescent antibody, neutralizing antibody and complement-enhanced neutralizing antibody assays for detection of serum antibody to respiratory syncytial virus. J Clin Microbiol 1981; 13: 957.

103. Fingeroth JD, Weiss JJ, Tedder TF, et al.: Epstein-Barr virus receptor of human B lymphocytes is the C3d receptor CR2. Proc Natl Acad Sci U S A 1984; 81: 4510–4516.

104. Domer JE, Lehrer RI: Introduction to candidiasis. In: Murphy JW, Friedman H, Bendinelli M (eds): Fungal Infections and Immune Response. New York: Plenum Press, 1993.

105. Lehner T, Wilton JMA, Ivanyi L: Immunodeficiencies in chronic mucocutaneous candidosis. Immunology 1972; 22: 755–787.

106. Pereira HA, Hosking CS: The role of complement and antibody in opsonization and intracellular killing of *Candida albicans*. Clin Exp Immunol 1984; 57: 307–314.

107. Laforce, FM, Mills DM, Iverson K, et al.: Inhibition of leukocyte candidacidal activity by serum from patients with disseminated candidiasis. J Lab Clin Med 1975; 86: 657–666.

108. Schaffner A, Douglas H, Braude A: Selective protection against conidia by mononuclear and against mycelia by polymorphonuclear phagocytes in resistance to Aspergillus: Observation on these two lines of defense *in vivo* and *in vitro* with human and mouse phagocytes. J Clin Invest 1982; 69: 617–631.

109. Diamond RD, Krzesicki R, Epstein B, et al.: Damage to hyphal forms of fungi by human leukocytes *in vitro:* A possible host defense mechanism against aspergillosis and mucormycosis. Am J Pathol 1978; 91: 313.

110. Daly AL, Velazquez LA, Bradley SF, et al.: Mucormycosis: Association with deferoxamine therapy. Am J Med 1989; 87: 468.

111. Boelaert JR, Fenves AZ, Coburn JW: Mucormycosis among patients on dialysis. N Eng J Med 1989; 321: 190.

112. Lim DJ: Functional morphology of the lining membranes of the middle ear and eustachian tube: An overview. Ann Otol Rhinol Laryngol Suppl 1974; 83: 5–22.

113. Bikhazi P, Ryan AF: Expression of cytokine during acute and chronic middle ear immune response. Laryngoscope 1995; 105: 629–634.

114. Yellon RF, Leonard G, Marucha PT, et al.: Characterization of cytokines present in middle ear effusions. Laryngoscope 1991; 101: 165–169.

115. Johnson MD, Fitzgerald JE, Leonard G, et al.: Cytokines in experimental otitis media with effusion. Laryngoscope 1994; 104: 191–196.

116. Okamoto Y, Kudo K, Ishikawa K, et al.: Presence of respiratory syncytial virus genomic sequences in middle ear fluid and its relationship to expression of cytokines and cell adhesion molecules. J Infect Dis 1993; 168: 1277–1281.

117. Lim DJ, Goro M: Mucosal immunology of the middle ear and eustachian tube. In: Ogra PL, Strober W, Mestecky J, et al. (eds): Handbook of Mucosal Immunology. San Diego: Academic Press, 1994.

118. Ogra PL, Bernstein JM, Yurchak AM, et al.: Characteristics of secretory immune system in human middle ear. J Immunol 1974; 112: 488–495.

119. Sloyer JL, Howie VM, Ploussard JH, Johnston RB: The immune response to acute otitis media in children. II: Serum and middle ear fluid antibody in otitis media due to *Haemophilus influenzae*. J Infect Dis 1975; 132: 685–688.

120. Faden H, Brodsky L, Bernstein J, Stanievich J, et al.: Otitis media in children: Local immune response to non-typable *Haemophilus influenzae*. Infect Immun 1989; 57: 3555–3559.

121. Faden H, Hong I, Murphy T: Immune response to outer membrane antigens of *Moraxella catarrhalis* in children with otitis media. Infect Immun 1992; 60: 3824–3829.

122. Faden H, Hong J, Pahade N: Immune response to *Moraxella catarrhalis* in children with otitis media: Opsonophagocytosis with antigen-coated latex beads. Ann Otol Rhinol Laryngol 1994; 103: 522–525.

123. Lund VJ, Henderson B, Song Y: Involvement of cytokines and vascular adhesion receptors in the pathology of fronto-ethmoidal mucocoeles. Acta Oto-Laryngol 1993; 113: L 540–546.

124. Tokushige E, Itoh K, Ushikai M, et al.: Localization of IL-1 beta mRNA and cell adhesion molecules in the maxillary sinus mucosa of patients with chronic sinusitis. Laryngoscope 1994; 104: 1245–1250.

125. Jousimies-Somer HR, Savolainen S, Yliskoski JS: Macroscopic purulence, leukocyte counts, and bacterial morphotypes in relation to culture findings for sinus secretions in acute maxillary sinusitis. J Clin Microbiol 1988; 26: 1926–1933.

126. Carenfelt C, Lundberg C, Karen K: Immunoglobulins in maxillary sinus secretion. Acta Otol 1976; 82: 123–130.

127. Rossen RD, Buttler WT, Cate TR, et al.: Protein composition of nasal secretion during respiratory virus infection. Proc Soc Exp Biol Med 1965; 119: 1169–1176.

128. Kurono Y, Mogi G: Secretory IgA and serum type IgA in nasal secretion and antibody activity against the M protein. Ann Otol Rhinol Laryngol 1987; 96: 419–424.

129. Harlin SW, Ansel DG, Lane SR, et al.: A clinical and pathologic study of chronic sinusitis: The role of the eosinophil. J Allergy Clin Immunol 1988; 81: 867–875.

130. Sawyer WD, Smith MR, Wood WB Jr: The mechanisms by which macrophages phagocytose encapsulated bacteria in the absence of antibody. J Exp Med 1954; 100: 417–424.

131. Michie C, Scott A, Cheesbrough J, et al.: Streptococcal toxic shock–like syndrome: Evidence of superantigen activity and its effect on T lymphocyte subsets *in vivo*. Clin Exp Immunol 1994; 98: 140–144.

132. Schooley RR: Epstein-Barr virus (infectious mononucleosis). In: Mandell GL, Bennett JE, Dolin R (eds): Principles and Practice of Infectious Diseases, 4th ed. New York: Churchill Livingstone, 1995.

133. Baum SG: *Mycoplasma pneumoniae* and atypical pneumonia. In: Mandell GL, Bennett JE, Dolin R (eds): Principles and Practice of Infectious Diseases, 4th ed. New York: Churchill Livingstone, 1995.

134. Keusch GT: Immunologic responses to infection. In: Feigin RD, Cherry JD (eds): Textbook of Pediatric Infectious Diseases, 3rd ed., vol 1. Philadelphia: WB Saunders Co., 1992.

135. Volanakis JE, Zhu ZB, Schaffer FM, et al.: Major histocompatibility complex class III genes and susceptibility to immunoglobulin A deficiency and common variable immunodeficiency. J Clin Invest 1992; 89: 1914–1922.

136. Plebani A, Monafo V, Ugazio AG, Burgio GR: Clinical heterogeneity and reversibility of selective immunoglobulin A deficiency in 80 children. Lancet 1986; 1: 829–831.

137. French MA, Denis KA, Dawkins R, Peter JB: Severity of infections in IgA deficiency: Correlation with decreased serum antibodies to pneumococcal polysaccharides and decreased serum IgG2 and/or IgG4. Clin Exp Immunol 1995; 100: 47–53.

138. Gross S, Blaiss MS, Herrod HG: Role of immunoglobulin and specific antibody determinations in the evaluation of recurrent infection in children. J Pediatr 1992; 121: 516–522.

139. Jefferis R, Kumararatne DS: Selective IgG subclass deficiency: Quantitation and clinical relevance. Clin Exp Immunol 1990; 81: 357–367.

140. Umetsu DT, Amrosino DM, Quinti I, et al.: Recurrent sinopulmonary infection and impaired antibody response to bacterial capsular polysaccharide antigen in children with selective IgG-subclass deficiency. N Engl J Med 1985; 313: 1247–1251.

141. Sirisinha S, Suskind R, Edelman R, et al.: Secretory and serum IgA in children with protein calorie malnutrition. Pediatrics 1975; 55: 166–170.

142. Semba RD: Vitamin A, immunity, and infection. Clin Infect Dis 1994; 19: 489–499.

143. Feigin RD, Sandberg ET: Interaction of infection and nutrition. In: Feigin RD, Cherry JD (eds): Textbook of Pediatric Infectious Diseases, 3rd ed., vol 1. Philadelphia: WB Saunders Co., 1992.

Gary V. Doern

Laboratory Diagnosis of Infectious Diseases

▼

The intent of this chapter is to summarize the role of the laboratory in establishing the etiology of infections of the sinuses, middle ear cavity, external auditory canal, epiglottis, pharynx, intermediate airways, and soft tissue of the head and neck. A variety of bacteria, viruses, mycobacteria, and fungi are recognized as causes of infections in these sites. The most common pathogens of individual disease entities are identified, as are the optimum clinical specimens for laboratory analysis. Transportation of specimens to the laboratory is considered, and specimen work-up elucidated. Lastly, the role of the laboratory in directing patient management is addressed.

GENERAL CONSIDERATIONS

The most common approach to determining the specific cause of an individual patient's infection, irrespective of the nature of that infection, is to examine representative clinical specimens microscopically and by culture for the presence of potential pathogens. The validity of this approach to infectious disease diagnosis is totally predicated on the quality of the specimens. Nowhere is this more true than in infections of the ears, nose, and throat (ENT).

ENT infections invariably arise on or contiguous to sites that harbor a commensal bacterial flora. The mucosal surfaces of the oral cavity, nasal passages, nasopharynx, and pharynx contain as many as 10^8 bacteria per milliliter of mucosal secretions.[1] Facultative saprophytic bacteria include viridans and microaerophilic streptococci, non-*aureus* species of staphylococci, aerobic diphtheroids, nonpathogenic *Neisseria* species, *Borrelia* species, certain nonpathogenic treponemes, and gram-negative bacilli such as *Eikenella corrodens*, *Haemophilus* species other than *Haemophilus influenzae*, *Actinobacillus actinomycetemcomitans*, *Cardiobacterium hominis*, *Kingella* species, and other miscellaneous gram-negative bacilli. Anaerobes outnumber aerobes by a factor of 10 in the upper respiratory tract commensal flora and typically include representatives of all genera and species except *Clostridium* species and the *Bacteroides fragilis* group.[2]

In patients with debilitating diseases, in individuals who are hospitalized or living in closed, often crowded environments with diminished mobility such as nursing homes, and in patients who have received antibiotics, especially broad-spectrum agents, the upper respiratory tract often becomes colonized with enteric gram-negative bacilli from the gastrointestinal tract and *Pseudomonas aeruginosa*.

In addition to these organisms that are usually present and rarely cause ENT disease, a variety of recognized causes of infection colonize the mucosal surfaces of the oral cavity and upper respiratory tract of asymptomatic individuals, in some cases transiently, in other cases persistently. They include *H. influenzae*, especially nontypable strains; *Streptococcus pneumoniae*; *Moraxella (Branhamella) catarrhalis*; *Staphylococcus aureus*; *Neisseria meningitidis*; groups A, C, F, and G beta-hemolytic streptococci; and *Bordetella pertussis*. Certain respiratory viruses colonize the upper respiratory tract asymptomatically, as do yeast such as *Candida* species and *Torulopsis glabrata*. With respect to defined causes of ENT infections, only *Neisseria gonorrhoeae* is not known to colonize the upper respiratory tract asymptomatically.

These observations underscore the necessity of obtaining representative clinical samples that are, as much as possible, free of contamination when one is attempting to establish an etiologic diagnosis of ENT infections. In addition, a knowledge of commensal flora and potential pathogens is essential.

With respect to ENT infections, it is important to recognize that in selected instances, for example, infections of the sinuses and middle ear cavities and soft tissue infections, the laboratory can actually establish the existence of infection by demonstrating the presence of microorganisms in representative clinical specimens, because the sites at which infection occur are normally sterile. In other cases, e.g., pharyngitis, epiglottitis, otitis externa, and intermediate airway infections, the results of laboratory analyses, even when performed on highly representative specimens, do not definitely establish a diagnosis of infection; they merely provide a clue as to the possible etiology of disease in individuals identified as having infection on clinical grounds. This is because these infections arise in nonsterile sites that may be asymptomatically colonized with disease-causing microorganisms.

SINUSITIS

Etiology

Among the paranasal sinuses, the maxillary sinuses represent the most common site for infection. Maxillary sinusitis, although primarily a pediatric infectious disease problem, may occur in patients of any age. With respect to etiology, it is convenient to consider maxillary sinusitis as having three forms: acute, chronic, and complicated. Acute maxillary sinusitis is most commonly caused by selected respiratory viruses (i.e., rhinovirus, adenovirus, respiratory syncytial virus [RSV], and parainfluenza viruses 1, 2, and 3), *S. pneumoniae, H. influenzae,* and *M. catarrhalis,* alone or in some combination.[3-6] Less commonly, *S. aureus* and beta-hemolytic streptococci are associated with this condition. Chronic maxillary sinusitis, however, is usually a polymicrobial infection involving the mixed aerobic and anaerobic sal bacterial flora of the upper respiratory tract.[3, 7-10, 14] In addition, the same bacteria noted as the principal causes of acute maxillary sinusitis can be associated with chronic infections. In patients with severe underlying immunocompromising conditions, filamentous fungi emerge as important etiologic agents of sinusitis.[15, 16] Any of the saprophytic molds can cause this condition, but two organisms, *Aspergillus* species and the phycomycetes, particularly *Rhizopus* and *Mucor* species, predominate.

Specimen Collection and Processing

The only nonsurgical specimen of consistent value in establishing the etiology of maxillary sinusitis is an aspirate of the involved sinus(es) collected after disinfection of the nasal mucosa and then antral needle puncture. Efforts to predict the etiology of sinusitis by analysis of the results of pharyngeal and nasopharyngeal swab cultures or examination of nasal discharge have largely been unrewarding.[4, 11-13] Aspirates should be transported to the laboratory in sterile screw-capped containers within 30 minutes. In circumstances in which anaerobes are considered, an anaerobic transport device should be used. Detection of viruses is enhanced by placing a portion of the specimen in a suitable viral transport medium and then cooling to 4° C on crushed ice.

A Gram's stain and aerobic culture should be performed routinely. When appropriate, a smear for fungi and specific cultures for anaerobes, fungi, and viruses may also be performed.

OTITIS MEDIA

Etiology

The etiology of acute otitis media is highly predictable; 20%–30% of cases appear to be nonbacterial and may be associated with a variety of respiratory viruses (noted previously) or characterized by sterile middle ear fluid (MEF).[18] The remaining 70%–80% of cases are typically found by tympanocentesis to yield one or more of a relatively few different bacteria in cultures of MEF. In order of prevalence, *S. pneumoniae,* nontypable *H. influenzae,* and *M. catarrhalis,* often in combination, are the most important bacterial causes of acute otitis media, accounting for 90%–95% of bacterial infections.[17-19] Group A beta-hemolytic streptococci and *S. aureus* also occur but much less commonly. Acute otitis media is usually a disease of children; however, it also occurs in adults and in this setting is characterized by the same etiology.

The same bacteria may be observed as pathogens in chronic otitis media, although in this disease process, infections are more commonly found to be mixed and often

contain representations of the commensal aerobic and anaerobic bacterial flora of the upper respiratory tract.[20] As a result, viridans streptococci, *Neisseria* species, aerobic diphtheroids, non-*aureus* staphylococci, and anaerobes such as *Peptostreptococcus, Fusobacterium,* non-*fragilis* group *Bacteroides, Prevotella, Porphyromonas,* and non–spore-forming, anaerobic, gram-positive bacilli may be found in the middle ear cavity. Finally, *P. aeruginosa* may also be associated with chronic otitis media.

Specimen Collection and Processing

The only definitive means of establishing the specific cause of otitis media in an individual patient is to examine MEF collected via tympanocentesis. As was the case in patients with sinusitis, examination of swabs from the nasopharynx or pharynx or of nasal discharge is of little value. In patients with frank otorrhea, examination of purulent drainage is probably warranted, although one must recognize that such specimens may be exogenously contaminated with organisms resident on the skin of the ear canal. In patients with bilateral disease in whom tympanocentesis is to be performed, only the most affected ear needs to be tapped. MEF specimens should be handled precisely as described for sinus aspirates.

OTITIS EXTERNA

Etiology

Infection of the external auditory canal is most commonly caused by *P. aeruginosa,* less commonly by *S. aureus* and anaerobic bacteria.[21]

Specimen Collection and Processing

Purulent drainage, if present in copious amounts, should be collected in a syringe and needle, the needle discarded, and the syringe capped and submitted in toto to the laboratory with a delay of no more than 30 minutes. Alternatively, especially in patients with sparse discharge, a swab specimen obtained by vigorous sampling of the infected site, collecting as much representative material as possible, should be submitted to the laboratory in a suitable bacterial transport medium. The specimen should be examined by Gram's stain and cultured aerobically.

ACUTE SUPRAGLOTTITIS (EPIGLOTTITIS)

Etiology

The vast majority of cases of epiglottitis in the past have been due to encapsulated type B strains of *H. influenzae.*[22-25] It is likely that this disease will become less common with the widespread application of *H. influenzae* type B conjugate antigen vaccines. Rare cases of this disease may also be caused by *S. pneumoniae*, *S. aureus*, non–type B *H. influenzae*, and beta-hemolytic streptococci.

Specimen Collection and Processing

In patients in whom access can be obtained without compromise of the airway, a swab of the epiglottis should be collected and submitted to the laboratory in a suitable transport medium. Notwithstanding the fact that the mucosal surface of the epiglottis harbors a commensal bacterial flora, the swab specimen should be gram-stained, insofar as a vast predominance of organisms that are morphologically compatible with *Haemophilus* (i.e., faintly staining, pleomorphic, gram-negative bacilli) in the presence of large numbers of polymorphonuclear leukocytes would be diagnostic. The swab specimen should also be cultured aerobically with inclusion of a chocolate agar plate rendered specifically selective for *Haemophilus* by the addition of 300 µg/mL bacitracin ± 5 µg/mL vancomycin ± 1 µg/mL clindamycin.[26] Finally, two blood cultures should be performed.

PHARYNGITIS

Etiology

Exudative pharyngitis may be caused by an extensive list of microorganisms.[23] They include a variety of bacteria: group A beta-hemolytic streptococci, groups C, F, and G beta-hemolytic streptococci, *Arcanobacterium haemolyticum, N. gonorrhoeae, Corynebacterium diphtheriae,* and *Corynebacterium ulcerans*. Vincent's angina, or ulcerative pharyngitis with pseudomembrane formation, is due to a combination of *Fusobacterium* species, saprophytic *Borrelia* of the oral cavity, and species of *Bacteroides* other than the *fragilis* group. *Mycoplasma pneumoniae* and *Chlamydia pneumoniae* apparently also cause pharyngitis, but infrequently. A variety of viral agents are associated with pharyngitis: the respiratory viruses previously noted as causes of acute sinusitis and otitis media; influenzaviruses A and B; selected viruses in the *Herpesviridae* family (i.e., Epstein-Barr virus [EBV], cytomegalovirus [CMV], and herpes simplex virus [HSV]); and certain serotypes of coxsackie A virus.

Among these many causes of pharyngitis, efforts to establish an etiologic diagnosis need be directed only at bacterial agents and viruses in the *Herpesviridae* family. From a practical point of view, with respect to routine diagnostic studies in patients with pharyngitis, only beta-hemolytic streptococci deserve consideration. In selected instances, based on either suggestive clinical findings or a contributory epidemiologic history, efforts to establish a diagnosis of infection due to *N. gonorrhoeae, C. diphtheriae* or *C. ulcerans, A. haemolyticum,* the herpes viruses, or mixed fusospirochetal disease can be undertaken. Laboratory studies directed at detecting respiratory viruses, coxsackie A virus, *Mycoplasma,* or *Chlamydia* are rarely necessary or justifiable. The procedures themselves are very expensive, and the clinical utility of an etiologic diagnosis is questionable, either because there exists no specific therapy or because the mere recovery of one of these agents in the laboratory does not conclusively establish it as being a cause of disease.

The laboratory is frequently asked to determine the presence of *S. pneumoniae, H. influenzae, N. meningitidis, S. aureus*, and even *M. catarrhalis* in swab specimens of the pharynx and nasopharynx. Such requests usually stem from the mistaken notion that these bacteria are the etiologic agents of pharyngitis or that their recovery from the URT serves to define their etiologic role in sinusitis or otitis media. Both of these assertions are without foundation. As a result, with the exception of epidemiologic studies in which carriage needs to be ascertained, there exists no reason for the laboratory to attempt to isolate these bacteria from throat or nasopharyngeal swab specimens.

Specimen Collection and Processing

Streptococcal Pharyngitis

A cotton-, Dacron-, or alginate-tipped swab should be used to vigorously sample the posterior pharynx, the pharynx, and the peritonsillar mucosa bilaterally. If purulent material is present, it too should be sampled. As a rule, unless the patient gags and the eyes start watering, the physician has not been aggressive enough in collecting the specimen. The swab should be sent to the laboratory in a suitable transport medium. In the laboratory, the contents of the swab are inoculated onto the surface of a 5% sheep blood agar (SBA) plate and incubated at 35° C in 5%–7% CO_2 for 16–24 hours prior to examining for the presence of beta-hemolytic colonies. A direct specimen Gram's stain is of no value. Use of selective medium containing various antibiotics, most commonly trimethoprim/sulfamethoxazole, has been found by some to enhance recovery rates; similarly, incubation of plates in a strictly anaerobic environment has been advocated.[27–29] Catalase-negative beta-hemolytic colonies consisting of gram-positive cocci in chains should be ruled out as group A beta-hemolytic streptococci. This is best accomplished by use of a rapid colorimetric spot test for production of a preformed enzyme, L-pyroglutamylpeptide hydrolase.[30–32] Other rapid identification tests are nucleic acid probe analysis of colonies and particle agglutination tests (Fig. 4–1) of colonies for the presence of the Lancefield group A antigen.

Alternatively, a disk diffusion test for susceptibility to bacitracin can be performed.[32, 33] This procedure, however, requires subculture and another 24 hours for availability of results. It is best performed using disks containing 0.02–0.04 units of bacitracin. Direct application of bacitracin disks to primary culture plates, as is often practiced, should be avoided, as it may result in both false-negative and false-positive results. When beta-hemolytic streptococci recovered in culture are ruled out as group A, they need not be further characterized as to their specific serogroup, i.e., group C, F, or G. Such isolates can simply be reported as "beta-hemolytic streptococci, not group A."

There now exist a variety of commercially available, non–culture-based diagnostic procedures that permit rapid detection of group A beta-hemolytic streptococci directly in swab specimens.[24] At least 20 such methods have been marketed.

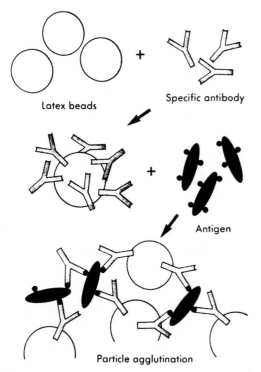

Figure 4–1. Latex particle agglutination test. Latex particles are coated with specific antibody. In the presence of soluble antigen, the latex particles agglutinate forming a visible clumping reaction. (From Baron EJ, Peterson LR, Finegold SM: Bailey and Scott's Diagnostic Microbiology, 9th ed. St. Louis, Mosby-Year Book, 1994, p 124.)

A swab specimen is obtained, the contents of the swab are eluted into a buffer solution, group A antigen is extracted either enzymatically, chemically with nitrous or acetic acid, or by heating, and antigen detection with group A–specific antibody is achieved by particle agglutination (see Fig. 4–1), enzyme immunoassay (EIA), or optical changes resulting from antigen-antibody complexes. EIAs may be solid or liquid phase (Fig. 4–2). Results are typically available in 10–30 minutes. Different assays have different performance characteristics, but in general, the following statements about direct "strep" detection tests appear to be true: In comparison with culture, direct detection tests achieve a sensitivity of 75%–95% and specificity of 85%–95%.[34] Direct tests almost always perform better in the hands of experienced laboratorians than when conducted by physicians, nurses, and office staff in outpatient clinics or private physicians' offices. Currently, in terms of sensitivity and specificity, ease of use, and cost, a group A streptococcal optical immunoassay (Strep A OIA; BioStar, Inc., Boulder, Colorado) is probably the preferred direct detection test for Group A beta-hemolytic streptococci.[35]

The obvious advantages of direct "strep" tests are the speed with which results are generated and the fact that positive results are invariably true positives because of high test specificity. Disadvantages include detection only of group A beta-hemolytic streptococci and, in some cases, relatively poor sensitivity. These observations underscore the necessity of performing cultures for patients with a negative direct "strep" test, to detect patients whose results are false-negative for group A streptococci, as well as to detect those

patients infected with serogroup C, F, or G beta-hemolytic streptococci. From a practical point of view, this means collecting a double throat swab specimen initially. The first swab is used for performance of the direct test; the second swab is used to perform culture if the direct test is negative. Another shortcoming of direct "strep" tests is the observation that test performance falls off when the tests are used by medical personnel in settings in which patients are seen. This is obviously the circumstance in which rapid "strep" tests could potentially be of greatest utility.

Serodiagnosis of group A streptococcal pharyngitis is largely a retrospective exercise. In general, 2–3 weeks following appearance of acute symptoms are required before diagnostic levels of antibody are found in the patient's serum.[36–38] The streptozyme procedure is a screening test with excellent sensitivity but limited specificity. It is simple to perform, quick, and inexpensive. Positive streptozyme results must be confirmed by use of either the anti–DNAse B procedure or determination of antistreptolysin (ASO) titers.[39–41] Both of these procedures, although more complex, time-consuming, and costly than the streptozyme test, have high specificity and, as a result, perform well as confirmatory procedures. Early administration of antibiotics, however, abrogates antibody responses, leading to false-negative results.[38, 39] The anti–DNAse B procedure detects antibody formed as a result of infection due to serogroup A, C, F, or G of beta-hemolytic streptococci.[38, 39] In contrast, the ASO test detects only group A–reactive antibody. Baseline levels of antibody detectable by all three procedures are often found in sera from patients with antecedent exposure to group A beta-hemolytic streptococci. For this reason, diagnostic titers on single specimens have been defined for the anti–DNAse B and ASO tests as 240. Antibody produced as a result of infection persists for up to 6–9 months.[38, 39, 41]

Gonococcal Pharyngitis

In situations in which gonococcal pharyngitis or asymptomatic pharyngeal colonization is suspected, a pharyngeal swab is the specimen of choice. Because the fatty acids found on cotton fibers may be deleterious to the survival of *N. gonorrhoeae*, a Dacron- or alginate-tipped swab should be used. The swab should be transported promptly to the laboratory in Amies or modified Stuart transport medium containing charcoal and then inoculated onto *Neisseria*-selective media (e.g., modified Thayer-Martin agar), which is incubated for up to 72 hours in 5%–7% CO_2 at 35° C and examined daily for the presence of colonies consisting of oxidase-producing, gram-negative diplococci. Alternatively, agar plates containing *Neisseria*-selective media can be inoculated directly by medical personnel at the time the swab specimen is obtained, and the plate transported to the laboratory in a sealed CO_2-containing vessel, for instance, a candle jar. Comparable approaches include direct inoculation and transport of John E. Martin Biologic Environmental Chamber plates or Transgrow bottles containing *Neisseria*-selective medium.[42–44] Gram's smears of pharyngeal swabs are of no value in the diagnosis of gonococcal pharyngitis, as commensal species of *Neisseria* normally colonize the pharynx.

Figure 4–2. Enzyme-linked immunosorbent assay (ELISA) for antigen detection. *A,* Direct assay in which the antibody specifically reactive with the target antigen (i.e., capture antibody) is immobilized on a solid support. Antigen, if present in a clinical specimen, binds to the capture antibody and is then detected with a second antibody also specifically reactive with the target antigen but one that is enzyme-labeled (i.e., detecting antibody). *B,* Indirect assay in which the detecting antibody is not enzyme-labeled. Rather, the presence of bound detecting antibody is ascertained by use of an enzyme-labeled antibody specific for immunoglobulin from the species of animal in which the detecting antibody was produced. In both the direct and indirect assays, results are usually predicated on substrate conversion by bound enzyme and measurement of reaction byproduct colorimetrically. (From Balows A, Hausler WJ, Herrmann KL, et al. Manual of Clinical Microbiology, 6th ed. Washington, D.C.: American Society for Microbiology, 1995, p 112.)

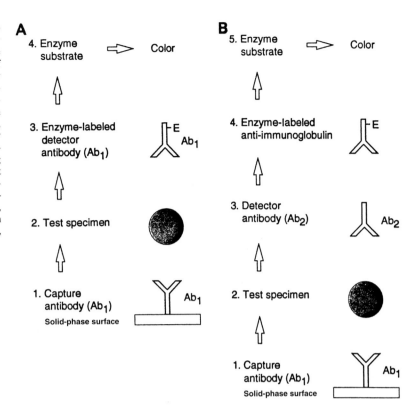

Definitive identification of colonies as *N. gonorrhoeae* can be achieved by use of any of a variety of biochemical, immunochemical, or nucleic acid probe–based assays. These procedures vary considerably in terms of length of time to a definitive result (i.e., minutes to days), logistical complexity, requirement for instrumentation, cost, and reliability of results. One useful approach is to test suspicious colonies for the presence of prolylaminopeptidase, an enzyme produced by *N. gonorrhoeae,* using a 30-minute, colorimetric assay for preformed enzyme.[44–46] Positive results permit presumptive identification of *N. gonorrhoeae* and can be confirmed by a 1-hour nonamplified probe–based assay (AccuProbe; Gen-Probe, Inc., San Diego, California).[47] If the probe assay is positive, a definitive identification of *N. gonorrhoeae* has been achieved. Direct detection of *N. gonorrhoeae* in pharyngeal swab specimens using either immunochemical methods or assays predicated on molecular methods is not yet possible. It is likely, however, that such procedures, especially those based on nucleic acid detection, will become available in the near future.

Diphtheria

In patients in whom diphtheria is suspected and a pseudomembrane is present, the pseudomembrane should be dislodged and sent in toto to the laboratory in a sterile, closed container. In the absence of a pseudomembrane, a pharyngeal swab should be obtained and placed in suitable transport medium prior to conveyance to the laboratory. In either case, specimens should be transported expeditiously.

A Gram's smear to look for abundant, small, pleomorphic gram-positive bacilli and a methylene blue preparation to examine for the presence of abundant pleomorphic, rod-shaped organisms containing metachromatic granules should be performed on pseudomembrane specimens.[48] These procedures are superfluous with swab specimens. A positive result obtained with tissue may be considered suggestive of infection due to either *C. diphtheriae* or *C. ulcerans.*

Culture is best accomplished by inoculation of specimens onto at least two different media. One such approach includes use of a slant containing Loeffler's or Pai's medium and a plate containing tellurite or Tindale's agar medium.[49] Media are incubated for up to 5 days at 35° C in 5%–7% CO_2 and examined daily for colonies containing catalase-positive, pleomorphic gram-positive bacilli, with metachromatic granules apparent following methylene blue stain. The latter characteristic is most conspicuous with colonies growing on Loeffler's or Pai's medium. Distinction of colony types *mitis, intermedius,* and *gravis* of *C. diphtheriae* based on colony morphology should not be attempted in the absence of extensive examiner experience, something that rarely exists today because of the current low prevalence of diphtheria. Species identification of suspicious colonies is accomplished using conventional biochemical tests, preferably in a public health reference laboratory.[51] Isolates of *C. diphtheriae* should be examined for the presence of toxin production using mouse, guinea pig, or rabbit neutralization studies, again in the setting of a reference laboratory.[49, 51]

Adjunctive diagnostic studies are directed at assessing patient immune status by detecting the presence of circulating protective antibody (i.e., antitoxin) as a result of immunization. Such antibody is best measured by use of a cell culture neutralization assay or by hemagglutination.[50] EIAs have been described, but their reliability is yet to be determined.

Other Bacterial Causes of Pharyngitis

A. haemolyticum can be recovered from the same throat swab used to detect beta-hemolytic streptococci. Small, beta-hemolytic colonies containing tiny, pleomorphic, catalase-negative, gram-positive bacilli appear on SBA plates following 24–48 hours of incubation at 35° C in 5%–7% CO_2.[49] Definitive species identification is based on conventional biochemical tests.

The diagnosis of Vincent's angina is best accomplished by Gram's stain of exudate collected by swabbing of the infected site(s). At least three smears on glass slides should be prepared at the time specimens are obtained, air dried, and then transported to the laboratory, where Gram's stain is performed and the slides are examined. The presence of at least moderate numbers of long, thin, faintly staining, gram-negative bacilli with pointed ends (i.e., *Fusobacterium*) and spiral, gram-negative bacilli with three to five large, conspicuous spirals (i.e., *Borrelia*) is diagnostic.

Viral Pharyngitis

Efforts to establish a viral etiology of pharyngitis are relevant only to EBV, CMV, and HSV. For suspicion of EBV in a patient with a compatible clinical illness, peripheral blood should be examined for the presence of relative and absolute lymphocytosis with varying numbers of atypical lymphocytes, which are present in 80%–95% of patients with EBV infectious mononucleosis.[52, 53] In addition, an EBV-specific heterophil agglutinin (EBV-sHA) test should be performed as a screening procedure. EBV-sHAs are antibodies that agglutinate sheep or horse erythrocytes following exposure to guinea pig kidney but are absorbed by beef red blood cells. In this respect, EBV-sHAs are readily distinguished from the heterophil agglutinins associated with serum sickness and Forssman's antibodies. A variety of commercial rapid, slide hemagglutination tests are available that reliably detect EBV-sHAs. If positive, these screening procedures strongly imply the presence of active or very recent disease. There are few recognized causes of false-positive test results: EBV-sHAs remain positive for about 6 months following an acute EBV infection.[55] A negative test does not exclude the diagnosis, as approximately 10% of adult patients and 20% of pediatric patients have a false-negative EBV-sHA test.[52, 54]

Alternatives to EBV-sHA tests, for purposes of serodiagnosis of acute EBV infection, are procedures that detect antibody reactive with fragments of the Epstein-Barr virus nuclear antigen (EBNA). This protein appears early during viral replication in B lymphocytes, and segments of it are highly immunogenic. The P62 peptide serves as the target antigen in several assays for immunoglobulin G (IgG) and IgM antibody that have become commercially available.[56] The most common test format is an EIA (Fig. 4–3). In general, P62-based procedures have slightly greater sensitivity than tests for EBV-sHAs and as a result identify at least some patients as having EBV infection in spite of a negative ESHA test. The presence of IgM but little or no IgG indicates current infection; the opposite pattern implies past infection. Definitive EBV serodiagnosis remains a product of indirect immunofluorescence tests for antibody reactive with several EBV antigens: EBNA (total antibody), viral capsid antigen (both IgG and IgM), and early antigen (IgG only).[55]

An etiologic diagnosis of the pharyngitis associated with CMV infectious mononucleosis is best accomplished by use of a serologic assay that detects CMV-reactive IgM. Direct detection of CMV antigens in respiratory secretions or culture of the virus is of little value, insofar as CMV is often shed in the upper respiratory tract of healthy individuals.

Lastly, a laboratory diagnosis of HSV 1 or 2 pharyngitis is best accomplished by shell vial culture of pharyngeal secretions obtained using a polyester- or alginate-tipped swab. When vesicular lesions are apparent, they should be unroofed and the base of the lesion sampled. A portion of the specimen should be smeared directly onto two segments of a glass slide and allowed to air-dry. The swab should then be placed in a suitable viral transport medium and, together with the slides, submitted to the laboratory. Unless transport time can be restricted to <30 minutes, the specimens should be placed on slush ice. With the use of fluorescein-labeled monoclonal antibodies reactive with HSV 1 and 2 and a direct immunofluorescence technique (direct fluorescent antibody; Fig. 4–4), the slide is examined directly for HSV antigens.[57] Optimum culture recovery of HSV is accomplished by use of shell vial cultures emphasizing a human diploid fibroblast cell line and viral antigen detection in cultures by use of fluorescein-labeled monoclonal antibodies reactive with antigens expressed early during viral replication.[58–62] Definitive positive results may be obtained with this procedure as soon as 16 hours following inoculation of cultures. Alternatively, especially in situations in which large volumes of specimens are to be processed, traditional tube cultures using any of a variety of cell lines may be performed, with characteristic cytopathic effect usually apparent within 24–48 hours. Useful cell lines include human embryonic kidney, rabbit kidney, human embryonic lung fibroblasts, and the human lung carcinoma cell line A549.[63]

LARYNGOTRACHEOBRONCHITIS AND BRONCHIOLITIS

Etiology

The most common causes of laryngotracheobronchitis and bronchiolitis are the respiratory viruses—respiratory syncytial virus (RSV), adenovirus, parainfluenza viruses 1, 2, and 3, and influenza viruses A and B—and *B. pertussis*.

Specimen Collection and Processing

Respiratory Viruses

Establishing an etiologic diagnosis of viral laryngotracheobronchitis or bronchiolitis is of epidemiologic value and, in some cases, therapeutically useful. For instance, management of RSV bronchiolitis with ribavirin is of proven benefit. The optimum specimen for detecting the respiratory viruses associated with infections of the intermediate airways is either a swab of the nasopharynx or saline washes of this

Figure 4–3. ELISA for antibody detection. *A*, A noncompetitive assay in which the purified target antigen is immobilized on a solid support. Human antibody reactive with the antigen that is present in the clinical specimen binds to the antigen and is then detected with an enzyme-labeled antihuman immunoglobulin. *B*, A competitive assay in which the bound antigen is exposed to clinical specimen. Antibody reactive with the antigen is bound. A second antibody, enzyme-labeled and of known reactivity with the target antigen, is then added and binds to uncovered sites on the antigen. The amount of binding of the second enzyme-labeled antibody is inversely proportional to the amount of specific antibody present in the clinical specimen. (From Balows A, Hausler WJ, Herrmann KL, et al.: Manual of Clinical Microbiology, 6th ed. Washington, D.C.: American Society for Microbiology, 1995, p 113.)

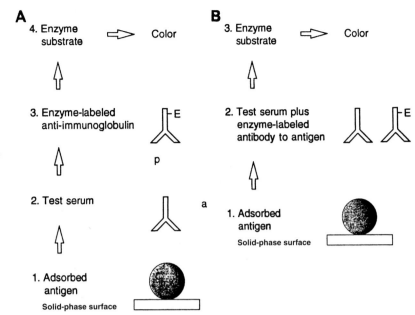

site. A vigorous attempt should be made to obtain columnar epithelial cells from the mucosal surface of the nasopharynx with both procedures, because respiratory viruses reside within these cells.

RSV, parainfluenza virus types 1 and 3, and influenza viruses A and B may be detected directly in nasopharyngeal specimens by use of a DFA procedure (see Fig. 4–4) using fluorescein-labeled monoclonal antibodies.[64, 65] In comparison with the results of virus cultures, if one assumes that high-quality, representative specimens are obtained, DFA procedures for respiratory viruses generally have a sensitivity of 75%–90%, and in the hands of experienced laboratory personnel using reagents of proven quality, such procedures have a specificity approaching 100%.[65] A desirable property of DFA tests is the opportunity to assess specimen quality microscopically.

RSV and influenza A may also be detected directly in clinical specimens by the use of commercially available EIAs.[66, 67] In general, these procedures have slightly lower sensitivity and specificity than DFA but benefit from objective assay endpoints that do not require subjective interpretation. A limitation of EIAs is their inability to permit assessment of specimen quality. The principal advantages of direct detection methods are speed (i.e., 1–2 h) and the lack of requirement for the facilities and expertise necessary to perform tissue culture.

Virus propagation does, however, remain the gold-standard method for diagnosing respiratory virus infections of the intermediate airway. Nasopharyngeal specimens are inoculated onto A549 cells and rhesus monkey kidney cells in the shell vial format; then they are examined for the presence of viral antigens at 48–72 hours using a pooled fluorescein-labeled monoclonal antibody reagent in a DFA format.[68, 69] The pooled reagent detects antigens of all of the respiratory viruses noted previously. When a positive result is obtained with the pool, the actual virus responsible for disease is elucidated by testing shell vial monolayers with antibodies specifically reactive with individual viral agents. If negative

Figure 4–4. Immunofluorescence. *A*, Direct detection of antigen on the slide with fluorescein-labeled antibody. *B*, Indirect detection of antigen on the slide with a primary antibody and then a secondary fluorescein-labeled antibody reactive with immunoglobulin from the species of animal from which the primary antibody was derived. (From Balows A, Hausler WJ, Herrmann KL, et al. Manual of Clinical Microbiology, 6th ed. Washington, D.C.: American Society for Microbiology, 1995, p 115.)

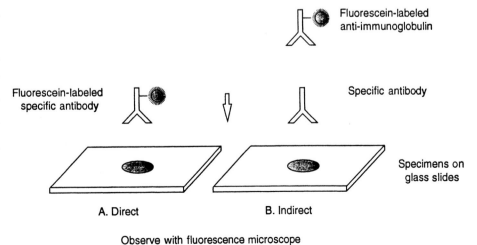

at 48–72 hours, the DFA test with pooled reagents is repeated after shell vials have incubated for 7 days.

Pertussis

The laboratory diagnosis of infection due to *B. pertussis* is best accomplished by examination of nasopharyngeal aspirates or calcium-alginate swab specimens. Aspirates may facilitate culture recovery.[70] If swabs are to be used, two specimens should be obtained, one through each nostril. Swabs or aspirates should be sent promptly to the laboratory in fluid transport medium (e.g., Casamino acid broth or half-strength Regan-Lowe medium).[71] Alternatively for swab specimens, culture plates can be inoculated and smears prepared directly at the patient's bedside. Because of the fastidious nature of the organism, this approach is preferred if the plates and slides can be transported to the laboratory immediately.

Smears should be examined by DFA testing (see Fig. 4–4) using a polyclonal fluorescein-labeled antibody reagent. A variety of agar media have been used for pertussis cultures. They include Bordet-Gengou potato agar containing 20% sheep blood cells and 2.5 μg/mL methicillin, Regan-Lowe agar, charcoal–horse blood agar, and Jones-Kendrick charcoal agar with 40 μg/mL cephalexin.[71] Two plates should be inoculated with one swab and two smears prepared from the other. Smears are examined immediately. Plates are incubated for up to 7 days at 35° C in a humidified chamber in ambient air. Colonies typically appear within 3–5 days. A combination of DFA testing and culture should be employed because neither technique has 100% sensitivity. The sensitivity of DFA testing has varied in different studies from 40% to 95%.[71] The likelihood that the DFA test will be positive appears to be inversely related to the length of time between onset of symptoms and collection of the specimen. Antibiotic therapy also causes the DFA test to be negative. The sensitivity of culture is also extremely variable (i.e., 20%–83%) and is influenced by similar factors.[71] Obviously, culture can be positive only in the presence of viable organisms.

In the absence of a definitive method for establishing an etiologic diagnosis of pertussis and in view of the time necessary to achieve a culture result, alternative diagnostic procedures have been sought. Polymerase chain reaction–based assays (Fig. 4–5) directed at either an insertion sequence (IS 481) present in 80–100 copies per cell or the promotor region of the gene for pertussis toxin have proved to be highly sensitive and specific.[72, 73]

SOFT TISSUE INFECTIONS OF THE HEAD AND NECK

Soft tissue infections of the head and neck may arise following contiguous seeding of organisms from primary sites of infection in the oral cavity, sinuses, middle ear, and pharynx. As a result, they may appear in the fascial spaces of the face as well as suprahyoid and infrahyoid areas.[74] The microbiology of these infections is highly variable. Infections are often mixed and may contain aerobic and anaerobic bacteria.[74]

Only tissue specimens and aspirates obtained using surgical technique, and then only when contamination with com-

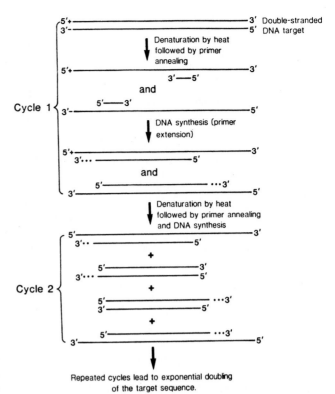

Figure 4–5. Polymerase chain reaction. Target DNA is denatured into single strands, both of which are replicated using short nucleotide primers, one from the 3′-end, the other from the 5′-end. The double-stranded segments of DNA that result are again denatured by heating and replicated with the same primers, resulting in a doubling of the amount of double-stranded DNA target. This amplification process is repeated automatically 20–40 times in a thermocycler during 1–2 h leading to logarithmically increased amounts of target DNA. (From Wolcott M: Advances in nucleic acid–based detection methods. Clin Microbiol Rev 1992; 5:370.)

mensal flora can be excluded, are acceptable for use in attempting to define the etiology of soft tissue infections of the head and neck. Tissue biopsy and aspirates are always superior to swab specimens of infected sites. Specimens should be transported directly to the laboratory in a sterile container, Gram's stains prepared and read immediately, and semiquantitative aerobic and anaerobic cultures performed. Fully quantitative cultures of tissue specimens need not be done, because this information adds nothing to establishing the cause of infection. Material draining from sinus tracts externally or internally is of little value. Similarly, swab specimens of purulent material accumulated on either mucosal surfaces or skin, even if contiguous with or part of the infection itself, should be avoided.

SUSCEPTIBILITY TESTING

A variety of procedures are available for determining the antimicrobial susceptibility patterns of bacteria recovered in the clinical laboratory.[76, 77] In general, test methods fall into one of two broad categories, quantitative and qualitative susceptibility tests. Quantitative procedures permit assessment of in vitro antibacterial activity in the form of minimum inhibitory concentrations (MICs).[76] MICs, which are expressed in the units μg/mL, may be determined (1) using a manual macrobroth tube dilution technique (Fig. 4–6), (2) in microdilution trays either manually or with instrument assistance, (3) by use of a gradient concentration strip agar diffusion method (the E-test), or (4) purely through instrumentation. Qualitative susceptibility tests generate results in the form of susceptibility categories, i.e., S, susceptible; I, intermediate; or R, resistant. The most popular qualitative susceptibility test is the Bauer-Kirby disk diffusion procedure (Fig. 4–7).[77] In addition, category susceptibility test results may be derived from various forms of instrumentation.

MIC values provide an estimate of the inhibitory activity of antimicrobials. Determination of MICs gives no assurance of microbe-killing (microbicidal) activity. This information is derived from determinations of minimum bactericidal concentrations (MBCs) of antimicrobials (Fig. 4–8). MBCs are a direct measure of killing activity. In ENT infections, however, knowledge of microbicidal activity is rarely necessary for predicting clinical outcome. Inhibitory activity, as estimated by either an MIC determination or a category susceptibility test, is nearly always sufficient for making therapeutic decisions. Similarly, the determination of the activity of antimicrobials in combination (i.e., synergy determinations) and the killing effect of serum on a patient's infecting pathogen (i.e., serum bactericidal titer), two other in vitro estimates of antibacterial activity, are of little or no predictive value in managing ENT infections.

Indeed, the role of the laboratory in the management of ENT infections is often limited, because most such infections are treated empirically without an etiologic diagnosis ever having been established. Furthermore, even when the cause of diseases such as maxillary sinusitis, otitis media, pharyngitis, and soft tissue infections of the head and neck can be established in an individual patient by recovering organism(s) in the laboratory from representative specimens, the actual clinical predictive value of in vitro susceptibility test results is questionable.[75]

Accepting the preceding caveats, the recommendations outlined here regarding in vitro susceptibility testing of organisms recovered from patients with ENT infections appear to be justified. In all cases, they are predicated on four fundamental assumptions:

1. Antimicrobial susceptibility tests (ASTs) should be performed only on isolates known to be or at least strongly suspected of being clinically significant. This necessitates careful attention to obtaining representative specimens free of contaminants.

2. A reliable (i.e., reproducible) AST should be performed in the laboratory. In most cases, this means use of a test method and results-interpretive criteria recommended by the National Committee for Clinical Laboratory Standards (NCCLS).[76, 77]

3. MICs as an estimate of antibacterial activity are inherently of no greater value in predicting therapeutic outcome than are category susceptibility test results (i.e., S, susceptible; I, intermediate; and R, resistant).

Figure 4–6. Minimum inhibitory concentration (MIC) determination.

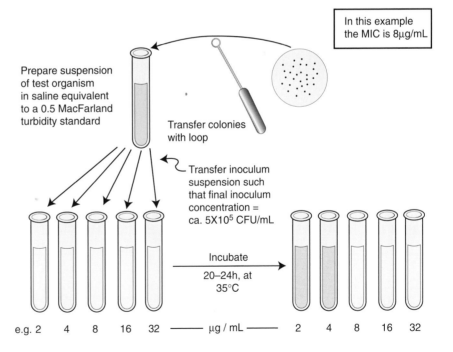

In this example the MIC is 8μg/mL

Prepare suspension of test organism in saline equivalent to a 0.5 MacFarland turbidity standard

Transfer colonies with loop

Transfer inoculum suspension such that final inoculum concentration = ca. 5X10⁵ CFU/mL

Incubate 20–24h, at 35°C

e.g.   2   4   8   16   32 ——— μg / mL ——— 2   4   8   16   32

Test tubes (or microtiter wells) containing broth growth medium and known concentrations of antimicrobial in serial two-fold concentration increments

Examine tubes and define MIC as the lowest concentration of antimicrobial tested that inhibits visible evidence of growth of the test organism

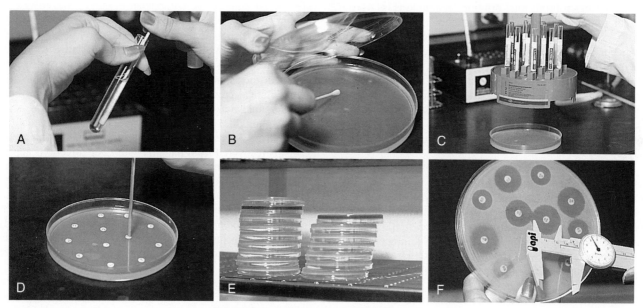

Figure 4–7. Disk diffusion susceptibility test *(A–F).*

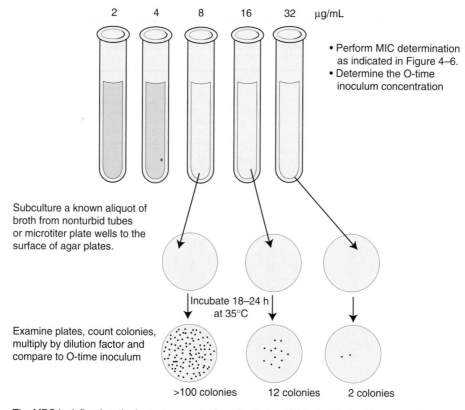

2   4   8   16   32   μg/mL

- Perform MIC determination as indicated in Figure 4–6.
- Determine the O-time inoculum concentration

Subculture a known aliquot of broth from nonturbid tubes or microtiter plate wells to the surface of agar plates.

Incubate 18–24 h at 35°C

Examine plates, count colonies, multiply by dilution factor and compare to O-time inoculum

>100 colonies   12 colonies   2 colonies

The MBC is defined as the lowest concentration of antimicrobial tested that achieves a ≥ 99.9% reduction (i.e., 3 log kill) of the O-time inoculum.

In this example, the MBC is 16 μg/mL

Figure 4–8. Minimum bactericidal concentration (MBC) determination.

4. There exists no reason to test organism-antimicrobial combinations in the laboratory that are known to be either uniformly active (i.e., susceptible) or uniformly inactive (i.e., resistant). In such cases, the laboratory can do one of only two things: generate a result that was known before the test was performed (hardly a cost-effective approach) or make a mistake.

Streptococcus pneumoniae

The emergence of penicillin resistance as a significant problem with the pneumococcus, combined with increasing rates of resistance to the macrolides, tetracyclines, and trimethoprim/sulfamethoxazole (TMP/SMX), underscores the need to perform ASTs routinely on all isolates of *S. pneumoniae*.[78, 84] Organisms should be screened for penicillin resistance using the oxacillin disk test.[77, 79] Isolates found to be resistant by this procedure should have MICs to penicillin determined for purposes of categorization—i.e., high-level resistance, penicillin MICs ≥2.0 μg/mL; intermediate resistance, MICs 0.12–1.0 μg/mL. Penicillin MICs are best determined using the gradient concentration strip method (i.e., E-test; Epsilometer, Inc., Solna, Sweden) on Mueller-Hinton agar containing 5% sheep blood.[80–83] Because of cross-resistance between other beta-lactams and penicillin, the penicillin result may also be used to predict the activity of ampicillin, amoxicillin, amoxicillin/clavulanate, and many cephalosporins. Exceptions include cefprozil, cefuroxime, cefpodoxime, ceftriaxone, and cefotaxime, which can be examined separately with the E-test. Macrolides and tetracyclines can be tested by the disk diffusion procedure. Results obtained with erythromycin are equivalent to those for azithromycin and clarithromycin. Similarly, results obtained with tetracycline, doxycycline, and minocycline are interchangeable. There exists no reliable, easy method for routine testing of trimethoprim/sulfamethoxazole versus *S. pneumoniae* short of a broth microdilution MIC in Mueller-Hinton broth containing 3% lysed horse blood.[76] Finally, there is no need currently to test quinolones against *S. pneumoniae*. High rates of intrinsic resistance pertain to currently licensed quinolones in the United States, and testing of these agents might serve unwittingly to encourage their inappropriate use.

Haemophilus influenzae

Currently in the United States, approximately one third of clinical isolates of nontypable *H. influenzae* produce a TEM-1 or ROB-1 beta-lactamase and as a result are resistant to ampicillin and amoxicillin.[84, 85] Beta-lactamase production is easily and reliably detected in the laboratory with the use of a 5-minute colorimetric assay that employs a chromogenic cephalosporin as a substrate.[86–88] A positive result denotes resistance to ampicillin and amoxicillin. The question arises, does a negative beta-lactamase test result mean that the isolate is ampicillin-susceptible? This question is relevant, insofar as strains of *H. influenzae* have been described that are resistant to ampicillin by mechanisms other than beta-lactamase production, i.e., altered permeability or altered penicillin-binding proteins.[89, 90] They have been termed beta-lactamase–negative, ampicillin-resistant strains. Such strains, however, are extremely uncommon, accounting for ≥0.1% of isolates in large surveillance studies.[84] Therefore, a negative test for beta-lactamase in the laboratory can be construed as indicating that the isolate is ampicillin-susceptible. Other antimicrobials need not be tested against *H. influenzae* because their activity is currently highly predictable: uniformly active, quinolones; ≤1% resistance, amoxicillin-clavulanate, cefuroxime, cefixime, cefpodoxime, ceftriaxone, cefotaxime, and azithromycin; 1%–5% resistance, cefprozil, cefaclor, loracarbef, tetracyclines, chloramphenicol, TMP/SMX, and clarithromycin.

Neisseria gonorrhoeae

Primary gonococcal isolates should probably be tested for beta-lactamase production, the most common mechanism of penicillin resistance, even though penicillin is no longer the 1st-line drug or drug of choice in treating gonococcal pharyngitis.[91] The test is easy to perform and provides information of epidemiologic value. Ceftriaxone, cefixime, and the quinolones ciprofloxacin and ofloxacin are currently the drugs of choice for treating uncomplicated gonococcal infections.[91] Resistance to the first two agents has not been described, and so tests need not be performed. Quinolone resistance has been recognized in certain geographic locations, such as Japan, Hawaii, and Ohio.[92, 93] Therefore, primary pharyngeal isolates of *N. gonorrhoeae* recovered in laboratories in areas known to be endemic for quinolone-resistant organisms should probably be tested against ciprofloxacin or ofloxacin using the disk diffusion procedure.[77]

Other Bacteria

Susceptibility tests need not be performed in the laboratory for *M. catarrhalis*, beta-hemolytic streptococci, *A. haemolyticum*, *C. diphtheriae*, and *B. pertussis*. Antimicrobial activity is highly predictable for most of these organisms, and in cases in which it is not, reliable susceptibility tests have not yet been developed, i.e., *A. haemolyticum*, *Corynebacterium* species, and *B. pertussis*.

Virtually all clinically significant isolates of *M. catarrhalis* produce a beta-lactamase and, as a result, are resistant to penicillin, ampicillin, and amoxicillin.[84, 85] This organism, however, remains nearly uniformly susceptible to other oral antimicrobials that might be used to treat the kinds of infections with which *M. catarrhalis* has been associated.

Similarly, group A beta-hemolytic streptococci, in the United States at least, appear to be highly susceptible to penicillin and the cephalosporins. Erythromycin resistance has been described with these organisms, but the prevalence is about 1%, hardly sufficient to justify routine susceptibility testing.[84, 94]

Susceptibility tests should, however, be performed on bacteria recovered from representative specimens obtained from patients who have closed-space infections of the head and neck. The agents to be tested should include those antimicrobials of consideration in managing these types of infection, i.e., penicillin, oxacillin when *S. aureus* is isolated, oral and parenteral beta-lactam/beta-lactamase inhibitor combinations, second- and third-generation oral and parenteral cephalosporins, a macrolide, clindamycin, imipenem, and gentamicin and tobramycin. The selection of a test method should be predicated on the individual organism being tested and should conform to NCCLS recommendations.

References

1. Tramont EC: General or non-specific host defense mechanisms. In: Mandell GL, Douglas RG, Bennett JE (eds): Principles and Practice of Infectious Disease. New York: Churchill Livingstone, 1994.
2. Gibbons RJ, Socransky SS, De Araujo WC, van Houte J: Studies of the predominant cultivable microbiota of dental plaque. Arch Oral Biol 1964; 9: 365.
3. Wald ER: Epidemiology, pathophysiology and etiology of sinusitis. Pediatr Infect Dis 1985; 4: S51.
4. Wald ER, Milmoe GJ, Bowen A, Delbert HT, et al.: Acute maxillary sinusitis in children. N Engl J Med 1980; 304: 749.
5. Jousimies-Somer HR, Savolainen S, Ylikoski JS: Bacteriological findings of acute maxillary sinusitis in young adults. J Clin Microbiol 1988; 26: 1919.
6. Jousimies-Somer HR, Savolainen S, Ylikoski JS: Macroscopic purulence, leukocyte counts, and bacterial morphotypes in relation to culture findings for sinus secretions in acute maxillary sinusitis. J Clin Microbiol 1988; 26: 1926.
7. Wald ER, Byers C, Guerra N, et al.: Subacute sinusitis in children. J Pediatr 1989; 115: 28.
8. Almadori G, Bastianini L, Bistoni F, et al.: Microbial flora of nose and paranasal sinuses in chronic maxillary sinusitis. Rhinology 1986; 24: 257.
9. Brook I: Bacteriologic features of chronic sinusitis in children. JAMA 1981; 246: 967.
10. Brook I: Bacteriology of chronic maxillary sinusitis in adults. Ann Otol Rhinol Laryngol 1989; 98: 426.
11. Evans FO, Sydnor B, Moore WEC: Sinusitis of the maxillary antrum. J Laryngol Otol 1963; 77: 1009.
12. Axelsson A, Brorson JE: The correlation between bacteriologic findings in the nose and maxillary sinus in acute maxillary sinusitis. Laryngoscope 1973; 83: 2003.
13. Jousimies-Somer HR, Savolainen S, Ylikoski JS: Comparison of the nasal bacterial floras in two groups of healthy subjects and in patients with acute maxillary sinusitis. J Clin Microbiol 1989; 27: 2736.
14. Tinkelman DG, Silk HJ: Clinical and bacteriologic features of chronic sinusitis in children. Am J Dis Child 1989; 143: 938.
15. Morgan MA, Wilson WR, Neel III HB, Roberts GD: Fungal sinusitis in healthy and immunocompromised individuals. Am J Clin Pathol 1984; 82: 597.
16. Daley CL, Saude M: The running nose infection of the paranasal sinuses. Infect Dis Clin North Am 1988; 2: 131.
17. Klein JO: State-of-the-art clinical article: Otitis media. Clin Infect Dis 1994; 19: 823.
18. Ruuskanen O, Arola M, Putto-Laurila A, et al.: Acute otitis media and respiratory virus infections. Pediatr Infect Dis J 1989; 8: 94.
19. Giebink GS: The microbiology of otitis media. Pediatr Infect Dis 1989; 8: S18.
20. Brook I, Finegold SM: Bacteriology of chronic otitis media. JAMA 1979; 241: 487.
21. Brook I, Frazier EH, Thompson DH: Aerobic and anaerobic microbiology of external otitis. Clin Infect Dis 1992; 15: 955.
22. Crysdale WS, Sendi K: Evolution in the management of acute epiglottitis: A 10-year experience with 242 children. Int Anesthesiol Clin 1988; 26: 32.
23. Baker AS, Beklan I, Tierney M: Infections of the pharynx, larynx, epiglottis, trachea and thyroid. In: Gorbach SL, Bartlett JG, Blacklow NR (eds): Infectious Disease. Philadelphia: WB Saunders Co, 1992.
24. Sheikh KH, Mostow SR: Epiglottitis—an increasing problem for adults. West J Med 1989; 151: 520.
25. Claesson BO, Trollfors B, Ekstrom-Jodal B, et al.: Incidence and prognosis of acute epiglottitis in children in a Swedish region. Pediatr Infect Dis 1984; 3: 534.
26. Chapin KC, Doern GV: Selective media for recovery of *Haemophilus influenzae* from specimens contaminated with upper respiratory tract microbial flora. J Clin Microbiol 1983; 17: 1163.
27. Kurzynski TA, Van Holten CM: Evaluation of techniques for isolation of group A streptococci from throat cultures. J Clin Microbiol 1981; 13: 891.
28. Gunn BA, Ohashi DK, Gaydos CA, Holt ES: Selective and enhanced recovery of group A and B streptococci from throat cultures with sheep blood agar containing sulfamethoxazole and trimethoprim. J Clin Microbiol 1977; 5: 650.
29. Lauer BA, Reller LB, Mirrett S: Effect of atmosphere and duration of incubation on primary isolation of group A streptococci from throat cultures. J Clin Microbiol 1983; 17: 338.
30. Ellner PD, Williams DA, Hosmer ME, Cohenford M: Preliminary evaluation of a rapid colorimetric method for the presumptive identification of a group A streptococci and enterococci. J Clin Microbiol 1985; 22: 880.
31. Facklam RR, Thacker LG, Fox B, Eriquez L: Presumptive identification of streptococci with a new test system. J Clin Microbiol 1982; 15: 987.
32. Yajko DM, Lawrence J, Nassos P, et al.: Clinical trial comparing bacitracin with Strep-a-Chek for accuracy and turnaround time in the presumptive identification of *Streptococcus pyogenes*. J Clin Microbiol 1986; 24: 431.
33. Maxted WR: The use of bacitracin for identifying group A haemolytic streptococci. J Clin Pathol 1953; 6: 224.
34. Todd JK, Radetsky M, Wheeler RC, Roe MH: Comparative evaluation of kits for rapid diagnosis of group A streptococcal disease. Pediatr Infect Dis 1985; 4: 274.
35. Harbeck RJ, Teague J, Crossen GR, et al.: Novel, rapid optical immunoassay technique for detection of group A streptococci from pharyngeal specimens: Comparison with standard culture methods. J Clin Microbiol 1993; 31: 839.
36. Whitnack E, Stollerman GH: Antistreptococcal antibodies in the diagnosis of rheumatic fever. In: Cohen AS (ed): Laboratory Diagnostic Procedures in Rheumatic Diseases, 3rd ed. Boston: Little, Brown, 1985.
37. Stollerman GH, Lewis AJ, Schultz I, et al.: Relationship of the immune response to group A streptococci to the course of acute, chronic and recurrent rheumatic fever. Am J Med 1956; 20: 163.
38. Ayoub EM, Harder E: Immune response to streptococcal antigens: Diagnostic methods. In: Rose NR, deMacario EC, Fakey II, et al. (eds): Manual of Clinical Immunology, 4th ed. Washington, D.C.: American Society for Microbiology, 1992.
39. James K: Immunoserology of infectious diseases. Clin Microbiol Rev 1990; 3: 132.
40. Klein GC, Jones WL: Comparison of the streptozyme test with the antistreptolysin O, antideoxyribonuclease B, and antihyaluronidase tests. Appl Microbiol 1971; 21: 257.
41. Bisno AL, Ofek I: Serologic diagnosis of streptococcal infection: Comparison of a rapid hemagglutination technique with conventional antibody tests. Am J Dis Child 1974; 127: 676.
42. Martin JE Jr, Jackson RL: A biological environment chamber for the culture of *Neisseria gonorrhoeae*. J Am Vener Dis Assoc 1975; 2: 28.
43. Martin JE Jr, Lester A: Transgrow, a medium for transport and growth of *Neisseria meningitidis*. HSNHA Health Rep 1977; 86: 30.
44. Evangelista AT, Beilstein HR: Laboratory diagnosis of gonorrhoea. Presented at Cumitech 4A, American Society for Microbiology, Washington, D.C., 1993.
45. Janda WM, Sobieski V: Evaluation of a ten-minute chromogenic substrate test for identification of pathogenic *Neisseria* species and *Branhamella catarrhalis*. Eur J Clin Microbiol Infect Dis 1988; 7: 25.
46. Dillon JR, Carballo M, Pauze M: Evaluation of eight methods for identification of pathogenic *Neisseria* species: Neisseria Kwik, RIM-N, Gonobio-Test, Minitek, Gonochek II, GonoGen, Phadebact Monoclonal GC OMNI test, and Syva Trak test. J Clin Microbiol 1988; 26: 493.
47. Lewis JS, Kranig-Brown D, Trainor DA: DNA probe confirmatory test for *Neisseria gonorrhoeae*. J Clin Microbiol 1990; 28: 2349.
48. Bannatyne RM, Clausen C, McCarthy LR: Laboratory diagnosis of upper respiratory tract infections. Presented at Cumitech 10, American Society for Microbiology, Washington, D.C., 1979.
49. Clarridge JE, Spiegel CA: *Corynebacterium* and miscellaneous irregular gram positive rods, *Erysipelothrix*, and *Gardnerella*. In: Murray PR, Baron EJ, Pfaller MA, et al. (eds): Manual of Clinical Microbiology. Washington, D.C.: American Society for Microbiology, 1994.
50. Craig JP: Immune response to *Corynebacterium diphtheriae* and *Clos-*

tridium tetani. In: Rose NR, deMacario EC, Fakey JL, et al. (eds): Manual of Clinical Immunology, 4th ed. Washington, D.C.: American Society for Microbiology, 1992.

51. Popovic T, Wharton M, Wenger JD, et al.: Are we ready for diphtheria? A report from the diphtheria diagnostic workshop. J Infect Dis 1995; 171: 765.

52. Henle W, Henle GE, Horowitz CA: Epstein-Barr virus–specific diagnostic tests in infectious mononucleosis. Hum Pathol 1974; 5: 551.

53. Fleisher G, Paradise J, Lennette E: Leukocyte response in childhood infectious mononucleosis. Am J Dis Child 1981; 135: 699.

54. Horwitz C, Henle G, Brown TL, et al.: Clinical and laboratory evaluation of infants and children with Epstein-Barr virus–induced infectious mononucleosis: Report of 32 patients (aged 10 months–48 months). Blood 1981; 57: 933.

55. Sumaya CV, Jenson HB: Epstein-Barr virus. In: Rose NR, deMacario EC, Fakey JL, et al. (eds): Manual of Clinical Immunology, 4th ed. Washington, D.C.: American Society for Microbiology, 1992.

56. Smith RS, Rhodes G, Vaughan JH, et al.: A synthetic peptide for detecting antibodies to Epstein-Barr virus nuclear antigen in sera from patients with infectious mononucleosis. J Infect Dis 1986; 154: 885.

57. Goldstein LC, Corey L, McDougall JK, et al.: Monoclonal antibodies to herpes simplex viruses: Use in antigenic typing and rapid diagnosis. J Infect Dis 1983; 147: 829.

58. Lipson SM, Salo RJ, Leonard GP: Evaluation of five monoclonal antibody–based kits or reagents for the identification and culture confirmation of herpes simplex virus. J Clin Microbiol 1991; 29: 466.

59. Seal LA, Toyama PS, Fleet KM, et al.: Comparison of standard culture methods, a shell vial assay, and a DNA probe for the detection of herpes simplex virus. J Clin Microbiol 1991; 29: 650.

60. Woods GL, Mills RD: Conventional tube cell culture compared with centrifugal inoculation of MRC-5 cells and staining with monoclonal antibodies for detection of herpes simplex virus in clinical specimens. J Clin Microbiol 1988; 26: 570.

61. MacDonald RL, Hughes BL, Aarnaes SL, et al.: Evaluation of a shell vial centrifugation method for the detection of herpes simplex virus. Diagn Microbiol Infect Dis 1988; 9: 51.

62. Gleaves CA, Wilson DJ, Wold AD, Smith TF: Detection and serotyping of herpes simplex virus in MRC-5 cells by use of centrifugation and monoclonal antibodies 16 h post-inoculation. J Clin Microbiol 1988; 21: 29.

63. Fayram SL, Aarnaes SL, Peterson EM, de la Maza LM: Evaluation of five cell types for the isolation of herpes simplex virus. Diagn Microbiol Infect Dis 1986; 5: 127.

64. Bell DM, Walsh EE, Hruska JF, et al.: Rapid detection of respiratory syncytial virus with a monoclonal antibody. J Clin Microbiol 1983; 17: 1099.

65. Grandien M, Pettersson C, Gardner PS, et al.: Rapid viral diagnosis of acute respiratory infections: Comparison of enzyme-linked immunosorbent assay and the immunofluorescence technique for detection of viral antigens in nasopharyngeal secretions. J Clin Microbiol 1985; 22: 757.

66. Waner JL, Whitehurst NJ, Jonas S, et al.: Isolation of viruses from specimens submitted for direct immunofluorescence test for respiratory syncytial virus. J Pediatr 1986; 108: 249.

67. Swenson PD, Kaplan MH: Rapid detection of respiratory syncytial virus in nasopharyngeal aspirates by a commercial enzyme immunoassay. J Clin Microbiol 1986; 23: 485.

68. Matthey S, Nicholson D, Ruhs S, et al.: Rapid detection of respiratory viruses by shell vial culture and direct staining by using pooled and individual monoclonal antibodies. J Clin Microbiol 1992; 30: 540.

69. Lee SHS, Boutilier JE, MacDonald MA, Forward KR: Enhanced detection of respiratory viruses using the shell vial technique and monoclonal antibodies. J Virol Methods 1992; 39: 39.

70. Hallander HO, Reizenstein E, Renemar B, et al.: Comparison of nasopharyngeal aspirates with swabs for culture of *Bordetella pertussis*. J Clin Microbiol 1993; 31: 50.

71. Friedman RL: Pertussis: The disease and new diagnostic methods. Clin Microbiol Rev 1988; 1: 365.

72. Grimprel E, Begue P, Anjak I, et al.: Comparison of polymerase chain reaction, culture, and western immunoblot serology for diagnosis of *Bordetella pertussis* infection. J Clin Microbiol 1993; 31: 2745.

73. He Q, Mertsola J, Soini H, et al.: Comparison of polymerase chain reaction with culture and enzyme immunoassay for diagnosis of pertussis. J Clin Microbiol 1993; 31: 642.

74. Chow AW: State-of-the-art clinical article: Life threatening infections of the head and neck. Clin Infect Dis 1992; 14: 991.

75. Doern GV: In vitro activity of loracarbef and effects of susceptibility test methods. Am J Med 1992; 92: 6A.

76. National Committee for Clinical Laboratory Standards: Methods for Dilution Antimicrobial Susceptibility Tests for Bacteria That Grow Aerobically, 3rd ed (approved standard, M7-A3). Philadelphia, PA: National Committee for Clinical Laboratory Standards, 1993.

77. National Committee for Clinical Laboratory Standards: Performance Standards for Antimicrobial Disk Susceptibility tests, 5th ed (approved standard, M2-A5). Philadelphia, PA: National Committee for Clinical Laboratory Standards, 1993.

78. Doern GV: Commentary: *S. pneumoniae* antibiotic resistance—an emerging problem. Infect Dis Clin Pract 1994; 3: 110.

79. Swenson JM, Hill BC, Thornsberry C: Screening pneumococci for penicillin resistance. J Clin Microbiol 1986; 24: 749.

80. Jorgensen JH, Ferraro MJ, McElmeel ML, et al.: Detection of penicillin and extended-spectrum cephalosporin resistance among *Streptococcus pneumoniae* clinical isolates by use of the E test. J Clin Microbiol 1994; 32: 159.

81. Macias EA, Mason Jr EO, Ocera HY, LaRocco MT: Comparison of E test with standard broth microdilution for determining antibiotic susceptibilities of penicillin-resistant strains of *Streptococcus pneumoniae*. J Clin Microbiol 1994; 32: 430.

82. Jacobs MR, Bajaksouzian S, Appelbaum PC, Bomstrom A: Evaluation of the E test for susceptibility testing of pneumococci. Diagn Microbiol Infect Dis 1992; 15: 473.

83. Jorgensen JH, Howell AW, Maher LA: Quantitative antimicrobial susceptibility testing of *Haemophilus influenzae* and *Streptococcus pneumoniae* by using the E test. J Clin Microbiol 1991; 29: 109.

84. Barry AL, Pfaller MA, Fuchs P, Packer RR: In vitro activities of 12 orally administered antimicrobial agents against four species of bacterial respiratory pathogens from U.S. medical centers in 1992 and 1993. Antimicrob Agents Chemo 1994; 38: 2419.

85. Doern GV: Resistance among problem respiratory pathogens in pediatrics. Pediatr Infect Dis J 1995; 14: 420.

86. O'Callaghan CH, Morris A, Kirby SM, Singler AH: Novel method for detecting penicillin resistance in *Staphylococcus aureus*. Antimicrob Agents Chemother 1972; 1: 283.

87. Montgomery K, Raymundo Jr L, Drew WL: Chromogenic cephalosporin spot test to detect beta-lactamase in clinically significant bacteria. J Clin Microbiol 1979; 9: 205.

88. Doern GV, Jones RN, Gerlach EH, et al.: Multicenter clinical laboratory evaluation of a β-lactamase disk assay employing a novel chromogenic cephalosporin, S1. J Clin Microbiol 1995; 33: 1665.

89. Markowitz SM: Isolation of an ampicillin-resistant, non-β-lactamase-producing strain of *Haemophilus influenzae*. Antimicrob Agents Chemother 1980; 17: 80.

90. Mendelman PM, Chaffin DO, Stull TL, et al.: Characterization of non-β-lactamase-mediated ampicillin resistance in *Haemophilus influenzae*. Antimicrob Agents Chemother 1984; 26: 235.

91. Centers for Disease Control: 1993 Sexually transmitted diseases treatment guidelines. MMWR 1993; 42: 1.

92. Knapp JS, Ohye R, Neal SW, et al.: Emerging in vitro resistance to quinolones in penicillinase-producing *Neisseria gonorrhoeae* strains in Hawaii. Antimicrob Agents Chemother 1994; 38: 2200.

93. Knapp JS, Washington JA, Doyle LJ, et al.: Persistence of *Neisseria gonorrhoeae* strains with decreased susceptibilities to ciprofloxacin and ofloxacin in Cleveland, Ohio, from 1992 through 1993. Antimicrob Agents Chemother 1994; 38: 2194.

94. Brown BA, Wallace Jr RJ, Flanagan CW, et al.: Tetracycline and erythromycin resistance among clinical isolates of *Branhamella catarrhalis*. Antimicrob Agents Chemother 1989; 33: 1631.

Richard Quintiliani
David P. Nicolau
Charles H. Nightingale

CHAPTER FIVE

Pharmacokinetic and Pharmacodynamic Principles in Antibiotic Usage

▼

The ultimate goal of antimicrobial therapy is to eradicate microbial pathogens at the specific sites of infection. To accomplish this goal, the clinician must become familiar with pharmacokinetics and pharmacodynamic concepts because an understanding of this information establishes the basis for appropriate dosing strategies to maximize clinical efficacy and minimize toxicity. In this chapter, we review these principles, showing how an appreciation of these concepts results in the dosing of antibiotics in a scientifically sound fashion rather than from style or habit.

PHARMACOKINETICS AND PHARMACODYNAMIC CONSIDERATIONS

The study of the movement of a drug from its administration site to the place of its pharmacologic activity and its elimination from the body is called pharmacokinetics. Factors affecting the movement (kinetics) and fate of a drug in the body are (1) release from the dosage form, (2) absorption from the site of administration into the blood stream, (3) distribution to various parts of the body, including the site of action, and (4) rate of elimination from the body via metabolism or excretion of the unchanged drug.

Pharmacodynamics correlates the concentration of the drug with its pharmacologic or clinical effect. For an antibiotic, the correlation refers to the ability of the drug to kill or inhibit the growth of microorganisms. Antibiotics elicit their activity against bacteria by binding to a specific protein or structure in the organism. For example, beta-lactams, fluoroquinolones, and aminoglycosides bind to penicillin-binding proteins, DNA gyrase, and the ribosome, respectively. It is necessary that the antibiotic occupy a sufficient number of binding sites for a sufficient length of time, so that the organism can no longer carry out essential biochemical reactions and, thereby, is inhibited or dies. This process is analogous to what is commonly termed the microbiologic activity of the antibiotic.

Although we cannot yet measure drug concentration directly at the site of attachment to the bacterium, we can measure drug levels in serum and other tissues as a function of time, thus using these surrogate concentrations to determine the minimum inhibitory concentration (MIC) or the minimum bactericidal concentration (MBC) of the antibiotic for microorganisms. Drug concentration in the blood (plasma, serum) has been correlated to in vivo bacterial eradication. Most bacteria reside on the outside membranes of the cell, thus exposed to interstitial fluids. Drug concentrations in interstitial fluid drive the antibiotic into the bacterium and ultimately to the binding site. Interstitial fluid drug concentrations are proportional to and in rapid equilibrium with blood, and therefore, antibiotic blood concentrations are correlated with bacterial eradication.

From a pharmacokinetics perspective, the product of concentration and time is defined as the area under the drug concentration–time curve (AUC). It follows that bacterial killing is a function of the drug's AUC. If this is indexed to microbiologic activity (e.g., MIC), one can develop a pharmacodynamic parameter such as AUC/MIC, which can be useful in correlating pharmacokinetics to bacterial killing. It should be emphasized that AUC is the product of concentration and time, and it is this product that affects bacterial killing. Fortunately, under certain conditions, one of the terms of the product (either concentration or time) makes a small or negligible contribution to the killing process and can therefore be ignored. The pharmacodynamic parameter can then be simplified to peak concentration/MIC or time the serum concentration is above the MIC. How this simplification occurs is based on whether the antibiotic eradicates bacteria via a concentration-dependent or -independent manner, which is discussed later in this chapter. The clinician should be aware that basing drug selection solely on the microbiologic activity (the MIC or MBC) or pharmacokinetics can lead to incorrect conclusions and inappropriate antimicrobial selection. Rather, the clinician should employ a pharmacodynamic approach by integrating the drug's microbiologic and pharmacokinetic properties.

VOLUME OF DISTRIBUTION

The experimentally observed changes in drug concentration in the body as a function of time can be empirically described by mathematical equations. It is possible to develop hypothetic models based on drugs moving between compartments (representing the body) that are consistent with the empirically obtained mathematical equations. Other techniques, such as statistical moment theory, use noncompartmental analysis of drug level versus time data.

One of the simplest compartmental models in pharmacokinetics describes the body as a single homogeneous compartment into which the drug appears to dissolve.[1] The volume of this compartment, called the apparent volume of distribution (V_D), rarely relates to physiologic volumes but serves as a proportionality constant between the dose of drug administered and the observed plasma or serum concentration. The equation that describes initial drug concentration just after an intravenous bolus dose is as follows:

$$\text{Conc(t0)} = \frac{\text{Dose}}{V_D} \qquad \text{(Equation 1)}$$

where

Conc(t0) = drug concentration at time = 0 (just after intravenous administration of bolus dose)

Dose = dose of drug administered

V_D = apparent volume of distribution.

This concept can be more easily understood using a hydrodynamic or "bathtub" model. In the bathtub model, we add a known quantity or amount of dye to a bathtub of known volume. The concentration of dye in the bathtub can be described by Equation 1.

Clearly, a large bathtub yields a smaller concentration than a smaller bathtub if the same quantity of dye is placed in each one. Drugs that distribute widely throughout the body tend to have large volumes of distribution and low serum concentrations. Drugs that tend to stay only in the blood volume (for example, those exhibiting a high level of serum protein binding) have small volumes of distribution and high serum concentrations.

Drugs that follow one-compartment kinetics exhibit log linear plasma concentrations as a function of time (Fig. 5–1). Most drugs do not exhibit log linear plasma concentration (C_p) versus time plots, and therefore, their movement in the body cannot be described by a simple one-compartment

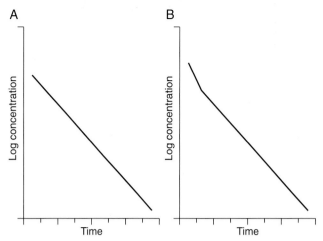

Figure 5–2. Concentration versus time plots for, *(A)*, one-compartment and, *(B)*, two-compartment model.

model. Models having two or more compartments are necessary to describe such behavior. These models feature a rapidly perfused compartment, usually composed of the blood volume and those tissues or organs receiving high blood flow, termed the central compartment V_c. In addition, one or more compartments, termed peripheral or tissue compartments (V_t), are needed to describe the movement of drug into less well perfused tissues or spaces. The time required to distribute to these tissue compartments (referred to as the distribution or alpha phase) is usually slower than that to the central compartment. After administration of a drug, the observed concentration is initially higher because the drug is only in the central compartment. As distribution to the tissue compartments occurs, drug concentration decreases because the same quantity of drug is now in a larger volume ($V_D = V_c + V_t$).

The value of V_D for the clinician is that this term roughly describes whether or not the antibiotic will be widely distributed in tissue. Drugs that reside in the interstitial fluid generally have $V_{D,SS}$ (volume of distribution at steady state) of less than 20 L, whereas agents with widespread tissue distribution, like the fluoroquinolones, have $V_{D,SS}$ greater than 100 L.

The distribution of drug from the central compartment to the tissue compartment results in the nonlinear curves in Figure 5–2. In the first portion of the graph (the distribution or beta phase), drug concentrations rapidly decline owing to elimination of the drug and distribution in tissue compartments. In the second or elimination phase, drug movement into the tissue reaches an equilibrium, and the decline in blood concentrations is due to removal from the central compartment.

Most drugs display a relationship between serum concentration and pharmacologic effect. For some drugs, such as quinidine and lidocaine, the pharmacologic receptor site appears to be located in the central compartment, V_c, and the rate of drug administration is important. If serum levels exceed therapeutic concentrations during the initial distribution phase before the drug has equilibrated with peripheral compartments, toxicity may occur. For many other drugs, the receptor site for pharmacologic activity appears to lie in

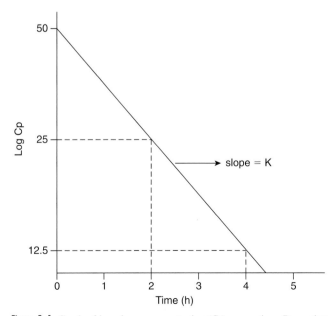

Figure 5–1. Graph of log plasma concentration (C_p) versus time. Drugs that display one-compartment model kinetics will exhibit a linear graph of log C_p versus time.

the tissue compartment. Thus, initially high serum concentrations resulting from rapid administration of drug are not related to pharmacologic effect or toxicity. This concept becomes important when monitoring clinical drug levels. For drugs whose pharmacologic effect is related to tissue compartment concentrations, distribution-phase drug samples are of limited value in predicting either pharmacologic effect or toxicity. Distribution to the peripheral compartment must be complete (that is, the initial and tissue compartments are in equilibrium) before serum samples are drawn.

CLEARANCE

Drug concentrations decline in the body as a result of elimination (usually from the kidneys or liver). The term clearance (Cl) is used to describe the intrinsic ability of the body to remove drug. Clearance represents a theoretic volume of blood or plasma that is cleared or completely removed of drug within a period of time. It is expressed as units of volume per time. The clearance volume for a drug is generally constant during a dosing interval.

The amount of drug removed per unit of time can be determined if we recall (Equation 1) that concentration and volume are related. Concentration = amount ÷ volume; thus, amount = concentration × volume. Dividing by time gives the following:

$$\frac{amount}{time} = \frac{concentration \times volume}{time}$$

Because clearance = volume ÷ time, the amount of drug removed per unit of time is equal to concentration × clearance.

Because the clearance of a drug remains constant after distribution is complete, but the serum concentration declines as drug is removed from the body, the amount of drug removed per unit of time is highest when the serum concentration is highest (just after administration of a dose).

HALF-LIFE

In the one-compartment model, distribution is assumed to be instantaneous, and elimination from the body follows first-order (log linear) decline. A semilogarithmic plot of drug concentration versus time yields a linear graph. During the elimination phase, the slope of the log C_p versus time plot is referred to as the elimination rate constant (k), which has units of time -1 (see Fig. 5–1).

This type of plot can also be used to determine the half-life ($t_{1/2}$) of a drug, which refers to the amount of time required for the drug concentration to decrease by 50%. The half-life is related to k by the following equation:

$$t_{1/2} = \frac{0.693}{k} \qquad \text{(Equation 2)}$$

The equation describing these kinetics after a bolus dose is as follows:

$$C_p(t_2) = C_p(t_1)e^{-K(t_2 - t_1)} \qquad \text{(Equation 3)}$$

e = exponential
t_1 = time of inital concentration
t_2 = time of 2nd concentration

In Figure 5–2, the half-life of 2 hours is the same for drug concentrations from 50 to 25 and from 25 to 12.5. The percentage of the original dose remaining in the body declines by 50% with every half-life (Table 5–1).

Because the concentration at any time follows a log linear decline, we can determine the concentration at any time t_2 if we know the time elapsed between t_1 and t_2. For example, if a drug follows a one-compartment model and has a V_D of 15 L and a $t_{1/2}$ of 2 hours, its initial concentration is 100 mg/L after a 1500 mg dose:

$$\text{Concentration} = \frac{dose}{volume} = \frac{1500 \text{ mg}}{15 \text{ L}} = 100 \text{ mg/L}$$

To determine the concentration of drug 6 hours after administration, we can substitute the drug parameters into Equation 2:

$$K = \frac{0.693}{t^{1/2}} = \frac{0.693}{2 \text{ hr}} = 0.3465 \text{ hrs} - 1$$

Then, using Equation 3, the concentration at 6 hours is:

$$C_{pt} = 6 \text{ hr} = C_{p6h} = Cp(t_1)e^{-K(t_2 - t_1)}$$
$$= 100^{e -0.3465(6)}$$
$$= 100^{e -2.076}$$
$$= 12.5 \text{ mg/L}$$

STEADY STATE

When a drug is administered as a constant intravenous infusion, two processes occur simultaneously: distribution and elimination. If the rate of administration exceeds the rate of elimination, drug accumulates in the body. As the serum concentration increases, the amount excreted per unit of time increases. When the rate of drug administration is equal to the rate of drug elimination, the serum concentration remains a constant value, called the steady-state concentration C_{pss} (Fig. 5–3).

If we know the half-life of a drug, we can predict the time required to reach steady state. Fifty percent of the final steady-state concentration accumulates during each half-life, so that after five half-lives, approximately 97% of the final

Table 5–1. PERCENTAGE OF THE ORIGINAL DOSE REMAINING IN THE BODY

Number of Half-Lives	Percentage of Original Concentration
0	100.0
1	50.0
2	25.0
3	12.5
4	6.25
5	3.125

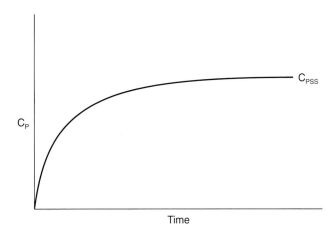

Figure 5–3. Drug administration by constant intravenous infusion. When the rate of drug administration is equal to the rate of drug elimination, the serum concentration remains a constant value (C_{PSS}).

steady-state concentration has been achieved (Table 5–2). For example, an antibiotic with a half-life of 2 hours (e.g., ceftazidime) would take about 10 hours to attain steady state, whereas an agent with an 8-hour half-life, like ceftriaxone, requires 40 hours or almost 2 days of dosing to achieve steady state. Note that this mirrors the effect shown for elimination in Table 5–1.

Clearly, the longer the half-life of a drug, the longer it will take to achieve a steady-state concentration. This can be particularly important for patients receiving drugs that have long half-lives and narrow therapeutic ranges of serum concentrations. In these patients, a loading dose is used in order to rapidly achieve therapeutic drug concentrations. The loading dose is determined by using Equation 1, as follows:

$$\text{Loading dose} = \frac{\text{desired serum concentration}}{V_c + V_t} \quad \text{(Equation 4)}$$

Drugs that are administered on an intermittent basis (for example, every 4 hours or every 6 hours) accumulate in the body and achieve steady-state concentrations similar to those of drugs administered by constant infusion. However, immediately after administration of a dose, the serum level is at maximal or peak concentration. The serum level declines in log linear fashion until just prior to the next dose, when it reaches its minimal or trough concentration. The peak and trough concentrations accumulate over time (Fig. 5–4) until, at steady state, all the peak concentrations are the same and all the trough concentrations are the same. The same princi-

Table 5–2. RELATIONSHIP BETWEEN NUMBER OF HALF-LIVES AND PERCENTAGE OF STEADY-STATE CONCENTRATION (C_{PSS})

Number of Half-Lives	Percentage of C_{PSS} Achieved
0	0.0
1	50.0
2	75.0
3	87.5
4	93.75
5	96.875

ples apply in this case as were described for drug administration by continuous infusion.

PROTEIN BINDING

The drug concentration reported by the laboratory represents the total concentration of agents that are bound to plasma proteins (e.g., albumin, α1-acid glycoprotein, lipoprotein) and unbound or free. Because only the unbound drug is in equilibrium with its target site(s) on the organism, the unbound drug is entirely responsible for the antibiotic's anti-infective action. Two major pharmacokinetics observations are dependent on protein binding: the ability of the drug to distribute in sufficient concentrations into body fluids and tissue, and the rapidity of elimination of the drug from the body.

Protein binding for most drugs has been shown to be a reversible phenomenon. A generally accepted model used to describe protein (P) binding of drug (D) is as follows:

$$D + P = D - P \quad \text{(Equation 5)}$$

Most antibiotics bind to serum albumin, and the strength of this attraction is described by the ratio of unbound drug, that is:

$$K_a = \frac{(D)(P)}{(D) - (P)} \quad \text{(Equation 6)}$$

where K_a is the dissociation constant for binding.

In general, drugs with a higher level of protein binding penetrate to a lesser extent into the interstitial spaces, produce higher peak serum concentrations, and exhibit a slower rate of elimination from the body, especially if the major elimination mode is by glomerulofiltration. There is no relationship between renal tubular secretion and protein binding. If a drug is highly albumin-bound, little of it distributes into tissue, and the volume it appears to dissolve into is small. If a drug is not greatly bound to albumin, it can distribute widely and rapidly into tissue, and the volume it appears to dissolve into is large. Thus, an inverse relationship exists between protein binding and volume of distribution. Protein

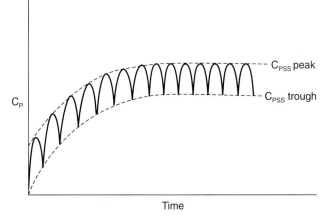

Figure 5–4. Administration of a drug by intermittent infusion results in peak and trough serum concentrations that accumulate over time. At steady state, serum concentration fluctuates between steady-state trough concentration.

binding usually does not play a clinically significant role unless it exceeds 90%, which can result in unusually low concentration of free or microbiologically active drug. High protein binding is not always a deleterious effect, for it can prolong the time that the serum concentration of an antibiotic remains above its MIC for an organism.

POSTANTIBIOTIC EFFECT

The postantibiotic effect (PAE) refers to the persistent suppression of bacterial growth after exposure of a microorganism to an antibiotic. The term should not be confused with the effects of bacterial suppression due to antibiotic subinhibitory concentrations. Antibiotics that kill bacteria either by interfering with protein synthesis (e.g., aminoglycosides) or through DNA replication (e.g., fluoroquinolones) usually demonstrate prolonged PAEs (e.g., 1 to 5 hours) against gram-negative bacteria, whereas agents that kill bacteria by interfering with cell-wall synthesis (e.g., beta-lactam antibiotics, glycopeptides) have little, if any, PAE against these types of organisms. Against gram-positive bacteria, both types of antibiotics typically exhibit short PAEs of about 1 hour. The clinical relevance of the PAE is related to its use in establishing dosage regimens that are directed against a specific pathogen. Although the clinical application of the PAE awaits more extensive investigation, appropriately designed dosage regimens that could minimize drug administration are desirable to reduce both toxicity and costs.

CONCENTRATION-DEPENDENT VERSUS CONCENTRATION-INDEPENDENT KILLING

Ever since intravenous antibiotics became available, there has been considerable controversy regarding the most appropriate way to administer them to maximize the killing of bacteria and yet to minimize toxicity. In only the past several years has adequate scientific information emerged from animal models of infection and toxicity, in vitro pharmacodynamic studies, and human clinical trials to enable us to establish the best mode of drug administration to achieve these goals.

Aminoglycosides (e.g., tobramycin, gentamicin) and fluoroquinolones (e.g., ciprofloxacin, ofloxacin) eliminate bacteria most rapidly when their concentrations are appreciably above their MICs for organisms; hence, their type of killing is referred to as concentration-dependent or dose-dependent killing. For these drugs, the rate of bacterial eradication rises with increasing concentration. If the concentration is high enough, most bacteria die within a short time. In these conditions, the effect of the drug exposure time is minimal and can be ignored. The pharmacodynamic parameter of AUC/MIC or $C_p \times t$/MIC simplifies to C_p/MIC. It has been shown that aminoglycosides eradicate organisms best when they achieve concentrations that are approximately 10 to 12 times above the MICs (i.e., C_p/MIC $\geq$ 10).[2, 3] In animal models of infection (including neutropenic animals), many more animals survive a potentially lethal challenge of bacteria if given the aminoglycosides as a single daily dose than when given the same amount of drug on an every-8-hour

basis. Moreover, pathologic examination of tissue, like the organ of Corti or the renal tubular cells, has shown less rather than more damage. The ototoxicity or nephrotoxicity of aminoglycosides correlates with tissue accumulation and not with peak concentration in serum. Because of these observations, there is a growing interest in once-daily aminoglycoside dosage (5–7 mg/kg) so that one can attain these preferable peak-to-MIC ratios (Fig. 5–5). Further advantages of once-daily aminoglycoside dosage include reduction in expensive ancillary service time. We have reported on our experience in approximately 2200 adult patients treated with once-daily aminoglycoside and observed excellent clinical outcomes with the lowest incidence (1.2%) of nephrotoxicity reported in our hospital, compared with historical data in which the incidence was 3%–5%.[4]

Although fluoroquinolones also exhibit concentration-dependent killing,[5] excessively high concentrations of these agents in serum can, unfortunately, be associated with seizures and other potentially serious central nervous system adverse reactions. Because the doses of quinolones cannot be safely increased, the only way to obtain C_p/MIC ratios of 10 or more is by targeting these drugs against very sensitive organisms (e.g., Enterobacteriaceae). When C_p/MIC ratios do not reach 10, then time of exposure cannot be ignored, and bacterial eradication is again a function of concentration and time of exposure, i.e., AUC/MIC. An indexing of the AUC with the MIC has been used to produce the pharmacodynamic relationship of AUC/MIC, or the so-called area under the inhibitory concentration (AUIC), to predict clinical outcomes with the fluoroquinolones (Fig. 5–6). Although this issue remains quite controversial, it is commonly believed that the AUC/MIC ratio should be equal to or greater than 125 to obtain good clinical responses.[6] Only one study has made such a correlation; the work was done in hospital-

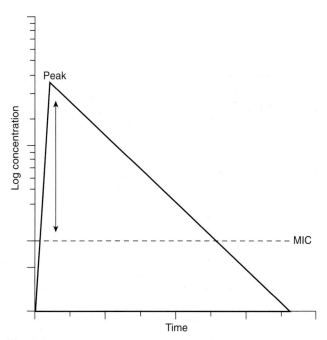

Figure 5–5. Integration of peak concentration with the minimum inhibitory concentration (MIC) to produce the pharmacodynamic relationship of peak/MIC.

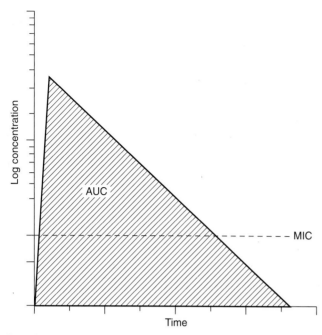

Figure 5–6. Integration of area under the concentration-time curve (AUC) with the minimum inhibitory concentration (MIC) to produce the pharmacodynamic relationship of AUC/MIC or AUIC.

ized patients mainly infected with nosocomial pathogens. A mismatch with this theory that the AUC/MIC must exceed 125 for good clinical response can be noted for some quinolones, like ofloxacin and levofloxacin. Clinical and microbiologic studies have demonstrated excellent results in infections when *Streptococcus pneumoniae* is a major pathogen, yet the AUC/MIC ratios for ofloxacin and levofloxacin are approximately 40 and 60, respectively. Obviously, the criterion that AUC/MIC must equal or exceed 125 is not universally applicable, and further studies are needed to clarify this issue.

In summary, for concentration-dependent killing antibiotics, the best, simplest pharmacokinetics parameter to use is C_p/MIC when this ratio is approximately 10. When it is not, such as in the use of quinolones against moderately susceptible organisms, the product of concentration and time (AUC) needs to be used for meaningful comparisons between drugs as well as designing dosing/treatment strategies.

Beta-lactam antibiotics (e.g., penicillins, cephalosporins, carbapenems, monobactams) and the glycopeptides (e.g., vancomycin) show little concentration-dependent bactericidal activity. Apparently, once the concentration exceeds a critical value, which appears to be about two to four times above the MIC for an organism, killing proceeds at a zero-order rate,[7] and increasing the drug concentration does not change the microbial death rate. In these conditions, little correlation with peak concentration in serum and its correlated parameter, AUC, is expected. In these conditions, the $C \times t$/MIC parameter reduces to time period of drug concentration above the MIC (T >MIC). Because the contribution of the concentration to the killing process is constant and, therefore, not a variable in the process, time of exposure becomes the major factor affecting bacterial killing. In essence, the contribution of concentration can be ignored. The

pharmacodynamic parameter AUC/MIC simplifies to time and MIC. In brief, beta-lactam and glycopeptide antibiotics exhibit time-dependent or concentration-independent killing, and hence, duration of the concentration of a drug above its MIC or MBC for the suspected or proven pathogens should be the best predictor of clinical outcome (Fig. 5–7). For beta-lactam antibiotics, the time above the MIC/MBC for the drug in serum is generally proportional to that in the fluid bathing the organism (i.e., the interstitial fluid, or wound fluid in tissues) because the antibiotics distribute to extracellular water, which is in dynamic equilibrium with serum. There are five major ways to prolong the duration of a beta-lactam drug's concentration above its MIC for bacteria in any dosing interval: (1) use another drug (e.g., probenecid) that interferes with its elimination, (2) dose frequently, (3) increase the dose of the antibiotic, (4) replace the drug with another therapeutically equivalent antibiotic that has a longer serum half-life, and (5) administer the drug by constant intravenous infusion.

Although probenecid blocks the tubular secretion of most beta-lactam antibiotics, it may also do the same for nonantibiotics, resulting in unexpected adverse reactions. Moreover, if a patient develops a hypersensitivity reaction, it would be difficult, if not impossible, to determine whether the reaction was caused by the antibiotic or by probenecid. Dosing frequently or increasing the dose is usually unacceptable in today's medical era of fiscal restraints, owing to excessive cost from high acquisition drug costs and greater burdens on ancillary service time. Increasing the dose of an antibiotic is generally inefficient, yielding an increase in time above MIC of only one half-life. For example, Figure 5–8 illustrates the concentration-time profile for ceftazidime after a 1-g or 2-g dose. The 1-g dose yields a time above MIC of 6.6 hours. Doubling the dose increases the time above MIC to 8.6

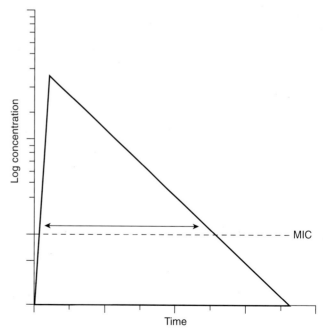

Figure 5–7. Integration of the time the concentration remains above the minimum inhibitory concentration (MIC) to produce the pharmacodynamic relationship of time > MIC.

INTRAVENOUS CEFTAZIDIME

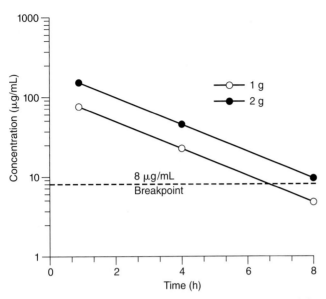

Figure 5–8. Simulated concentration versus time profile of 1- and 2-g intravenous bolus doses of ceftazidime. Doubling the dose increases the time > minimum inhibitory concentration by 30%, which may not be clinically useful and is more expensive.

hours, a 30% increase in the peak serum concentrations (not needed for efficacy) with a 100% increase in cost. Using an antibiotic with a longer half-life is sensible as long as it is not appreciably more expensive than the shorter-acting agent. By using constant infusion, one can optimize the time the antibiotic levels remain above the MIC (Fig. 5–9) by using the lowest daily dose and the least amount of nursing and pharmacy time. Constant infusion is merely another method of once daily dosing.

For antibiotics with concentration-independent killing, the often-mentioned advice in package inserts that antibiotics should be given in larger and more frequent doses for infections considered severe than for those deemed mild makes little, if any, pharmacodynamic or pharmacoeconomic sense, unless the site of infection exists in a body area (e.g., cerebrospinal fluid, vitreous humor of the eye) where the higher serum levels may improve drug penetration. The high serum levels of beta-lactam antibiotics do not drive more drugs intracelluarly or into tissue because these drugs exhibit insignificant intracellular penetration. The higher serum levels merely result in similar levels in the interstitial fluid that surrounds the cells, and the same pharmacodynamic concepts that apply to serum levels apply to interstitial concentrations. Although there typically exists a slight lag period before interstitial and serum levels attain equilibrium, there is a close parallel with beta-lactam antibiotics between their concentrations in the serum and the interstitial fluid compartments.[8]

How long the concentration of a beta-lactam antibiotic in serum should remain above its MICs for pathogens is unknown. It is likely that this time may vary with different pathogens, the site of infection, and the immunocompetence of the host. Certainly, levels above the MIC for the entire dosing interval should ensure the best clinical results. At the

moment, it appears from animal models of infection and clinical trials that beta-lactam antibiotic levels should remain above the MIC for a pathogen for at least 50% of the dosing interval in order to ensure the highest level of bacterial eradication.

POTENTIAL PROBLEMS ENCOUNTERED IN THERAPEUTIC DRUG LEVEL MONITORING

In the clinical setting, predicted and measured drug levels do not always coincide. Some of the more common and often predictable reasons are presented here. For most drugs, pharmacokinetics variables such as volume, clearance, and half-life are well described in the literature, but they are often based on population data from normal volunteer studies. Therefore, it is important to realize that patient-specific factors may cause a patient's pharmacokinetics parameters to be different from those in normal volunteers. For example, the volume of distribution of water-soluble drugs, such as aminoglycosides, is affected by alterations in total body water. Patients with ascites or those receiving peritoneal dialysis may require adjustments in V_D for the extra fluid volume present.

Drugs such as theophylline that are metabolized by the liver may require adjustments in clearance in patients with poor liver function (for example, those with cirrhosis), who are unable to metabolize drugs as quickly. Conversely, smokers have an increased metabolism of theophylline.

Similarly, drugs that are eliminated renally are affected by changes in renal function. Therapeutic drug-level monitoring is especially important in this patient population. Drug-drug interactions can alter one or more pharmacokinetics variables concurrently. For example, quinidine alters both the volume of distribution and the clearance of digoxin.

In theoretic pharmacokinetics, patients always receive the correct dose at the appropriate time of administration. In the clinical setting, this is not necessarily true. The administered

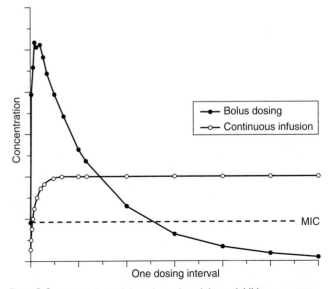

Figure 5–9. Optimization of time above the minimum inhibitory concentration (MIC) with continuous infusion.

dose may not be exact or may even be missed entirely. Dosing intervals may vary because of busy nursing schedules.

Even if the patient receives the correct dose at the correct time, sampling errors can occur. Drug levels drawn during the distribution phase are of little value except for drugs whose toxicity is related to high serum concentrations in the central compartment (V_c). For most other drugs, distribution-phase levels are not useful for predictions of clearance, half-life, or toxicity. Therefore, it is useful to know the duration of the distribution phase for each drug and to ensure that drug level samples are drawn after completion of this phase.

Drug levels may be interpreted incorrectly if the exact time of drug administration and serum collection are not properly recorded. Often, a dose is increased because a peak concentration appears to be subtherapeutic, when in fact the sample was merely drawn late (and is therefore not the peak concentration but a lower value). Similarly, a trough concentration may appear elevated if the sample was drawn too early. If the correct sampling times are recorded, the true peak or trough concentration can be determined by using Equation 3.

CONCLUSIONS

The variables that influence antimicrobial activity form a multifactorial system complex. Components such as microorganism susceptibility, host defenses, and toxicity factors affect the therapeutic outcome in the treatment of infections. The eradication of the infection, however, occurs only if the antibiotic reaches the site of the pathogen in adequate concentrations for an appropriate length of time. To predict whether an antibiotic will achieve this goal, one must be familiar with pharmacokinetics and pharmacodynamic principles.

References

1. Gibaldi M, Perrier D: Noncompartmental analysis based on statistical moment theory. In: Swarbrick J (ed): Pharmacokinetics, 2nd ed. New York: Marcel Dekker, 1982, pp 409–417.
2. Moore RD, Lietman PS, Smith CR: Clinical response to aminoglycoside therapy: Importance of the ratio of peak concentration to minimal inhibitory concentration. J Infect Dis 1987; 155: 93–99.
3. Gilbert DN: Once-daily aminoglycoside therapy. Antimicrob Agents Chemother 1991; 35: 399–405.
4. Nicolau PD, Freeman CD, Belliveau PP, et al.: Experience with a once-daily aminoglycoside program administered to 2,184 adult patients. Antimicrob Agents Chemother 1995; 39: 650–655.
5. Dudley MN: Pharmacodynamics and pharmacokinetics of antibiotics with special reference to the fluoroquinolones. Am J Med 1991; 91(suppl 6a): 455–505.
6. Forest A, Nix DE, Ballow CH, et al.: Pharmacodynamics of intravenous ciprofloxacin in seriously ill patients. Antimicrob Agents Chemother 1993; 37: 1073–1081.
7. Nishida M, Murakawa T, Kaminura T, et al.: Bactericidal activity of cephalosporins in an in-vitro model simulating serum levels. Antimicrob Agents Chemother 1978; 14: 6–12.
8. Nicolau DP, Quintiliani R: Choosing among the new cephalosporin antibiotics. Pharmacoeconomics 1994; 5(suppl 2): 34–39.

SECTION II

ANTIMICROBIAL AGENTS

CHAPTER SIX

Beta-Lactam Antibiotics

William A. Petri, Jr.
Gerald L. Mandell

PART 1

Penicillins and Cephalosporins

▼

The beta-lactam antibiotics are important natural and synthetic compounds that exert their antibacterial effect via inhibition of bacterial peptidoglycan cell-wall synthesis (Fig. 6–1). The targets of the penicillins, known as penicillin-binding proteins (PBPs), include carboxypeptidases, endopeptidases, and transpeptidases and vary widely among bacterial species. Penicillins (Fig. 6–2) are derived from the *Penicillium* fungus. Important classes of penicillins are the natural penicillins G and V, which are highly active against susceptible gram-positive cocci; penicillinase-resistant penicillins, such as dicloxacillin and nafcillin, which are active against penicillinase-producing *Staphylococcus aureus*; the aminopenicillins amoxicillin and ampicillin, with an improved gram-negative spectrum; and finally, the extended-spectrum penicillins, including ticarcillin and piperacillin,

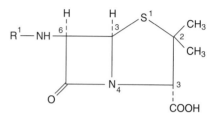

Figure 6–2. Basic penicillin structure. Substitutions at the R^1 site create the extended-spectrum penicillins.

with activity against *Pseudomonas aeruginosa*. Beta-lactamase inhibitors such as clavulanate are used to extend the spectrum of penicillins to include some beta-lactamase–producing organisms.

Cephalosporins are derivatives of cephalosporin C produced by the fungus *Cephalosporium acremonium* (Fig. 6–3). The cephalosporin antibiotics are classified by generation, with the 1st-generation agents having excellent gram-positive and modest gram-negative activity; the 2nd-generation agents having slightly improved gram-negative activity and some having anti–*Bacteroides fragilis* activity; the 3rd-generation agents with less activity against gram-positive organisms but much more activity against the Enterobacteriaceae, and a subset active against *P. aeruginosa*; and the 4th generation, which has a 3rd-generation spectrum of activity but increased stability to hydrolysis by beta-lactamases.

MECHANISMS OF BACTERIAL RESISTANCE TO BETA-LACTAM ANTIBIOTICS

Major mechanisms of resistance to beta-lactam antibiotics include changes in drug permeability in the bacterial outer

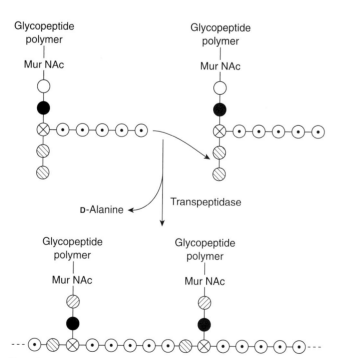

Figure 6–1. Transpeptidation reaction in bacterial cell-wall synthesis inhibited by the beta-lactams. (From Mandell GL, Petri WA: Antimicrobial agents: Penicillins, cephalosporins and other beta-lactam antibiotics. In Hardman JG, Limbird LE [eds]: Goodman and Gilman's The Pharmacologic Basis of Therapeutics. New York: McGraw-Hill, 1996.)

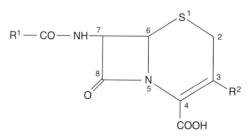

Figure 6–3. Basic cephalosporin structure. Substitutions at positions 1, R^1, R^2, and C^7 create the therapeutically important classes.

membrane (for example, ampicillin resistance of *Pseudomonas* species), changes in PBPs to prevent drug binding (for example, penicillin-resistant pneumococci), and production of beta-lactamases to degrade the drug (for example, penicillin-resistant *S. aureus*).

Destruction of the beta-lactam antibiotics by beta-lactamases is a common mechanism of resistance (Fig. 6–4). There are a wide variety of beta-lactamases with different substrate specificities produced by microorganisms, with most bacteria producing only a single enzyme. Beta-lactamases can be plasmid or chromosomally encoded and of narrow (penicillinases or cephalosporinases) or extended spectrum in their substrate specificity. The beta-lactamases of gram-positive bacteria such as staphylococci and *Enterococcus faecalis* are secreted extracellularly, and most are penicillinases. The gram-positive penicillinases are for the most part plasmid encoded, facilitating transfer to other bacteria. The beta-lactamases of gram-negative bacteria are located in the periplasmic space between the outer and inner membranes.

Treatment of infections caused by aerobic gram-negative bacteria with 3rd-generation cephalosporins is being hampered by extended-spectrum beta-lactamases (ESBLs) that can be either plasmid-encoded or induced (type I) chromosomal enzymes. Treatment of infections due to the Enterobacteriaceae (especially *Enterobacter* species, *Citrobacter freundii*, *Morganella*, *Serratia*, *Providencia*, and *P. aeruginosa*) with a 2nd- or 3rd-generation cephalosporin and/or imipenem may result in the induction of type I beta-lactamases and resistance to all 3rd-generation cephalosporins. For example, such induction occurred in 19% of patients receiving 3rd-generation cephalosporins for *Enterobacter* bacteremia. Induction may also be seen with use of beta-lactamase inhibitors such as clavulanate, tazobactam, and sulbactam, which have no inhibitory activity against the chromosomal type I beta-lactamases. The soon-to-be-released 4th-generation cephalosporins, such as cefepime, are poor inducers of type I beta-lactamases and are also less susceptible to hydrolysis by type I beta-lactamases. Imipenem is also less susceptible to hydrolysis by ESBLs, although metallo beta-lactamases that hydrolyze carbapenems are a growing threat. Induction of chromosomal ESBLs or selection for plasmid-encoded ESBLs should be suspected in patients with aerobic gram-negative rod infections that either fail to respond to or relapse with 3rd-generation cephalosporin therapy. Pending results of cultures, consideration should be given to replacing the cephalosporin with another class of agent predicted to be active, such as imipenem or a fluoroquinolone.

The development of high-molecular-weight (HMW) PBPs that have decreased affinity for the antibiotic is the explanation for the emergence of beta-lactam resistance in the pneumococcus. Because the beta-lactam antibiotics inhibit many different PBPs in a single bacterium, change in the affinity for beta-lactam antibiotics of several PBPs must occur for the organism to be resistant. Altered PBPs with decreased affinity for beta-lactam antibiotics are acquired by homologous recombination between PBP genes of different bacterial species. Four of the five HMW PBPs of the most highly penicillin-resistant *Strepococcus pneumoniae* isolates have decreased affinity for beta-lactam antibiotics as a result of interspecies homologous recombination events (Fig. 6–5). In contrast, pneumococcal isolates with high-level resistance to 3rd-generation cephalosporins contain alterations of only two of the five HMW PBPs, as the other PBPs have inherently low affinity for the 3rd-generation cephalosporins. Penicillin resistance in *Streptococcus sanguis* apparently emerged as a result of replacement of its PBPs with resistant PBPs from *S. pneumoniae*. Methicillin-resistant *S. aureus* is resistant via acquisition of an additional HMW PBP (via a

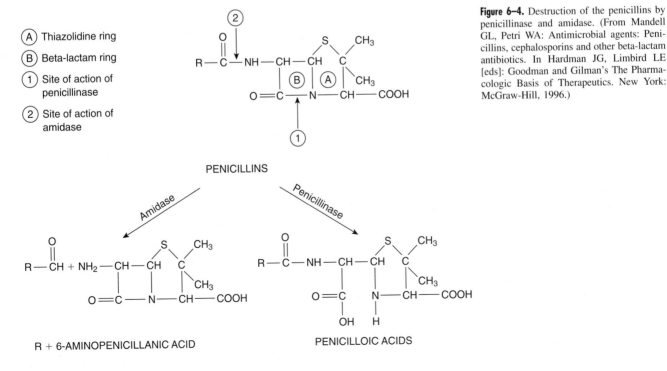

(A) Thiazolidine ring
(B) Beta-lactam ring
(1) Site of action of penicillinase
(2) Site of action of amidase

PENICILLINS

Amidase *Penicillinase*

R + 6-AMINOPENICILLANIC ACID

PENICILLOIC ACIDS

Figure 6–4. Destruction of the penicillins by penicillinase and amidase. (From Mandell GL, Petri WA: Antimicrobial agents: Penicillins, cephalosporins and other beta-lactam antibiotics. In Hardman JG, Limbird LE [eds]: Goodman and Gilman's The Pharmacologic Basis of Therapeutics. New York: McGraw-Hill, 1996.)

Figure 6–5. Production of novel penicillin-binding protein 2B genes with decreased affinity for penicillin in *S. pneumoniae* by homologous recombination with genes from other bacteria. The location of the active site (transpeptidase) in the parental and recombinant genes is indicated. (From Spratt BG: Resistance to antibiotics mediated by target alterations. Science 1994; 264: 388–393.)

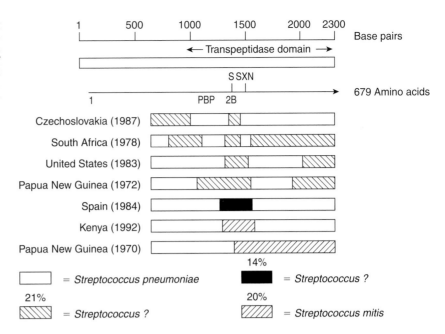

transposon from an unknown organism) with a very low affinity for all beta-lactam antibiotics. The gene encoding this new PBP is also present in, and responsible for, methicillin resistance in the coagulase-negative staphylococci.[1]

Gram-negative bacterial resistance to beta-lactam antibiotics can also be due to failure of the antibiotic to penetrate to the PBP targets or to rapid efflux of the penicillin from the site of action. The outer membrane of gram-negative bacteria forms an effective barrier against the diffusion of macromolecules to the periplasmic space, where PBPs are located (Fig. 6–6). Even when the antibiotics successfully penetrate into the periplasmic space, they may be subjected to hydrolysis by beta-lactamases present there. An important channel for entry of antibiotics into the periplasmic space is the outer membrane porins that selectively allow diffusion of nutrients into the bacterium. *P. aeruginosa* is a good example of a gram-negative bacterium that is resistant to most beta-lactam antibiotics by virtue of the failure of antibiotics to transverse the outer membrane porins. Only beta-lactam antibiotics, such as ceftazidime and imipenem, that

can diffuse through the *P. aeruginosa* porins can reach the PBPs in the periplasmic space to exert their antibacterial action. Resistance to these antibiotics is associated with changes in or loss of outer membrane porins.

PENICILLINS

Summary of the Pharmacologic and Antimicrobial Activities of the Penicillins

Several generalizations can be made about the pharmacologic properties of the penicillins as a class. Upon administration, the penicillins are distributed throughout the body, with therapeutic concentrations achieved in serum, bile, tissues, and joint and pleural fluids. In contrast, central nervous system, intraocular, and prostatic concentrations are relatively low. Concentrations of penicillins in the cerebrospinal fluid (CSF) increase from 1% or less of serum values in the absence of inflammation up to 5%–10% with inflammation.

Figure 6–6. Cell envelopes of the gram-positive and gram-negative bacteria. The gram-positive bacteria (left) are covered by a peptidoglycan layer that in most bacteria does not exclude beta-lactams from access to the penicillin-binding proteins in the cytoplasmic membrane. The gram-negative bacteria (right) are surrounded by an outer membrane that restricts the access of many beta-lactams to penicillin-binding proteins in the periplasmic space and cytoplasmic membrane. (Reprinted with permission from Nikaido H: Prevention of drug access to bacterial targets: Permeability barriers and active efflux. Science 1994; 264: 388–393. Copyright 1994 American Association for the Advancement of Science.)

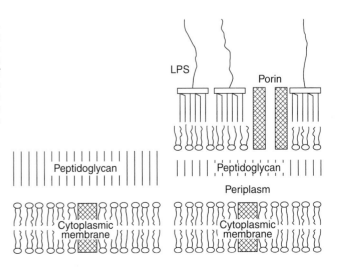

Glomerular filtration and renal tubular secretion of the penicillins rapidly remove them from the circulation, resulting in short plasma half-lives and high urinary concentrations.

Classification

Penicillins are logically classified by their antimicrobial activity (Tables 6–1 and 6–2).

Natural penicillins, such as penicillin G, are excellent for streptococci, *Listeria, Enterococcus* (although enterococcal endocarditis requires combining penicillin with an aminoglycoside), and spirochetes, including *Treponema pallidum* and *Borrelia burgdorferi.* In most areas of the United States, at least 25% of *S. pneumoniae* isolates are relatively to highly resistant to penicillin, so penicillin is no longer the 1st choice for empiric treatment of bacterial meningitis. Natural penicillins are active against gram-negative bacteria such as *Neisseria meningitidis* as well as non–penicillinase-producing *Neisseria gonorrhoeae* and *Haemophilus influenzae.* Natural penicillins are active against many gram-positive and some gram-negative anaerobes, including *Actinomyces israelii, Peptococcus, Peptostreptococcus, Fusobacterium,* and some strains of *Bacteroides.* Penicillin also has activity against some aerobic gram-negative bacilli, including *Streptobacillus moniliformis, Spirillum minus,* and *Pasteurella multocida* but is inactive against Enterobacteriaceae and *P. aeruginosa.* Penicillin G is destroyed by the beta-lactamases produced by most staphylococci and *B. fragilis.*

Antistaphylococcal penicillins, such as dicloxacillin and nafcillin, are resistant to beta-lactamases produced by staphylococci and are excellent for most *S. aureus* (except methicillin-resistant *S. aureus,* or MRSA, isolates). This class is inactive against *Enterococcus* and *Listeria* and lacks activity for Enterobacteriaceae, *Pseudomonas, B. fragilis,* and most coagulase-negative staphylococci. These drugs are generally less active than the natural penicillins against other bacteria, restricting their usefulness to the beta-lactamase–producing staphylococci.

Aminopenicillins, such as ampicillin and amoxicillin, have an expanded spectrum compared with penicillin, including some *Escherichia coli, Proteus, Salmonella,* and *Shigella.* They are inactive against other Enterobacteriaceae, *B. fragilis,* and *Pseudomonas.* With the exception of the enterococci, the aminopenicillins are less active than the natural penicillins against gram-positive organisms and spirochetes. The addition of a beta-lactamase inhibitor (sulbactam or clavulanic acid) extends the activity of the aminopenicillins to include many beta-lactamase–producing *E. coli, H. influenzae, Proteus, Klebsiella,* and *B. fragilis.*

Extended-spectrum penicillins have the best activity against the Enterobacteriaceae of all the penicillins. They are less active than the natural penicillins and aminopenicillins against gram-positive aerobic and anaerobic bacteria. Piperacillin is superior to carbenicillin or ticarcillin in this class in its activity against *Pseudomonas.* Addition of a beta-lactamase inhibitor (piperacillin-tazobactam or ticarcillin–clavulanic acid) does not improve anti-*Pseudomonas* activity but improves Enterobacteriaceae coverage and offers activity (albeit inferior to that of nafcillin) against *S. aureus.*

Table 6–1. PENICILLIN CLASSES

Class	Examples	Useful Spectrum
Natural penicillins	Penicillin G Penicillin V	*Streptococcus species*[1] Enterococci[1] *Listeria* *Neisseria meningitidis*[1] Anaerobes (not *Bacteroides fragilis* or some *Bacteroides melaninogenicus*) Spirochetes *Actinomyces*
Penicillinase-resistant	Methicillin, nafcillin Oxacillin Dicloxacillin	*Staphylococcus aureus*[2] *Staphylococcus epidermidis*[2]
Aminopenicillins	Ampicillin Amoxicillin Bacampicillin	Extends penicillin spectrum to Enterobacteriaceae (*Escherichia coli,*[3] *Proteus mirabilis,*[3] *Salmonella,*[3] *Shigella*[3]), *Haemophilus influenzae,*[3] and *Helicobacter pylori*[4]
Extended-spectrum	Piperacillin Ticarcillin Mezlocillin	Extends ampicillin spectrum to *Pseudomonas aeruginosa,* Enterobacteriaceae, *Bacteroides* species, and *B. fragilis* group[5]
Beta-lactamase inhibitor combinations	Amoxicillin-clavulanate Ampicillin-sulbactam	Extend ampicillin spectrum to beta-lactamase–producing strains of *H. influenzae, Moraxella* (*Branhamella*) *catarrhalis, S. aureus,* Enterobacteriaceae, *Neisseria,* and *Bacteroides*
	Ticarcillin-clavulanate Piperacillin-tazobactam	Extend ticarcillin-piperacillin spectrum to beta-lactamase–producing strains of *H. influenzae, M. catarrhalis, S. aureus,* Enterobacteriaceae, *Neisseria,* and *Bacteroides*[6]

[1]Except for penicillin-resistant isolates.
[2]Except for methicillin-resistant isolates.
[3]Except for beta-lactamase–producing isolates.
[4]In combination with bismuth salt and metronidazole.
[5]Except for some beta-lactamase–producing isolates. Piperacillin is the most potent agent of this class against *P. aeruginosa.*
[6]Except for chromosomally and some plasmid-encoded beta-lactamases. The currently recommended dose of piperacillin-tazobactam may be inadequate to treat *P. aeruginosa.*

Table 6–2. PHARMACOLOGY OF SELECTED PENICILLINS

Antibiotic	Usual Adult Dose	Peak Serum Levels, μg/mL	Dosage Adjustment Needed for	
			Renal Insufficiency?	Hepatic Impairment?
Penicillin G	20 million units continuous infusion over 24h (high dose)	20 (3 million units IV)	Yes	Yes
Procaine penicillin G	300,000–600,000 units IM q12h			
Benzathine penicillin G	1.2–2.4 million units q15–20d			
Penicillin V	125–500 mg PO q6h	2.1–2.8 (250 mg PO)	Yes	No
Nafcillin	1–2 g IV q4h	40 (500 mg IV)	No	Yes
Cloxacillin	250–500 mg PO q6H	7.7 (500 mg PO)	No	Yes
Dicloxacillin	125–500 mg PO q6h	10–18 (500 mg PO)	No	Yes
Oxacillin	500 mg PO q6h	2.6–3.9 (500 mg PO)	No	Yes
Ampicillin	40–50 mg/kg IV q6h	3–6 (500 mg PO)	Yes	Yes
Amoxicillin	250 mg PO q6h	5.5–11 (500 mg PO)	Yes	Yes
Bacampicillin	400 mg PO q12h	5.8–8.3 (400 mg PO)	Yes	Yes
Piperacillin	3–4 g IV q4–6h	389–484 (2 g IV)	Yes	Yes
Ticarcillin	3 g IV q3–6h	200–218 (2 g IV)	Yes	Yes
Mezlocillin	3 g IV q4h	161–364 (2 g IV)	Yes	Yes
Carbenicillin indanyl	382–764 mg PO q6h	6.8–17 (764 mg PO)	Avoid	Yes
Amoxicillin-clavulanate	250–500 mg PO q6h	3.7–4.8 (250 mg PO)	Yes	Yes
Ampicillin-sulbactam	1.5–3 g IV/IM q6h	40–71 (1.5 g IV)	Yes	Yes
Ticarcillin-clavulanate	3.1 g IV q4–6h	324 (3.1 g IV)	Yes	Yes
Piperacillin-tazobactam	3.375 g IV q6h–4.5 g IV q8h	389–484 (2 g IV)	Yes	Yes

Individual Agents

Natural Penicillins

Penicillin G and penicillin V are active against many aerobic gram-positive cocci, including viridans streptococci, group D nonenterococcal streptococci, and other streptococci, as well as some isolates of *S. pneumoniae*, enterococci (for which penicillin is effective only in combination with an aminoglycoside), and non–penicillinase-producing staphylococci. Sensitive gram-positive bacilli include *Listeria monocytogenes, Corynebacterium diphtheriae, Erysipelothrix rhusiopathiae*, and *Bacillus anthracis*. Gram-negative aerobic bacteria susceptible to penicillin include most *N. meningitidis*, non–penicillinase-producing *N. gonorrhoeae* and *Haemophilus* species, *Bordetella pertussis*, and *Eikenella corrodens*. Gram-positive anaerobic bacteria are generally sensitive to the natural penicillins; of the gram-negative anaerobes, the *B. fragilis* group is most commonly resistant. Spirochetes that are susceptible include *T. pallidum, B. burgdorferi, Borrelia recurrentis*, and *Leptospira*.

Penicillin V is more acid stable than penicillin G and therefore has better oral absorption, resulting in two to five times higher peak serum concentrations. Peak serum levels are achieved approximately 30–60 minutes after an oral dose and are undetectable within 6 hours of the dose. Intramuscular administration of penicillin G benzathine and penicillin G procaine results in detectable serum levels of penicillin for 1–4 weeks and 1–2 days, respectively. Penicillins are widely distributed following absorption into tissue; ascitic, synovial, pleural, and pericardial fluids; placenta; and breast milk. Penicillin concentrations are low but detectable in tonsils, maxillary sinus secretions, and saliva. Penetration into CSF ranges from 1% to 10% of serum concentrations in inflamed meninges. With normal renal function, the half-lives of the natural penicillins are on the order of 30–60 minutes; with anuria, the half-lives increase to about 10 hours. The drugs are metabolized to some extent by the liver into penicilloic acids. Penicillin G is removed by hemodialysis.

Therapeutic Uses. Increasing resistance to the natural penicillins limits their usefulness, but several important primary indications remain.

Pneumococcal Infections. *S. pneumoniae* is an important cause of community-acquired pneumonia, meningitis, sinusitis, otitis media, and bacteremia. The Centers for Disease Control and Prevention (CDC) have conducted surveillance for penicillin-resistant pneumococci in invasive isolates from sentinel hospitals in 13 states. From 1979 to 1987, high-level penicillin resistance was seen in 0.02% of isolates; during 1992, 1.3% of isolates had high-level penicillin resistance. In some pediatric populations, the incidence of penicillin resistance approaches 30%, with many strains multiplying as drug resistant. *S. pneumoniae* is resistant to penicillin because of alterations in its PBPs and not from beta-lactamase production. Addition of a beta-lactamase inhibitor to a penicillin therefore does not overcome penicillin resistance. Penicillin resistance is defined as a minimum inhibitory concentration (MIC) ≥ 0.1 μg/mL with high-level penicillin resistance defined as an MIC ≥ 2.0 μg/mL. The same breakpoints should be used for 3rd-generation cephalosporins. Pneumococcal isolates associated with disease should be screened for penicillin resistance with a 1-μg oxacillin disk; for isolates with zone sizes ≤ 19 mm, penicillin MICs should be determined. Because some penicillin-resistant pneumococci are also resistant to 3rd-generation cephalosporins, ceftriaxone or cefotaxime sensitivity should be tested (screen with a 30-μg ceftizoxime disk and then determine MICs if zone diameter is <15 mm).

Cefotaxime or ceftriaxone, and not penicillin, is the agent of choice for empiric therapy of bacterial meningitis in nonimmunocompromised children if the CSF Gram's stain does not show gram-positive cocci. For a patient with a CSF Gram's stain positive for gram-positive cocci, vancomycin plus ceftriaxone is a recommended regimen until the organism and its antibiotic sensitivity are determined. There have been many examples of failure of monotherapy with 3rd-generation cephalosporins for meningitis by pneumococci with MICs for cefotaxime-ceftriaxone of 2.0 μg/mL, and two reported failures when the MICs were 0.5–1.0 μg/mL.

Achievable serum concentrations of beta-lactam antibiotics are many times the MICs for intermediate and many highly penicillin-resistant pneumococci, and experience suggests that for pneumococcal pneumonia and bacteremia, high-dose penicillin (20 million units/day via continuous infusion in the adult) or 3rd-generation cephalosporin treatment should be successful. However, when highly penicillin-resistant pneumococcal infections are suspected, the prudent course may be to treat with a combination of a 3rd-generation cephalosporin plus vancomycin or with imipenem.

The current practice of administering empiric therapy with amoxicillin for community-acquired otitis media and sinusitis is unlikely to be changed by the emergence of penicillin-resistant pneumococci, again because of the excellent drug levels achieved in the affected organs by the penicillins. In cases in which initial therapy fails, use of a beta-lactamase–resistant oral antibiotic (to treat beta-lactamase–producing *H. influenzae* or *Moraxella (Branhamella) catarrhalis* can be tailored to also cover the possibility of a resistant pneumococcus by choosing an oral cephalosporin such as cefuroxime axetil, which has good in vitro activity against most strains of penicillin-resistant pneumococci.

Other Infections by Streptococci. No penicillin-resistant isolates of *Streptococcus pyogenes* (the group A beta-hemolytic streptococci) have been identified, so penicillin V, 500 mg every 6 hours for 10 days, remains the drug of choice for streptococcal pharyngitis (including scarlet fever). Parenteral therapy with a single injection of 1.2 million units of benzathine penicillin G is equally effective and may be preferable when patient compliance with the 10-day oral regimen cannot be ensured. Penicillin treatment of streptococcal pharyngitis decreases the duration of symptoms and reduces the risk of subsequent acute rheumatic fever, but it may not affect the rate of poststreptococcal glomerulonephritis. Ten days of penicillin treatment eradicated *S. pyogenes* from the pharynx in 82% of patients in one study. *Streptococcus agalactiae* (the group B streptococci) infections in neonates and adults (including meningitis and bacteremia) should be treated with high-dose intravenous penicillin G in combination with an aminoglycoside, because of penicillin tolerance in some isolates of group B streptococci. Endocarditis caused by penicillin-sensitive (MIC < 0.1 μg/mL) viridans streptococci (the most common cause of endocarditis) can be successfully treated with intravenous high-dose penicillin G, normally in combination with an aminoglycoside.

Enterococcal Endocarditis. Enterococcal endocarditis is optimally treated with two antibiotics—an increasingly difficult proposition because of the emergence of enterococcal strains resistant to all available antibiotics (88% of vancomycin-resistant enterococci are resistant to all licensed antibiotics). For a sensitive isolate, the optimum therapy is 20 million units a day of penicillin G via constant infusion (or ampicillin 12 g IV in divided doses) in combination with an aminoglycoside, usually for a total of 6 weeks. Treatment of serious infection due to multidrug-resistant enterococci (resistant to ampicillin, aminoglycosides, and vancomycin) may be unsuccessful, as evidenced by the 87% mortality reported in patients with resistant enterococci isolated from more than one site. Penicillin resistance in the enterococci in most cases is due to altered PBPs and not to beta-lactamase production; in the rare case of resistance due to beta-lactamase production, the addition of a beta-lactamase inhibitor should be useful.

Anaerobic Infections. The natural penicillins are drugs of choice for many anaerobic infections caused by *Actinomyces, Peptococcus,* and *Peptostreptococcus.* Most *B. fragilis* group bacteria are resistant, as are some other *Bacteroides* species. Periodontal and pulmonary infections respond well to penicillin G in most cases, although clindamycin is more effective than penicillin for lung abscess. Mild infections at these sites can be treated with oral penicillin, whereas more severe infections should be treated with high-dose intravenous penicillin G. Brain abscesses commonly contain several species of anaerobes, with the most commonly accepted regimen combining 20 million units/day of penicillin G via continuous infusion with metronidazole. Some experts prefer cefotaxime or ceftriaxone plus metronidazole.

Meningococcal Infections. High-dose intravenous penicillin G remains the drug of choice for meningococcal disease. Penicillin-resistant *N. meningitidis* has been reported from Great Britain and Spain but is uncommon at present. Its occurrence should be suspected in patients with slow response to treatment. Penicillin G does not eradicate the meningococcal carrier state.

Syphilis. Penicillin is the drug of choice for all stages of syphilis. Primary, secondary, and latent syphilis of less than 1 year's duration can be treated with a single intramuscular dose of 2.4 million units of penicillin G benzathine. In a patient with human immunodeficiency virus (HIV) infection, repeating this treatment for an additional two doses is recommended. High-dose intravenous penicillin G therapy for 10 days is recommended for patients with neurosyphilis, cardiovascular syphilis, and late latent syphilis. Infants with congenital syphilis should receive a minimum of 10 days of treatment with 50,000 units/kg/day of intramuscular procaine penicillin G or 100,000–150,000 units/kg/day of intravenous or intramuscular penicillin G in two divided doses for 10 days. Most patients with secondary syphilis who are treated with penicillin develop a Jarisch-Herxheimer reaction, which manifests as chills, fever, headache, myalgias, and/or arthralgias several hours after the first injection of penicillin. This reaction should be treated symptomatically, and penicillin treatment continued.

Actinomycosis. Penicillin G is the drug of choice for treatment of systemic and cervicofacial actinomycosis. Intravenous penicillin G (12–20 million units/day via continuous infusion) should be continued for 4–6 weeks, followed by several months of oral penicillin V. Intrauterine device (IUD)–associated pelvic actinomycosis limited to the endometrium can be treated, upon removal of the IUD, with oral penicillin V for several weeks.

Clostridial Infections. Parenteral penicillin G (12–20 million units/day via continuous infusion) remains the drug of choice for treatment of gas gangrene, in combination with aggressive surgical débridement.

Acute Necrotizing Ulcerative Gingivitis. This entity, also known as trench mouth and Vincent's disease, is due to *Leptotrichia buccalis* and spirochetes in the mouth. It responds readily to penicillin V (500 mg PO q6h) plus local débridement.

Listeriosis. Penicillin G or ampicillin with or without gentamicin is the drug of choice for infections due to *L. monocytogenes.* Penicillin G is recommended to be given intravenously, 15–20 million units/day for at least 2 weeks (4 weeks for endocarditis).

Erysipeloid. Uncomplicated *E. rhusiopathiae* infection responds to a single dose, 1.2 million units, of penicillin G benzathine. When endocarditis is present, high-dose intravenous penicillin G for 4–6 weeks has been effective.

Prophylactic Uses. The penicillins are of proven effectiveness in the prevention of *S. pyogenes* infection, rheumatic fever (primary and recurrent disease), and endocarditis. Detailed recommendations for endocarditis prophylaxis are published by the American Heart Association.[2]

Penicillinase-Resistant Penicillins

Antimicrobial activity of the penicillinase-resistant penicillins such as dicloxacillin and nafcillin is excellent against most *S. aureus* (except MRSA isolates) and some *Staphylococcus epidermidis.* Their use should be restricted to situations in which beta-lactamase–producing staphylococci are known or suspected to be involved, because penicillinase-resistant penicillins are less active than the natural penicillins against other penicillin-sensitive microorganisms. Methicillin-resistant *S. aureus* and *S. epidermidis* are resistant to the penicillinase-resistant penicillins by virtue of the production of an additional HMW PBP with a very low affinity for beta-lactam antibiotics.

Absorption of the isoxazolyl penicillins oxacillin, cloxacillin, and dicloxacillin is excellent with oral dosage, as all of these agents are acid stable. Absorption is better when they are taken on an empty stomach. Serum half-lives are 30–60 minutes, with rapid renal excretion and hepatic metabolism. Dosages do not need to be adjusted for renal insufficiency but do for hepatic insufficiency. Nafcillin, which is erratically absorbed when given orally, should be used parenterally only.

Aminopenicillins

Aminopenicillins, such as ampicillin and amoxicillin, have an expanded spectrum compared with penicillin, including some *E. coli* as well as *Proteus, Salmonella,* and *Shigella.* They are inactivated by beta-lactamases and lack activity against other Enterobacteriaceae, *B. fragilis,* and *Pseudomonas.* With the exception of the enterococci, the aminopenicillins are less active than the natural penicillins against gram-positive organisms and spirochetes. The addition of a beta-lactamase inhibitor (sulbactam or clavulanic acid) extends the activity of the aminopenicillins to include many beta-lactamase–producing *E. coli, Proteus, Klebsiella,* and *B. fragilis.*

Both ampicillin and amoxicillin are orally bioavailable, but amoxicillin is more rapidly and completely absorbed from the gastrointestinal tract than ampicillin. The drugs have the same antimicrobial spectrum. Bacampicillin is a 1-ethoxy-carbonyloxyethyl ester of ampicillin that is hydrolyzed to ampicillin during absorption from the gastrointestinal tract. Its drug concentrations are approximately 50% higher in serum than those of amoxicillin, and bacampicillin has been effective clinically in twice-daily dosing.

Therapeutic indications for the aminopenicillins are limited because of the emergence of resistance, especially via beta-lactamase production. However, they are still considered excellent drugs for uncomplicated otitis media, sinusitis, and exacerbations of chronic bronchitis, because they are well tolerated and of low cost. A beta-lactamase inhibitor (clavulanate or sulbactam) expands indications for these agents to include sinusitis, recurrent or severe otitis media, and certain chronic bronchitis exacerbations. Ampicillin has excellent activity against *L. monocytogenes* and against sensitive strains of *Enterococcus,* and it may be preferable to the natural penicillins for these infections. Amoxicillin with or without probenecid is effective oral therapy for stage 1 Lyme disease and, in combination with bismuth salts and metronidazole, for *Helicobacter pylori* disease.

Extended-Spectrum Penicillins

Extended-spectrum penicillins have the best activity against the Enterobacteriaceae of the penicillins. They are useful agents for the treatment of serious infections such as sepsis, respiratory tract infections, intraabdominal infections, skin and soft tissue infections, and urinary tract infections due to susceptible bacteria. They are less active than the natural penicillins and aminopenicillins against gram-positive aerobic and anaerobic bacteria, and are susceptible to destruction by beta-lactamases. Piperacillin is superior to mezlocillin or ticarcillin in this class in its in vitro activity against *Pseudomonas* and may be effective against *Pseudomonas* isolates resistant to mezlocillin and ticarcillin. Addition of a beta-lactamase inhibitor (piperacillin-tazobactam or ticarcillin–clavulanic acid) does not improve anti-*Pseudomonas* activity (in fact, the currently recommended dose of piperacillin-tazobactam is too low to be reliably effective for treatment of severe *P. aeruginosa* infections) but improves coverage against some beta-lactamase–producing Enterobacteriaceae and offers activity (albeit inferior to that of nafcillin) against *S. aureus.*

Ticarcillin is a semisynthetic penicillin very similar to carbenicillin but with somewhat greater activity against *P. aeruginosa.* Mezlocillin is more active than ticarcillin against *E. faecalis, Citrobacter,* and *Klebsiella,* and in the absence of biliary tract obstruction mezlocillin achieves high concentrations in bile. Piperacillin has activity similar to that of mezlocillin against *Klebsiella* and *Citrobacter* and increased activity against *Pseudomonas.* High biliary concentrations are achieved, similar to those for mezlocillin.

The only oral agent in this class is indanylcarbenicillin. Because of the low serum levels achieved after an oral dose, however, its usefulness is restricted to the treatment of urinary tract infections by susceptible strains of bacteria and perhaps acute or chronic prostatitis. It has mostly been replaced by the quinolones for these indications.

Toxicities With and Hypersensitivity Reactions to the Penicillins

Allergic reactions to the penicillins are the most common (0.7%–10% overall incidence) adverse effects noted with the penicillins. Manifestations of allergic reactions to the penicillins, in approximate order of decreasing frequency, are maculopapular rash, urticarial rash, fever, bronchospasm, vasculitis, serum sickness, exfoliative dermatitis, Stevens-Johnson syndrome, and anaphylaxis. No one of the penicillins is any more or less likely to cause a severe allergic reaction. Allergy to one penicillin makes it more likely that the patient will be allergic to another penicillin. Antipenicillin antibodies can be detected in almost all patients who have received the drug. Penicillins and their breakdown products covalently attach to proteins and act as haptens, generating antibodies against major and minor penicillin determinants. The major determinant (major because this is a more common site of antibody reactivity, not because a more severe reaction may result from an antibody against this region) is the penicilloyl moiety formed when the beta-lactam ring is opened. Minor determinants include penicilloate and the intact molecule.

Ampicillin (and probably amoxicillin) appears to cause the highest incidence of skin rashes (as high as 9%, including virtually all patients with infectious mononucleosis given the drug). Skin rashes can be maculopapular, morbilliform, scarlatiniform, vesicular, or bullous. Exfoliative and exudative eruptions of the skin are seen in the Stevens-Johnson syndrome. Fever with or without eosinophilia can sometimes be the only sign of penicillin allergy.

Angioedema and anaphylaxis are life-threatening hypersensitivity reactions to the penicillins. Angioedema can manifest as swelling of the tongue, lips, face, and periorbital area accompanied by hives and wheezing. Anaphylactic reactions are estimated to occur in 0.004%–0.04% of patients treated with penicillins and are fatal in 5%–10% of reported cases. Only 70% of patients dying of anaphylaxis had a history of prior penicillin use, and only one third had a prior history of penicillin allergy. Anaphylaxis most commonly follows intravenous administration of a penicillin and ranges in clinical severity from rapid hypotension and death to bronchoconstriction or abdominal pain, nausea, and vomiting.

A serum sickness–like reaction, also an unusual allergic reaction to penicillins, develops after 1 week or more of exposure to a penicillin. It is characterized clinically by fever, arthralgias/arthritis, urticaria, splenomegaly, and lymphadenopathy; in most cases, the reaction is mild and self-limiting. Positive direct Coombs's tests occur in up to 3% of patients receiving penicillins; the incidence of hemolytic anemia is much lower, and this reaction is most commonly seen during the administration of intravenous penicillin G.

Acute interstitial nephritis (in up to 17% of patients receiving intravenous methicillin but rare with other penicillinase-resistant penicillins), hepatotoxicity (especially with high doses of oxacillin), and reversible neutropenia (seen in up to 30% of patients receiving 8–12 g nafcillin a day for longer than 3 weeks) also may be allergic manifestations of penicillin exposure.

Penicillin G, carbenicillin, and ticarcillin have been associated with hemostasis defects apparently due to inhibition of platelet aggregation. Central nervous system toxicity (lethargy, confusion, seizures) is seen with intravenous administration of high doses of penicillin G, especially in patients with renal insufficiency. Severe or fatal hyperkalemia has occurred with intravenous administration of high doses of penicillin G potassium, which contain 34 mEq of K^+ in 20 million units. Intrathecal administration of penicillin should be avoided because of the possibility of causing a chemical arachnoiditis or encephalitis. Intramuscular injection of penicillin G procaine may lead to immediate dizziness, tinnitus, headache, hallucinations, and sometimes seizures owing to rapid liberation of toxic quantities of procaine.

Pseudomembranous colitis due to the overgrowth of *Clostridium difficile* in the intestine is a common problem with oral and sometimes with parenteral administration of beta-lactam antibiotics. It should be suspected in patients who have diarrhea and a recent history of beta-lactam antibiotic use.

Precautions for and Management of Penicillin Allergies

Most patients who report a history of penicillin, cephalosporin, or cephamycin allergy should be treated with a non–beta-lactam antibiotic. If there is a strong reason for using a penicillin in a patient with a history of penicillin allergy (such as syphilis during pregnancy), skin testing is a useful method to determine the risk of penicillin treatment. Individuals with a negative skin reaction to benzylpenicilloyl polylysine have been shown to have a 1%–4% risk of a cutaneous reaction; in contrast, two thirds of individuals with a positive skin test may have an allergic reaction to subsequent penicillin administration. Penicillin can be cautiously administered to patients with a negative skin test. It would be optimum to test also for sensitivity to the minor antigenic determinants to further identify individuals more likely to suffer an allergic reaction, because 25% of patients who test positive to the minor antigenic determinant mixture do not react with penicillin G and could be at risk for an anaphylactic reaction. Unfortunately, a commercially prepared mixture of minor antigenic determinants is not available.

In the unusual situation in which penicillin must be administered to a penicillin-allergic patient, rapid desensitization to penicillin can be performed. An intravenous line should be in place, and the patient should be continuously observed, with epinephrine and intubation equipment and expertise available at the bedside. Rapid desensitization involves giving gradually increasing doses of penicillin intradermally or orally (finally increasing it to the therapeutic dose), with the goal of inducing a state of antigen-specific mast cell unresponsiveness. In the limited numbers of patients who have been desensitized, this procedure, compared with historical controls, has been effective in preventing anaphylactic reactions. Desensitization is lost, however, within a few days of completion of penicillin therapy.

CEPHALOSPORINS

Summary of the Pharmacologic and Antimicrobial Activities of the Cephalosporins

The chemistry of the cephalosporins differs from that of the penicillins in that the beta-lactam ring is attached to a dihydrothiazine six-membered ring, as opposed to the thiazolidine five-membered ring of the penicillins. The targets of the cephalosporins are the PBPs involved in peptidoglycan cell-wall synthesis; mechanisms of resistance to the cephalosporins include modification of PBPs, decreased entry of the antibiotic into or increased efflux of the antibiotic from the periplasmic space, and destruction by beta-lactamases. New plasmid-encoded, extended-spectrum beta-lactamases (especially in *Klebsiella pneumoniae*) and chromosomally inducible beta-lactamases (first noted in *Enterobacter* species and *C. freundii*), which mediate resistance to all cephalosporins, have emerged.

One rational approach to classifying the cephalosporins is to divide them into generations. The spectrum of antimicrobial activity of a cephalosporin places it into a generation (Tables 6–3 and 6–4).

All cephalosporins lack activity against *Listeria*, enterococci, methicillin-resistant *S.aureus* and *S. epidermidis*, some strains of penicillin-resistant *S. pneumoniae*, *Legionella*, *C. difficile*, *Campylobacter jejuni*, *Acinetobacter* species, and *Stenotrophomonas (Xanthomonas) maltophilia*.

Pharmacologic Properties of the Cephalosporins

The orally absorbed cephalosporins are cephalexin, cephradine, cefadroxil, cefaclor, cefuroxime axetil, cefprozil, loracarbef, cefixime, and cefpodoxime proxetil. Because of pain from intramuscular administration of cephalothin and cephapirin, these agents are used only intravenously; the other parenteral formulations of cephalosporins can be given intramuscularly and intravenously. Renal elimination is the major path of cephalosporin clearance; in patients with renal failure the dosage must be adjusted. Cefoperazone and ceftriaxone are exceptions: Their dosages do not need to be adjusted for renal failure, as their elimination is primarily biliary or hepatic.

Cephalosporins that penetrate into CSF in sufficient quantities for the treatment of meningitis due to susceptible bacteria include cefotaxime, ceftriaxone, ceftizoxime, ceftazidime, and cefepime. Cephalosporins are found in high concentrations in urine, in synovial and pericardial fluids, and in the aqueous humor of the eye, but their concentrations in the vitreous are low. Cephalosporins cross the placenta and achieve high concentrations in bile, especially cefoperazone.

The Generations of Cephalosporins

The 1st-generation cephalosporins (for example, cephalexin and cefazolin) have good activity against gram-positive cocci, including *S. pyogenes* and *S. aureus*, limited activity against *M. catarrhalis*, *E. coli*, and *Proteus mirabilis*, and no activity against methicillin-resistant *S. aureus* or *S. epidermidis*, enterococci, and *Listeria*. Oral cavity anaerobes are sensitive, but most *B. fragilis* are resistant, to the 1st-generation cephalosporins. These agents are widely distributed in tissue upon administration but do not penetrate the CSF in appreciable quantities. They are commonly used for perioperative prophylaxis as well as for skin and soft tissue infec-

Table 6–3. CEPHALOSPORIN GENERATIONS

Generation	Examples	Useful Spectrum[1]
1st	Cefazolin Cephalothin Cephalexin	Streptococci[2] *Staphylococcus aureus*[3] No activity against enterococci, *Listeria*, or MRSA
2nd	Cefuroxime Cefaclor	Expands 1st-generation spectrum to include greater gram-negative activity (*Haemophilus influenzae*, including ampicillin-resistant strains, as well as *Escherichia coli*, *Neisseria*, *Klebsiella*, *Acinetobacter*, *Enterobacter*, *Citrobacter*, *Proteus*, *Providencia*, and *Moraxella (Branhamella) catarrhalis*) Not as active against gram-positive organisms as 1st generation; no activity against enterococci, *Listeria*, MRSA, or *Pseudomonas*
	Cefoxitin Cefotetan	Spectrum similar to that of cefuroxime, but with added activity against *Bacteroides fragilis*, *Bacteroides* species, and other anaerobes
3rd	Cefotaxime Ceftriaxone Ceftazidime	Achieves therapeutic concentrations in CSF, unlike 1st and 2nd generations Less active than 1st generation against gram-positive bacteria[4]; less active than cefoxitin or cefotetan against anaerobes Expanded gram-negative spectrum[5] compared with 1st and 2nd generations, including *Citrobacter*, *E. coli*, *Klebsiella*, *Enterobacter*, *Pseudomonas aeruginosa*,[6] *Proteus*, *Morganella*, *Providencia*, *Serratia*, *Neisseria gonorrhoeae* No activity against enterococci, or *Listeria*, or MRSA Oral 3rd-generation antibiotics (cefixime, cefpodoxime) lack useful activity against most strains of *Enterobacter* and *Pseudomonas* and have limited antianaerobic activity
4th	Cefepime	Comparable with that of 3rd generation but more resistant to some extended-spectrum beta-lactamases

[1]CSF, cerebrospinal fluid; MRSA, methicillin-resistant *S. aureus*.
[2]Except for some penicillin-resistant strains.
[3]Except for methicillin-resistant strains.
[4]Cefotaxime is most active in class against *S. aureus* and *Streptococcus pyogenes*.
[5]Resistance to cephalosporins may be rapidly induced during therapy by de-repression of bacterial chromosomal beta-lactamases, which destroy the cephalosporins, especially in the case of *Enterobacter* species and *Citrobacter freundii*.
[6]Ceftazidime and cefoperazone only.

tions (although a penicillin may be the drug of 1st choice for skin and soft tissue infections).

The 2nd-generation cephalosporins (for example, cefuroxime, cefoxitin, cefaclor, cefotetan) have an expanded gram-negative spectrum compared with the 1st-generation agents but are much less active than the 3rd-generation. There is some loss of activity against *S. pyogenes* and *S. aureus* compared with the 1st generation, but improved activity against *E. coli, Klebsiella, Proteus, H. influenzae, and M. catarrhalis*. A subset of the 2nd-generation agents are the cephamycins cefoxitin and cefotetan, which have the best activity against *B. fragilis* and other *Bacteroides* of any of the cephalosporins.

The 3rd-generation cephalosporins (including cefotaxime,

Table 6–4. PHARMACOLOGY OF SELECTED CEPHALOSPORINS

Cephalosporin	Usual Adult Dosage	Peak Serum/CSF Levels, μg/mL	Dosage Adjustment Needed for	
			Renal Insufficiency?	Hepatic Impairment?
1st generation				
Parenteral				
Cephalothin (Keflin, Seffin)	0.5–2 g IV q4–6h	67 (1)/—	Yes	No
Cefazolin (Ancef, Kefzol)	0.5–1.5 g IV/IM q6–8h	188 (1)/—	Yes	No
Cephapirin (Cefadyl)	0.5–2 g IV/IM q4–6h	67 (1)/—	Yes	No
Cephradine (Velosef)	0.5–2 g IV/IM q4–6h	18 (0.5)/—	Yes	No
Oral				
Cephalexin (Keflex, Keftab, Biocef)	0.25–1 g PO q6h	18 (0.5)/—	Yes	No
Cephradine (Velosef, Anspor)	0.25–1 g PO q6h	18 (0.5)/—	Yes	No
Cefadroxil (Duricef, Ultracef)	1–2 g PO q12–24h	10–18 (0.5)/—	Yes	No
2nd generation				
Parenteral				
Cefamandole (Mandol)	0.5–2 g IV/IM q4–6h	214 (2)/—	Yes	No
Cefonicid (Monocid)	0.5–2 g IV/IM q24h	221 (2)/—	Yes	No
Cefuroxime (Kefurox, Zenacef)	0.75–1.5 g IV/IM q6–8h	100 (1.5)/1.10	Yes	No
Parenteral, antianaerobic				
Cefoxitin (Mefoxin)	1–2 g IV/IM q6h	221 (2)/—	Yes	No
Cefotetan (Cefotan)	1–2 g IV/IM q12h	230 (2)/—	Yes	No
Cefmetazole (Zefazone)	2 g IV q6–12h	140 (2)/—	Yes	No
Oral				
Cefaclor (Ceclor)	0.25–0.5 g PO q8h	13 (0.5)/—	Yes	No
Cefuroxime axetil (Ceftin)	0.25–0.5 g PO q12h	8 (0.5)/—	Yes	No
Cefprozil (Cefzil)	0.25–0.5 g PO q12–24h	10 (0.5)/—	Yes	No
Loracarbef (Lorabid)	0.2–0.4 g PO q12h	15 (0.4)/—	Yes	No
3rd generation				
Parenteral				
Cefotaxime (Claforan)	1–2 g IV/IM q4–8h	214 (2)/5.6–44	Yes	No
Ceftizoxime (Cefizox)	1–4 g IV/IM q8–12h	130 (2)/0.5–29	Yes	No
Ceftriaxone (Rocephin)	0.5–2 g IV/IM q12–24h	250 (2)/1.2–39	No	Yes[1]
Parenteral, anti-Pseudomonas				
Cefoperazone (Cefobid)	2–4 g IV/IM q8–12	250 (2)/—	No	Yes
Ceftazidime (Fortaz, Tazidime, Tazicef)	0.5–2 g IV/IM q8–12h	160 (2)/0.5–30	Yes	Yes[1]
Oral				
Cefixime (Suprax)	0.2 g PO q12h	4.3 (0.4)/—	Yes	No
Cefpodoxime proxetil (Vantin)	0.2–0.4 g PO q12h	4 (0.4)/—	Yes	No
4th generation				
Cefepime	1–2 g IV q12h	130 (2)/—	Yes	No

[1]Adjust dose only if hepatic impairment is accompanied by renal impairment.

ceftriaxone, and ceftazidime) are 1st-line agents for the treatment of bacterial meningitis due to susceptible bacteria. They are much more active than the 2nd-generation agents against gram-negative bacteria. They also have excellent activity against sensitive strains of *S. pneumoniae, S. pyogenes,* and other streptococci and, with the exception of ceftazidime, have activity against methicillin-sensitive *S. aureus.* Most Enterobacteriaceae should be susceptible; ceftazidime and, to a lesser extent, cefoperazone also have activity against *P. aeruginosa;* ceftriaxone has the longest serum half-life of the cephalosporins. Concentrations of the 3rd-generation cephalosporins in CSF are usually high enough to achieve therapeutic levels for many infections.

Cefotaxime and ceftriaxone are 1st-line agents for empiric treatment of community-acquired meningitis (in combination with ampicillin if *Listeria* is suspected and in combination with vancomycin if penicillin-resistant pneumococci are suspected). Ceftazidime is useful in the treatment of nosocomial meningitis. Cefotaxime and ceftriaxone are effective for community-acquired pneumonia, pneumonia and sepsis (in combination with an aminoglycoside), and *N. gonorrhoeae* infections. The appearance of chromosomally encoded beta-lactamases (in *Enterobacter* species and *C. freundii*) and plasmid-mediated ESBLs is resulting in a rising frequency of resistance to the 3rd-generation cephalosporins.

The 4th-generation cephalosporins (such as the investigational agent cefepime) are less susceptible to hydrolysis by the chromosomally induced and plasmid-encoded ESBLs, but otherwise they have a spectrum of activity similar to that of the 3rd-generation agents. The 4th-generation cephalosporins may be especially useful in the treatment of aerobic gram-negative bacilli resistant to the 3rd-generation agents.

Individual Agents in Each Class

1st-Generation Cephalosporins

Cephalothin, the most resistant of the 1st-generation agents to the *S. aureus* beta-lactamase, is the cephalosporin of choice for treatment of serious *S. aureus* infections. It has a short plasma half-life (30–40 minutes) and, in common with all 1st-generation cephalosporins, does not penetrate into the CSF. Cephapirin is similar to cephalothin in its antimicrobial activity and pharmacokinetics. Cefazolin is similar in antibacterial spectrum to cephalothin, being more active against *E. coli* and *Klebsiella* but somewhat more sensitive to *S. aureus* beta-lactamase. It has a half-life of 1.8 hours and is well tolerated upon intramuscular and intravenous administration. The longer half-life, and subsequently longer dosing intervals, of cefazolin make it a preferred 1st-generation agent.

Cephalexin is an oral 1st-generation cephalosporin with a 50-minute half-life that shares the antibacterial spectrum of the other 1st-generation agents, but it is less active against beta-lactamase–producing *S. aureus* than cephalothin. Cephradine is similar in structure and activity to cephalexin, has a 30- to 40-minute half-life, and can be administered orally or parenterally. Its oral absorption is so complete that serum levels are equivalent to those achieved with intramuscular administration. Cefadroxil has the longest half-life (1.2 h) of the orally administered 1st-generation cephalosporins, permitting once- or twice-daily treatment of pharyngeal, urinary tract, and mild skin or soft tissue infections.

2nd-Generation Cephalosporins

Cefamandole has a half-life of 45–50 minutes and is excreted unchanged in the urine. It is more active than 1st-generation agents against *Enterobacter* species, indole-positive *Proteus*, *E. coli*, and *Klebsiella*. *H. influenzae* that produces the plasmid beta-lactamase TEM-1 is resistant to cefamandole. Cefamandole contains the methylthiotetrazole (MTT) side chain and its associated toxicities (see later). Cefonicid is similar in antibacterial spectrum and pharmacodynamic properties to cefamandole but has a much longer half-life (4.4 h). It is effective for once-daily treatment of mild infections due to susceptible bacteria. Cefuroxime is similar to cefamandole in activity and structure but is significantly more resistant to beta-lactamases of *H. influenzae* and *N. gonorrhoeae* and has a longer serum half-life (1.7 h), enabling every-8-hour administration.

Cefoxitin is a cephamycin that is resistant to some beta-lactamases produced by gram-negative rods. It shares the unfortunate property with the 3rd-generation cephalosporins of inducing chromosomally encoded type I beta-lactamases,

which confer resistance to all cephalosporins (with the possible exception of 4th-generation agents). Cefoxitin is less active than cefamandole against *Enterobacter* species and *H. influenzae* as well as gram-positive bacteria, but it is more active against anaerobes, particularly *B. fragilis*. Cefotetan is also a cephamycin with good activity against *B. fragilis* and other *Bacteroides* species and better activity against gram-negative aerobic bacteria than cefoxitin. Coadministration of vitamin K prevents the cefotetan MTT side chain–associated bleeding due to hypoprothrombinemia that is seen in malnourished patients. The role of cefoxitin and cefotetan may be for the treatment of mild to moderate, mixed aerobic-anaerobic infections, including pelvic inflammatory disease and lung abscess.

Cefaclor, cefuroxime axetil, cefprozil, and loracarbef are orally administered 2nd-generation cephalosporins. Cefprozil and cefuroxime axetil have greater in vitro activity against the pneumococcus (penicillin-sensitive and penicillin-resistant) than cefaclor and loracarbef. Of the oral 2nd-generation cephalosporins, cefaclor is the least resistant to beta-lactamases produced by *H. influenzae* and *M. catarrhalis*. Cefaclor has a half-life of 0.8 hours and should be administered every 8 hours. Cefprozil has an antibacterial spectrum similar to that of cefaclor, with the best activity of the 2nd-generation oral cephalosporins against *S. pneumoniae*, *S. pyogenes*, and other streptococci. Its serum half-life is 1.2–1.4 hours. Cefuroxime axetil is hydrolyzed to cefuroxime during oral absorption; its serum half-life, 1.3–1.5 hours, allows twice-daily dosing. Loracarbef has activity similar to that of cefaclor but greater stability against the beta-lactamases of *H. influenzae* and *M. catarrhalis*. Loracarbef, as is the case for many cephalosporins, is destroyed by the ESBLs; it has a half-life of 1.1 hours.

3rd-Generation Cephalosporins

Cefotaxime is resistant to many (but not the type I chromosomally encoded and plasmid-encoded, extended-spectrum) beta-lactamases and has good activity against gram-positive and gram-negative aerobic bacteria. It has poor activity against *B. fragilis* and no activity against *P. aeruginosa*. The half-life of cefotaxime is 1 hour, requiring administration every 4–8 hours. Cefotaxime, at a dose of 2 g every 4 hours, has been effective in the treatment of meningitis due to *H. influenzae*, *N. meningitidis*, and sensitive strains of *S. pneumoniae*. However, there are many examples of failure of monotherapy with 3rd-generation cephalosporins for meningitis by pneumococci, with MICs for cefotaxime/ceftriaxone of 2.0 μg/mL, and two reported failures when the MICs were 0.5–1.0 μg/mL. Therefore, until the sensitivity of the responsible pneumococcus is known, suspected pneumococcal meningitis should be treated with a combination of vancomycin plus a 3rd-generation cephalosporin. Ceftizoxime has a similar spectrum of activity to that of cefotaxime with a slightly longer half-life of 1.8 hours, allowing less frequent dosing (every 8–12 h), and better activity than cefotaxime (but worse than cefoxitin) against *B. fragilis*. Data suggest that ceftizoxime is less active than cefotaxime or ceftriaxone for penicillin-resistant pneumococci. Ceftriaxone's in vitro antibacterial activity is also very similar to that of cefotaxime. Its half-life of 8 hours permits treatment of meningitis with once- or twice-daily dosing. The drug appears to be eliminated equally by renal and biliary routes. Moxalactam has a spectrum similar to that of ceftizoxime except for inferior gram-positive activity; bleeding complications due in part to the MTT group as well as a drug-induced platelet aggregation defect have led to the recommendation that moxalactam not be used.

A subset of the 3rd-generation cephalosporins, including cefoperazone and ceftazidime, have excellent activity against *P. aeruginosa*. Ceftazidime has the best anti–*P. aeruginosa* activity of the beta-lactams. Because resistant strains emerge with monotherapy, serious *P. aeruginosa* infections are treated with ceftazidime in combination with an aminoglycoside. Cefoperazone is eliminated predominantly via the biliary route; biliary concentrations are higher than with other cephalosporins. Its serum half-life is 2 hours. Cefoperazone has inferior gram-negative and gram-positive activity compared with cefotaxime, with the exception of its modest activity against *P. aeruginosa*. For *P. aeruginosa* infection, ceftazidime has much better activity than cefoperazone and is the preferred treatment. Cefoperazone-associated bleeding due to hypoprothrombinemia can be prevented by coadministration of vitamin K. Ingestion of alcohol can result in a disulfiram reaction–like effect in patients who are taking cefoperazone as well as other cephalosporins containing the MTT group. Cefoperazone has little activity against *B. fragilis* and poor anti–*S. aureus* activity. Its half-life is 1.5 hours in serum.

Oral 3rd-generation cephalosporins include cefixime and cefpodoxime proxetil. Compared with the orally administered 2nd-generation cephalosporins, cefixime is less active against gram-positive cocci and more active against beta-lactamase–producing *H. influenzae*, *N. gonorrhoeae*, and Enterobacteriaceae. Its activity against *S. aureus* is poor; its serum half-life is 3.7 hours. Cefixime has a role in the treatment of otitis media, pharyngitis, tonsillitis, bronchitis, and uncomplicated urinary tract infections caused by susceptible organisms, especially when longer dosing intervals are desired. Its lack of activity against *S. aureus*, *P. aeruginosa*, and enterococci limits its usefulness in many settings. Cefpodoxime proxetil has a spectrum of antimicrobial activity similar to that of cefixime, a slightly better *S. aureus* activity, and a serum half-life of 2.2 hours. It may be useful as oral treatment for some penicillin-resistant pneumococcal infections.

4th-Generation Cephalosporins

Cefepime, a 4th-generation cephalosporin, is active against many Enterobacteriaceae that are resistant to other cephalosporins via induction of type I beta-lactamases. It is currently not available for use in the United States. Cefepime is stable to hydrolysis by many of the older plasmid-encoded beta-lactamases (TEM-1, TEM-2, and SHV-1) and is a poor inducer of, and relatively resistant to, the type I chromosomally encoded beta-lactamases. This agent remains susceptible to many bacteria expressing extended-spectrum plasmid beta-lactamases (such as TEM-3 and TEM-10). Against the fastidious gram-negative bacteria (*H. influenzae*, *N. gonorrhoeae*, and *N. meningitidis*), cefepime has greater in vitro activity than cefotaxime. For *P. aeruginosa* infection, cefe-

pime has activity comparable to that of ceftazidime, although it is less active than ceftazidime for other *Pseudomonas* species and *S. maltophilia*. Cefepime has higher activity than ceftazidime, and comparable activity to cefotaxime, for streptococci and methicillin-sensitive *S. aureus*. It is not active against methicillin-resistant *S. aureus*, penicillin-resistant pneumococci, enterococci, *B. fragilis*, *L. monocytogenes*, *Mycobacterium avium* complex, or *Mycobacterium tuberculosis*. Cefepime is almost 100% renally excreted, and doses should be adjusted for renal failure. Cefepime has excellent penetration into the CSF in animal models of meningitis. When this agent is given at the recommended dosage for adults, 2 g intravenously every 12 hours, peak serum concentrations in humans range from 126 to 193 μg/mL. The serum half-life is 2 hours.

Untoward Reactions to the Cephalosporins

Allergic reactions to the cephalosporins are the most common side effects and are similar to those seen with the penicillins, likely owing to the shared beta-lactam structure of the two classes of antibiotics. Anaphylactic and urticarial reactions are less common than with the penicillins. Cross-reactivity to cephalosporins in penicillin-allergic patients has been demonstrated immunologically in up to 20% of cases, but clinically significant hypersensitivity reactions appear less frequently. There is a low risk of an allergic reaction to a cephalosporin in patients with a history of mild or distant allergic reactions to penicillins. However, if the patient has had a severe immediate reaction to a penicillin, cephalosporins should be avoided, if possible, or should be administered with great caution. Unlike for the penicillins, skin test reagents are not commercially available or reliable for the prediction of the likelihood of a hypersensitivity reaction to cephalosporins. A common manifestation of hypersensitivity is a maculopapular rash that develops after several days of therapy. More severe but much less common reactions include anaphylaxis, bronchospasm, and urticaria.

Important toxicities for these antibiotics include vitamin K abnormalities and disulfiram reaction–like effect with cephalosporins containing the MTT side chain (cefamandole, cefotetan, cefmetazole, cefoperazone, and others), gallbladder sludge mimicking cholecystitis with ceftriaxone, and rare instances of bone marrow depression accompanied by neutropenia. Cephalosporins also can cause an isolated eosinophilia. Elevations in transaminases and alkaline phosphatase can occur with cephalosporin therapy but are usually minor. A positive Coombs's test is common in patients receiving large doses of cephalosporin, although hemolysis is unusual. Nephrotoxicity is also unusual but has occurred with large doses of cephalothin, especially when it is given in combination with an aminoglycoside and in patients with preexisting renal disease. Antibiotic-associated colitis due to *C. difficile* can be a side effect of treatment with any of the cephalosporins.

Therapeutic Uses of the Cephalosporins

Cephalosporins are therapeutically important and widely used antibiotics. Unfortunately, their overuse in situations in which a more narrow-spectrum antibiotic would suffice has been associated with the emergence of resistance, most recently and most ominously through the induction of the chromosomally encoded beta-lactamases.

A single dose of cefazolin "on call" for the operating room is the preferred perioperative prophylaxis for procedures in which skin flora are the likely pathogens. Cephalosporins with or without aminoglycosides are the preferred treatment for serious infections caused by *Klebsiella, Enterobacter, Proteus, Providencia, Serratia*, and *Haemophilus* species. Ceftriaxone is the 1st-line agent for therapy of gonorrhoeae.

The 3rd-generation cephalosporins are the drugs of choice for the empiric treatment of community-acquired meningitis but should be part of combined therapy with ampicillin when *L. monocytogenes* is part of the differential diagnosis (in young, elderly, and immunocompromised individuals) and should be combined with vancomycin for suspected penicillin-resistant pneumococcal meningitis. Ceftazidime plus an aminoglycoside is the most active treatment for *Pseudomonas* meningitis and is useful for other serious infections due to *P. aeruginosa*.

Cephalosporins are useful alternatives to penicillins for patients who cannot tolerate the penicillins because of a history of mild penicillin allergy or for other reasons.

Ceftriaxone or cefotaxime is the treatment of choice for late neurologic and musculoskeletal manifestations of Lyme disease. The good antianaerobic activity of cefoxitin and cefotetan makes these agents useful in the treatment of certain mixed infections. Community-acquired pneumonia due to pneumococci, *S. aureus*, or *H. influenzae* can be treated with cefuroxime, cefotaxime, ceftriaxone, or ceftizoxime.

The 3rd- and 4th-generation cephalosporins are important agents for treatment of nosocomial infections caused by resistant microorganisms, although this is less the case now with the emergence of inducible chromosomally encoded beta-lactamases and the plasmid-encoded ESBLs in gram-negative aerobic bacilli. The 4th-generation agents may prove useful in this situation of growing resistance in nosocomially acquired bacterial infections.

CLINICAL USE OF SOME COMMON EAR, NOSE, AND THROAT INFECTIONS WITH BETA-LACTAM ANTIBIOTICS

Bacterial pharyngitis is caused by group A (*S. pyogenes*) and group C beta-hemolytic streptococci and is treated optimally with oral penicillin V for 10 days or a single injection of 1.2 million units of benzathine penicillin G. A 1st-generation cephalosporin, such as cephalexin, cephradine, or cefadroxil, is an effective alternative to penicillin. Erythromycin is an alternative for treatment of bacterial pharyngitis in the penicillin-allergic patient, although some group A streptococci are resistant to it. Only penicillin has been shown to reduce the incidence of poststreptococcal rheumatic fever, but since eradication rates are similar with alternative therapies, they are assumed to be equivalent.

Acute otitis media is caused predominantly by *S. pneumoniae, H. influenzae*, and *M. catarrhalis*, with respiratory viruses implicated in approximately one quarter of cases.

Amoxicillin remains a 1st-line agent for the treatment of otitis media on the basis of its low cost and excellent tolerance. It should be effective for all but the minority of infections (at present) due to beta-lactamase–producing *H. influenzae* and *M. catarrhalis*. Failure of response or recurrent otitis media can be treated with trimethoprim-sulfamethoxazole, amoxicillin-clavulanate, erythromycin-sulfisoxazole, or an oral cephalosporin with good in vitro activity against amoxicillin-resistant *H. influenzae* and *M. catarrhalis* and against penicillin-resistant pneumococci, such as cefprozil, cefuroxime axetil, or cefpodoxime proxetil.

Invasive (malignant) otitis externa is caused in almost all cases by *P. aeruginosa* and can be treated with an antipseudomonal beta-lactam antibiotic (such as ceftazidime or piperacillin) in combination with an aminoglycoside.

Empiric antibiotic therapy for community-acquired sinusitis should cover the most likely etiologies—*S. pneumoniae, H. influenzae*, and *M. catarrhalis*. Less common etiologies include anaerobic bacteria and *S. aureus*. Therapy with amoxicillin is one approach, if beta-lactamase–producing *H. influenzae* and *M. catarrhalis* and penicillin-resistant pneumococci are uncommon in the community. Amoxicillin-clavulanate overcomes resistance due to beta-lactamase production; the oral cephalosporins cefprozil, cefuroxime axetil, and cefpodoxime proxetil are attractive agents because of their activity against both amoxicillin-resistant *H. influenzae* and *M. catarrhalis* and penicillin-resistant pneumococci.

Acute epiglottitis in children is most commonly due to *H. influenzae* infection. Parenteral antibiotic therapy is usually with a 3rd-generation cephalosporin that is active against beta-lactamase–producing *H. influenzae*, such as cefotaxime or ceftriaxone.

Odontogenic infections are polymicrobial with a preponderance of anaerobic bacteria, reflecting the indigenous oral flora. At present, penicillin V remains a 1st-line agent for this infection, although there has been an increase in beta-lactamase–producing *Bacteroides* species and *Prevotella melaninogenica* associated with penicillin treatment failure. Amoxicillin-clavulanate should be an effective agent even if beta-lactamase–producing anaerobes are present in the infection. Clindamycin and erythromycin are alternative agents for the penicillin-allergic patient.

Ludwig's angina is a potentially life-threatening infection of the sublingual, submaxillary, and submandibular space that originates in a dental source. Parenteral antibiotic therapy should be with agents active against anaerobes, facultative gram-negative bacilli, and streptococci. Suggested regimens include penicillin G plus metronidazole, imipenem, and, in less severe infections, clindamycin or cefoxitin.

References

1. Spratt BG: Resistance to antibiotics mediated by target alterations. Science 1994; 264: 388–393.
2. Dajani AS, Bisno AL, Chung KJ, et al.: Prevention of bacterial endocarditis: Recommendations by the American Heart Association. JAMA 1990; 264: 2919–2922.

Further Readings

Anonymous: Antimicrobial prophylaxis in surgery. Med Letter 1993; 35: 91–94.

Anonymous: The choice of antibacterial drugs. Med Letter 1994; 36: 53–60.

Barradell LB, Bryson HM: Cefepime: A review of its antibacterial activity, pharmacokinetic properties and therapeutic use. Drugs 1994; 47: 471–505.

Chambers HF, Neu HC: Penicillins. In: Mandell GL, Bennett JE, Dolin R (eds): Mandell, Douglas and Bennett's Principles and Practice of Infectious Diseases, 4th ed. New York: Churchill Livingstone, 1995, pp 233–246.

Donowitz GR, Mandell GL: Beta-lactam antibiotics. N Engl J Med 1988; 318: 419–426, 490–500.

Drug Information: American Hospital Formulary Service. Bethesda, Maryland: American Society of Health-System Pharmacists, 1995, pp 54–375.

John CC: Treatment failure with use of a third generation cephalosporin for penicillin-resistant pneumococcal meningitis: Case report and review. Clin Infect Dis 1994; 18: 188–193.

Karchmer AW: Cephalosporins. In: Mandell GL, Bennett JE, Dolin R (eds): Mandell, Douglas and Bennett's Principles and Practice of Infectious Diseases, 4th ed. New York: Churchill Livingstone, 1995, pp 247–263.

Medeiros AA: Nosocomial outbreaks of multiresistant bacteria: Extended-spectrum beta-lactamases have arrived in North America. Ann Intern Med 1993; 119: 428–431.

Nikaido H: Prevention of drug access to bacterial targets: Permeability barriers and active efflux. Science 1994; 264: 382–387.

Thornsberry C, Brown SD, Yee YC, et al.: Increasing penicillin resistance in *Streptococcus pneumoniae* in the U.S. Infections in Medicine 1995; suppl: 15–24.

S. Ragnar Norrby

PART 2

Monobactams

▼

Monobactams are beta-lactam antibiotics characterized by a simple chemical structure in which the beta-lactam nucleus lacks a cyclic structure. Several monobactams have been investigated but only one, aztreonam, has been licensed for clinical use. Aztreonam has many similarities to ceftazidime. It has a side chain identical to the one in ceftazidime, which confers broad-spectrum activity against gram-negative bacteria, including *Pseudomonas aeruginosa*, and a high degree of beta-lactamase stability. Aztreonam typically lacks activity against gram-positive bacteria.

PHARMACOLOGY AND PHARMACOKINETICS

Aztreonam is water soluble, lipid insoluble, and about 55% protein bound. As reviewed by Swabb,[1] aztreonam has uncomplicated pharmacokinetics. It is not absorbed after oral administration and must be given intravenously or intramuscularly. After bolus infusions, high serum concentrations are achieved: 125, 50, 13, and 3 mg/L at 5 minutes 1 and 4, and 8 hours, respectively, after a 1-g dose. The corresponding values after a 2-g dose are approximately twice as high. The plasma half-life in healthy subjects is 1.5–2 hours, and aztreonam is eliminated renally, mainly by glomerular filtration. In patients who are elderly or have renal impairment, the half-life increases to up to 8 hours.[1-3]

Aztreonam's penetration to peripheral compartments seem to be predictable from its relatively low protein binding and low molecular weight. Few studies have been performed on the penetration of aztreonam into ear, nose, and throat (ENT)-related tissues. In one study, the concentration in mastoid cell mucosa in patients with suppurative otitis was 7.5 mg/kg following a 1-g dose.[4] Low and variable concentrations were found in saliva, but the concentrations achieved exceeded the minimal inhibitory concentrations (MICs) of aztreonam-susceptible bacteria.[5] The penetration into cerebrospinal fluid of patients with meningeal inflammation has been studied and 2–8 hours after single doses of 2 g, concentrations ranging between 0.8 and 17 mg/L were recorded.[6] In individuals without meningeal inflammation, considerably lower concentrations were achieved.[7]

SPECTRUM OF ACTIVITY AND MODE OF ACTION

Like other monobactams, aztreonam is inactive against gram-positive bacteria and anaerobes but is highly active against gram-negative aerobic bacteria.[8, 9] The activity against Enterobacteriaceae and *Pseudomonas* species is similar to or slightly inferior to that of ceftazidime, with MICs below 1 mg/L for most strains that do not produce certain beta-lactamases (see later). These concentratons are exceeded for more than 8 hours after a 1-g dose of aztreonam.

To some extent, the spectrum of aztreonam is limited by its susceptibility to class I cephalosporinase and to so-called extended-spectrum beta-lactamases.[10, 11] In this respect, this agent is similar to 3rd-generation cephalosporins; i.e., both types of enzyme hydrolyze aztreonam.

Aztreonam acts by binding to penicillin-binding protein 3 (PBP-3) in Enterobactericeae, resulting in filament formation.[12] This may in turn increase the amount of endotoxin released from dying cells in comparison with beta-lactams, which acts on other PBPs.[13, 14] The clinical significance of this feature is not known.

CLINICAL USE IN EAR, NOSE, AND THROAT INFECTIONS

Only one study has been found in which aztreonam was used for treating ENT infections.[4] In that study, patients with suppurative otitis media caused by *Pseudomonas* or *Proteus* showed good response to 1–2 g given three times daily.

Aztreonam has been used in combination with other antibiotics for treatment of infections in low-risk neutropenic patients, and the results reported were similar to those obtained with other combinations.[15] One small, uncontrolled study reported positive results of aztreonam used in children with meningitis caused by *Haemophilus influenzae*.[16]

Several reports have pointed out that if aztreonam is used in patients with systemic infections of the respiratory tract or skin and soft tissue infections, it should be combined with another antibiotic that has gram-positive activity to avoid superinfections.[17, 18]

SAFETY

Aztreonam has a very high level of safety.[19] An important advantage is that aztreonam seems to lack cross-reactivity with penicillins and cephalosporins in patients who have reacted to such antibiotics with immunoglobulin E–mediated reactions.[20, 21] Aztreonam is occasionally used in place of aminoglycosides as a less toxic alternative.

DOSAGE

Aztreonam is given as 1–2 g every 8 hours.

References

1. Swabb EA: Clinical pharmacology of aztreonam in healthy recipients and patients: A review. Rev Infect Dis 1985; suppl 4: S605–612.
2. el Guinaidy MA, Nawishy S, Abd el Bary M, Sabbour MS: Single-dose pharmacokinetics of aztreonam in healthy volunteers and renal failure patients. K Chemother 1989; 1: 164–169.
3. Meyers BR, Wilkinson P, Mendelson MH, et al.: Pharmacokinetics of aztreonam in healthy elderly and young adults. J Clin Pharmacol 1993; 33: 470–474.
4. Baba S, Kinoishita H, Mori Y, et al.: Efficacy evaluation of aztreonam for suppurative otitis media. Jpn J Antibiot 1986; 39: 159–176.
5. Pterikkos G, Androulakis M, Goumas P, Giamarellou H: A comparative

study of cefoxitin, cefotaxime, moxalactam and aztreonam kinetics in saliva. Chemother (Florens) 1987; 6: 355–358.
6. Greenman RL, Arcey SM, Dickinson GM, et al.: Penetration of aztreonam into human cerebrospinal fluid in the presence of meningeal inflammation. J Antimicrob Chemother 1985; 15: 637–640.
7. Duma RJ, Berry AJ, Smith SM, et al.: Penetration of aztreonam into cerebrospinal fluid of patients with and without inflamed meninges. Antimicrob Agents Chemother 1984; 26: 730–733.
8. Rylander M, Gezelius L, Norrby SR: Comparative in vitro activity of tigemonam, a new monobactam, J Antimicrob Chemother 1988; 22: 307–314.
9. Martinez-Beltran J, Canton R, Linarez J, et al.: Multicentre comparative study on the antibacterial activity of FK-037, a new parenteral cephalosporin. Eur J Clin Microbiol Infect Dis 1995; 14: 244–252.
10. Jett BD, Ritchie DJ, Reichley R, et al.: In vitro activities of various beta-lactam antimicrobial agents against clinical isolates of *Escherichia coli* and *Klebsiella* spp. resistant to oxyamino cephalosporins. Antimicrob Agents Chemother 1995; 39: 1187–1190.
11. Ramadan MA, Tawfik AF, Shibl AM: Effects of beta-lactamase susceptibility of local isolates of *Enterobacter cloacae, Serratia marcescens* and *Pseudomonas aeruginosa* to beta-lactam antibiotics. Chemother 1995; 41: 193–119.
12. Satta G, Cornaglia G, Mazzariol A, et al.: Target for bacteriostatic and bactericidal activities of beta-lactam antibiotics against *Escherichia coli* resides in different pencillin-binding proteins. Antimicrob Agents Chemother 1995; 39: 812–818.
13. Dofferhoff AS, Esselink MT, de Vries-Hospers HG, et al.: The release of endotoxin from antibiotic treated *Escherichia coli* and the production of tumor necrosis factor by human monocytes. J Antimicrob Chemother 1993; 31: 373–384.
14. Enf RH, Smith SM, Fan-Havard P, Ogbara T: Effects of antibiotics on endotoxin release from gram-negative bacteria. Diagn Microbiol Infect Dis 1993; 16: 185–189.
15. Rubinstein EB, Rolston K, Benjamin RS, et al.: Outpatient treatment of febrile episodes in low-risk neutropenic patients with cancer. Cancer 1993; 71: 3640–3666.
16. Girgis NI, Abu el Alla AH, Farid Z, et al.: Parenteral aztreonam in the treatment of *Haemophilus influenzae* type b meningitis in Egyptian children. Scand J Infect Dis 1988; 20: 111–112.
17. Norrby SR: Clinical experience with aztreonam in Europe: A summary of studies performed in Belgium, Eire, England, Finland, Holland, Norway, Portugal and Sweden. Rev Infect Dis 1985; 7: S836–S839.
18. Davies BI, Maesen FP, Teengs JP: Aztreonam in patients with acute purulent exacerbations of chronic bronchitis: Failure to prevent emergence of pneumococcal infections. J Antimicrob Chemother 1985; 15: 375–384.
19. Alvan G, Nord CE: Adverse effects of monobactams and carbapenems. Drug Safety 1995; 12: 305–313.
20. Adkinson NF, Jr, Swabb EA, Sugerman AA: Immunology of the monobactam aztreonam. Antimicrob Agents Chemother 1984; 25: 93–97.
21. Vega JM, Blanca M, Garcia JJ, et al.: Tolerance of aztreonam in patients allergic to beta-lactam antibiotics. Allergy 1991; 46: 196–202.

PART 3

S. Ragnar Norrby

Carbapenems

▼

The carbapenem group of antibiotics includes imipenem/cilastatin, which is licensed in most countries; meropenem, which is licensed in many European countries and is being considered for licensure by the U.S. Food and Drug Administration; and panipenem/betamipron, which is registered in Japan. Other carbapenems, e.g., biapenem, are not likely to be registered widely. Still other derivatives are being investigated but will not reach large-scale clinical trials before 1997.

Carbapenems are beta-lactam antibiotics with a nucleus structure containing a carbon instead of a sulfur in the 1-position and an unsaturated bond between carbons 2 and 3 in the five-membered ring structure.

PHARMACOLOGY AND PHARMACOKINETICS

Like other beta-lactam antibiotics, carbapenems are water-soluble, lipid-insoluble drugs. Imipenem dissolves poorly and requires a volume of 200 mL per gram to dissolve. One gram of meropenem is easily dissolved in 5 mL of water or saline.

Imipenem and meropenem are not absorbed from the gastrointestinal tract after oral administration, so are given by the intravenous or intramuscular route. If imipenem is given intramuscularly, it is administered as a suspension. Intravenous imipenem is given as intermittent infusion with the drug dissolved in 100 mL of saline per 500 mg of imipenem. Meropenem can be given as an intramuscular injection, an intravenous bolus in 5 mL of water, or an intermittent infusion.

Imipenem is metabolized in the kidneys by a dipeptidase, dehydropeptidase-I (DHP-I), which hydrolyses the beta-lactam bond and renders imipenem inactive.[1] This metabolism leads to low and highly varying concentrations of imipenem in the urine if the drug is given alone. Moreover, imipenem given alone to rabbits is nephrotoxic.[2] These factors resulted in the development of cilastatin, an inhibitor of DHP-I that in a 1:1 combination with imipenem blocks the renal metabolism of imipenem and inhibits its nephrotoxicity.[3, 4] Meropenem is less susceptible to DHP-I and also less nephrotoxic in rabbits and therefore does not require a DHP-I inhibitor.[5]

The plasma pharmacokinetics of imipenem and meropenem are summarized in Table 6–5. Cilastatin as well as the open-lactam metabolites of imipenem and meropenem ("imipenemoyl" and "meropenemoyl," respectively) have pharmacokinetics very similar to those of imipenem, with the exception that they are excreted more slowly than imipenem and meropenem in patients with renal impairment.[7–9]

Table 6–5. PHARMACOKINETICS OF IMIPENEM* AND MEROPENEM†

Kinetic Parameter	Imipenem	Meropenem
Maximal plasma concentration	68 mg/L	55 mg/L
Elimination half-life	1.0 h	1.0 h
Plasma clearance	185 mL/min	254 mL/min
Renal clearance	134 mL/min	199 mL/min
Urinary excretion of parent compound	75%	79%

Modified from Norrby SR: Carbapenems. Med Clin North Am 1995; 79: 745–759.
*Given in a 1:1 combination with cilastatin
†After single 1 g dose

Also in such patients, the plasma half-lives of imipenem and meropenem are increased, although to a lesser extent.[8, 9]

Both imipenem and meropenem are less than 20% protein bound in plasma.[5, 10] This feature, in combination with the fact that the molecules are relatively small with a molecular weight of less than 400, should result in relatively good tissue penetration. However, limited data are available on the tissue penetration of imipenem, because of the instability of the compound and the complicated assay method that must be used. As reviewed by Buckley and colleagues[10] and Hutchison and colleagues,[11] tissue concentrations of imipenem and meropenem are in agreement with what can be expected, i.e., high concentrations are achieved in tissues that are well perfused, and both drugs pass poorly over biologic membranes with tight junctions, e.g., into cerebrospinal fluid of individuals with uninflamed meninges. Table 6–6 summarizes the available data on penetration of imipenem and meropenem into tissues and body fluids of interest for the ENT specialist.

SPECTRUM OF ACTIVITY AND MODE OF ACTION

Carbapenems inhibit bacterial cell-wall synthesis by binding to penicillin-binding proteins (PBPs). In Enterobacericeae, imipenem binds primarily to PBP-2 and PBP-1 and meropenem binds to PBP-2 and PBP-3. This is in contrast to the aminopenicillins and cephalosporins, for which PBP-3 is the prime target. In gram-positive bacteria, carbapenems seem to have better affinity than penicillins for PBP-2′, the PBP responsible for penicillin resistance in staphylococci and pneumococci.[15] Carbapenems are bactericidal and rapidly lyse susceptible bacterial cells without filament formation. A theoretic advantage of this feature is that less endotoxin is released than after lysis of filaments resulting from the actions of penicillins or cephalosporins.[16]

Table 6–6. TISSUE PENETRATION OF IMIPENEM AND MEROPENEM

Tissue	Antibiotic and Dose	Mean Concentration (mg/kg or L) and Time	Reference
Tonsil	Imipenem 0.5 g	2.2 after 17–50 min	12
Mastoid	Imipenem 0.5 g	3.6 after 40 min	12
mucosa	Imipenem 0.5 g	10.7 after 30–40 min	12
Sinus mucosa	Imipenem 0.1 g	0.6–0.9 after 1–8 h	13
Cerebrospinal fluid			
Normal	Meropenem 1 g	0.1–0.2 after 0.5–2 h	11
Meningitis	Imipenem 1 g	1.1–2.3 after 1–6 h	13
	Meropenem 40 mg/kg	0.3–3.3 after 1.5–3.5 h	14

The antibacterial spectra of imipenem and meropenem are very broad and include most pathogenic aerobic and anaerobic, gram-negative and gram-positive rods and cocci.[17] Resistance is seen mainly in *Stenotrophomas (Xanthomonas) maltophilia, Burkholderia (Pseudomonas) cepacia, Corynebacterium jeikeium, Enterococcus faecium*, and occasionally in other enterococcal species. Methicillin-resistant staphylococci vary in their susceptibility to carbapenems, as do pneumococci with reduced susceptibility or resistance to penicillin.[15] Generally, meropenem and imipenem are more active than cephalosporins, including cefotaxime, against these organisms but may still not be sufficiently more active than imipenem against gram-negatives (aerobes and anaerobes), whereas imipenem is more active against gram-positive aerobes and anaerobes. For most species, these differences are not clinically important. However, that may not be the case for *H. influenzae, Proteus* species, and *P. aeruginosa*, which are considerably more susceptible to meropenem than to imipenem, and for enterococci and highly penicillin-resistant pneumococci, which may be easier to treat with imipenem than with meropenem, although carbapenems may not be the antibiotics of choice for the latter infections.

One reason for the broad spectrum of activity of meropenem and imipenem is their high degree of beta-lactamase stability. Only zinc-containing enzymes have been shown to hydrolyze carbapenems, and such enzymes have so far been seen mainly in *S. maltophilia*. When resistance emerges against carbapenems, something that has been seen most commonly in *P. aeruginosa*, it is mediated by altered outer membrane proteins (porins) of the bacterial cell wall. Since carbapenems seem to use different porins from other beta-lactam antibiotics, carbapenem resistance in *P. aeruginosa* is usually not indicative of cross-resistance against cephalosporins or penicillins.

CLINICAL USE IN EAR, NOSE, AND THROAT INFECTIONS

Imipenem/cilastatin and meropenem are not commonly used in the treatment of ENT infections. However, the antibacterial spectrum of these drugs, which includes a majority of pathogenic bacteria, makes them suitable for treatment of serious hospital-acquired infections, especially when mixed aerobic-anaerobic flora are causing the infections. Also, in the treatment of chronic suppurative otitis or necrotizing otitis externa due to *P. aeruginosa*, the carbapenems are alternative antimicrobial agents.

Both imipenem/cilastatin and meropenem have been evaluated as empiric monotherapy in patients with neutropenia after treatment with cytostatic drugs and have been found to be equally as effective as classic combinations of beta-lactams and aminoglycosides.[6, 18]

Meropenem has been evaluated in the treatment of bacterial meningitis and has been found to be as effective as cefotaxime or ceftriaxone, although clinical experience is still rather limited.[19, 20] Imipenem/cilastatin, on the other hand, cannot be used for this indication because of a high frequency of seizures in children with meningitis treated with that drug.[21]

SAFETY

The safety documentation for both imipenem/cilastatin and meropenem indicates that the two drugs have a high level of safety.[10, 22] With imipenem/cilastatin, two adverse reactions, nausea and neurotoxicity, have been reported at higher than usual frequencies. Animal studies indicate that imipenem/cilastatin is about 10 times more neurotoxic than benzylpenicillin and that meropenem is less neurotoxic than imipenem/cilastatin.[23, 24] In clinical studies of meropenem, no significant differences were found between imipenem/cilastatin and meropenem with respect to these reactions. However, patients with neurologic diseases were excluded from these studies, and imipenem was administered over long periods to avoid nausea.

Hypersensitivity reactions have been reported in low frequencies with both imipenem/cilastatin and meropenem. However, because the metabolites of both drugs, "imipenemoyl" and "meropenemoyl," are chemically similar to penicilloyl, it should be assumed that the risk of cross-allergenicity is high in patients who have reacted to penicillin with IgE-mediated (type I) reactions (urticaria, anaphylactic reaction) and that penicillin allergy contraindicates carbapenems and vice versa.

DOSAGE

Imipenem is given at 0.5–1 g every 6–8 hours. The lower dose is recommended for treatment of infections originating from the urinary tract, whereas the higher dose should be employed in patients with *Pseudomonas* infections or neutropenia.

Meropenem doses are 0.5–2 g every 8 hours, with the 6 g/day dose being intended for treatment of bacterial meningitis in adults.

References

1. Kropp H, Sundelof JG, Hajdu R, et al.: Metabolism of thienamycin and related carbapenem antibiotics by the renal dipeptidase: Dehydropeptidase-I. Antimicrob Agents Chemother 1982; 22: 62–70.
2. Kahan FM, Kropp H, Sundelof JG, et al.: Thienamycin; development

of imipenem-cilastatin. J Antimicrob Chemother 1983; 12 (suppl D): 1–35.

3. Norrby SR Alestig K, Björnegård B, Burman LÅ, et al.: Urinary recovery of N-formimidoyl thienamycin (MK0787) as affected by coadministration of N-formimidoyl thienamycin dehydropeptidase inhibitors. Antimicrob Agents Chemother 1983; 23: 300–307.

4. Norrby SR: Imipenem/cilastatin: Rationale for a fixed combination. Rev Infect Dis 1985; 7 (suppl): S477–S481.

5. Bax RP, Bastain W, Featherstone A, et al.: The pharmacokinetics of meropenem in volunteers. J Antimicrob Chemother 1980; 24 (suppl A): 311–320.

6. Norrby SR: Carbapenems. Med Clin North Am 1995; 79: 745–759.

7. Norrby SR, Rogers JD, Ferber F, et al.: Disposition of radiolabeled imipenem and cilastatin in normal human volunteers. Antimicrob Agents Chemother 1984; 26: 707–714.

8. Gibson TP, Demetriades Jl, Bland JA: Imipenem/ cilastatin: Pharmacokinetic profile in renal insufficiency. Am J Med 1985; 78 (suppl 6A): 54.

9. Christensson BA, Nilsson-Ehle I, Hutchison M, et al.: Pharmacokinetics of meropenem in subjects with various degree of renal impairment. Antimicrob Agents Chemother 1992; 36: 1532–1537.

10. Buckley MM, Brogden RN, Barradell LB, Goa KL: Imipenem/cilastatin: A reappraisal of its antibacterial activity, pharmacokinetic properties and therapeutic efficacy. Drugs 1992; 44: 408–444.

11. Hutchison M, Faulkner KL, Turner PJ, et al.: A compilation of meropenem tissue distribution data. J Antimicrob Chemother 1995; 36 (suppl A): 43–46.

12. Suzuki K, Baba S, Kiroshita H, et al.: Laboratory and clinical studies of imipenem in the field of otorhinolaryngology. Chemother (Tokyo) 1985; 33 (suppl 4): 1109–1117.

13. Dealy DH, Duma RJ, Tartaglione TA, et al.: Penetration of Primaxin (N-formidoyl thienamycin and cilastatin) into human cerebrospinal fluid [abstract S-78-4]. Presented at 14th International Congress of Chemotherapy; June, 23–28, 1985; Kyoto, Japan.

14. Dagan R, Velghe L, Rodda JL, Klugman KP: Penetration of meropenem into the cerebrospinal fluid of patients with inflamed meninges. J Antimicrob Chemother 1994; 31: 175–179.

15. Kayser FH, Morenzoni G, Strassle A, et al.: Activity of meropenem against gram-positive bacteria. J Antimicrob Chemother 1989; 24 (suppl A): 101.

16. Jackson JJ, Kropp H: Beta-lactam antibiotic-induced release of free endotoxin: In vitro comparison of penicillin-binding protein (PBP) 2–specific imipenem and PBP 3–specific ceftazidime. J Infect Dis 1992; 165: 1033–1038.

17. Edwards JR: Meropenem: A microbiological overview. J Antimicrob Chemother 1995; 36 (suppl A): 1–17.

18. Boogaerts MA: Anti-infective strategies in neutropenia. J Antimicrob Chemother 1995; 36 (suppl A): 167–178.

19. Schmutzhard E, Williams KJ, Vukmirovits G, et al.: A randomised comparison of meropenem with cefotaxime or ceftriaxone for the treatment of bacterial meningitis in adults. J Antimicrob Chemother 1995; 36 (suppl A): 85–97.

20. Klugman KP, Dagan R: The Meropenem Meningitis Study Group: Randomized comparison of meropenem with cefotaxime for treatment of bacterial meningitis. Antimicrob Agents Chemother 1995; 39: 1140–1146.

21. Wong VK, Wright HT Jr, Ross LA, et al.: Imipenem/cilastatin treatment of bacterial meningitis in children. Pediatr Infect Dis J 1991; 10: 122–125.

22. Norrby SR, Newell PA, Faulkner KL, Lesky W: Safety profile of meropenem: International clinical experience based on the first 3125 patients treated with meropenem. J Antimicrob Chemother 1995; 36 (suppl A): 207–223.

23. Schliamser SE, Broholm KA, Norrby SR: Comparative neurotoxicity of benzylpenicillin, imipenem/cilastatin and FCE 22101, a new injectable penem. J Antimicrob Chemother 1988; 22: 687–696.

24. Patel JB, Giles RE: Meropenem: Evidence of lack of proconvulsive tendency in mice. J Antimicrob Chemother 1989: 24 (suppl A): 307–309.

Diane M. Cappelletty
Lisbeth K. Nordstrom-Lerner
Stephen A. Lerner

CHAPTER SEVEN

Aminoglycosides

DESCRIPTION OF DRUG

Aminoglycoside antibiotics have been available since the development of streptomycin in the late 1940s. Streptomycin, the only available member of the streptidine group of aminoglycosides, has been replaced by members of the 2-deoxystreptamine group for the treatment of infections caused by aerobic gram-negative bacilli. However, streptomycin retains some utility in the treatment of tuberculosis and enterococcal infections as well as for various uncommon infections, such as tularemia, plague, and brucellosis. The toxicity of neomycin precludes its systemic use, but it is used topically in the gastrointestinal tract, on the skin, and in the ear and eye. Kanamycin has been superseded by the more recently introduced aminoglycosides gentamicin, tobramycin, netilmicin, and amikacin because of their improved activity against *Pseudomonas aeruginosa* and other kanamycin-resistant strains of gram-negative bacilli, especially hospital strains that have acquired resistance to many antibacterial agents.

Highly polar, water-soluble polycations, aminoglycosides are generally stable to heat and to pH change within the range 5–8. They interact with penicillins, resulting in mutual inactivation of the two drugs.[1] Amikacin and netilmicin are reported to be less susceptible than gentamicin or tobramycin to such inactivation. Because of the potential for inactivation, aminoglycosides should be infused separately from penicillins, and serum specimens for aminoglycoside assay should be assayed promptly or kept frozen prior to assay if a penicillin is present.

MECHANISM OF ACTION

Aminoglycosides bind to the smaller subunit of bacterial ribosomes and cause both irreversible cessation of protein synthesis and mistranslation of messenger RNA into false proteins. Aminoglycosides are bactericidal, and killing takes place fairly rapidly. The cidal effect is concentration-dependent (i.e., the higher the concentration of the drug, the more rapid and extensive the killing).[2–4] Aminoglycosides also exhibit a postantibiotic effect against gram-negative bacilli; the surviving bacteria continue to be inhibited for hours after the concentration of the drug has declined below the minimum inhibitory concentration.[5] Aminoglycosides enter bacteria by active uptake. Because this uptake of aminoglycosides requires oxidative metabolism and is diminished by acidic conditions, it is clear why anaerobic bacteria are intrinsically resistant to aminoglycosides, and even facultative aerobic bacteria are relatively resistant when growing under anaerobic conditions. In combination with agents that interfere with bacterial cell-wall biosynthesis, such as the beta-lactams and vancomycin, aminoglycosides may exhibit synergistic activity against some bacteria, as a result of mutual enhancement of penetration of the drugs into the cell.

SPECTRUM OF ACTIVITY

Aminoglycosides are active against a broad spectrum of aerobic and facultative bacteria, including gram-positive cocci and gram-negative bacilli, but there is no useful activity against anaerobes. The principal activity of aminoglycosides is directed against gram-negative bacilli, including *Pseudomonas, Acinetobacter,* and other nonfermentative bacteria. Against gram-positive cocci, aminoglycosides are used adjunctively for their synergistic action with anti–cell-wall antibiotics, such as ampicillin or vancomycin for enterococci and nafcillin or vancomycin for staphylococci.

The utility of streptomycin is restricted practically to mycobacterial infections, enterococcal infections, plague, tularemia, and brucellosis. Although kanamycin has activity against mycobacteria, enterococci, and Enterobacteriaceae, it has generally been replaced by other aminoglycosides for each of these classes of bacteria.

The principal aminoglycosides for systemic therapy today are gentamicin, tobramycin, and amikacin. Netilmicin is rarely used in the United States and is not considered further. Against Enterobacteriaceae, the three most widely used agents are generally equivalently active, although gentamicin is often more potent than tobramycin against isolates of *Serratia marcescens.* Gentamicin, tobramycin, and amikacin are all active against *P. aeruginosa,* although tobramycin is generally more potent than gentamicin against this organism. Amikacin is less potent on a molar basis than gentamicin or tobramycin, but the higher serum levels allowable by its lower molar toxicity compensate for this feature and produce activity equivalent to that of the other aminoglycosides against susceptible strains.

PHARMACOKINETICS

Absorption

Aminoglycosides administered as an intramuscular injection achieve peak serum concentrations 30–90 minutes after the injection that are similar to those achieved 30 minutes after a 30-minute intravenous infusion. Poor vascular perfusion impedes absorption from intramuscular administration. Aminoglycosides are poorly absorbed from the gastrointestinal tract.

Distribution

The volume of distribution of aminoglycosides is similar to that of the extracellular fluid space[6, 7]; thus, the presence of edema and/or ascites may markedly increase the volume of distribution. Protein binding is less than 10% and is considered negligible.[8] The alpha phase or distributive phase for aminoglycosides occurs rapidly following intravenous administration and is considered negligible by approximately 30 minutes after the end of a 30-minute infusion.

Elimination

Aminoglycosides are excreted unchanged and almost completely by the kidneys. They are filtered by the glomerulus, and only a very small fraction is actively absorbed into the proximal tubular cells.[9] The beta phase or excretory phase represents renal excretion due primarily to glomerular filtration; thus, aminoglycoside clearance correlates with glomerular filtration rate. The half-life of aminoglycosides in adults with normal renal function ranges from 1.5 to 3.5 hours.[10, 11] A decrease in renal function prolongs the half-life of aminoglycosides, so dosages need to be reduced in patients with renal impairment. There is also a gamma phase of excretion that is very slow, with a half-life of 30–700 hours,[12] and that probably represents release of the aminoglycosides from the proximal tubular cells.

Penetration Into Cerebrospinal Fluid and Perilymph

Aminoglycosides are highly polar compounds and do not penetrate the blood-brain barrier well, even in the presence of meningeal inflammation. If aminoglycosides are needed to treat meningitis, intraventricular (per reservoir) or intrathecal administration is recommended along with systemic aminoglycoside therapy. The average volume of cerebrospinal fluid in an adult is 160 mL, and administration of 4 mg of a preservative-free aminoglycoside would yield a therapeutic concentration of approximately 25 μg/mL. The dose is repeated daily.

Pharmacokinetic parameters of aminoglycosides in the inner ear (perilymph) are significantly different from those in plasma. It was once thought that aminoglycosides accumulate in the inner ear, but this theory has been disproved.[13, 14] Entry into perilymph from the blood stream is slow, and peak concentrations in perilymph never exceed peak plasma concentrations. Furthermore, the elimination half-life is longer in perilymph than in plasma. In studies by Tran Ba Huy and colleagues,[15, 16] a dose of 4 mg/kg intramuscularly in rats or 100 mg/kg intramuscularly in guinea pigs yielded peak perilymph concentrations of only 0.143 μg/mL and 0.06 μg/mL, respectively. The half-life of the drug in the perilymph ranged from 3.2 to 13 hours.[15, 16]

CLINICAL USES OF AMINOGLYCOSIDES

General

Aminoglycosides are used to treat a variety of conditions, including nosocomial aerobic gram-negative bacillary infec-

tions. For topical use, both neomycin and gentamicin are available. Both are directed against *Staphylococcus aureus* and aerobic gram-negative bacilli; among the latter, *P. aeruginosa* is treated by gentamicin but not by neomycin. Systemic therapy with gentamicin, tobramycin, or amikacin is generally by intravenous infusion, although aminoglycosides may also be injected intramuscularly.

Traditionally, aminoglycosides formed the bulwark of chemotherapy against infections caused by aerobic gram-negative bacilli. Because of the usage patterns of aminoglycosides in the United States and the enzymatic mechanisms of resistance against these drugs, the probability of resistance to these drugs among strains of gram-negative bacilli is generally: gentamicin > tobramicin > amikacin. Because the patterns of aminoglycoside resistance are fairly stable for a given medical center, aminoglycoside therapy is initiated presumptively, according to probabilities of resistance, and then the therapeutic regimen can be altered, if necessary, on the basis of definitive susceptibility results when they are available.

For therapy of gram-negative bacillary infections, gentamicin is usually employed as the first-line aminoglycoside, unless the clinical and epidemiologic setting suggests a high probability of *P. aeruginosa* or other organisms for which another aminoglycoside is likely to have superior activity. Amikacin is generally restricted to use against organisms that are resistant to both gentamicin and tobramycin, in an attempt to preserve the activity of this "ultimate" aminoglycoside. For synergistic use in the treatment of enterococcal or staphylococcal infections, gentamicin is generally the preferred aminoglycoside because strains that are resistant to synergism with gentamicin are resistant to tobramycin and amikacin as well. Occasional strains of gentamicin-resistant enterococci may be susceptible to the synergistic activity of streptomycin with ampicillin or vancomycin. With the advent of alternative, less toxic agents for aerobic gram-negative bacilli, such as extended-spectrum beta-lactams (e.g., antipseudomonal penicillins, third-generation cephalosporins, aztreonam, and imipenem) and fluoroquinolones (e.g., ciprofloxacin), the role of aminoglycosides against these organisms has diminished. Therefore, one must question in which situations one might still rely on aminoglycosides for therapy.

Current use of aminoglycosides depends principally on two attributes of these drugs. Although the efficacy of aminoglycosides has been compromised over time by the development of resistance in the target pathogens, this resistance has generally appeared slowly, and resistance levels are fairly stable and predictable within the organisms of individual medical centers.[17] In contrast, resistance to extended-spectrum beta-lactams and fluoroquinolones has emerged rapidly, even during the treatment of individual patients.[18–20] Whereas one can generally select an aminoglycoside for initial, presumptive therapy with reasonable confidence of activity against aerobic gram-negative bacilli, the activity of a beta-lactam or fluoroquinolone may be less assured because susceptibility to these agents is less predictable. Therefore, in practice, if a serious infection requires urgent, effective treatment against aerobic gram-negative bacilli, such as in life-threatening gram-negative bacteremia, one would likely use an aminoglycoside in addition to a beta-lactam for initial therapy. After several days, when the patient has presumably improved and the situation has clarified, therapy can be shifted to an appropriate alternative regimen without an aminoglycoside.

The other principal indication for the use of an aminoglycoside is for synergistic activity with an anti–cell-wall agent against a therapeutically problematic organism, such as *Enterococcus* (gentamicin plus ampicillin or vancomycin) or *P. aeruginosa* (usually tobramycin or amikacin plus an antipseudomonal beta-lactam, such as ceftazidime or piperacillin). Alternatively, a fluoroquinolone may be used to treat *P. aeruginosa,* but there is a risk of emergence of resistance, especially if a large number of organisms are present at the site of infection.

Otolaryngology

Some of the clinical indications for use of aminoglycosides in otolaryngology are malignant and other external otitis, chronic otitis media, sinusitis in cystic fibrosis patients, and Meniere's disease.

Otitis externa is often treated with aural toilet, followed by administration of ototopical antibiotic preparations.[21, 22] The choice of ototopical preparation varies among physicians; however, the most commonly prescribed are Cortisporin (neomycin; polymyxin B; hydrocortisone) suspension and gentamicin.[23] Malignant external otitis can be treated by high-dose systemic therapy with an aminoglycoside and an antipseudomonal penicillin or cephalosporin.[24–26] Ioannides-Demos and colleagues[26] examined high-dose (single daily dose) tobramycin plus several different antipseudomonal beta-lactams in the long-term treatment of malignant external otitis. All patients underwent long-term oral therapy with ciprofloxacin after their course of therapy with tobramycin and a beta-lactam. The six patients who were assessed were all cured. The duration of tobramycin therapy ranged from 58 to 154 days. Audiometric and renal function tests were performed weekly. The mean peak tobramycin concentration ($\pm$ SD) was 10.8 $\pm$ 3.1 μg/mL. Ototoxicity was not detected in any of the patients. Two patients had transient increases in serum creatinine concentrations, reflecting modest, reversible nephrotoxicity. Aminoglycoside/beta-lactam therapy was once the only available therapeutic regimen, but as in the study just described, such therapy is often followed by an oral fluoroquinolone. In fact, malignant external otitis may be treated successfully with long-term fluoroquinolone therapy alone[24] (see Chapter 9), although the probability of selection of quinolone-resistant mutant strains exists.

Chronic otitis media is often managed medically by any combination of aural toilet, systemic antibiotics, and/or ototopical antibiotics with or without steroids. The most prevalent pathogens are staphylococci, coliforms, and *Pseudomonas.* Instillation of a topical aminoglycoside into an ear with a perforated tympanic membrane is theoretically hazardous because of ototoxicity induced in animal models. However, neither hearing loss nor vestibular dysfunction has been documented in the literature as a result of ototopical aminoglycoside instillation in humans. Therefore, such therapy is occasionally prescribed for the patient who has chronic otitis media with otorrhea that is unresponsive to other therapies.

Commonly prescribed ototopical preparations contain neomycin, which is not active against *Pseudomonas,* and this lack of activity may account for treatment failures.[27] Browning and colleagues[28] reported in 1983 that efficacy of aural toilet, systemic antibiotics, or ototopical neomycin without steroids was approximately 30%, which was no better than spontaneous resolution of the infection. However, the use of ototopical aminoglycosides with steroids has been found to be superior to steroid alone or to placebo. In 1988, Browning and colleagues[29] compared gentamicin plus hydrocortisone with placebo ear drops. After 4–6 weeks of therapy, they demonstrated 51% efficacy in the gentamicin/hydrocortisone-treated patients and only 24% efficacy in the placebo group. Crowther and Simpson[30] compared the efficacy of gentamicin plus hydrocortisone with betamethasone alone. After 2–4 weeks of therapy, an efficacious response of 80% was observed in the gentamicin/hydrocortisone treatment group and only 29% in the steroid-only group.

Chronic sinusitis is a common problem in patients with cystic fibrosis. Routine medical management of sinusitis in this patient population often fails because of poor penetration of antibiotics into the sinus cavities, which contain characteristically thick secretions, and/or because of the recovery of antibiotic-resistant organisms. Davidson and colleagues[31] reported that endoscopic sinus surgery followed by tobramycin and saline nasal irrigations appeared to be effective in treating chronic sinusitis in cystic fibrosis patients who have undergone lung transplantation. However, more controlled prospective studies are needed to confirm that *P. aeruginosa* colonization is eradicated from the nasal passage by this procedure.

Intratympanic instillation of aminoglycosides is one method used in the treatment of recalcitrant, incapacitating Meniere's disease. Gentamicin and streptomycin are the two most commonly used agents. Nedzelski and colleagues[32] treated 67 patients with unilateral disease with 1 mL of 26.7 mg/mL gentamicin solution three times daily intratympanically for a maximum of 12 doses. Vertigo was eliminated in 83% of patients and controlled in the rest. Hearing loss occurred in approximately 10%. Pyykkö and colleagues[33] injected one to four 0.5 mL doses of gentamicin, 30 mg/mL, intratympanically in patients with bilateral disease. They found that 2 years after treatment, vertigo was still eliminated in 11 of 14 patients and controlled in the other 3. Two ears showed mild auditory deficits after therapy, and three ears showed mild improvement. Magnusson and colleagues[34, 35] also studied the use of two doses of intratympanic gentamicin (0.5–0.9 mL of 30 mg/mL) in five patients with Meniere's disease. They found that all patients had complete elimination of their vertigo. No relief from tinnitus was observed, and auditory testing revealed no significant change following therapy. Because of the delayed onset and progressive nature of the vestibular effect observed with gentamicin, these authors suggest cautious use of low doses to reduce the likelihood of auditory toxicity.

Streptomycin perfusion of the labyrinth directly was examined by Shea and Ge,[36, 37] during the 1980s, but they have since abandoned this approach. They perfused 25 μg of streptomycin directly into the perilymph of the lateral semicircular canal. The rate of relief from dizzy spells was high; however, the incidence of hearing loss was also unacceptably high. Shea and Ge[37] have since reported administering 1 g of streptomycin intravenously as well as 0.5 mL of hyaluronan containing 60 mg of streptomycin through the drum and into the round window niche, once daily for 3 consecutive days. Three to eight months posttreatment of their 24 patients, 96% had complete relief from dizzy spells, and only one had impairment of hearing.

ADVERSE EFFECTS

The principal types of toxicity associated with aminoglycoside therapy are neuromuscular blockade, nephrotoxicity, and ototoxicity. The neuromuscular blockade is reversible and is considered to result from an antagonistic relationship between calcium and aminoglycosides.[38] The incidence of neuromuscular blockade is rare, and this phenomenon can be reversed more rapidly by administration of calcium gluconate. Hypersensitivity reactions to aminoglycosides are also rare. These drugs are not hepatotoxic or phototoxic, and they do not produce inflammation in tissues.

Nephrotoxicity

Nephrotoxicity from aminoglycosides has been associated with uptake and long-term retention of these agents by the proximal tubular cells of the kidney. Accumulation of aminoglycosides in the lysosomes of these cells eventually leads to cell death. Clinically, nephrotoxicity is manifested as azotemia, usually without oliguria. The decline in renal function is generally mild, especially if serum levels of the aminoglycoside and serum creatinine levels are monitored and the dosing is adjusted to avoid excessive accumulation of the drug. Nephrotoxicity is almost always reversible to the baseline pretreatment level of renal function, as a result of regeneration of the proximal tubular cells.[39, 40] The incidence of nephrotoxicity has been reported in the range 0%–50%[41–43]; naturally, the absolute incidence depends on the definition of nephrotoxicity that is used.[44, 45] Factors that have been associated with increased risk of nephrotoxicity include older age, hypotension, the presence of liver disease, duration of therapy, and concomitant treatment with other nephrotoxic agents.[41–46]

Ototoxicity

All aminoglycosides have the potential for both auditory and vestibular toxicity, but vestibular toxicity is certainly more prominent with streptomycin and perhaps also with gentamicin. This differential toxic potential forms the basis of the use of these agents to obliterate vestibular function in the treatment of Meniere's disease.

Histopathologic studies of aminoglycoside ototoxicity in animals have revealed that the principal targets are the sensory hair cells of the organ of Corti and of the vestibular epithelia.[47, 48] Similar reports in humans are few, but the findings of cochlear hair cell loss parallel those in animals.[49–52] One histopathologic study of two cases with ototoxicity reported preservation of hair cells but reduction in cochlear ganglion cells.[53]

The subcellular mechanisms by which aminoglycosides cause hair cell damage are still unknown. Several theories exist and are as follows: the slow elimination of aminoglycosides from the sensory cells and a saturation of the detoxification capabilities of the cells[54]; binding of aminoglycosides to polyphosphoinositides[55]; inhibition of ornithine decarboxylase[55]; and cytopathic effect of a metabolite of the aminoglycoside.[55–59] There may also be a hereditary component to hearing loss associated with aminoglycosides, which is due to a mutation of mitochondrial DNA.[60]

Symptoms of auditory toxicity include hearing loss, tinnitus, and a feeling of fullness in the ear. Symptoms of severe vestibular toxicity may appear as nausea, vomiting, vertigo, nystagmus, and difficulty with gait, especially in the dark or on an uneven surface. Furthermore, some patients may report difficulty in fixating visually on objects, especially when the head is moving.

Cochlear and vestibular damage may occur in the same patient,[61, 62] and ototoxicity may appear unilaterally or bilaterally.[61, 62] The ototoxic effect may progress after cessation of therapy, and symptoms may not appear until after treatment.[62] Severe otototoxicity is generally irreversible because cochlear and vestibular hair cells do not regenerate.[62, 63] However, reversibility can be demonstrated in some cases, which are usually mild or even subclinical.[61–64]

Cochlear toxicity is generally assessed by pure-tone audiometric testing of air and bone conduction at doubling frequencies from 0.5 to 8.0 kHz.[62, 65] To improve the testing at the higher frequencies, 3.0 and 6.0 kHz are often also included.[66] Although criteria for defining auditory toxicity have not been standardized, an increase in threshold from baseline of at least 15 dB in either ear is considered significant, and such a change is often required for at least two frequencies in the same ear.[67] Typically, the earliest effects of auditory toxicity are detectable at the higher frequencies. Therefore, testing at frequencies above the 8.0-kHz limit of conventional audiometers may increase sensitivity for early detection, but because of technical problems and lack of standardization, such high-frequency audiometry is not applied routinely in aminoglycoside toxicity.[62, 65, 67]

Because the testing of vestibular function is more arduous and poorly standardized, relatively few patients have been evaluated objectively for vestibular toxicity in clinical studies.[41, 62] Responses to caloric stimulation with water or air are recorded on an electronystagmogram.[62, 66, 68]

Although prospective clinical studies of aminoglycoside toxicity have yielded a broad range of incidences, surveys of the literature have estimated an overall incidence of cochlear toxicity in the range 5%–15%,[41, 69] and for vestibular toxicity a similar[69] or somewhat lower[41] incidence. Comparative studies suggest that the relative potentials for ototoxicity are comparable for gentamicin, tobramycin, and amikacin, but netilmicin appears to be associated with somewhat lower rates of ototoxicity.[41, 69, 70] It has been estimated that symptomatic ototoxicity occurs in less than 0.5% of patients treated parenterally with gentamicin, tobramycin, or amikacin.[71] Various analyses of risk factors for aminoglycoside ototoxicity have implicated age, elevation of trough levels of aminoglycoside in serum (suggesting impairment of renal excretion), development of nephrotoxicity, and duration of therapy.[61, 72–74] Although use of ethacrynic acid appears to increase the risk of ototoxicity with aminoglycosides,[75, 76] and one study suggested that treatment with furosemide was a risk factor,[74] other studies have failed to implicate furosemide use as a risk factor.[77] Vancomycin therapy enhances the nephrotoxic potential for aminoglycosides, but it appears to have no effect on the ototoxicity of these drugs in humans. The effects of prolonged duration of therapy on risk of ototoxicity and correlation with higher trough levels in serum suggest that the area under the aminoglycoside serum concentration–time curve may be important for the development of ototoxicity, perhaps by fostering the penetration of drug into the inner ear.

The risk of toxicity from ototopical preparations containing aminoglycosides is not clear and is controversial. Two factors that make assessment of toxicity difficult are (1) most ototopical preparations contain several different agents that are ototoxic, such as propylene glycol, alcohol, and an aminoglycoside (neomycin or gentamicin)[78] and (2) the risk of hearing impairment from the underlying disease. In a 1992 survey of otolaryngologists, 80% agreed with the statement, "The risk for ototoxicity of otitis media is as great as or greater than the risk for ototoxicity of an ototopical preparation."[79] Several animal studies have demonstrated sensorineural hearing loss with ototopical administration of neomycin and gentamicin.[80–82]

Extrapolation of results concerning ototoxicity of aminoglycosides from animal studies to humans should be viewed with caution because the round window is more exposed in experimental animals than in humans, owing to differences in orientation of the round window and in the surrounding structures. Additionally, the thickness of the round window membrane differs between the animals tested (13–15 μm) and humans (50–60 μm). Studies that examine ototoxicity of topical aminoglycosides in humans have not supported the results from the animal models. Welling and colleagues[83] studied 50 patients receiving neomycin/polymyxin B/hydrocortisone for 4 weeks following typanostomy tube insertion. Audiograms prior to insertion and following treatment did not reveal any statistical difference with respect to hearing loss between the treated and untreated ears. Merifield and colleagues[84] studied the ototoxic effects of five different preparations, four containing neomycin and one containing gentamicin, in 44 children with chronic suppurative otitis media. The results did not demonstrate any hearing loss, and the authors concluded that ototopical aminoglycosides are safe and that the risk of toxicity is either quite small or nonexistent. Browning and colleagues[29] compared gentamicin/hydrocortisone drops to placebo ear drops in patients with chronic otitis media. After 4–6 weeks of therapy, they found no difference in hearing between the treated ears and either the contralateral ears or the placebo-treated ears. In contrast to the preceding studies, Podoshin and colleagues[85] found an apparent association between the duration of treatment with topical neomycin and hearing loss. They treated 124 patients with neomycin/polymyxin B/dexamethasone and grouped them according to the following regimens: continuous treatment (no duration indicated); prolonged treatment with 3-month intermissions (not more than 9 months of treatment); and prolonged treatment with 6-month intermissions (not more than 6 months of treatment). Hearing loss was statistically greater in patients who were treated continuously (10.9 dB) than in the second and third groups (3.6 dB and 1.8 dB, respectively).

DOSING OF AMINOGLYCOSIDES AND MONITORING OF PATIENTS

Aminoglycosides are dosed to achieve the peak serum concentrations considered therapeutically effective for the type and site of infection and to allow trough concentrations in serum to fall below 2 μg/mL before the next dose is given in order to reduce the risk of ototoxicity. By conventional administration, gentamicin and tobramycin peak concentrations in serum should be in the range 4–10 μg/mL. Patients with normal renal function can be given 1.5–2.0 mg/kg every 8–12 hours to achieve these ranges of serum levels. Amikacin peak concentrations in serum should be in the range of 15–35 μg/mL and trough concentrations below 10 μg/mL. For this drug, patients with normal renal function can be treated with 7.5 mg/kg every 8–12 hours.

The dosing regimen for all patients with abnormal renal function, and even for patients with normal renal function who are treated with an aminoglycoside for more than 3 days, should be monitored by a pharmacokinetics-based dosing service that is available in most hospitals. Monitoring of serum creatinine should be performed one to three times a week, as long as the patient's renal function appears to be stable, and more often in patients with unstable renal function. Serum concentrations of the aminoglycoside are usually measured within the first 48 hours of therapy, and the dosage is adjusted as needed to achieve the desired range of serum levels. Once the peak and trough levels are in the desired ranges, trough levels are rechecked once or twice a week because a rising trough level is a sensitive indicator of declining renal function. In addition, serum levels should be rechecked within a day or two after any dosage adjustment or in situations of changing renal function or volume of distribution.

Patients treated with aminoglycosides do not generally undergo routine testing of inner ear function. Audiometric or vestibular function testing may be undertaken to confirm a possible symptom of cochlear or vesibular toxicity, although interpretation without a baseline test may be problematic. Patients who are at greater risk for ototoxicity, especially those who undergo long-duration therapy, are receiving a higher dosage to achieve high serum levels, or have marked renal impairment, should be alerted to the possibility of ototoxic symptoms. Such patients may be considered for periodic audiometry, if feasible.

Once-daily administration of high doses of aminoglycosides is challenging the conventional approach to aminoglycoside dosing. The microbiologic rationale for once-daily dosing is based on the concentration-dependent killing and postantibiotic effect associated with aminoglycosides. Indeed, in animal models of infection, once-daily dosing has been shown to be at least as effective as conventional divided dosing, either with adjunctive beta-lactam treatment or in the presence of adequate neutrophils.[4, 86–89] Experiments in animals have shown that the entry of aminoglycosides into the organ of Corti from the general circulation is dose-dependent, with rapid saturation kinetics as in the proximal tubular cells of the kidney.[49, 90] From this observation, it was postulated that the shorter exposure of inner ear tissues to drug in animals treated with larger but less frequent doses should be associated with less ototoxicity. Indeed, less cochlear damage has been observed in animals with once-daily therapy than with multiple divided doses.[91, 92] In other animal experiments, the results have been inconsistent,[93, 94] but in no case has once-daily dosing been associated with increased ototoxicity.

Various investigators have compared once-daily dosing with aminoglycosides with conventional dosing in clinical trials. The dosages of gentamicin, tobramycin, or netilmicin have ranged from 4 to 6 mg/kg every 24 hours, yielding peak serum levels of 12–20 µg/mL, and for amikacin, from 15 to 20 mg/kg every 24 hours yielding 30–60 µg/mL.[95–101] Predose serum levels should be less than with conventional dosing, but the optimal duration for concentrations to be less than 1 µg/mL have yet to be determined. The results suggest that once-daily administration is at least as efficacious as conventional dosing in most patient populations. The incidences of nephrotoxicity and of ototoxicity have been either comparable between the two dosage regimens[95, 98–101] or lower in patients treated with the once-daily regimen.[96, 97]

References

1. McLaughlin JE, Reeves DS: Clinical and laboratory evidence for inactivation of gentamicin and carbenicillin. Lancet 1971; 1: 261–264.
2. Vogelman BS, Craig WA: Postantibiotic effects. J Antimicrob Chemother 1985; 15 (suppl A): 37–46.
3. Vogelman BS, Craig WA: Kinetics of antimicrobial activity. J Pediatr 1986; 108: 835–840.
4. Kapusnik JE, Hackbarth CJ, Chambers HF, et al.: Single, large, daily dosing versus intermittent dosing of tobramycin for treating experimental pseudomonas pneumonia. J Infect Dis 1988; 158: 7–12.
5. Bundtzen RW, Gerber AU, Chon DL, Craig WA: Postantibiotic suppression of bacterial growth. Rev Infect Dis 1981; 3: 28–37.
6. Riff LJ, Jackson GG: Pharmacology of gentamicin in man. J Infect Dis 1971; 124 (suppl): S98–S105.
7. Siber GR, Echeverria P, Smith AL, et al.: Pharmacokinetics of gentamicin in children and adults. J Infect Dis 1975; 132: 637–651.
8. Gordon RC, Regamey C, Kirby WMM: Serum protein binding of the aminoglycoside antibiotics. Antimicrob Agents Chemother 1972; 2: 214–216.
9. Silverblatt FJ, Kuehn C: Autoradiography of gentamicin uptake by the rat proximal tubular cell. Kidney Int 1979; 15: 335–345.
10. Gyselynck A-M, Forrey A, Cutler R: Pharmacokinetics of gentamicin: Distribution and plasma and renal clearance. J Infect Dis 1971; 124 (suppl): S70–S76.
11. Plantier J, Forrey AW, O'Neill MA, et al.: Pharmacokinetics of amikacin in patients with normal or impaired renal function: Radioenzymatic acetylation assay. J Infect Dis 1976; 134 (suppl): S323–S330.
12. Schentag JJ, Jusko WJ: Renal clearance and tissue accumulation of gentamicin. Clin Pharmacol Ther 1977; 22: 364–370.
13. Tran Ba Huy P, Manuel C, Meulemans A: Kinetics of aminoglycoside antibiotics in perilymph and endolymph in animals. In: Lerner SA, Matz GJ, Hawkins JE Jr (eds): Aminoglycoside Ototoxicity. Boston: Little, Brown, 1981, pp 81–97.
14. Federspil P: Pharmacokinetics of aminoglycoside antibiotics in the perilymph. In: Lerner SA, Matz GJ, Hawkins JE Jr (eds): Aminoglycoside Ototoxicity. Boston: Little, Brown, 1981, pp 99–108.
15. Tran Ba Huy P, Manuel C, Meulemans A, et al.: Pharmacokinetics of gentamicin in perilymph and endolymph of the rat as determined by radioimmunoassay. J Infect Dis 1981; 143: 476–486.
16. Tran Ba Huy P, Deffrennes D: Aminoglycoside ototoxicity: Influence of dosage regimen on drug uptake and correlation between membrane binding and some clinical features. Acta Otolaryngol (Stockh) 1988; 105: 511–515.
17. Shimizu K, Kumada T, Hsieh W-C, et al.: Comparison of aminoglycoside resistance patterns in Japan, Formosa, Korea, Chile and the United States. Antimicrob Agents Chemother 1985; 28: 282–288.
18. Hooper DC, Wolfson JS, Ng EY, et al.: Mechanism of action of and resistance to ciprofloxacin. Am J Med 1987; 82 (suppl 4A): 12–20.
19. Dudley MN: Pharmacodynamics and pharmacokinetics of antibiotics with special reference to the fluoroquinolones. Am J Med 1991; 91: 45S–50S.
20. Peloquin CA, Cumbo TJ, Nix DE, et al.: Evaluation of intravenous ciprofloxacin in patients with nosocomial lower respiratory tract infections. Arch Intern Med 1989; 149: 2269–2273.
21. Raza SA, Denholm SW, Wong JCH: An audit of the management of acute otitis externa in an ENT casualty clinic. J Laryngol Otol 1995; 109: 130–133.
22. Barr GD, AL-Khabori M: A randomized prospective comparison of two methods of administering topical treatment in otitis externa. Clin Otolaryngol 1991; 16: 547–548.
23. Lundy LB, Graham MD: Ototoxicity and ototopical medications: A survey of otolaryngologists. Am J Otol 1993; 14: 141–146.
24. Giamarellou H: Malignant otitis externa: The therapeutic evolution of a lethal infection. J Antimicrob Chemother 1992; 30: 745–751.
25. Lucente FE, Parisier SC, Som PM, Arnold LM: Malignant external otitis: A dangerous misnomer? Otolaryngol Head Neck Surg 1982; 90: 266–269.
26. Ioannides-Demos LL, Li SC, Bastone EB, et al.: Absence of toxicity in patients with malignant otitis externa following long-term treatment with high dosage tobramycin. J Antimicrob Chemother 1994; 34: 267–274.
27. Esposito S, Noviello S, D'Errico G, Montanaro C: Topical ciprofloxacin vs. intramuscular gentamicin for chronic otitis media. Arch Otolaryngol Head Neck Surg 1992; 118: 842–844.
28. Browning GG, Picozzi GL, Calder IT, Sweeney G: Controlled trial of medical treatment of active chronic otitis media. Br Med J 1983; 287: 1024.
29. Browning GG, Gatehouse S, Calder IT: Medical management of chronic otitis media: A controlled study. J Laryngol Otol 1988; 102: 491–495.
30. Crowther JA, Simpson D: Medical treatment of chronic otits media: Steroid or antibiotic with steroid ear-drops? Clin Otolaryngol 1991; 16: 142–144.
31. Davidson TM, Murphy C, Mitchell M, et al.: Management of chronic sinusitis in cystic fibrosis. Laryngoscope 1995; 105: 354–358.
32. Nedzelski JM, Chiong CM, Fradet G, et al.: Intratympanic gentamicin instillation as treatment of unilateral Meniere's disease: Update of an ongoing study. Am J Otol 1993; 14: 278–282.
33. Pyykkö I, Ishizaki H, Kaasinen S, Aalto H: Intratympanic gentamicin in bilateral Meniere's disease. Otolaryngol Head Neck Surg 1994; 110: 162–167.
34. Magnusson M, Padoan S: Delayed onset of ototoxic effects of gentamicin in treatment of Meniere's disease. Acta Otolaryngol (Stockh) 1991; 111: 671–676.
35. Magnusson M, Padoan S, Karlberg M, Johansson R: Delayed onset of ototoxic effects of gentamicin in patients with Meniere's disease. Acta Otolaryngol Suppl (Stockh) 1991; 485: 120–122.
36. Shea JJ, Ge X: Factors influencing results with streptomycin perfusion of the labyrinth. Am J Otol 1993; 14: 570–575.
37. Shea JJ, Ge X: Streptomycin perfusion of the labyrinth through the round window plus intravenous streptomycin. Otolaryngol Clin North Am 1994; 27: 317–324.
38. Corrado AP, Demorais IP, Prado WA: Aminoglycoside antibiotics as a tool for the study of the biological role of calcium ions: Historical overview. Acta Physiol Pharmacol Lat Am 1989; 39: 419–430.
39. Lortholary O, Tod M, Cohen Y, Petitjean O: Aminoglycosides. Med Clin North Am 1995; 79: 761–787.
40. Kaloyanides GJ: Renal pharmacology of aminoglycoside antibiotics. Contrib Nephrol 1984; 42: 148–167.
41. Kahlmeter G, Dahlager JI: Aminoglycoside toxicity—a review of clinical studies published between 1975 and 1982. J Antimicrob Chemother 1984; 13 (suppl A): 9–22.
42. Lietman PS, Smith CR: Aminoglycoside nephrotoxicity in humans. Rev Infect Dis 1983; 5 (suppl 2): 284–292.

43. Bertino JS, Booker LA, Franck PA, et al.: Incidence of and significant risk factors for aminoglycoside-associated nephrotoxicity in patients dosed by using individualized pharmacokinetic monitoring. J Infect Dis 1993; 167: 173–179.

44. Lerner SA, Schmitt BA, Seligsohn R, Matz GJ: Comparative study of ototoxicity and nephrotoxicity in patients randomly assigned to treatment with amikacin or gentamicin. Am J Med 1986; 80 (suppl 6B): 98–104.

45. Moore RD, Lerner SA, Levine DP: Nephrotoxicity and ototoxicity of aztreonam versus aminoglycoside therapy in seriously ill nonneutropenic patients. J Infect Dis 1992; 165: 683–688.

46. Sawyers CL, Moore RD, Lerner SA, Smith CR: A model for predicting nephrotoxicity in patients treated with aminoglycosides. J Infect Dis 1986; 153: 1062–1068.

47. Hawkins JE Jr, Johnsson L-G: Histopathology of cochlear and vestibular ototoxicity in laboratory animals. In: Lerner SA, Matz GJ, Hawkins JE Jr (eds): Aminoglycoside Ototoxicity. Boston: Little, Brown, 1981, pp 175–195.

48. Wersäll J: Structural damage to the organ of Corti and the vestibular epithelia caused by aminoglycoside antibiotics in the guinea pig. In: Lerner SA, Matz GJ, Hawkins JE Jr (eds): Aminoglycoside Ototoxicity. Boston: Little, Brown, 1981, pp 197–214.

49. Johnsson L-G, Hawkins JE Jr, Kingsley TC, et al.: Aminoglycoside-induced inner ear pathology in man, as seen by microdissection. In: Lerner SA, Matz GJ, Hawkins JE Jr (eds): Aminoglycoside Ototoxicity. Boston: Little, Brown, 1981, pp 389–408.

50. Nadol JB Jr: Histopathology of human aminoglycoside ototoxicity. In: Lerner SA, Matz GJ, Hawkins JE Jr (eds): Aminoglycoside Ototoxicity. Boston: Little, Brown, 1981, pp 409–434.

51. Backus RM, De Groot JCMJ, Tange RA, Huizing EH: Pathological findings in the human auditory system following long-standing gentamicin ototoxicity. Arch Otorhinolaryngol 1987; 344: 69–73.

52. Huizing EH, De Groot JCMJ: Human cochlea pathology in aminoglycoside ototoxicity—a review. Acta Otolaryngol Suppl (Stockh) 1987; 436: 117–125.

53. Hinojosa R, Lerner SA: Cochlear neural degeneration without hair cell loss in two patients with aminoglycoside ototoxicity. J Infect Dis 1987; 156: 449–455.

54. Aran JM: Current perspectives on inner ear toxicity. Otolaryngol Head Neck Surg 1995; 112: 133–144.

55. Schacht J: Biochemical basis of aminoglycoside ototoxicity. Otolaryngol Clin North Am 1993; 26: 845–856.

56. Takada A, Bledsoe Jr S, Schacht J: An energy-dependent step in aminoglycoside ototoxicity: Prevention of gentamicin ototoxicity during reduced endolymphatic potential. Hear Res 1985; 19: 245–251.

57. Hoffman DW, Whitworth CA, Jones-King KL, Rybak LP: Potentiation of ototoxicity by glutathione depletion. Ann Otol Rhinol Laryngol 1988; 97: 36–41.

58. Huang MY, Schacht J: Formation of a cytotoxic metabolite from gentamicin by liver. Biochem Pharmacol 1990; 40: 11–14.

59. Crann SA, Huang MY, McLaren JD, Schacht J: Formation of a toxic metabolite from gentamicin by a hepatic cytosolic fraction. Biochem Pharmacol 1992; 43: 1835–1839.

60. Hutchin T, Cortopassi G: Proposed molecular and cellular mechanism for aminoglycoside ototoxicity. Antimicrob Agents Chemother 1994; 38: 2517–2520.

61. Lerner SA, Schmitt BA, Seligsohn R, Matz GJ: Comparative study of ototoxicity and nephrotoxicity in patients randomly assigned to treatment with amikacin or gentamicin. Am J Med 1986; 80 (suppl 6B): 98–104.

62. DeOliveira JAA: Audiovestibular Toxicity of Drugs, vols I and II. Boca Raton, Florida: CRC Press, 1989.

63. Tran Ba Huy P, Bernard P, Schacht J: Kinetics of gentamicin uptake and release in the rat: Comparison of inner ear tissues and fluid with other organs. J Clin Invest 1986; 77: 1492–1500.

64. Black FO, Peterka RJ, Elardo SM: Vestibular reflex changes following aminoglycoside-induced ototoxicity. Laryngoscope 1987; 97: 582–586.

65. Thompson PL, Northern JL: Audiometric monitoring of patients treated with ototoxic drugs. In: Lerner SA, Matz GJ, Hawkins JE Jr (eds): Aminoglycoside Ototoxicity. Boston: Little, Brown, 1981, pp 237–245.

66. Mowry HJ, Roeder JW, Matz GJ, Lerner SA: Auditory and vestibular assessment of patients receiving aminoglycosides. In: Lerner SA, Matz GJ, Hawkins JE Jr (eds): Aminoglycoside Ototoxicity. Boston: Little, Brown, 1981, pp. 249–254.

67. Brummett RE, Fox KE: Aminoglycoside-induced hearing loss in humans. Antimicrob Agents Chemother 1989; 33: 797–800.

68. Roeder JW, Mowry HJ, Matz GJ, Lerner SA: Serial vestibular testing in normal subjects. In: Lerner SA, Matz GJ, Hawkins JE Jr (eds): Aminoglycoside Ototoxicity. Boston: Little, Brown, 1981, pp 309–319.

69. Govaerts PJ, Claes J, Van De Heyning PH, et al.: Aminoglycoside-induced ototoxicity. Toxicol Lett 1990; 52: 227–251.

70. Buring JE, Evans DA, Mayreut SL, et al.: Randomized trials of aminoglycoside antibiotics: Quantitative overview. Rev Infect Dis 1988; 10: 951–957.

71. Lietman PS: Aminoglycosides and spectinomycin: Aminocyclitols. In: Mandell GL, Douglas RG Jr, Bennett JE (eds): Principles and Practice of Infectious Diseases, 3rd ed. New York: Churchill Livingstone, 1990, pp 269–284.

72. Moore RD, Smith CR, Lietman PS: Risk factors for the development of auditory toxicity in patients receiving aminoglycosides. J Infect Dis 1984; 149: 23–30.

73. Gatell JM, Ferran F, Araujo V, et al.: Univariate and multivariate analyses of risk factors predisposing to auditory toxicity in patients receiving aminoglycosides. Antimicrob Agents Chemother 1987; 31: 1383–1387.

74. Lerner SA, Matz GJ, Schmitt BA: Prospective, randomized, blinded assessment of nephro- and ototoxicity in patients treated with gentamicin, netilmicin, and tobramycin [abstract 488]. 24th Interscience Conference on Antimicrobial Agents and Chemotherapy, Washington, D.C., 1984.

75. Mathog RH, Klein WJ Jr: Ototoxicity of ethacrynic acid and aminoglycoside antibiotics in uremia. N Engl J Med 1969; 280: 1223–1224.

76. Brummett RE, Brown RT, Himes DL: Quantitative relationships of the ototoxic interaction of kanamycin and ethacrynic acid. Arch Otolaryngol 1979; 105: 240–246.

77. Smith CR, Lietman PS: Effect of furosemide on aminoglycoside-induced nephrotoxicity and auditory toxicity in humans. Antimicrob Agents Chemother 1983; 23: 133–137.

78. Rohn GN, Meyerhoff WL, Wright CG: Ototoxicity of topical agents. Otolaryngol Clin North Am 1993; 26: 747–758.

79. Lundy LB, Graham MD: Ototoxicity and ototopical medications: A survey of otolaryngologists. Am J Otol 1993; 14: 141–146.

80. Meyerhoff WL, Morizono T, Wright CG, et al.: Tympanostomy tubes and otic drops. Laryngoscope 1983; 93: 1022–1026.

81. Smith, BM, Myers MG: The penetration of gentamicin and neomycin into perilymph across the round window membrane. Otolaryngol Head Neck Surg 1978; 87: 888–891.

82. Wright CG, Meyerhoff WL: Ototoxicity of otic drops applied to the middle ear in the chinchilla. Am J Otolaryngol 1984; 5: 166–176.

83. Welling DB, Forrest LA, Goll F: Safety of ototopical antibiotics. Laryngoscope 1995; 105: 472–474.

84. Merifield DO, Parker NJ, Nicholson NC: Therapeutic management of chronic suppurative otitis media with otic drops. Otolaryngol Head Neck Surg 1993; 109: 77–82.

85. Podoshin L, Fradis M, David JB: Ototoxicity of ear drops in patients suffering from chronic otitis media. J Laryngol Otol 1989; 103: 46–50.

86. Vogelman B, Gundmundsson S, Turnidge J, et al.: In vivo postantibiotic effect in a thigh infection in neutropenic mice. J Infect Dis 1988; 157: 287–298.

87. Gerber AU, Craig WA, Brugger HP, et al.: Impact of dosing intervals on activity of gentamicin and ticarillin against *Pseudomonas aeruginosa* in granulocytopenic mice. J Infect Dis 1983; 147: 910–917.

88. Herscovici L, Grise G, Thauvin C, et al.: Efficacy and safety of once daily versus intermittent dosing of tobramycin in rabbits with acute pyelonephritis. Scand J Infect Dis 1988; 20: 205–212.

89. Wood CA, Norton DR, Kohlhepp SJ, et al.: The influence of tobramycin dosage regimens on nephrotoxicity, ototoxicity and antibacterial efficacy in a rat model of subcutaneous abscess. J Infect Dis 1988; 158: 13–22.

90. Tulkens PM: Nephrotoxicity of aminoglycoside antibiotics. Toxicol Lett 1989; 46: 107–123.

91. Brummett RE: Ototoxicity of aminoglycoside antibiotics in animal models. In: Fillastre J-P (ed): Nephrotoxicity and Ototoxicity of Drugs. Rouen: INSERM, 1982, p 359.

92. Pechere JC, Bernard PA: Gentamicin ototoxicity can be avoided if a

new therapeutic regimen is used [abstract 484]. 24th Interscience Conference on Antimicrobial Agents Chemotherapy, Washington, D.C., 1984.

93. Bamonte F, Dionisotti S, Gamba M, et al.: Relation of dosing regimen to aminoglycoside ototoxicity: Evaluation of auditory damage in the guinea pig. Chemotherapy 1990; 36: 41–50.

94. Davis RR, Brummett RE, Bendrick TW, Himes DL: Dissociation of maximum concentration of kanamycin in plasma and perilymph from ototoxic effect. J Antimicrob Chemother 1984; 14: 291–302.

95. Maller R, Isaksson B, Nilsson L, Soren L: A study of amikacin given once versus twice daily in serious infections. J Antimicrob Chemother 1988; 22: 75–79.

96. Tulkens PM: Efficacy and safety of aminoglycosides once-a-day: Experimental and clinical data. Scand J Infect Dis 1991; 74: 249–257.

97. Prins JM, Buller HR, Kuijper EJ, et al.: Once versus thrice daily gentamicin in patients with serious infections. Lancet 1993; 341: 335–339.

98. Ter Braak EW, deVries PJ, Bouter KP, et al.: Once-daily dosing regimen for aminoglycoside plus β-lactam combination therapy of serious bacterial infections: Comparative trial with netilmicin plus ceftriaxone. Am J Med 1990; 89: 58–66.

99. de Vries PJ, Verkooyen RP, Leguit P, Verbrugh HA: Prospective randomized study of once-daily versus thrice-daily netilmicin regimens in patients with intraabdominal infection. Eur J Clin Microb Infect Dis 1990; 9: 161–168.

100. Nordström L, Ringberg H, Cronberg S, et al.: Does administration of an aminoglycoside in a single daily dose affect its efficacy and toxicity? J Antimicrob Chemother 1990; 25: 159–173.

101. Mendes da Costa P, Kaufman L: Amikacin once daily plus metronidazole versus amikacin twice daily plus metronidazole in colorectal surgery. Hepatogastroenterology 1992; 39: 350–354.

George M. Eliopoulos

CHAPTER EIGHT

Vancomycin

DESCRIPTION, SOURCE, CHEMISTRY

Vancomycin was discovered in fermentation broths of an organism, originally called *Streptomyces orientalis* (subsequently *Nocardia orientalis*) and now named *Amycolatopsis orientalis,* which was isolated in 1956 from a soil specimen collected in Borneo.[1, 2] Early lots were termed "Mississippi mud," reflecting the substantial impurities retained in the preparation process.[3] In contrast, current preparations are an off-white color and of greater than 90% purity.[4] Approval for use in the United States was granted expeditiously in 1958 because of increasing concerns about staphylococci resistant to penicillin, erythromycin, and tetracycline.[1, 3] Use of vancomycin decreased substantially with the introduction of methicillin 2 years later[1] but rose again later because of infections due to methicillin-resistant staphylococci.

Vancomycin is a large (approximately 1450 D) glycopeptide molecule, consisting of a heptapeptide core arranged in a tricyclic structure to which is attached a disaccharide consisting of glucose and the amino sugar vancosamine.[5] The sugars contribute both to the antimicrobial activities and pharmacologic properties of the molecule.[2]

MECHANISM OF ACTION

Vancomycin inhibits peptidoglycan synthesis. The glycopeptide binds tightly via hydrogen bonds to the terminal D-alanine-D-alanine dipeptide of UDP-*N*-acetylmuramyl-pentapeptide cell-wall precursors. By virtue of its bulk, attachment of vancomycin to the precursor prevents the transglycosylation reaction that normally adds this building block to the growing cell-wall peptidoglycan polymer.[2] Because the terminal D-alanine-D-alanine is also the site of the final cross-linking step of peptidoglycan synthesis, binding of vancomycin to the dipeptide probably interferes with this transpeptidation reaction as well.

PHARMACOLOGY

Routes of Administration

Vancomycin is poorly absorbed following oral administration and reaches high concentrations in the intestine, a fact that is exploited in the treatment of *Clostridium difficile* colitis. In occasional patients with severe colitis and renal insufficiency, significant levels of vancomycin can accumulate in the serum.[6, 7] Intramuscular injections are extremely painful, and this route must be avoided. Therefore, intrave-

nous administration is required for therapy of nonenteric infections.

Serum Pharmacokinetics Following Intravenous Administration

Vancomycin is administered by slow intravenous infusion, usually more than 60 minutes, because of adverse effects encountered with more rapid infusions (see later). The kinetics is complex. There is a rapid distribution phase with a half-life of about 8 minutes; this is followed by an intermediate distribution phase of variable length ($t_{1/2}$ = 0.5–1.5 h) and a subsequent terminal elimination phase.[8] The terminal elimination half-life in adults with normal renal function averages 6 hours but varies widely (3–9 h).[8–10] Steady-state distribution volumes have been estimated from ≤0.5 to ≥0.9 L/kg.[8, 9, 11] Because of the complex pharmacokinetics, serum levels measured in early periods after drug administration are highly dependent on actual sampling time. In adults with normal renal function, administration of a 1-g dose over 1 hour results in serum levels of about 25 μg/mL at 2 hours after the end of infusion and trough levels at 11 hours of approximately 8 μg /mL.[1, 8] Doses of 500 mg every 6 hours given to normal adult volunteers resulted in mean (±SD) peak serum concentrations at 1 hour of 22.6 ± 3.2 μg/mL and trough concentrations of 11.2 ± 2.2 μg/mL.[12] In this same group, 1-g infusions resulted in peak (1 h) and trough serum concentrations of 33.7 ± 3.8 μg/mL and 11.2 ± 2.2 μg/mL, respectively.

Distribution Into Tissues

The drug penetrates well into several body fluids, including ascites as well as pericardial, pleural, and synovial fluids, achieving concentration ratios of 0.38–0.78 those of corresponding serum levels.[1] Vancomycin penetrates poorly into the aqueous humor and across uninflamed meninges. Even in the presence of meningeal inflammation, the drug crosses into the cerebrospinal fluid unreliably.[1, 13, 14] Supplemental intrathecal or intraventricular dosing has been employed in the treatment of central nervous infections.[14–17] Parenteral vancomycin is not effective in eradicating nasal carriage of *Staphylococcus aureus*.[18] Information is lacking concerning penetration of vancomycin into ear, nose, and throat tissues and fluids.

Drug Elimination

Vancomycin is eliminated almost exclusively by renal mechanisms, and its clearance from blood is highly correlated with creatinine clearance.[19] Elimination half-life increases with decreasing renal function and in functionally anephric patients may exceed 7 days. The linear relationship between vancomycin and creatinine clearances has permitted construction of dosing nomograms based on actual measurement of creatinine clearance or on estimates, subject to certain limitations, derived from age, weight, sex, and serum creatinine levels in adults according to the formula of Cockcroft and Gault,[20] which is

$$\text{Creatinine clearance} = \frac{(140 - \text{age}) \times \text{weight} \ (\times \ 0.85 \text{ for females})}{72 \times \text{serum creatinine}}$$

(Equation 1)

where the weight is in kilograms, the creatinine in milligrams per deciliter, and the age in years. The nomogram developed by Moellering and colleagues[19] is commonly used to calculate a daily vancomycin dose for various levels of renal function. That nomogram was derived from studies of adults and older children and is based on a desired mean steady-state serum concentration of 15 μg/mL (see later). Modifications of this approach have yielded dosing interval recommendations for various levels of renal dysfunction.[11] Vancomycin is inefficiently removed by peritoneal dialysis or by conventional hemodialysis, but dialysis with newer membrane materials or by continuous arteriovenous hemofiltration or hemodialysis techniques may result in greater drug removal and require individualized dosing assessments.[21, 22]

Antibacterial Spectrum

Susceptible Bacteria

With rare exceptions, the activity of vancomycin is limited to gram-positive bacteria (Table 8–1).[23–35] Organisms inhibited by vancomycin at concentrations ≤4 μg/mL are considered fully susceptible, whereas those with minimal inhibitory concentrations (MICs) >16 μg/mL are considered resistant.[36] It is evident that vancomycin is active against staphylococci, streptococci, and other organisms relevant to head and neck infections. Because mechanisms of action of and resistance to beta-lactam antibiotics differ from those for vancomycin, methicillin-resistant staphylococci and penicillin-resistant pneumococci remain susceptible to the glycopeptide. Although vancomycin inhibits many anaerobic gram-positive bacteria in vitro, resistant strains are encountered.

Resistant Gram-Positive Organisms

Resistance to vancomycin is a common feature of *Leuconostoc* species, *Pediococcus* species, and many lactobacilli, which are occasionally encountered as pathogens, especially in immunocompromised patients.[37] Inhibitory concentrations of vancomycin against these organisms often exceed 256

Table 8–1. REPRESENTATIVE MINIMAL INHIBITORY CONCENTRATIONS (MICs) OF VANCOMYCIN AGAINST GRAM-POSITIVE BACTERIA

Organism	Usual MIC Range[a]	Range of MIC₉₀[b]
Aerobic and Facultative Bacteria		
Staphylococcus aureus (Methicillin-susceptible)	0.5–2	1–2
Staphylococcus aureus (Methicillin-resistant)	0.5–2	1–2
Coagulase-negative staphylococci (Methicillin-susceptible)	0.5–4	1–2
Coagulase-negative staphylococci (Methicillin-resistant)	0.25–4	2–4
Streptococci, groups A, C, or G	0.25–1	0.5–1
Streptococcus agalactiae (group B)	0.25–1	0.5–1
Streptococcus pneumoniae	0.06–0.5	0.5
Streptococci, viridans group	0.125–2	1
Corynebacteria (JK group)	0.25–2	0.5–1
Listeria monocytogenes	0.5–4	1–2
Enterococcus faecalis[c]	0.5–4	1–4
Enterococcus faecium[c]	0.5–4	2
Anaerobic Bacteria		
Propionibacterium acnes	0.05–1	0.5–1
Pepto(strepto)cocci	0.12–8[d]	2–8[d]
Actinomyces species	0.5–2	2
Clostridium difficile	0.5–4	1–2
Clostridium perfringens	0.25–32	0.5–2
Clostridium species	0.25–≥128	1–64

Data derived from references 23–35.
[a]MIC in μg/mL.
[b]MIC₉₀ is the concentration of drug required to inhibit 90% of the strains of any species determined in any study.
[c]Excludes vancomycin-resistant strains (see text).
[d]Some strains reported with MICs ≥128 μg/mL.

μg/mL.[38] Since the late 1980s, vancomycin resistance in enterococci has emerged as a significant clinical problem. By 1993, almost 14% of enterococcal isolates from patients in intensive care units in the United States exhibited resistance to vancomycin.[39] This observation has the following implications:

1. Increasing numbers of enterococcal wound infections, urinary tract infections, and nosocomial bacteremias will be caused by vancomycin-resistant enterococci, many of which will also be resistant to penicillins and other antibiotics.

2. There is a risk that vancomycin resistance genes may spread to other organisms, such as staphylococci, group A streptococci, and viridans group streptococci, because transfer of resistance has been demonstrated under laboratory conditions in vitro.[40]

3. Concern that vancomycin resistance will spread has led health authorities to recommend that use of the drug be constrained by guidelines designed to minimize its excessive or inappropriate use.[41]

CLINICAL USE

Indications and Clinical Experience

The resurgence of interest in vancomycin came about largely because of the need for an alternative antistaphylococcal antimicrobial. The drug has been used effectively to treat staphylococcal bacteremia, endocarditis, lower respiratory tract infections, as well as infections of bone, skin, and skin structures.[1, 42] It has become the agent of choice for most infections due to methicillin-resistant staphylococci and various bacteria (e.g., diphtheroids, enterococci) resistant to other agents. Because it is chemically unrelated to beta-lactams, vancomycin can be used in most penicillin- and cephalosporin-allergic patients with infections due to susceptible organisms. Vancomycin is administered orally for the treatment of *C. difficile* colitis.[43] Because of poor penetration into the eye or across the meninges, intravenous therapy alone may be inadequate for infections at those sites.

Vancomycin is recommended by the American Heart Association (AHA) as an alternative in the prophylaxis of patients at high risk for developing infective endocarditis who undergo dental, oral, or upper respiratory tract procedures requiring prophylaxis and who are allergic to penicillins.[44] The AHA's recommendation for adults is 1-g infused over 1 hour, and for children 20 mg/kg (not to exceed adult dose), administered prior to the procedure. Although the drug has activity against most aerobic gram-positive upper respiratory flora, gram-negative bacteria and some gram-positive anaerobes are resistant. Hence, vancomycin is not generally considered an alternative prophylactic agent in head and neck surgery to decrease risk of wound infection.[45–47] In the patient intolerant of other agents, however, vancomycin could constitute part of a multidrug regimen designed to provide such prophylaxis.

Adverse Reactions

As with all other antimicrobials, side effects occur with use of vancomycin in some patients. The following potential adverse reactions to this agent have received the greatest attention.

Ototoxicity

Hearing loss or abnormal audiometry was reported as a potential side effect of vancomycin in early clinical experience.[48, 49] However, many of the patients described had received concurrent treatment with aminoglycosides or erythromycin or prior courses of ototoxic drugs. For example, Hook and Johnson[49] noted minimal changes on serial audiograms in 3 of 10 patients who received vancomycin for endocarditis for 3–5 weeks. Two of these patients had received streptomycin previously, and the third had an abnormal baseline examination. Hearing loss was not apparent clinically in any, and in one patient, the audiogram returned to normal with continued therapy at a reduced dose. Tinnitus without apparent hearing loss has been described in several patients with improvement within 24 hours of stopping vancomycin, but the relationship of this symptom to other concurrent medications is often not described.[50–52] Vertigo or dizziness with rapid resolution on stopping vancomycin was noted in 1 of 100 patients reviewed by Farber and Moellering[53] and in 2 of 34 followed prospectively by Mellor and colleagues.[52] In the latter study, the two patients had clinically inapparent hearing loss at one or multiple frequencies.

In several cases, apparent auditory toxicity was associated with high peak serum levels (>45 μg/mL) of vancomycin.[49, 54–56] In one report,[56] a 21-year-old man being treated with vancomycin plus rifampin for endocarditis due to methicillin-resistant *S. aureus* developed tinnitus in one ear on day 7 of treatment. Two days later, an audiogram confirmed a profound unilateral sensorineural hearing loss. Serum vancomycin peak and trough levels were 46.5 μg/mL and 32 μg/mL, respectively. The dose of vancomycin was reduced, but treatment was continued to 4 weeks. Repeat audiography on the 18th day of therapy showed a 20-dB improvement in sensory thresholds in the affected ear. Reversible hearing loss due to the inadvertent administration of excessive vancomycin was reported in a 29-year-old man on chronic hemodialysis.[57] Peak serum levels reached only 35–40 μg/mL, but he developed nausea, bilateral tinnitus, and a 60- to 80-dB neurosensory high-tone hearing loss. Hemoperfusion was instituted, and in 2 days the tinnitus resolved, at which time vancomycin levels had decreased to approximately 10 μg/mL. His audiogram returned largely to normal in 6 weeks. Inadvertent vancomycin overdosage in a 35-week-old infant resulted in peak serum levels in excess of 400 μg/mL.[58] Exchange transfusions were initiated; nevertheless, serum vancomycin concentrations remained above 50 μg/mL for more than 5 days. Despite this event having occurred after 16 days of aminoglycoside therapy, brain-stem auditory evoked responses were normal when tested about 10 days later.

Animal studies have not revealed any convincing evidence of ototoxicity from vancomycin as a single agent.[59] Vancomycin administered to gerbils at 80 mg/kg/day[60] or to guinea pigs at 100–200 mg/kg/day[61] caused no evidence of diminished auditory function and no microscopic evidence of cochlear injury. In the latter study, however, when combined with gentamicin, vancomycin greatly enhanced the loss of outer cochlear hair cells that was seen to a limited extent with gentamicin alone.[61]

Although a few of the reported cases of ototoxicity ascribed to vancomycin seem convincing, most of the evidence suggests that ototoxicity due to vancomycin alone must be uncommon. This seems to be particularly true when peak levels are <40 μg/mL,[62, 63] but lack of apparent toxicity in some patients with even higher levels, the common concurrent use of other potentially ototoxic agents, and the limited number of cases reported make it impossible to predict the risk of ototoxicity at any specific level of the drug accurately. There would be reason to believe that vancomycin could augment the ototoxic potential of aminoglycosides in humans, but this has not been established.[64] Tinnitus or vertigo may sometimes be early symptoms of ototoxicity that may be rapidly reversible and that may precede recognizable hearing loss, which in some cases may also be at least partially reversible.[59, 65, 66] Chromatographically purified preparations of vancomycin are, apparently, not devoid of ototoxic potential,[67] but it is not possible to estimate their risk relative to older preparations. Some observations relevant to ototoxicity of vancomycin are shown in Table 8–2.

Nephrotoxicity

Vancomycin appears to enhance the nephrotoxicity of aminoglycosides in animal models.[69–71] Analysis of vancomycin

Table 8–2. EXAMPLES OF OBSERVATIONS RELEVANT TO THE OTOTOXIC POTENTIAL OF VANCOMYCIN

Study	Observations
Woodley and Hall (1961)[48]	Patient 1: Vancomycin 2–6 g daily for circa 5 weeks + erythromycin + brief course streptomycin. Audiogram normal except moderate acuity loss bilaterally at 4000 Hz.
	Patient 2: Vancomycin, 2 g daily for 5 days. Developed "moderate nerve deafness" 2 months later.
Hook and Johnson (1978)[49]	3 of 10 patients developed hearing loss beyond social range after 3–5 weeks of vancomycin, with peak levels of 25, 25, and 50 μg/mL. Vancomycin continued in all: one audiogram reverted to normal, loss progressed slightly in one, and remained unchanged in the third.
Sorrell et al. (1982)[50]	1 of 19 patients developed tinnitus (peak = 37.5 μg/mL), which disappeared within 24 hours of stopping vancomycin.
Farber and Moellering (1983)[53]	Vertigo in 1 of 100 patients; rapidly resolved after stopping therapy.
Mellor et al. (1985)[52]	2 of 34 patients developed tinnitus or dizziness, which resolved within 24 hours of stopping vancomycin. One had acute asymptomatic loss of 30 dB at one frequency in one ear. The other had a delayed loss of 20 dB at several frequencies, but improved and remained asymptomatic.
Sorrell and Collignon (1985)[55]	1 of 11 patients tested by audiometry had loss at multiple frequencies unilaterally. Levels were peak = 51.3 μg/mL, trough = 17.8 μg/mL. Also received an aminoglycoside.
Levine et al. (1982)[54]	"Mild, transient ototoxicity" in 5 of 24 patients, 2 of whom were also on aminoglycosides; 2 others had peak levels of 49 and 62 μg/mL.
Meyerhoff et al. (1989)[68]	19 patients had biweekly audiologic monitoring during long courses of vancomycin (≥8 weeks). No patients had symptoms. No unequivocal ototoxicity was encountered. Patients with hearing loss of ≥5 dB in either ear tended to be older.

For additional cases, see references 59, 62, and 66.

nephrotoxicity in humans is compromised by the multiplicity of potential variables and cofactors involved, but most studies suggest that toxicity would occur in <10% of therapeutic courses of vancomycin alone,[52, 53, 55, 72–74] although some studies quote higher rates (15%–19%).[75–77] In most studies, nephrotoxicity is defined as increases in the serum creatinine (generally by 0.5 mg/dL above baseline) and thus does not necessarily reflect severe compromise of function or imply irreversibility. One group observed a 14% incidence of nephrotoxicity when two 1-g doses were administered 4 hours apart for prophylaxis of vascular surgery procedures (versus 2% in the placebo group).[78, 79] Age, serum levels, severity of comorbid conditions, and other nephrotoxic agents (aminoglycosides, loop diuretics, amphotericin B) are cited as potential risk factors for nephrotoxicity.[53, 74, 75, 80] Nephrotoxicity occurred in 30%–40% of patients treated with vancomycin plus an aminoglycoside in some series.[53, 75, 81] Toxicity has occurred three to seven times more frequently with combined therapy than with the aminoglycoside alone; although interesting, such differences are not necessarily statistically significant.[53, 72, 75] Other studies suggest equivalent nephrotoxicities for vancomycin with or without aminoglycosides.[76, 77] Although nephrotoxicity has been seen in children receiving vancomycin with aminoglycosides,[82] the overall added risk of such combinations does not appear to be great.[83–85]

A 1993 meta-analysis demonstrated a statistically significant 13% greater incidence of nephrotoxicity with vancomycin plus an aminoglycoside than with vancomycin alone, and a 4.3% greater risk than with aminoglycosides alone.[77] It is not clear whether these observations are of sufficient magnitude to be clinically important. In experimental animals, endotoxin amplifies the nephrotoxicity of vancomycin plus gentamicin combinations.[86] Such an effect has not been proven in humans. Acute interstitial nephritis due to vancomycin has also been convincingly demonstrated in patients.[87]

Infusion-Related Syndrome

In some individuals, infusion of vancomycin results in flushing (particularly of the head and upper body), pruritus, and,

in severe cases, dyspnea, chest pain, muscle spasms, and hypotension.[1, 88] This reaction has been termed red man or red neck syndrome. It is thought to be due to histamine release, as some have found a correlation between severity and plasma histamine levels (although others have not[88, 89]) and the reaction can be at least partially blocked by hydroxyzine.[90] This phenomenon has been reported in as many as 75%–90% of healthy volunteers,[89, 90] but in <10% of patients.[1, 88, 89] It is generally believed that such reactions can be minimized by slow (>1 h) infusion or more dilute solutions, or both. Rapid infusion has been associated with cardiac arrest,[1] possibly owing to exaggerated histamine release.

Other Related Syndromes

Other skin rashes that likely represent true allergic or hypersensitivity phenomena have been described, including maculopapular rashes occurring well into courses of therapy.[53] They have been estimated to occur in 2%–3% of patients.[22] Stevens-Johnson syndrome temporally related to vancomycin administration has been reported,[91] as has toxic epidermal necrolysis,[92] but in the latter case, multiple other potentially offending drugs were administered concurrently. Neutropenia has occurred with vancomycin use, but additional factors probably contribute in many cases.[63, 93–95] Phlebitis at peripheral vein infusion sites occurs at rates that vary widely.[1, 53, 55, 63]

Vancomycin Dosing and Therapeutic Monitoring

The usual dose of oral vancomycin for treatment of *C. difficile*–related colitis in adults is 125–500 mg four times daily.[43] Except in rare cases, significant systemic absorption is not expected from oral administration.

Recommended dosing regimens for intravenous vancomy-

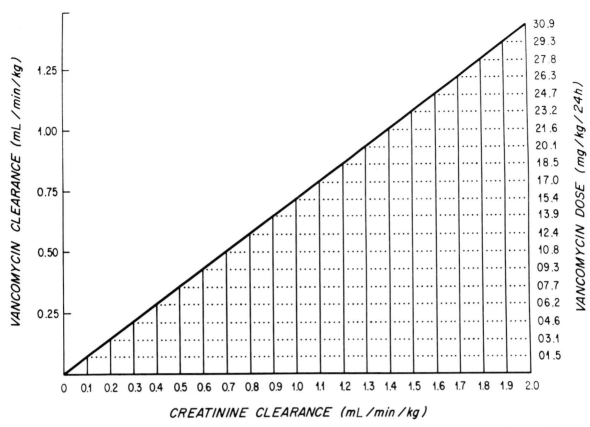

Figure 8–1. Dosage nomogram, developed by Moellering and colleagues, for vancomycin in patients with impaired renal function. This nomogram is intended to yield mean steady-state serum levels of approximately 15 μg/mL. The nomogram is not valid for functionally anephric patients on dialysis. (From Moellering RC Jr, Krogstad DJ, Greenblatt DJ: Vancomycin therapy in patients with impaired renal function: A nomogram for dosage. Ann Intern Med 1981; 94: 343–346.)

cin are derived from early clinical experience, which indicated that in normal-size adults with intact renal function, a total daily dose of 2 g, administered as 1 g twice daily or 500 mg every 6 hours, was usually effective and resulted in acceptably low rates of adverse reactions.[1, 96] The ranges of serum vancomycin concentrations obtained with these regimens have served as the basis for generally accepted "therapeutic ranges" for peak and trough serum levels. Peak concentrations of 30–35 μg/mL,[62] 30–40 μg/mL,[63] and 20–40 μg/mL[21] have been considered desirable, with trough concentrations of 5–10 μg/mL[21, 62, 63] or 5–15 μg/mL[97] recommended. The timing at which trough levels are sampled does not appear to be critical (usually within 1 h of next dose), but sampling for peak measurements is delayed until 1 or 2 hours after completion of vancomycin infusions to allow time for the initial and intermediate distribution phases to occur.[1, 96] For selection of initial regimens in patients with impaired renal function after an initial loading dose, a dosing nomogram designed to achieve mean steady-state serum concentrations of 15 μg/mL has been widely used[19] (Fig. 8–1). For functionally anephric patients on dialysis, the authors recommended an initial maintenance dose of 1.9 mg/kg daily. Initial dosing regimens for infants and children depend on age.[42]

The routine use of serum vancomycin determinations in patients treated with this agent has been called into question.[96, 97] Cantú and colleagues[97] suggest that data correlating therapeutic outcome with specific serum levels are nonexistent, that putative relationships between serum concentrations and risks of ototoxicity or nephrotoxicity are largely conjectural, and that the pharmacokinetics of the drug are sufficiently predictable that dosing regimens calculated on the basis of age, weight, and renal function result in serum concentrations within or acceptably close to the target range. This approach seems reasonable if carried out by individuals skilled in clinical pharmacokinetics. For others, verification that serum levels fall within generally accepted limits during therapy with empirically selected regimens will probably remain a useful way of ensuring appropriate drug dosing. Measurement of serum levels may be particularly useful in patients on various forms of dialysis, in those whose renal function is unstable or difficult to assess, and in those receiving higher-than-usual doses of vancomycin or vancomycin together with an aminoglycoside.[96]

References

1. Cooper GL, Given DB: Vancomycin: A Comprehensive Review of 30 Years of Clinical Experience. Park Row Publishers, Inc, 1986.
2. Nagarajan R: Antibacterial activities and modes of action of vancomycin and related glycopeptides. Antimicrob Agents Chemother 1991; 35: 605–609.

3. Griffith RS: Vancomycin use—an historical review. J Antimicrob Chemother 1984; 14 (suppl D): 1–5.

4. Anonymous: New preparations of vancomycin. Med Let Drugs Ther 1986; 28: 121–122.

5. Pfeiffer RR: Structural features of vancomycin. Rev Infect Dis 1981; 3 (suppl): S205–S209.

6. Spitzer PG, Eliopoulos GM: Systemic absorption of enteral vancomycin in a patient with pseudomembranous colitis. Ann Intern Med 1984; 100: 533–534.

7. Matzke GR, Halstenson CE, Olson PL, et al.: Systemic absorption of oral vancomycin in patients with renal insufficiency and antibiotic-associated colitis. Am J Kidney Dis 1987; 9: 422–425.

8. Moellering RC Jr: Pharmacokinetics of vancomycin. J Antimicrob Chemother 1984; 14 (suppl D): 43–52.

9. Farber BB: Vancomycin: Renewed interest in an old drug. Eur J Clin Microbiol 1984; 3: 1–3.

10. Rotschafer JC, Crossley K, Zaske DE, et al.: Pharmacokinetics of vancomycin: Observations in 28 patients and dosage recommendations. Antimicrob Agents Chemother 1982; 22: 391–394.

11. Brown DL, Mauro LS: Vancomycin dosing chart for use in patients with renal impairment. Am J Kidney Dis 1988; 11: 15–19.

12. Healy DP, Polk RE, Garson ML, et al.: Comparison of steady-state pharmacokinetics of two dosage regimens of vancomycin in normal volunteers. Antimicrob Agents Chemother 1987; 31: 393–397.

13. Viladrich PF, Gudiol F, Liñares J, et al.: Evaluation of vancomycin for therapy of adult pneumococcal meningitis. Antimicrob Agents Chemother 1991; 35: 2467–2472.

14. Gump DW: Vancomycin for treatment of bacterial meningitis. Rev Infect Dis 1981; 3 (suppl): S289–S292.

15. McLaurin RL, Frame PT: Treatment of infections of cerebrospinal fluid shunts. Rev Infect Dis 1987; 9: 595–603.

16. Reesor C, Chow AW, Kureishi A, Jewesson PF: Kinetics of intraventricular vancomycin in infections of cerebrospinal fluid shunts. J Infect Dis 1988; 158: 1142–1143.

17. Hirsch BE, Amodio M, Einzig AI, et al.: Instillation of vancomycin into a cerebrospinal fluid reservoir to clear infection: Pharmacokinetic considerations. J Infect Dis 1991; 163: 197–200.

18. Yu VL, Goetz A, Wagener M, et al.: Staphylococcus aureus nasal carriage and infection in patients on hemodialysis. N Engl J Med 1986; 315: 91–96.

19. Moellering RC Jr, Krogstad DJ, Greenblatt DJ: Vancomycin therapy in patients with impaired renal function: A nomogram for dosage. Ann Intern Med 1981; 94: 343–346.

20. Cockroft DW, Gault MH: Prediction of creatinine clearance from serum creatinine. Nephron 1976; 16: 31–41.

21. Wilhelm MP: Vancomycin. Mayo Clinic Proc 1991; 66: 1165–1170.

22. Matzke GR: Vancomycin. In: Evans WE, Schentag JJ, Jusko WJ, et al. (eds): Applied Pharmacokinetics: Principles of Therapeutic Drug Monitoring, 3rd ed. Vancouver, WA: Applied Therapeutics, 1992, pp 15-2–15-31.

23. Biavasco F, Lupidi R, Varaldo PE: In vitro activities of three semisynthetic amide derivatives of teicoplanin, MDL 62208, MDL 62211, and MDL 62873. Antimicrob Agents Chemother 1992; 36: 331–338.

24. Chin N-X, Neu HC: In vitro activity of LY264826 compared to other glycopeptides and daptomycin. Diagn Microbiol Infect Dis 1991; 14: 181–184.

25. Chow AW, Cheng N: In vitro activities of daptomycin (LY146032) and paldimycin (U-70,138F) against anaerobic gram-positive bacteria. Antimicrob Agents Chemother 1988; 32: 788–790.

26. Glupczynski Y, Labbe M, Crokaert F, et al.: In vitro activity of teicoplanin and vancomycin against anaerobes (letter). Eur J Clin Microbiol 1984; 3: 50–51.

27. Korten V, Tomayko JF, Murray BE: Comparative in vitro activity of DU-6859a, a new fluoroquinolone agent, against gram-positive cocci. Antimicrob Agents Chemother 1994; 38: 611–615.

28. Malanoski G, Collins L, Eliopoulos CT, et al.: Comparative in vitro activities of L-695, 256, a novel carbapenem, against gram-positive bacteria. Antimicrob Agents Chemother 1995; 39: 990–995.

29. McWhinney PHM, Patel S, Whiley RA, et al.: Activities of potential therapeutic and prophylactic antibiotics against blood culture isolates of viridans group streptococci from neutropenic patients receiving ciprofloxacin. Antimicrob Agents Chemother 1993; 37: 2493–2495.

30. Niu W-W, Neu HC: Activity of mersacidin, a novel peptide, compared with that of vancomycin, teicoplanin, and daptomycin. Antimicrob Agents Chemother 1991; 35: 998–1000.

31. Pankuch GA, Jacobs MR, Appelbaum PC: Study of comparative antipneumococcal activities of penicillin G, RP59500, erythromycin, sparfloxacin, ciprofloxacin and vancomycin by using time-kill methodology. Antimicrob Agents Chemother 1994; 38: 2065–2072.

32. Soriano F, Zapardiel J, Nieto E: Antimicrobial susceptibilities of Corynebacterium species and other non-spore-forming gram-positive bacilli to 18 antimicrobial agents. Antimicrob Agents Chemother 1995; 39: 208–214.

33. Spangler SK, Jacobs MR, Appelbaum PC: Susceptibilities of 177 penicillin-susceptible and -resistant pneumococci to FK037, cefpirome, cefepime, ceftriaxone, ceftazidime, imipenem, biapenem, meropenem and vancomycin. Antimicrob Agents Chemother 1994; 38: 898–900.

34. Testa RT, Petersen PJ, Jacobus NV, et al.: In vitro and in vivo antibacterial activities of the glycylcyclines, a new class of semisynthetic tetracyclines. Antimicrob Agents Chemother 1993; 37: 2270–2277.

35. Wise R, Andrews JM: In vitro activities of two glycylcyclines. Antimicrob Agents Chemother 1994; 38: 1096–1102.

36. National Committee for Clinical Laboratory Standards: Performance Standards for Antimicrobial Susceptibility Testing; Third Information Supplement. [NCCLS Document M100-S3.] Villanova, Pennsylvania: NCCLS, 1991.

37. Ruoff KL, Kuritzkes DR, Wolfson JS, et al.: Vancomycin-resistant gram-positive bacteria isolated from human sources. J Clin Microbiol 1988; 26: 2064–2068.

38. Swenson JM, Facklam RR, Thornsberry C: Antimicrobial susceptibility of vancomycin-resistant Leuconostoc, Pediococcus, and Lactobacillus species. Antimicrob Agents Chemother 1990; 34: 543–549.

39. Centers for Disease Control and Prevention: Nosocomial enterococci resistant to vancomycin—United States, 1989–1993. Morb Mortal Wkly Rep 1993; 42: 597–599.

40. Courvalin P: Resistance of enterococci to glycopeptides. Antimicrob Agents Chemother 1990; 34: 2291–2296.

41. Centers for Disease Control and Prevention: Preventing the spread of vancomycin resistance. Federal Register 1994; 59: 25758–25763.

42. Anonymous: Physicians' Desk Reference. Montvale, New Jersey: Medical Economics Data Production Co, 1995.

43. Fekety R, Shah AB: Diagnosis and treatment of Clostridium difficile colitis. JAMA 1993; 269: 71–75.

44. Dajani AS, Bisno AL, Chung KJ, et al.: Prevention of bacterial endocarditis: Recommendations by the American Heart Association. JAMA 1990; 264: 2919–2922.

45. Page CP, Bohnen JMA, Fletcher R, et al.: Antimicrobial prophylaxis for surgical wounds. Arch Surg 1993; 128: 79–88.

46. Anonymous: ASHP therapeutic guidelines on antimicrobial prophylaxis in surgery. Clin Pharm 1992; 11: 483–513.

47. Anonymous: Antimicrobial prophylaxis in surgery. Med Lett Drugs Ther 1993; 35: 91–94.

48. Woodley DW, Hall WH: The treatment of severe staphylococcal infections with vancomycin. Ann Intern Med 1961; 55: 235–249.

49. Hook EW, Johnson WD Jr: Vancomycin therapy of bacterial endocarditis. Am J Med 1978; 65: 411–415.

50. Sorrell TC, Packham DR, Shanker S, et al.: Vancomycin therapy for methicillin-resistant Staphylococcus aureus. Ann Intern Med 1982; 97: 344–350.

51. Mellor JA, Kingdom J, Cafferkey M, et al.: Vancomycin ototoxicity in patients with normal renal function. Br J Audiol 1984; 18: 179–180.

52. Mellor JA, Kingdom J, Cafferkey M, et al.: Vancomycin toxicity: A prospective study. J Antimicrob Chemother 1985; 15: 773–780.

53. Farber BF, Moellering RC Jr: Retrospective study of the toxicity of preparations of vancomycin from 1974 to 1981. Antimicrob Agents Chemother 1983; 23: 138–141.

54. Levine DP, Cushing RD, Jui J, et al.: Community-acquired methicillin-resistant Staphylococcus aureus endocarditis in a Detroit medical center. Ann Intern Med 1982; 97: 330–338.

55. Sorrell TC, Collignon PJ: A prospective study of adverse reactions associated with vancomycin therapy. J Antimicrob Chemother 1985; 16: 235–241.

56. Traber PG, Levine DP: Vancomycin ototoxicity in a patient with normal renal function. Ann Intern Med 1981; 95: 458–460.

57. Ahmad R, Raichura N, Kilbane V, et al.: Vancomycin: A reappraisal (letter). Lancet 1982; 284: 1953.

58. Burkhart KK, Metcalf S, Shurnas E, et al.: Exchange transfusion and multidose activated charcoal following vancomycin overdose. J Toxicol Clin Toxicol 1992; 30: 285–294.

59. Brummett RE: Ototoxicity of vancomycin and analogs. Otolaryngol Clin North Am 1993; 26: 821–828.

60. Tange RA, Kieviet HL, v Marle J, et al.: An experimental study of vancomycin-induced cochlear damage. Arch Otorhinolaryngol 1989; 246: 67–70.

61. Brummett RE, Fox KE, Jacobs F, et al.: Augmented gentamicin ototoxicity induced by vancomycin in guinea pigs. Arch Otolaryngol Head Neck Surg 1990; 116: 61–64.

62. Bailie GR, Neal D: Vancomycin ototoxicity and nephrotoxicity. Med Toxicol 1988; 3: 376–386.

63. Rybak SC: Monitoring vancomycin therapy. Drug Intell Clin Pharm 1986; 20: 757–760.

64. Brummett RE, Fox KE: Vancomycin- and erythromycin-induced hearing loss in humans. Antimicrob Agents Chemother 1989; 33: 791–796.

65. Matz GJ: Clinical perspectives on ototoxic drugs. Ann Otol Rhinol Laryngol 1990; 99 (suppl 148): 39–41.

66. Duffull SB, Begg EJ: Vancomycin toxicity: What is the evidence for dose dependency? Adverse Drug React Toxicol Rev 1994; 13: 103–114.

67. Wang L-S, Liu C-Y, Wang F-D, et al.: Chromatographically purified vancomycin: Therapy of serious infections caused by *Staphylococcus aureus* and other gram-positive bacteria. Clin Ther 1988; 10: 574–584.

68. Meyerhoff WL, Maale GE, Yellin W, et al.: Audiologic threshold monitoring of patients receiving ototoxic drugs: Preliminary report. Ann Otol Rhinol Laryngol 1989; 98: 950–954.

69. Wood CA, Kohlhepp SJ, Kohnen PW, et al.: Vancomycin enhancement of experimental tobramycin nephrotoxicity. Antimicrob Agents Chemother 1986; 30: 20–24.

70. Beauchamp D, Pellerin M, Gourde P, et al.: Effects of daptomycin and vancomycin on tobramycin nephrotoxicity in rats. Antimicrob Agents Chemother 1990; 34: 139–47.

71. Fauconneau B, DeLemos E, Pariat C, et al.: Chrononephrotoxicity in rat of a vancomycin and gentamicin combination. Pharmacol Toxicol 1992; 71: 31–36.

72. Rybak MJ, Albrecht LM, Boike SC, et al.: Nephrotoxicity of vancomycin, alone and with an aminoglycoside. J Antimicrob Chemother 1990; 25: 679–687.

73. Eng RHK, Wynn L, Smith SM, et al.: Effect of intravenous vancomycin on renal function. Chemotherapy 1989; 35: 320–325.

74. Pauly DJ, Musa DM, Lestico MR, et al.: Risk of nephrotoxicity with combination vancomycin-aminoglycoside antibiotic therapy. Pharmacotherapy 1990; 10: 378–382.

75. Downs NJ, Neihart RE, Dolezal JM, et al.: Mild nephrotoxicity associated with vancomycin use. Arch Intern Med 1989; 149: 1777–1781.

76. Cimino MA, Rotstein C, Slaughter RL, et al.: Relationship of serum antibiotic concentrations to nephrotoxicity in cancer patients receiving concurrent aminoglycoside and vancomycin therapy. Am J Med 1987; 83: 1091–1097.

77. Goetz MB, Sayers J: Nephrotoxicity of vancomycin and aminoglycoside therapy separately and in combination. J Antimicrob Chemother 1993; 32: 325–334.

78. Gudmundsson GH, Jensen LJ: Vancomycin and nephrotoxicity (letter). Lancet 1989; 1: 625.

79. Jensen LJ, Aagaard MT, Schifter S: Prophylactic vancomycin versus placebo in arterial prosthetic reconstructions. Thorac Cardiovasc Surg 1985; 33: 300–303.

80. Vance-Bryan K, Rotschafer JC, Gilliland SS, et al.: A comparative assessment of vancomycin-associated nephrotoxicity in the young versus the elderly hospitalized patient. J Antimicrob Chemother 1994; 33: 811–821.

81. Sheftel TG, Mader JT, Pennick JJ, et al.: Methicillin-resistant *Staphylococcus aureus* osteomyelitis. Clin Orthop 1985; 198: 231–239.

82. Odio C, McCracken GH, Nelson JD: Nephrotoxicity associated with vancomycin-aminoglycoside therapy in four children. J Pediatr 1984; 105: 491–493.

83. Goren MP, Baker DK, Shenep JL: Vancomycin does not enhance amikacin-induced tubular nephrotoxicity in children. Pediatr Infect Dis 1989; 8: 278–282.

84. Nahata MC: Lack of nephrotoxicity in pediatric patients receiving concurrent vancomycin and aminoglycoside therapy. Chemotherapy 1987; 33: 302–304.

85. Swinney VR, Rudd CC: Nephrotoxicity of vancomycin-gentamicin therapy in pediatric patients (letter). J Pediatr 1987; 110: 497–498.

86. Ngeleka M, Beauchamp D, Tardif D, et al.: Endotoxin increases the nephrotoxic potential of gentamicin and vancomycin plus gentamicin. J Infect Dis 1990; 161: 721–727.

87. Codding CE, Ramseyer L, Allon M, et al.: Tubulointerstitial nephritis due to vancomycin. Am J Kidney Dis 1989; 14: 512–515.

88. O'Sullivan TL, Ruffing MJ, Lamp KC, et al.: Prospective evaluation of red man syndrome in patients receiving vancomycin. J Infect Dis 1993; 168: 773–776.

89. Rybak MJ, Bailey EM, Warbasse LH: Absence of "red man syndrome" in patients being treated with vancomycin or high dose teicoplanin. Antimicrob Agents Chemother 1992; 36: 1204–1207.

90. Sahai J, Healy DP, Garris R, et al.: Influence of antihistamine pretreatment on vancomycin-induced red-man syndrome. J Infect Dis 1989; 160: 876–881.

91. Laurencin CT, Horan RF, Senatus PB, et al.: Stevens-Johnson-type reaction with vancomycin treatment. Ann Pharmacother 1992; 26: 1520–1521.

92. Hannah BA, Kimmel PL, Dosa S, Turner ML: Vancomycin-induced toxic epidermal necrolysis. South Med J 1990; 83: 720–722.

93. Chandrasekar PH, Rybak MS: White blood cell count and vancomycin (letter). Am J Med 1986; 81: 1114.

94. Strikas R, Studlo J, Venezio FR, et al.: Vancomycin-induced neutropenia. J Infect Dis 1982; 146: 575.

95. Adrouny A, Meguerditchian S, Koo CH, et al.: Agranulocytosis related to vancomycin therapy. Am J Med 1986; 81: 1059–1061.

96. Moellering RC Jr: Monitoring serum vancomycin levels: Climbing the mountain because it is there? (editorial) Clin Infect Dis 1994; 18: 544–546.

97. Cantú TG, Yamanaka-Yuen NA, Lietman PS: Serum vancomycin concentrations: Reappraisal of their clinical value. Clin Infect Dis 1994; 18: 533–543.

CHAPTER NINE

Jennifer Rubin Grandis
Suzanne Belfiglio
Victor L. Yu

Quinolones

▼

The availability of the quinolones has dramatically improved our ability to treat certain otolaryngologic infections. The oral route of administration, the low toxicity profile, and the excellent penetration into nares secretions, saliva, and bone are noteworthy advantages.[1] Unfortunately, objective data from well-controlled studies of infections of the ear, nose, and throat (ENT) are scanty; the major weakness in the few studies that have been reported is the failure to document adequately the type of infection being treated and the response being measured. Thus, the widespread empirical use of oral quinolones as first-line therapy for ENT infections is inappropriate.

DESCRIPTION OF THE DRUG

The quinolones are analogues of an earlier antibiotic used for urinary tract infection called nalidixic acid. Potency was greatly improved by the addition of a fluorine on the quinolone ring; hence the use of the word fluoroquinolones. Other chemical substitutions broadened the antimicrobial spectrum and improved the pharmacokinetic properties.

PHARMACOLOGY AND PHARMACOKINETICS

The quinolones are well absorbed from the gastrointestinal tract with excellent bioavailability. Peak serum concentrations are usually obtained within 1 to 3 hours after administration, and serum concentrations increase proportionately with dose. Food does not substantially reduce quinolone absorption but may delay the time to reach peak concentrations in the serum. Administration of quinolones with antacids containing calcium, magnesium, or aluminum or with cations such as iron or zinc may reduce the bioavailability of the quinolone by as much as 90%.

Most quinolones are primarily eliminated renally (Table 9–1). About 40%–50% of an oral dose of ciprofloxacin is excreted unchanged in the urine. Four metabolites of ciprofloxacin have been identified in the urine, which together account for approximately 15% of an oral dose. The metabolites have antimicrobial activity but are less active than unchanged ciprofloxacin.[2] Although bile concentrations of ciprofloxacin are higher than serum concentrations after oral dosing, only a small amount of the dose administered is recovered from the bile as unchanged. An additional 1%–2% of the dose is recovered from the bile in the form of metabolites. Approximately 20%–35% of the oral dose is recovered from feces within 5 days.[3]

The presence of a pyridobenzoxazine ring appears to decrease the metabolism of the parent compound; 60%–85% of ofloxacin is excreted unchanged in the urine, and 4%–8% is excreted in the feces (see Table 9–1). Pefloxacin is primarily cleared by the liver, and studies suggest a saturability of this nonrenal clearance pathway. Urinary excretion of unchanged pefloxacin is higher in patients with cirrhosis.[4]

The terminal half-lives for elimination of quinolones from serum range from 3 hours for ciprofloxacin to 11 hours for fleroxacin, allowing for once- or twice-daily dosing (see Table 9–1). Clearance of renally cleared quinolones is reduced in patients with impaired renal function (creatinine clearance < 50 mL/min), and dosage adjustment is necessary (Table 9–2).

The duration of postantibiotic effect for quinolones has been in the range of 1 to 2 hours and tends to increase with increasing drug concentration and length of drug exposure.

Penetration into ENT Secretions and Cerebrospinal Fluid

The quinolones are widely distributed throughout the body, with tissue concentrations, including those in the middle ear (cartilage, bone, inflamed mucosa) often exceeding serum concentrations[5] (Table 9–3). The mean concentration of ciprofloxacin in the maxillary sinus mucosa has been found to be almost twice that of simultaneous mean drug level in the serum. Pefloxacin accumulates in inflamed sinus fluid at

Table 9–1. PHARMACOKINETICS OF QUINOLONES IN HEALTHY VOLUNTEERS

Drug	Dose	Route	Bioavail-ability (%)	T_{max} (h)	C_{max} (mg/L)	$T_{1/2}$ (h)	AUC (mg h/L)	Primary Route of Elimination	Urinary Excretion (% of dose/24 h)	Protein Binding %	Reference(s)
Ciprofloxacin	500	PO	80–85	1.13 ± 0.06	2.56 ± 1.2	4.12 ± 0.62	12 ± 3.39	Renal	30–60	20–40	3, 64
Lomefloxacin	400	PO	>95		4.2	8	26.1	Renal	65	10	55
Ofloxacin	400	PO	85–95	1.92 ± 0.65	3.51 ± 0.7	4.9 ± 0.75	28 ± 4.9	Renal	73.3 ± 6.9	10–20	3, 4
Pefloxacin	400	PO	90		4–5	10.5 ± 2	54.5 ± 11.2	Hepatic	11.8 ± 4	20–30	3, 4
Fleroxacin	400	PO	96	1.3 ± 1.1	4.36 ± 1.15	9.2 ± 1.7	48.3 ± 9.3	Renal	49.8 ± 9.2	23	4, 55
Levofloxacin	200	PO		1.05 ± 0.17	3.27 ± 0.2	4.13 ± 0.21	18.67 ± 1.41	Renal	57.04 ± 15.46		65

Table 9–2. DOSAGE OF QUINOLONES IN PATIENTS WITH NORMAL AND IMPAIRED RENAL FUNCTION

Quinolone	Dosage with Normal Renal Function		Dosage with Impaired Renal Function with GFR (mL/mm)	
	Oral	Intravenous	10–50	<10
Ciprofloxacin	250–750 mg q12h	200–400 mg q12h	1 × dose q18h	1 × dose q24h
Ofloxacin	200–400 mg q12h	200–400 mg q12h	1 × dose q24h	½ × dose q24h
Pefloxacin	400 mg q12h	400 mg q12h	No change	No change
Lomefloxacin	400 mg q24h	—	½ × dose q24h	½ × dose q24h

concentrations exceeding blood levels.[6] Ciprofloxacin distributes into the cerebrospinal fluid; however, cerebrospinal fluid concentrations are generally less than 10% of peak serum concentrations. Ofloxacin and pefloxacin penetrate the central nervous system better than do the other quinolones. Low levels of quinolones have been detected in the aqueous and vitreous humors of the uninflamed human eye[1] (see Table 9–2).

The quinolones penetrate into cells and accumulate in human leukocytes to levels 10 times the serum concentration. This result may promote killing of intracellular pathogens such as *Legionella, Brucella, Salmonella,* and *Mycobacterium.*[3]

SPECTRUM OF ACTIVITY

Quinolones are most active against aerobic gram-negative bacilli, including members of the Enterobacteraceae family and *Haemophilus* species, and against aerobic gram-negative cocci, including *Neisseria* species and *Moraxella (Branhamella) catarrhalis* (Table 9–4).

Among gram-positive organisms, staphylococci, including most methicillin-sensitive *Staphylococcus aureus* and coagulase-negative staphylococci, are variably susceptible to the quinolones. On the other hand, streptococci, particularly *Streptococcus pneumoniae* and *Enterococcus faecalis,* are less susceptible to most quinolones.[3] Newer agents such as clinafloxacin, trovafloxacin, and levofloxacin have enhanced

activity against some gram-positive cocci, including *S. pneumoniae,* that may be clinically significant.

Ciprofloxacin has excellent activity against *Pseudomonas aeruginosa* and marginal activity against staphylococci. It is the quinolone most potent against gram-negative bacteria, although ofloxacin has better activity against both streptococci and oropharyngeal anaerobes. Successful eradication of organisms with high minimum inhibitory concentrations (MICs) (MIC values higher than 0.25 μg/mL) can be achieved by selectively raising dosages; however, many organisms with MIC values of 1 to 2 μg/mL failed to respond even to higher dosages[7] (see Table 9–3).

Quinolones also have activity against mycobacterial species, with both ciprofloxacin and ofloxacin being active against not only *Mycobacterium tuberculosis* but also many of the atypical mycobacterium species, including *Mycobacterium avium-intracellulare.* Ofloxacin has activity against *Mycobacterium leprae* in animal models. Ciprofloxacin and ofloxacin have activity against many of the atypical agents of pneumonia, including *Legionella pneumophila, Mycoplasma pneumoniae,* and *Chlamydia pneumoniae.*

Combinations of quinolones with aminoglycosides and beta-lactam agents have been found to be indifferent or additive in in vitro studies. The combination of ciprofloxacin and rifampin was indifferent in in vitro studies of *P. aeruginosa.*[8]

MECHANISM OF ACTION

For prokaryotic DNA, enzymes called DNA gyrases allow DNA unwinding and supercoiling to be performed effi-

Table 9–3. TISSUE AND FLUID KINETICS OF QUINOLONES

Drug	Tissue or Fluid	Dosage (mg)	Route	n	Sampling Time (h)	Tissue (t) or Fluid (f) Concentration	Serum Concentration(s)	Ratio (t/s or f/s)	Reference
Ciprofloxacin	Tonsils	250 SD	PO	8	3	2.3	1.28	1.8	64
Ciprofloxacin	Tonsils	200 SD	IV	10	1.5–4	0.26–0.88	0.2–0.6	1.53	64
Ciprofloxacin	CSF	200 q12h × 3	IV	23	2	0.56	1.44	0.37	64
Ciprofloxacin	Middle ear mucosa	500 q12h	PO	16	3–4	5.54 ± 3.46	2.8	2–3	5
Ciprofloxacin	Cortical bone of mastoid	500 q12h	PO	21	4	1.07 ± 1.29		0.63	5
Ciprofloxacin	Aqueous humor	50 mg/kg SD	PO	21		0.32	1.5	0.21	4
Pefloxacin	Aqueous humor	50 mg/kg SD	IM	29		2.6	8.9	0.29	4
Pefloxacin	Sinus fluid	400 q12h × 2	PO	6	3	6.9 ± 1.8	3.1 ± 1	>2	6
Pefloxacin	Cystic sinus fluid	400 q12h × 2	PO	2	3	7.1 ± 1.34	3.1 ± 1	>2	6
Pefloxacin	Nasal secretions	400 q12h × 2	PO	2	3	9.1 ± 0.21	3.1 ± 1	>2	6
Sparfloxacin	Aqueous humor	50 mg/kg SD	PO	18		0.74	4	0.19	4

SD = single dose; PO = orally; IV = intravenous; IM = intramuscular; CSF = cerebrospinal fluid.

Table 9–4. ANTIBACTERIAL ACTIVITY OF QUINOLONES

	Ciprofloxacin			Ofloxacin			Lomefloxacin			Pefloxacin			Sparfloxacin			Fleroxacin		
	MIC_{50}	MIC_{90}	MIC Range	MIC_{50}	MIC_{90}	MIC Range	MIC_{50}	MIC_{90}	MIC Range	MIC_{50}	MIC_{90}	MIC Range	MIC_{50}	MIC_{90}	MIC Range	MIC_{50}	MIC_{90}	MIC Range
S. aureus	0.25	0.5	0.25–2	0.25	0.5	0.1–2		2	0.5–4		0.5	0.1–2	0.25	0.12	0.06–0.25	0.5	1	0.125–4
S. pneumoniae	1	2	0.78–6.2	2	4	2–8	4	8	4–16		12	8–16		0.5	0.25–1	8	8	4–16
P. pyogenes	0.5	1	0.5–4	1	2	0.5–2		8	4–12.5		8	8–16		1	0.5–2	8	8	4–12.5
H. influenzae	0.004	0.008	0.002–0.03	0.015	0.03	0.015–0.3		0.12	0.06–0.12		0.06		0.015	0.1	0.01–0.1	0.06	0.12	0.06–1
M. catarrhalis	0.03	0.03	0.03–0.25	0.06	0.12	0.06–0.5			0.1–1		0.25		0.015	0.015	0.01–0.12			0.25–1
Bacteroides spp. (non-fragilis)	1	8	1–32	4	8	2–32			8–32					0.4	1–4			2–64
E. coli	0.008	0.01	0.004–0.06	0.1	0.125	0.06–0.25		0.5	0.06–1		0.125			0.12	0.01–0.12		0.125	0.03–2
K. pneumoniae	0.03	0.06	0.004–0.5	0.1	0.25	0.03–1		0.5	0.2–6.25		2	0.5–2		0.25	0.06–0.5		0.25	0.12–6.25
P. aeruginosa	0.12	0.5	0.25–8	2	8	2–>32		12.5	4–>20		2–8			2	1–8	2	8	0.5–>32

Data from references 4, 55, 66.
Entries represent µg/mL.

ciently. The DNA gyrase is essential for DNA replication.[9] Quinolones bind to and inhibit DNA gyrase and subsequently damage the DNA of the bacterial cell, producing a bactericidal effect.[3] In order to interact with DNA gyrase in the gram-negative bacterial cell cytoplasm, quinolones must traverse both outer and inner membranes. The quinolones diffuse through porin channels of the outer membrane; the mechanism by which they penetrate the inner membrane is unknown. Some bacteria may possess an energy-dependent efflux mechanism.[2] Spontaneously occurring mutations in bacterial chromosome genes that alter the target enzyme DNA gyrase and drug permeation across the bacterial cell membranes are responsible for quinolone resistance. Alterations in the subunits of the DNA gyrase cause the resistance.

CLINICAL USE IN EAR, NOSE, AND THROAT INFECTIONS

Necrotizing (Malignant) External Otitis

Necrotizing external otitis is an invasive infection of the external ear canal, mastoid, and base of skull caused almost universally by *P. aeruginosa* (>98%).[10, 11] Prior to the introduction of systemic antipseudomonal antibiotics in the early 1970s, necrotizing external otitis was fatal in the majority of cases despite extensive surgical débridement of infected tissues. This was primarily due to the multiple cranial neuropathies associated with extensive skull base involvement. With the introduction of aminoglycosides and antipseudomonal penicillins, the mortality rate was reduced to approximately 15%–30%, although recurrences remained a significant problem (20%–25%).[10] Prolonged combination parenteral antibiotic therapy for this disease has been associated with long-term hospitalization as well as vestibular and renal toxicity.

Quinolone agents, especially ciprofloxacin, have proved to represent a major therapeutic advance in the treatment of necrotizing external otitis, for a number of reasons. Quinolones have an extensive antimicrobial spectrum but are particularly active against *P. aeruginosa*. They can be administered orally with high bone and soft tissue penetration,[12–16] thereby obviating prolonged hospitalization. The dose need not be adjusted in elderly patients without renal failure,[17] and side effects of ototoxicity and nephrotoxicity seen with aminoglycosides are not problematic with the quinolones. These latter side effects can be particularly troublesome for the patient who characteristically contracts necrotizing external otitis—the elderly diabetic.

Numerous reports have chronicled the successful treatment of patients with necrotizing external otitis using quinolone agents.[18–25] Ciprofloxacin alone (750 mg twice daily orally) has been the most widely used regimen, with one report of ciprofloxacin plus rifampin (600 mg twice daily).[8] Prolonged treatment (6–12 weeks) is recommended despite rapid relief of symptoms (pain and otorrhea) because of the traditionally recalcitrant nature of the infection. A high rate of success (>95%) has been universally reported, with only a few cases of recurrence or persistent disease. In addition to symptomatic relief, the erythrocyte sedimentation rate

appears to be an accurate objective indicator of disease activity and response to antimicrobial agents. To date, the emergence of quinolone resistance has not yet been a problem in cases of necrotizing external otitis, although there are scattered reports of ciprofloxacin resistance in *P. aeruginosa* in patients with presumed but undocumented necrotizing external otitis.[26] Anecdotal reports of emergence of resistance to ofloxacin and pefloxacin in *P. aeruginosa* isolates in necrotizing external otitis have appeared.[27] Thus, ciprofloxacin has emerged as the drug of choice in patients with this disease, and the oral route of administration seems to be successful.

We emphasize that when one is reporting and evaluating cases of necrotizing external otitis, it is important to detail the diagnostic criteria, since there is no single sign or symptom that clearly distinguishes the disease. Some reports in the literature of patients with necrotizing external otitis are difficult to interpret because the diagnostic criteria are not explicitly given.[22, 26] For example, one study reported that less than half (41%) of the patients had diabetes mellitus.[22] This study is difficult to interpret because it has been the exception to find this disease in the nondiabetic adult.

Auricular Perichondritis

Perichondritis of the auricle caused by *P. aeruginosa* can occur in the burn patient as well as the patient with malignant external otitis. Because of its excellent soft tissue and cartilage penetration and the prolonged duration of therapy, ciprofloxacin seems to be an ideal agent. Oral ciprofloxacin has been successfully used for individuals with auricular perichondritis.[28]

Chronic Ear Disease

In discussing the utility of quinolones in the treatment of chronic otitis, one must define the disease process under scrutiny. Specifically, the status of the middle ear and tympanic membrane, the presence of cholesteatoma, and prior mastoid surgery are all important parameters in delineating the population being studied. Too often, in the few reports of quinolone usage for ear disease other than malignant external otitis, patients with different processes are grouped together for evaluation, thus clouding interpretation of the data.[29–32] Furthermore, the assessment of the efficacy of fluoroquinolones for these diseases would benefit from comparison with results either of another drug or in untreated control subjects, a study design feature that is absent from most reports. *P. aeruginosa* is commonly recovered from the patient with a chronic draining ear; however, its pathogenicity is uncertain because in many patients without underlying cholesteatoma the otorrhea resolves without antipseudomonal therapy. Most studies have combined all patients with "ear infections" and compared topical with oral ciprofloxacin. In general, although about 50%–70% of patients respond to oral cirprofloxacin, topical ciprofloxacin also appears to be most efficacious.[32, 33] These results are encouraging and confirm the numerous reports suggesting that topical antimicrobial agents as monotherapy are effective for uncomplicated otorrhea. Furthermore, topical ciprofloxacin is unlikely to lead to systemic toxicities and, as such, may be an ideal candidate for the treatment of chronic otorrhea in the pediatric population unresponsive to traditional therapies.

There are two reports of randomized trials comparing a fluoroquinolone with another agent in adults who had chronic otitis media and otorrhea.[34, 35] In one study, enoxacin was found to be more effective than amoxicillin in eradicating the organism as well as improving bone conduction thresholds on audiogram.[34] Both enoxacin and cirprofloxacin have been found in relatively high concentrations in middle ear and mastoid mucosa after oral dosing.[5, 31] The other study noted a more favorable clinical response to topical ciprofloxacin than to intramuscular gentamicin.[35]

Despite these reports, the use of quinolones in the treatment of chronic otitis remains unestablished. Although *P. aeruginosa* can be isolated from a large number of chronic draining ears, its pathogenicity in this setting is questionable. The efficacy of systemic therapy for uncomplicated chronic otorrhea was debated prior to the introduction of the quinolones. Prospective, randomized trials that outline rigorous criteria for entry, specify the disease process being studied, include a comparative antimicrobial agent or placebo-treated control group, and evaluate objective endpoints are needed.

Sinusitis

It is essential to differentiate between acute and chronic sinusitis when evaluating therapies. Most cases of acute sinusitis are believed to be the result of bacterial infections, but chronic sinusitis is more commonly associated with allergic rhinitis and polypoid hypertrophy of the sinus mucosa resulting in mucosal edema and obstruction of the osteomeatal complex. A bacteriologic diagnosis in acute sinusitis requires sterile puncture of the maxillary antrum. Although radiography can provide a noninvasive means of diagnosis, therapy is most often instituted empirically on the basis of clinical history and physical examination. Aspiration of the maxillary sinus in a number of studies reveals that more than 50% of the isolates are *S. pneumoniae* and unencapsulated strains of *Haemophilus influenzae,* with anaerobic bacteria, *S. aureus, S. pyogenes, M. catarrhalis,* and gram-negative bacteria being recovered less often.[36–38] Despite the excellent penetration of fluoroquinolones into the tissues of the upper respiratory tract, including the nasal and sinus mucosa, their relatively weak activity against gram-positive cocci argues against their use as first-line agents in treating sinus infections.

Ofloxacin has been evaluated in two studies totaling only 18 patients with acute sinusitis.[39, 40] In both studies, there was no control group, the duration of treatment was relatively short, three cultures were sterile, and the recovery of *S. aureus* was unusually high (10/18). Oral ciprofloxacin (500 mg twice daily for 10 days) was equivalent to cefuroxime for acute sinusitis in a double-blind multicenter study[41]; all patients underwent sinus puncture or aspiration. Oral ciprofloxacin has also been evaluated for chronic sinusitis, but results were indeterminant.[42–44] These studies were limited by their failure to use antral puncture for obtaining pretreatment and posttreatment cultures. Moreover, ci-

profloxacin proved no better than amoxicillin plus clavulanate, an agent whose antimicrobial spectrum justifies its empirical use in patients with chronic sinusitis for whom amoxicillin therapy has failed. *P. aeruginosa* is a rare cause of sinusitis in immunocompetent patients.

Acute Pharyngotonsillitis

There have been several reports concerning the efficacy of fluoroquinolones for acute pharyngotonsillitis.[45–47] When compared with amoxicillin (250 mg three times daily), ofloxacin (200 mg three times daily) was found to be equally effective.[47] The other studies did not use comparative control groups but reported good results using either ciprofloxacin (250 mg twice daily) or ofloxacin (600 mg daily). Despite the general success reported in these studies, there is little rationale for employing fluoroquinolones as first-line agents in acute bacterial tonsillitis given the efficacy of other, less expensive agents.

Nasal Carriage of Bacteria

Neisseria meningitidis

Ciprofloxacin has excellent in vitro activity against *N. meningitidis,* and its concentration in nasal secretions exceeds the MIC_{90} of this organism by 70-fold.[48] Nasal secretion concentrations were as high as 0.40 μg/mL (mean of about 0.14 μg/mL), approximately 10% of that in serum, whereas the MIC^{90} of *N. meningitidis* was about 0.004 μg/mL.

Short courses of ciprofloxacin, ranging from 2 to 5 days at doses of 250–500 mg twice daily, were effective in eradicating meningococcal carriage in chronic carriers.[49–51] Furthermore, a single oral dose of 750 mg of ciprofloxacin was evaluated in a placebo-controlled, double-blind trial of healthy volunteers.[52] One dose proved to be effective in eradicating the organism in 96% of subjects at 7 and 21 days after therapy. Of note, one of the subjects who was successfully treated carried a minocycline-resistant strain. Thus, ciprofloxacin may prove to be particularly useful in nasopharyngeal carriers of sulfonamide- or minocycline-resistant organisms.

Staphylococcus aureus

Ciprofloxacin concentration in nasal secretions failed to reach concentrations sufficient to inhibit *S. aureus,* either methicillin-sensitive or methicillin-resistant strains.[48] In a study of staphylococcal nasal carriage in hemodialysis patients given ciprofloxacin, 750 mg a day for 6 days, 54% of the patients were free of staphylococci 1 day after therapy; however, the percentage had declined to only 27% 4 weeks later.[53] Not only has prolonged usage of ciprofloxacin been relatively ineffective in eradicating carriage by methicillin-resistant *S. aureus,* but also, emergence of resistance in vitro has been commonplace following therapy.[54]

ADVERSE REACTIONS

In general, the quinolones are relatively safe, and severe toxic effects are rare. Adverse reactions seem to occur at similar rates among various quinolones (4%–15%), and most have been mild to moderate in severity.[2] Prolonged use of the quinolones has been well tolerated, a factor that has allowed oral administration for 6–12 weeks or even long-term suppressive treatment.[4, 8]

The most common adverse effects are gastrointestinal symptoms, including nausea, dyspepsia, vomiting, abdominal pain, and diarrhea. These have been reported in 1%–8% of patients. *Clostridium difficile* enterocolitis has been reported infrequently. Symptoms involving the central nervous system, including headache, dizziness, confusion, restlessness, tremors, hallucinations, and seizures, have been reported in 0.9%–7.4% of patients in clinical trials.[4] Seizures may occur more commonly in patients with underlying brain disorders than in other patients.[3]

Like other antibiotics, the quinolones can cause hypersensitivity reactions, including rashes, pruritus, fever, urticaria, and anaphylaxis. With widespread use, other adverse reactions have been reported: acute renal failure, vasculitis, serum sickness. Leukopenia and eosinophilia generally occur in less than 1% of patients, and mild elevations in serum transaminases occur in less than 1%–3% of patients receiving quinolones; these abnormalities are rarely sufficient to require cessation of therapy.[55]

Ciprofloxacin has been implicated in damage to developing cartilage in immature animals. Such damage, however, has not been shown in children treated with ciprofloxacin.[56–58] Nevertheless, quinolones should be used selectively in children and reserved for microorganisms refractory to other antimicrobial agents. The most common indication in children has been outpatient therapy for chronic lower respiratory infection due to *P. aeruginosa* in selected children with cystic fibrosis.

DRUG INTERACTIONS

Gastrointestinal absorption of all quinolones is substantially reduced with concurrent administration of aluminum, mag-

nesium, or calcium containing antacids, sucralfate (which contains a large amount of aluminum), oral iron preparations, oral zinc salts and zinc in multivitamin preparations, and the buffered formulation of didanosine. Spacing the administration times of the quinolones and the interacting substance by at least 2 to 4 hours may reduce this interaction, although expecting patient compliance with exact dosing times may be unreasonable. The bioavailability of quinolones may also be decreased by enteral feedings.[4]

Quinolones vary in the extent to which they impair the elimination of the methylxanthine alkaloids theophylline, caffeine, and theobromine. The effects come from inhibition by some quinolones of hepatic microsomal enzymes involved in theophylline and caffeine metabolism. There is a 30% reduction in clearance and a 20%–90% increase in serum concentrations of theophylline with ciprofloxacin and pefloxacin, but only 2%–11% increases in serum concentrations of theophylline with ofloxacin and fleroxacin. Lomefloxacin does not appear to inhibit theophylline metabolism. Ciprofloxacin has also been shown to reduce the clearance of caffeine by about one third. In general, theophylline concentrations should be closely monitored, and caffeine consumption evaluated or minimized, when treatment with a quinolone is initiated.[59]

Ciprofloxacin may increase cyclosporine levels and thereby lead to additional toxicity. Nonsteroidal anti-inflammatory drugs may affect the central nervous stimulant effects of quinolones. Enoxacin, when administered with fenbufen, has been associated with seizures. Cimetidine and probenecid reduce the renal clearance of ciprofloxacin, norfloxacin, lomefloxacin, and fleroxacin by competing for tubular secretion.[3] Interactions with other drugs have been studied less extensively (Table 9–5).

DOSING

Only a few studies have assessed the dosing of quinolones in otorhinolaryngeal infections. Ciprofloxacin, 500 mg ad-

Table 9–5. QUINOLONE DRUG INTERACTIONS

Precipitant Drug	Object Drug(s)	Object Drug Increased or Decreased	Description	Reference
Antacids Didanosine Iron salts Sucralfate Zinc salts	Quinolones	Decreased	Interference of gastrointestinal absorption of the quinolones, resulting in decreased serum levels. Avoid concurrent use; separate administration times by at least 2–4 hours.	4
Cimetidine	Quinolones	Increased	Cimetidine may interfere with the elimination of the quinolone.	3
Probenecid	Quinolones	Increased	Ciprofloxacin renal clearance is reduced by 50%, and its serum concentration is increased 50%; diminished urinary excretion of lomefloxacin and fleroxacin.	3
Ciprofloxacin Pefloxacin	Caffeine	Increased	Total-body clearance of caffeine is reduced, possibly resulting in increased pharmacologic effect. Ofloxacin and lomefloxacin do not appear to affect caffeine.	59
Ciprofloxacin	Cyclosporine	Increased	The nephrotoxic effect of cyclosporine may be increased.	3
Ciprofloxacin	Hydantoins	Decreased	Phenytoin serum concentrations may be reduced, producing a decrease in therapeutic effect.	4
Quinolones	Anticoagulants	Increased	The effect of the anticoagulant may be increased. Monitor prothrombin time.	2
Quinolones excluding lomefloxacin	Theophylline	Increased	Decreased clearance and increased plasma levels and toxicity of theophylline have occurred. Monitor theophylline levels.	59
Nonsteroidal anti-inflammatory drugs	Quinolones	Increased	May increase the risk of CNS stimulation and seizures.	3

ministered orally every 12 hours for 9 days, was effective in the treatment of chronic suppurative otitis in adults.[5] Lang and colleagues[56] used ciprofloxacin, 30 mg/kg/day, in children for the treatment of chronic suppurative otitis media without cholesteatoma. More than 100 patients have been treated with a quinolone alone for malignant otitis externa, most commonly ciprofloxacin given by mouth in a dosage of 750 mg twice daily for 6 to 12 weeks; at least 90% of the patients were cured.[8, 60] In another study, ciprofloxacin, 250 mg given by mouth twice daily for 7 to 10 days, was clinically effective in 100% of patients with paranasal sinusitis or pharyngitis/pharyngolaryngitis, in 90% of patients with otitis media, and in 85.7% of patients with tonsillitis.[61] Pefloxacin, 400 mg administered by mouth every 12 hours, has been shown to be effective in the treatment of chronic maxillary sinusitis.[6]

SUMMARY

Although ENT infections are among the most common outpatient maladies in the world, fluoroquinolones are inappropriate agents for initial therapy of most infections, for a number of reasons. They possess only intermediate activity against the most commonly isolated bacterial pathogens and thus may only suppress rather than eradicate the organism. Reports of pneumococcal bacteremia and meningitis following ciprofloxacin therapy for acute otitis media support this hypothesis.[62, 63] Ciprofloxacin appears to be an ideal drug for infections caused by *P. aeruginosa* (such as malignant external otitis and auricular perichondritis). The quinolones may be useful as alternative agents for treatment of nasal carriage of *N. meningitidis*. They have proved disappointing against nasal carriage of *S. aureus*. The use of newer quinolones for ENT therapy remains to be evaluated.

References

1. Barza M: Use of quinolones for treatment of ear and eye infections. Eur J Clin Microbiol Infect Dis 1991; 10: 296–303.
2. Maddix DS, Warner L: Do we need an intravenous fluoroquinolone? West J Med 1992; 157: 55–59.
3. Walker RC, Wright AJ: The fluoroquinolones: Symposium on antimicrobial agents—part IV. Mayo Clin Proc 1991; 66: 1249–1259.
4. Hooper DC, Wolfson JS: Quinolone Antimicrobial Agents, 2nd ed. Washington, D.C.: American Society of Microbiology, 1993.
5. Massias L, Buffe P, Cohen B, et al.: Study of the distribution of oral ciprofloxacin into the mucosa of the middle ear and the cortical bone of the mastoid process. Chemotherapy 1994; 40 (suppl): 3–7.
6. Petrikkos G, Goumas P, Moschovakis E, Giamarellou H: Penetration of pefloxacin into maxillary sinus cavity and nasal secretions. Eur J Clin Microbiol Infect Dis 1992; 11: 828–830.
7. Evans WE, Schentag JJ, Jusko WJ, Relling MV (eds): Applied Pharmacokinetics. Principles of Therapeutic Drug Monitoring. 3rd ed. Vancouver, Washington: Applied Therapeutics, 1992.
8. Rubin J, Stoehr G, Yu VL, et al.: Efficacy of oral ciprofloxacin plus rifampin for treatment of malignant external otitis. Arch Otolaryngol Head Neck Surg 1989; 115: 1063–1069.
9. Hooper DC: Quinolone mode of action. Drugs 1995; 49 (suppl 2): 10–15.
10. Rubin J, Yu VL: Malignant external otitis: Insights into pathogenesis, clinical manifestations, diagnosis, and therapy. Am J Med 1988; 85: 391–397.
11. Rubin J, Yu VL, Stool SE: Malignant external otitis in children. J Pediatr 1988; 113: 965–970.

12. Gilbert D, Tice AD, Marsh PK, et al.: Oral ciprofloxacin therapy for chronic contiguous osteomyelitis caused by aerobic gram-negative bacilli. Am J Med 1987; 82: S254–S258.
13. Hessen MT, Ingerman MJ, Kaufman OH, et al.: Clinical efficacy of ciprofloxacin therapy for gram-negative bacillary osteomyelitis. Am J Med 1987; 83: S262–S265.
14. Leese AJ, Freer C, Salata RA, et al.: Oral ciprofloxacin therapy for gram-negative bacillary osteomyelitis caused by aerobic gram-negative bacilli. Am J Med 1987; 82: 255–262.
15. Slama TG, Misinski J, Sklar S: Oral ciprofloxacin therapy for osteomyelitis caused by aerobic gram-negative bacilli. Am J Med 1987; 82: S259–S261.
16. Wise R, Donovan IA: Tissue penetration and metabolism of ciprofloxacin. Am J Med 1987; 182: S103–S107.
17. Hirata CA, Hirata I, Guay DRP, et al.: Steady-state pharmacokinetics of intravenous and oral ciprofloxacin in elderly patients. Antimicrob Agents Chemother 1989; 33: 1927–1931.
18. Hickey SA, Ford GR, O'Connor AF, et al.: Treating malignant otitis with oral ciprofloxacin. Br Med J 1989; 299: 550–551.
19. Joachims HZ, Danino J, Raz R: Malignant external otitis: Treatment with fluoroquinolones. Am J Otolaryngol 1988; 9: 102–105.
20. Leggett JM, Prendergast K: Clinical records: Malignant external otitis: The use of oral ciprofloxacin. 1988; 102: 53–54.
21. Levenson MJ, Parisier SC, Dolitsky J, Bindra G: Ciprofloxacin: Drug of choice in the treatment of malignant external otitis (MEO). Laryngoscope 1991; 101: 821–824.
22. Levy RT, Shpitzer J, Shvero, Pitlik SD: Oral ofloxacin as treatment of malignant external otitis: A study of 17 cases. Laryngoscope 1990; 100: 548–551.
23. Morrison GAJ, Bailey CM: Relapsing malignant otitis externa successfully treated with ciprofloxacin. J Laryngol Otol 1988; 102: 872–876.
24. Sade J, Lang R, Goshen S, Kitzes-Cohen R: Ciprofloxacin treatment of malignant external otitis. Am J Med 1989; 87: 5A138S–5A141S.
25. Zikk D, Rapport Y, Shalit I, et al.: Oral ciprofloxacin therapy for invasive external otitis. Ann Otol Rhinol Laryngol 1991; 100: 632–637.
26. Cooper MA, Andrews JM, Wise R: Ciprofloxacin resistance developing during treatment of malignant otitis externa. J Antimicrob Chemother 1993; 32: 163–164.
27. Giamarellou H: Malignant otitis externa: The therapeutic evolution of a lethal infection. J Antimicrob Chemother 1992; 30: 745–751.
28. Noel SB, Scallan P, Meadors MC, et al.: Treatment of *Pseudomonas aeruginosa* auricular perichondritis with oral ciprofloxacin. J Dermatol Surg Oncol 1989; 6: 633–637.
29. Giamarellou H, Galanakis N, Daphnis E, et al.: Treating acute and chronic otitis with ciprofloxacin: A step toward a better prognosis? (extended abstract). Rev Infect Dis 1988; 10 (suppl 1): S248.
30. Piccirillo JF, Parnes SM: Ciprofloxacin for the treatment of chronic ear disease. Laryngoscope 1989; 99: 510–513.
31. Sundberg L, Eden T: Penetration of enoxacin into middle ear fluid effusion. Acta Otolaryngol 1990; 109: 438–443.
32. Esposito S, D'Errico G, Montanaro C: Topical and oral treatment of chronic otitis media with ciprofloxacin: A preliminary study. Otolaryngol Head Neck Surg 1990; 116: 557–559.
33. Rodriguez JAG, Sanchez JEG, Garcia MIG, et al.: Efficacy of topical ciprofloxacin in the treatment of ear infections in adults. J Antimicrob Chemother 1993; 31: 452–453.
34. Krajewski MJ: Effectiveness of enoxacin in the treatment of chronic suppurative otitis media. Rev Infect Dis 1988; 10 (suppl 1): S248.
35. Esposito S, Noviello S, D'Errico G, Monteraro C: Topical ciprofloxacin versus intramuscular gentamicin for chronic otitis media. Arch Otolaryngol Head Neck Surg 1992; 118: 842–844.
36. Jousimies-Somer HR, Sarolainen S, Ylikoski JS: Bacteriologic findings of acute maxillary sinusitis in young adults. J Clin Microbiol 1985; 26: 1919–1925.
37. Hamory BH, Sande MA, Sydnor A Jr, et al.: Etiology and antimicrobial therapy of acute maxillary sinusitis. J Infect Dis 1979; 139: 192–202.
38. Evans FO Jr, Sydor JB, Moore WEC, et al.: Sinusitis of the maxillary antrum. N Engl J Med 1975; 293: 735–739.
39. Sanbe B, Yoshihama H, Veda R, et al.: Experimental and clinical studies on DL-8280 in the field of otorhinolaryngology. Chemotherapy (Tokyo) 1984; 32 (suppl): 1019–1029.
40. Sugita R, Kawamura S, Fujimaki Y, Deguchi K: Clinical experience of DL-8280 in the otorhinolaryngological infections. Chemotherapy (Tokyo) 32 (suppl 1): 1013–1018.

41. Heyd A, Echols R, Shan M, et al.: Oral ciprofloxacin vs. cefuroxime axetil in the treatment of acute sinusitis [abstract]. Presented at the 35th Interscience Conference on Antimicrobial Agents and Chemotherapy; 1995; LM31, San Francisco.

42. Fombeur JP, Barrault S, Kaubbi G, et al.: Study of the efficacy and safety of ciprofloxacin in the treatment of chronic sinusitis. Chemotherapy 1994; 40 (suppl): 24–28.

43. Legent F, Bordure PH, Beauvillain C, Berchep P: A double-blind comparison of ciprofloxacin and amoxicillin/clavulanate acid in the treatment of sinusitis. Chemotherapy 1994; 40 (suppl 1): 8–15.

44. Scully BE, Parry MF, Neu HC, Mandell W: Oral ciprofloxacin therapy of infections due to *Pseudomonas aeruginosa*. Lancet 1986; 1: 819–822.

45. Esposito S, D'Errico G, Montanaro C: Oral ciprofloxacin for treatment of acute bacterial pharyngotonsillitis. J Chemother 1990; 2: 108–112.

46. Iwasawa T: Fundamental and clinical studies on DL-8280 in the otorhinolaryngologic field. Chemotherapy (Tokyo) 1984; 32 (suppl 1): 1001–1012.

47. Sasaki T, Unno T, Tomiyama T, et al.: Evaluation of clinical effectiveness and safety of DL-8280 in acute lacunar tonsillitis. Otol Fukuoka 1984; 30: 484–513.

48. Darouiche R, Perkins B, Musher D, et al.: Levels of rifampin and ciprofloxacin in nasal secretions: Correlation with MIC 90 and eradication of nasopharyngeal carriage of bacteria. J Infect Dis 1990; 162: 1124–1127.

49. Piercy EA, Bawdon R, MacKowiak MPA: Penetration of ciprofloxacin into saliva and nasal secretion and effect of the drug on the oropharyngeal flora of all subjects. Antimicrob Agents Chemother 1989; 33: 1645–1646.

50. Pugsley MP, Dworzack DL, Horowitz E, et al.: Efficacy of ciprofloxacin in the treatment of nasopharyngeal carriers of *Neisseria meningitidis*. J Infect Dis 1987; 156: 211–213.

51. Renkonen OV, Sivonen A, Visakorpi R: Effect of ciprofloxacin on carrier rate of *Neisseria meningitidis* in army recruits in Finland. Antimicrob Agents Chemother 1987; 31: 962–963.

52. Dworzack DL, Sanders CC, Horowitz EA, et al.: Evaluation of a single dose ciprofloxacin in the eradication of *Neisseria meningitidis* from nasopharyngeal carriers. Antimicrob Agents Chemother 1988; 32: 1740–1741.

53. Chow JW, Yu VL: Failure of oral ciprofloxacin in suppressing *Staphylococcus aureus* carriage in hemodialysis patients. J Antimicrob Chemother 1992; 29: 88–89.

54. Peterson L, Quick J, Jensen B, et al.: Emergence of ciprofloxacin resistance in nosocomial methicillin-resistant *Staphylococcus aureus* isolation: Resistance during ciprofloxacin plus rifampin therapy for methicillin-resistant *S. aureus* colonization. Arch Intern Med 1990; 150: 2151–2155.

55. Hooper DC: Quinolones. In: Mandell GL, Bennett JE, Dolin R (eds): Principles and Practice of Infectious Diseases. New York: Churchill-Livingstone, 1995.

56. Lang R, Goshen S, Raas-Rothschild A, et al.: Oral ciprofloxacin in the management of chronic suppurative otitis media without cholesteatoma in children: Preliminary experience in 21 children. Pediatr Infect Dis J 1992; 11: 925–929.

57. Orenstein DM, Pattishall EN, Noyes B, et al.: Safety of ciprofloxacin in children with cystic fibrosis. Clin Pediatr 1993; 32: 504–506.

58. Schaad UB, Salam MA, Aujard Y, et al.: Use of fluoroquinolones in pediatrics: Consensus report of an International Society of Chemotherapy Commission. Pediatr Infect Dis J 1995; 14: 1–9.

59. Robson RA: The effects of quinolones on xanthine pharmacokinetics. Am J Med 1992; 92 (suppl 4A): 4A–22S.

60. Barza M: Pharmacokinetics and efficacy of the new quinolones in infections of the eye, ear, nose, and throat. Rev Infect Dis 1988; 10: S241–S247.

61. Speciale A, Blandino G, Caccamo F, Serra A: In vitro activity and clinical efficacy of ciprofloxacin in otorhinolaryngeal infections. Drugs 1995; 49 (suppl 2): 403–405.

62. Frieden TR, Mangi RJ: Inappropriate use of oral ciprofloxacin. JAMA 1990; 264: 1438–1440.

63. Marane C, Quadri F: Beware of ciprofloxacin in acute otitis media [letter]. Br Med J 1992; 305: 870.

64. Sorgel F, Naber KG, Kinzig M, et al.: Comparative pharmacokinetics of ciprofloxacin and temafloxacin in humans: A review. Am J Med 1991; 91: 6A–51S.

65. Miao J, Zhang G, Sun C, Zhang X: Clinical and pharmacokinetics studies of levofloxacin tablet on respiratory tract infections [abstract]. Presented at International Congress of Chemotherapy; 1995.

66. Barry AL, Jones RN: In-vitro activities of temafloxacin, tosufloxacin (A-61827) and five other fluoroquinolone agents. J Antimicrob Chemother 1989; 23: 527–535.

Lutfiye Mulazimoglu
Lowell S. Young

CHAPTER TEN

Macrolides

▼

DESCRIPTION

The macrolide (macro = large; olide = lactone) antibiotics are a group of antimicrobial drugs with generally similar chemical structures, antibacterial spectra, mechanism of action and resistance, but different pharmacokinetic properties. The structure consists of a large lactone ring with 12 to 16 atoms to which sugars moieties are attached. The natural compound of the 14-membered ring is erythromycin, produced by *Streptomyces erythreus,* a soil organism, and is the prototype of the macrolide class antibiotics.[1] In the azalides, the lactone ring has a nitrogen atom inserted, and lancacidin derivatives have a 17-membered ring without attached sugars.[2]

CHEMISTRY

The large lactone ring with attached sugar is the main chemical structure of macrolides. This lactone ring is substituted by hydroxyl or alkyl groups: one ketone at C7 in 12-membered macrolides and at C9 in 14-membered macrolides, one aldehyde group in 16-membered compounds.[2] The macrolides can be classified according to the size of lactone ring and whether they are natural compounds or semisynthetic derivatives[2, 3] (Fig. 10–1).

Erythromycin and oleandomycin are naturally occurring 14-membered compounds of macrolide class antibiotics. The chemical modifications designed to prevent the acid-catalyzed decomposition of erythromycin lead to the creation of new agents. Erythromycin acistrate and rikamycin were developed through esterification or salt formation of the natural compound erythromycin. Roxithromycin, clarithromycin, dirithromycin, and flurithromycin are semisynthetic compounds with 14-membered lactone nuclei. Other new macrolides are under development.[4]

The azalides, a new structure, have a methyl-substituted nitrogen atom in the lactone ring expanded to a 15-membered structure. Azithromycin is the only member of this subclass that is commercially available. The nitrogen substitution enhances the activity of azalide against gram-negative species as well as improving the stability of the compound in acid.[3, 5, 6]

MECHANISM OF ACTION

Although erythromycin has been in clinical use for four decades, the precise mode of action of macrolides is still uncertain. All macrolides bind to 50S subunit of procaryotic ribosomes with a specific target in the 23S ribosomal RNA

molecule. The 14-membered macrolides block the translocation of peptidyl transfer RNA (tRNA), whereas the 16-membered macrolides inhibit the peptidyl transfer reaction, resulting in different inhibitory effects on the elongation phase of bacterial protein synthesis.[3] Two competing theories have been proposed for the precise mechanism of inhibition of protein synthesis: (1) Bound macrolides in the ribosome tunnel inhibit peptide bond formation and/or translocation shortly after initiation of the polypeptide chain, leading to blocking of protein synthesis.[7] (2) Bound macrolides stimulate the dissociation of peptidyl tRNA from ribosome during the elongation phase, resulting in accumulation of peptidyl tRNA, which blocks protein synthesis.[8]

MECHANISM OF RESISTANCE

Erythromycin inhibits protein synthesis by its effects on ribosome function. The metabolic modifications that enable bacteria to overcome the inhibitory action of erythromycin can be classified as follows: (1) target site alteration, (2) antibiotic modification, and (3) altered antibiotic transfer.[9] Alterations in the 23S ribosomal RNA by methylation of adenine confer resistance to all macrolides.[10, 11] This form of resistance can have either a chromosomal or a plasmid basis and can be inducible or constitutive.[12] Gram-negative bacteria are intrinsically resistant to the macrolides because the outer cell membrane is relatively impermeable to these compounds. Although relative in vitro susceptibilities to the different macrolides vary with individual bacteria, bacteria susceptible to one macrolide are usually susceptible to the other macrolides, and bacteria resistant to one macrolide are generally resistant to the other macrolides.[13, 14]

SPECTRUM OF ACTIVITY

The antimicrobial activity of the different macrolides for bacteria often associated with ear, nose, and throat (ENT) infections is listed in Table 10–1. In general, the macrolides show a fairly uniform activity against pyogenic bacteria such as streptococci and staphylococci.[15–17] Methicillin-resistant *Staphylococcus aureus* is resistant to the macrolides.[18] Clarithromycin is the most active against the *Bacteroides* species, but the least active against *Haemophilus influenzae;* however, when clarithromycin is combined with its metabolite, it has an additive activity against *H. influenzae.*[12] Azithromycin is the most active macrolide against *H. influenzae, Moraxella catarrhalis, Pasteurella multocida, Neisseria gonorrhoeae,* and *Fusobacterium* species, and the least active

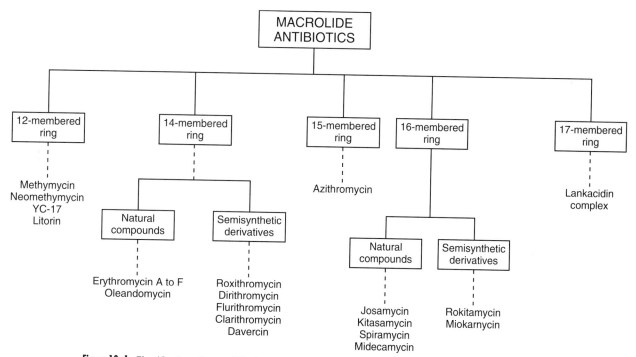

Figure 10–1. Classification of macrolides based on the lactone structure and the natural or semisynthetic origin.

macrolide against *Streptococcus* species and *Enterococcus* species. The macrolides have little activity against Enterobacteriaceae, although azithromycin at 4 mg/L is inhibitory to some of these species, especially *Escherichia coli* and *Citrobacter diversus.*[13, 15, 17] All macrolides showed excellent activity against *Bordetella pertussis,*[19] the causative agent of whooping cough. *B. pertussis* is virtually always sensitive to erythromycin (minimum inhibitory concentration [MIC] = 0.02–0.1 μg/mL); however, a strain resistant to erythromycin (MIC>64 μg/mL) was isolated from a baby who failed to respond to prolonged oral and intravenous erythromycin.[20] Clarithromycin has excellent in vitro and in vivo activity against atypical mycobacteria, including *Mycobacterium avium-intracellulare.*[21, 22] Azithromycin has excellent activity

against *Chlamydia* species,[23] *Legionella* species,[24] and *Mycoplasma pneumoniae.*[25] The in vivo activity of azithromycin against *M. avium-intracellulare* appears comparable to that of clarithromycin.[26]

The prevalence of resistance to macrolides varies for different countries. Erythromycin resistance for beta-hemolytic group A streptococci was 44% in Finland,[27] 3% in Spain,[28] and 0.5% in Japan.[29] Resistance for erythromycin was not seen in the United States against 187 isolates of group A streptococci.[30] Resistance of *Streptococcus pneumoniae* to macrolides was about 17% in Spain, 25% in France and Belgium, 20% in Greece,[31, 32] and 5%–23% in the United States.[32, 33] Acquired resistance of *H. influenzae* to macrolides has not been reported.[32] Low-level (MIC>0.5 mg/L but <8

Table 10–1. ANTIBACTERIAL ACTIVITY OF MACROLIDES

	Erythromycin		Roxithromycin		Clarithromycin		Dirithromycin		Azithromycin	
	MIC Range	*MIC90*	*MIC Range*	*MIC90*	*MIC Range*	*MIC90*	*MIC Range*	*MIC90*	*MIC Range*	*MIC90*
S. aureus	0.13–4	4	0.13–0.16	4	0.13–4	1	0.25–8	4	0.25–8	4
S. pneumoniae Penicillin-sensitive	0.03–0.5	0.06	0.06–1	0.06	0.008–0.25	0.06	0.25–1	0.25	0.06–0.5	0.25
S. pneumoniae Penicillin-resistant	0.03–2	2	0.06–4	4	0.03–1	1	0.25–8	8	0.13–8	8
S. pyogenes	0.03–0.06	0.06	0.13–0.25	0.25	0.03–0.06	0.03	0.13–0.5	0.25	0.03–0.5	0.5
H. influenzae Ampicillin-sensitive	2–4	4	2–8	8	1–4	4	4–8	8	0.13–2	1
H. influenzae Ampicillin-resistant	0.5–4	4	1–16	8	1–8	8	8–16	16	0.06–2	1
M. catarrhalis	0.03–0.25	0.25	0.06–0.25	0.25	0.03–0.13	0.13	0.06–0.25	0.25	0.03–0.125	0.125
Bacteroides spp.	0.03–4	2	0.25–16	2	0.06–1	0.5	2–32	32	0.25–2	2

Data tallied from references 15, 16
MIC = minimum inhibitory concentration

Table 10–2. PHARMACOKINETICS OF MACROLIDES

Antibiotic	Dose (mg)	t_{max} (h)	C_{max} (mg/L)	$t_{1/2}$ (h)	AUC (mg.h/l)	Primary Route of Elimination	Reference Number
Erythromycin	500	1.2	2.1	1.6	7.3	Bile	35
Erythromycin acistrate	250	0.6	2.31	1.9	8.1	Bile	36
Roxithromycin	150	1.9	7.9	10.5	8.1	Bile	37
Clarithromycin[a]	400	2	2.41	4.9	18.9	Bile and urine	12
14-OH-Clarithromycin			0.66	7.2	6.0		
Dirithromycin	500	3.9	0.3	28	1.4	Bile	38
Azithromycin[b]	500	1.7	0.4	11	3.4	Bile	39

[a]Dose modification in severe renal failure is required for clarithromycin.
[b]Dosage modifications for azithromycin may not be required for patients with class A or B liver cirrhosis.[40]

mg/L) macrolide resistance was evident in less than 5% of the *M. catarrhalis* strains.[34] *Corynebacterium diphtheriae* resistance to erythromycin has been reported.[12] Resistance for *M. pneumoniae* has not been documented.[12, 32]

PHARMACOKINETICS AND PENETRATION INTO THE ENT SECRETIONS

The pharmacokinetics and penetration into the ENT secretions are shown in Table 10–2[35-40] and Table 10–3,[41-48] respectively. The new macrolides have good tissue penetration and favorable pharmacokinetic profiles such that once- or twice-daily dosage is possible. One drawback of all macrolides is their poor penetration into the cerebrospinal fluid.[1, 12] Although erythromycin crosses the placenta, no adverse effects on the human fetus have been reported.[49] Macrolides are excreted in breast milk.

CLINICAL USE IN ENT INFECTIONS

Macrolides can be considered as ideal antimicrobial agents for ENT infections, with good penetration into oropharyn-geal and respiratory secretions and minimal ecologic disturbance to the normal flora. In addition, the new macrolides appear to have only minor side effects, can be administered only once or twice a day, and require shorter duration of therapy. Treatment failures with penicillin for group A streptococci,[50] increasing resistance of *S. pneumoniae* against penicillin,[51] and emergence of ampicillin-resistant *H. influenzae* and beta lactamase–producing *M. catarrhalis*[32, 34, 52, 53] are factors that make macrolides unusually attractive alternative therapy for the treatment of ENT infections. Table 10–4 shows dosages for macrolides.

Major Indications

Erythromycin is one of the most effective antimicrobial agents for treatment of nonstreptococcal pharyngitis due to *Chlamydia pneumoniae*[54-56] and *M. pneumoniae*.[57] It is very effective for pertussis infection as well as decreasing transmission in pertussis outbreaks.[58] For diphtheria and for carrier state with *Corynebacterium diphtheriae*, erythromycin is the antibiotic of choice.[59]

Table 10–3. TISSUE AND FLUID KINETICS OF MACROLIDES

Antibiotic	Tissue or Fluid	Dose	Sampling Time (h)	Peak Serum Concentration	Tissue (t) or Fluid (f) Concentration	Ratio t/s or f/s	Reference Number
Erythromycin ethylsuccinate	Sinus mucosa	1000 mg	1.5–2	1.60 ± 0.50	1.2 ± 0.4	0.80	41
	Tonsils	1000 mg	2	3.39 ± 0.28	1.20	0.35	42
Roxithromycin	Nasal mucosa	300 mg	12	2.00 ± 0.28	0.52 ± 0.26	0.26	43
	Tonsils	300 mg	12	2.36 ± 0.60	1.26 ± 0.66	0.53	43
Clarithromycin	Middle ear effusion	7.5 mg/kg twice daily	2.5[b]	1.7 ± 1.2	2.5 ± 2.3	2.5 ± 3.6	44
14-OH-metabolite	Middle ear effusion	7.5 mg/kg twice daily	2.5[b]	0.8 ± 0.3	1.3 ± 1.0	1.7 ± 1.4	44
Dirithromycin[a]	Nasal mucosa	500 mg	12	0.07 ± 0.03	1.86 ± 0.54	26.5	45
	Tonsils	500 mg	15	0.08	1.8	22	45
Azithromycin	Tonsils	500 mg	13	0.03 ± 0.04	4.5 ± 2.6	> 150	46
	Leukocytes	0.5 mg/mL	2			> 270	47
	Macrophages	0.5 mg/mL	2			> 300	47
	Sinus fluid (acute)	500 mg	24		1.34		48
	Sinus fluid (chronic)	500 mg	24		0.25		48

[a]Data on file, Eli-Lilly.
[b]After the 5th dose.

Table 10–4. DOSAGES FOR MACROLIDES

	Adult	Child
Erythromycin base	250–1000 mg every 6 h	30–50 mg/kg day 4 times daily
Roxithromycin	150 mg every 12 h or 300 mg daily	5–8 mg/kg day 2 times daily
Clarithromycin[a]	250–500 mg every 12 h	15 mg/kg day 2 times daily
Dirithromycin	250–500 mg/daily	N/A
Azithromycin	250–500 mg/daily	5–10 mg/kg daily

Consult packages for definitive recommendations.

[a]Dosage modification is required for severe renal failure.

Pharyngitis

Erythromycin is the alternative therapy of choice for penicillin-allergic patients with group A beta-hemolytic streptococcal pharyngitis, the most common bacterial cause of pharyngitis.[60] All macrolides appear efficacious for therapy of streptococcal pharyngitis, with one exception—the efficacy of roxithromycin remains uncertain. Two open studies found roxithromycin (300 mg once daily for 9 days and 150 mg twice daily for 7–14 days) effective for the treatment of tonsillopharyngitis with 100% and 97% clinical success rates respectively.[61, 62] However, one study of 31 evaluable patients[63] showed a comparable clinical response rate (83% for 300 mg daily for 10 days and 100% for 150 mg twice daily for 10 days) but an unacceptable bacteriologic cure rate (33%) for both roxithromycin dosing regimens. This study excluded patients considered to be carriers rather than infected. Tissue (tonsil) concentrations of roxithromycin are somewhat lower compared to those of the other macrolides.[43, 64]

Comparative studies with clarithromycin (250 mg twice daily for 10 days) versus penicillin V[65, 66] and versus erythromycin (500 mg twice daily for 10 days)[67] in adults showed clinical and bacteriologic cure rates at about 90% without significant differences between the two drugs. In children with streptococcal pharyngitis, clarithromycin (7.5 mg/kg twice daily for 10 days) was significantly more likely to produce bacteriologic cure than penicillin V (92% versus 81%, p < .004), although clinical cure rates were identical (96% versus 94%).[68] The gastrointestinal side effects were significantly greater for clarithromycin (14%) as compared to those for penicillin V (5%) (p < .001).

In adults with streptococcal pharyngitis, dirithromycin (500 mg once daily for 10 days) had comparable clinical and bacteriologic response to erythromycin (250 mg four times daily for 10 days).[69, 70] Cure rates were more than 79% for both macrolides; however, adverse effects, mainly gastrointestinal, were significantly more frequent for erythromycin in the first study (54% versus 44%, p < .015).[69]

Azithromycin (10 mg/kg/day for 3 days, 500 mg initially, then 250 mg daily for 5 days) compared with penicillin V (125 or 250 mg four times daily for 10 days) and erythromycin (30–50 mg/kg/day for 10 days) in adults and children with streptococcal pharyngitis showed efficacy of more than 90%, both clinically and bacteriologically for all drugs.[71–73] The side effects, mainly gastrointestinal, were significantly more frequent for azithromycin than penicillin V in one study of adults (17% versus 2%, p < .001).[71] However, azithromycin (12 mg/kg/day for 5 days) was statistically superior to penicillin V (250 mg three times daily for 10 days) both clinically (97% versus 82%, p < .001) and bacteriologically (95% versus 69%, p < .001) in one study of children.[74] On the other hand, azithromycin (10 mg/kg/day for 3 days) had more frequent bacteriologic (46% versus 14%, p < .0001) and clinical recurrences (25% versus 9%, p <.01) than penicillin V (25,000 units/kg twice daily for 10 days) in another study of children.[75]

Otitis Media

Erythromycin-sulfisoxazole has long been standard therapy for acute otitis media.[52, 76, 77] Clarithromycin (7.5 mg/kg twice daily for 10 days) compared with amoxicillin in the treatment of acute otitis media in children showed clinical success rates of more than 90% for both drugs without any significant differences between the two antibiotics.[78] Clarithromycin and amoxicillin/clavulanate showed clinical response rates above 90% in two comparative studies;[53, 79] diarrhea (32% versus 12%, p < .001 and 40% versus 12%, p < .001)[53, 79] and diaper rash[53] (12% versus 1%, p < .004) were significantly more common for patients treated with amoxicillin/clavulanate.

Azithromycin (10 mg/kg/day for 3 days) compared with amoxicillin[80] and amoxicillin/clavulanate[81] showed comparable clinical success (more than 95%) with a low incidence of side effects for either antibiotic. Two other comparative studies of azithromycin versus amoxicillin/clavulanate reported clinical response rates higher than 90% for both antibiotics;[82, 83] however, a significantly higher incidence of diarrhea was found in the amoxicillin/clavulanate group in the second study (16% versus 2.5%, p < .001).[83] Azithromycin (10 mg/kg once initially, then 5 mg/kg daily for 4 days) was comparable to amoxicillin/clavulanate in another study, with 61% and 65% clinical response rates, respectively. Side effects—mostly diarrhea—were more common in the amoxicillin/clavulanate group (17% versus 7%, p < .001).[84] Long-term erythromycin (erythromycin base 600 mg/day for more than 4 months) was effective for the treatment of sinobronchial syndrome–associated otitis media with effusion.[85]

Sinusitis

Clarithromycin (500 mg twice daily for 10–14 days) was comparable to amoxicillin and amoxicillin/clavulanate for therapy of acute maxillary sinusitis in adults.[86, 87] Clinical success rates were about 90%, with comparable radiologic and bacteriologic outcomes for all drugs. However, amoxicillin/clavulanate had significantly more gastrointestinal side effects compared with clarithromycin (38% versus 21%, p < .001).

Azithromycin (500 mg initially, then 250 mg/day for 5 days) (74% and 81%) was comparable to amoxicillin (73% and 72%) for therapy of acute maxillary and frontal sinusitis as defined by radiologic and bacteriologic criteria.[88, 89] Azithromycin (500 mg daily for 3 days) was comparable to clarithromycin (250 mg twice daily for 10 days), with greater than 90% clinical and bacteriologic response rates for both drugs for the treatment of adult patients with acute sinusitis.[90]

ADVERSE EFFECTS

Macrolides are among the safest antimicrobial agents, and serious adverse effects are rare. Gastrointestinal adverse effects are the most prominent. Abdominal pain (16%), nausea and vomiting (14%), and diarrhea (4%) are reported most frequently with erythromycin, and their overall incidence is about 30%.[91] Erythromycin acts as a motilin receptor agonist in the gastrointestinal tract and stimulates motility.[92] Macrolide-induced emesis may be partially due to 5-hydroxytryptamine receptors. This side effect is dose-dependent and probably structurally related. The presence of the dimethylamino group on the neutral sugar at C3 of the lactone ring appeared necessary for the motor stimulating activity.[93] Gastrointestinal adverse effects can occur with any route of administration, including parenteral.[94]

The new derivative, erythromycin acistrate, causes fewer gastrointestinal side effects (7%) compared with erythromycin base (50%).[95] The newer macrolides have fewer gastrointestinal adverse effects than erythromycin (about 30%)[91]: 3% for roxithromycin,[96] 9% for clarithromycin,[97] 16% for dirithromycin, and 10% for azithromycin.[98]

Hepatotoxicity

Overall hepatotoxicity is very rare, but is the most serious side effect of erythromycin. The incidence of patients developing acute symptomatic liver disease resulting in hospitalization after treatment with a 10-day course of erythromycin was estimated at 2.3 per million patients,[99] and the risk of cholestatic jaundice was estimated at 0.4 per million patients.[100] Although not fully understood, the mechanism of this injury may represent a hypersensitivity and toxic reactions resulting from formation of nitrosoalkanes.[101] Troleandomycin, erythromycin, and its pro-drugs form nitrosoalkanes, which are hepatotoxic. The semisynthetic macrolides rarely or never form nitrosoalkanes and therefore are less likely to cause hepatotoxicity.[5]

Hepatotoxicity can occur with any erythromycin formulation, including erythromycin ethylsuccinate, propionate, and estolate,[102–104] although most of the initial reports implicated the estolate formulation.[105]

Hepatotoxicity occurs most commonly in adults and usually after 1 to 2 weeks of drug administration. Nausea and abdominal pain are initial symptoms followed by fever (50%). Jaundice with pruritus has been reported in 20% of patients. Sixty-seven percent of patients have eosinophilia, with total eosinophil counts exceeding 500 cells/mm³. Serum bilirubin and alkaline phosphatase concentrations are increased in about 50% of patients, and transaminase levels are uniformly elevated. Liver function tests reverted to normal within days after discontinuation of drug but may recur on rechallenge.[105]

Ototoxicity

The hearing loss due to erythromycin was first reported in 1973 following high-dose intravenous administration of the drug;[106] since then more than 50 anecdotal cases have been reported. The incidence of ototoxicity is uncertain but is likely underestimated. Eleven cases of hearing loss attributed to erythromycin ototoxicity were reported from one hospital in 20 months, once clinicians were informed of this potential adverse effect.[107] A prospective case-control study found evidence of ototoxicity in 21% of patients receiving a 4 g/day dose, when audiograms were performed and patients were closely monitored.[108]

The mechanism of erythromycin ototoxicity is not known, but it may occur by an effect on the central auditory pathways.[109] Auditory dysfunction is most common;[109] however, vestibular dysfunction may also occur.[110, 111] Erythromycin causes low tonal tinnitus, and hearing loss ranges from bilateral flat to high-frequency sensorineural loss, which can be detected on audiograms at both conventional (0.25–8.0 kHz) and extended high frequencies (8–14 kHz). Ototoxicity can occur with all formulations, including the lactobionate and stearate.[107, 112]

Subjective symptoms begin within the first week of drug administration,[107, 108] but are usually reversible within 1 to 30 days upon discontinuation of the drug.[109] However, irreversible tinnitus unilaterally has been reported with intravenous administration of erythromycin lactobionate 4 g/day in an elderly patient after 24 hours of therapy.[113] Irreversible hearing loss after 5 days of therapy with intravenous erythromycin lactobionate 2 g/day occurred in one elderly patient with underlying liver disease. Persistent labyrinthitis occurred in an elderly patient given intravenous erythromycin lactobionate 4 g/day after five doses.[114]

Erythromycin ototoxicity is probably dose-dependent, as high plasma and serum concentrations have been documented in patients with hearing loss.[108, 115, 116] Preexisting hepatic or renal abnormalities, advanced age, and dosages exceeding 4 g/day and concurrent ototoxic medications are predisposing factors.[117–119] In a prospective study, erythromycin ototoxicity occurred significantly more often in patients who received erythromycin 4 g/day versus 2 g/day, with peak erythromycin concentrations exceeding 12µg/mL for patients experiencing ototoxicity. Ototoxicity was found significantly related to high-peak concentration and high area under the serum concentration time curve 0–infinity as a function of decreased total systemic clearance.[108] On the other hand, ototoxicity has been reported in patients with no recognized risk factors and no overt renal or hepatic dysfunction.[107, 114]

Decreased hearing was documented in a patient with acquired immunodeficiency syndrome (AIDS) with disseminated *M. avium-intracellulare* disease while receiving clarithromycin 2000 mg/day.[120] Increased tinnitus was reported in four elderly patients with chronic mycobacterial lung disease treated with clarithromycin 2000 mg/day for 3 months. Three of these four patients had been previously treated for at least 6 months with streptomycin.[121] Reversible bilateral hearing loss occurred in three AIDS patients with *M. avium-intracellulare* infection given azithromycin 500 mg/day. The duration of therapy was 30 to 90 days.[122]

Reversible otologic complaints occurred in 17% of AIDS patients given azithromycin 600 mg/day after an average of 7.6 weeks.[123]

Other Adverse Reactions

Allergic reactions are rare (0.5%–6%) for all macrolides.[5] Erythromycin administered intramuscularly can cause pain at the injection site and when administered intravenously causes thrombophlebitis (4%).[108] Ventricular tachycardia with Qtc-interval prolongation caused by intravenous erythromycin has been reported.[124]

DRUG INTERACTIONS

Erythromycin is oxidized by cytochrome P-450 to its major metabolite and forms a stable inactive complex with reduced cytochrome P-450.[125] This may induce inhibition of metabolism of other drugs also oxidized by P-450, resulting in increased concentrations of these drugs. Interactions by this mechanism occur with the following drugs: terfenadine,[126] theophylline,[127] cyclosporin,[128, 129] warfarin,[130] carbamazepine,[131] triazolam,[132] alfentanil,[133] methylprednisolone,[134] and bromocriptine[135].

The potential for drug interaction varies with the individual macrolides. Erythromycin is more prone to form cytochrome P-450 complexes, which leads to higher concentration of drugs metabolized by the liver. Clarithromycin, flurithromycin, and roxithromycin are less potent inhibitors, and drug interactions are less frequent. Azithromycin and dirithromycin do not form complexes and therefore do not have the preceding drug interactions.[136]

Accelerated metabolism of all macrolides is seen with rifampin and rifabutin, resulting in lower serum concentrations.[137] However, concomitant use of rifabutin, clarithromycin, and fluconazole has been associated with increased levels of rifabutin in AIDS patients, resulting in hypopyon uveitis.[138] Erythromycin inhibits digoxin degradation in the gut and can induce digoxin toxicity.[139, 140]

References

1. Griffith RS, Black HR: Erythromycin. Med Clin North Am 1970; 54: 1199–1215.
2. Bryskier A, Labro MT, Chantot JF, Gasc JC: New trends in macrolide research. Chemioterapia 1987; 6: 343–345.
3. Mazzei T, Mini E, Novelli A, Periti P: Chemistry and mode of action of macrolides. J Antimicrob Chemother 1993; 31 (supp C): 1–9.
4. Asaka T, et al.: A new marcolide antibiotic, TE-802, synthesis and biological properties. 35th Intersci Conf Antimicrob Ag Chemother, San Francisco, 1995; Abstract F126, p 143.
5. Periti P, Mazzei T, Mini E, Novelli A: Adverse effects of macrolide antibacterials. Drug Sat 1993; 9: 346–364.
6. Williams JD: The new azalide antimicrobials. Curr Opin Infect Dis 1994; 7: 653–657.
7. Vazquez D: Inhibitors of protein synthesis. FEBS Lett 1974; 40: S63–84.
8. Menninger JR: Functional consequences of binding macrolides to ribosomes. J Antimicrob Chemother 1985; 16: 23–24.
9. Weisblum B: Erythromycin resistance by ribosome modification. Antimicrob Agents Chemother 1995; 39: 577–585.
10. Leclercq R, Courvalin P: Bacterial resistance to macrolide, lincosamide, and streptogramin antibiotics by target modification. Antimicrob Agents Chemother 1991; 35: 1267–1272.
11. Leclercq R, Courvalin P: Intrinsic and unusual resistance to macrolide, lincosamide, and streptogramin antibiotics in bacteria. Antimicrob Agents Chemother 1991; 35: 1273–1276.
12. Neu HC: The development of macrolides: clarithromycin in perspective. J Antimicrob Chemother 1991; 27: 1–9.
13. Fass RJ: Erythromycin, clarithromycin, and azithromycin: Use of frequency distribution curves, scattergrams, and regression analyses to compare in vitro activities and describe cross-resistance. Antimicrob Agents Chemother 1993; 37: 2080–2086.
14. Porter B, Irizarry L, Massie L: Cross resistance to macrolides among Streptococcus pneumoniae. 35th Intersci Conf Antimicrob Ag Chemother, San Francisco, 1995; Abstract E28, p 90.
15. Bauernfeind A: In vitro activity of dirithromycin in comparison with other new and established macrolides. J Antimicrob Chemother 1993; 31: 39–49.
16. Barry AL, Fuchs PC: In vitro activities of a streptogramin (RP59500), three macrolides, and an azalide against four respiratory tract pathogens. Antimicrob Agents Chemother 1995; 39: 238–240.
17. Williams JD: Spectrum of activity of azithromycin. Eur J Clin Microbiol Infect Dis 1991; 10: 813–820.
18. Hardy DJ, Hensey DM, Beyer JM, et al.: Comparative in vitro activities of new 14-, 15- and 16–membered macrolides. Antimicrob Agents Chemother 1988; 32: 1710–1719.
19. Hoppe JE, Eichhorn A: Activity of new macrolides against Bordetella pertussis and Bordetella parapertussis. Eur J Clin Microbiol Infect Dis 1989; 8: 653–654.
20. Centers for Disease Control and Prevention: Erythromycin-resistant Bordetella pertussis—Yuma County, Arizona, May–October 1994. JAMA 1995; 273: 13–14.
21. Brown BA, Wallace RJ Jr., Onyi GO: Activities of clarithromycin against eight slowly growing species of nontuberculous mycrobacteria, determined by using a broth microdilution MIC system. Antimicrob Agents Chemother 1992; 36: 1987–1990.
22. Dautzenberg B, Saint Marc T, Meyohas MC, et al.: Clarithromycin and other antimicrobial agents in the treatment of disseminated Mycobacterium avium infections in patients with acquired immunodeficiency syndrome. Arch Intern Med 1993; 153: 368–372.
23. Agacfidan A, Moncada J, Schachter J: In vitro activity of azithromycin (CP-62,993) against Chlamydia trachomatis and Chlamydia pneumoniae. Antimicrob Agents Chemother 1993; 37: 1746–1748.
24. Arnold B, Ta A, Stout JE, Yu VL: Erythromycin, dirithromycin, azithromycin, clarithromycin, and roxithromycin activity against Legionella by broth dilution and intracellular penetration. 34th Intersci Conf Antimicrob Ag Chemother, Orlando, 1994; Abstract E29, p 156.
25. Ishida K, Kaku M, Irifune K, et al.: In vitro and in vivo activities of macrolides against Mycoplasma pneumoniae. Antimicrob Ag Chemother 1994; 38: 790–798.
26. Young LS: Macrolides as antimycobacterial agents. In: Neu HC, Young LS, Zimmer SZ, Acar JF (eds): New Macrolides, Azalides, and Streptogramins in Clinical Practice. New York: Marcel Dekker, 1995.
27. Seppala H, Nissinen A, Jarvinen H, et al.: Resistance to erythromycin in group A streptococci. N Engl J Med 1992; 5: 292–297.
28. Betriu C, Sanchez A, Gomez M: Antibiotic susceptibility of group A streptococci: A 6-year follow-up study. Antimicrob Agents Chemother 1993; 37: 1717–1719.
29. Bass JW, Weisse ME, Plymyer MR, et al.: Decline of erythromycin resistance of group A beta-hemolytic streptococci in Japan: Comparison with worldwide reports. Arch Pediatr Adolesc Med 1994; 148: 67–71.
30. Kelley R, Langley G, Bates L: Erythromycin: Still a good choice for strep throat. Clin Pediatr 1993; 744–745.
31. Kanavaki S, Karabela S, Marinis E, Legakis NJ: Antibiotic resistance of clinical isolates of Streptococcus pneumoniae in Greece. J Clin Microbiol 1994; 32: 3056–3058.
32. Baquero F, Loza E: Antibiotic resistance of microorganisms involved in ear, nose, and throat infections. Pediatric Infect Dis J 1994; 13: S9–S14.
33. Lonks JR, Medeiros AA: High rate of erythromycin and clarithromycin resistance among Streptococcus pneumoniae isolates from blood cultures from Providence, R.I. Antimicrob Agents Chemother 1993; 37: 1742–1745.

34. Fernandez-Roblas R, Jimenez-Arriero M, Rodriguez-Tudela JL, Soriano F: In-vitro activity of amoxicillin/clavulanate acid and five other oral antibiotics against isolates of *Haemophilus influenzae* and *Branhamella catarrhalis*. J Antimicrob Chemother 1988; 22: 867–72.

35. Kavi J, Webberley JM, Andrews JM, Wise R: A comparison of the pharmacokinetics and tissue penetration of spiramycin and erythromycin. J Antimicrob Chemother 1988; 22 (suppl B): 105–110.

36. Mannisto PT, Taskinen J, Ottoila P: Fate of single oral doses of erythromycin acistrate, erythromycin stearate and pelleted erythromycin base analyzed by mass-spectrometry in plasma of healthy human volunteers. J Antimicrob Chemother 1988; 21 (suppl D): 33–43.

37. Tremblay D, Jaeger H, Fountillani JB, Manuel C: Pharmacokinetics of three single doses (150, 300, 450 mg) of roxithromycin in young volunteers. Br J Clin Pract 1988; 42 (suppl)55: 49–50.

38. Sides GD, Cerimele BJ, Black HR, et al.: Pharmacokinetics of dirithromycin. J Antimicrob Chemother 1993; 31 (suppl C): 65–75.

39. Foulds G, Shepard RM, Johnson RB: The pharmacokinetics of azithromycin in human and serum tissues. J Antimicrob Chemother 1990; 25 (suppl A): 73–82.

40. Mazzei T, Surrenti C, Novelli A, et al.: Pharmacokinetics of azithromycin in patients with impaired hepatic function. J Antimicrobial Chemother 1993; 31 (suppl E): 57–63.

41. Blenk H, Simm K, Blenk B, Jahnake G: Vergleich von Erythromycin und Sinusgewebe bei Patienten mit Tonsillitis und Sinusitis. Infection 1982; 10 (suppl 2): 108–112.

42. Falchi M, Teodori F, Carraro A, et al.: Penetration of erythromycin into tonsillar tissue. Curr Med Res Opin 1985; 9: 611–615.

43. Fraschini F, Scaglione F, Pintucci G, et al.: The diffusion of clarithromycin and roxithromycin into nasal mucosa, tonsil and lung in humans. J Antimicrob Chemother 1991; 27: 61–65.

44. Sundberg L, Cederberg A: Penetration of clarithromycin and its 14-hydroxy metabolite into middle ear effusion in children with secretory otitis media. J Antimicrob Chemother 1994; 33: 299–307.

45. Bergogne-Berezin E: Tissue distribution of dirithromycin: Comparison with erythromycin. J Antimicrob Chemother 1993; 31 (suppl C): 77–87.

46. Foulds G, Chan KH, Johnson JT, et al.: Concentrations of azithromycin in human tonsillar tissue. Eur J Clin Microbiol Infect Dis 1991; 10: 853–859.

47. Panteix G, Guillaumond B, Harf R, et al.: In vitro concentration of azithromycin in human phagocytic cells. J Antimicrob Chemother 1993; 31 (suppl E): 1–4.

48. Karma P, Pukander J, Penttila M: Azithromycin concentrations in sinus fluid and mucosa after oral administration. Eur J Clin Microbiol Infect Dis 1991; 10: 856–859.

49. Rothman KF, Pochi PE: Use of oral and topical agents for acne in pregnancy. J Am Acad Dermatol 1988; 19: 431–442.

50. Holm SE: Reasons for failures in penicillin treatment of streptococcal tonsillitis and possible alternatives. Pediatr Infect Dis J 1994; 13: S66–S69.

51. Klugman KP: Pneumococcal resistance to antibiotics. Clin Microbiol Rev 1990; 3: 171–196.

52. Wald ER: Antimicrobial therapy of pediatric patients with sinusitis. J Allergy Clin Immunol 1992; 90: 469–473.

53. Aspin MM, Hoberman A, McCarty J, et al.: Comparative study of the safety and efficacy of clarithromycin and amoxicillin-clavulanate in the treatment of acute otitis media in children. J Pediatr 1994; 125: 136–141.

54. McDonald CJ, Tierney WM, Hui SL, et al.: A controlled trial of erythromycin in adults with nonstreptococcal pharyngitis. J Infect Dis 1985; 152: 1093–1094.

55. Grayston JT: *Chlamydia pneumoniae,* strain TWAR: Review. Chest 1989; 95: 664–669.

56. Ogawa K, Hashiguchi K, Kazuyama Y, et al.: Respiratory tract diseases due to *Chlamydia pneumoniae*. Nippon Jibiinkoka Gakkai Kaiho 1991; 94; 351–356.

57. Martin RE, Bates JH: Atypical pneumonia. Infect Dis Clin North Am 1991; 5: 585–601.

58. Steketee RW, Wassilak SGF, Adkins WN, et al.: Evidence for a high attack rate and efficacy of erythromycin prophylaxis in a pertussis outbreak in a facility for the developmentally disabled. J Infect Dis 1988; 157: 434–440.

59. Stein GE, Havlichek DH: The new macrolide antibiotics, azithromycin and clarithromycin. Postgrad Med 1992; 92: 269–280.

60. Klein JR: Current issues in upper respiratory tract infections in infants and children: rationale for antibacterial therapy. Pediatric Infect Dis J 1994; 13: S5–8.

61. deCampora E, Camaioni A, Leonardi M, et al.: Comparative efficacy and safety of roxithromycin and clarithromycin in upper respiratory tract infections. Diagn Microbiol Infect Dis 1992; 15: 119S–122S.

62. Marsac JH: An international clinical trial on the efficacy and safety of roxithromycin in 40,000 patients with acute community-acquired respiratory tract infections. Diagn Microbiol Infect Dis 1992; 15: 81S–84S.

63. Melcher GP, Hadfield TL, Gaines JK, Winn RE: Comparative efficacy and toxicity of roxithromycin and erythromycin ethylsuccinate in the treatment of streptococcal pharyngitis in adults. J Antimicrob Chemother 1988; 22: 549–556.

64. Galioto GB, Ortisi G, Mevio E, Sassella D, et al.: Roxithromycin disposition in tonsils after single and repeated administration. Antimicrob Agents Chemother 1988; 32: 1461–1463.

65. Levenstein JH: Clarithromycin versus penicillin in the treatment of streptococcal pharyngitis. J Antimicrob Chemother 1991; 27: 67–74.

66. Bachand RT Jr: A comparative study of clarithromycin and penicillin VK in the treatment of outpatients with streptococcal pharyngitis. J Antimicrob Chemother 1991; 27: 75–82.

67. Scaglione F: Comparison of the clinical and bacteriological efficacy of clarithromycin and erythromycin in the treatment of streptococcal pharyngitis. Curr Med Res Opin 1990; 12: 25–53.

68. Still JG, Hubbard WC, Poole JM, et al.: Comparison of clarithromycin and penicillin VK suspensions in the treatment of children with streptococcal pharyngitis and review of currently available alternative antibiotic therapies. Pediatr Infect Dis J 1993; 12: S134–41.

69. Derriennic M, Conforti PM, Sides GD: Dirithromycin in the treatment of streptococcal pharyngitis. J Antimicrob Chemother 1993; 31: 89–95.

70. Muller O, Wettich K: Clinical efficacy of dirithromycin in pharyngitis and tonsillitis. J Antimicrob Chemother 1993; 31: 97–102.

71. Hooton TM: A comparison of azithromycin and penicillin V for the treatment of streptococcal pharyngitis. Am J Med 1991; 91: 3A–23S.

72. Weippl G: Multicentre comparison of azithromycin versus erythromycin in the treatment of paediatric pharyngitis or tonsillitis caused by Group A streptococci. J Antimicrob Chemother 1993; 31: 95–101.

73. Hamill J: Multicentre evaluation of azithromycin and penicillin V in the treatment of acute streptococcal pharyngitis and tonsillitis in children. J Antimicrob Chemother 1993; 31: 89–74.

74. Still JG: Treatment of streptococcal pharyngitis in children with five days of azithromycin suspension. 34th Intersci Conf Antimicrob Ag Chemother, Orlando, 1994; Abstract M67, p 246.

75. Pacifico L, Orefici G, Ranucci A, et al.: Comparison of three-day azithromycin versus ten-day penicillin V in the treatment of children with streptococcal group A pharyngitis. 35th Intersci Conf Antimicrob Ag Chemother, San Francisco, 1995; Abstract LM47, p 335.

76. Rodriguez WJ, Schwartz RH, Sait T, et al.: Erythromycin-sulfisoxazole vs. amoxicillin in the treatment of acute otitis media in children: A double-blind, multiple-dose comparative study. Am J Dis Child 1985; 139: 766–770.

77. Giebink GS, Canafax DM: Antimicrobial treatment of otitis media (review). Semin Respir Infect 1991; 6: 85–93.

78. Pukander JS, Jero JP, Kaprio EA, Sorri MJ: Clarithromycin versus amoxicillin suspensions in the treatment of pediatric patients with acute otitis media. Pediatr Infect Dis J 1993; 12: S118–21.

79. McCarty JM, Philips A, Wiisanen R: Comparative safety and efficacy of clarithromycin and amoxicillin/clavulanate in the treatment of acute otitis media in children. Pediatr Infect Dis J 1993; 12 (suppl 3): S122–127.

80. Mohs E, Rodriguez-Solares A, Rivas E, El Hoshy Z: A comparative study of azithromycin and amoxycillin in paediatric patients with acute otitis media. J Antimicrob Chemother 1993; 31 (suppl E): 73–79.

81. Pestalozza G, Cioce C, Facchini M: Azithromycin in upper respiratory infections: A clinical trial in children with otitis media. Scand J Infect Dis 1992; 83: 22–25.

82. Daniel RR: Comparison of azithromycin and co-amoxiclav in the treatment of otitis media in children. J Antimicrob Chemother 1993; 31: 65–71.

83. Schaad UB: Multicentre evaluation of azithromycin in comparison with co-amoxiclav for the treatment of acute otitis media in children. J Antimicrob Chemother 1993; 31 (suppl E): 81–88.

84. Khurana C, McLinn S, Block S, Pichichero M: Trial of azithromycin (AZ) versus Augmentin (AUG) for treatment of acute otitis media (AOM). 34th Intersci Conf Antimicrob Ag Chemother, Orlando, 1994; Abstract M61, p 246.

85. Iino Y, Sugita K, Toriyama M, Kudo K: Erythromycin therapy for otitis media with effusion in sinobronchial syndrome. Arch Otolaryngol Head Neck Surg 1993; 119: 648–651.

86. Karma P, Pukander J, Penttila M, et al.: The comparative efficacy and safety of clarithromycin and amoxycillin in the treatment of outpatients with acute maxillary sinusitis. J Antimicrob Chemother 1991; 27: 83–90.

87. Dubois J, Saint-Pierre C, Tremblay C: Efficacy of clarithromycin versus amoxicillin/clavulanate in the treatment of acute maxillary sinusitis. Ear Nose Throat J 1993; 72: 804–810.

88. Casiano RR: Azithromycin and amoxicillin in the treatment of acute maxillary sinusitis. Am J Med 1991; 91: 3A-27S–3A-30S.

89. Felstead SJ, Daniel R: European Azithromycin Study Group. Short-course treatment of sinusitis and other upper respiratory tract infections with azithromycin: a comparison with erythromycin and amoxycillin. J Int Med Res 1991; 19: 363–372.

90. Muller O: Comparison of azithromycin versus clarithromycin in the treatment of patients with upper respiratory tract infections. J Antimicrob Chemother 1993; 31: 137–146.

91. Ellsworth AJ, Christensen DB, Volpone-McMahon MT: Prospective comparison of patient tolerance to enteric-coated vs nonenteric-coated erythromycin. J Fam Pract 1990; 31: 265–270.

92. Kondo Y, Torii K, Itoh Z, Omura S: Erythromycin and its derivatives with motilin-like biological activities inhibit the specific binding of 125I-motilin to duodenal muscle. Biochem Biophys Res Commun 1988; 150: 877–882.

93. Omura S, Tsuzuki K, Sunazuka T, et al.: Gastrointestinal motor-stimulating activity of macrolide antibiotics and the structure activity relationship. J Antibio (Tokyo) 1985; 38: 1631–1632.

94. Seifert CF, Swaney RJ, Bellanger-McCleery RA: Intravenous erythromycin lactobionate-induced severe nausea and vomiting. Ann Pharmacother 1989; 23: 40–44.

95. Wuolijoki E, Flygare U, Hilden M, et al.: Treatment of respiratory tract infections with erythromycin acistrate and two formulations of erythromycin base. J Antimicrob Chemother 1988; 21: 107–112.

96. Blanc F, D'Enfert J, Fiessinger S, et al.: An evaluation of tolerance of roxithromycin in adults. J Antimicrob Chemother 1987; 20: 179–183.

97. Hardy DJ, Guay DRP, Jones RN: Clarithromycin, a unique macrolide: A pharmacokinetic, microbiological, and clinical overview. Diagn Microbiol Infect Dis 1992; 15: 39–53.

98. Hopkins S. Clinical toleration and safety of azithromycin. Am J Med 1991; 91: 40S–45S.

99. Carson JL, Strom BL, Duff A, et al.: Acute liver disease associated with erythromycin, sulfonamides, and tetracyclines. Ann Intern Med 1993; 119: 576–583.

100. Derby LE, Jick H, Henry DA, Dean AD: Erythromycin-associated cholestatis hepatitis. Med J Aust 1993; 158: 600–602.

101. Pessayre D, Larrey D, Funck-Brentano C, Benhamou JP: Drug interactions and hepatitis produced by some macrolide antibiotics. J Antimicrob Chemother 1985; 16: 181–194.

102. Diehl AM, Latham P, Boitnott JK, et al.: Cholestatic hepatitis from erythromycin ethylsuccinate: Report of two cases. Am J Med 1984; 76: 931–934.

103. Ortuno JA, Olaso V, Berenguere J: Cholestatic hepatitis caused by erythromycin propionate (letter). Med Clin (Barc) 1984; 82: 912.

104. Inman WH, Rawson NS: Erythromycin estolate and jaundice. BMJ 1983; 286: 1954–1955.

105. Eichenwald HF: Adverse reactions to erythromycin. Pediatr Infect Dis J 1986; 5: 147–150.

106. Mintz U, Amir J, Pinkhas J, DeVries A: Transient perceptive deafness due to erythromycin lactobionate. JAMA 1973; 225: 1122–1123.

107. Sacristan JA, Soto JA, deCos MA: Erythromycin-induced hypoacusis: 11 new cases and literature review. Ann Pharmacother 1993; 27: 950–955.

108. Swanson DJ, Sung RJ, Fine MJ, et al.: Erythromycin ototoxicity: Prospective assessment with serum concentrations and audiograms in a study of patients with pneumonia. Am J Med 1992; 92: 61–68.

109. Brummett RE: Ototoxic liability of erythromycin and analogues. Otolaryngol Clin North Am 1993; 26: 811–819.

110. Lornoy W, Steyaert J: Ototoxicity of erythromycin lactobionate. Acta Clin Belg 1979; 34: 11.

111. Ouinnan GV, McCabe WR: Ototoxicity of erythromycin. Lancet 1978; 1: 1160–1161.

112. Dylewski J: Irreversible sensorineural hearing loss due to erythromycin. Can Med Assoc J 1988; 139: 230–231.

113. Levin G, Behrenth E: Irreversible ototoxic effect of erythromycin. Scand Audiol 1986; 15: 41–42.

114. Agusti C, Ferran F, Gea J, Picado C: Ototoxic reaction to erythromycin. Arch Intern Med 1991; 151: 380.

115. Taylor R, Schofield IS, Ramos JM, et al.: Ototoxicity of erythromycin in peritoneal dialysis patients. Lancet 1981; 2: 935–936.

116. Kroboth PD, McNeil MA, Kreeger A, et al.: Hearing loss and erythromycin pharmacokinetics in a patient receiving hemodialysis. Arch Intern Med 1983; 143: 1263–1265.

117. Haydon RC, Thelin JW, Dawis WE: Erythromycin ototoxicity: Analysis and conclusions based on 22 case reports. Otolaryngol Head Neck Surg 1984; 92: 678–684.

118. Umstaed GS, Neumann KH: Erythromycin ototoxicity and acute psychotic reaction in cancer patients with hepatic dysfunction. Arch Intern Med 1986; 146: 897–899.

119. Vasquez EM, Maddux MS, Sanchez J, Pollak R: Clinically significant hearing loss in renal allograft recipients treated with intravenous erythromycin. Arch Intern Med 1993; 153: 879–882.

120. Dautzenberg B, Saint-Marc T, Averous V, et al.: Clarithromycin containing regimens in the treatment of 54 AIDS patients with disseminated *Mycobacterium avium*-intracellular infection. 31st Intersci Conf Antimicrob Ag Chemother 1991; Abstract 293, p 148.

121. Wallace RJ, Brown BA, Griffith DE: Drug intolerance to high-dose clarithromycin among elderly patients. Diagn Microbiol Infect Dis 1993; 16: 215–221.

122. Wallace MR, Miller LK, Nguyen MT, Shields AR: Ototoxicity with azithromycin. Lancet 1994; 343: 241.

123. Tseng A, Dolovich L, Salit I: Azithromycin ototoxicity in HIV patients. 35th Intersci Conf Antimicrob Ag Chemother, San Francisco, 1995; Abstract LM19, p 330.

124. Joslin S, Guay D, Straka R, et al.: Qtc-interval (Qtc) prolongation and intravenous (IV) erythromycin lactobionate (E) infusions in critically ill patients (pts). 34th Intersci Conf Antimicrob Ag Chemother, Orlando, 1994; Abstract M63, p 246.

125. Periti P, Mazzei T, Mini E, Novelli A: Pharmacokinetic drug interactions of macrolides. Clin Pharmacokinet 1992; 23: 106–131.

126. Cortese LM, Bjornson DC: Potential interaction between terfanadine and macrolide antibiotics. Clin Pharm 1992; 11: 675.

127. Rieder MJ, Spino M: The theophylline-erythromycin interaction. J Asthma 1988; 25: 195–204.

128. Martell R, Heinrichs D, Stiller CR, et al.: The effects of erythromycin in patients treated with cyclosporine. Ann Intern Med 1986; 104: 660–661.

129. Fabre I, Fabre G, Maurel P, et al.: Metabolism of cyclosporin A. III: Interaction of the macrolide antibiotic, erythromycin, using rabbit hepatocytes and microsomal fractions. Drug Metab Dispos Biol Fate Chem 1988; 16: 296–301.

130. Hassell D, Utt JK: Suspected interaction: warfarin and erythromycin. South Med J 1985; 78: 1015–1016.

131. Mitsch RA: Carbamazepine toxicity precipitated by intravenous erythromycin. DICP 1989; 23: 878–879.

132. Phillips JP, Antal EJ, Smith RB: A pharmacokinetic drug interaction between erythromycin and triazolam. J Clin Psychopharmacol 1986; 6: 297–299.

133. Bartkowski RR, Goldberg ME, Larijani GE, Boerner T: Inhibition of alfentanil metabolism by erythromycin. Clin Pharmacol Ther 1989; 46: 99–102.

134. LaForce CF, Szefler SJ, Miller MF, et al.: Inhibition of methylprednisolone elimination in the presence of erythromycin therapy. J Allergy Clin Immunol 1983; 72: 34–39.

135. Nelson MW, Berchou RC, Kareti T, et al.: Pharmacokinetic evaluation of erythromycin and caffeine administered with bromocriptine. Clin Pharmacol Ther 1990; 47: 694–697.

136. Lode H: The pharmacokinetics of azithromycin and their clinical significance. Eur J Clin Microbiol Infect Dis 1991; 10: 807–812.

137. Wallace RJ, Brown BA, Griffith DE, et al.: Reduced serum levels of clarithromycin in patients on multidrug regimens including rifampin or rifabutin for treatment of *Mycobacterium avium-intracellulare* (MAI). 34th Intersci Conf Antimicrob Ag Chemother, Orlando, 1994; Abstract M60, p 246.

138. Saran BR, Maguire AM, Nichols C, et al.: Hypopyon uveitis in patients with acquired immunodeficiency syndrome treated for systemic *Mycobacterium avium* complex infection with rifabutin. Arch Ophthalmol 1994; 112: 1159–1165.

139. Maxwell DL, Gilmour-White SK, Hall MR: Digoxin toxicity due to interaction of digoxin with erythromycin. BMJ 1989; 298: 572.

140. Morton MR, Cooper JW: Erythromycin-induced digoxin toxicity. Ann Pharmacother 1989; 23: 668–670.

Miscellaneous Antibacterial Agents

Stephen C. Threlkeld
Maureen R. Tierney

P A R T 1

Trimethoprim-Sulfamethoxazole

▼

The combination antimicrobial agent trimethoprim-sulfamethoxazole (TMP-SMX) first became available in oral form in Europe in 1968 and in the United States in 1973. Since that time, it has found a prominent place in the treatment of many common infections because of its convenience and its effectiveness against a wide variety of pathogens. Also known as co-trimoxazole, it is marketed under the trade names Bactrim (Roche Laboratories) and Septra (Burroughs-Wellcome). The chemical structure of TMP-SMX is shown in Figure 11–1.

MECHANISM OF ACTION

Trimethoprim and the sulfonamide agents inhibit sequential enzymatic steps in microbial synthesis of tetrahydrofolic acid (folinic acid). Sulfonamide agents inhibit an enzyme responsible for the synthesis of the immediate precursor of dihydrofolic acid (folic acid), which must be synthesized by bacteria but is acquired preformed in the diet in humans. TMP, a diaminopyrimidine, blocks the subsequent conversion of folic acid to folinic acid, a necessary cofactor for nucleic acid synthesis. The avidity of TMP for the bacterial enzyme catalyzing this step is many thousand–fold higher than that for humans. This sequential inhibition is believed to be responsible for TMP-SMX in vitro synergistic activity against many microorganisms, though corresponding in vivo synergy has never been clearly demonstrated.

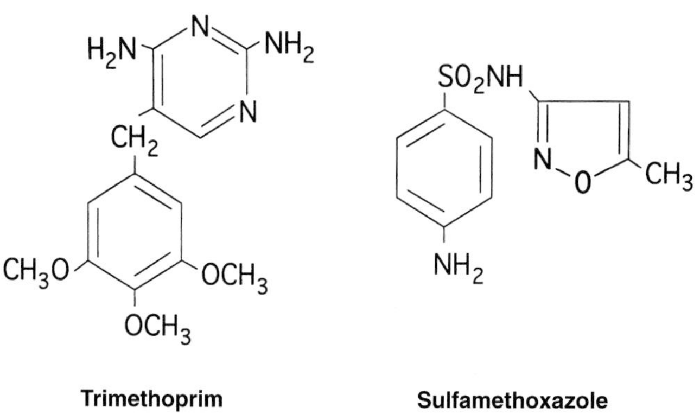

PHARMACOKINETICS

The common oral and intravenous formulations available for TMP-SMX are listed in Table 11–1. All preparations of TMP-SMX contain fixed-dose ratios of 1 part TMP to 5 parts SMX, designed to achieve serum ratios for TMP to SMX of 1:20. This value has been shown to be optimal for in vitro synergy in susceptible bacteria, though ratios found in tissues may vary from this significantly.

SMX was chosen as the sulfonamide agent for combination with TMP in part because of its similar pharmacokinetic properties, though important differences such as tissue penetration remain. Both agents are well absorbed from the upper gastrointestinal tract, with peak serum levels occurring approximately 1–4 hours after administration and serum half-lives of 8–12 hours in patients with normal creatinine clearance. TMP reaches higher concentrations in upper respiratory tract secretions than SMX, with levels in saliva frequently exceeding serum levels. Cerebrospinal fluid levels approach 50% of those in serum for both agents, and both cross the placenta quite well.

TMP and SMX are excreted through the kidney, SMX largely as inactive liver metabolites. Impaired creatinine clearance is associated with decreased excretion of the drugs and requires appropriate dose adjustment. Both agents are removed by hemodialysis but not by peritoneal dialysis.

ANTIMICROBIAL SPECTRUM

Table 11–2 lists the in vitro TMP-SMX susceptibility pattern by disk diffusion for a variety of bacterial clinical isolates at the Massachusetts General Hospital from January to December 1994. *Streptococcus pneumoniae* has not been routinely tested to TMP-SMX in our clinical laboratory and has historically been more than 90% sensitive. There are, however, increasing reports of regional pneumococcal resistance, and this may continue to become a more important clinical problem in specific geographic areas.[1, 2] TMP-SMX shows excellent activity against a wide variety of common gram-positive and gram-negative bacteria, and it is also the treatment of choice for many less common infections, including *Nocardia, Pneumocystis carinii,* and *Isospora belli* in immunocompromised individuals.

Figure 11–1. Chemical structures of trimethoprim and sulfamethoxazole.

Table 11–1. AVAILABLE FORMULATIONS OF TRIMETHOPRIM-SULFAMETHOXAZOLE

Formulation	Amount of Trimethoprim	Amount of Sulfamethoxazole
Single-strength tablet	80 mg	400 mg
Double-strength tablet	160 mg	800 mg
Oral suspension, 5 mL (1 tsp)	40 mg	200 mg
Injectable (1 ampule)	80 mg	400 mg

Also not listed in Table 11–2 is *Pseudomonas aeruginosa.* Unlike other pseudomonads and many other common gram-negative rods, *P. aeruginosa* is routinely resistant to TMP-SMX. TMP-SMX likewise has almost no activity against anaerobes and is not reliable against *Enterococcus faecalis.*

CLINICAL USE IN EAR, NOSE, AND THROAT INFECTIONS

The broad activity of TMP-SMX against most common pathogens of the ear, nose and throat, including the pneumococcus and *H. influenzae,* has made it an attractive agent for treatment of these infections. TMP-SMX has been shown to attain sufficient concentrations in middle ear effusions to inhibit *S. pneumoniae,* beta-lactamase–producing *Haemophilus influenzae,* and *Moraxella (Branhamella) catarrhalis,*[3] and multiple clinical trials have shown TMP-SMX to be effective in treatment of acute otitis media. These data combined with its very low cost, convenient twice-daily dosing, and its minimal gastrointestinal irritation make it an agent of choice for these infections. In chronic otitis media with effusion, TMP-SMX, either alone or in combination with prednisone, has been shown to speed resolution of effusion and to prevent recurrent acute episodes, but no significant difference has been demonstrated in antibiotic-treated patients over longer periods of follow-up to date.[4]

Although many patients with acute sinusitis may improve without therapy or with decongestants alone, TMP-SMX has been shown to be effective in improving clinical response rates and radiographic findings in acute bacterial sinusitis. One trial showed that radiographic and clinical response to a 3-day regimen of TMP-SMX with decongestants was

Table 11–2. IN VITRO SUSCEPTIBILITY BY DISK DIFFUSION OF CLINICAL ISOLATES

Organism	No. Strains	% Susceptible
Staphylococcus aureus	1779	93
Coagulase-negative *Staphylococcus*	1928	67
Haemophilus influenzae	519	87
Klebsiella pneumoniae	1183	89
Pseudomonas cepacia	51	94
Xanthomonas maltophilia	183	94
Acinetobacter calcoaceticus (anitratus)	153	87
Enterobacter aerogenes	201	98
Escherichia coli	3995	92
Serratia marcescens	192	96
Citrobacter freundii	162	85
Proteus mirabilis	478	91

*At the Massachusetts General Hospital, January–December 1994

equivalent to a 10-day course of therapy,[5] but treatment has generally consisted of at least a 14-day course, and we recommend at least 2 to 3 weeks of therapy for true bacterial sinusitis. There is little role for TMP-SMX in the treatment of chronic sinusitis because of the prevalence of anaerobic organisms involved. TMP-SMX has occasionally been used as an alternative for the treatment of meningitis in patients with serious hypersensitivity reaction to both penicillins and cephalosporins. Although TMP-SMX can achieve inhibitory concentrations in the cerebrospinal fluid against *S. pneumoniae, H. influenzae, Neisseria meningitidis,* and *Listeria monocytogenes,* increasing resistance in pneumococci raises serious concerns about the use of TMP-SMX for treatment of meningitis (as well as for serous otitis media and sinusitis), and it should be used for this purpose only in consultation with an infectious disease specialist. Also, other agents with more limited spectra and with even higher percentage susceptibility for group A streptococci should be used for pharyngitis believed to be bacterial in origin.

In addition to a number of more common uses, TMP-SMX has been used effectively in conjunction with topical agents and chlorhexidine soap baths in the eradication of carriage of methicillin-resistant *Staphylococcus aureus* from the nasopharynx.[6] TMP-SMX has also been cited in multiple case reports to be effective, either alone or as an immunosuppressive-sparing agent, in the treatment of Wegener's granulomatosis. Its role in disease modulation is not certain at this time, and determination of a defined role for TMP-SMX in the treatment of this disease awaits further controlled trials.[7, 8]

TOXICITIES AND DRUG REACTIONS

A high prevalence of adverse reactions to TMP-SMX has been reported since it has gained widespread use in patients infected with the human immunodeficiency virus (HIV). Although patients with HIV infection experience a substantially higher rate of adverse reactions, TMP-SMX is generally tolerated quite well with very few serious complications in non–HIV-infected individuals.

The most common side effects of TMP-SMX are skin rash (noted in approximately 3% of non–HIV-infected patients) and gastrointestinal tract irritation, including nausea, vomiting, and, less commonly, diarrhea.[9] More severe adverse reactions are infrequently noted, including anaphylaxis, erythema multiforme, hepatitis, renal tubular acidosis and crystalluria, central nervous system toxicity, and hematologic effects such as bone marrow suppression and hemolysis. In addition to its potential for true renal toxicity, TMP-SMX also causes a reversible increase in serum creatinine owing to decreased renal tubular creatinine secretion. The hematologic effects of TMP-SMX can be severe in patients with folic acid deficiency, and TMP-SMX is contraindicated in patients with megaloblastic anemia. TMP-SMX can also lead to hemolysis in patients with glucose-6-phosphate dehydrogenase (G6PD) deficiency, although at least one study failed to demonstrate this.[10]

Both TMP and SMX cross the placenta and are contraindicated in women who are pregnant. TMP may have teratogenic effects, and sulfa agents can cause kernicterus by displacing bilirubin from albumin, dramatically increasing indirect bilirubin levels.

Drug interactions should be carefully considered with TMP-SMX use. TMP can dramatically increase levels of phenytoin and rifampin, and sulfa agents can decrease the protein binding of other drugs, including warfarin and oral hypoglycemic agents. TMP-SMX can also cause decreased clearance of methotrexate with resultant marked pancytopenia. TMP-SMX should be used with extreme caution in transplant patients receiving cyclosporine because of possible combined effects to decrease creatinine clearance in patients receiving both agents.

DOSING

Whereas considerably higher doses must be given for treatment of *P. carinii* infection (20 mg/kg/day TMP component), a dose of 1 double-strength TMP-SMX tablet every 12 hours can be given for most mild bacterial infections of the ear, nose, and throat in adults (8–10 mg/kg/day TMP component). Dosing every 6 hours is generally preferred for more severe infections. In children with routine otitis media or other upper respiratory tract infection, TMP-SMX can be administered in liquid oral form in a dose of 8–10 mg/kg/day TMP component divided into twice-daily doses.

The dose of TMP-SMX must be reduced in patients with impaired creatinine clearance, and the drug should be avoided in individuals with creatinine clearance lower than 10 mL/min. In patients with creatinine clearance lower than 50 mL/min, a normal loading dose can be given, followed by a maintenance dose of ~2 mg/kg TMP component every 12 hours. Sulfamethoxazole levels can be obtained, and blood specimens should be drawn 3–4 hours after an oral dose or 1 hour after an intravenous dose.

References

1. Henderson F, Gilligan P, Wait K, Goff D: Nasopharyngeal carriage of antibiotic-resistant pneumococci by children in group day care. J Infect Dis 1988; 157: 256–263.
2. Linares J, Perez J, Garau J, et al.: Comparative susceptibility of penicillin-resistant pneumococcus to co-trimoxazole, vancomycin, rifampicin and fourteen beta-lactam antibiotics. J of Antimicrob Chemother 1984; 13: 353–359.
3. Krause P, Owens N, Nightingale C, et al.: Penetration of amoxicillin, cefaclor, erythromycin-sulfisoxazole, and trimethoprim-sulfamethoxazole into the middle ear fluid of patients with chronic serous otitis media. J Infect Dis 1982; 145: 815–821.
4. Giebink G, Batalden P, Le C, Lassman G, et al.: A controlled trial comparing three treatments for chronic otitis media with effusion. Pediat Infect Dis J 1990; 9: 33–40.
5. Williams J, Holleman D, Samsa G, Simel D: Randomized controlled trial of 3 vs 10 days of trimethoprim/sulfamethoxazole for acute maxillary sinusitis. JAMA 1995; 273: 1015–1021.
6. Parras F, Guerrero C, Bouza E, et al.: Comparative study of mupirocin and oral co-trimoxazole plus topical fusidic acid in eradication of nasal carriage of methicillin-resistant *Staphylococcus aureus*. Antimicrob Agents Chemother 1995; 39: 175–179.
7. McRae D, Buchanan G: Long-term sulfamethoxazole-trimethoprim in Wegener's granulomatosis. Arch Otoloaryngol Head Neck Surg 1993; 119: 103–105.
8. Valeriano-Marcet J, Spiera H: Treatment of Wegener's granulomatosis with sulfamethoxazole-trimethoprim. Arch Intern Med 1991; 151: 1649–1652.
9. Jick H: Adverse reactions to trimethoprim-sulfamethoxazole in hospitalized patients. Rev Infect Dis 1982; 4: 426–428.
10. Markowitz N, Saravolatz L: Use of trimethoprim-sulfamethoxazole in a glucose-6-phosphate dehydrogenase-deficient population. Rev Infect Dis 1987; 9: S218–S225.

Stephen C. Threlkeld
Maureen R. Tierney

PART 2
The Tetracyclines

▼

The tetracycline family, originally isolated from *Streptomyces aureofaciens,* is a class of antibiotics whose members are bacteriostatic and possess a broad spectrum of activity. Only four members of the tetracyclines have widespread clinical use today, and only three are regularly used in the treatment of infections. Over the past 20 years, increasing resistance of bacteria to the tetracyclines and the development of new antimicrobial agents have limited their routine use.

Tetracyclines have traditionally been divided into three groups on the basis of their pharmacokinetic characteristics. Of the short-acting tetracyclines, including chlortetracycline (the original agent isolated), only tetracycline hydrochloride (tetracycline) remains in active use today. No intermediate-acting agent currently plays a role in antimicrobial therapy, but demeclocycline does serve in the treatment of the syndrome of inappropriate antidiuretic hormone production. Finally, the long-acting agents doxycycline and minocycline remain useful antimicrobial agents.

MECHANISM OF ACTION AND PHARMACOKINETICS

After accumulating in the bacterial cytoplasm, all tetracyclines act by reversibly binding the 30S ribosomal subunit, blocking the binding of aminoacyl-transfer RNA. This action halts the elongation of the growing peptide chain and thus inhibits bacterial protein synthesis.[1]

Tetracycline is 60%–80% absorbed from the upper gastrointestinal tract and reaches peak serum concentrations 1–3 hours after administration; its serum half-life is 8 hours.[2] The long-acting agents, doxycycline and minocycline, are almost completely absorbed from the gastrointestinal tract and have serum half-lives of 16–18 hours.[2]

The absorption of tetracycline from the gut is dramatically reduced by milk and other foodstuffs, by divalent and trivalent cations such as magnesium, calcium, and iron, and, possibly, by decreased gastric acidity. Absorption of doxycycline and minocycline is not affected by these interactions, and they can be given with food if necessary to decrease gastrointestinal irritation.

Tetracyclines penetrate into many tissues in low levels, and levels in sinus mucosa are nearly equivalent to those in serum.[3] Minocycline reaches very high levels in saliva and tears because of its high lipophilicity. Penetration into the cerebrospinal fluid is marginal, and these agents in general should no longer be used for routine treatment of central nervous system infections.

The tetracyclines should not be used in pregnancy, as they cross the placenta well and are concentrated in fetal teeth and bones. They are also excreted in breast milk and should, therefore, be avoided in nursing mothers. Tetracyclines are eliminated by the kidney and should not be used in patients with renal insufficiency. The exception is doxycycline, which is excreted via the gastrointestinal tract in patients with renal insufficiency and requires no dose adjustment for decreased creatinine clearance. All the tetracyclines are cleared slowly by hemodialysis and are not cleared by peritoneal dialysis.

ANTIMICROBIAL SPECTRUM AND CLINICAL USE IN EAR, NOSE, AND THROAT INFECTIONS

At the time of their introduction, the tetracyclines had broad activity against aerobic gram-positive and gram-negative organisms, as well as anaerobes, Chlamydia, spirochetes, and others, but the gradual emergence of resistance has progressively limited the use of these agents against many pathogens commonly encountered in otolaryngology. Increasing plasmid-mediated tetracycline resistance in pneumococcal isolates has been particularly problematic for the use of these agents in respiratory infections. Resistance to one member of the class generally corresponds to resistance to the other agents as well. In addition, other antibiotics have arisen with better activity against most aerobic and facultatively anaerobic bacteria. Despite these limitations, tetracyclines do maintain activity against several common pathogens.

The tetracyclines remain a therapy of choice for chlamydial infections, including urethritis, trachoma, and psittacosis. Tetracyclines are also effective alternatives for treatment of Mycoplasma infections in patients who are intolerant of macrolides and as alternative treatment in patients with Vincent's angina. Many spirochetes, including Borrelia burgdorferi, are susceptible to tetracyclines, and they provide effective treatment for early Lyme disease when there is no meningeal involvement. Rickettsial diseases are also treated

effectively with tetracyclines, but chloramphenicol is sometimes preferred in the treatment of life-threatening cases such as advanced Rocky Mountain spotted fever. In addition, minocycline has good activity against Nocardia and Mycobacterium marinum, and it finds most of its limited use in these less common infections. Tetracyclines rarely serve as alternative therapy for bacterial pharyngitis in patients with allergies to beta-lactam and macrolide antibiotics. This therapy, however, should be undertaken with caution, as treatment failures do occur with group A streptococci, possibly putting patients at risk for rheumatic fever.

TOXICITIES AND DRUG INTERACTIONS

The most common adverse reaction to the tetracyclines is mild gastrointestinal irritation, but photosensitivity rashes, fixed drug eruptions, and hypersensitivity reactions also occur. Hypersensitivity to one member of this class precludes use of the others as well. More serious gastrointestinal side effects include life-threatening fatty hepatic necrosis at high doses, but in pregnant women, this can occur even at lower doses. The irritative quality of tetracycline is often utilized in sclerosis of the pleural space, and use of the less irritative doxycycline is favored for intravenous therapy in order to avoid phlebitis at injection sites.

A well-known side effect of the tetracyclines is their effect on teeth and bones. Administration of tetracyclines in children has been associated with permanent yellow-brown discoloration of teeth and can lead to hypoplasia of the enamel[4] as well as inhibition of skeletal development in premature infants.[5] Tetracyclines, therefore, should be strongly avoided in pregnant mothers and children till approximately age 9 years. However, these effects seem to be related to total duration of therapy with tetracyclines, and a tetracycline should not be withheld in serious infections in which it would be the chosen therapy.

Minocycline is uncommonly associated with vestibular toxicity and skin and nail pigmentation, and because of its toxicity, its use is generally limited to special circumstances such as nocardial infection in the immunocompromised host who is allergic to trimethoprim-sulfamethoxazole. Central nervous toxicity in the form of pseudotumor cerebri can also rarely occur with any of the tetracyclines.

In addition to the food interactions described earlier, several drugs, including phenytoin, carbamazepine, and ethanol, decrease the half-life of doxycycline by inducing hepatic metabolism. Failure of oral contraceptives has been reported in patients taking tetracyclines,[6] and tetracyclines can potentiate the effects of oral anticoagulants, requiring close monitoring of prothrombin times in patients receiving these agents simultaneously. Tetracyclines have also been associated with nephrotoxicity in patients receiving methoxyflurane anesthesia.

DOSING

Tetracycline is given in an oral dose of 500 mg every 6 hours without food. It can be given in the same dose by intravenous route, but doxycycline is favored for intravenous use for the reasons already mentioned. Doxycycline is given in an oral dose of 100 mg every 12–24 hours. Dosing of doxycycline is not changed for intravenous use, but this is generally not required because of its excellent oral bioavailability. Minocycline is available orally and is given in a dose of 100 mg every 12 hours.

Doxycycline is the only agent of the tetracycline family that is safely used in renal insufficiency, and it requires no dose adjustment. Although no dose adjustment is required in the presence of hepatic insufficiency, the tetracyclines should be used with caution in this setting because of their potential hepatotoxic effects.

References

1. Craven G, Gavin R, Fanning T: The transfer RNA binding site of the 30S ribosome and the site of tetracycline inhibition. Symp Quant Biol 1969; 34: 129.
2. Standiford H: Tetracyclines and chloramphenicol. In: Mandell G, Douglas RJ, Bennett J (eds): Principles and Practice of Infectious Disease, 4th ed. New York: Churchill Livingstone, 1995, pp 306–317.
3. Lundberg C, Malmburg A, Ivemark B: Antibiotic concentrations in relation to structural changes in maxillary sinus mucosa following intramuscular or peroral treatment. Scand J Infect Dis 1974; 6: 187.
4. Witkop C, Wolf R: Hypoplasia and intrinsic staining of enamel following tetracycline therapy. JAMA 1963; 185: 1008.
5. Cohan S, Bevelander G, Tiamsic T: Growth inhibition of prematures receiving tetracycline. Am J Dis Child 1963; 105: 453.
6. Bacon J, Chenfield G: Pregnancy attributable to interaction between tetracycline and oral contraceptives. Br Med J 1980; 280: 293.

Itzhak Brook

PART 3

Chloramphenicol

Chloramphenicol is a broad-spectrum antibiotic originally isolated from *Streptomyces venezuelae*.[1] It was commercially available in 1949, but widespread publicity of aplastic anemia as an extremely rare side effect has limited its use in ear, nose, and throat infections as an alternative antimicrobial agent for ampicillin-resistant *H. influenzae* and anaerobic bacteria.

PHARMACOLOGY AND PHARMACOKINETICS

Encapsulated chloramphenicol is well absorbed from the gastrointestinal tract, although variable absorption is seen in children. The achieved peak serum level in adults is 12 μg/mL after a 1-g dose.[2] There is wide variation in the metabolism and excretion in children, and the dose requirement may vary. The slow metabolism in newborns requires a decrease in the dose and monitoring of serum levels. Chloramphenicol palmitate in suspension form is hydrolyzed in the intestine to active chloramphenicol.

The intravenous chloramphenicol succinate is hydrolyzed into active chloramphenicol, which produces serum levels that are 25%–33% of those produced by oral chloramphenicol. This is due to the slow hydrolysis of the drug.[2] Intramuscular route of administration was not recommended because of inadequate serum levels achieved. It is metabolized primarily in the liver, where it is conjugated with glucuronic acid, and is excreted in the urine in this inactive form. Biotransformation also occurs by oxidation and reduction in children.[3] Urine concentration is reduced in renal failure. Chloramphenicol concentration rises in neonates and adults with liver disease. This high level can induce dose-related bone marrow suppression.

Serum level measurements are often advocated for infants, for young children, and occasionally for adults, owing to wide variations noted.[2] The usual objective is therapeutic levels of 10–25 μg/mL. Levels exceeding 25 μg/mL are considered potentially toxic in terms of reversible bone marrow suppression, and levels of 40–200 μg/mL have been associated with gray baby syndrome in neonates and encephalitis in adults.[2]

Chloramphenicol half-life is 4.1 hours after a single intravenous injection. It is widely distributed in body fluids and tissues. The drug has a unique property of lipid solubility that permits penetration across lipid barriers. A consistent observation is the high concentrations achieved in the central nervous system, even in the absence of inflammation. The cerebrospinal fluid concentration is 30%–50% of the serum in noninflamed meninges, and about 70% in inflamed meninges. Levels in brain tissue may be substantially higher than serum levels.[4]

The drug also shows rather unique properties for penetration across the blood-ocular barrier and the placenta. Joint fluid levels are generally low in the absence of inflammation, but are relatively high—50% or more of serum concentration—in the presence of septic arthritis. Studies in experimental animals with subcutaneous abscesses show peak levels within abscesses that approximate 15%–20% of the peak serum concentration.[2] This is comparable to the levels achieved with other antimicrobials, including virtually all beta-lactam compounds, but is substantially lower compared with abscess levels achieved with clindamycin.

The plasma half-life in renal failure is not prolonged. Thus, chloramphenicol can be given in normal doses in patients with renal failure. However, partially metabolized inactive nontoxic products accumulate in renal failure.[5]

SPECTRUM OF ACTIVITY

Chloramphenicol has a broad spectrum of activity against a variety of organisms, including many gram-positive and gram-negative bacteria, rickettsiae, *Chlamydia,* and *Mycoplasma.*[6]

Although most gram-positive and gram-negative aerobic bacteria are inhibited by chloramphenicol, more active or less toxic antimicrobial agents are available for most of these pathogens. *H. influenzae, N. meningitis,* and *S. pneumoniae,* the most common causes of bacterial meningitis, are susceptible to chloramphenicol. However, *H. influenzae* and *S. pneumoniae* strains resistant to both chloramphenicol and amoxicillin have increased in frequency.

Chloramphenicol has excellent activity against gram-positive and gram-negative anaerobic bacteria. These include *Peptostreptococcus, Clostridium, Fusobacterium, Prevotella* and *Porphypomonas* species, and *Bacteroides fragilis* group.[7]

Although it is a bacteriostatic agent, chloramphenicol is one of the antimicrobial agents most active against anaerobes. Resistance to this drug is rare, although it has been reported in some *Bacteroides* species.[8] Although several failures to eradicate anaerobic infections, including bacteremia, with chloramphenicol have been reported, this drug has been used for more than 25 years for treatment of anaerobic infections. Chloramphenicol is often regarded as the drug of choice for treatment of serious anaerobic infections when the nature and susceptibility of the infecting organisms are unknown and of infections of the central nervous system.

MECHANISM OF ACTION

Chloramphenicol enters the bacterial cell by an energy-dependent process. It inhibits protein synthesis by reversibly binding to the 50S subunit of the 70S ribosomes at a locus that prevents the aminoacyl-transfer RNA attachment to its binding site.[9] This block in protein synthesis is bacteriostatic in most susceptible isolates. Bactericidal activity is generated, however, against *H. influenzae, S. pneumoniae,* and *N. meningitidis.* The effect of chloramphenicol on the human mitochondria that also contain 70S particles may explain its dose-related bone marrow suppression. Bacteria become resistant to chloramphenicol by development of impermeability to the drug or by production of acetyltransferase enzyme, which inactivates the drug.

CLINICAL USE IN EAR, NOSE, AND THROAT INFECTIONS

Potential indications for chloramphenicol are life-threatening *H. influenzae, S. pneumoniae,* and *N. meningitidis* infections in which resistance to other drugs may exist. These include acute epiglotitis, bacteremia, and meningitis. The excellent penetration of chloramphenicol into the central nervous system makes it a preferred agent for the treatment of brain abscess.[4] It can also be used for the treatment of severe otolaryngologic anaerobic infections, including chronic otitis media, sinusitis, and mastoiditis, as well as abscesses and wounds of the head and neck.[8, 10] The good gastrointestinal absorption and the ease of oral administration are advantages. However, the benefits of chloramphenicol must be weighed against its well-known adverse effects.

ADVERSE REACTIONS

Chloramphenicol can occasionally cause hypersensitivity reaction (rash and fever) and, rarely, optic neuritis. Its most notable side effect is bone marrow toxicity. A dose-related reversable bone marrow suppression is especially likely to occur in patients who are taking high doses or prolonged courses and who have free serum concentrations of chloramphenicol more than 20–25 μg/mL. Anemia, neutropenia, reticulocytopenia, and thrombocytopenia can occur. Rarely, an unexplained aplastic anemia occurs, in every 25,000–40,000 courses of chloramphenicol.[11] Because of the direct bone marrow toxicity, a complete blood and platelet count should be done every 3 days while the patient is on chloramphenicol. The gray baby syndrome occurs in premature infants and neonates. Cyanosis and shock lead to grayish discoloration of the skin. The syndrome results from accumulation of chloramphenicol because of the lesser ability of neonates to excrete the drug. The syndrome has also been described in children and adults with high levels of serum chloramphenicol. Chloramphenicol should therefore be avoided in premature infants during the first 2 weeks of life, except in extreme life-threatening situations, in which decreased doses should be used and serum levels monitored. Chloramphenicol can also induce hemolysis in patients with (G6PD) deficiency, and optic neuritis in individuals who take the drug for a prolonged time.

DRUG INTERACTIONS

Chloramphenicol can prolong the half-life of cyclophosphamide, phenytoin, chlorpropamide, tolbutamide, and derivatives of warfarin.[6] Phenytoin, rifampin, and phenobarbital decrease serum concentration and increase the total body clearance of chloramphenicol.

Because of the bacteriostatic activity of chloramphenicol, it may antagonize the activity of bactericidal agents such as penicillins, cephalosporins, and aminoglycosides. Combination of such agents with chloramphenical should be used with care.

DOSING

The oral or intravenous dosage in newborn (younger than 7 days) is 25 mg/kg once daily, and in infants (1–4 weeks) 25 mg/kg once every 12 hours. The dosage for older children and adults is 50 mg/kg/day given in individual doses every 6 hours. The dosage used in older children and adults with meningitis is 100 mg/kg/day. Serum levels should be monitored to avoid toxicity, especially in newborns and premature infants and in patients with hepatic dysfunction. Peak serum concentration should be between 15 and 30 μ/mL. Intramuscular administration of chloramphenicol generates unpredictable serum levels, and monitoring of levels should be done in this situation.

References

1. Woodward TE, Wisseman CL: Chloromycetin (Chloramphenicol). New York: Medical Encyclopedia, 1958.
2. Smith AL, Weber A: Pharmacology of chloramphenicol. Pediatr Clin North Am 1983; 30: 309–326.
3. Holt DE, Hurley R, Harvey D: A reappraisal of chloramphenicol metabolism: Detection and quantification of metabolites in the sera of children. J Antimicrob Chemother 1995; 35: 115–127.
4. Kramer PW, Griffith RS, Campbell RL, et al.: Antibiotic penetration of the brain: A comparative study. J Neurosurg 1969; 31: 295–311.
5. Kunin CM: A guide to use of antibiotics in patients with renal disease. Ann Intern Med 1967; 67: 151–156.
6. Standiford HC: Tetracyclines and chloramphenicol. In: Mandell GI, Douglas RG Jr, Bennett JE (eds): Principles and Practice of Infectious Diseases, 4th ed. New York: Churchill-Livingstone, 1995, pp 306–317.
7. Sutter VL, Finegold SM: Susceptibility of anaerobic bacteria to 23 antimicrobial agents. Antimicrob Agents Chemother 1976; 10: 736–752.
8. Finegold SM: Anaerobic Bacteria in Human Disease. New York: Academic Press, 1977.
9. Abdel-Sayed S: Transport of chloramphenicol into sensitive strains of *Escherichia coli* and *Pseudomonas aeruginosa*. J Antimicrob Chemother 1987; 19: 7–20.
10. Brook I: Pediatric Anaerobic Infections, Diagnosis, and Management, 2nd ed. Philadelphia: Mosby Company, 1989.
11. Feder HM Jr, Osier C, Maderazo EG: Chloramphenicol: A review of its use in clinical practice. Rev Infect Dis 1981; 3: 479–491.

Itzhak Brook

P A R T   4
Clindamycin

Clindamycin is a semisynthetic antibiotic produced by a 7(S) chloro-substitution of the 7(R) hydroxyl group of the parent compound lincomycin.[1] Lincomycin was isolated in 1962 from an actinomycete, *Streptomyces lincolnensis,* found in soil in Lincoln, Nebraska. Although the biologic properties of lincomycin are similar to those of erythromycin, it is unrelated chemically and consists of an amino acid linked to an amino sugar. The chemical modification of lincomycin into clindamycin increased the antibacterial activity and gastrointestinal absorption.

Clindamycin is prepared as the hydrochloride salt of the base as a capsule, and as the palmitate ester for pediatric suspension. It is also available as a phosphate ester for intramuscular or intravenous use in topical solution, gel, lotion, and cream.

PHARMACOLOGY AND PHARMACOKINETICS

Clindamycin hydrochloride is rapidly and almost completely (90%) absorbed from the gastrointestinal tract. Absorption is slightly delayed but not reduced by food.[2]

In children receiving 2 mg/kg, the mean peak serum concentrations were 2.1 μg/mL at 30 minutes and 0.3 μg/mL at 6 hours.[3] In adults, mean peak serum concentration after single oral doses of 150 and 300 mg occurred in 1 hour and were 2.5 and 3.6 μg/mL, respectively.

Clindamycin palmitate is also absorbed rapidly and efficiently after oral administration, but serum concentrations are slightly lower than after clindamycin hydrochloride. Food does not affect absorption. In healthy children, a dose of 4 mg/kg gave mean peak serum concentrations of 0.5 μg/mL with a half-life of 2.2 hours. After repeated doses, the serum concentrations increased until they reached equilibrium. Infants younger than 6 months of age who received doses of 3 mg/kg had serum concentrations up to 2.7 μg/mL. Following intravenous administration of 7mg/kg clindamycin phosphate to infected children over 1 hour, a mean serum concentrations of 9 and 2 μg/mL were reached at 1 and 8 hours, respectively.[3]

Following intramuscular injection in healthy adults, mean peak serum levels occurred at 3 hours and were about 6 μg/mL after 300 mg and 9 μg/mL after 600 mg.[2] Serum levels were 10, 11, and 14 μg/mL immediately after intravenous infusion of 600, 900, and 1200 mg of clindamycin phosphate, respectively. Continuous intravenous infusions of 900–1350 mg/day maintained serum concentrations of 4–6 μg/mL. The normal half-life of clindamycin is 2.4 hours. The half-life increases to 6 hours in patients with severe renal failure and to 8–12 hours in the presence of severe liver disease. This drug is not removed by hemodialysis or peritoneal dialysis.

About 5%–10% of clindamycin and its metabolites are excreted in the urine of adults and 10%–20% are excreted in the urine of children. Most of the drug is inactivated by metabolism in the liver to *N*-demethyl clindamycin, which has three times the bioactivity of the parent compound and clindamycin sulfoxide, both of which are excreted in the urine and bile.[2] The drug and its metabolites persist in the stool because of its enterohepatic circulation, which causes changes in the gut flora for up to 2 weeks after its discontinuation.

Clindamycin is rapidly removed from serum to body tissues and fluids, and it penetrates well into saliva, sputum, tonsils, adenoids, pleural fluid, soft tissues, prostate, semen, bones, and joints. The concentration in bone compared with serum level is particularly high (1.3 µg/mL). The concentration achieved in respiratory tissues is 5.1–9.3 µg/g.

Clindamycin achieved a concentration in the cerebrospinal fluid of approximately 10% of its serum concentration in a model of experimental *S. pneumoniae* meningitis and in sterilized cerebrospinal fluid cultures after three doses.[4] Clindamycin is actively transported into polymorphonuclear leukocytes and macrophages and is present in relatively high concentrations in experimental abscesses.[5, 6]

SPECTRUM OF ACTIVITY

Clindamycin is considered a bacteriostatic antibiotic; however, it has bactericidal activity for strains of streptococci, staphylococci, and anaerobes.

Gram-Positive Aerobic Bacteria

Clindamycin is active against streptococci, including group A beta-hemolytic *Streptococcus* (GABHS), *S. pneumoniae, Streptococcus bovis,* microaerophilic streptococci, and penicillin-susceptible viridans streptococci.[5] More than 90% of intermediately resistant *S. pneumoniae* are susceptible to clindamycin. However, resistance to clindamycin by GABHS has been reported. Methicillin-susceptible but not methicillin-resistant *S. aureus* and *Staphylococcus epidermidis* are generally susceptible to clindamycin. Emergence of clindamycin-resistant *S. aureus* has been noted, especially in erythromycin-resistant isolates.

Clindamycin is active against *Corynebacterium diphtheriae* and has intermediate activity against *L. monocytogenes, Bacillus cereus,* and *Bacillus anthracis,* and has poor activity against *Enterococcus* species.

Gram-Negative Aerobic Bacteria

Clindamycin has poor activity against most species of gramnegative aerobic bacteria, including the Enterobacteriaceae and *P. aeruginosa.* It has moderate activity against *M. catarrhalis, H. influenzae,* and *N. meningitidis,* and has in vitro activity against *Campylobacter* species, *Gardnerella vaginalis,* and *Neisseria gonorrhoeae.*

Gram-Positive Anaerobic Bacteria

Clindamycin is highly active against *Actinomyces, Eubacterium, Lactobacillus, Propionobacterium,* and *Peptostreptococcus* species. Resistance has been observed in about 10% of streptococci. Clostridia are generally more resistant, and 10%–20% of clostridia other than *Clostridium perfringens* are resistant. Variable susceptibility is seen within some *Clostridia* species. The highest variability is seen for *Clostridium difficile,* the causative agent of antibiotic-associated colitis, in which many isolates are resistant. However, other clinically important clostridia are generally susceptible.

Gram-Negative Anaerobic Bacteria

Clindamycin is one of the most active antimicrobial agents against *B. fragilis* group.[5] Resistance of *B. fragilis* to clindamycin has been observed and has been associated with increased use of the drug.[7] Resistance was especially noted with *Bacteroides thetaiotaomicron* and *Bacteroides vulgatus* (rates of about 9%). Pigmented *Prevotella* and *Porphyromonas* species (previously called *Bacteroides melaninogenicus* group), *Fusobacterium* species, and *Veillonella* species are very susceptible to clindamycin. Most *Fusobacterium varium* and *Eikenella corrodens* are resistant.

Miscellaneous Organisms

Significant activity was noted against *Chlamydia trachomatis, Mycoplasma* species, and *Toxoplasma gondii.* Although clindamycin alone has poor activity against *P. carinii,* its combination with primaquine is effective in prophylaxis and treatment.[5]

MECHANISM OF ACTION

The antibiotics bind preferentially to the 50S ribosomal subunit, at the same binding site as macrolides and chloramphenicol. Clindamycin inhibits bacterial protein synthesis in the early chain elongation by interference with the transpeptidation reaction. It also exerts prolonged postantibiotic effect against some pathogens, probably because of its persistence at the ribosomal binding site. Clindamycin enhances opsonization and phagocytosis of bacteria at subinhibitory concentrations,[6] reduces bacterial adherence to host cells, and inhibits production of staphylococcal and streptococcal toxins.

CLINICAL USE IN EAR, NOSE, AND THROAT INFECTIONS

Clindamycin's major role in otolaryngologic infections is in the treatment of polymicrobial infections that are caused by polymicrobial aerobic-anaerobic bacteria. The bacterial origin of these infections is generally the oropharyngeal flora, in which anaerobic bacteria outnumber the aerobic bacteria in ratio of 100:1.[3]

The dual activity of clindamycin against gram-positive aerobic bacteria (i.e., streptococci and staphylococci) and anaerobes is its main virtue. Because of its ability to bind toxins produced by staphylococci and streptococci, its use has been advocated for patients with toxic shock syndrome. It also can reduce toxin production by *Clostridium* species and M protein and capsule generation by GABHS.[6, 8, 9]

Many of these polymicrobial infections are chronic and include ear and sinus infections.[3, 10] Other indications are Ludwig's angina, chronic mastoiditis, wounds and abscesses of the head and neck (i.e., retropharyngeal and tonsillar abscesses), postsurgical wound infections, dental infections and their complications, and other polymicrobial infections.

Clindamycin has been found superior to amoxicillin, erythromycin, and cefaclor (which are not effective against anaerobes) for therapy of chronic otitis media[11] and sinusitis.[12] When organisms resistant to clindamycin are also recovered in the infection (e.g., *P. aeruginosa*), antimicrobials effective against these bacteria should be added.[3]

Clindamycin is generally reserved for the therapy of acute GABHS tonsillitis in penicillin-allergic patients. However, clindamycin was found superior to penicillin in the treatment of recurrent GABHS pharyngotonsillitis. The presence in the tonsils of beta-lactamase–producing *S. aureus* and anaerobic gram-negative bacilli (mostly *Prevotella* and *Fusobacterium* species) was associated with penicillin failure in eradication of GABHS.[13] It is postulated that these organisms "shield" GABHS from penicillin but cannot protect them from clindamycin. Following clindamycin therapy, GABHS, as well as most of the beta-lactamase–producing bacteria, were eradicated from these patients.[13] Clindamycin was also found to be superior to penicillin in the therapy of pleuropulmonary infection due to aspiration of oral flora.[14, 15] This includes the therapy of aspiration pneumonia, lung abscess, and empyema. Clindamycin is also effective as a prophylactic agent for oncologic and other major head and neck surgery.[16]

The worldwide increase in the recovery rate of penicillin-resistant *S. pneumoniae* from respiratory infections creates a new potential use for clindamycin. Its in vitro efficacy against more than 90% of intermediately resistant strains (but not highly resistant) merits its consideration in infections caused by these organisms.[17] However, clinical studies are needed for evaluation of efficacy.

ADVERSE REACTIONS

Clindamycin allergy includes morbilliform rash, fever, and, rarely, erythema multiforme and anaphylaxis. Minor reversible elevations of transaminase, reversible neutropenia, and thrombocytopenia have also been noted. Rapid intravenous administration has rarely been associated with cardiopulmonary arrest and hypotension.

Diarrhea may occur in 2%–20% of patients and is more common with oral therapy. The side effect of most concern is colitis,[18] which can occur during or after discontinuation of therapy. The rate of colitis was estimated to occur in about 1 in 50,000 patients. It should be noted that colitis has been associated with a number of other antimicrobial agents, such as penicillins and cephalosporins, and was even noted in seriously ill patients in the absence of previous antimicrobial therapy. Colitis following clindamycin therapy was associated with recovery of toxin-producing *C. difficile* strains.[18] The risk of colitis increases with age and has rarely been observed in children. Discontinuation of clindamycin therapy and administration of vancomycin or metronidazole is effective therapy. Relapses may occur and are more common with metronidazole therapy.

DRUG INTERACTIONS

Blockage of neuromuscular transmission by clindamycin may enhance action of other blocking agents. Clindamycin

phosphate solution is incompatible with ampicillin, barbiturates, phenytoin, aminophylline, calcium gluconate, and magnesium sulfate.

DOSING

Clindamycin dose, route of administration, and duration of treatment depend on the severity of the infection. Oral doses for adults are usually 150–450 mg every 6 hours, and parenteral doses, 150–900 mg every 8 hours (total 450–2700 mg/day). The oral and parenteral (intramuscular or intravenous) dose of clindamycin in children is 10–20 mg/kg/day given as individual doses every 6–8 hours. For serious infection, the daily dose can be increased to 40 mg/kg/day.

References

1. Birkenmeyer RD, Kagan F: Lincomycin XI: Synthesis and structure of clindamycin, a potential antibacterial agent. J Med Chem 1970; 13: 616–619.
2. Dhawan VK, Thadepalli H: Clindamycin: A review of fifteen years of experience. Rev Infect Dis 1982; 4: 1133–1953.
3. Brook I: Pediatric Anaerobic Infection: Diagnosis and Management, 2nd ed. St Louis: CV Mosby, 1989.
4. Paris MM, Ramilo O, McCracken GH Jr: Management of meningitis caused by penicillin-resistant *Streptococcus pneumoniae*. Antimicrob Agents Chemother 1995; 39: 2171–2175.
5. Van Landuyt HW: Spectrum of clindamycin: In-vitro effects and efficacy. Acta Therapeutica 1987; 13: 541–551.
6. Gemmell CG, Peterson PK, Schmeling D, et al.: Potentiation of opsonization and phagocytosis of *Streptococcus pyogenes* following growth in the presence of clindamycin. J Clin Invest 1981; 67: 1249–1256.
7. Sutter VL: In vitro susceptibility of anaerobes: Comparison of clindamycin and other antimicrobial agents. J Infect Dis 1977; 135 (suppl): S7–S12.
8. Stevens D: Invasive Group A streptococcal infection: The past, present, and future. Pediat Infect Dis J 1994; 13: 561–566.
9. Brook I, Gober AE, Leyra F: *In vitro* and *in vivo* effects of penicillin and clindamycin on expression of group A beta-hemolytic streptococcal capsule. Antimicrob Agents Chemother 1995; 39: 1565–1568.
10. Nord CE: The role of anaerobic bacteria in recurrent episodes of sinusitis and tonsillitis. Clin Infect Dis 1995; 20: 1512–1524.
11. Brook I: Management of chronic suppurative otitis media: Superiority of therapy effective against anaerobic bacteria. Pediatr Infect Dis J 1994; 13: 188–193.
12. Brook I, Yocum P: Antimicrobial management of chronic sinusitis in children. J Laryngol Otol 1995; 109: 1159–1162.
13. Brook I: The role of beta-lactamase-producing bacteria in the persistence of streptococcal infection. Rev Infect Dis 1984; 6: 601–607.
14. Levison ME, Mangura CT, Lorber B, et al.: Clindamycin compared with penicillin for the treatment of anaerobic lung abscess. Ann Intern Med 1983; 98: 466–471.
15. Gudiol F, Manresa F, Pallares R, et al.: Clindamycin versus penicillin for anaerobic lung infections: High failure rate of penicillin, failures associated with penicillin-resistant *Bacteroides melaninogenicus*. Arch Intern Med 1990; 150: 2525–2529.
16. Johnson JT, Yu VL, Myers EN, Wagener RL: An assessment of the need for gram-negative bacterial coverage in antibiotic prophylaxis for oncological head and neck. J Infect Dis 1987; 155: 331–333.
17. Nelson CT, Mason EO, Kaplan SL: Activity of oral antibiotics in middle ear and oral sinus infections caused by penicillin resistant *Streptococcus pneumoniae*: Impact for treatment. Pediatr Infect Dis J 1994; 13: 585–589.
18. Knoop FC, Owens M, Crocker IC: *Clostridium difficile*: Clinical disease and diagnosis. Clin Microbiol Rev 1993; 6: 251–265.

Itzhak Brook

PART 5

Metronidazole

▼

Metronidazole is a nitroimidazole with a formula 1-(2-hydroxyethyl)-2 methyl-5-nitroimidazole. It is the first 5-nitroimidazole derivative introduced as an antimicrobial agent.[1] Other 5-nitroimidazoles (tinidazole, ornidazole, nimorazole, etc.) are less commonly used and differ in their pharmacokinetics and pharmacologic properties but not in their mode of antimicrobial action. Metronidazole was first used in 1959 for the treatment of *Trichomonas vaginalis,* but later, its spectrum of efficacy was expanded to cover other parasitic infections as well as infections caused by anaerobic bacteria.

PHARMACOLOGY AND PHARMACOKINETICS

Metronidazole is absorbed rapidly and almost completely when given orally. Peak serum levels following single doses of 250 mg and 500 mg are approximately 6 μg/mL and 12 μg/mL, respectively. Multiple 500-mg oral doses given four times daily result in peak serum levels of 20 to 30 μg/mL. The recommended dosage of the intravenous preparation for serious anaerobic infections is 15 mg/kg infused over 1 hour (approximately 1 g for a 70-kg adult) with maintenance dosage of 7.5 mg/kg every 6 hours (approximately 500 mg for a 70-kg adult). The peak blood levels achieved with intravenous administration approximate those noted with oral administration, indicating that the oral formulation is nearly completely absorbed.[2] Thus, parenteral administration appears to offer no additional benefit for patients who can receive oral treatment; furthermore, the intravenous form is substantially more expensive. The serum half-life is approximately 8 hours. Metronidazole can also be given rectally through an enema or suppository.

The drug diffuses well into nearly all tissue, including the central nervous system, brain abscess, middle ear discharge and mucosa, saliva, abscesses, bile, bone, pelvic tissue, breast milk, and placenta. Metronidazole is extensively metabolized in the liver by oxidation, hydroxylation, or conjugation of side chains on the imidazole ring. The major metabolic products are the acid or alcohol metabolites. The major route of elimination of the parent compound and its metabolites (60%–80%) is in the urine. The clearance of metronidazole is not altered in renal failure, but accumulation of metabolites may be noted with repeated doses. Dosages reduced by at least 50% are recommended in patients with severe hepatic disease. Newborns have decreased elimination capacity. Peritoneal dialysis and hemodialysis are effective in removing metronidazole.

SPECTRUM OF ACTIVITY

Metronidazole is active against certain protozoa, including *T. vaginalis, Entamoeba histolytica, Balantidium coli,* and *Giardia lamblia.* Also susceptible to metronidazole are *Treponema pallidum,* oral spirochetes, *Campylobacter fetus, Gardnerella vaginalis,* and *Helicobacter pylori.* This drug is bactericidal and shows excellent in vitro activity against most obligate anaerobic bacteria, such as *B. fragilis* group and *Prevotella, Porphyromonas,* and *Fusobacterium* species. It is effective against most species of *Peptostreptococcus* and *Clostridium* (including *C. difficile*). Occasional strains of anaerobic gram-positive cocci and nonsporulating bacilli are highly resistant. Microaerophilic streptococci, *Propionibacterium acnes, Arachnia,* and *Actinomyces* species are almost uniformly resistant. Aerobic and facultative anaerobes, such as Enterobacteriaceae, are usually highly resistant. Over 90% of obligate anaerobes are susceptible to less than 2 μg/mL metronidazole.[3]

Resistant to metronidazole by anaerobic gram-negative bacilli and *T. vaginalis* is rare and is caused by several mechanisms, both plasma-mediated and chromosomally mediated. Slower uptake and decreased intracellular reduction of the drug were found in resistant *B. fragilis.*

MECHANISM OF ACTION

Metronidazole enters the cell by passive diffusion only in cells that possess the required enzymatic system.[1] The nitro group accepts electrons given by a ferredoxin-like cell protein. Toxic short-lived derivatives are produced intracellularly, whose target is probably DNA.

CLINICAL USE IN OTOLARYNGOLOGY

The main advantages of metronidazole are its bactericidal activity and low potential for *C. difficile* overgrowth. The main disadvantage of metronidazole is its narrow spectrum. Metronidazole is useful for most orofacial and odontogenic anaerobic infections, except those caused by *Actinomyces* and *Propionibacterium* species. Metronidazole can also be used for the treatment of head and neck, skin and soft tissue, bone, joint, and blood-borne infection due to susceptible organisms. However, because most anaerobic infections are polymicrobial aerobic-anaerobic in nature, coverage against the aerobic or facultative components of the infection is warranted.[4, 5] This type of polymicrobial infection is very common in the oral and pulmonary regions. Such extra coverage can be achieved by adding a beta-lactam or a glycopeptide (i.e., vancomycin) to cover *Streptococcus* species; a penicillinase-resistant penicillin, a macrolide, or a glycopeptide to cover *Staphylococcus* species; or an aminoglycoside, ceftazidime, or a quinolone to cover aerobic gram-negative bacilli (i.e., *Haemophilus* species, Enterobacteriaceae, or *P. aeruginosa*).

The excellent penetration of metronidazole into the central nervous system allows its use for the treatment of brain abscess and other intracranial infections due to anaerobes. However, it should be combined with agent(s) effective against microaerophilic streptococci and other potential pathogens that can also be recovered in these sites.

Metronidazole in an oral or parenteral form is effective in the management of pseudomembranous colitis due to *C. difficile*.[6] It is also more effective than penicillin in therapy of *Clostridium tetani* infection.[7]

Metronidazole in combination with other agents has been used effectively in the treatment of peridontitis, soft tissue infection, aspiration pneumonia, chronic otitis media, chronic sinusitis, and intracranial abscess.[4, 5, 8, 9]

ADVERSE REACTIONS

Tolerance to metronidazole in patients is generally very good. Adverse reactions are rare and include symptoms such as nervous system toxicity, peripheral neuropathy, ataxia, vertigo, headaches, encephalopathy, and convulsions. Gastrointestinal side effects include nausea, vomiting, epigastric discomfort, pancreatitis, metallic taste, glossitis, anorexia, and diarrhea. Pseudomembranous colitis has been rarely observed. Other adverse reactions are reversible neutropenia, phlebitis at intravenous infusion site, and drug fever. Minor adverse reactions include dark or red brown urine, maculopapular rash, urethral or vaginal burning, and gynecomastia. Metronidazole also interferes with liver function tests, resulting in falsely low levels of the drug.

Some studies in mice have shown possible mitogenic activity associated with administration of metronidazole for prolonged periods and in high doses.[10] Metronidazole showed mutagenic activity in some in vitro assay systems but not in mammalian systems. Other experiments have shown that administration of metronidazole to hamsters does not induce any pathologic condition.[10] No evidence of mutagenicity was ever found in women who received metronidazole for *T. vaginalis*. However, the development of breast and colon cancer in patients with Crohn's disease treated for an extended period with metronidazole has been noted.[10]

DRUG INTERACTIONS

Disulfiram (Antabuse) reaction–like symptoms can occur in patients ingesting alcohol. These include nausea, vomiting, abdominal cramps, headaches, and strange taste sensation. Metronidazole inhibits the metabolism of warfarin and other oral coumarin-type anticoagulants, thus increasing their anticoagulant effect. The dosage of anticoagulants should therefore be adjusted to maintain adequate prothrombin time. Phenobarbital and phenytoin, which induce microsomal liver enzymes, enhance the metabolism of metronidazole and thus decrease its effectiveness. Conversely, the clearance of phenytoin is decreased.

DOSING

The recommended intravenous dosage of metronidazole for the therapy of anaerobic infection in children and adults is a loading dose of 15 mg/kg, then 7.5 mg/kg q6h. The oral dose in adults is 1–2 g/d given in two to four doses q6–12h. The daily adult dose should not exceed 4.0 g. The pediatric oral dose is 15–35 mg/kg/day given in individual doses every 8 hours.

References

1. Muller M: Action of clinically utilized 5-nitromidazoles on microorganisms. Scand J Infect Dis Suppl 1981; 26: 31–41.
2. Fredricsson B, Hagstrom B, Nord C-E, et al.: Systemic concentrations of metronidazole and its main metabolites after intravenous, oral and vaginal administration. Gynecol Obstet Invest 1987; 24: 200–207.
3. Sutter VL, Finegold SM: Susceptibility of anaerobic bacteria to 23 antimicrobial agents. Antimicrob Agents Chemother 1976; 10: 736–752.
4. Finegold SM: Anaerobic Bacteria in Human Disease. New York: Academic Press, 1977.
5. Brook I: Pediatric Anaerobic Infections: Diagnosis and Management, 2nd ed. St. Louis: Mosby Company, 1989.
6. Bolton RP, Culshaw MA: Faecal metronidazole concentrations during oral and intravenous therapy for antibiotic associated colitis due to *Clostridium difficile*. Gut 1986; 27: 1169–1172.
7. Ahmadsyah I, Salim A: Treatment of tetanus: An open study to compare the efficacy of procaine penicillin and metronidazole. Br Med J 1985; 291: 648–650.
8. Brook I: Treatment of anaerobic infections in children with metronidazole. Dev Pharmacol 1983; 6: 187–198.
9. Brook I: Aerobic and anaerobic bacteriology of intracranial abscess. Pediatr Neurol 1992; 8: 210–214.
10. Rosenblatt JE, Edson RS: Metronidazole. Mayo Clin Proc 1987; 62: 1013–1017.

CHAPTER TWELVE

Irmgard Behlau
Thomas M. Daniel

Antimycobacterial Agents

I have been horribly ill the last few weeks. I had a bit of a relapse, then they had another go with the streptomycin, which previously did me a lot of good, at least temporarily. This time only one dose of it had ghastly results, as I had built up an allergy or something.

GEORGE ORWELL

▼

Robert Koch discovered the tubercle bacillus in 1882, yet today we continue to struggle with the control, treatment, management, and cure of tuberculosis. Prior to 1985, there was hope that tuberculosis was soon to be eradicated, at least in the wealthier countries of Western Europe and the United States. This was an overly simplistic hope, given the plethora of newly recognized risk factors and the breakdown of geographical barriers. Tuberculosis is a global problem requiring a comprehensive approach.

In his Nobel Prize lecture in 1905, Koch laid down guidelines for tuberculosis control: prevention of infection by isolation of the patient in hospitals or screening at home; disinfection of the patient's excretions; care of the patients in organized dispensaries; circulation of information to and health education of the population and, above all, of the patients and their families; and compulsory registration of all cases as the basis of coverage for statistical purposes. The semantics may have changed but the message and guidelines remain valid even today.

ANTITUBERCULOSIS DRUGS

In approaching the treatment of a patient with tuberculosis, it is useful to recognize that patients harbor two populations of *Mycobacterium tuberculosis,* both of which must be eradicated.[1] The first is an actively multiplying population containing about 10^8 or perhaps 10^9 tubercle bacilli. The second is a slowly or intermittently multiplying population of about 10^4–10^5 organisms. The first population takes up drugs readily and is readily killed by bactericidal agents. However, about 1 in every 10^5–10^7 bacilli in this population is resistant to one of the major bactericidal drugs used in treating tuberculosis. Thus, treatment exerts a selection pressure favoring the emergence of drug-resistant bacillary populations. This problem is avoided by always using two or more bactericidal drugs in combination during an initial, intensive phase of treatment. The second population, although small enough to be unlikely to harbor drug-resistant bacilli, takes up drugs only slowly or intermittently. Treatment must be continued for many months in a consolidation phase to eradicate this bacillary population.

All initial isolates of *M. tuberculosis* should be tested for antimicrobial susceptibility, but because results do not become available for at least 3–8 weeks, empiric initial therapy must often be initiated. The resurgence of tuberculosis has been accompanied by a dramatic increase in drug resistance in some areas of the United States.[2, 3] Because poor compliance is the most important cause of treatment failure and is associated with emergence of drug resistance, some experts now recommend that patients with tuberculosis take their drugs under direct observation.[4, 5] Table 12–1 lists the most commonly used drugs for the treatment of tuberculosis. Of the drugs used for the treatment of tuberculosis, isoniazid and rifampin are by far the most active.[1, 6] Table 12–2 and 12–3 outline treatment regimens for tuberculosis based on risk for drug resistance. An excellent summary of treatment regimens has been published as a joint statement of the American Thoracic Society and the Centers for Disease Control and Prevention and subsequently endorsed by the American Academy of Pediatrics and the Infectious Disease Society of America.[7]

First-Line Antituberculosis Drugs

Isoniazid

Isoniazid (INH) is the hydrazide of isonicotinic acid, a synthetic compound with specific antimycobacterial activity. It is readily absorbed from the gastrointestinal tract and penetrates well into all tissues, including the cerebrospinal fluid (CSF). It is metabolized in the liver through the action of *N*-acetyltransferase. A relative deficiency of this enzyme leads to slow inactivation and prolongation of the usual serum half-life from 1 hour up to 4 hours. INH acts by inhibiting the synthesis of mycolic acid, an important constituent of the bacterial cell wall. It is bactericidal against both extracellular and intracellular, actively multiplying tubercle bacilli. Resistance develops in 1 out of 10^6 organisms. INH remains the most widely used drug in the treatment of tuberculosis. It is used in combination with other agents for active disease (see Tables 12–2 and 12–3) and is also used singly as preventive treatment in infected patients who do not yet have active disease (see Table 12–6). INH is also included routinely in the treatment of *Mycobacterium kan-*

Table 12–1. ANTIMYCOBACTERIAL AGENTS

Drug	Adult Daily Dosage (Alternative Twice-Weekly Dosage)	Pediatric Daily Dosage (Alternative Twice-Weekly Dosage)	Major Toxicity	Monitor
1st-Line drugs				
Isoniazid[1,2]	5 mg/kg to 300 mg PO, IM, or IV (15 mg/kg to 900 mg PO)	10–20 mg/kg to 300 mg PO (20–40 mg/kg to 900 mg PO)	Peripheral neuropathy Hepatitis, drug fever	Symptoms, signs monthly
Rifampin[1]	10 mg/kg to 600 mg PO or IV (same)	10–20 mg/kg to 600 mg PO (same)	Hepatitis, cytopenias Immune reactions Interaction with many drugs Orange discoloration of secretions Possible teratogen	SGOT every 2, 4, 6 months Levels of other drugs Symptoms, signs monthly
Pyrazinamide[1]	15–30 mg/kg to 2.5 g PO (50–70 mg/kg to 4 g PO)	15–30 mg/kg to 2 g PO (50–70 mg/kg to 4 g PO)	Hepatitis, arthralgias Hyperuricemia	SGOT Uric acid
Ethambutol	15 mg/kg PO (50 mg/kg to 2.5 g PO)	15–25 mg/kg PO (50 mg/kg to 2.5 g PO); not recommended in children younger than 6 years	Optic neuritis	Symptoms, visual acuity Color vision testing monthly
Streptomycin	15 mg/kg to 1 g IM (25–30 mg/kg to 1.5 g IM)	20–30 mg/kg IM (25–30 mg/kg to 1.5 g IM)	8th nerve damage Nephrotoxicity (uncommon)	Auditory and vestibular function BUN/creatinine
2nd-Line Drugs				
Capreomycin	15 mg/kg to 1 g IM	15–30 mg/kg IM	8th nerve damage, nephrotoxicity	Same as for streptomycin
Kanamycin	15 mg/kg to 1 g IM, IV	15–30 mg/kg IM	Auditory toxicity, nephrotoxicity	Same as for streptomycin
Amikacin	15 mg/kg to 1 g IM, IV	15–30 mg/kg IM	Auditory toxicity, nephrotoxicity	Same for streptomycin
Ethionamide[2]	15–20 mg/kg to 1g PO	15–20 mg/kg PO	Gastrointestinal disturbance Neurotoxicity, hepatotoxicity	
Cycloserine[2]	10–20 mg/kg to 1 g PO	10–20 mg/kg PO	Central nevous system effects, interactions with phenytoin	Symptoms, signs Drug levels
Thiacetazone[1] (not marketed in U.S.)	2.5 mg/kg to 150 mg PO (450 mg PO)		Gastrointestinal upset Cutaneous reactions Hematologic toxicities Hepatitis	
Para-aminosalicylic acid	200 mg/kg to 12 g PO	75–100 mg/kg BID PO	Diarrhea, hepatitis Hypersensitivity reactions	
Ciprofloxacin	1.0–1.5 g PO	Not recommended	Nausea, abdominal pain	
Ofloxacin	600–800 mg PO	Not recommended	Nausea, abdominal pain	
Rifabutin	150–300 mg PO		Hepatitis, cytopenias	
Clofazimine	50 mg PO	1 mg/kg PO	Skin pigmentation, ichthyosis Gastrointestinal disturbance	
Dapsone	100 mg PO	1–1.5 mg/kg	Anemia	

[1]Combination capsules of isoniazid 150 mg and rifampin 300 mg (Rifamate, 2 tablets/day); isoniazid 50 mg, rifampin 120 mg, and pyrazinamide 300 mg (Rifater, 4–6 tablets/day); and isoniazid and thiacetozone are available.
[2]Pyridoxine supplementation recommended.

sasii, *Mycobacterium szulgai,* and *Mycobacterium xenopi.* It is often ineffective against many of the other mycobacteria.

Hepatitis and peripheral neuropathy are the principal adverse effects. Serum aspartate aminotransferase (AST, SGOT) activity increases in 10%–20% of patients taking INH, especially in the early weeks of treatment, but often returns to normal even when the drug is continued. Severe liver damage due to INH can occur and is more common in older patients.[8] Therefore, it is wise to obtain baseline hepatic enzyme and bilirubin determinations and to monitor patients clinically for signs and symptoms of hepatitis during treatment. Routine laboratory monitoring is not useful, because normal values may be falsely reassuring and may not give warning of impending hepatitis and because moderate

Table 12–2. TREATMENT OPTIONS FOR SUSCEPTIBLE TUBERCULOSIS

Regimen	Initial Phase (1 to 2 Months)		Consolidation Phase (4–7 Months)	
	Drugs	Doses	Drugs	Doses
Short 6-month	Isoniazid	300 mg qd	Isoniazid	300 mg qd
	Rifampin	600 mg qd	Rifampin	600 mg qd
	Pyrazinamide	15–30 mg/kg qd		
Intermittent 9-month[1]	Isoniazid	300 mg qd	Isoniazid	900 mg twice weekly
	Rifampin	600 mg qd	Rifampin	600 mg twice weekly
Rifampin intolerance[2]	Isoniazid	300 mg qd	Isoniazid	300 mg qd
	Ethambutol	15 mg/kg qd	Ethambutol	15 mg/kg qd
	± Streptomycin	0.75–1 g qd		
During pregnancy[3]	Isoniazid	300 mg qd	Isoniazid	300 mg qd
	Ethambutol	15 mg/kg qd	Ethambutol	15 mg/kg qd

[1]All intermittent regimens must be monitored by directly observed therapy (DOT) for the duration of treatment.
[2]Continue for 12–18 months.
[3]Change to rifampin-containing regimen after delivery.

enzyme elevations do not predict clinical liver disease. INH should always be discontinued in the presence of symptoms of hepatitis or jaundice; continuation of INH in patients with drug hepatitis can have a fatal outcome. A peripheral neuritis, characterized initially by paresthesia of the hands and feet, is due to induction of pyridoxine deficiency by INH and occurs more commonly in undernourished patients. Small doses of pyridoxine can prevent or ameliorate the neuritis without interfering with the antimycobacterial effect. It is wise to use pyridoxine (25–50 mg/day) prophylactically in patients predisposed to peripheral neuritis, such as those who have diabetes, are elderly, or are malnourished or alcoholic. Occasionally, INH causes a hypersensitivity drug fever and skin rash. Rare side effects include encephalopathy, convulsions, optic atrophy, purpura, and a lupus-like syndrome. In glucose-6-phosphate dehydrogenase (G6PD) deficiency, INH can precipitate hemolytic anemia. INH also reduces the metabolism of several anticonvulsants (phenytoin, carbamazepine, primidone), potentiating their toxicities.

Rifampin

Rifampin is a semisynthetic derivative of rifamycin B, a macrocyclic antibiotic produced from *Streptomyces mediter-*

ranei. Rifampin is well absorbed when taken orally in a fasting state. It is distributed throughout tissues and cells. Its cerebrospinal fluid (CSF) concentrations are 10%–50% of the concurrent plasma concentrations when the meninges are inflamed. Rifampin is excreted principally in the bile after deacetylation to an active metabolite in the liver. Rifampin is reabsorbed well from the intestine after biliary excretion, whereas its metabolite is not. Excretion is primarily into the gastrointestinal tract, with lesser amounts in the urine. Rifampin acts by inhibiting bacterial DNA-dependent RNA polymerase, thereby interfering with bacterial RNA synthesis. It has a wide spectrum of activity. Rifampin is bactericidal against all extracellular and intracellular populations of tubercle bacilli. It is also active against many other mycobacteria, including *Mycobacterium leprae, M. kansasii, Mycobacterium marinum, Mycobacterium haemophilum,* and *M. xenopi.* Only one half of *Mycobacterium scrofulaceum* or *Mycobacterium avium-intracellulare* complex (MAI) strains are sensitive to rifampin. *Mycobacterium fortuitum* strains are usually resistant. In addition, rifampin is active against many gram-positive and gram-negative bacteria. Resistance to rifampin emerges so quickly as to preclude its use alone.

Several adverse effects can limit the use of rifampin.

Table 12–3. TREATMENT OPTIONS FOR POSSIBLY DRUG-RESISTANT TUBERCULOSIS[1]

Regimen	Initial Phase (1–2 Months)		Consolidation Phase (4–7 Months)	
	Drugs	Doses	Drugs	Doses
Option 1	Isoniazid (INH)	300 mg qd	Isoniazid	300 mg qd
	Rifampin (RIF)	600 mg qd	Rifampin	600 mg qd
	Pyrazinamide	15–30 mg/kg qd		
	Ethambutol	15 mg/kg qd		
	or Streptomycin	0.75–1 g/d until susceptibility to INH and RIF is shown		
Option 2[2]	Isoniazid	300 mg qd	Isoniazid	900 mg twice weekly
	Rifampin	600 mg qd	Rifampin	600 mg twice weekly
	Pyrazinamide	15–30 mg/kg qd	(Continue until susceptibility to INH and RIF is documented.)	
	Ethambutol	15 mg/kg qd		
	or Streptomycin	0.75–1 g qd		

[1]When tuberculosis infection occurs with human immunodeficiency virus infection, options 1 and 2 should be continued for a total of 12 months and at least 6 months beyond culture conversion.
[2]All intermittent regimens must be monitored by directly observed therapy (DOT) for the duration of treatment.

Hepatotoxicity with transient elevations of the transaminases as seen with INH occur not uncommonly; toxic hepatitis may be seen in 1% of patients. Rifampin may increase the risk of hepatitis from INH, because rifampin is a potent enzyme inducer and increases the binding of the acetyl isoniazid metabolite in the liver. Monitoring for hepatotoxicity should be as described for INH (see Table 12–1). Severe hypersensitivity reactions, including thrombocytopenia, purpura, transient leukopenia, hemolysis, and acute renal failure, can occur with rifampin. An immune-mediated, systemic, flu-like syndrome has been described almost exclusively with intermittent, high-dose rifampin therapy. Patients should be warned about orange pigmentation of the urine, tears, and sweat, and that soft contact lenses will also become discolored. Rifampin is not recommended for use during pregnancy, especially the first trimester, because of possible teratogenic effects and its ability to cross the placental barrier. Rifampin is a potent hepatic microsomal cytochrome P-450 enzyme inducer that increases the metabolism of many substances, including warfarin sodium, oral contraceptives, corticosteroids, phenytoin, quinidine, methadone, zidovudine, clarithromycin, oral hypoglycemics, and the azoles.

Pyrazinamide

Pyrazinamide (PZA) is a synthetic analog of nicotinic acid. It is well absorbed when given orally, is widely distributed in body fluids and passes freely into the cerebrospinal fluid. It is hydrolyzed to pyrazinoic acid in the liver, which is then excreted by the kidneys. It is active only at a pH less than 5.5 in vitro, yet it penetrates cells well and is bactericidal against intracellular growing mycobacteria. Because metabolically inactive tubercle bacilli are resistant to PZA, it is inappropriate for long-term therapy. This agent's antibacterial activity is restricted to *M. tuberculosis.* Its mechanism of action remains unknown.

The most common side effects are nausea and vomiting. Dose-related hepatotoxicity is the major side effect. Hyperuricemia is common and is due to the inhibition of the renal excretion of urate; clinical gout is rare. Pyrazinamide also inhibits the hypouricemic action of allopurinol. Rarely, thrombocytopenia and sideroblastic anemia have been reported. There is insufficient information about the use of PZA in pregnancy; therefore, it would be prudent to avoid its use.

Ethambutol

Ethambutol is a synthetic derivative of ethylenediamine. Approximately 75% of ethambutol is absorbed after oral administration. It is widely distributed through all body fluids, and in the presence of inflamed meninges, it achieves 10%–50% of the serum levels in the CSF. At least 50% of the drug is excreted unchanged in the urine; therefore, dosage reduction must be made in the presence of renal failure. Ethambutol is specific for mycobacteria, is bacteriostatic to both intracellular and extracellular bacteria, and acts by inhibiting nucleic acid synthesis. It blocks the ability of bacilli to build and maintain cell walls. Ethambutol's principal role is its use in combination therapy to curtail resistance.

Ethambutol's major toxicity is dose-related optic neuritis, which is rare unless the ethambutol dose exceeds 15 mg/kg/day. Some workers recommend tuberculosis treatment regimens employing a larger dose of ethambutol (25 mg/kg/day) during the first 2 months of treatment, then a maintenance dose (15 mg/kg/day) for the remainder of the treatment; there is no evidence to indicate that this initially higher dose increases treatment efficacy. Tests for visual acuity should be performed monthly, and symptoms followed closely and promptly. Optic neuritis may result in decreased visual acuity, constriction of visual fields, and loss of red-green discrimination. The optic neuritis may be slowly and partially reversible if it is detected early and therapy is discontinued immediately; often, though, much of the damage is irreversible.

Streptomycin

Streptomycin is an aminoglycoside derived from *Streptomyces griseus.* It is poorly absorbed from the gastrointestinal tract and therefore is usually given intramuscularly. There is little penetration across membranes into cells, and the drug is distributed extracellularly. It does penetrate most inflamed body fluids and spaces (synovial fluid, pleural and pericardial spaces, and peritoneal cavity), achieving concentrations close to those in serum. Penetration of systemically administered streptomycin into bronchial secretions, the eye (cornea, aqueous humor, and vitreous humor), and the CSF is poor, and administration of streptomycin endotracheally, topically, or by direct injection is recommended in addition to systemic injection. Streptomycin is excreted unchanged and almost completely by the kidneys. It is important that the dosage be reduced in patients with impaired renal function. Streptomycin has a wide spectrum of activity; in addition to its bactericidal activity against extracellular mycobacteria, it inhibits a wide variety of gram-negative and gram-positive organisms. Streptomycin is active in neutral to alkaline pH in vitro (optimal pH is 7.8). It acts by binding to the 30S subunit of ribosomes, thereby producing inhibition of protein synthesis. Resistance emerges rapidly with streptomycin, with an initial resistance of 1 in 10^6 organisms seen. Therefore, the use of streptomycin is recommended only for multidrug therapy.

The toxicity of streptomycin is similar to that of other aminoglycosides, but with less renal and acoustic toxicity and greater vestibular toxicity. The major site of toxicity is the eighth cranial nerve, both the vestibular and the auditory branches. Dysfunction of the labyrinth results in the inability to maintain equilibrium; symptoms are ataxia, vertigo, tinnitus, and nerve deafness. Monthly monitoring of vestibular function and hearing is recommended. Symptoms may be reversible if they are recognized promptly and streptomycin is discontinued. Streptomycin should be avoided in pregnancy, because damage to the fetal eighth nerve has been reported. Hypersensitivity reactions occur in 4%–5% of patients. Paresthesias may occur, especially at the site of injection, and transient lightheadedness following injection is common. Rarely, nephrotoxicity and peripheral neuropathy can occur.

Second-Line Antituberculosis Agents

Second-line agents tend to be more difficult to use, are less effective, and/or are more toxic than the 1st-line drugs for treatment of mycobacteria. In addition, the dosages, pharmacokinetics, mechanisms of action, emergence of resistance, and long-term toxicity of 2nd-line drugs are less well understood. The following alternative drugs are usually considered only if there is resistance to 1st-line agents or if conventional therapy fails. The use of these 2nd-line agents should be guided by the expertise of a specialist in the treatment of tuberculosis.

Capreomycin, Kanamycin, Amikacin

Because streptomycin tends to have less renal toxicity and ototoxicity than other aminoglycosides, capreomycin, kanamycin, and amikacin are used only if a person cannot tolerate streptomycin or if the infecting organisms are resistant to it. Capreomycin is a macrocyclic polypeptide derived from *Streptomyces capreolus.* Its antimicrobial activity is similar to that of streptomycin, but there is no cross-resistance to streptomycin. Capreomycin is used in multiple-drug regimens for treatment of drug-resistant tuberculosis, especially when streptomycin resistance is present. Kanamycin is much less effective than streptomycin against mycobacteria and has greater toxicity. Its advantage is cost, and it is used in the treatment of streptomycin-resistant *M. tuberculosis.* Amikacin is the most active aminoglycoside against *M. tuberculosis* in vitro and in animals, but there is little experience with its use in the treatment of human tuberculosis. It is also more costly than the other aminoglycosides and more toxic than streptomycin.

Ethionamide

Ethionamide is a synthetic derivative of isonicotinic acid. It is well absorbed orally and widely distributed in body fluids, including the CSF. It is metabolized by the liver to active and inactive metabolites and is excreted renally. Ethionamide appears to be active against most multiple-drug–resistant *M. tuberculosis* isolates. The major limiting side effect of this drug is gastrointestinal upset, which affects at least one half of all patients and leads to poor compliance and discontinuation of therapy. Neurotoxicity can also be seen and may be alleviated by concomitant administration of pyridoxine. Hypersensitivity reactions manifested as hepatoxicity may also occur.

Cycloserine

Cycloserine is a structural analogue of D-alanine. It is produced synthetically. Cycloserine is well absorbed from the gastrointestinal tract and widely distributed to cells and tissues, including the CSF. Only a small percentage of the drug is metabolized; two thirds of it is excreted unchanged in the urine. In the presence of renal dysfunction, the dosage of cycloserine must be modified. Cycloserine has a wide spectrum of activity. It is bacteriostatic against both intracellular and extracellular tubercle bacilli, it has moderate in vitro activity against several other mycobacteria, and it is active against many gram-negative and gram-positive organisms. It probably acts by competitive inhibition with D-alanine in the synthesis of the cell wall. Currently, cycloserine has demonstrated no cross-resistance with any drug used to treat

mycobacterial infections. It appears to have only moderate activity in multiple-drug–resistant tuberculosis (MDR-TB). Significant central nervous system (CNS) toxicity is associated with cycloserine, including major convulsions and psychoses in 5%–10% of patients receiving 1 g/day. Suicidal depression may be severe. This agent is contraindicated in epileptics. The CNS effects may be partially counteracted by concomitant high-dose pyridoxine (100 mg/day). Like INH, cycloserine inhibits the hepatic metabolism of phenytoin.

Para-Aminosalicylic Acid

Para-aminosalicylic (*p*-aminosalicylic) acid (PAS) is usually administered as its calcium or sodium salt. It is incompletely absorbed and is mostly excreted in the urine as various degradation products. It inhibits folate synthesis and is bacteriostatic for tubercle bacilli. The major limiting side effect is severe gastrointestinal disturbance, which occurs in the majority of patients. Coupled with the large dose (up to 12 g daily), this side effect leads to poor compliance. A new enteric-coated formulation of *p*-aminosalicylic acid has been licensed and may be tolerated better than older formulations. PAS has a short shelf life, hydrolyzing to meta-amino phenol, which is severely toxic to the gastrointestinal tract. PAS can also cause multiple hypersensitivity reactions, including a drug-induced lupus-like syndrome, toxic hepatitis, fever, and rash. Owing to its low cost, PAS has retained a limited role in multidrug therapy.

Thiacetazone

Thiacetazone is a synthetic compound identified chemically as *p*-acetaminobenzaldehyde thiosemicarbazone. It is also known as amithiozone, conteben, and tibione. It is well absorbed orally but there is little information regarding its distribution. About one fourth of the drug is excreted unchanged in the urine. It was removed from the U.S. market shortly after its introduction, when it was given at a 300 mg/day dosage, owing to its excess toxicity. It is now given in an adult dosage of 150 mg/day. In this dosage, it is combined with 300 mg INH to provide an inexpensive (circa 1 cent per tablet) combination therapy that is widely used in developing countries. Cutaneous toxicity is not common but may include toxic epidermal necrolysis. Thiacetazone has been reported to cause skin reactions in 20% of human immunodeficiency virus (HIV)–positive patients, with a 3% mortality.[9] Less commonly, this agent has been associated with bone marrow suppression, hepatitis, and renal toxicity.

Quinolones

Ciprofloxacin and ofloxacin are quinolones that have demonstrable in vitro activity against *M. tuberculosis* and appear to have considerable efficacy in vivo. These quinolones enter cells well but have poor CSF penetration. They act by inhibition of the A subunit of DNA gyrase, which shuts down DNA synthesis. The quinolones are generally well tolerated, with only occasional mild gastrointestinal disturbances reported. Resistance rapidly emerges when they are used alone. There appears to be antagonism between ciprofloxacin and rifampin, which may hamper the former's clinical usefulness. Preliminary trials suggest that these quinolones are useful in combination with other 2nd-line agents in the treatment of resistant tuberculosis.

DRUGS USED FOR OTHER MYCOBACTERIA

Other mycobacteria vary in their susceptibility to antimicrobial agents (Table 12–4). Rational therapy is currently based on susceptibility testing in vitro; the important exception is the *M. avium-intracellulare* complex (MAI) infections, for which the results of in vitro susceptibility testing is not predictive of clinical response. In general, *M. kansasii* tends to be susceptible to the same drugs used to treat *M. tuberculosis,* the rapid growers (*Mycobacterium chelonae, M. fortuitum*) tend to respond to drugs used to treat more typical pyogenic bacterial infections, and MAI is broadly more resistant to most antimicrobial agents.

Rifabutin

Rifabutin is a new semisynthetic derivative of rifamycin S, which is produced by *S. mediterranei.* It is well absorbed orally, penetrates well into cells, and concentrates in the tissues. It is excreted partly in the urine and in the bile. Its mechanism of action and antimicrobial activity in vitro are similar to those of rifampin. Rifabutin appears more active in vitro and more effective in experimental animals against *M. tuberculosis,* and appears no more toxic in animals. In addition, although this agent shares some cross-resistance with rifampin, one fourth of rifampin-resistant strains remain sensitive to rifabutin, a feature that may prove clinically useful. With more experience in its use, rifabutin may well become a 1st-line agent against tuberculosis. Currently, rifabutin is most valuable in its role in the treatment of most strains of *M. avium-intracellulare.* Rifabutin has been shown to reduce the incidence and rate of dissemination of MAI infections in patients with the acquired immunodeficiency syndrome (AIDS) whose CD_4 counts are less than 200.[10]

Its toxicity profile is similar to that of rifampin and includes rash, hepatitis, leukopenia, thrombocytopenia, gastrointestinal disturbance, and orange discoloration of secretions. In addition, musculoskeletal discomfort and uveitis have occurred in persons taking higher doses of rifabutin and/or

concurrent azole or macrolide antibiotics, which appear to increase plasma rifabutin concentrations. Rifabutin decreases zidovudine plasma levels.

Macrolides

Clarithromycin and azithromycin are macrolides and semisynthetic derivatives of the erythromycin base, which is produced by *Streptomyces erytheus.* Nearly all strains of other mycobacteria, including MAI, are inhibited by clarithromycin. These drugs should not be used as monotherapy because of the rapid emergence of resistance. They hold new promise, however, for the combination treatment of the other mycobacteria, especially MAI. They are undergoing clinical trials in multidrug treatment of disseminated MAI infections and as single drugs for chemoprophylaxis in AIDS patients.

TREATMENT OF LEPROSY

Multidrug therapy is recommended for all forms of leprosy (Table 12–5). The major drugs currently in use are dapsone, rifampin, and clofazimine. Combination treatment is for a minimum of 6 months in paucibacillary disease and for a minimum of 2 years in multibacillary disease.

Dapsone

Diaminodiphenylsulfone (DDS) is a synthetic compound. It is well absorbed orally, distributed throughout body fluids, and has a long half-life of 28 hours. It is acetylated in the liver, and then its metabolites are excreted into the urine. Dosage should be reduced in the presence of renal failure. It acts by probably inhibiting bacterial folate synthesis. Dapsone is weakly bactericidal against susceptible leprosy bacilli. It is also used as prophylaxis and treatment of *Pneumocystis carinii* pneumonia. Resistance to dapsone can emerge in large populations of *M. leprae.* Previous monotherapy of lepromatous leprosy with dapsone alone resulted in a 20% rate of secondary resistance that emerged 5–24 years after the beginning of therapy.[11]

The most common side effect of dapsone is hemolytic anemia, especially in patients with G6PD deficiency. Erythema nodosum leprosum is seen in one half of patients

Table 12–4. TREATMENT POSSIBILITIES FOR OTHER MYCOBACTERIA

Runyon Group	Mycobacterial Species	Antimicrobials to Which Species is Likely to Be Susceptible	Number and Duration
I	*M. kansasii*	Rifampin, ethambutol, (isoniazid), clarithromycin, streptomycin, ethionamide, amikacin, cycloserine, sulfamethoxazole, quinolones	3 drugs × 9 months
	M. marinum	Rifampin, minocycline, ethambutol, clarithromycin, amikacin, kanamycin	2 drugs × 6 weeks–18 months
II	*M. scrofulaceum*	Amikacin, erythromycin, rifampin, streptomycin, sulfonamides (Surgical excision is the treatment of choice)	
III	*M. avium-intracellulare*	Clarithromycin, azithromycin, rifabutin, clofazamine, amikacin	3–5 drugs × 18–36 months
IV	*M. fortuitum*	Amikacin, cefoxitin, imipenem-cilastin, sulfamethoxazole, clarithromycin, ciprofloxacin	2 drugs × 6 months
	M. chelonae	Clarithromycin, azithromycin, tobramycin, amikacin	2–3 drugs × 6 months

Table 12–5. POSSIBLE TREATMENT REGIMENS FOR LEPROSY

Type	Drug Regimen and Dose	Number and Duration
Multibacillary	Dapsone 100 mg PO qd Clofazimine 50 mg PO qd plus 300 mg every month Rifampin 600 mg PO every month (or 100 mg qd if resources permit)	Three drugs × at least 2 years
Paucibacillary	Dapsone 100 mg PO qd Rifampin 600 mg PO every month (or 100 mg qd if resources permit)	Two drugs × 6–12 months, then dapsone alone × 2–5 years
Erythema nodosum leprosum	Prednisone 60–80 mg PO qd, then taper Thalidomide 200 mg PO bid, taper to 50–100 mg PO qd[1] Clofazimine 300 mg PO qd (for long-term use)	

[1]Contraindicated in women of childbearing age due to teratogenicity.

during the 1st year and may be suppressed by corticosteroids or by thalidomide.

Clofazimine

Clofazimine is a synthetic substituted phenazine dye derived from phenylenediamine. It is also known as B663 and Lamprene. It is slowly and incompletely absorbed orally, with a half-life of 70 days. Clofazimine is lipophilic, widely distributed throughout the body, and taken up by cells but does not penetrate the CSF. It is minimally metabolized and excreted via the biliary system. It is weakly bactericidal against *M. leprae*. Its current role is in combination therapy with rifampin and dapsone against leprosy. Clofazimine is also used in combination with other antimycobacterial agents against disseminated MAI infection in HIV-infected patients; it is not effective against MAI when used alone. In addition, it is active against a few gram-positive organisms. Its precise mechanism of action remains unknown.

Dose-related gastrointestinal intolerance is the most common side effect. In addition, the vast majority of patients acquire a progressive reddish to purple-black hue to the skin and body fluids, owing to a deposition of red crystals and accompanied by dryness and itching. This pigmentation usually clears up 6–12 months after therapy ends, but in some patients, it may take up to 4 years. No mutagenic or teratogenic effects have been demonstrated, but clofazimine is not recommended for use in pregnancy because it crosses the placenta and colors the infant red, and because there is concern regarding an increased incidence of spontanous abortions.

Newer Agents Against Leprosy

Promising new drugs that have shown activity against *M. leprae* in mouse footpad models and in early clinical trials include minocycline, clarithromycin, and the fluorinated quinolones, especially sparfloxacin.[12] These may prove useful in multidrug combinations in the future.

DRUG REGIMENS AGAINST TUBERCULOSIS

Susceptible Organisms

It can generally be assumed that infecting organisms are susceptible to all major therapeutic agents when the patient is not HIV-infected, has no history of prior treatment, and is not living in or an immigrant from an area where drug resistance is common (>4%). Older persons initially infected at a time when drug resistance was rare can also be assumed to harbor susceptible bacilli. Treatment can be begun for such patients using one of the regimens outlined in Table 12–2, with modifications being made if necessary when the results of drug susceptibility testing are available.

Possibly Resistant Organisms

For treatment of most patients with pulmonary or extrapulmonary tuberculosis, particularly in areas with substantial (>4%) or unknown prevalence of bacillary resistance to INH or when the patient has other risk factors for INH-resistant tuberculosis, an initial four-drug combination of INH, rifampin, pyrazinamide, and either ethambutol or streptomycin is recommended, as described in Table 12–3.[7] If full drug susceptibility is documented, ethambutol or streptomycin can be stopped and pyrazinamide continued for at least 2 months. INH and rifampin are continued for at least 6 months in all, and at least 3 months after culture conversion. Tuberculosis resistant only to INH (the most common form of resistance) should be treated with rifampin, pyrazinamide, and either ethambutol or streptomycin for 6 months, or with rifampin and ethambutol for 12 months. In patients with HIV infection and in those with disseminated disease or meningitis, treatment should be continued for at least 12 months in all, and at least 6 months after culture conversion.

Multiple-Drug–Resistant Organisms

Effective treatment for multiple-drug–resistant tuberculosis should include at least three drugs to which the organism is susceptible and should be continued for 18–24 months or at least 12 months after conversion of cultures to negative. A single drug should never be added to a failing regimen. In settings in which multiple-drug–resistant tuberculosis is likely or in patients with a history of previous tuberculosis therapy, treatment may be started with combinations of five, six, or seven drugs before laboratory susceptibility data are available.[13, 14] Directly observed therapy (DOT) is recommended for all patients with drug-resistant tuberculosis.

Intermittent Treatment

Intermittent high-dose, four-drug regimens with two doses per week after at least 2 weeks of daily therapy (see Table 12–3) can be effective for treatment of tuberculosis.[15, 16] With intermittent treatment, most experts recommend direct observation of the patient taking each dose of the drug; this is a particularly useful regimen in patients at high risk for noncompliance. Intermittent treatment is not recommended for treatment of multiple-drug–resistant tuberculosis.

PREVENTIVE THERAPY

The main application of chemoprophylaxis (Table 12–6) is to prevent the development of clinical tuberculosis from latent infection. Currently, INH is the only antituberculosis drug shown to be effective for preventive therapy. INH therapy has reduced the prevalence of disease by 54%–88% (USPHS study).[16a] The major determinant of efficacy in different studies has been the compliance rate. In fact, success rates can be 90%–98% in very compliant infected persons.[7] Dosage of INH is 300 mg daily for 6–12 months in adults and 10 mg/kg to 300 mg daily for 9 months in children; at least 12 months is suggested for patients with HIV infection, other immunosuppression, or radiographic evidence of healed tuberculosis. Tuberculin-positive persons exposed to patients infected with organisms resistant to INH alone should be treated with rifampin (600 mg daily) with or without ethambutol for 6–12 months. For those with known exposure to multiple-drug–resistant tuberculosis, pyrazinamide (25–30 mg/kg daily) concurrently with ethambutol (15 mg/kg daily), ofloxacin (400 mg bid), or ciprofloxacin (750 mg bid) may be effective.[17]

Tuberculin-reactive persons at high risk should receive preventive therapy regardless of age (see Table 12–6). The management of low-risk persons is more controversial. For patients less than 35 years old with a positive tuberculin test in the absence of recent exposure or other risk factors (see Table 12–6), the benefits of INH preventive therapy outweigh the risk of drug-associated hepatitis.[18] Because the risk of serious liver damage from INH increases with age, generally the drug should not be given to tuberculin-positive patients more than 35 years old unless other factors, such as recent tuberculin conversion, a chest radiograph consistent with healed tuberculosis, or immunosuppression or other medical condition, suggest a higher risk of developing active tuberculosis. Treatment is also recommended for children younger than 5 years who are tuberculin negative and have recently had contact with persons with active disease.[7] The tuberculin skin test is repeated in such children after 3 months, and treatment is continued only if the result is positive.

VACCINATION

Because tuberculosis is a major cause of death and morbidity worldwide, finding a vaccine that prevents tuberculosis has long been a high-priority goal. Emergence of drug-resistant strains has reemphasized the importance of finding an effective vaccine. Even in the case of treatable tuberculosis, the cost of therapy (cost of the drugs and the staff to ensure compliance) is so high that a vaccine provides the only realistic hope of controlling tuberculosis, especially in poorer countries.

Immunization against tuberculosis in endemic areas is currently effected using an attenuated strain of *Mycobacterium bovis,* bacille Calmette-Guérin (BCG). This strain enters macrophages and replicates briefly before being killed. BCG can be administered intracutaneously or orally and is safe enough to be given to infants. Billions of doses have been administered worldwide, and the lack of toxic side effects makes this one of the safest vaccines known. The only reported problems have occurred in patients with AIDS; there have been a few reports of patients developing an infection caused by BCG itself. BCG is also a very inexpensive vaccine, about 10 cents per dose. Unfortunately, its effectiveness in preventing tuberculosis remains controversial. It has reported efficacy rates ranging from 0%–80%. It does prevent dissemination of tuberculosis infection, especially in children.

BCG vaccination may be used selectively in the United States for certain populations at excessive risk of exposure or disease, and in individuals uninfected but exposed to drug-resistant cases. BCG should not be administered to persons who have symptomatic HIV infection, as it may lead to disseminated BCG infection. Immunization results in a positive tuberculin skin test and may obscure further assessment of newly infected cases.

Table 12–6. INDICATIONS FOR CHEMOPROPHYLAXIS IN PERSONS WITH POSITIVE TUBERCULIN SKIN REACTIONS

With Risk Factors (chemoprophylaxis irrespective of age)

≥ 5 mm	Household contacts of persons with recently diagnosed tuberculous disease
	HIV infection
	Roentogenographic evidence of nonprogressive tuberculous disease
≥ 10 mm	Recent skin test conversion (within the past two years)
	Intravenous drug abuse
	Predisposing medical conditions (silicosis, postgastrectomy, diabetes mellitus, chronic obstructive pulmonary disease, renal failure, immunosuppressive therapy, malignancies of the lymphatic system)

No risk factors, high-incidence group (chemoprophylaxis only if less than 35 years of age)

≥ 10 mm	Recent immigrants from high-incidence areas
	Medically underserved populations
	Residents and staff of long-term care facilities

No risk factors, low-incidence group (chemoprophylaxis only if less than 35 years of age)

≥ 15 mm	

References

1. Grosset J: Bacteriologic basis of short-course chemotherapy for tuberculosis. Clin Chest Med 1980; 1: 232–241.

2. Bloch AB, Cauthen GM, Onorator IM, et al.: Nationwide survey of drug-resistant tuberculosis in the United States. JAMA 1994; 271: 665–671.

3. Centers for Disease Control and Prevention: Tuberculosis Morbidity—United States, 1994. MMWR 1995; 44: 387–395.

4. Weis SE, Slocum PC, Blais FX, et al.: Effect of directly observed therapy on the rates of drug resistance and relapse in tuberculosis. N Engl J Med 1994; 330: 1179.

5. Bayer R, Wilkinson D: Directly observed therapy for tuberculosis: History of an idea. Lancet 1995; 345: 1545–1548.

6. Heifets LB: Antimycobacterial drugs (review). Semin Respir Infect 1994; 9: 84–103.

7. American Thoracic Society: Treatment of tuberculosis and tuberculosis infection in adults and children. Am J Respir Crit Care Med 1994; 149: 1359–1374.

8. Centers for Disease Control and Prevention: Severe INH-associated hepatitis—New York, 1991–1993. MMWR 1993; 42: 545–547.

9. Nunn P, Kibuga D, Gathua S, et al.: Cutaneous hypersensitivity reactions due to thiacetazone in HIV-1 seropositive patients treated for tuberculosis. Lancet 1991; 337: 627–630.

10. Nightingale SD, Cameron DW, Gordin FM, et al.: Two controlled trials of rifabutin prophylaxis against *Mycobacterium avium* complex infection in AIDS. N Engl J Med 1993; 329: 828–833.

11. Pearson JMH, Rees RJW, Waters MFR: Sulphone resistance in leprosy: A review of one hundred proven clinical cases. Lancet 1975; 2: 69–72.

12. Gelber RH, Iranmanesh A, Murray L, Siu P, Tsang M: Activities of various quinolone antibiotics against *Mycobacterium leprae* in infected mice. Antimicrob Agents Chemother 1992; 36: 2544–2547.

13. Goble M, Iseman M, Madsen LA, et al.: Treatment of 171 patients with pulmonary tuberculosis resistant to INH and rifampin. N Engl J Med 1993; 328: 527–532.

14. Iseman MD: Treatment of multidrug-resistant tuberculosis. N Engl J Med 1993; 329: 784–791.

15. Cohn DL, Catlin BJ, Peterson KL, et al.: A 62-dose, 6-month therapy for pulmonary and extrapulmonary tuberculosis. Ann Intern Med 1990; 112: 407–415.

16. Hong Kong Chest Service/British Medical Research Council: Controlled trial of 2, 4, and 6 months of pyrazinamide in 6 month, 3-times-weekly regimens for smear-positive pulmonary tuberculosis, including an assessment of a combined preparation of INH, rifampin, and pyrazinamide. Am Rev Respir Dis 1991; 143: 700–706.

16a. Ferebee SH: Controlled chemoprophylaxis trials in tuberculosis: a general review. Adv Tuberc Res 1970; 17: 28–106.

17. Stevens JP, Daniel TM: Chemoprophylaxis of multidrug-resistant tuberculosis infection in HIV-uninfected individuals with ciprofloxacin and pyrazinamide: A decision analysis. Chest 1995; 108: 712–717.

18. Comstock GW, Edwards PQ: The competing risks of tuberculosis and hepatitis for adult tuberculin reactors. Am Rev Respir Dis 1975; 111: 573–577.

Carol A. Kauffman

Antifungal Agents

Several different types of drugs are now available for the treatment of fungal infections. Amphotericin B has been the standard for years, but with the advent of azole antifungal agents, safer and more easily administered antifungal therapy is now available. For several life-threatening infections, amphotericin B remains the treatment of choice, whereas for other infections that are chronic or localized, azoles clearly have replaced amphotericin B as therapy.

AMPHOTERICIN B (FUNGIZONE)

Amphotericin B is a product of *Streptomyces nodosus* and a member of the polyene macrolide family of drugs. The mechanism of action is via its binding to the ergosterol component of the fungal cell membrane. Changes in membrane permeability occur, leading to leakage of cell components and ultimately fungal cell death.[1]

Pharmacology

Amphotericin B is available only as an intravenous formulation. The drug is not water soluble and is prepared in sodium desoxycholate, yielding a colloidal dispersion for intravenous infusion.[2] Amphotericin B is highly protein bound and consequently distributes poorly to various body compartments. Drug levels are very low in cerebrospinal fluid, urine, synovial fluid, aqueous humor, and vitreous body.[3] Serum levels are low because the drug avidly attaches to cell membranes; however, tissue levels, especially kidney, liver, spleen, and lung, are high, and the drug is effective in the treatment of localized infections, such as meningitis and urinary tract infections.[2–4] The metabolic pathways of amphotericin B have not been detailed. It is only very slowly eliminated, and active drug can be found in tissues and urine for as long as a month after the drug has been stopped.[5]

Spectrum of Antifungal Activity

Amphotericin B has a very broad spectrum of activity. It is active against the dermatophytes; yeasts, including *Candida* species, *Torulopsis glabrata, Cryptococcus neoformans,* and others; filamentous fungi, including *Aspergillus* species, *Rhizopus* species, *Mucor* species, and others; the dimorphic endemic mycoses, *Histoplasma capsulatum, Blastomyces dermatitidis, Coccidioides immitis, Paracoccidioides brasiliensis;* and *Sporothrix schenckii.*[4] It is not active against *Pseudallescheria boydii* or *Fusarium* species.[6, 7]

Clinical Use in Otolaryngologic Infections

The major use of amphotericin B for head and neck infections is in the treatment of life-threatening sinusitis, orbital apex syndrome, and cavernous sinus thrombosis due to the zygomycetes, *Aspergillus,* and a variety of other filamentous fungi.[8–15] In addition, *Aspergillus* species may cause invasive external otitis that requires treatment with amphotericin B.[16, 17] For these infections, infusion of 1 mg/kg of amphotericin B daily beginning on the first day of therapy is usually required. Surgical débridement is an essential component of treatment for most of these infections.

The other major use of amphotericin B is in treatment of the endemic mycoses.[18–20] However, these infections are often subacute to chronic and frequently can be treated with azoles rather than amphotericin B. When amphotericin B is required, treatment can begin at lower daily doses and increase to maximal daily doses of 0.5–0.7 mg/kg over several days.

Dosing and Administration

Amphotericin B is supplied as a powder that is reconstituted in sterile water, giving a concentration of 5 mg/mL; the drug is further diluted in 5% dextrose in water to give a concentration of 0.1 mg/mL for infusion. Because of the rare occurrence of anaphylaxis, the initial 1 mg (in 10 mL) can be infused slowly over 20 minutes as a test dose. If the patient tolerates this dose, the rest of the infusion can be given. The drug is usually administered slowly over 2–4 hours.[4] The daily dose and total cumulative dose depend on the infection being treated.

Amphotericin B has been used as an irrigating fluid in patients with fungal sinusitis.[21] It is difficult to evaluate the effectiveness of this method of administration. The dose is not standardized, nor is this use of amphotericin B approved by the U.S. Food and Drug Administration (FDA).

Adverse Reactions

Nephrotoxicity, the major side effect associated with the use of amphotericin B, is experienced by almost every patient receiving the drug.[4, 22–26] The nephrotoxic effects are primarily related to the drug's actions on the afferent arterioles of the kidney and are reflected by a rising serum creatinine level.[25] In addition, tubular loss of potassium and magnesium is common and may be pronounced in some individuals.[26] Renal tubular acidosis and nephrogenic diabetes insipidus have also been reported. Infusion of 500 mL 0.9% NaCl prior to the infusion can decrease amphotericin B–induced nephrotoxicity.[22] The nephrotoxic effects of amphotericin B are reversible unless the total amount of drug administered exceeds 5 g, at which point irreversible decreases in glomerular filtration may occur.[23]

Adverse reactions frequently accompany the infusion of amphotericin B. Rigors, fever, nausea, and vomiting are common and may be severe.[23] Phlebitis is also common when the drug is infused through a peripheral vein. For patients who experience infusion-related side effects, premedication with acetaminophen, diphenhydramine, and/or prochlorperazine can be given. For the occasional patient with rigors unresponsive to antipyretics, intravenous meperidine is useful.[27]

Anemia is seen in almost every patient receiving amphotericin B. Rarely are transfusions required, and red blood cell production returns to normal after the drug is stopped.[28] Uncommonly, thrombocytopenia, hepatotoxicity, and arrhythmias may also occur.[4]

Drug interactions are not a major problem with the administration of amphotericin B. However, one should try to avoid other nephrotoxic drugs, such as aminoglycosides, when amphotericin B is used. Additionally, as renal function decreases during amphotericin B use, other drugs that have dose-related toxicities and that are cleared by the kidneys, such as flucytosine and cyclosporine, must be monitored carefully.

New Formulations of Amphotericin B

Over the last decade, much work has gone into packaging amphotericin B within liposomes, globules, or sheets of fat in an attempt to decrease the toxicity. Three preparations are currently used: liposomal amphotericin B (AmBisome), amphotericin B lipid complex (Abelcet), and amphotericin B colloidal dispersion (ABCD or Amphocil). It appears that all of these preparations are less nephrotoxic than amphotericin B; infusion-related reactions are still seen. The amount of amphotericin B able to be given with these preparations is threefold to sixfold greater than possible with the parent compound. In some patients, clinical and microbiologic success has been noted with one of these newer preparations when amphotericin B therapy has failed, but the ultimate role of these drugs has not yet been defined.

FLUCYTOSINE (5-FLUOROCYTOSINE, ANCOBON)

Flucytosine is a synthetic fluorinated pyrimidine compound. The drug acts on both fungal RNA and DNA synthesis, but the major mechanism of inhibition of fungal cell growth is through its effects on RNA metabolism after conversion to 5-fluorouracil (5-FU). Mammalian cells are less able to take up the drug, so the toxic effects are directed primarily toward the fungal cell.[1, 29]

Pharmacology

Flucytosine is available in the United States only as an oral formulation. Flucytosine is well absorbed from the gastroin-

testinal tract, distributes into all body fluids, and is excreted almost wholly unchanged by the kidneys.[30] The serum half-life is short (3–6 hours), and high levels are achieved in synovial fluid, cerebrospinal fluid, aqueous humor, and vitreous body.[30] Because active drug is excreted unchanged in the urine, decreases in glomerular filtration lead to accumulation in the serum. This feature has important implications, because toxicity is directly related to flucytosine serum levels.[31]

Spectrum of Antifungal Activity

Flucytosine has limited antifungal activity.[1] It is used primarily for treating infections due to *Candida* species, *T. glabrata,* and *C. neoformans.* When it is used alone, resistance develops rapidly. When it is used with amphotericin B, synergistic killing of *Candida* species and *C. neoformans* has been described.[32, 33] When flucytosine is used with fluconazole, synergy may also occur against *Candida* and *Cryptococcus.*

Clinical Use in Otolaryngologic Infections

Flucytosine has limited usefulness in infections of the head and neck. The major use of the drug is for treating cryptococcal meningitis and *Candida* infections.[32, 34] For both of these indications, flucytosine should be used with amphotericin B. Although in vitro activity against filamentous fungi is limited, some workers recommend adding flucytosine to amphotericin B for treatment of life-threatening aspergillosis.[10, 11]

Dosing and Administration

Flucytosine is supplied as 250-mg and 500-mg capsules. Although the package insert recommends a total daily dose of 150 mg/kg, most authorities now consider this dose excessive and almost certain to produce toxic serum levels. Currently, most workers recommend a total of 100 mg/kg daily, given in four divided doses. When the creatinine clearance falls below 40 mL/min, the dosing interval should be stretched to every 12 hours (thus giving a total daily dose of 50 mg/kg); for a creatinine clearance <20 mL/min, a single daily dose of 25 mg/kg should be given.

Adverse Reactions

The major side effect of flucytosine is bone marrow suppression. This effect is reversible when the drug is stopped, but fatal marrow aplasia has been reported.[31] Toxicity is related to flucytosine serum levels >100 µg/mL.[1, 31] Other side effects are nausea, vomiting, rash, and hepatotoxicity. When flucytosine is used, careful monitoring of serum levels should be performed. Peak serum levels should be kept between 50 and 75 µg/mL. If drug monitoring is not available, it is prudent to avoid using flucytosine.

AZOLE DRUGS: KETOCONAZOLE (NIZORAL), ITRACONAZOLE (SPORANOX), FLUCONAZOLE (DIFLUCAN), MICONAZOLE (MONISTAT)

Azole antifungal drugs are multiringed compounds that have a five-membered azole ring with either two nitrogen atoms, in the case of the imidazoles, ketoconazole, and miconazole, or three nitrogen atoms, in the case of the triazoles, itraconazole and fluconazole.[35] The azoles act to inhibit ergosterol synthesis in the fungal cell membrane via the fungal cytochrome P-450 enzyme system. The binding of each drug to various components of the P-450 complex varies, and thus, both toxicity for mammalian cells and the antifungal spectrum vary.[36–38]

Pharmacology (Table 13–1)

Ketoconazole is available only as an oral formulation. The drug is insoluble in water, and the tablet requires gastric acid in order to be broken down and absorbed.[39] Ketoconazole is highly protein bound and consequently distributes poorly into various compartments. Drug levels can be measured, but are low, in cerebrospinal fluid, urine, aqueous humor, vitreous body, and saliva.[40] Ketoconazole is metabolized by the liver, and once-daily dosing is possible because the serum half-life is long.[2]

Itraconazole has many similarities in pharmacologic attributes to ketoconazole.[41] Currently, itraconazole is available only as a capsule, but it is likely that an intravenous formulation and a suspension will be available in the future. The agent is insoluble in water and requires gastric acidity for absorption to occur. The serum levels of the drug are twofold to threefold higher when given with food.[38] A saturation phenomenon appears to occur, in that single doses above 200 mg do not result in the expected increase in serum levels. Thus, higher doses should be given as multiple 200-mg doses rather than a large single dose. The drug is metabolized almost entirely by the liver, and steady state is reached only after several weeks. Itraconazole accumulates in tissues

with high lipid content, such as skin and nails,[41] but distributes poorly into cerebrospinal fluid, eye, and urine.[42]

Miconazole is mentioned only briefly here because it has limited clinical use. It is available only as an intravenous formulation. Because of its insolubility in water, it is dissolved in polyethoxylated castor oil. Miconazole distributes into many body fluids, but generally, levels in cerebrospinal fluid, saliva, and brain tissue are low. Usually, the drug is administered three to four times daily for serious infections.[43]

Fluconazole differs in almost every pharmacologic characteristic from the other azoles.[35–38] Fluconazole is water soluble, and both intravenous and oral formulations are available. Oral absorption is excellent, not requiring gastric acid for absorption.[44] Fluconazole, unlike itraconazole and ketoconazole, is not highly protein bound and distributes well into all body fluids, including aqueous humor, vitreous body, synovial fluid, cerebrospinal fluid, brain tissue, and saliva.[44–47] The drug is excreted almost entirely through the kidneys. Because of its long serum half-life, the drug can be given once daily.

Spectrum of Antifungal Activity

The azoles are active against a diverse group of fungi—dermatophytes, filamentous fungi, yeastlike organisms, and dimorphic endemic fungi.[38] However, important differences in activity exist among the azoles. Itraconazole is the only azole with activity against *Aspergillus* species.[48] Itraconazole and ketoconazole appear to have the best activity against the endemic mycoses *H. capsulatum, B. dermatitidis,* and *P. brasiliensis,*[49–51] whereas all three oral azole agents have good activity against *C. immitis.*[52] Although all the available azoles have excellent activity against yeasts, there are several *Candida* species, especially *Candida krusei,* and *T. glabrata* that are either totally or relatively resistant to fluconazole.[53] No clinically available azole agent has activity against the zygomycetes *Mucor* and *Rhizopus.*

Table 13–1. CLINICALLY IMPORTANT FEATURES OF THE PHARMACOLOGY OF AZOLES

	Ketoconazole	Itraconazole	Fluconazole
Formulation	200-mg tablets	100-mg capsules	50-, 100-, 150-, 200-mg tablets 2 mg/mL IV solution 50-mg or 200-mg/5 mL suspension
Absorption	Requires acid; decreased with antacids, omeprazole, histamine$_2$ blockers, sucralfate	Requires acid; decreased with blockers, omeprazole, histamine$_2$ blockers, (?) sucralfate	Excellent; not affected by antacids, omeprazole, histamine$_2$ blockers, sucralfate
Distribution	Minimal in CSF, eye, and other sites	Minimal in CSF, eye, and other sites	Excellent in CSF, eye, and other sites
Protein binding	High (~99%)	High (~99%)	Low (~10%)
Metabolism	Almost entirely hepatic	Almost entirely hepatic	Minimal hepatic metabolism
Excretion in urine	Little unchanged drug in urine	Little unchanged drug in urine	>80% excreted by kidneys
Reduction of dose in renal failure	Not necessary	Not necessary	20–50 mL/min: ↓ by 50% <20 mL/min: ↓ by 75% Hemodialysis: dose after dialysis
Dosing regimen	Once-daily dosing	Once daily for 200 mg; twice daily if higher dose required	Once-daily dosing
Usual daily dose	200–800 mg	100–400 mg	100–800 mg

Clinical Use in Otolaryngologic Infections

The azoles are used for localized infections of the head and neck due to *Candida, Aspergillus,* and other filamentous fungi and for disseminated endemic mycoses.

For histoplasmosis, blastomycosis, and paracoccidioidomycosis (South American blastomycosis), itraconazole is the drug of choice.[49, 51, 54] Almost always, the head and neck manifestations are indicative of disseminated infection. For most patients, a minimum of 6 months of therapy is required, and some patients may require therapy for years. Ketoconazole also is effective, but side effects are greater[50]; fluconazole is not as effective for these infections and should remain a 2nd-line drug.[51, 55] Coccidioidomycosis can be treated with any of the three oral azoles, although fluconazole is preferred if meningitis is present.[52]

When it is not life-threatening, sinusitis due to *Aspergillus* or other filamentous fungi often can be treated with itraconazole.[48, 54, 56–58] In many patients, initial therapy should be instituted with amphotericin B and then can be followed by long-term oral therapy with itraconazole. In the case of life-threatening invasive sinusitis due to *P. boydii*, which is resistant to amphotericin B, miconazole should be given initially, followed by itraconazole or ketoconazole.[57]

The most widespread use of azoles is for treatment of mucocutaneous candidiasis.[59–63] Although all three oral azoles are effective in treating thrush, most experience has been obtained with fluconazole. Fluconazole appears to be superior to both clotrimazole troches and ketoconazole for treating patients with acquired immunodeficiency syndrome (AIDS).[61, 63] It is better than ketoconazole for neutropenic patients[59] and has been very effective for denture-associated candidiasis.[60] Less experience is available regarding the use of itraconazole for thrush.[62] Development of a suspension yielding high local levels of itraconazole appears promising for the treatment of fluconazole-resistant thrush.

Dosing and Administration

Ketoconazole is available as 200-mg tablets. Simple infections, such as thrush, can be treated with 200 mg daily, whereas serious systemic infections, such as histoplasmosis or coccidioidomycosis, are treated with 400–800 mg daily.[50] Doses as high as 1200 mg and 1600 mg have been given for the treatment of coccidioidomycosis,[52] but most physicians use a different azole agent rather than giving such a high dose of ketoconazole. The drug is given once daily unless very high doses are required, in which case multiple-dose regimens are often better tolerated by the patient. It is important that the patient not take antacids, histamine 2 (H_2) blockers, or omeprazole, as these agents would markedly decrease absorption of ketoconazole.[38]

Itraconazole is supplied as 100-mg capsules. For simple tinea or *Candida* infections, 100–200 mg daily is adequate. For serious systemic fungal infections, such as histoplasmosis or blastomycosis, 200–400 mg is usually given.[49] Patients with aspergillosis require a minimum daily dose of 400 mg.[48] A loading dose of 200 mg three times daily is usually given for the first 3 days in order to achieve steady-state levels more quickly. Daily doses beyond 200 mg require splitting the dose, and the drug should always be given with food. Itraconazole should not be used with antacids, H_2 blockers, or omeprazole.[38]

Miconazole is an intravenous formulation with a concentration of 10 mg/mL. The drug is diluted further and infused slowly over an hour. The patient should be watched carefully during the first infusion, since hypersensitivity reactions may occur.

Fluconazole is available in a variety of formulations: 50-, 100-, 150-, and 200-mg tablets; suspensions containing either 50 mg/5 mL or 200 mg/5 mL; and an intravenous preparation with a concentration of 2 mg/mL. The bioavailability of fluconazole is almost 100%. Thus, if the patient has a functional gastrointestinal tract, the oral preparations can almost always be used, and intravenous infusion is rarely required. For minor infections, such as thrush, 100 mg of fluconazole is adequate. For more serious infections doses of 400–800 mg daily are used. Doses as high as 2000 mg daily have been used, but this high dose is rarely indicated. In patients with renal insufficiency, the dose should be reduced by 50% for a creatinine clearance <50 mL/min and by 75% for a creatinine clearance <20 mL/min.

Table 13–2. EFFECTS OF AZOLE ANTIFUNGAL DRUGS ON SERUM LEVELS OF CONCOMITANTLY ADMINISTERED DRUGS

Drug Affected	Effect on Serum Level[1]		
	Ketoconazole	*Itraconazole*	*Fluconazole*
Cyclosporine	↑[2]	↑[2]	↑[2]
Warfarin	↑[2]	↑[2]	↑[2]
Phenytoin	↑[2]	↑[2]	↑[2]
Loratadine	↑	None known	None known
Terfenadine	↑[3]	↑[3]	None known
Astemizole	↑[3]	↑[3]	None known
Cisapride	↑[3]	↑[3]	None known
Digoxin	None known	↑[2]	None known
Triazolam	↑	None known	None known
Oral hypoglycemics	↑	↑	↑[2]
Isoniazid	↓	None known	None known
Rifampin	↓	None known	None known
Rifabutin	None known	None known	↑
Zidovudine (AZT)	None known	None known	↑

[1] ↑ = increase; ↓ = decrease.
[2] Significant interaction; serum levels of drug and/or clinical status should be monitored.
[3] Life-threatening interaction causing arrhythmias; the combination should be avoided.

Table 13–3. EFFECTS OF CONCOMITANTLY ADMINISTERED DRUGS ON AZOLE ANTIFUNGAL DRUG LEVELS

Drug Affecting Azole Level	Effect on Azole Level[1]		
	Ketoconazole	*Itraconazole*	*Fluconazole*
Rifampin	↓	↓	↓
Rifabutin	None known	↓	None known
Isoniazid	↓	None known	None known
Phenytoin	↓	↓	None known
Carbamazepine	None known	↓	None known
Didanosine (ddI)	↓	↓	None known
Antacids	↓	↓	None known
Histamine₂ blockers	↓	↓	None known
Omeprazol	↓	↓	None known
Sucralfate	↓	None known	None known

[1] ↑ = increase; ↓ = decrease.

Adverse Reactions

Side effects occur more often with ketoconazole than with the other two oral azole drugs and are most common when daily doses of 800 mg or more are given.[64] Decreased libido, gynecomastia, and oligospermia are related to the effects of ketoconazole on androgenic hormones.[65] Ketoconazole has rarely been associated with the development of adrenal suppression.[66] Other side effects include nausea, vomiting, rash, and fatigue. The most serious side effect is hepatitis, which appears to be idiosyncratic and has been estimated to occur in 1 in every 15,000 patients.[67] This effect is reversible if the drug is stopped; however, fatal hepatocellular necrosis has occurred when the drug was continued in the presence of rising liver enzyme values.

Itraconazole has fewer side effects than ketoconazole. It produces much less inhibition of mammalian steroid synthesis. However, at daily doses ≥600 mg, effects on steroid metabolism have been noted.[68] Other side effects are nausea, vomiting, rash, hypokalemia, edema, and hypertension.[69] Hepatitis has been reported rarely.[70]

In comparison with ketoconazole and itraconazole, fluconazole is relatively nontoxic. Side effects that have been seen include nausea, vomiting, fatigue, hepatitis, and rash, which progressed to Stevens-Johnson syndrome in several patients with AIDS.[71] Alopecia has been noted with prolonged used of fluconazole.[72]

Miconazole toxicity is almost entirely due to the vehicle in which it is suspended. Phlebitis, pruritus, nausea and vomiting, headache, and bitter taste may occur with infusion. Hyperlipidemia, hyponatremia, arrhythmias, and anemia also can occur.[43, 73]

Drug interactions are common with all the azoles because of their actions on the P-450 enzyme system (Tables 13–2 and 13–3). Ketoconazole and itraconazole have several serious drug interactions. The most important interactions are with the antihistamines terfenadine (Seldane), astemizole (Hismanal), and possibly loratadine (Claritin) and with the motility drug cisapride (Propulsid). Serum levels of all of these drugs are markedly increased when ketoconazole is used concomitantly and also appear to increase when itraconazole is used. This increase has led to ventricular arrhythmias, including torsades de pointes, and subsequent death in several patients.[74] Additionally, itraconazole may increase serum digoxin levels and lead to digoxin toxicity.[75] Fluconazole has several important drug interactions but does not interact with the previously mentioned antihistamines or cisapride.

NONABSORBABLE DRUGS FOR LOCALIZED INFECTIONS

Two nonabsorbable drugs are available for use in the treatment of thrush: nystatin, a polyene antibiotic similar to amphotericin B, and clotrimazole, an azole agent. Neither of these drugs is absorbed systematically, and thus they are used only for treating localized mucous membrane infections.

Nystatin is available as a suspension with a concentration of 100,000 units/mL. It is generally given as a swish-and-swallow regimen at a dose of 500,000 units four times daily. In addition, nystatin oral lozenges can also be used to treat thrush. No significant side effects are noted with the use of nystatin oral suspension or lozenges, nor are there adverse drug interactions that need be sought.

Clotrimazole is available as 10-mg troches or lozenges. The usual dose is 10 mg four or five times daily. No significant adverse events or drug interactions occur. However, the constant use of clotrimazole troches over several years can lead to periodontal disease because of their high sugar content.

References

1. Medoff G, Kobayashi GS: Strategies in the treatment of systemic fungal infections. N Engl J Med 1980; 302: 145.
2. Daneshmend TK, Warnock DW: Clinical pharmacokinetics of systemic antifungal drugs. Clin Pharmacokinet 1983; 8: 17.
3. Bindschadler DD, Bennet JE: A pharmacologic guide to the clinical use of amphotericin B. J Infect Dis 1969; 120: 427.
4. Gallis HW, Drew RH, Pickard WW: Amphotericin B: 30 years of clinical experience. Rev Infect Dis 1990; 12: 308.
5. Atkinson AJ, Bennet JE: Amphotericin B pharmacokinetics in humans. Antimicrob Agents Chemother 1978; 13: 271.
6. Patterson TF, Andriole VT, Zervos MJ, et al.: The epidemiology of pseudallescheriasis complicating transplantation: Nosocomial and community-acquired infection. Mycoses 1990; 33: 297.
7. Nelson PE, Dignani MC, Anaissie EJ: Taxonomy, biology, and clinical aspects of *Fusarium* species. Clin Microbiol Rev 1994; 7: 479.

8. Parfrey NA: Improved diagnosis and prognosis of mucormycosis. Medicine 1986; 65: 113.

9. Saah D, Drakos PE, Elidan J, et al.: Rhinocerebral aspergillosis in patients undergoing bone marrow transplantation. Ann Otol Rhinol Laryngol 1994; 103: 306.

10. Bradley SF, McGuire NM, Kauffman CA: Sino-orbital and cerebral aspergillosis: Cure with medical therapy. Mykosen 1987; 30: 379.

11. Yu VL, Wagner GE, Shadomy S: Sino-orbital aspergillosis treated with combination antifungal therapy. JAMA 1980; 244: 814.

12. Viollier A-F, Peterson DE, DeJongh CA, et al.: *Aspergillus* sinusitis in cancer patients. Cancer 1986; 58: 366.

13. Morrison VA, Weisdorf DJ: *Alternaria:* A sinonasal pathogen of immunocompromised hosts. Clin Infect Dis 1993; 16: 265.

14. Adam RD, Paquin ML, Petersen EA, et al.: Phaeohyphomycosis caused by the fungal general *Bipolaris* and *Exserohilum:* A report of 9 cases and review of the literature. Medicine 1986; 65: 203.

15. Washburn RG, Kennedy DW, Begley MG, et al.: Chronic fungal sinusitis in apparently normal hosts. Medicine 1988; 67: 237.

16. Bickley LS, Betts RF, Parkins CW: Atypical invasive external otitis from *Aspergillus*. Arch Otolaryngol Head Neck Surg 1988; 114: 1024.

17. Gordon G, Giddings NA: Invasive otitis externa due to *Aspergillus* species: Case report and review. Clin Infect Dis 1994; 19: 866.

18. Mikaelian AK, Varkey B, Grossman TW: Blastomycosis of the head and neck. Otolaryngol Head Neck Surg 1989; 101: 489.

19. Goodwin RA, Shapiro JL, Thurman GH, et al.: Disseminated histoplasmosis: Clinical and pathologic correlations. Medicine 1980; 59: 1.

20. Drutz DJ: Amphotericin B in the treatment of coccidioidomycosis. Drugs 1983; 26: 337.

21. Robb PJ: Aspergillosis of the paranasal sinuses: A case report and historical perspective. J Laryngol Otol 1986; 100: 1071.

22. Branch RA: Prevention of amphotericin B induced renal impairment. Arch Intern Med 1981; 148: 2389.

23. Butler WT, Bennett JE, Alling DW, et al.: Nephrotoxicity of amphotericin B: Early and late effects in 81 patients. Ann Intern Med 1964; 61: 175.

24. Clements JS, Peacock JE: Amphotericin B revisited: Reassessment of toxicity. Am J Med 1990; 88: 22N.

25. Sawaya BP, Weihprecht M, Campbell WR, et al.: Direct vasoconstriction as a possible cause for amphotericin B–induced nephrotoxicity in rats. J Clin Invest 1991; 87: 2097.

26. Burgess JL, Bircholl R: Nephrotoxicity of amphotericin B, with emphasis on changes in tubular function. Am J Med 1972; 53: 77.

27. Burks LC, Aisner J, Fortner CL, et al.: Meperidine for the treatment of shaking chills. Ann Intern Med 1980; 140: 483.

28. Lin AC, Goldwasser E, Bernard EM, et al.: Amphotericin B blunts erythropoietin response to anemia. J Infect Dis 1990; 161: 348.

29. Diasio RB, Lakings DE, Bennett JE: Evidence for conversion of 5-fluorocytosine to 5-fluorouracil in humans: Possible factor in 5-fluorocytosine clinical toxicity. Antimicrob Agents Chemother 1978; 14: 903.

30. Schonebeck J, Polak A, Fernax M, et al.: Pharmacokinetic studies on the oral antimycotic agent 5-fluorocytosine in individuals with normal and impaired renal function. Chemotherapy (Basel) 1973; 18: 321.

31. Kauffman CA, Frame PT: Bone marrow toxicity associated with 5-fluorocytosine therapy. Antimicrob Agents Chemother 1977; 11: 244.

32. Bennett JE, Dismukes WE, Duma RJ, et al.: A comparison of amphotericin B alone and combined with flucytosine in the treatment of cryptococcal meningitis. N Engl J Med 1979; 301: 126.

33. Montgomerie JZ, Edwards JE, Guze LB: Synergism of amphotericin B and 5-fluorocytosine for *Candida* species. J Infect Dis 1975; 132: 82.

34. Edwards JE, Filler SG: Current strategies for treating invasive candidiasis: Emphasis on infections in nonneutropenic patients. Clin Infect Dis 1992; 14 (suppl 1): S106.

35. Saag MS, Dismukes WE: Azole antifungal agents: Emphasis on new triazoles. Antimicrob Agents Chemother 1988; 32: 1.

36. Fromtling RA: Overview of medically important antifungal azole derivatives. Clin Microbiol Rev 1988; 1: 187.

37. Bodey GP: Azole antifungal agents. Clin Infect Dis 1992; 14 (suppl 1): S161.

38. Como JA, Dismukes WE: Oral azole drugs as systemic antifungal therapy. N Engl J Med 1994; 330: 263.

39. Lelawongs P, Barone JA, Colaizzi JL, et al.: Effect of food and gastric acidity on absorption of orally administered ketoconazole. Clin Pharm 1988; 7: 228.

40. Heel RC, Brogdan RN, Carmine A, et al.: Ketoconazole: A review of its therapeutic efficacy in systemic fungal infections. Drugs 1980; 19: 7.

41. Heykants J, Van Peer A, Van de Velde V, et al.: The clinical pharmacokinetics of itraconazole: An overview. Mycoses 1989; 32(suppl 1): 67.

42. Perfect J, Durack DT: Penetration of imidazoles and triazoles into cerebrospinal fluid of rabbits. J Antimicrob Chemother 1985; 16: 81.

43. Stevens DA: Miconazole in the treatment of systemic fungal infections. Am Rev Respir Dis 1977; 116: 801.

44. Brammer KW, Farrow PR, Faulkner JW: Pharmacokinetics and tissue penetration of fluconazole in humans. Rev Infect Dis 1990; 12(suppl 3): S318.

45. Arndt CA, Walsh TJ, McCulley CL, et al.: Fluconazole penetration into cerebrospinal fluid: Implications for treating fungal infections of the central nervous system. J Infect Dis 1988; 157: 178.

46. Oliary J, Tod M, Louchahi K, et al.: Influence of local radiotherapy on penetration of fluconazole into human saliva. Antimicrob Agents Chemother 1993; 37: 2674.

47. Thaler F, Bernard B, Tod M, et al.: Fluconazole penetration in cerebral parenchyma in humans at steady state. Antimicrob Agents Chemother 1995; 39: 1154.

48. Denning DW, Lee JY, Hostetler JS, et al.: NIAID Mycoses Study Group multicenter trial of oral itraconazole therapy for invasive aspergillosis. Am J Med 1994; 97: 135.

49. Dismukes WE, Bradsher RW, Cloud GA, et al.: Itraconazole therapy of blastomycosis and histoplasmosis. Am J Med 1992; 93: 489.

50. NIAID Mycoses Study Group: Treatment of blastomycosis and histoplasmosis with ketoconazole: Results of a prospective randomized clinical trial. Ann Intern Med 1985; 103: 861.

51. Kauffman CA: New therapies for endemic mycoses. Clin Infect Dis 1994; 19(suppl 1): S28.

52. Galgiani JN: Coccidioidomycosis. West J Med 1993; 159: 153.

53. Rex J, Rinaldi MG, Pfaller MA: Resistance of *Candida* species to fluconazole. Antimicrob Agents Chemother 1995; 39: 1.

54. Ganer A, Arathoon E, Stevens DA: Initial experience in therapy for progressive mycoses with itraconazole, the first clinically studied triazole. Rev Infect Dis 1987; 9(suppl 1): S77.

55. Pappas PG, Bradsher RW, Chapman SW, et al.: Treatment of blastomycosis with fluconazole: A pilot study. Clin Infect Dis 1995; 20: 267.

56. McGinnis MR, Campbell G, Gourley WK, et al.: Phaeohyphomycosis caused by *Bipolaris specifera:* An informative case. Eur J Epidemiol 1992; 8: 383.

57. Grigg AP, Phillips P, Durham S, et al.: Recurrent *Pseudallescheria boydii* sinusitis in acute leukemia. Scand J Infect Dis 1993; 25: 263.

58. Ismail Y, Johnson RH, Wells MV, et al.: Invasive sinusitis with intracranial extension caused by *Curvularia lunata*. Arch Intern Med 1993; 153: 1604.

59. Meunier F, Aoun M, Gerard M: Therapy for oropharyngeal candidiasis in the immunocompromised host: A randomized double-blind study of fluconazole vs. ketoconazole. Rev Infect Dis 1990; 12(suppl 3): S364.

60. Budtz-Jorgensen E, Holmstrup P, Krogh P: Fluconazole in the treatment of *Candida*-associated denture stomatitis. Antimicrob Agents Chemother 1988; 32: 1859.

61. Sangeorzan JA, Bradley SF, He X, et al.: Epidemiology of oral candidiasis in HIV-infected patients: Colonization, infection, treatment, and emergence of fluconazole resistance. Am J Med 1994; 97: 339.

62. Blatchford NR: Treatment of oral candidosis with itraconazole: A review. J Am Acad Dermatol 1990; 23: 565.

63. Laine L, Dretler RH, Conteas CN, et al.: Fluconazole compared with ketoconazole for the treatment of *Candida* esophagitis in AIDS: A randomized trial. Ann Intern Med 1992; 117: 655.

64. Dismukes WE, Stamm AE, Graybill JR, et al.: Treatment of systemic mycoses with ketoconazole: Emphasis on toxicity and clinical response in 52 patients. Ann Intern Med 1983; 8: 13.

65. Feldman D: Ketoconazole and other imidazole derivatives as inhibitors of steroidogenesis. Endocr Rev 1986; 7: 409.

66. Khosla S, Wolfson JS, Demerjian Z, et al.: Adrenal crisis in the setting of high-dose ketoconazole therapy. Arch Intern Med 1989; 149: 802.

67. Lewis JH, Zimmerman HJ, Benson GD, et al.: Hepatic injury associated with ketoconazole therapy. Gastroenterology 1984; 86: 503.

68. Sharkey PK, Rinaldi MG, Dunn JF, et al.: High-dose itraconazole in the treatment of the severe mycoses. Antimicrob Agents Chemother 1991; 35: 707.

69. Tucker RM, Haq Y, Denning DW, et al.: Adverse events associated

with itraconazole in 189 patients on chronic therapy. J Antimicrob Chemother 1990; 26: 561.

70. Lavrijsen APM, Balmus KJ, Nugteren-Huying WM, et al.: Hepatic injury associated with itraconazole. Lancet 1992; 340: 251.

71. Gussenhoven MJE, Haak A, Peereboom-Wynia JDR, et al.: Stevens-Johnson syndrome after fluconazole. Lancet 1991; 338: 120.

72. Pappas PG, Kauffman CA, Perfect J, et al.: Alopecia associated with fluconazole therapy. Ann Intern Med 1995; 123: 354–357.

73. Bagnarello AG, Lewis LA, McHenry MC, et al.: Unusual serum lipoprotein abnormality induced by the vehicle of miconazole. N Engl J Med 1977; 296: 497.

74. Honig PK, Wortham DC, Zamani K, et al.: Terfenadine-ketoconazole interaction. JAMA 1993; 269: 1513.

75. Kauffman CA, Bagnasco FA: Digoxin toxicity associated with itraconazole therapy. Clin Infect Dis 1992; 15: 886.

CHAPTER FOURTEEN

Eurico Arruda

Antiviral Agents

▼

Viruses are among the most common causes of infections of the ears, nose, and throat (ENT). However, only a few therapeutic or preventive interventions with antiviral drugs are available for these infections. An overview of the antivirals currently in use for ENT infections is presented in the following paragraphs: amantadine and rimantadine for influenza A, acyclovir and valacyclovir for herpes simplex virus (HSV), and interferon for juvenile laryngeal papillomatosis. The reader is referred to previously published reviews on antiviral therapy.[1, 2]

INFLUENZA A: AMANTADINE AND RIMANTADINE

Influenza A and B viruses cause outbreaks practically every winter. Although the most common clinical manifestations of influenza are myalgias, cough, and fever, influenza viruses may produce respiratory syndromes such as colds, pharyngitis, croup, tracheobronchitis, bronchiolitis, and pneumonia.[3] In the United States, amantadine and rimantadine are approved for the treatment and prophylaxis of influenza A virus infections.

During an outbreak of influenza A, specific therapy can frequently be instituted for a suggestive case on clinical and epidemiologic grounds.[3] In nonoutbreak situations, laboratory diagnosis may be necessary. Rapid, type-specific methods for the detection of influenza viruses in clinical samples, including polymerase chain reaction (PCR)–based assays and tests that can produce same-day results such as antigen detection, have become increasingly available.[4, 5] The application of such tests in primary care facilities is likely to increase the use of antiviral therapy for influenza virus infections.

The preferred method for influenza prophylaxis is vaccination; however, amantadine and rimantadine are approved for use in the prophylaxis of influenza A for selected groups of susceptible individuals during outbreak situations. Groups such as elderly persons who were not vaccinated, immunodeficient patients, patients in long-term care institutions, and individuals who received a vaccine strain substantially different from the outbreak strain may receive prophylaxis with amantadine or rimantadine.[1, 3]

Description of the Agents

The tricyclic amine amantadine (1-aminoadamantane hydrochloride) and its α-methyl derivative, rimantadine, are petroleum hydrocarbon derivatives that are active against influ-

enza A viruses. Both compounds consist of tricyclic 10 carbon rings with an amine side chain.[6]

Spectrum of Activity

Amantadine and rimantadine are active against influenza A viruses at concentrations <1 μg/mL but have little activity against influenza B and C or against other respiratory viruses at clinically achievable concentrations. Rimantadine exhibits greater activity than amantadine against influenza A in vitro, but both are effective clinically.[1, 6]

Mechanism of Action

At low, clinically attainable concentrations, the adamantanamines inhibit influenza A virus at the level of uncoating and, for some strains, also at the level of assembly. They inhibit the intracellular viral uncoating by blocking the ion channel function of the transmembrane domain of the M2 membrane protein, thus interfering with the acid-dependent dissociation of the matrix protein.[7]

Pharmacology and Pharmacokinetics

Although amantadine and rimantadine have the same spectrum and mechanism of action, they are metabolized differently. They are both water soluble and well absorbed orally, with peak plasma levels occurring 2–4 and 2–6 hours after oral administration for amantadine and rimantadine, respectively. The half-lives of amantadine and rimantadine are approximately 12–18 hours and 24–36 hours, respectively.[1, 6] Amantadine is excreted in an unchanged state in the urine, and elderly persons require only half of the dose needed for young adults to achieve similar plasma levels, mainly because of reduced renal function. Rimantadine is extensively metabolized after absorption, and less than 10% of the dose is excreted unchanged in the urine. Dose reductions of amantadine proportional to the creatinine clearance are suggested for patients with renal insufficiency. Nasal secretions and salivary levels of amantadine are similar to the serum levels, whereas rimantadine is present in respiratory secretions in higher concentrations than in the serum.[1, 6]

Clinical Studies

Several studies have documented the efficacy of amantadine and rimantadine in the treatment and prophylaxis of influenza A virus illness.[1, 3]

In placebo-controlled studies, both drugs have been shown to reduce the duration of signs and symptoms of influenza by approximately 50% if started within 48 hours of the onset of symptoms and continued for 5–10 days or for 48 hours after resolution of symptoms. Comparisons of amantadine and rimantadine have shown no major differences in therapeutic benefits.[1–3]

Both drugs are 70%–90% effective in preventing influenza A virus illness, a level similar to the protective efficacy of vaccine, but rimantadine induces fewer side effects.[1–3] Both drugs are more effective in preventing illness than in preventing infection by influenza A, a feature that is probably beneficial because it allows for the development of antibodies without the development of frank illness. Amantadine or rimantadine can be considered for seasonal prophylaxis of influenza A at doses of 200 mg/day (100 mg/day for elderly persons) for 5–7 weeks during an influenza A outbreak.[3, 8–11] Prophylaxis is usually continued for 10 days after a known exposure or, in outbreak situations, until 10 days after the last case is identified.

Resistance

Amantadine- and rimantadine-resistant mutants of influenza A virus have been selected in vitro and in vivo.[7, 12] The resistant variants, which occur in heterogeneous cell culture-grown virus populations with a frequency of 1 in 10^3–10^4, contain mutations in the region of gene M that encodes the transmembrane domain of the M2 protein. No obvious differences in pathogenicity and infectiousness have been documented between sensitive and resistant influenza A viruses.[7, 12, 13] Resistant influenza A virus can be recovered from up to 30% of treated patients.[7, 14] Treated individuals shedding resistant virus clear their infections, but the transmission of resistant virus to household contacts is associated with failure of drug prophylaxis and development of typical influenza.[12] It has been recommended that contact between treated patients and high-risk contacts and the use of treatment and prophylaxis in the same household be avoided.[1, 13]

Adverse Reactions

Amantadine or rimantadine in low doses (200 mg/day) have few serious renal, hepatic, or hematopoietic adverse effects. The widespread use of amantadine in the influenza season over the years has established a good safety profile, which indicates that these drugs are very safe. Transient mild neurologic adverse effects can occur in up to one third of the treated patients and include insomnia, dizziness, restlessness, anxiety, and difficulty concentrating.[1–3] Amantadine use has been associated with an increased incidence of falls in nursing home patients.[10] Patients with seizure disorders are at greater risk for these neurologic side effects.[2] Gastrointestinal complaints include dry mouth, anorexia, and nausea.[15] Side effects usually develop within the first week, are reversible upon discontinuation, and frequently even despite continuation, of treatment.[1] Rimantadine produces comparatively fewer central nervous system (CNS) side effects and more gastrointestinal side effects than amantadine.[1, 15] Side effects are more common in the presence of renal or hepatic insufficiency and are more common (20%–40%) in the elderly, even at lower doses.[1] Extrapyramidal side effects of antipsychotic drugs can be additive with those of amantadine. The antimuscarinic effects of amantadine such as dry mouth may be exacerbated by drugs with similar effects, including trihexyphenidyl, benzatropine, orphenadrine, procyclidine, ipratropium bromide, hyoscine, and propantheline. Rimantadine interacts comparatively less with these drugs.[15] Rare serious neurotoxic reactions occur with overdose or in the presence of renal insufficiency; they include tremor, seizures, coma, cardiac arrhythmias, and death.[1] Amantadine is a teratogen for laboratory animals and should not be used during pregnancy.[15]

Dosing

Amantadine (Symmetrel) and rimantadine (Flumadine) are marketed as 100-mg tablets and 10 mg/ml syrup. The recommended dosage is 100 mg twice daily, with reduction to 100 mg/day for individuals older than 65 years.[1] For children less than 10 years old, a dose of 4.4 mg/kg/day (maximum, 150 mg/day) has been suggested, but optimal pediatric dosage has not been established.[1]

For the prophylaxis of influenza A during outbreaks for selected individuals, amantadine or rimantadine can be used at the preceding dosages for 5–7 weeks. Patients with severe renal insufficiency should have dose reductions proportional to the creatinine clearance (Table 14–1). Patients in hemodialysis do not require additional doses. Prophylaxis for 2–4 weeks can be considered when vaccine is administered during an outbreak to protect the individual until antibodies develop.[1, 3]

HERPES SIMPLEX VIRUS: ACYCLOVIR AND VALACYCLOVIR

Acyclovir is indicated for the treatment of the different forms of HSV infection. Although the use of systemic acyclovir in primary and recurrent genital herpes has been extensively evaluated, its use in the treatment of HSV gingivostomatitis and pharyngitis has been less well studied.[1, 16]

Table 14–1. SUGGESTED DOSAGE REDUCTIONS FOR AMANTADINE IN RENAL INSUFFICIENCY

Creatinine Clearance (mL/min/1.73 m²)	Dosage[1]
60–80	200 mg/100 mg on alternate days
40–60	100 mg/day
30–40	200 mg twice weekly
20–30	100 mg three times a week
10–20	200 mg/100 mg on alternate weeks

[1]Data from Hayden FG: Antiviral agents. In: Mandell GL, Bennett JE, Dolin R (eds): Principles and Practice of Infectious Diseases. New York: Churchill Livingstone, 1995, pp 411–450.

Description of the Agents

Acyclovir, 9-(2-hydroxyethoxy)methylguanine, is an acyclic analogue of the natural nucleoside guanine deoxyribose, with antiviral activity against herpesviruses.[1, 7, 17]

Valacyclovir is an L-valyl ester of acyclovir, which functions as an acyclovir pro-drug. It is rapidly converted to acyclovir by first-pass intestinal and hepatic hydrolysis, thus substantially increasing acyclovir oral bioavailability.[18]

Spectrum of Activity

Acyclovir is a potent inhibitor of herpesvirus replication and is 10 times more active against HSV than against varicella-zoster virus (VZV).[1, 17] In descending order of susceptibility, the herpesviruses against which acyclovir exhibits antiviral activity are HSV-1 and HSV-2, VZV, Epstein-Barr virus (EBV), human herpesvirus 6 (HHV-6) and cytomegalovirus (CMV).[19] CMV does not encode a thymidine kinase and is the least susceptible of the herpesviruses. Although acyclovir inhibits EBV DNA replication, it does not preclude the establishment of latency.[17]

Mechanism of Action

Acyclovir inhibits DNA replication of herpesviruses with low host cell toxicity. In infected cells, the drug is phosphorylated to acyclovir monophosphate by a virus-specific thymidine kinase and, subsequently, to diphosphate and triphosphate by cellular enzymes.[1, 2, 17] Acyclovir triphosphate, the active form, is incorporated into the viral DNA during DNA replication. It has higher affinity for the viral DNA polymerase than the natural substrate, 2-deoxyguanosine-5'-triphosphate (dGTP), so it outcompetes dGTP during the DNA replication. Once it is incorporated in the DNA chain, further elongation by the viral DNA polymerase is prevented, terminating the DNA replication. The complex formed between the acyclovir-containing DNA chain and the viral DNA polymerase inactivates the enzyme, which becomes incapable of any further DNA synthesis. In addition, acyclovir triphosphate has higher affinity for the viral DNA polymerase compared with the cellular enzyme.[17] These properties make acyclovir highly selective for the viral DNA replication, with little effect on the host cell function.

Pharmacology and Pharmacokinetics

Absorption of oral acyclovir is slow, resulting in low bioavailability (15%–30%), with peak plasma concentration after 1.5–2.5 hours.[19] A liquid suspension has even lower bioavailability.[1]

Plasma protein binding occurs with 9%–33% of the plasma concentration, and acyclovir distributes to a wide range of tissues and fluids, crossing the placenta and being eliminated in breast milk. Cerebrospinal fluid (CSF) and salivary concentrations are approximately 50% and 10% of the plasma values, respectively.[1, 19]

The elimination half-life of acyclovir after intravenous administration is 2–3 hours. The kidneys are the main route of acyclovir elimination, responsible for the elimination of 60%–90% of a dose. Therefore, dose reductions are indicated in patients with renal insufficiency in whom creatinine clearance is less than 50 mL/min. Acyclovir is readily removed by hemodialysis and less efficiently by peritoneal dialysis.[1, 19] There is no systemic absorption of acyclovir from topical doses of 5% ointment.[19]

Valacyclovir administered orally is rapidly converted to acyclovir and results in threefold to fourfold higher acyclovir levels than those achievable by oral acyclovir.[18] This may permit the use of less frequent dosing.

Clinical Studies

Primary infections of the oral cavity by HSV are usually asymptomatic but may produce gingivostomatitis and pharyngitis, the latter being specially common in young adults.[14–16, 20–25] In a longitudinal study carried out among college students with pharyngitis, of the 613 patients cultured for viruses, 35 (5.7%) had positive cultures for HSV, and group A *Streptococcus* and EBV were concomitant in only 2 and 3 of them, respectively.[21] Occasionally, primary HSV infections may produce tonsillitis, epiglottitis, or laryngotracheobronchitis.[26–28]

Oral acyclovir (30–60 mg/kg/day) given prophylactically to children in early stages of three daycare HSV outbreaks significantly reduced the frequency of seroconversion and gingivostomatitis in comparison with two outbreaks in which no treatment was given.[29] One small controlled trial of the efficacy of acyclovir in primary HSV gingivostomatitis found modest reductions in pain and hypersalivation in the acyclovir recipients.[30] Because HSV gingivostomatitis may cause severe discomfort, it would not be unreasonable to try an antiviral therapy with few side effects such as acyclovir. Acyclovir is not approved by the U.S. Food and Drug Administration (FDA) for these indications.

The efficacy of acyclovir for acute HSV pharyngitis has not been evaluated in controlled trials, and the reports on its use remain anecdotal. The development of accurate and rapid tests for the detection of HSV in throat samples will provide opportunities to determine whether oral acyclovir can reduce the morbidity associated with HSV pharyngitis.

On the other hand, the efficacy of systemic acyclovir for the prevention and treatment of oropharyngeal manifestations of recurrent HSV infection in immunocompromised patients is well established. Intravenous and oral acyclovir are effective for the prevention of mucocutaneous HSV infection in bone marrow transplant patients.[1]

Oral acyclovir (200–400 mg five times daily for 5 days) has modest clinical benefits in the treatment of an episode of recurrent orolabial herpes.[31] Topical acyclovir reduces virus shedding but is not associated with clinical benefit in recurrent herpes labialis.[1, 20]

Valacyclovir is being evaluated for many of the conditions for which acyclovir is indicated.

Resistance

Acyclovir-resistant strains of HSV can be selected readily in vitro. Resistance can occur by the lack of the thymidine kinase gene (TK-deficient), production of a thymidine kinase that phosphorylates acyclovir less efficiently, or production of an altered viral DNA polymerase that is less inhibited by acyclovir triphosphate.[19] The emergence of acyclovir-resistant HSV strains occurs during prolonged treatment, mainly in immunocompromised patients, and its incidence has been increasing as the population of patients with AIDS increases. TK-deficient mutants are generally less pathogenic and less able to reactivate from latency.[1]

Adverse Reactions

On the basis of adverse effects reported among the more than 20 million people estimated to have been treated worldwide and the published literature in the first decade of widespread acyclovir use, acyclovir seems to be a safe drug.[32] Oral acyclovir is generally well tolerated, and nausea, diarrhea, and headache seldom develop.[15] Intravenous acyclovir is sometimes associated with local inflammation and phlebitis, and rarely with nausea, hypotension, headache, skin rashes, and hematuria. Reversible encephalopathy occurs in only 1% of patients treated with high doses and, in most cases, is associated with renal insufficiency.[1, 15] Long-term oral acyclovir may cause neutropenia in infants.[1] Approximately 5% of patients treated with intravenous acyclovir develop reversible renal dysfunction. This renal toxicity may be enhanced in patients receiving aminoglycosides, cyclosporine, and other nephrotoxic agents.[15]

On the basis of safety data from studies in normal volunteers and phase I trial in patients with advanced AIDS, valacyclovir has a safety profile similar to that of acyclovir and permits higher plasma levels to be achieved than with oral acyclovir.[18, 33, 34]

Dosing

Acyclovir (Zovirax) and valacyclovir (Valtrex) are marketed for oral and intravenous use. For the long-term suppression of recurring orolabial herpes, oral acyclovir, 400 mg twice daily for 4 months, reduces clinical recurrences by approximately 50%.[1] For the prevention of mucocutaneous HSV infections in patients who will undergo immunosuppression, acyclovir can be administered intravenously (250 mg/m^2/8h), begun prior to transplantation and continued for 5 weeks. Patients who can tolerate oral medication can receive oral acyclovir (400 mg five times daily for 5 weeks).[1] Established oral lesions in immunosuppressed patients can be treated intravenously or orally with similar doses for 1–2 weeks, but recurrences after cessation of therapy are common.

JUVENILE LARYNGEAL PAPILLOMATOSIS: INTERFERON-α

Clinical use of interferon (IFN) for the treatment of viral infections has generally met with limited success because of lack of potency, dose-limiting toxicity, and available alternative treatments. Approved indications currently are condyloma acuminatum, chronic hepatitis B and C, and Kaposi's sarcoma in AIDS. Among the ENT infections, interferon-α (IFN-α) has been studied as an adjunctive in the treatment of juvenile laryngeal papillomatosis.[35]

Description of the Agent

IFNs are cytokines produced by animal cells in response to a broad range of stimuli, such as double-stranded RNA, bacterial toxins, cytokines, and, most importantly, viral infections.[1, 36] They constitute an important part of the early immune response to viruses by inducing an antiviral state on a host species–specific basis. IFNs are classified into α, β, and γ according to their physicochemical properties, antigenicity, and molecular structure. IFN-α and IFN-β are the main antiviral interferons, whereas IFN-γ is mainly an immunoregulatory cytokine. Human IFN-αs are a family of proteins that share a >70% sequence homology and have similar biologic effects. IFNs can be purified from stimulated leukocytes or produced by recombinant (r) DNA methods.[1, 35–37]

Spectrum of Activity

IFN-α has a broad antiviral spectrum, but DNA viruses are generally less susceptible than RNA viruses. Despite their broad antiviral spectrum, IFNs have had limited success as antiviral agents, because of lack of potency, toxicity, and availability of alternative antiviral agents.[35]

Mechanisms of Action

IFNs bind to specific receptors on the cell surface, forming complexes that are endocytosed and triggering nuclear events that culminate with the transcription of IFN-responsive genes. Several IFN-induced proteins are synthesized, such as 2′-5′ oligodenylate synthetase, protein kinase, and phosphodiesterase, among others. These proteins lead, by multiple mechanisms, to the establishment of an antiviral state. In addition to the induction of an antiviral state within susceptible cells, IFNs also modulate the host's immune response to the infecting virus.[35]

Pharmacology and Pharmacokinetics

The forms of IFN-α that have been studied as antiviral agents in clinical studies in the United States include recombinant IFN alpha-2a (Roferon A), recombinant IFN alpha-2b (Intron A), lymphoblastoid IFN alpha-nl (Wellferon), and leukocyte IFN alpha-n3 (Alferon N).

More than 80% of a parenterally administered IFN dose is absorbed, with plasma peak levels in 4–8 hours and return to baseline in 18–36 hours.[38] Low levels of IFN are detected in respiratory secretions, CSF, and the eye following systemic administration. IFN levels are cleared rapidly by inactivation and metabolism by different tissues and urinary excretion of active IFN is minimal. Serum levels are not detectable following oral administration.[1]

Clinical Studies

A study of surgical long-term intramuscular administration of leukocyte-derived IFN-α (2 MU/m² thrice weekly for 12 months) compared with surgery alone found that IFN-α reduced the growth rates and the need for surgical removal of the papillomas in the first 6 months. However, high rates of recurrence were common, and the long-term response variable.[39] Another study with lymphoblastoid IFN-α (5 MU/m² daily for 28 days plus the same dose thrice weekly for 5 months) found that one third of patients who required surgery every 2–3 months developed remission lasting more than 500 days.[40]

Adverse Reactions

Systemic administration of IFN is associated with dose-related adverse reactions. Doses of 3–5 MU/day induce an influenza-like syndrome 6–72 hours after administration, with fever, chills, myalgias, headache, and arthralgia, which tends to subside with time. Other adverse effects at low doses include bone marrow suppression, hypotension, chest pain, mild elevation of liver enzymes, and proteinuria, which are usually not dose-limiting.[15] Severe neurologic and gastrointestinal toxicity is seen only with higher doses, of 18 MU/day or more. Administration during pregnancy is not recommended.[15]

Dosing

Therapeutic benefit of IFN-α for patients with juvenile laryngeal papillomatosis who require surgery more frequently than every 3 months may be achieved with a dose of 5 MU/m²/day for 28 days followed by the same dose thrice weekly for 5–6 months.[40]

References

1. Hayden FG: Antiviral agents. In: Mandell GL, Bennett JE, Dolin R (eds): Principles and Practice of Infectious Diseases. New York: Churchill-Livingstone, 1995, pp 411–450.
2. Hirsch MS, Kaplan JC: Antiviral agents. In: Fields BN, Knipe DM (eds): Virology, 2nd ed. New York: Raven Press, 1990, pp 441–468.
3. Betts RF. Influenza virus. In: Mandell GL, Bennett JE, Dolin R (eds): Principles and Practice of Infectious Diseases. New York: Churchill-Livingstone, 1995, pp 1546–1567.
4. Leonardi GP, Leib H, Birkhead GS, et al.: Comparison of rapid detection methods for influenza A virus and their value in health-care management of institutionalized geriatric patients. J Clin Microbiol 1994; 32: 70–74.
5. Zhang W, Evans DH: PCR detection and differentiation of influenza virus A, B and C strains. In: Persing DH, Smith TF, Tenover FC, White TJ: Diagnostic Molecular Microbiology Principles and Applications. Washington, D.C.: American Society for Microbiology, 1993, pp 374–388.
6. Tominack RL, Hayden FG: Rimantadine hydrochloride and amantadine hydrochloride use in influenza A virus infections. Infect Dis Clin North America 1987; 1: 459–478.
7. Hay AJ: The action of adamantanamines against influenza A viruses: Inhibition of the M2 ion channel protein. Semin Virol 1992; 3: 21–30.
8. Monto AS: Using antiviral agents to control outbreaks of influenza A infection. Geriatrics 1994; 49: 30–34.
9. LaForce FM, Nichol KL, Cox NJ: Influenza: Virology, epidemiology, disease and prevention. Am J Preven Med 1994; 10(suppl): 31–44.
10. Gravenstein S, Miller BA, Drinka P: Prevention and control of influenza A outbreaks in long-term care facilities. Infect Control Hosp Epidemiol 1992; 13: 49–54.
11. Gomolin IH, Leib HB, Arden NH, Sherman FT: Control of influenza outbreaks in nursing homes: Guidelines for diagnosis and management. J Am Geriatr Soc 1995; 43: 71–74.
12. Hayden FG, Couch RB: Clinical and epidemiologic importance of influenza A viruses resistant to amantadine and rimantadine. Rev Med Virol 1992; 2: 89–96.
13. Monto AS, Arden NH: Implications of viral resistance to amantadine in control of influenza A. Clin Infect Dis 1992; 15: 362–367.
14. Hayden FG, Sperber SJ, Belshe RB, et al.: Recovery of drug-resistant influenza A virus during therapeutic use of rimantadine. Antimicrob Agents Chemother 1991; 35: 1741–1747.
15. Morris DJ: Adverse effects and drug interactions of clinical importance with antiviral drugs. Drug Safety 1994; 10: 281–291.
16. Hirsch MS: Herpes simplex virus. In: Mandell GL, Bennett JE, Dolin R (eds): Principles and Practice of Infectious Diseases. New York: Churchill-Livingstone, 1995, pp 1336–1337.
17. Elion GB: Acyclovir: Discovery, mechanism of action, and selectivity. J Med Virol 1993; Suppl 1: 2–6.
18. Jacobson MA. Valaciclovir (BW256U87): The L-valyl ester of acyclovir. J Med Virol 1993; Suppl 1: 150–153.
19. Wagstaff AJ, Faulds D, Goa KL: Aciclovir: A reappraisal of its antiviral activity, pharmacokinetic properties and therapeutic efficacy. Drugs 1994; 47: 153–205.
20. Higgins CR, Schofield JK, Tatnall FM, Leigh IM: Natural history, management and complications of herpes labialis. J Med Virol 1993; Suppl 1: 22–26.
21. McMillan JA, Weiner LB, Higgins AM, Lamparella VJ: Pharyngitis associated with herpes simplex virus in college students. Pediatr Infect Dis J 1993; 12: 280–284.
22. Glezen WP, Fernald GW, Lohr JA: Acute respiratory disease of university students with special reference to the etiologic role of herpesvirus hominis. Am J Epidemiol 1975; 101: 111–121.
23. Smith TF, Martin WJ, Washington JA: Isolation of viruses from single throat swabs processed for diagnosis of group A β-hemolytic streptococci by fluorescent antibody technique. Am J Clin Pathol 1973; 60: 707–710.
24. Ross PW, Chisty SMK, Knox JDE: Sore throat in children: Its causation and incidence. Br Med J 1971; 2: 624–626.
25. Glezen WP, Fernald GW, Lohr JA: Acute respiratory disease of university students with special reference to the etiologic role of herpesvirus hominis. Am J Epidemiol 1975; 101: 111–121.
26. Inglis AF: Herpes simplex virus infection, a rare cause of prolonged croup. Arch Otolaryngol Head Neck Surg 1993; 119: 551–552.
27. Wat PJ, Strickler JG, Myers JL, Nordstrom MR: Herpes simplex infection causing acute necrotizing tonsillitis. Mayo Clin Proc 1994; 69: 269–271.
28. Bogger-Goren S: Acute epiglottitis caused by herpes simplex virus. Pediatr Infect Dis J 1987; 6: 1133–1134.
29. Kuzushima K, Kudo T, Kimura H, et al.: Prophylactic oral acyclovir in outbreaks of primary herpes simplex virus type 1 infection in a closed community. Pediatrics 1992; 89: 379–383.
30. Ducoulombier H, Cousin J, Dewilde A, et al.: La stomato-gingivite herpétique de l'enfant: Essai contrôlé aciclovir versus placebo. Ann Pédiatr (Paris) 1988; 35: 212–216.
31. Spruance SL, Stewart JCB, Rowe NH, et al.: Treatment of recurrent herpes simplex labialis with oral acyclovir. J Infect Dis 1990; 161: 185–190.
32. Tilson HH, Engle CR, Andrews EB: Safety of acyclovir: A summary of the first 10 years experience. J Med Virol 1993; Suppl 1: 67–73.
33. Weller S, Blum MR, Doucette M, et al.: Pharmacokinetics of the acyclovir pro-drug valaciclovir after escalating single- and multiple-dose administration to normal volunteers. Clin Pharmacol Ther 1993; 54: 595–605.

34. Jacobson MA, Gallant J, Wang LH, et al.: Phase I trial of valaciclovir, the L-valyl ester of acyclovir, in patients with advanced human immunodeficiency virus disease. Antimicrob Agents Chemother 1994; 38: 1534–1540.

35. Arruda E, Hayden FG: Role of cytokines in viral infections. In: Oppenheim JJ, Rossio JL, Gearing AJH (eds): Clinical Applications of Cytokines. New York: Oxford University Press, 1993, pp 79–92.

36. Joklik WK. Interferons. In: Fields BN, Knipe DM (eds): Virology, 2nd ed. New York: Raven Press, 1990, pp 383–410.

37. Taylor JL, Grossberg SE: Recent progress in interferon research: Molecular mechanisms of regulation, action, and virus circumvention. Virus Res 1990; 15: 1–26.

38. Wills RJ: Clinical pharmacokinetics of interferons. Clin Pharmacokinet 1990; 19: 390–399.

39. Healy GB, Gelber RD, Trowbridge AL, et al.: Treatment of recurrent respiratory papillomatosis with human leukocyte interferon. N Engl J Med 1988; 319: 401–407.

40. Leventhal BG, Kashima HK, Mounts P, et al.: Long-term response of recurrent respiratory papillomatosis to treatment with lymphoblastoid interferon N1. N Engl J Med 1991; 325: 613–617.

SECTION III

MICROORGANISMS

▼ *Bacteria*

▼ *Fungi*

▼ *Miscellaneous Organisms*

Dennis L. Stevens

▼ *Bacteria*

CHAPTER FIFTEEN

Streptococcus pyogenes

▼

DESCRIPTION

History

Group A streptococcal infections of the throat, sinuses, ears, and soft and bony structures of the head and neck have been described since the time of Hippocrates. Severe forms of pharyngitis occurring in Spain in the sixteenth century were referred to as *garittilo,* and in England in the eighteenth century were known as Fothergills sore throat. Complications of pharyngitis, such as mastoiditis and thrombosis of the cavernous sinus, tonsillar vein, and lateral sinus, were still reported as complications of group A streptococcal infections in the 1930s and carried a mortality rate of 55%.[1] Perhaps the earliest clinical evidence of mastoiditis was found in pre-Columbian skulls (8000–6500 B.C.) recovered from an archeologic excavation in the Americas in 1930.[2] Throughout history, there have been numerous epidemics of other forms of group A streptococcal infections, such as scarlet fever, rheumatic fever, impetigo, and erysipelas, demonstrating that (1) group A streptococcus causes a variety of clinical illnesses, (2) the severity of each type of infection can independently wax and wane, and (3) an epidemic of only one type of group A streptococcal infection may materialize in a specific time. In contrast, the annual prevalence of group A streptococcal pharyngitis has remained quite constant over decades. Thus, these historical perspectives provide solid clues that many different strains of group A streptococci may be present in a given geographic site at a specific point in time. Over a 10-year period, one strain may emerge as a dominant strain, only to be replaced by one or more different strains.[3] That this dynamic process affects the expression of disease with a regular periodicity is suggested by the work of Kohler and colleagues,[4] who demonstrated that the severity of scarlet fever varied in 6- to 7-year cycles and was correlated with the appearance of M-1 strains producing streptococcal pyrogenic exotoxin A.[4]

Over the last 40 years in the Western world, streptococcal pharyngitis has become a very mild disease, and during this time, the prevalence of acute rheumatic fever has reached an all-time low. Thus, some have argued that antibiotics should no longer be prescribed for streptococcal pharyngitis. Several epidemics of rheumatic fever[5] and severe invasive group A streptococcal infections have been described from many areas around the world.[6] Thus, at present, it seems prudent to aggressively diagnose and treat group A streptococcal infections of the throat to prevent rheumatic fever, extension of infection into the vital structures of the head and neck, and life-threatening invasive infections such as bacteremia, necrotizing fasciitis, and streptococcal toxic shock syndrome (strep TSS).

The Pathogen

Streptococcus pyogenes, or group A streptococcus, is a facultative, gram-positive coccus that grows in chains and causes numerous infections in humans, including pharyngitis, tonsillitis, scarlet fever, cellulitis, erysipelas, rheumatic fever, poststreptococcal glomerulonephritis, necrotizing fasciitis, myonecrosis, and lymphangitis. Its only known niche is the skin and mucous membranes of the human host. Though the clinical diseases produced by group A streptococci have been well described, the pathogenic mechanisms underlying these diverse clinical entities are poorly understood.

Microbiologic Characteristics

Group A streptococci require complex media containing blood products and 10% CO_2 for optimal growth. On blood agar plates, these organisms produce pinpoint colonies surrounded by a zone of complete (beta) hemolysis. The exhaustive work of Rebecca Lancefield[7] established the classification of streptococci into types A through O on the basis of acid-extractable antigens of cell-wall material.

Virulence Factors

Capsule

Some strains of *S. pyogenes* possess luxuriant capsules of hyaluronic acid, resulting in large mucoid colonies on blood agar. Luxuriant production of M protein may also impart a mucoid colony morphology, a trait that has been associated most commonly with M-18 strains.[8]

Cell Wall

The cell wall consists of a peptidoglycan backbone with integral lipoteichoic acid components. Both peptidoglycan and lipoteichoic acid play important roles in adherence of group A streptococci to pharyngeal epithelial cells.[9]

M Proteins

More than 80 different M-protein types of group A streptococcus are currently described. The protein is a coiled coil consisting of four regions of repeating amino acids (A–D), a proline/glycine-rich region that serves to intercalate the protein into the bacterial cell wall, and a hydrophobic region that acts as a membrane anchor.[10] Region A near the *N*-terminus is highly variable, and antibodies to this region confer type-specific protection. Within the more conserved B–D regions lies an area that binds one of the complement regulatory proteins (factor H), stearically inhibiting antibody binding and complement-derived opsonin deposition, and effectively camouflaging the organism against humoral immune surveillance. M protein also protects the organism against phagocytosis by polymorphonuclear leukocytes, though this property can be overcome by type-specific antisera.[7, 10, 11] Observations by Lancefield[7] suggest that the quantity of M protein produced decreases with passage on artificial media but increases rapidly with passage through mice.[7] In humans, the quantity of M protein produced by an infecting strain progressively decreases during convalescence and with prolonged carriage.[7] Nontypable strains of group A streptococcus may express minute amounts of M protein, may lack M protein altogether, or may be of a totally new M type.

Streptolysin O

Streptolysin O belongs to a family of oxygen-labile, thiol-activated cytolysins and causes the broad zone of beta hemolysis surrounding colonies of *S. pyogenes* on blood agar plates.[12] Thiol-activated cytolysins bind to cholesterol on eukaryotic cell membranes, creating toxin-cholesterol aggregates that contribute to cell lysis via a colloid-osmotic mechanism. Cholesterol inhibits toxicity in isolated myocytes and hemolysis of red blood cells in vitro. In situations in which serum cholesterol is high (i.e., nephrotic syndrome), falsely elevated anti–streptolysin O (ASO) titers may occur, because both cholesterol and anti-ASO antibody will neutralize streptolysin O. Striking amino acid homology exists between streptolysin O and thiol-activated cytolysins from other gram-positive bacteria.

Streptolysin S

Streptolysin S is a cell-associated hemolysin from *S. pyogenes* that does not diffuse into the agar media. Purification and characterization of this protein have been difficult, and its only role in pathogenesis may be direct, contact-dependent cytotoxicity.

Deoxyribonucleases A, B, C, and D

Expression of deoxyribonucleases (DNases) by *S. pyogenes* in vivo, especially DNase B, elicits production of anti-DNase antibody following either pharyngeal or skin infection.

Hyaluronidase

The extracellular enzyme hyaluronidase hydrolyzes hyaluronic acid in deeper tissues, facilitating the spread of infection along fascial planes. Antihyaluronidase titers rise following *S. pyogenes* infections, especially those involving the skin.

Pyrogenic Exotoxins

Streptococcal pyrogenic exotoxins type A, B, and C, also called scarlatina or erythrogenic toxins, induce lymphocyte blastogenesis, potentiate endotoxin-induced shock, induce fever, suppress antibody synthesis, and act as superantigens.[13] The identification of these three different types of pyrogenic exotoxins may in part explain why some individuals may have multiple attacks of scarlet fever. The gene for pyrogenic exotoxin A (*speA*) is transmitted by bacteriophage, and stable production depends upon lysogenic conversion in a manner analogous to toxin production by *Corynebacterium diphtheriae*.[14] Control of streptococcal pyrogenic exotoxin A production is not yet understood, though the quantity of streptococcal pyrogenic exotoxin A produced by strains varies dramatically from decade to decade. Historically, streptococcal pyrogenic exotoxin A–producing strains have been associated with severe cases of scarlet fever and, later, with streptococcal toxic shock syndrome.[15, 16]

All strains of group A streptococci are endowed with genes for streptococcal pyrogenic exotoxin B (*speB*), but as with streptococcal pyrogenic exotoxin A, the quantity of toxin produced varies greatly from strain to strain.[4, 14, 15, 17]

Pyrogenic exotoxin C, like streptococcal pyrogenic exotoxin A, is bacteriophage-mediated and its expression is likewise highly variable. Mild cases of scarlet fever in England and the United States have been associated with streptococcal pyrogenic exotoxin C–positive strains.[17] Two new superantigens, mitogenic factor[18, 19] and streptococcal superantigen,[20] have been described; however, their roles in pathogenesis have not been fully investigated.

EPIDEMIOLOGY

Natural Reservoir

Group A streptococcus is purely a human pathogen. This statement is based on the following observations:

1. Natural group A streptococcal infection in animals is rare.

2. Laboratory animals are not useful models for streptococcal pharyngitis, scarlet fever, erysipelas, rheumatic fever, or poststreptococcal glomerulonephritis.

3. The inoculum needed to cause infection in laboratory animals is greater than that estimated to cause infection in humans.

4. Group A streptococci have developed highly sophisticated defensive molecules that bind, inactive, or destroy human immune response molecules, such as immunoglobulin[10] and complement.[21]

Relationship to Humans

The highest incidence of most group A streptococcal infections is in children younger than age 10.[8] The asymptomatic prevalence is also higher (15%–20%) in children compared with adults (<5%). Age is not the only factor, because crowded conditions in temperate climates during the winter months are associated with epidemics of pharyngitis in military recruits as well as in schoolchildren. Impetigo is most common in children from ages 2–5 years and may occur throughout the year in tropical areas or largely in the summer in temperate climates. Similarly, 90% of cases of scarlet fever occur in children 2–8 years old, and like pharyngitis, scarlet fever is most common in temperate regions during the winter months.

In contrast to pharyngitis, impetigo, and scarlet fever, the age-specific attack rate of bacteremia is highest in the elderly and in neonates.[22] However, between 1986 and 1988, the prevalence of bacteremia increased 800%–1000% in adolescents and adults in Western countries.[23] Though some of this increase is attributable to intravenous drug abuse and puerperal sepsis, most involves cases of streptococcal toxic shock syndrome.[22] This clinical manifestation of streptococcal infection may be related in part to the emergence of more virulent strains.[15, 24–26]

COLONIZATION, TRANSMISSION, AND IMMUNITY

Human skin and mucous membranes serve as the natural reservoirs of *S. pyogenes*. Pharyngeal and cutaneous acquisition is person-to-person, spread via aerosolized microdroplets or by direct contact. Epidemics of pharyngitis and scarlet fever have also occurred following ingestion of contaminated nonpasteurized milk or food. Epidemics of impetigo have been reported, particularly in tropical areas, in daycare centers, and among underprivileged children. Group A streptococcal infections in hospitalized patients occur during child delivery (puerperal sepsis), times of war (epidemic gangrene), or surgical convalescence (surgical wound infection, surgical scarlet fever) or as a result of burns (burn wound sepsis). Thus, in most clinical streptococcal infections, the mode of transmission and portal of entry are easily ascertained. In contrast, among patients with strep TSS, the portal of entry is obvious in only 50% of cases.[26]

PATHOGENESIS

Adherence of cocci to the pharyngeal mucosal epithelium is necessary but not sufficient to cause disease in all cases, since prolonged asymptomatic carriage is well documented. Complex interactions between host epithelium and streptococcal factors such as M protein, lipoteichoic acid, peptidoglycan, and fimbriae are necessary for adherence.[9, 27] Fibronectin-binding protein (protein F) also contributes to adherence, since protein F–deficient mutants are incapable of binding to epithelial cells.[28]

On the surface of respiratory epithelial cells or within the tissues, streptococci may evade opsonophagocytosis by destroying or inactivating complement-derived chemoattractants and opsonins (C5a peptidase) and by binding immunoglobulins. Expression of M protein, in the absence of type-specific antibody, also protects the organism from phagocytosis by polymorphonuclear leukocytes and monocytes. In tissues, streptolysin O secreted in high concentration destroys approaching phagocytes. Distal to the focus of infection, lower concentrations of streptolysin O stimulate polymorphonuclear leukocyte adhesion to endothelial cells, effectively preventing continued granulocyte migration and promoting vascular damage.[29] In the nonimmune host, streptolysin O, streptococcal pyrogenic exotoxin A, and other streptococcal components stimulate host cells to produce tumor necrosis factor (TNF) and interleukin-1 (IL-1), cytokines that mediate hypotension and stimulate leukostasis, resulting in shock, microvascular injury, multiorgan failure, and, if excessive, death.[22] A unique feature of the pyrogenic exotoxins[30] and some M protein fragments[31] is their ability to interact with certain V_β regions of the T-cell receptor in the absence of classic antigen processing. Such antigens are called superantigens, and they induce massive clonal proliferation of T lymphocytes and production of the lymphokines TNF-β, interferon gamma, and interleukin-2.[32] Streptococcal pyrogenic exotoxin B, which is related to the proteinase precursor, may play a role in the pathogenesis of necrotizing fasciitis and myositis and may also contribute to shock in strep TSS through its ability to cleave pre–IL-1β into active IL-1β.[33] Thus, in strep TSS, both lymphokines and monokines may mediate shock and microvascular injury.[22]

CLINICAL TYPES OF INFECTION

Pharyngitis and the Asymptomatic Carrier

Group A streptococcus may be isolated from the throats of 1%–70% of the population, many of whom are asymptomatic. The lowest carriage rates are in adults, whereas children living in crowded conditions in temperate climates during the winter months are highly affected. Patients with pharyngitis have abrupt onset of sore throat, submandibular adenopathy, fever, and chilliness but usually not frank rigors. Cough and hoarseness are rare, but pain on swallowing is characteristic. The uvula is edematous, tonsils are hypertrophied, and the pharynx is erythematous with exudates that may be punctate or confluent. Uncomplicated pharyngitis is usually self-limited, and pain, swelling, and fever resolve spontaneously in 3–4 days even without treatment. Since the late 1940s, the main reason to treat streptococcal throat was to prevent rheumatic fever. However, depending upon the nature of the infecting strain and on the immunologic state of the host, pharyngitis may progress to scarlet fever, bacteremia, suppurative head and neck infections, rheumatic fever, poststreptococcal glomerulonephritis, or strep TSS. Definitive diagnosis of streptococcal pharyngitis is difficult when based solely upon clinical parameters, especially in infants, in whom rhinorrhea may be the dominant manifestation. Even in older children with all of the preceding physical findings, the correct clinical diagnosis is made in only 75%

of cases. Absence of any one of the classic signs greatly reduces the diagnostic specificity (see also Chapter 46).

Scarlet Fever

During the last 30–40 years, scarlet fever in the Western world has been infrequent and of such a mild nature that some have referred to it as pharyngitis with a rash or benign scarlet fever. In contrast, in the latter half of the 19th century, mortalities of 25%–35% were common in the United States, Western Europe, and Scandinavia.[34] The fatal or malignant forms of scarlet fever have been described as either septic or toxic. Understanding of septic scarlet fever is particularly germane to this chapter on ear, nose, and throat infections, since patients with this form of scarlet fever subsequently develop local invasion of the soft tissues of the neck. Children with septic scarlet fever had prolonged courses and succumbed 2–3 weeks after the onset of pharyngitis, frequently owing to complications such as upper-airway obstruction, otitis media with perforation, meningitis, mastoiditis, invasion of the jugular vein or carotid artery, and bronchopneumonia. The second form of severe or malignant scarlet fever, referred to as toxic scarlet fever, was associated with profound hyperpyrexia (temperatures of 107–113° F), delirium, convulsions, and death. All these suppurative complications of streptococcal pharyngitis as well as the malignant forms of scarlet fever have been markedly less common since the advent of antibiotics.

Erysipelas

Erysipelas is usually caused by *S. pyogenes,* although groups C, G, and B have also been isolated from patients with this illness.[35] Distinctive features are an abrupt onset; fiery red, salmon, or scarlet rash with well defined margins, particularly along the nasolabial fold; rapid progression; and intense pain. Flaccid bullae may develop during the 2–3 day of illness, yet extension to deeper soft tissues is rare. Surgical débridement is rarely necessary, and treatment with penicillin is effective. Swelling may progress despite treatment, though fever, pain, and the intense redness diminish. Desquamation of the involved skin occurs 5–10 days into the illness. Infants and elderly adults are most commonly afflicted, and historically, erysipelas, like scarlet fever, was more severe prior to the turn of the century. Though erysipelas is most common on the face, it may occur anywhere in the body. The portal of entry is usually the skin when it occurs on an extremity, though even here, no portal of entry can be found in 26% of cases. The oropharynx serves as the source of bacteria and portal of entry when erysipelas occurs on the face.

Streptococcal Pyoderma (Impetigo Contagiosa)

Impetigo is most common in patients with poor hygiene or malnutrition. It may occur on the face but is more common on the extremities. Colonization of the unbroken skin occurs first; then intradermal inoculation is initiated by minor abrasions, insect bites, and so on. Single or multiple, thick-crusted, golden-yellow lesions develop within 10–14 days. Penicillin used orally or parenterally and bacitracin or mupuricin used topically are effective treatments for impetigo and also reduce transmission of streptococci to susceptible individuals. None of these treatments, including penicillin, prevents poststreptococcal glomerulonephritis.

Cellulitis

Group A streptococcus is the most common cause of cellulitis; however, alternative diagnoses may be obvious when cellulitis is associated with a primary focus, such as an abscess or boil (*Staphylococcus aureus*), dog bite (*Capnocytophaga canimorsus*), cat bite (*Pasteurella multocida*), freshwater injury (*Aeromonas hydrophila*), or seawater injury (*Vibrio vulnificus*).[36] Clinical clues to diagnosis are important, because aspiration of the leading edge or punch biopsy yields a causative organism in only 15% or 40% of cases, respectively.[37] Patients with lymphedema of any cause, such as lymphoma, filariasis, or postsurgical regional lymph node dissection (mastectomy, carcinoma of the prostate, etc.) are predisposed to developing streptococcal cellulitis, as are patients with chronic venous stasis. Recurrent saphenous vein donor site cellulitis has also been attributed to group A, C, or G streptococci. Group A streptococci may invade the epidermis and subcutaneous tissues, resulting in local swelling, erythema, and pain. The skin becomes indurated and, unlike the brilliant redness seen in erysipelas, is a pinkish color. Streptococcal cellulitis responds quickly to penicillin, though in some cases in which Staphylococcus is of concern, nafcillin or oxacillin may be a better choice.

Lymphangitis

Cutaneous infection such as cellulitis or erysipelas with bright red streaks ascending proximally is invariably due to group A streptococcus. Prompt parenteral antibiotic treatment is mandatory, since bacteremia and systemic toxicity develop rapidly once streptococci reach the blood stream via the thoracic duct.

Necrotizing Fasciitis

Necrotizing fasciitis, originally called streptococcal gangrene, is a deep-seated infection of the subcutaneous tissue that results in progressive destruction of fascia and fat but may spare the skin itself. Subsequently, necrotizing fasciitis has become the preferred term, because *Clostridium perfringens, Clostridium septicum, Staphylococcus aureus,* and mixed aerobic-anaerobic flora of the mouth or gastrointestinal tract can produce a similar pathologic process. Infection may begin at the site of trivial or inapparent trauma. Within the first 24 hours, swelling, heat, erythema, and tenderness develop and rapidly spread proximally and distally from the original focus. During the next 24 to 48 hours, the erythema darkens, changing from red to purple and then to blue, and blisters and bullae form that contain clear yellow fluid. On the 4th or 5th day, the purple areas become frankly gangrenous.

Myositis

Historically, streptococcal myositis has been an extremely uncommon infection, only 21 cases being documented from 1900 to 1985. The prevalence of streptococcal myositis has increased in the United States, Norway, and Sweden. Translocation of streptococci from the pharynx to the site of deep trauma (muscle) must occur hematogenously. Symptomatic pharyngitis or penetrating trauma is uncommon. Severe pain may be the only presenting symptom, and swelling and erythema may be the only signs of infection. In most cases, a single muscle group is involved; however, because patients are frequently bacteremic, multiple sites of myositis or abscess can occur. Distinguishing streptococcal myositis from spontaneous gas gangrene due to *C. perfringens* or *C. septicum* may be difficult, although the presence of crepitus or gas in the tissue would favor clostridial infection. Myositis is easily distinguished from necrotizing fasciitis anatomically by surgical exploration or incisional biopsy, although clinical features of the two conditions overlap. In published reports, the case-fatality rate of necrotizing fasciitis is between 20% and 50%, whereas that of streptococcal myositis is between 80% and 100%. Aggressive surgical débridement is extremely important because of the poor efficacy of penicillin described in human cases as well as in experimental models of streptococcal myositis (see section on treatment below).

Pneumonia

Pneumonia caused by group A streptococcus is most common in women in the 2nd and 3rd decades of life and is associated with the rapid appearance of large pleural effusions and empyema. Chest tube drainage is mandatory, though management is complicated by multiple loculations and fibrinous effusions, resulting in restrictive lung disease. Prolonged penicillin therapy, thoracoscopy, and decortication of the pleura may be necessary.

Streptococcal Toxic Shock Syndrome (Strep TSS)

In the late 1980s, invasive group A streptococcal infections associated with bacteremia, deep soft-tissue infection, shock, multiorgan failure, and death in 30%–70% of cases were reported from North America and Europe (reviewed by Stevens[6]). Such cases have been defined as strep TSS.[38] Though all age groups may be affected, most cases have occurred sporadically in previously healthy individuals between the ages of 20 and 50 years. More than 50% of patients have experienced a viral-like prodrome, minor trauma, recent surgery, or varicella infection. In cases that progress to necrotiz-

ing fasciitis, the infection may begin at the site of a break in the skin and extend deep in the soft tissue, or alternatively, infections may begin deep at the site of blunt trauma, such as a hematoma or muscle strain, and extend through muscle and fascia to the superficial skin layers. Though preceding symptomatic pharyngitis is rare, the pharyngeal mucosa is the likely bacterial source. Presumably, a transient bacteremia from a pharyngeal colonization seeds the site of trauma.

The abrupt onset of severe pain is a common initial symptom of strep TSS. The pain most commonly involves an extremity, but may also mimic peritonitis, pelvic inflammatory disease, acute myocardial infarction, headache, toothache, meningitis, or sinus infection. Treatment with nonsteroidal anti-inflammatory agents may mask the presenting symptoms or predispose to more severe complications such as shock.

Fever is the most common presenting sign, though some patients present with profound hypothermia secondary to shock. Confusion is present in over half of the patients and may progress to coma or combativeness. On admission, 80% of patients have tachycardia and more than half have systolic blood pressure of <110 mm Hg. Of those with normal blood pressure on admission, most become hypotensive within 4 hours. Soft tissue infection evolves to necrotizing fasciitis or myositis in 50%–70% of patients, requiring emergent surgical débridement, fasciotomy, or amputation. An ominous sign is progression of soft tissue swelling to violaceous or bluish vesicles or bullae. Invariably, this development indicates necrotizing fasciitis or myonecrosis and demands immediate surgical exploration. Many other clinical presentations may be associated with strep TSS, including endophthalmitis, myositis, perihepatitis, peritonitis, myocarditis, meningitis, septic arthritis, and overwhelming sepsis. Patients with shock and multiorgan failure without signs or symptoms of local infections have a worse prognosis, since definitive diagnosis and surgical débridement may be delayed. In addition, infection involving the soft tissues of the head and neck are problematic, because surgical débridement may be disfiguring or impossible.

LABORATORY DIAGNOSIS

Rapid antigen detection tests in the office setting have a sensitivity and specificity of 40%–90% (see Chapter 46). A popular approach in clinical practice is to obtain two throat swab samples from the posterior pharynx or tonsillar surface. A rapid strep test is performed on the 1st sample; if it is positive, the patient is treated with antibiotics and the second swab is discarded. If the rapid strep test is negative, the 2nd sample is sent to the laboratory for culture, and treatment is withheld pending a positive culture. Bacitracin susceptibility remains an excellent presumptive test for group A streptococcus. Alternatively, rapid Lancefield group typing can be performed using latex agglutination tests. Acute pharyngitis results in sufficient antigenic stimulation to induce antibody production directed against M protein, streptolysin O, DNase and hyaluronidase, and, if present, pyrogenic exotoxins. An increase in titer of any of these is indicative of a recent streptococcal infection. The antihyaluronidase test is the best test for infections involving the skin.

TREATMENT

Group A streptococci remain exquisitely sensitive to penicillin, though resistance to sulfonamides and erythromycin has been a significant problem since the 1940s and 1970s, respectively. Numerous studies have demonstrated the clinical efficacy of penicillin, cephalosporins, erythromycin, and clindamycin in the treatment of streptococcal pharyngitis, erysipelas, impetigo, and cellulitis. In addition, Wannamaker and colleagues[39] demonstrated that penicillin therapy prevented the development of rheumatic fever following streptococcal pharyngitis if therapy was begun within 8–10 days of the onset of sore throat. Nonetheless, some clinical failures of penicillin treatment of streptococcal infection do occur (see also Chapter 46). One problem with penicillin treatment of S. pyogenes has been the inability of that drug to eradicate bacteria from the pharynx of 5%–20% of patients with documented streptococcal pharyngitis.[40–42] In addition, more aggressive group A streptococcal infections (such as necrotizing fasciitis, empyema, burn wound sepsis, subcutaneous gangrene, and myositis) respond less well to penicillin and continue to be associated with high mortality and extensive morbidity.[16, 22, 43] For example, in a 1985 report of 25 cases of streptococcal myositis, the overall mortality was 85% in spite of penicillin therapy.[43] Finally, several studies in experimental infection suggest that penicillin fails when large numbers of organisms are present.[44, 45] In addition, experimental data for group A streptococcal myositis demonstrate that penicillin is ineffective when treatment is delayed ≥2 hours after initiation of infection.[45] Interestingly, erythromycin and clindamycin have significantly greater efficacy.[45, 46] Eagle[44] suggested that penicillin fails in this type of infection because of the "physiologic state of the organism." My colleagues and I[47, 48] have attributed this phenomenon to both in vitro and in vivo inoculum effects.[47, 48]

Penicillin and other beta-lactam antibodies are most efficacious against rapidly growing bacteria. We hypothesized that large inocula reach the stationary phase of growth sooner than smaller inocula both in vitro and in vivo. That high concentration of S. pyogenes accumulate in deep seated infection is supported by data from Eagle.[44] We compared the penicillin-binding protein (PBP) patterns from membrane proteins of group A streptococci isolated from different stages of growth, i.e., mid–log phase and stationary phase. Binding of radiolabeled penicillin by all PBPs was decreased in stationary cells; however, PBPs 1 and 4 were undetectable at 36 hours.[47] Thus, the loss of certain PBPs during stationary phase growth in vitro may be responsible for the inoculum effect observed in vivo and may account for the failure of penicillin in both experimental and human cases of severe streptococcal infection.

The greater efficacy of clindamycin is likely multifactorial. First, its efficacy is not affected by inoculum size or stage of growth.[47, 49] Second, clindamycin is a potent suppressor of bacterial toxin synthesis.[50, 51] Third, clindamycin facilitates phagocytosis of S. pyogenes by inhibiting M-protein synthesis.[51] Fourth, clindamycin suppresses synthesis of penicillin-binding proteins, which in addition to being targets for penicillin are also enzymes involved in cell-wall synthesis and degradation.[49] Fifth, clindamycin has a longer postan-

tibiotic effect than beta-lactams such as penicillin. Lastly, my colleagues and I[52] have shown that clindamycin causes suppression of lipopolysaccharide-induced monocyte synthesis of TNF-α. Thus, clindamycin's efficacy may also be related to its ability to modulate the immune response.

Though antibiotic selection is critically important, other measures, such as prompt and aggressive exploration and débridement of suspected deep-seated S. pyogenes infection, are mandatory and provide material for gram stain and culture. Thus, it is critical that our surgical colleagues be involved early in such cases, because later in the course, surgical intervention may be impossible owing to toxicity or because infection has extended to vital areas that are impossible to débride.

Anecdotal reports suggest that hyperbaric oxygen has been used in a handful of patients, but no controlled studies are under way, nor is it clear whether this treatment is useful.

Because of intractable hypotension and diffuse capillary leak, massive amounts of intravenous fluids (10–20 L/day) are often necessary. Pressors such as dopamine are used frequently, though no controlled trials have been performed in strep TSS. In patients with intractable hypotension, vasoconstrictors such as epinephrine have been used, but symmetric gangrene of digits seems to result frequently (my own unpublished observations, 1995), often with loss of limb. In these cases, it is difficult to determine whether symmetric gangrene is due to pressors or infection or both.

Neutralization of circulating toxins would be a desirable therapeutic modality, yet appropriate antibodies are not commercially available in the United States or Europe. Several small, nonrandomized studies describe successful use of intravenous gamma globulin in the treatment of strep TSS.[53–56]

References

1. Keefer CS, Ingelfinger FJ, Spink WW: Significance of hemolytic streptococcic bacteremia; a study of two hundred and forty-six patients. Arch Intern Med 1937; 60: 1084–1097.
2. Brothwell D, Sandison AT: Antiquity of diseases caused by bacteria and viruses. In: Brothwell D, Sandison AT (ed): Diseases in Antiquity: A Survey of the Diseases, Injuries and Surgery of Early Populations. Springfield, Illinois: Charles C Thomas, 1967, pp 122–124.
3. Gaworzewska E, Colman G: Changes in the patterns of infection caused by Streptococcus pyogenes. Epidemiol Infect 1988; 100: 257–269.
4. Kohler W, Gerlach D, Knoll H: Streptococcal outbreaks and erythrogenic toxin type A. Zentralbl Bakteriol Hyg 1987; 266: 104–115.
5. Veasy LG, Wiedmeier SE, Orsmond GS: Resurgence of acute rheumatic fever in the intermountain area of the United States. N Engl J Med 1986; 316: 421–427.
6. Stevens D: Streptococcal toxic shock syndrome: Spectrum of disease, pathogenesis and new concepts in treatment. Emerging Infect Dis 1995; 1: 69–78.
7. Lancefield RC: Current knowledge of type specific M antigens of Group A streptococci. J Immunol 1962; 89: 307–313.
8. Stevens DL: Group A streptococcal infections. In: Stern JH (ed): Internal Medicine. St. Louis, MO: Mosby, 1993, pp 2078–2087.
9. Hasty DL, Ofek I, Courtney HS, Doyle RJ: Minireview: Multiple adhesins of streptococci. Infect Immun 1992; 60: 2147–2152.
10. Fischetti VA: Streptococcal M protein. Sci Amer 1991; 264: 58–65.
11. Dale J, Chiang E: Intranasal immunization with recombinant group A streptococcal M protein fragment fused to the B subunit of Escherichia coli labile toxin protects mice against systemic challenge infections. J Infect Dis 1995; 171: 1038–1041.
12. Alouf JE, Geoffroy C: Structure activity relationships in sulfhydryl-

activated toxins. In: Freer JH, Jeljaszewicz J (ed): Bacterial Protein Toxins. London: Academic Press, 1984, pp 165–171.

13. Barsumian EL, Schlievert PM, Watson DW: Non-specific and specific immunological mitogenicity by group A streptococcal pyrogenic exotoxins. Infect Immun 1978; 22: 681–688.

14. Nida SK, Ferretti JJ: Phage influence on the synthesis of extracellular toxins in group A streptococci. Infect Immun 1982; 36: 745–750.

15. Hauser AR, Stevens DL, Kaplan EL, Schlievert PM: Molecular analysis of pyrogenic exotoxins from *Streptococcus pyogenes* isolates associated with toxic shock-like syndrome. J Clin Microbiol 1991; 29: 1562–1567.

16. Stevens DL, Tanner MH, Winship J, et al.: Reappearance of scarlet fever toxin A among streptococci in the Rocky Mountain West: Severe group A streptococcal infections associated with a toxic shock-like syndrome. N Engl J Med 1989; 321: 1–7.

17. Hallas G: The production of pyrogenic exotoxins by group A streptococci. J Hyg (Camb) 1985; 95: 47–57.

18. Iwasaki M, Igarashi H, Hinuma Y, Yutsudo T: Cloning, characterization and overexpression of a *Streptococcus pyogenes* gene encoding a new type of mitogenic factor. FEBS Lett 1993; 331: 187–192.

19. Norrby-Teglund A, Newton D, Kotb M, et al.: Superantigenic properties of the group A streptococcal exotoxin SpeF (MF). Infect Immun 1994; 62: 5227–5233.

20. Mollick JA, Miller GG, Musser JM, et al.: A novel superantigen isolated from pathogenic strains of *Streptococcus pyogenes* with amino-terminal homology to staphylococcal enterotoxins B and C. J Clin Invest 1993; 92: 710–719.

21. Cleary PP, Peterson J, Chen C, Nelson C: Virulent human strains of group G streptococci express a C5a peptidase enzyme similar to that produced by group A streptococci. Infect Immun 1991; 59: 2305–2310.

22. Stevens DL: Invasive group A streptococcus infections. Clin Infect Dis 1992; 14: 2–13.

23. Martin PR, Hoiby EA: Streptococcal serogroup A epidemic in Norway 1987–1988. Scand J Infect Dis 1990; 22: 421–429.

24. Cleary PP, Kaplan EL, Handley JP, et al.: Clonal basis for resurgence of serious *Streptococcus pyogenes* disease in the 1980s. Lancet 1992; 339: 518–521.

25. Musser JM, Hauser AR, Kim MH, et al.: *Streptococcus pyogenes* causing toxic-shock-like syndrome and other invasive diseases: Clonal diversity and pyrogenic exotoxin expression. Proc Natl Acad Sci U S A 1991; 88: 2668–2672.

26. Stevens DL, Tanner MH, Winship J, et al.: Group A streptococcal infections and a toxic shock-like syndrome. N Engl J Med 1989; 321: 2545–2546.

27. Caparon MG, Stephens DS, Olsen A, Scott JR: Role of M protein in adherence of group A streptococci. Infect Immun 1991; 59: 1811–1817.

28. Hanski E, Caparon M: Protein F, a fibronectin-binding protein, is an adhesin of the group A streptococcus *Streptococcus pyogenes*. Proc Natl Acad Sci U S A 1992; 89: 6172–6176.

29. Bryant AE, Kehoe MA, Stevens DL: Streptococcal pyrogenic exotoxin A and streptolysin O enhance PMNL binding to protein matrixes. J Infect Dis 1992; 166: 165–169.

30. Marrack P, Kappler JW: The staphylococcal enterotoxins and their relatives. Science 1990; 248: 705–711.

31. Kotb M, Ohnishi H, Majumdar G, et al.: Temporal relationship of cytokine release by peripheral blood mononuclear cells stimulated by the streptococcal superantigen pep M5. Infect Immun 1993; 61: 1194–1201.

32. Hackett SP, Stevens DL: Superantigens associated with staphylococcal and streptococcal toxic shock syndromes are potent inducers of tumor necrosis factor beta synthesis. J Infect Dis 1993; 168: 232–235.

33. Kappur V, Majesky MW, Li LL, et al.: Cleavage of Interleukin 1B (IL-1B) precursor to produce active 1L-1B by a conserved extracellular cysteine protease from *Streptococcus pyogenes*. Proc Natl Acad Sci U S A 1993; 90: 7676–7680.

34. Rotch TM: Pediatrics: The Hygienic and Medical Treatment of Children. Philadelphia: JB Lippincott, 1896.

35. Bernard P, Bedane C, Mounier M, et al.: Streptocococcal cause of erysipelas and cellulitis in adults. Arch Dermatol 1989; 125: 779–782.

36. Stevens DL: Soft tissue infections. In Isselbacher KJ, Braunwald E, Wilson JD, Martin JB, Fauci AS, Kasper DL (eds): Harrison's Principles of Internal Medicine. New York: McGraw–Hill, Inc., 1994, pp 561–563.

37. Duvanel T, Auckenthaler R, Rohner P, et al.: Quantitative cultures of biopsy specimens from cutaneous cellulitis. Arch Intern Med 1989; 149: 293–296.

38. The Working Group on Severe Streptococcal Infections: Defining the group A streptococcal toxic shock syndrome: Rationale and consensus definition. JAMA 1993; 269: 390–391.

39. Wannamaker LW, Rammelkamp CH Jr, Denny FW, et al.: Prophylaxis of acute rheumatic fever by treatment of the preceding streptococcal infection with various amounts of depot penicillin. Am J Med 1951; 10: 673–695.

40. Kim KS, Kaplan EL: Association of penicillin tolerance with failure to eradicate group A streptococci from patients with pharyngitis. J Pediatr 1985; 107: 681–684.

41. Gatanaduy AS, Kaplan EL, Huwe BB, et al.: Failure of penicillin to eradicate group A streptococci during an outbreak of pharyngitis. Lancet 1980; 2: 498–502.

42. Brook I: Role of beta-lactamase-producing bacteria in the failure of penicillin to eradicate group A streptococci. Pediatr Infect Dis 1985; 4: 491–495.

43. Adams EM, Gudmundsson S, Yocum DE, et al.: Streptococcal myositis. Arch Intern Med 1985; 145: 1020–1023.

44. Eagle H: Experimental approach to the problem of treatment failure with penicillin I: Group A streptococcal infection in mice. Am J Med 1952; 13: 389–399.

45. Stevens DL, Gibbons AE, Bergstrom R, Winn V: The Eagle effect revisited: Efficacy of clindamycin, erythromycin, and penicillin in the treatment of streptococcal myositis. J Infect Dis 1988; 158: 23–28.

46. Stevens DL, Bryant AE, Yan S: Invasive group A streptococcal infection: New concepts in antibiotic treatment. Int J Antimicrob Agents 1994; 4: 297–301.

47. Stevens DL, Yan S, Bryant AE: Penicillin binding protein expression at different growth stages determines penicillin efficacy in vitro and in vivo: An explanation for the inoculum effect. J Infect Dis 1993; 167: 1401–1405.

48. Yan S, Mendelman PM, Stevens DL: The in vitro antibacterial activity of ceftriaxone against *Streptococcus pyogenes* is unrelated to penicillin-binding protein 4. FEMS Microbiol Lett 1993; 110: 313–318.

49. Yan S, Bohach GA, Stevens DL: Persistant acylation of high-molecular weight penicillin binding proteins by penicillin induces the post antibiotic effect in *Streptococcus pyogenes*. J Infect Dis 1994; 170: 609–614.

50. Stevens DL, Maier KA, Mitten JE: Effect of antibiotics on toxin production and viability of *Clostridium perfringens*. Antimicrob Agents Chemother 1987; 31: 213–218.

51. Gemmell CG, Peterson PK, Schmeling D, et al.: Potentiation of opsonization and phagocytosis of *Streptococcus pyogenes* following growth in the presence of clindamycin. J Clin Invest 1981; 67: 1249–1256.

52. Stevens DL, Bryant AE, Hackett SP: Antibiotic effects on bacterial viability, toxin production, and host response. Clin Infect Dis 1995; 20: S154–S157.

53. Barry W, Hudgins L, Donta S, Pesanti E: Intravenous immunoglobulin therapy for toxic shock syndrome. JAMA 1992; 267: 3315–3316.

54. Yong JM: Letter. Lancet 1994; 343: 1427.

55. Norby-Teglund A, Kaul R, Low DE, McGeer A, Kotb M: Intravenous immunoglobulin and superantigen-neutralizing activity in streptococcal toxic shock syndrome patients [abstract]. 35th Annual Interscience Conference on Antimicrobial Agents and Chemotherapy (ICAAC), San Francisco, Sept. 1995.

56. Kaul R, McGeer A, Norby-Teglund A, et al.: Intravenous immunoglobulin therapy in streptococcal toxic shock syndrome: Results of a matched case-controlled study [abstract]. 35th Annual Interscience Conference on Antimicrobial Agents and Chemotherapy (ICAAC), San Francisco, Sept. 1995.

Ian R. Friedland
George H. McCracken

CHAPTER SIXTEEN

Streptococci Including *S. pneumoniae*

▼

STREPTOCOCCAL SPECIES IN ORAL FLORA

There are more than 25 species of streptococci, most of which populate the mouth and nasopharyngeal passages. *Streptococcus pneumoniae* and group A *Streptococcus* (*Streptococcus pyogenes*) are the two most important streptococcal species responsible for ear, nose, and throat (ENT) infections. Most other streptococci form part of the normal oral flora but are seldom responsible for ENT infections. The classification of streptococci is complex and is based on the type of hemolysis produced on blood agar, the antigenic composition of the cell wall, growth and biochemical characteristics, and, most recently, genetic traits. A simplified classification of streptococci and their usual sites of colonization is shown in Table 16–1.

STREPTOCOCCUS PNEUMONIAE

History

The pneumococcus was discovered concurrently in 1881 by Pasteur and Sternberg and was soon recognized as a major cause of lobar pneumonia.[1] It was previously termed *Diplococcus pneumoniae* because of its appearance on Gram staining but was classified with the streptococci in 1974. Soon after the discovery of the pneumococcus, it was found that (1) serum from infected patients afforded protection in models of pneumococcal infection and (2) there were several types of pneumococci[2] to which specific serologic responses developed. In the 1920s, the polysaccharide capsule of the pneumococcus was found to be responsible for the type-specific immunologic response.[3] Vaccines based on capsular serotypes were soon produced and found to be immunogenic and protective in humans.[4]

Microbiology

Pneumococci, like all streptococci, are gram-positive cocci that grow in chains. Pneumococci produce a hemolysin, resulting in green discoloration around colonies on blood agar (termed alpha hemolysis). In gram-stained smears of clinical specimens, the characteristic extracellular encapsulated diplococci can be seen. *S. pneumoniae* is distinguished from other alpha-hemolytic streptococci by its susceptibility to optochin (although optochin-resistant strains have been described)[5] and by its solubility in bile.

Knowledge of the structure of the pneumococcus (Fig. 16–1) is vital to the understanding of the pathogenesis of pneumococcal disease. The outermost structure is the polysaccharide capsule, which is anchored to the underlying cell wall. Except for occasional conjunctival isolates, all pneumococcal strains obtained from clinical specimens are encapsulated. Currently, more than 80 different capsular types are recognized, and the prevalence of particular serotypes varies from country to country. The Danish numbering system is the most widely used method of classifying pneumococcal capsular serotypes into antigenically related groups. Some serogroups that commonly infect adults, such as serogroups 3, 1, and 7, are uncommon in children, in whom serogroups 6, 14, 19F, and 23F usually predominate. Serotyping is a useful epidemiologic tool but is generally not clinically important.

Beneath the capsule is the cell wall, which consists of interlinking molecules of peptidoglycan and teichoic acid. In the cell wall are peptidases responsible for the cross-linking and subsequent elongation of the peptidoglycan chain. These enzymes are inhibited by penicillin (and other beta-lactam antibiotics) and are thus termed penicillin-binding proteins (PBPs). Pneumococci produce an autolysin, an enzyme that disrupts the integrity of the cell wall. Autolysis may render pneumococci that have been growing for more than 18–24 hours nonviable. This is sometimes a problem in older blood culture systems that are read only once daily.

Epidemiology and Antimicrobial Resistance

Pneumococci are human pathogens and are ubiquitous in both temperate and tropical environments. Exposure occurs early in life, and pneumococcal disease is most prevalent in the first 2 years of life, a time when the immunologic response to pneumococcal polysaccharide is especially poor. Factors predisposing to pneumococcal disease include the extremes of age, crowding (including daycare centers as well as nursing, military, and correctional institutions), alcoholism, cigarette smoking, sickle cell disease (and other causes of splenic dysfunction), nephrotic syndrome, immunodeficiencies (especially agammaglobulinemia, disorders of complement, and human immunodeficiency virus [HIV] infection), and preceding viral infections, especially influenza.[6–11] The incidence of pneumococcal disease is especially high in Native American populations.[7, 12] Pneumococcal infections are generally more prevalent in winter.[13, 14]

Table 16–1. CLASSIFICATION OF MEDICALLY IMPORTANT STREPTOCOCCI ACCORDING TO TYPE OF HEMOLYSIS AND LANCEFIELD GROUP[1]

Hemolysis	Group or Species	Subspecies	Sites of Colonization
Beta (clear hemolysis)	*S. pyogenes* (Group A)		Pharynx, skin
	S. agalactiae (Group B)		Genital tract, lower GI tract
Gamma (nonhemolytic)	Group D	*S. bovis*	GI tract
		Enterococcus faecalis, Enterococcus faecium	GI tract
Alpha (green hemolysis)	Viridans streptococci	*S. mitis, S. mutans, S. sanguis, S. salivarius, S. intermedius*	Oropharynx, teeth, GI tract
	S. pneumoniae		Nasopharynx

[1]GI = gastrointestinal; *S.* = *Streptococcus*.

Pneumococcal resistance to penicillin was first recognized as a clinical problem in South African children in the late 1970s.[15, 16] Subsequently, penicillin-resistant pneumococci have been recognized worldwide and are particularly prevalent in Spain, France, Eastern Europe, Israel, parts of Asia, South Africa, and parts of the United States. Penicillin-resistant pneumococci are much more common in children than adults and have emerged as important causes of treatment failure in children with otitis media in parts of the United States.[17–19] Resistance to penicillin results from alteration of one or more penicillin-binding proteins; the greater the number of changes in the PBPs, the higher the level of resistance to both penicillin and the cephalosporins.

Pneumococcal resistance to other antibiotics, particularly erythromycin and trimethoprim/sulfamethoxazole (TMP/SMX), has also increased in areas where penicillin resistance is prevalent. Resistance to the latter two agents and to the cephalosporins frequently coexists in highly penicillin-resistant strains, severely limiting the number of effective oral antimicrobial agents.

Colonization

The success of the pneumococcus as a pathogen is related to its ability to colonize the human upper respiratory tract. Pneumococci adhere to mucosal epithelium by binding to the cell-surface glycolipids.[20] The highest concentrations of pneumococci are found in the nasopharynx, where colonization rates in young children frequently exceed 40%. On average, 20%–40% of adults are colonized at any time. Individuals may carry more than one different serotype.[21]

In daycare center settings, a single clone can spread and become the predominant colonizing strain,[22] or multiple clones can be present, each clone usually being confined to

a specific area or room within the center. Development of resistance occurs through transfer of genetic material from taxonomically related streptococci residing in the nasopharynx and is independent of antibiotic pressure. Antibiotic exposure, however, favors the selection of antibiotic-resistant strains, which can spread, resulting in disease in some patients.[17, 23] For example, in a daycare center in Kentucky, more than 50% of nasopharyngeal isolates were penicillin-resistant, of which most were highly penicillin-resistant and half were multidrug resistant.[18]

Virulence, Pathogenesis, and Host Defense

The pathogenesis of pneumococcal disease is the result of a complex interaction between the organism and the host. Infections of the ENT are a result of direct invasion, and local defense mechanisms are important in preventing or limiting such infections.

Abnormalities of host defenses may predispose to severe or recurrent infections of the upper respiratory tract. These include alterations in local defenses (cleft palate or uvula, patulous eustachian tube, abnormal cilia function) and systemic immunity (e.g., immunoglobulin deficiencies). Defense mechanisms protecting against blood stream or deep tissue invasion have been reviewed.[24]

The cell wall is probably the most important part of the pneumococcus responsible for inflammatory damage in acute otitis media.[25, 26] Penicillin therapy results in lysis of the cell wall and release of cell-wall fragments (especially peptidoglycan), which are proinflammatory, thereby initially enhancing the inflammatory cascade in the middle ear induced by the pneumococcus.[27] The inflammatory reaction is enhanced if cell-wall fragments contain teichoic acid. Teichoic acid contains phosphorylcholine, which is also a critical moiety

Figure 16–1. Schematic representation of the outer structures of *Streptococcus pneumoniae*.

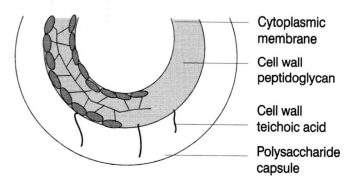

Cytoplasmic membrane

Cell wall peptidoglycan

Cell wall teichoic acid

Polysaccharide capsule

of platelet-activating factor, a cytokine that plays an important role in the inflammatory cascade.[28] The increased inflammation after antibiotic therapy appears to be more important early in the course of middle ear infection and is not observed once high bacterial concentrations develop.[29]

Pneumococci produce a number of polypeptide toxins. Pneumolysin is an intracellular toxin that is released only following lysis of the bacterial cell wall.[30] Pneumolysin has deleterious effects on leukocytes, platelets, respiratory epithelium, the hair cells of the cochlea, and other cells and tissues[31, 32, 33] and is thought to be important in the pathogenesis of pneumococcal pneumonia.[34] Pneumolysin may induce inflammation by stimulating the release of tumor necrosis factor and interleukin-1 from monocytes.[35] Another enzyme produced by pneumococci is neuraminidase, an enzyme that damages the glycoprotein and glycolipid components of the mammalian cell-wall membrane. The pathogenetic role of pneumolysin, neuraminidase, and other pneumococcal toxins, including autolysin, is currently unclear. Pneumococci also produce proteases that destroy secretory immunoglobulin A (IgA) and other immunoglobulins, facilitating long periods of colonization.

Clinical Manifestations

S. pneumoniae is the most important bacterial cause of acute otitis media and acute sinusitis in all age groups. In children, pneumococci can be isolated from the middle ear in 30%–40% of cases of acute otitis media, and pneumococcal antigens can be detected from one third of sterile middle ear fluid specimens.[36–38] Similarly, *S. pneumoniae* can be isolated by sinus aspiration from 25%–36% of both children and adults with acute sinusitis.[39–42] Although isolated less frequently, pneumococci are also important causes of chronic otitis media.[43]

In addition to their role in upper respiratory diseases, pneumococci are currently among the most common bacterial causes of pneumonia, meningitis, and bacteremia, especially in children.

Diagnosis

Pneumococcal otitis media or sinusitis is clinically indistinguishable from that caused by other organisms, and a specific diagnosis can be made only by isolation of the organism from middle ear or sinus aspirates. Because this requirement involves invasive procedures, such as tympanocentesis and sinus needle aspiration, the causative organisms of otitis media or sinusitis are seldom identified in routine management. Pneumococcal strains isolated from the nasopharynx do not reliably predict the organism isolated from middle ear or sinus aspirates but may be of value in epidemiologic surveys of antimicrobial resistance patterns. Serologic methods for diagnosis of pneumococcal disease are not widely available and are seldom helpful in management.

Because of the spread of resistance to many parts of the world (including most of the United States), antimicrobial susceptibility testing should be routine where *S. pneumoniae* has been isolated. The determination of susceptibility to

penicillin is a minimum; susceptibility testing for other agents should be determined by therapeutic options being considered. The identification of penicillin resistance should alert the clinician to the possiblity of resistance to other agents, especially the oral cephalosporins (discussed in more detail later).

Treatment

Penicillin or amoxicillin is the antibiotic of choice for penicillin-susceptible pneumococcal infections. The oral cephalosporins, macrolides (including erythromycin, clarithromycin, and azithromycin), trimethoprim-sulfamethoxazole (TMP/SMX), and erythromycin-sulfamethoxazole are also active against most penicillin-susceptible pneumococci.

Because penicillin resistance among pneumococcal strains has become a problem in many parts of the world, beta-lactam therapy for otitis media or sinusitis may not be reliable. Pneumococcal resistance is subdivided according to the minimal inhibitory concentration (MIC) of penicillin; intermediate resistance is defined by MICs of $>0.06–1$ μg/mL, whereas strains with MICs ≥ 2 μg/mL are regarded as highly resistant. Ampicillin and amoxicillin have activity similar to that of penicillin; the definitions for penicillin resistance are thus relevant for these agents. The distinction between intermediate and high levels of resistance is important, because strains of intermediate resistance usually respond to oral amoxicillin or intravenous penicillin therapy.[44] Limited data available suggest that highly resistant strains also frequently respond to amoxicillin therapy, especially if large dosages (70–80 mg/kg/day) are used. However, treatment failures associated with highly resistant pneumococcal strains have become a problem in areas with a high prevalence of such strains. Because all beta-lactam antibiotics bind to penicillin-binding proteins, pneumococcal strains with decreased susceptibility to penicillin have roughly proportional decreases in susceptibility to the cephalosporins. The cephalosporins can be divided into three groups according to their activity against penicillin-resistant pneumococci (Table 16–2).[45, 46] Because all the currently available oral cephalosporins are less active than amoxicillin, failure

Table 16–2. COMPARATIVE IN VITRO ACTIVITY FOR CEPHALOSPORINS, RELATIVE TO PENICILLIN, AGAINST PENICILLIN-RESISTANT PNEUMOCOCCI

Greater Activity[1]	Similar or Slightly Reduced Activity[2]	Poor Activity[3]
Ceftriaxone	Cefuroxime	Cephalexin
Cefotaxime	Cefpodoxime	Cefaclor
		Cefixime
		Ceftibuten
		Cefprozil
		Loracarbef
		Ceftazidime

[1]These agents are likely to retain useful activity against penicillin-resistant pneumococci.

[2]These agents are likely to be effective for intermediately penicillin-resistant pneumococcal infections but not for many highly resistant infections.

[3]These agents are poorly active against even intermediately penicillin-resistant infections and should be avoided in areas with a high prevalence of penicillin-resistant pneumococci.

of amoxicillin therapy in pneumococcal infections necessitates a change to a non–beta-lactam oral antimicrobial agent or a parenteral cephalosporin, such as ceftriaxone. The addition of clavulanate to amoxicillin does not improve activity against pneumococci because pneumococci do not produce beta-lactamase.

Penicillin-resistant infections may be treated with non–beta-lactam antibiotics, such as a macrolide or TMP-SMX. However, resistance to these agents frequently coexists in penicillin-resistant pneumococci and can involve more than 40% of penicillin-resistant isolates in some geographical areas.[18, 46, 47] Clindamycin remains active against most penicillin-resistant pneumococci in the United States,[48] but resistance is a problem in some parts of Europe. Vancomycin, cefotaxime, ceftriaxone, and imipenem are recommended for serious highly penicillin-resistant pneumococcal infections[49] but are rarely necessary for treatment of upper respiratory infections. A possible exception is daily ceftriaxone therapy, which can be administered intramuscularly (for 3–5 days) as outpatient therapy. Although one dose of ceftriaxone has been shown to be effective for acute otitis media in children,[50] the efficacy of this therapy in otitis media due to penicillin-resistant pneumococci (with associated reduced cephalosporin susceptibility) is unknown. The current definition for resistance to ceftriaxone or cefotaxime is specific for meningitis and is unlikely to be relevant in treating respiratory infections.

Recommendations for therapy of pneumococcal upper respiratory tract infections are summarized in Table 16–3. Even in areas where penicillin-resistant pneumococci are common, amoxicillin remains a suitable choice for empirical therapy of acute otitis media or sinusitis, because (1) it is effective against many resistant pneumococcal strains, (2) it is inexpensive, and (3) acute otitis media has a high natural recovery rate. However, in cases not improving with amoxicillin therapy, the possibility that the infection is caused by a resistant pneumococcus should be considered. Because of the unpredictable antimicrobial susceptibility patterns of penicillin-resistant pneumococci, tympanocentesis and isolation of the causative organism should be considered in poorly responsive cases of otitis media in areas where such strains are prevalent.

For the penicillin-allergic patient, the macrolides, cephalosporins, clindamycin, and TMP/SMX are suitable alternatives to amoxicillin therapy. However, as described previously, resistance to these agents is a problem in some

areas. In addition, erythromycin and clindamycin alone are unsuitable for the empirical therapy of otitis media or sinusitis, because they have limited activity against *Haemophilus*, an important cause of these infections.

Prevention

Prophylactic oral penicillin has proved effective in reducing the incidence of overwhelming pneumococcal infections in children with sickle cell disease, for whom such therapy is currently recommended.[51] Determination of when to discontinue penicillin prophylaxis in such children has not been studied, but in most instances, prophylaxis is continued throughout early childhood, and polyvalent pneumococcal vaccine is also given. Selection of penicillin-resistant strains has occasionally occurred as a result of prolonged prophylactic administration of penicillin to children with sickle cell disease.

Passive immunization with intramuscular or intravenous immunoglobulin preparations is recommended in patients with congenital or acquired immunodeficiencies. Monthly intravenous immunoglobulin therapy is effective in preventing pneumococcal sepsis in children with symptomatic HIV infection. Chemoprophylaxis with trimethoprim-sulfamethoxazole is similarly effective, and intravenous immunoglobulin therapy offers no additional benefit in HIV-infected children receiving trimethoprim-sulfamethoxazole chemoprophylaxis for *Pneumocystis* pneumonia.

Active immunization can be achieved with the currently available pneumococcal polysaccharide vaccine. This vaccine contains antigens from 23 pneumococcal serotypes, which cause approximately 90% of pneumococcal infections in adults and 85% of cases of pneumococcal otitis media in children. As with other polysaccharide vaccines, the 23-valent pneumococcal vaccine is poorly immunogenic in children less than 2 years of age, the age group in which pneumococcal infections are most common. The vaccine is recommended in children 2 years and older with sickle cell disease, asplenia, nephrotic syndrome, cerebrospinal fluid (CSF) leaks, and symptomatic HIV infection and in those receiving immunosuppressive therapy.[52] It is recommended for adults with chronic lung disease, advanced cardiac disease, diabetes mellitus, alcoholism, chronic renal failure, cirrhosis, and CSF leaks and those older than 65 years of age.[53] The vaccine should also be considered for adults with

Table 16–3. RECOMMENDED THERAPY FOR PNEUMOCOCCAL UPPER RESPIRATORY TRACT INFECTIONS ACCORDING TO PENICILLIN SUSCEPTIBILITY[1]

Penicillin-Susceptible (MIC ≤ 0.06 μg/mL)		Intermediately Penicillin-Resistant (MIC > 0.06–1.0 μg/mL)		Highly Penicillin-Resistant (MIC > 2 μg/mL)	
Agent of Choice	**Alternatives**	**Agent of Choice**	**Alternatives[2]**	**Agents of Choice**	**Alternatives**
Amoxicillin	Trimethoprim-sulfamethoxazole (TMP/SMX), oral cephalosporin, macrolide, erythromycin-SMX, amoxicillin-clavulanate[4]	Amoxicillin	TMP/SMX, macrolide, cefuroxime, cefpodoxime, amoxicillin-clavulanate[4]	Amoxicillin[3], clindamycin, ceftriaxone	Depends on susceptibility

[1]MIC = minimum inhibitory concentration.
[2]Resistance to the agents listed frequently coexists in penicillin-resistant pneumococci.
[3]High dosage recommended, e.g., 70–80 mg/kg/day for children.
[4]The addition of clavulanate does not improve the activity of amoxicillin for pneumococci.

immunodeficiency secondary to HIV infection, asplenia, malignancies such as lymphoma, and organ transplantation. Revaccination every 3–7 years is recommended for patients at especially high risk, such as those with anatomic or functional asplenia and those over 65 years of age.

Protein conjugated pneumococcal vaccines similar to the conjugate *Haemophilus* vaccines are currently under evaluation in children less than 2 years of age. Unlike the *Haemophilus* conjugate vaccines, which contain only type b polysaccharide, pneumococcal conjugate vaccines need to contain polysaccharide from multiple serotypes. The actual number of serotypes that can be included is limited because of the large volume required.

VIRIDANS STREPTOCOCCI

A number of streptococcal species produce partial or green hemolysis (alpha hemolysis). Once such strains have been differentiated from pneumococci (by the optochin disk or bile solubility tests), they are referred to as viridans or alpha-hemolytic streptococci (see Table 16–1). Some laboratories may report the actual species, but this is seldom necessary, as these organisms produce similar clinical diseases. The one group that deserves special mention is the *Streptococcus anginosus* (*Streptococcus milleri*) group of organisms. These bacteria have a propensity to abscess formation; bacteremia with these organisms may herald an inapparent deep tissue abscess.[54]

The usual habitats of the viridans streptococci are the oropharynx and the digestive tract. They are found in high concentrations on the gums and teeth surfaces and constitute roughly half of the oral bacterial flora. They are of low virulence but contribute to dental caries, especially *Streptococcus mutans*. The only serious disease commonly associated with viridans streptococci is infective endocarditis. Patients with underlying cardiac disease should receive chemoprophylaxis when undergoing procedures involving trauma to the oral cavity or teeth. Immunocompromised hosts with mucositis resulting from chemotherapy may develop bacteremia and sepsis with viridans streptococci. The viridans streptococci may be isolated from sites with mixed infection, such as abscesses, but with the exception of *S. anginosis,* are unlikely to be the primary pathogen.

The viridans streptococci are usually highly susceptible to penicillin. However, it is important to test for susceptibility to penicillin, because resistance is a problem in some areas.[55, 56] Penicillin-resistant infections can be treated with clindamycin or vancomycin.

OTHER STREPTOCOCCI

Group D streptococci, *Streptococcus bovis* and *Streptococcus equinus,* are usually nonhemolytic but occasionally produce alpha or beta hemolysis. They are found in small numbers in the mouth but increase in number along the alimentary canal and are present in large concentrations in the feces. They are not important pathogens in ENT infections but may be found in mixed infections such as abscesses. Group

D streptococci are generally susceptible to penicillin, which is the antibiotic of choice.

Group B streptococci (*Streptococcus agalactiae*) produce beta hemolysis and are important genitourinary and neonatal pathogens. They are seldom isolated from the nasopharynx. They are not recognized ENT pathogens but have been described as a cause of epiglottic abscess[57] and occasionally of pharyngitis in adolescent patients.

References

1. Watson DA, Musher DM, Jacobson JW: A brief history of the pneumococcus in biomedical research: A panoply of discovery. Clin Infect Dis 1993; 17: 913–924.
2. Dochez AR, Gillespie LJ: A biologic classification of pneumococci by means of immunity reactions. JAMA 1913; 61: 727–730.
3. Heidelberger M, Goebel WF, Avery OT: The soluble specific substance of pneumococcus. J Exp Med 1925; 42: 727–745.
4. Smillie WG, Wornock GH, White HJ: A study of a type I pneumococcus epidemic at the state hospital at Worcester, Mass. Am J Publ Health 1938; 28: 293–302.
5. Muñoz R, Fenoll A, Vicioso D, et al.: Optochin-resistant variants of *Streptococcus pneumoniae.* Diagn Microbiol Infect Dis 1990; 13: 63–66.
6. Cherian T, Steinhoff MC, Harrison LH, et al.: A cluster of invasive pneumococcal disease in young children in child care. JAMA 1994; 271: 695–697.
7. Davidson M, Parkinson AJ, Bulkow LR, et al.: The epidemiology of invasive pneumococcal disease in Alaska, 1986–1990: Ethnic differences and opportunities for prevention. J Infect Dis 1994; 170: 368–376.
8. Broome CV, Facklam RR: Epidemiology of clinically significant isolates of *Streptococcus pneumoniae* in the United States. Rev Infect Dis 1981; 3: 277–280.
9. Bruyn GAW, van der Meer JWM, Hermans J, et al.: Pneumococcal bacteremia in adults over a 10-year period at University Hospital, Leiden. Rev Infect Dis 1988; 10: 446–450.
10. Breiman RF, Spika JS, Navarro, et al.: Pneumococcal bacteremia in Charleston County, South Carolina: A decade later. Arch Intern Med 1990; 150: 1401–1405.
11. Burman LA, Norrby R, Trollfors B: Invasive pneumococcal infections: Incidence, predisposing factors, and prognosis. Rev Infect Dis 1985; 7: 133–142.
12. Cortese MM, Wolff M, Almeido-Hill L, et al.: High incidence rates of invasive pneumococcal diseases in the White Mountain Apache population. Arch Intern Med 1992; 152: 2277–2282.
13. Eskola J, Takala AK, Kela E, et al.: Epidemiology of invasive pneumococcal infections in children in Finland. JAMA 1992; 268: 3323–3327.
14. Gray BM, Converse GM, Dillon HC Jr: Serotypes of *Streptococcus pneumoniae* causing disease. J Infect Dis 1979; 140: 979–983.
15. Appelbaum PC, Bhamjee A, Scragg JN, et al.: *Streptococcus pneumoniae* resistant to penicillin and chloramphenicol. Lancet 1977; 2: 995–997.
16. Jacobs MR, Koornhof HJ, Robins-Browne RM, et al.: Emergence of multiple resistant pneumococci. N Engl J Med 1978; 299: 735–740.
17. Morbidity and Mortality Weekly Report: Drug-resistant *Streptococcus pneumoniae*—Kentucky and Tennessee, 1993. MMWR 1994; 43: 23–25.
18. Duchin JS, Breiman RF, Diamond A, et al.: High prevalence of multi-drug-resistant *Streptococcus pneumoniae* among children in a rural Kentucky community. Pediatr Infect Dis J 1995; 14: 745–750.
19. Block SL, Harrison CJ, Hedrick JA, et al.: Penicillin-resistant *Streptococcus pneumoniae* in acute otitis media: Risk factors, susceptibility patterns and antimicrobial management. Pediatr Infect Dis J 1995; 14: 751–759.
20. Andersson B, Dahmen T, Frejd T, et al.: Identification of an active disaccharide unit of a glycoconjugate receptor for pneumococci attaching to human pharyngeal epithelial cells. J Exp Med 1983; 158: 559–570.
21. Austrian R: Some aspects of the pneumococcal carrier state. Antimicrob Chemother 1968; 18 (suppl A): S35–S45.

22. Cherian T, Steinhoff MC, Harrison LH, et al.: A cluster of invasive pneumococcal disease in young children in child care. JAMA 1994; 271: 695–697.

23. Reichler MR, Allphin AA, Breiman RF, et al.: The spread of multiply resistant *Streptococcus pneumoniae* at a day care center in Ohio. J Infect Dis 1992; 166: 1346–1353.

24. Bruyn GAW, Zegers BJM, van Furth R: Mechanisms of host defense against infection with *Streptococcus pneumoniae*. Clin Infect Dis 1992; 14: 251–262.

25. Carlsen BD, Kawana M, Kawana C, et al.: Role of the bacterial cell wall in middle ear inflammation caused by *Streptococcus pneumoniae*. Infect Immun 1992; 60: 2850–2854.

26. Ripley-Petzold ML, Giebink GS, Juhn SK, et al.: The contribution of the pneumococcal cell wall to the pathogenesis of experimental otitis media. J Infect Dis 1988; 157: 245–255.

27. Kawana M, Kawana C, Giebink GS: Penicillin treatment accelerates middle ear inflammation in experimental otitis media. Infect Immun 1992; 60: 1908–1912.

28. Tuomanen EI, Austrian R, Masure HR: Pathogenesis of pneumococcal infection. N Engl J Med 1995; 332: 1280–1284.

29. Sato K, Quartey MK, Liebeler CL, et al.: Timing of penicillin treatment influences the course of *Streptococcus pneumoniae*–induced middle ear inflammation. Antimicrob Agents Chemother 1995; 39: 1896–1898.

30. Johnson KK: Cellular location of pneumolysin. FEMS Microbiol Lett 1987; 2: 243–245.

31. Johnson MK, Boes-Marrazzo D, Rierce WA: Effects of pneumolysin on human polymorphonuclear leukocytes and platelets. Infect Immun 1981; 34: 171–176.

32. Comis SD, Osborne MP, Stephen J, et al.: Cytotoxic effects on hair cells of guinea pig cochlea produced by pneumolysin, the thiol activated toxin of *Streptococcus pneumoniae*. Acta Otolaryngol 1993; 113: 152–159.

33. Paton JC, Andrew PW, Boulnois GJ, Mitchell TJ: Molecular analysis of the pathogenicity of *Streptococcus pneumoniae:* The role of pneumococcal proteins. Annu Rev Microbiol 1993; 47: 89–115.

34. Feldman C, Munro NC, Jeffery PK, et al.: Pneumolysin induces the salient histologic features of pneumococcal infection in the rat lung in vivo. Am J Respir Cell Mol Biol 1991; 5: 416–423.

35. Houldsworth S, Andrew PW, Mitchell TJ: Pneumolysin stimulates production of tumor necrosis factor alpha and interleukin-1 beta by human mononuclear phagocytes. Infect Immun 1994; 62: 1501.

36. Bluestone CD, Stephenson JS, Martin LM: Ten-year review of otitis media pathogens. Pediatr Infect Dis J 1992; 11: S7–S11.

37. Giebink GS: The microbiology of otitis media. Pediatr Infect Dis J 1989; 8: S18–S20.

38. Del Baccaro MA, Mendelman PM, Inglis AF, et al.: Bacteriology of acute otitis media: A new perspective. J Pediatr 1992; 120: 81–84.

39. Wald ER: Sinusitis in children. N Engl J Med 1992; 326: 319–323.

40. Gwaltney JM Jr, Scheld WM, Sande MA, et al.: The microbial etiology and antimicrobial therapy of adults with acute community-acquired sinusitis: A fifteen-year experience at the University of Virginia and review of other selected series. J Allergy Clin Immunol 1992; 90: 457–462.

41. Hamory BH, Sande MA, Sydnor A Jr, et al.: Etiology and antimicrobial therapy of acute maxillary sinusitis. J Infect Dis 1979; 139: 197–202.

42. Giebink GS: Childhood sinusitis: Pathophysiology, diagnosis and treatment. Pediatr Infect Dis J 1994; 13: S55–S58.

43. Giebink GS, Juhn SK, Weber ML, et al.: The bacteriology and cytology of chronic otitis media with effusion. Pediatr Infect Dis J 1982; 1: 98–103.

44. Friedland IR, McCracken GH: Management of infections caused by *Streptococcus pneumoniae*. N Engl J Med 1994; 331: 377–382.

45. Thornsberry C, Brown SD, Cheung Yee Y, et al.: Increasing penicillin resistance in *Streptococcus pneumoniae* in the USA: Effect on susceptibility to oral cephalosporins. Infect Med 1993; 10 (suppl D): 14–23.

46. Baquero F, Loza E: Antibiotic resistance of microorganisms involved in ear, nose and throat infections. Pediatr Infect Dis J 1994; 13: S9–S14.

47. Appelbaum PC: Antimicrobial resistance in *Streptococcus pneumoniae:* An overview. Clin Infect Dis 1992; 15: 77–83.

48. Nelson CT, Mason EO, Kaplan SL: Activity of oral antibiotics in middle ear and sinus infections caused by penicillin-resistant *Streptococcus pneumoniae:* Implications for treatment. Pediatr Infect Dis J 1994; 13: 585–589.

49. Friedland IR: Treatment of pneumococcal infections in the era of increasing penicillin resistance. Curr Opin Infect Dis 1995; 8: 213–217.

50. Green SM, Rothrock SG: Single-dose intramuscular ceftriaxone for otitis media in children. Pediatrics 1993; 91: 23–29.

51. Wong WY, Overturf GD, Powars DR: Infection caused *Streptococcus pneumoniae* in children with sickle cell disease: Epidemiology, immunologic mechanisms, prophylaxis, and vaccination. Clin Infect Dis 1992; 14: 1124–1136.

52. American Academy of Pediatrics: Pneumococcal infections. In: Peter G (ed): 1994 Red Book: Report of the Committee on Infectious Diseases, 23rd ed. Elk Grove Village, Illinois: American Academy of Pediatrics; 1994, pp 371–375.

53. Advisory Committee on Immunization Practices, Centers for Disease Control and Prevention: Pneumococcal polysaccharide vaccine. MMWR 1989; 38: 64–74.

54. Gossling J: Occurrence and pathogenicity of the *Streptococcus milleri* group. Rev Infect Dis 1988; 10: 257–275.

55. Quinn JP, DiVincenzo CA, Luck A, et al.: Serious infections due to penicillin-resistant viridans streptococci with altered penicillin-binding proteins. J Infect Dis 1988; 157: 764–769.

56. Lewis MAO, Parkhurst CL, Douglas CWI, et al.: Prevalence of penicillin resistant bacteria in acute suppurative oral infection. J Antimicrob Chemother 1995; 35: 785–791.

57. Ridgeway NA, Perlman PE, Verghese A: Epiglottic abscess due to group B *Streptococcus*. Ann Otol Rhinol Laryngol 1984; 93: 277–278.

Enterococci

▼

Enterococci are facultatively anaerobic, gram-positive, catalase-negative cocci that occur in pairs or short chains.[1] For many years they were classified as streptococci. In 1937,[2] it was proposed that streptococci be divided into four groups, namely the pyogenic, viridans, lactic acid, and enterococcal groups. The enterococcal streptococci comprised organisms capable of growth at 10° C and 45° C, at pH 9.6, and in the presence of 6.5% salt. Enterococcal streptococci were also capable of hydrolyzing esculin in the presence of 40% bile, contained the enzyme pyrrolidonyl arylamidase, and reacted with antisera to streptococci of Lancefield group D.[1,2] However, during the 1980s, chemotaxonomic and nucleic acid hybridization studies indicated that there are sufficient differences between enterococci and true streptococci to merit classification of enterococci as a separate genus. The enterococci were thus assigned to the new genus *Enterococcus*, which currently comprises 19 species (Table 17–1).[1] In many laboratories, the majority of enterococcal isolates are either *Enterococcus faecalis* (85%–90%) or *Enterococcus faecium* (5%–10%), although there have been increasing numbers of reports of infection caused by *Enterococcus avium*, *Enterococcus casseliflavus*, *Enterococcus durans*, *Enterococcus gallinarum*, and *Enterococcus raffinosus*.[3] The other species in the genus have rarely, if ever, been found in clinical material, and are usually isolated from agricultural or veterinary sources.

CLINICAL FEATURES OF ENTEROCOCCAL INFECTION

Enterococci cause a range of diseases including bacteremia, endocarditis, urinary tract infection, and neonatal sepsis. They may also be found (often in association with other organisms) in intraabdominal and pelvic infections and infections of skin and soft tissues, such as those affecting burns, diabetic ulcers, or wounds. Although it may be difficult to assess the pathogenic role played by enterococci in mixed infections, treatment of such infections may sometimes be unsuccessful if the antimicrobial agents used fail to eradicate the enterococci.[3]

Among patients with enterococcal bacteremia, common sources of blood-borne organisms include infections of the urinary tract, the abdomen, or intravascular lines.[2,3] Recent studies suggest that the frequency of enterococcal endocarditis among patients with bacteremia varies depending on the clinical setting, with about 33% of patients with community-acquired bacteremia having endocarditis, as opposed to about 1% of patients with nosocomial enterococcal bacteremia.[3] Mortality among patients with enterococcal bacteremia is high, although it is unclear if this reflects the vascular dissemination of enterococci per se, or the presence of underlying disease, which is often noted in such patients.[4–6]

PATHOGENICITY OF ENTEROCOCCI

Although enterococci appear relatively less virulent than many other pathogenic bacteria, there is, nonetheless, increasing evidence that they exhibit phenotypic traits that facilitate their ability to produce infection.[7,8] In vitro studies have shown that enterococci produce surface adhesins that mediate adherence to intestinal, urinary tract, and heart cells, which may explain, at least in part, the ability of enterococci to colonize intestinal and urinary tract mucosal surfaces and the lining of the endocardium in cases of endocarditis. It is of particular interest to note that enterococci have been found to modulate their expression of surface adhesins depending on their growth conditions. For example, organisms grown in human serum showed an increased ability to adhere to heart cells, which correlated with the production of an adhesin containing D-lactose and L-fucose.[7,8] Furthermore, organisms grown in serum showed reduced interaction with polymorphonuclear leukocytes (PMNLs) in phagocytosis assays, suggesting a possible mechanism by which enterococci may evade the host's nonspecific defense mechanisms.

The acute inflammatory reaction, which can occur at sites of enterococcal infection, may result from the production of enterococcal factors that are chemotactic for PMNLs. Such factors include both sex pheromones and pheromone inhibitors that are secreted by *E. faecalis* to mediate the interstrain transfer of genetic material. Many strains of enterococci also produce a plasmid-encoded hemolysin (also referred to as a cytolysin), which is associated with increased severity of infection both in humans and in experimentally infected animals.[7,8] However, the fact that nonhemolytic enterococci can cause clinical infection indicates that hemolysin production is not a prerequisite for enterococcal pathogenicity.

Table 17–1. SPECIES OF THE GENUS *Enterococcus*

E. faecalis	E. hirae
E. faecium	E. malodoratus
E. avium	E. mundtii
E. casseliflavus	E. pseudoavium
E. cecorum	E. raffinosus
E. columbae	E. saccharolyticus
E. dispar	E. seriolicida
E. durans	E. solitarius
E. flavescens	E. sulfureus
E. gallinarum	

ENTEROCOCCI AS NOSOCOMIAL PATHOGENS

Although enterococci may occasionally cause infections in the community, their major significance lies in their role as nosocomial pathogens. Data from the National Nosocomial Infections Surveillance (NNIS) system organized by the Centers for Disease Control and Prevention (CDC) showed that between 1986 and 1989, enterococci were the second most common pathogen associated with nosocomial infections in the United States.[9] The increased isolation of enterococci from nosocomial infections appears to be part of a general shift toward an increasing role for gram-positive bacterial pathogens in the hospital setting.[10]

For many years nosocomial infections caused by enterococci were thought to be endogenous, involving the patient's own flora, particularly that of the intestinal tract.[2] However, investigations of clusters of nosocomial enterococcal infections using molecular methods to differentiate between strains have provided evidence of patient-to-patient transmission and, in some instances, of interhospital spread of strains.[11, 12] Further epidemiologic investigations will be needed to clarify the relative importance of endogenous and acquired infections in hospitalized patients.

ANTIMICROBIAL RESISTANCE IN ENTEROCOCCI

Intrinsic Resistance

Enterococci show intrinsic low-level resistance to a range of antimicrobial agents including aminoglycosides, beta-lactams, and lincosamides.[2, 3, 13] Although enterococci may appear sensitive to trimethoprim-sulfamethoxazole in vitro, this agent is of little therapeutic use, possibly because enterococci use exogenous sources of folic acid.[3] Low-level resistance to aminoglycosides appears to be due to low-level uptake of these agents, whereas reduced sensitivity to penicillins and resistance to cephalosporins is due to a reduction in the affinity of enterococcal penicillin-binding proteins.[2, 13] In addition to showing reduced sensitivity to the growth inhibitory activity of beta-lactams, almost all clinical isolates of enterococci show tolerance to the bactericidal activity of beta-lactams and glycopeptides.[2, 13] Interestingly, the tolerance of enterococci to beta-lactams may be a trait that has evolved after their clinical exposure to penicillin. Enterococci isolated from patients in the Solomon Islands who had never received antibiotics exhibited penicillin minimal inhibitory concentrations (MICs) comparable to those seen in enterococci isolated in the United States but were readily killed by concentrations of penicillin just above their MICs. However, exposure of these organisms to penicillin in vitro resulted in the development of tolerance, which persisted even when the organisms were subcultured in the absence of antibiotic.[13]

Acquired Resistance

In addition to the intrinsic low-level resistance to certain antimicrobial agents described above, some strains of enterococci have developed high-level resistance to aminoglycosides and/or penicillin and ampicillin. High-level resistance to aminoglycosides (which abrogates the synergy normally seen between aminoglycosides and cell wall–active agents) most commonly reflects the production of aminoglycoside-modifying enzymes. For example, high-level resistance to gentamicin is mediated by a bifunctional enzyme that has both 2″-phosphotransferase and 6′-acetyltransferase activity and is active against all currently available aminoglycosides except streptomycin. Unfortunately, high-level resistance to streptomycin mediated by an adenylyltransferase enzyme also occurs commonly in clinical isolates of enterococci. Enzymes may also occasionally be involved in resistance to beta-lactams, as some strains of enterococci have the ability to inactivate penicillin and ampicillin because of the production of beta-lactamase.[13] DNA hybridization studies have shown that the gene encoding beta-lactamase production in enterococci is highly homologous to a beta–lactamase-encoding gene found in *Staphylococcus aureus,* suggesting that beta-lactamase activity in enterococci may have arisen following intergeneric transfer of the relevant genetic determinant.

Enterococci have also shown remarkable propensity to acquire or develop resistance to a range of other agents including tetracyclines, macrolides, chloramphenicol, quinolones, and glycopeptides.[3, 13–15] Resistance to glycopeptides, which is of particular concern, was first documented in enterococci isolated in the United Kingdom and France in the late 1980s, but subsequently spread to other parts of the world including the United States, where it has increased in prevalence.[16] Data from the NNIS system showed a 20-fold increase in the proportion of nosocomial isolates of enterococci that were resistant to vancomycin between 1989 and 1993, with many isolates resistant to all available antimicrobial agents.[17]

The first reports of glycopeptide resistance in enterococci described isolates of *E. faecalis* and *E. faecium* that were characterized by high-level resistance to vancomycin (MICs >256 mg/L) and cross-resistance to teicoplanin.[16] Shortly thereafter, however, isolates were described that exhibited resistance to lower levels of vancomycin (MICs up to 128 mg/L) and remained sensitive to teicoplanin.[16] These two types of glycopeptide resistance were designated VanA and VanB respectively. Low-level resistance to vancomycin and sensitivity to teicoplanin was later also found in isolates of *E. casseliflavus, E. flavescens,* and *E. gallinarum.* However, in these species, the resistance to vancomycin (designated VanC) appears to be an intrinsic rather than an acquired trait, as it has been noted in almost all strains tested to date. Molecular studies have shown that all three types of glycopeptide resistance have a similar mechanism involving biochemical modification of the D-alanine–D-alanine component of cell wall peptidoglycan, which constitutes the vancomycin-binding site.[18]

THERAPY AND CONTROL OF ENTEROCOCCAL INFECTIONS

Although many cases of enterococcal infection are still amenable to treatment with antibiotics, the widespread occurrence of resistance makes it essential that therapy of individual patients be guided by laboratory results of sensitivity testing. As enterococci exhibit diverse patterns of multiresistance, it is clearly important that the antibiotics to which individual isolates are sensitive be identified and their suitability for use in particular clinical settings be evaluated.

Many infections caused by enterococci may be treated successfully with bacteriostatic agents, provided the patient's immune system is functioning adequately and the infecting strain is sensitive to the agent being used. For example, urinary tract or intraabdominal infections may be treated with penicillin or ampicillin alone, whereas in patients allergic to beta-lactams, vancomycin may be used. Other therapeutic options for the treatment of urinary tract infections include nitrofurantoin and fluoroquinolones, although relapses have been noted with the latter agents, particularly in infections involving relatively resistant organisms.[3]

Cases of enterococcal bacteremia may also be treated with bacteriostatic agents alone, although there is some evidence that combination therapy may be more effective.[3] In patients with endocarditis a combination of a cell wall–active agent such as a beta-lactam or glycopeptide together with an aminoglycoside should be considered, as historically such a combination of agents has exhibited synergistic bactericidal activity. The effectiveness of such combination therapy has been compromised, however, by the emergence of high-level aminoglycoside resistance, which abolishes the synergy seen between aminoglycosides and cell wall–active agents.[2, 3, 13] For this reason, when combination therapy is being considered, isolates should be screened for high-level aminoglycoside resistance, using either high-content disks or breakpoint plates containing aminoglycosides at a concentration of 2000 mg/L.[2] The screening procedure should include both gentamicin and streptomycin, as the genes encoding resistance to these agents are distinct and may occur independently of each other. The current absence of alternative bactericidal antibiotic regimens for patients with endocarditis caused by enterococci with high-level resistance to all aminoglycosides raises the specter of surgical intervention becoming a key component of therapy in such patients.[13]

Antibacterial agents that have been given for vancomycin-resistant enterococci (VRE) with mixed success in anecdotal reports include novobiocin, minocycline, doxycycline, chloramphenicol, ciprofloxacin, and quinupristin/dalfopristin. In vitro susceptibility testing with infectious disease specialist consultation is recommended for therapy of VRE.

The rising prevalence of antimicrobial resistance among enterococci and the recognition that resistant strains are capable of both interpatient and interhospital spread has focused attention on possible ways of controlling nosocomial infections caused by such organisms. In 1995, the CDC Hospital Infection Control Practices Advisory Committee (HICPAC) issued recommendations for the control of VRE, which included the isolation or cohorting of patients infected or colonized with VRE, the cohorting of staff nursing such patients, the screening of patients and staff for carriage of VRE, and the microbiologic assessment of the hospital environment to ensure that cleaning procedures are adequate.[19] In addition, the committee highlighted a number of clinical settings, such as routine surgical prophylaxis, in which they considered the use of vancomycin to be inappropriate, and in which unnecessary use created a selective pressure for the emergence of resistance.[19] However, there have been mixed reports of the efficacy of certain guidelines. Although it was reported early on that strict application of the infection control procedures stopped the transmission of VRE in one hospital unit facing an outbreak, other workers felt that the prospective screening of patients highlighted the fact that many patients were already colonized with VRE at the time of admission to the hospital.[20] It is evident that further work is needed to improve our understanding of the epidemiology of nosocomial enterococcal infections, if attempts at control are to applied rationally rather than empirically. The HICPAC clearly recognized this need, recommending that further research using molecular typing techniques be undertaken to define reservoirs and patterns of transmission of enterococci.[19]

FUTURE PROSPECTS

Problems with the therapy of enterococcal infections related to the widespread occurrence of antimicrobial resistance may be expected to get worse in the future. Over the half century that antimicrobial agents have been in clinical use, the problem of the emergence of bacterial resistance to particular drugs has been counterbalanced by the regular development of new compounds. The signs are, however, that these days are drawing to a close, as a recent survey of large pharmaceutical companies in the United States and Japan revealed that about half had reduced or phased out research on new antibacterial agents in the belief that bacterial infections are being successfully controlled.[21] However, recent reports of enterococci and other bacteria that are resistant to all or virtually all currently available antimicrobial agents[14, 17, 22] clearly indicate the fallacy of such a view. Although treatment of infections due to multiresistant enterococci using the pristinamycins has been reported,[23, 24] the paucity of other new antimicrobial agents in the near future is a cause for concern. If insufficient new antibacterial drugs are forthcoming, future generations of patients may face a return to the days of untreatable bacterial infections. In light of the current clinical situation, the enterococci may be at the forefront of any such threat.

References

1. Devriese LA, Pot B, Collins MD: Phenotypic identification of the genus *Enterococcus* and differentiation of phylogenetically distinct enterococcal species and species groups. J Appl Bacteriol 1993; 75: 399–408.
2. Murray BE: The life and times of the enterococcus. Clin Microbiol Rev 1990; 3: 46–65.
3. Moellering RC Jr: Emergence of enterococcus as a significant pathogen. Clin Infect Dis 1992; 14: 1173–1176.
4. Gray J, Marsh PJ, Stewart D, Pedler SJ: Enterococcal bacteraemia: A prospective study of 125 episodes. J Hosp Infect 1994; 27: 179–186.
5. Antalek MD, Mylotte JM, Lesse AJ, Sellick JA Jr: Clinical and molecular epidemiology of *Enterococcus faecalis* bacteremia, with special reference to strains with high-level resistance to gentamicin. Clin Infect Dis 1995; 20: 103–109.
6. Noskin GA, Peterson LR, Warren JR: *Enterococcus faecium* and *Enterococcus faecalis* bacteremia: Acquisition and outcome. Clin Infect Dis 1995; 20: 296–301.
7. Johnson AP: The pathogenicity of enterococci. J Antimicrob Chemother 1994; 33: 1083–1089.

8. Jett BD, Huycke MM, Gilmore MS: Virulence of enterococci. Clin Microbiol Rev 1994; 7: 462–478.

9. Schaberg DR, Culver DH, Gaynes RP: Major trends in the microbial etiology of nosocomial infection. Am J Med 1991; 91(suppl 3B): 72–75.

10. Sanders WE Jr: New infective problems with old gram-positive pathogens: Setting the stage. Eur J Clin Microbiol Infect Dis 1995; 14(suppl 1): 1–2.

11. Murray BE, Singh KV, Markowitz SM et al.: Evidence for clonal spread of a single strain of β-lactamase-producing *Enterococcus (Streptococcus) faecalis* to six hospitals in five states. J Infect Dis 1991; 163: 780–785.

12. Woodford N, Morrison D, Johnson AP, et al.: Application of DNA probes for rRNA and *vanA* genes to investigation of a nosocomial cluster of vancomycin-resistant enterococci. J Clin Microbiol 1993; 31: 653–658.

13. Moellering RC Jr: The enterococcus: A classic example of the impact of antimicrobial resistance on therapeutic options. J Antimicrob Chemother 1991; 28: 1–12.

14. Eliopoulos GM: Increasing problems in the therapy of enterococcal infections. Eur J Clin Microbiol Infect Dis 1993; 12: 409–412.

15. Nicoletti G, Stefani S. Enterococci: Susceptibility patterns and therapeutic options. Eur J Clin Microbiol Infect Dis 1995; 14(suppl 1): 33–37.

16. Johnson AP, Uttley AHC, Woodford N, George RC: Resistance to vancomycin and teicoplanin: An emerging clinical problem. Clin Microbiol Rev 1990; 3: 280–291.

17. Nosocomial enterococci resistant to vancomycin—United States, 1989–1993: MMWR Morb Mortal Wkly Rep 1993; 42: 597–599.

18. Woodford N, Johnson AP: Glycopeptide resistance in gram-positive bacteria: From black and white to shades of grey. J Med Microbiol 1994; 40: 375–378.

19. Hospital Infection Control Practices Advisory Committee: Recommendations for preventing the spread of vancomycin resistance. Infect Control Hosp Epidemiol 1995; 16: 105–113.

20. Are final VRE guidelines too little too late? Hosp Infect Control 1995; 22: 33–35.

21. Shlaes D, Levy S, Archer G: Antimicrobial resistance: New directions. ASM News 1991; 57: 455–458.

22. Tomasz A: Multiple-antibiotic-resistant pathogenic bacteria. N Engl J Med 1994; 330: 1247–1251.

23. Wade J, Baillie L, Rolando N, Casewell M: Pristinamycin for *Enterococcus faecium* resistant to vancomycin and gentamicin. Lancet 1992; 339: 312–313.

24. Lynn WA, Clutterbuck E, Want S, et al.: Treatment of CAPD-peritonitis due to glycopeptide-resistant *Enterococcus faecium* with quinupristin/dalfopristin. Lancet 1994; 344: 1025–1026.

CHAPTER EIGHTEEN

Robert D. Arbeit

Staphylococcus aureus

▼

DESCRIPTION OF THE ORGANISM

Microbiologic Characteristics

Staphylococcus aureus is an aerobic, gram-positive coccus that is readily identified in clinical microbiology laboratories. The organism is distinguished among normal oral flora by the production of pigment (classically golden), hemolysin, catalase, and coagulase. On Gram's stains of infected material, organisms are characteristically in clusters but may also be found singly, in pairs, and in short chains. *S. aureus* infections typically elicit a strong polymorphonuclear leukocyte response, and intracellular organisms are often seen.

Species identification is based on the expression of coagulase, which can be detected by various well-established methods as well as recent rapid techniques. Coagulase-negative staphylococci, which include *Staphylococcus epidermidis* and other species, are generally considered nonpathogenic commensal flora except in the presence of a foreign body.

Virulence Factors

S. aureus secretes a series of enzymes—coagulase, hyaluronidase, proteases, nucleases, cytolysins (hemolysins)—that contribute to local pathogenicity by killing host cells and digesting extracellular materials. These enzymes can persist after organisms are killed by antibiotics and/or host defenses; consequently, the clinical response to treatment may be relatively slow for established infections. Extracellular toxins also mediate systemic reactions including epidermal necrolysis and toxic shock syndrome; the latter has been associated with a wide variety of infections, including pharyngitis, tonsillitis, and laryngotracheitis.[1] Surface capsular polysaccharides are present on most clinical isolates of *S. aureus* and may mediate resistance to phagocytosis and facilitate invasive, bacteremic infection. These polysaccharides are being investigated as the basis for passive and active immunization strategies. Despite this repertoire of virulence factors, *S. aureus* infections occur predominantly in patients with decreased host defenses or with acute breaks in the skin or mucous membranes due to trauma or surgery.

S. aureus is able to persist intracellularly within host phagocytes. Such organisms may be quiescent and clinically occult for indefinite periods but may serve as the basis for chronic recurrent infections, especially in the bone (osteomyelitis).[2] These infections are often particularly difficult to eradicate and can be associated with considerable morbidity, suggesting that it is prudent to seek to diagnosis acute *S.*

aureus infection quickly and accurately and to institute effective treatment promptly.

Characteristics of Typical Infection

Infections due to *S. aureus* are generally focal, with a tendency to local tissue destruction and the formation of abscesses consisting of a purulent exudate and necrotic tissue. Established infections typically require drainage as well as antimicrobial therapy. Focal infection may progress to invasive disease with bacteremia, which can in turn lead to potentially catastrophic metastatic infections (e.g., osteomyelitis, endocarditis). There is some risk of bacteremia with any *S. aureus* infection, although it appears to be an uncommon consequence of ear, nose, and throat (ENT) infections. Nevertheless, regardless of the site of primary infection, *S. aureus* bacteremia always carries a real risk for seeding cardiac valves (especially in patients with preexisting valvular abnormality, but also in patients with normal valves), other internal sites (e.g., bone, visceral organs, and foreign bodies, such as prostheses), and sites of preexisting abnormality (e.g., fractures, operative wounds, tumors). Because of the potential for these complications, *S. aureus* bacteremia typically requires 2–4 weeks of intravenous therapy and perhaps is best managed with appropriate infectious diseases consultation.

COLONIZATION OF THE SKIN AND MUCOUS MEMBRANES

S. aureus is a natural colonizer of skin and mucous membranes; the anterior nasal vestibule is the primary reservoir in older children and adults. The nasal carriage rate among adults is approximately 30% but varies with season and geographic locale. About 30% of individuals experience prolonged carriage, and about 50% intermittent carriage; the remaining 20% have very low, if any, risk of colonization. Among patients with rhinosinusitis, ~35% are colonized with *S. aureus*.[3] Carriage is associated with the intranasal use of cocaine, topical decongestants, and steroid sprays. In addition, increased frequency of nasal carriage has been noted in patients with various dermatologic conditions, human immunodeficiency virus 1 infection, hemodialysis, and the use of percutaneous needles for injecting either insulin or illicit drugs. Patients with active focal *S. aureus* infection frequently carry the organisms in the nares and at multiple cutaneous sites; in patients with chronic mucocutaneous defects (e.g., lower extremity ulcers in diabetics), carriage may persist until the defect is resolved.[4]

S. aureus is frequently transferred from persons with infection or carriage to close contacts, such as family members. Health care workers are at increased risk for becoming colonized with *S. aureus* because of regular contact with colonized or infected patients. In addition, health-care workers who do become colonized may serve as a source of organisms that can infect the highly susceptible patient populations found in health-care facilities. Boyce and coworkers described an outbreak of nosocomial infections due to methicillin-resistant *S. aureus* for which the source was a respiratory therapist with sinusitis.[5] Eradication of the sinusitis and carriage was the major factor in terminating the epidemic.

The prevalence of colonization in children does not appear to be increased in uncomplicated pharyngitis. *S. aureus* was recovered from throat and tonsillar pillar swabs from about 15% of ambulatory children (aged 2–12 years), including subjects complaining of sore throat and those without any upper or lower respiratory symptoms.[6]

S. AUREUS AS A PATHOGEN IN EAR, NOSE, AND THROAT INFECTIONS

Sinusitis

S. aureus is rarely the causative pathogen in acute sinusitis. In two recent studies, *S. aureus* was isolated from less than 1% of aspirates obtained from patients with acute maxillary sinusitis, and even when it was present there were typically only small numbers of the organisms.[7, 8]

Chronic sinusitis in both adults and children is most commonly associated with strict anaerobes; however, *S. aureus* has been cultured from 15%–20% of aspirates from well-characterized patients.[9, 10] It is important to appreciate that although *S. aureus* is typically considered an aerobic pathogen, it is fully capable of growing and causing disease under anaerobic conditions (e.g., visceral abscesses). There are anecdotal reports of chronic sinusitis associated with *S. aureus* small colony variants, which are fastidious forms that grow poorly on routine aerobic media and respond poorly to treatment with cell-wall antibiotics.[11] Consideration of such variants may be warranted in particularly recurrent or recalcitrant cases.

Complications of Sinusitis

Because *S. aureus* has a particular propensity to cause locally invasive infection with tissue destruction, the organism is responsible for a disproportionately high frequency of complications associated with sinusitis. Although it is estimated that <1% of children with sinusitis develop intracranial complications (excluding meningitis), Rosenfeld and Rowley observed that four of nine such episodes were associated with *S. aureus*.[12] Similarly, of 649 adults hospitalized for sinusitis, 24 (3.7%) had intracranial complications; among these *S. aureus* was the single most common organism and caused five (21%) infections, including abscesses, venous sinus thromboses, and osteomyelitis.[13] Mortality and serious

morbidity, including long-term neurologic sequelae, were appreciably more common in the adults than in the children. A substantial fraction of the adults had significant comorbid illness, such as chronic renal failure and diabetes mellitus, which may have increased their overall risk.

Tonsillopharyngitis

S. aureus is not considered a cause of acute tonsillopharyngitis,[6] but it is isolated relatively frequently from children with recurrent or chronic tonsillitis. Accurate assessment of those infections requires aspirates of the tonsillar core or cultures of the deep cut surface of extirpated tonsils since organisms obtained by such procedures are often considerably different from those recovered from superficial mucosal surfaces.[14] Several careful studies indicate that *S. aureus* is present within tonsillar tissue in 30%–40% of patients with recurrent or chronic tonsillitis.[14–17] In addition, *S. aureus* has been implicated in ~5% of patients with frank peritonsillar abscess.[18]

Otitis Media with Effusion

Acute otitis media with purulent (polymorphonuclear leukocytic) effusion typically involves aerobic bacterial pathogens, as assessed by tympanocentesis of the middle ear exudate. Although the frequency of *S. aureus* as a cause of this problem varies from 5% to 25% in different series, it is consistently the third most common bacterial species isolated, following *Haemophilus influenzae* and *Streptococcus pneumoniae*.[19–21] Similarly, *S. aureus* has been implicated in about 10% of episodes of both acute otitis media occurring during the first 6 weeks of life[22] and of chronic otitis media with effusion requiring the placement of tympanostomy tubes.[23]

Otitis Externa

Diffuse otitis externa is typically an acute bacterial infection of the skin lining the external auditory canal and is most commonly precipitated by factors that result in maceration of that skin, such as prolonged swimming. *S. aureus* is variably present among the normal flora of the external auditory canal in up to 15% of healthy individuals, but is consistently cultured from 15% to 20% of patients with otitis externa, with only *Pseudomonas* species being more frequent.[24]

Malignant otitis externa is a progressive, necrotizing infection occurring predominantly in diabetic patients and involving soft tissue, cartilage, and bone of the external ear. The disease is most commonly caused by *Pseudomonas aeruginosa* and is associated with considerable morbidity and mortality. A recent case report described a patient who was infected concurrently with *P. aeruginosa* and *S. aureus*.[25]

Bacterial Tracheitis

In 1979, Jones and colleagues described eight infants and children with acute, infectious, upper airway obstructive disease with features common to both croup and epiglottitis.[26] Direct laryngoscopy revealed only marked subglottic mucosal edema with copious mucus secretions from below that level. In all eight patients, smear and culture of the tracheal secretions implicated bacterial infection; six cases yielded *S. aureus,* and one each gave group A streptococcus and *H. influenzae.* In all cases, the problem resolved with periodic tracheal suctioning and appropriate antibiotics.

THE TREATMENT OF EAR, NOSE, AND THROAT INFECTIONS DUE TO *S. AUREUS*

At the beginning of the antibiotic era, virtually all *S. aureus* were susceptible to penicillin; currently, essentially all hospital isolates and most community isolates produce beta-lactamase and are resistant to penicillin, ampicillin, and amoxicillin. Beta-lactam-class antibiotics resistant to staphylococcal beta-lactamases are now widely available, both as beta-lactamase-resistant penicillins (e.g., oxacillin, nafcillin) and as beta-lactamase-resistant cephalosporins, particularly the "first- and second-generation" cephalosporins, e.g., cephalothin, cefazolin, cefoxitin, and cefuroxime. Although later-generation cephalosporins typically have increased potency and an extended spectrum against gram-negative species, they may be less effective against gram-positive organisms and less resistant to gram-positive beta-lactamases.

Beta-lactamase-producing *S. aureus* can also be effectively treated by ampicillin or amoxicillin in combination with highly effective beta-lactamase inhibitors, such as clavulanic acid or sulbactam (e.g., amoxicillin and clavulanic acid [Augmentin]; ampicillin and sulbactam [Unasyn]). In recent years, several authorities have suggested that beta-lactamase-producing organisms present in the upper respiratory flora—including not only *S. aureus,* but also *Moraxella* and *Bacteroides* species—may adversely influence the outcome of ENT infections even if the organisms themselves are not directly pathogenic or involved in the infection.[27-31] The mechanism proposed is that the beta-lactamases produced by colonizing organisms inactivate beta-lactamase-susceptible antibiotics being given for treatment of otherwise susceptible pathogens, e.g., group A beta-hemolytic streptococci or penicillin-sensitive anaerobes. A corollary of this concept is that with the increasing prevalence of beta-lactamase-producing organisms among the normal or colonizing flora in the community, there is an increasing need to treat ENT infections with beta-lactamase-resistant antibiotics. Both the second-generation cephalosporins and the combinations that include beta-lactamase inhibitors are effective against beta-lactamase-producing *S. aureus* and gram-negative oral flora and have proved highly effective for a range of ENT infections.

Extended-spectrum macrolides (azithromycin and clarithromycin) represent a recently introduced class of drugs that are frequently active against *S. aureus* as well as *Streptococcus, Haemophilus,* and *Moraxella* species, and have proved effective in ENT infections.[32] These drugs are discussed in detail in Chapter 10.

During the 1960s, methicillin-resistant (or oxacillin-resistant) *S. aureus* (MRSA) appeared. These organisms have new chromosomal genes, apparently acquired from other species, that permit the assembly of staphylococcal cell walls in the presence of penicillins and cephalosporins and thus render the organisms resistant to all members of both these classes of drugs. MRSA became widespread in hospitals of developed countries during the 1980s and are now appearing even in developing countries. Community-acquired MRSA infections, previously seen only in patients with recent hospitalizations and in intravenous drug users, are also now being seen in some areas in patients without such specific risk factors.[33] Typically, MRSA has also acquired resistance to other classes of antibiotics and are thus often "multidrug resistant." Among hospitalized patients, MRSA infections are generally treated with intravenous vancomycin. Outpatient treatment of MRSA with oral drugs must be based on specific knowledge of the susceptibilities of the infecting strain and often requires combinations of drugs, including macrolides, quinolones, rifampin, and trimethoprim-sulfamethoxazole.

MANAGEMENT OF *S. AUREUS* CARRIAGE

Eradication of *S. aureus* carriage is frequently a challenging and difficult task. Experience suggests that in patients with active infection or persistent mucocutaneous problems (e.g., chronic dermatitis, peripheral vascular ulcers), carriage is likely to continue despite treatment until the primary problem is resolved. Even in persons without such factors, the treatment of carriage often requires multiple agents.

Mupirocin (Bactroban) is a bacteriocin with a broad spectrum of activity against gram-positive organisms. Intranasal application of a 2% ointment twice daily for 5 days is an effective topical regimen. This can be supplemented by rifampin (300 mg orally twice daily) and trimethoprim-sulfamethoxazole (one double strength tablet orally twice daily); these agents are particularly useful because both rifampin and trimethoprim are secreted at mucosal surfaces. Rifampin should not be used in any patient who may have undiagnosed tuberculosis, nor should it be used alone because of the potential for the rapid emergence of resistance staphylococci. Because organisms are easily transferred between the nares and cutaneous sites, the addition of twice daily chlorhexidine (Hibiclens) showers may be useful. Ciprofloxacin has been evaluated in hemodialysis patients and minocycline in nursing home patients; neither proved useful in eradicating *S. aureus* carriage.[34, 35]

Patients who fail to clear carriage after treatment should be carefully reexamined for occult mucocutaneous defects or infections. Occasionally the primary site of carriage may be the vagina or rectum. Although the above regimens can be effective against either methicillin-sensitive or methicillin-resistant *S. aureus,* isolates may be resistant to any of the antibiotics mentioned above. Finally, patients with recurrent carriage may be recolonized from an exogenous close contact, such as a family member, or in the case of health-care workers, a patient or patients.

References

1. Dann EJ, Weinberger M, Gillis S, et al.: Bacterial laryngotracheitis associated with toxic shock syndrome in an adult. Clin Infect Dis 1994; 18: 437–439.

2. Proctor R, van Langevelde P, Kristjansson M, et al.: Persistent and relapsing infections associated with small colony variants of *Staphylococcus aureus*. Clin Infect Dis 1995; 20: 95–102.

3. Gittelman PD, Jacobs JB, Lebowitz AS, Tierno PM Jr: *Staphylococcus aureus* nasal carriage in patients with rhinosinusitis. Laryngoscope 1991; 101: 733–737.

4. Maslow J, Brecher S, Gunn J, et al.: Persistance and variation of methicillin-resistant *Staphylococcus aureus* strains among individual patients over extended periods of time. Eur J Clin Microbiol Infect Dis 1995; 14: 282–290.

5. Boyce JM, Opal SM, Potter-Bynoe G, Medeiros AA: Spread of methicillin-resistant *Staphylococcus aureus* in a hospital after exposure to a health care worker with chronic sinusitis. Clin Infect Dis 1993; 17: 496–504.

6. Reed BD, Huck W, Lutz LJ, Zazove P: Prevalence of *Chlamydia trachomatis* and *Mycoplasma pneumoniae* in children with and without pharyngitis. J Fam Pract 1988; 26: 387–392.

7. Jousimies-Somer H, Savolainen S, Ylikoski J: Bacteriological findings of acute maxillary sinusitis in young adults. J Clin Microbiol 1988; 26: 1919–1925.

8. Sydnor A, Gwaltney J, Cocchetto D, Scheld M: Comparative evaluation of cefuroxime axetil and cefaclor for treatment of acute bacterial maxillary sinusitis. Arch Otolaryngol Head Neck Surg 1989; 115: 1430–1433.

9. Frederick J, Braude A: Anaerobic infection of the paranasal sinuses. N Engl J Med 1974; 290: 135–137.

10. Brook I: Bacteriologic features of chronic sinusitis in children. JAMA 1981; 246: 967–969.

11. Proctor RA: Microbial pathogenic factors: Small colony variants. In: Bisno AL, Waldvogel FA (eds): Infections Associated with Indwelling Medical Devices, 2nd ed. Washington, DC: American Society for Microbiology, 1994: 79–90.

12. Rosenfeld E, Rowley A: Infectious intracranial complications of sinusitis, other than meningitis, in children: 12-year review. Clin Infect Dis 1994; 18: 750–754.

13. Clayman G, Adams G, Paugh D, Koopmann C: Intracranial complications of paranasal sinusitis: A combined institutional review. Laryngoscope 1991; 101: 234–239.

14. Timon CI, Cafferkey MT, Walsh M: Fine-needle aspiration in recurrent tonsillitis. Arch Otolaryngol Head Neck Surg 1991; 117: 653–656.

15. Brook I, Yocum P: Comparison of the microbiology of group A and non-group A streptococcal tonsillitis. Ann Otol Rhinol Laryngol 1988; 97: 243–246.

16. Timon CI, McAllister VA, Walsh M, Cafferkey MT: Changes in tonsillar bacteriology of recurrent acute tonsillitis: 1980 vs. 1989. Respir Med 1990; 84: 395–400.

17. Gaffney RJ, Freeman DJ, Walsh MA, Cafferkey MT: Differences in tonsil core bacteriology in adults and children: A prospective study of 262 patients. Respir Med 1991; 85: 383–388.

18. Snow DG, Campbell JB, Morgan DW: The microbiology of peritonsillar sepsis. J Laryngol Otol 1991; 105: 553–555.

19. Kurono Y, Tomonaga K, Mogi G: *Staphylococcus epidermidis* and *Staphylococcus aureus* in otitis media with effusion. Arch Otolaryngol Head Neck Surg 1988; 114: 1262–1265.

20. Schwartz R, Rodriguez WJ, Mann R, et al.: The nasopharyngeal culture in acute otitis media. A reappraisal of its usefulness. JAMA 1979; 241: 2170–2173.

21. Lim DJ, Lewis DM, Schram JL, Birck HG: Otitis media with effusion. Cytological and microbiological correlates. Arch Otolaryngol 1979; 105: 404–412.

22. Shurin PA, Howie VM, Pelton SI, et al.: Bacterial etiology of otitis media during the first six weeks of life. J Pediatr 1978; 92: 893–896.

23. Liu YS, Lang R, Lim DJ, Birck HG: Microorganisms in chronic otitis media with effusion. Ann Otol Rhinol Laryngol 1976; 85: 245–249.

24. Cassisi N, Cohn A, Davidson T, Witten BR: Diffuse otitis externa: Clinical and microbiologic findings in the course of a multicenter study on a new otic solution. Ann Otol Rhinol Laryngol Suppl 1977; 86: 1–16.

25. Britigan BE, Blythe WB: Malignant external otitis in a diabetic renal transplant patient. Successful treatment without discontinuation of immunosuppressive therapy. Transplantation 1987; 43: 769–771.

26. Jones R, Santos JI, Overall JC Jr: Bacterial tracheitis. JAMA 1979; 242: 721–726.

27. Brook I: Beta-lactamase-producing bacteria recovered after clinical failures with various penicillin therapy. Arch Otolaryngol 1984; 110: 228–231.

28. Brook I: Emergence and persistence of beta-lactamase-producing bacteria in the oropharynx following penicillin treatment. Arch Otolaryngol Head Neck Surg 1988; 14: 667–670.

29. Brook I, Heyning PH: Microbiology and management of otis media. Scand J Infect Dis Suppl 1994; 93: 20–32.

30. Bluestone C: Update on antimicrobial therapy for otitis media and sinusitis in children. Cutis 1985; 36: 7–12.

31. Brook I, Gober AE: Emergence of beta-lactamase-producing aerobic and anaerobic bacteria in the oropharynx of children following penicillin chemotherapy. Clin Pediatr (Phila) 1984; 23: 338–341.

32. Muller O: Comparison of azithromycin versus clarithromycin in the treatment of patients with upper respiratory tract infections. J Antimicrob Chemother 1993; 31: 137–146.

33. Gottlieb RD, Shah MK, Perlman DC, Kimmelman CP: Community-acquired methicillin-resistant *Staphylococcus aureus* infections in otolaryngology. Otolaryngol Head Neck Surg 1992; 107: 434–437.

34. Chow JW, Yu VL: Failure of oral ciprofloxacin in suppressing *Staphylococcus aureus* carriage in haemodialysis patients. J Antimicrob Chemother 1992; 29: 88–89.

35. Muder RR, Boldin M, Brennen C, et al.: A controlled trial of rifampicin, minocycline, and rifampicin plus minocycline for eradication of methicillin-resistant *Staphylococcus aureus* in long-term care patients. J Antimicrob Chemother 1994; 34: 188–190.

CHAPTER NINETEEN

Jerome O. Klein

Haemophilus influenzae

DESCRIPTION

History

Haemophilus influenzae was first identified as a pathogen in 1883 by Koch, who described small gram-negative rods in pus from cases of conjunctivitis in Egypt. The organism was later called the Koch-Weeks bacillus or *Haemophilus aegyptius*. In 1893 Pfeiffer determined that the "influenza bacillus" was the cause of epidemic influenza; this concept persisted through the pandemic of World War I and remained until the viral cause of influenza was demonstrated in 1933. In 1929 Fleming used the *Penicillium* mold for the isolation of *Bacillus influenza*. In 1930 Pittman indicated the importance of the capsule and type B as the cause of invasive disease and classified capsulated strains into six serotypes (types A through F). Nonencapsulated strains were subsequently documented as the cause of sinusitis, otitis media, and pneumonia. In 1985 a polysaccharide *H. influenzae* type B vaccine was approved for use in children older than 2 years of age. The efficacy of the vaccine in reducing the burden of *Haemophilus* disease was limited because the highest attack rate for invasive disease was in early infancy. In October 1990 the first of a series of conjugated polysaccharide vaccines was introduced in the United States. The conjugated vaccines are immunogenic in infants beginning at 2 months of age. Widespread usage of this vaccine has resulted in almost complete eradication of disease due to type B organisms, but the incidence of disease due to nontypable strains has been unaffected. Interested readers are referred to the proceedings of a symposium on the epidemiology, pathogenesis, and prevention of *H. influenzae* disease.[1] For current information about the epidemiology of infection and disease, the reader should refer to the Morbidity and Mortality Weekly Reports published by the Centers for Disease Control and Prevention in Atlanta; for recommendations for treatment and control measures, the reader should refer to the most recent Report of the Committee on Infectious Diseases (The Red Book) published by the American Academy of Pediatrics, Elk Grove Village, Illinois.

Description of Pathogen

Nonencapsulated strains of *H. influenzae* are important causes of otitis media, sinusitis, conjunctivitis, chronic bronchitis, and pneumonia. The nonencapsulated organisms rarely invade the bloodstream, although sepsis in the newborn infant has been associated with these strains. *H. influenzae* type B organisms are invasive and may result in meningitis, arthritis, osteomyelitis, and pericarditis. Type B strains may also cause disease in contiguous areas—cellulitis, uvulitis, and epiglottitis. Types A, C, D, and E are uncommon causes of sepsis and suppurative disease.

Microbiology

The genus *Haemophilus* consists of facultatively anaerobic gram-negative bacilli. *H. influenzae* organisms appear as coccobacilli in Gram-stained smears of clinical materials. They are pleomorphic and may occur as long filamentous or stout rods and, on occasion, as short chains or pairs of cocci simulating the appearance of streptococci.

Encapsulated strains responsible for invasive disease may be serotyped with specific antiserums. The type-specific substance of the capsule is a polysaccharide. Most strains that colonize the upper respiratory tract do not have capsular material. Nonencapsulated strains of *H. influenzae* may be classified on the basis of biochemical and antigenic markers. Biochemical profiles have been used to classify strains isolated from middle ear fluids; the majority of strains belong to two biotypes based on assays of indole, urease, and ornithine decarboxylase. Current studies of outer membrane proteins aim to develop a serotyping system based on antigenic patterns.[2]

Both encapsulated and nonencapsulated strains produce a plasmid-mediated beta-lactamase that breaks the beta-lactam ring of susceptible penicillins. Resistance to ampicillin and other penicillins may also be due to a permeability defect or alteration in penicillin-binding proteins. Resistant strains were first reported in the early 1970s. At present in the United States approximately 10%–30% of strains of type B and nontypable *H. influenzae* isolated from children with otitis media are beta-lactamase-positive.[3]

Virulence Factor

Nonencapsulated organisms colonize the respiratory tract and cause disease by contiguous spread into the sinuses, the middle ear, or the lung. Encapsulated organisms invade the blood stream and may cause disease at distant foci including the meninges, bones and joints, and pericardium or may invade local tissues causing cellulitis, epiglottitis, or uvulitis. Both capsular polysaccharide and lipopolysaccharide are important microbial virulence factors for type B organisms.[4]

EPIDEMIOLOGY

The human respiratory tract is the only source for *H. influenzae*. The incubation period and period of communicability are uncertain, but infants may carry the organism for months[5] and may be communicable as long as the organism is present in the upper respiratory tract. Epidemic disease may occur in infants in closed communities such as households and day care centers.

The highest age-specific attack rates for sepsis and meningitis due to *H. influenzae* type B disease occur between the ages of 3 and 12 months. In contrast, the highest age-specific incidence of epiglottis and uvulitis occurs between the ages of 2 and 4 years. Other host factors influencing susceptibility to invasive disease due to *H. influenzae* type B include sex (males are affected more frequently than females), the presence of congenital or acquired asplenia, sickle cell disease and other hemoglobinopathies, and racial or ethnic factors. Patients with acquired immunodeficiency syndrome or human immunodeficiency virus infection are at risk for invasive *H. influenzae* disease. A high incidence of disease in Native Americans and Alaskan Eskimos may be associated with genetic predisposition and/or factors of poverty and difficult environmental factors. The incidence of type B disease has significantly declined in the United States since introduction of the conjugate polysaccharide vaccine in the fall of 1990.

Host and environmental factors associated with disease due to nonencapsulated strains has been best documented for otitis media.[6] Acute otitis media is a disease of infancy and early childhood with a peak age-specific incidence among children from the ages of 6 to 18 months. Children who have few episodes of acute otitis media before the age of 3 years are unlikely to develop recurrent middle ear infections subsequently. Factors of sex, race, and poverty are similar to those of type B disease. Familial aggregation is a risk factor for recurrent acute otitis media. Breast-feeding is an important factor in the prevention of respiratory infections, including otitis media, in infancy. Protection during the first year of life appears to result from some component of breast milk rather than the position or development of facial musculature, or some deleterious quality of formula or cow's milk.[6]

The transmission of respiratory pathogens in day care centers has been associated with an increased risk of acute otitis media and of invasive *H. influenzae* type B disease. Each infant brings to the day care center a microflora acquired in the household, and these organisms are spread by coughing, sneezing, and touching. Longitudinal studies of children attending the Frank Porter Graham Day Care Center in Chapel Hill, North Carolina, revealed almost one episode of respiratory infection a month during the first year of life with decreased incidence during the second through fifth years; acute otitis media was diagnosed in almost half the episodes of respiratory illness.[7]

Passive smoking and environmental pollutants have come under increased scrutiny as agents of structural and physiologic changes in the respiratory tree. The availability of a biochemical marker, cotinine, has made documentation of passive exposure to tobacco smoke far more reliable than that provided by history alone. Cotinine concentrations in urine or serum were related to the number of smokers in the household, and high concentrations of serum cotinine were associated with an increased incidence of acute otitis media and the duration of middle ear effusion after acute infection.[8]

COLONIZATION, TRANSMISSION, AND PATHOGENESIS

Asymptomatic colonization of the upper respiratory tract by nonencapsulated strains begins within the first months of life.[9] During infancy and early childhood, nonencapsulated strains were recovered from the throats of 60%–90% of children; colonization by type B strains was less than 5% in infants and young children.[5, 9] Carriage may persist for months.[5] Colonization of type B strains is now uncommon in populations immunized with the conjugate polysaccharide vaccine.[10, 11] Rates of carriage of older children and adults are lower than those of infants.

The transmission of *H. influenzae* is person to person by direct contact or by the inhalation of droplets of secretions from the respiratory tract.

Pathogenesis of invasive *H. influenzae* type B disease in the human host includes colonization of the mucosal surfaces of the upper respiratory tract; transport of the organism across epithelial and endothelial cells; entry of the organism into the blood; multiplication of organisms in the blood; and localization in tissue and tissue injury. Concurrent viral infection may increase inflammation of the upper respiratory tract and encourage invasion by encapsulated *H. influenzae*.[12] Patients with immune deficiency are susceptible to severe invasive disease, but the reason for invasive disease in some among the many who are colonized remains uncertain.

The pathogenesis of otitis media and sinusitis due to *H. influenzae* is associated with anatomic or physiologic obstruction of the eustachian tube or the ostia of the sinuses. Acute infection usually follows an antecedent viral infection or allergic reaction that results in congestion of the respiratory mucosa. Congestion of the mucosa may result in obstruction of the tube or ostia. Secretions of the sinuses or middle ear have no egress and accumulate; if pathogenic bacteria, including *H. influenzae,* that colonize the nasopharynx are present in the secretions before obstruction, they multiply, and an acute suppurative infection results. Bacterial cell wall components of the organism including peptidoglycan, induce inflammation and histopathologic changes in the tympanic membrane and the middle ear mucosa in experimental models.[13]

IMMUNOLOGY

Immune Response to Infection

A wide variety of antibodies, including agglutinins and complement-fixing, capsular-swelling, and bactericidal antibodies, appear in the blood of patients after infection. Bactericidal antibodies persist for prolonged periods. The appearance of protective antibodies is age-dependent and is correlated with the age-specific pattern of disease. In 1933 Fothergill and Wright measured the bactericidal effect of blood of persons of various ages against a virulent strain of *H. influenzae* type B.[14] In the first months of life, the infant was protected by passively transferred maternal antibodies. The absence of bactericidal activity in serums before the second birthday was correlated with the known susceptibility of young children to serious influenzal disease. Only after 2 years of age is the child's immune system mature enough to respond to naturally occurring type B polysaccharide.

Natural defense mechanisms protect against some infections due to *H. influenzae.* Approximately half of middle ear infections due to nontypable *H. influenzae* clear from the middle ear without antibacterial drug intervention.[15] Of invasive type B strains, approximately one third of untreated patients with bacteremia clear the organism from the blood stream and recover clinically without antimicrobial drug intervention.[16] The reasons for spontaneous clearance are unknown but probably include clearance by the reticuloendothelial system and humoral and cellular mechanisms.

Type B Polysaccharide Vaccines

The stimulation of protective antibodies is the basis for the successful development of vaccines against type B *H. influenzae.* In 1985 a vaccine prepared from capsular polysaccharide of type B organisms was introduced in the United States. Because it was a poor immunogen in children 2 years of age and younger, the vaccine could be recommended only for older children. In retrospective analyses, the efficacy of the vaccine in the United States varied between 45%–88%, but a study of vaccine use in Minnesota indicated an absence of any protective effect.[17]

The first conjugate vaccine, a capsular polysaccharide of *H. influenzae* conjugated to diphtheria toxoid, was licensed for use in the United States in December 1987. One year later two additional conjugate vaccines incorporating a nontoxic mutant diphtheria toxin protein and an outer membrane protein were licensed. The conjugate vaccines resulted in significantly higher titers of type-specific antibody than was achieved by the polysaccharide vaccines in the infant age groups. In 1996 four *H. influenzae* type B vaccines and one combination *H. influenzae* type B conjugate diphtheria-tetanus-pertussis vaccine were licensed in the United States. The licensed products consist of type B capsular polysaccharide or oligosaccharide covalently linked to a carrier protein directly or by means of an intervening spacer molecule. Protein carriers include diphtheria toxoid, a nontoxic mutant diphtheria toxin, an outer membrane protein complex prepared from group B *Neisseria meningitidis,* and tetanus toxoid. Vaccine efficacy is attributable not only to the stimulation of protective antibodies but to the decrease in carriage, leading to a reduced reservoir of organisms for transmission to susceptible children.[10, 11]

Nontypable Vaccines

Vaccines for the prevention of disease due to nontypable strains are under investigation. Vaccine candidates include pili, surface proteins that occur as filamentous appendages on the bacterial cell surface[18] and outer membrane proteins and lipo-oligosaccharides.[19] Nontypable vaccines are still in early phases of investigation of antigens for an optimal vaccine.

PATHOGENS IN EAR, NOSE, AND THROAT INFECTIONS

Otitis Media

Microbiologic diagnosis of otitis media is made by the aspiration of middle ear fluid through the tympanic membrane (tympanocentesis). *H. influenzae* is isolated from middle ear fluids of children with acute otitis media in about one-quarter of cases; the mean of cases studied in 12 reports published between 1952 and 1981 was 21% (range 14%–31%); the mean of 12 reports published between 1985 and 1992 was 27% (range 16%–52%).[20] Otitis media due to *H. influenzae* is associated with nontypable strains in the vast majority of patients. Before the introduction of the conjugate *H. influenzae* type B vaccines, approximately 10% of cases of otitis media due to *H. influenzae* were due to type B strains; approximately a quarter of these children had concurrent sepsis or meningitis. Cases of otitis media due to types A, E, and F are infrequent. *H. influenzae* occurs in all age groups in approximately equivalent proportions of the bacterial cause of otitis media.

H. influenzae is the primary pathogen of the conjunctivitis-otitis syndrome. Bodor and colleagues obtained *H. influenzae* from simultaneous cultures of conjunctivae and middle ear fluids of 18 of 20 episodes of the syndrome. Biotyping and outer membrane protein analyses identified that isolates obtained from the sites were concordant.[21]

Sinusitis

Microbiologic diagnosis of sinusitis is made by needle or catheter aspiration of sinus fluids. The microbiology of acute sinusitis in children and adults parallels that of acute otitis media. Almost all of the strains of *H. influenzae* are nonencapsulated. The mean percentage of cultures of aspirates of sinus fluids from patients with acute sinusitis was 21% for adults[22] and 23% for children.[23]

Epiglottitis

Acute epiglottitis or supraglottitis is usually due to *H. influenzae* type B. Although most cases occur in children between 1 and 5 years of age, epiglottitis due to *H. influenzae* also occurs in older children and adults. Cultures of the posterior pharynx, epiglottis, and blood usually reveal the pathogen of epiglottitis. Daum and Smith summarized 33 pediatric series of epiglottitis and found that bacteremia due to *H. influenzae* type B occurred in 77% of children and 23% of adults.[24] Supraglottitis may be accompanied by suppurative foci at other sites including meningitis.[25]

Uvulitis

The bacterial pathogens of uvulitis include *H. influenzae* type B and group A *Streptococcus*. Uvulitis caused by *H. influenzae* may occur with or without epiglottitis. The epidemiology, diagnosis, and management are similar to those of epiglottitis.

Cellulitis

Cellulitis due to *H. influenzae* type B may occur as an extension from an upper respiratory focus, as in periorbital cellulitis after localization of disease in the ethmoid sinus, or by the hematogenous route after bacteremia. The disease is restricted almost exclusively to children younger than 4 years of age. The cheek, head, and neck are the site of three quarters of cases of cellulitis due to *H. influenzae*. A unique dusky or reddish-purple discoloration is characteristic and distinguishes *H. influenzae* cellulitis from that caused by other suppurative bacteria. Microbiologic diagnosis may be made by needle aspiration of the central indurated area and culture of blood.

Conjunctivitis

H. influenzae biogroup *aegyptius* (the Koch-Weeks bacillus) is a frequent cause of acute catarrhal conjunctivitis. Seasonal outbreaks of conjunctivitis occur in California and in the southeastern United States. The conjunctivitis may be an initial sign of a fulminant childhood Brazilian purpuric fever infection caused by *H. influenzae* biogroup *aegyptius*. The disease was first recognized in 1984 in São Paulo after a description of deaths due to an acute febrile illness in children with purpura and vascular collapse.[26]

LABORATORY DIAGNOSIS

Gram's stain of pus or infected fluid may suggest the organism, but the pleomorphic nature of *H. influenzae* may mislead; gram-negative cocci may be misinterpreted as inadequately stained streptococci. Specimens need to be processed quickly because the organism is fastidious. Optimal growth of *H. influenzae* is achieved on chocolate agar or in special preparations including heme and nicotinamide adenine dinucleotide. Colonies are pinpoint and transparent and may be flat or convex. Enhanced growth of colonies of *H. influenzae* occurs in the immediate vicinity of colonies of *Staphylococcus aureus*. This phenomenon results from the diffusion of metabolic products from the growing *Staphylococcus*. *H. influenzae* may occur in either rough, nonencapsulated forms or smooth, encapsulated forms. Organisms possessing capsules may be serotyped with specific antiserums. Latex particle agglutination for the detection of capsular antigen is of value for the diagnosis of *H. influenzae* type B in serum or cerebrospinal fluid but is of limited value in the diagnosis of focal infection of the ears, nose, and throat.

TREATMENT

In Vitro Activity of Antimicrobial Agents

Strains of *H. influenzae* responsible for otolaryngologic infections may be subdivided on the basis of the production of beta-lactamase and susceptibility to amoxicillin. Most amoxicillin-resistant strains of *H. influenzae* produce the enzyme beta-lactamase, which breaks open the beta-lactam ring, rendering the drug inactive. In most communities in the United States, approximately 10%–30% of nontypable and type B strains of *H. influenzae* responsible for otitis media produce beta-lactamase and are resistant to amoxicillin. The addition of a beta-lactamase inhibitor, clavulanic acid, to oral amoxicillin, or sulbactam to parenteral ampicillin, protects the drug from inactivation by the enzyme. Although first-generation cephalosporins (cephalexin, cefazolin) have limited activity against *H. influenzae*, activity is enhanced in second-generation cephalosporins (cefaclor, cefixime, cefuroxime, cefpodoxime, and loracarbef) and is excellent in third-generation cephalosporins (ceftriaxone, cefotaxime, and ceftazidime). Other drugs that are effective in vitro include sulfonamides, trimethoprim-sulfamethoxazole, chloramphenicol, and aminoglycosides. Macrolides and tetracyclines have variable activity.

Antimicrobial Therapy

Otitis Media. Differences in microbiologic efficacy are apparent among the various antibacterial agents available in the United States. To determine the efficacy of antibacterial drugs in eradicating bacterial pathogens in middle ear fluids of children with acute otitis media, investigators have aspirated middle ear fluid before therapy was begun and 2 or more days after therapy was initiated. The microbiologic results for the various drugs are consistent with data on in vitro activity and concentrations of drug achieved in the middle ear.[15] Amoxicillin is no better than placebo against beta-lactamase-producing strains of *H. influenzae*, but amoxicillin clavulanate and active cephalosporins eradicate most strains from the middle ear. In studies in which placebo was used, approximately one half of nontypable *H. influenzae* cleared (in contrast, only 19% of pneumococci cleared from the middle ear fluid).[15] Thus, many children with acute otitis media due to *H. influenzae* have spontaneous microbiologic resolution of the infection (and are clinically improved).

Amoxicillin remains the current drug of choice because it continues to be effective and is safe and relatively inexpensive. However, the anticipated failure rate of approximately 10% (based on resistant pneumococci as well as beta-lactamase-producing *H. influenzae*) warrants continued surveillance and a possible change to beta-lactamase-stable drugs if the incidence of resistant strains of *H. influenzae* significantly increases.[27]

Sinusitis. Because the microbiology of sinusitis parallels that of otitis media, the same considerations of choice of antimicrobial agent apply to acute sinusitis. For the patient who is toxic and requires parenteral therapy, a cephalosporin with activity against the major pathogens such as cefuroxime, ceftriaxone, or cefotaxime is appropriate.

Epiglottitis and Uvulitis. Maintenance of the airway remains the major concern in the management of epiglottitis, but appropriate antibacterial therapy should be administered because of the frequency of bacteremia as well as locally invasive disease. The choice of parenteral therapy includes second- and third-generation cephalosporins or chloramphenicol.

Cellulitis. Since most children with *H. influenzae* cellulitis are toxic and may have concurrent bacteremia, initial therapy should include a parenteral drug that is active against *H. influenzae* as well as other possible pathogens such as group A *Streptococcus, Streptococcus pneumoniae,* and *N. meningitidis.*

Control Measures

Infants who are exposed to patients with invasive disease due to type B *H. influenzae* are at risk and should be carefully observed. Prophylaxis is recommended for all household contacts when an unvaccinated child younger than 48 months is present and in child care homes including unvaccinated children younger than 2 years of age. Rifampin eradicates *H. influenzae* type B from the upper respiratory tract and is the only effective drug for prophylaxis. Rifampin is administered orally once daily for 4 days in a dosage of 20 mg/kg/day (maximum dose, 600 mg).

References

1. Daum RS (guest editor): Epidemiology, pathogenesis, and prevention of *Haemophilus influenzae* disease, Veldhoven, Netherlands, September 24–28, 1990. J Infect Dis 1992; 165(suppl 1): S1.
2. Murphy TF, Apicella MA: Antigenic heterogenicity of outer membrane proteins of nontypable *Haemophilus influenzae* is a basis for serotyping system. Infect Immun 1985; 50: 15–21.
3. Bluestone CD, Stephenson JS, Martin LM: Ten-year review of otitis media pathogens. Pediatr Infect Dis J 1992; 11: S7–S11.
4. Moxon ER: Session III: Pathogenesis of invasive *Haemophilus influenzae* disease molecular basis of invasive *Haemophilus influenzae* type b disease. J Infect Dis 1992; 165(suppl 1): S77–S81.
5. Faden H, Duffy L, Williams A, et al.: Epidemiology of nasopharyngeal colonization with nontypeable *Haemophilus influenzae* in the first 2 years of life. J Infect Dis 1995; 172: 132–135.
6. Teele DW, Klein JO, Rosner B, the Greater Boston Otitis Media Study Group: Epidemiology of otitis media during the first seven years of life in children in greater Boston: A prospective, cohort study. J Infect Dis 1989; 160: 83–94.
7. Schwartz B, Giebink GS, Henderson FW, et al.: Respiratory infections in day care. Pediatrics 1994; 84: 1018–1020.
8. Etzel RA, Pattishall EN, Haley NJ, et al.: Passive smoking and middle ear effusion among children in day care. Pediatrics 1992; 90: 228–232.
9. Aniansson G, Alm B, Andersson B, et al.: Nasopharyngeal colonization during the first year of life. J Infect Dis 1992; 165(suppl 1): S38–S42.
10. Mohle-Boetani JC, Ajello G, Breneman E, et al.: Carriage of *Haemophilus influenzae* type b in children after widespread vaccination with conjugate *Haemophilus influenzae* type b vaccines. Pediatr Infect Dis J 1993; 12: 589–593.
11. Barbour ML, Mayon-White RT, Coles C, et al.: The impact of conjugate vaccine on carriage of *Haemophilus influenzae* type b. J Infect Dis 1995; 171: 93–98.
12. Feigin RD, McCracken GH Jr, Klein JO: Diagnosis and management of meningitis. Pediatr Infect Dis J 1992; 11: 785–814.
13. Leake ER, Holmes K, Lim DJ, DeMaria TF: Peptidoglycan isolated from nontypeable *Haemophilus influenzae* induces experimental otitis media in the chinchilla. J Infect Dis 1994; 170: 1532–1538.
14. Fothergill LD, Wright J: Influenzal meningitis: The relation of age incidence to the bactericidal power of blood against the causal organism. J Immunol 1933; 24: 273–284.
15. Klein JO: Microbiologic efficacy of antibacterial drugs for acute otitis media. Pediatr Infect Dis J 1993; 12: 973–975.
16. Marshall R, Teele DW, Klein JO: Unsuspected bacteremia due to *Haemophilus influenzae*: Outcome in children not initially admitted to hospital. Pediatrics 1979; 95: 690–695.
17. Granoff DM, Sheetz K, Pandey JP, et al.: Host and bacterial factors associated with *Haemophilus influenzae* type b disease in Minnesota children vaccinated with type b polysaccharide vaccine. J Infect Dis 1989; 159: 908–916.
18. Brinton CC Jr, Carter MJ, Derber DB, et al.: Design and development of pilus vaccines for *Haemophilus influenzae* diseases. Pediatr Infect Dis 1989; 8: S54–S61.
19. Murphy TF, Campagnari AA, Nelson MB, Apicella MA: Somatic antigens of *Haemophilus influenzae* as vaccine components. Pediatr Infect Dis 1989; 8: S66–S68.
20. Bluestone CD, Klein JO (eds): Otitis Media in Infants and Children, 2nd ed. Philadelphia: WB Saunders Co, 1995, p 56.
21. Bodor FF, Marchant CD, Shurin PA, Barenkamp SJ: Bacterial etiology of conjunctivitis-otitis media syndrome. Pediatrics 1985; 76: 26–28.
22. Gwaltney JM Jr, Scheld WM, Sande MA, et al.: The microbial etiology and antimicrobial therapy of adults with acute community-acquired sinusitis: A fifteen-year experience at the University of Virginia and review of other selected studies. J Allergy Clin Immunol 1992; 90: 457–462.
23. Wald ER, Milmoe GJ, Bowen AD, et al.: Acute maxillary sinusitis in children. N Engl J Med 1981; 304: 749.
24. Daum RS, Smith AL: Epiglottitis (supraglottis). In: Feigin RD, Cherry JD (eds): *Textbook of Pediatric Infectious Diseases,* 3rd ed. Philadelphia: WB Saunders Co, 1992, p 197.
25. Friedman EM, Damion J, Healy GB, McGill TJI: Supraglottitis and concurrent *Hemophilus* meningitis. Ann Otol Rhinol Laryngol 1985; 94: 470–472.
26. Tondella MLC, Quinn FD, Perkins BA: Brazilian purpuric fever caused by *Haemophilus influenzae* biogroup aegyptius strains lacking the 3031 plasmid. J Infect Dis 1995; 171: 209–212.
27. Klein JO: Otitis media. Clin Infect Dis 1994; 19: 823–833.

Abraham Verghese

CHAPTER TWENTY

Moraxella (Branhamella) catarrhalis

▼

Moraxella (Branhamella) catarrhalis is an organism that is part of the normal oral flora. As many as 50% of children may be colonized with *M. catarrhalis*. In addition to being an important cause of otitis media, the organism causes acute exacerbations of chronic bronchitis and pneumonia, primarily in persons with underlying chronic obstructive lung disease.[1]

DESCRIPTION

History

M. catarrhalis was at various times considered a pathogen or a normal commensal.[2] Speculation that *M. catarrhalis* could be the cause of the common cold led J. E. Gordon to perform an elegant study sequentially examining patients with and without cold symptoms; he proved the organism was a common oral commensal.[3] Gordon's study may have led to the widespread belief that the organism was never a pathogen. In the pneumococcal era, *M. catarrhalis* faded from the American literature despite continued interest in Europe. It failed to be mentioned in Osler's Principles and Practice of Medicine (1892),[4] but an entry from Osler's diary near the time of his death suggests that Osler may have believed the organism to be a pathogen, at least in his own illness:

No fever since the 16th but cough persists with an occasional paroxysm—bouts as bad as senile whooping cough, one night they nearly blew my candle out. No. 3 pneumococcus with *M. catarrhalis*.

CUSHING[5]

In 1970 the organism was assigned to the genus *Branhamella* in honor of Dr. Sarah Branham, who made many contributions to the taxonomy of the *Neisseria* species. For a detailed discussion of nomenclature, the reader is referred to the review by Catlin.[6] From Osler's time (when the organism was referred to as *Micrococcus catarrhalis*), this gram-negative coccus has undergone a number of name changes. The designation *Neisseria catarrhalis* (which followed *Micrococcus catarrhalis*) reflected the resemblance of this organism in both appearance and habitat to *Neisseria meningitidis*. Given the lack of DNA relatedness between the two organisms, it was proposed that the genus be transferred to *Moraxella*, a genus within the family Neisseriaceae,

since it shared more in common with *Moraxella* than with *Neisseria*. The species name *Branhamella catarrhalis* was proposed.[7] Bovre found it expedient to divide the genus *Moraxella* into the subgenus *Branhamella* (to contain coccal organisms) and *Moraxella* (to contain rod-shaped organisms) and therefore suggested the terminology *Moraxella (Branhamella) catarrhalis*.[8, 9]

Description of Pathogen

M. catarrhalis on Gram's stain is a gram-negative diplococcus with a tendency to resist decolorizing.[8, 9] The organism is often larger than the meningococcus or gonococcus.

Microbiologic Characteristics

On blood agar, the organism forms small, opaque, gray-white colonies, 1–3 mm in diameter, that are circular and nonhemolytic. They can be pushed over the surface of the agar like a hockey puck on ice.[10, 11] *M. catarrhalis* typically is oxidase-positive and fails to ferment glucose, maltose, sucrose, and lactose. Only *Neisseria flavescens* (among species that may be recovered from the same site) shares these biochemical characteristics, and *M. catarrhalis* may be distinguished by its reduction of nitrates, its lack of colony pigmentation, and its production of deoxyribonuclease.[7, 10] Hydrolysis of DNA and tributyrin are valuable differentiating tests for *M. catarrhalis*. The B.CAT CONFIRM (Scott Laboratories, Fiskeville, Rhode Island) is a rapid test for the detection of tributyrin hydrolysis. Louie and colleagues compared five rapid methods of identification: the 4-methyl-umbelliferyl butyrate (MUB), API quadFerm, B.CAT CONFIRM, Gonochek II, and the tributyrin disc.[12] All five tests reliably and accurately identified 31 *M. catarrhalis* isolates. However, the MUB test was the least expensive and least labor-intensive and did not require overnight purity plates for performance. The MUB test provided same-day identification of *M. catarrhalis* isolates from the initial primary isolation culture.[12]

Virulence Factors and Pathogenesis

Bacterial colonization of mucosal surfaces depends on the attachment of bacteria to mucosal epithelium, a process often mediated by pili or fimbriae.[13] Piliation has been observed on clinical stains[14, 15] but not on ATCC strains 8193,[15] 25238[T],[16] and 8176.[15]

The cell wall of *M. catarrhalis* is similar to that of *Neisseria gonorrhoeae.* The lipopolysaccharide (LOS) present in the outer membrane lacks the long repeating units that characterize the O antigen of enteric gram-negative bacteria. Much as with *N. gonorrhoeae,* vesicles or blebs are released from the outer membrane and can be visualized on electron microscopy.[17]

As discussed below, there appears to be a correlation between increased nasopharyngeal colonization with *M. catarrhalis* and otitis media; the reasons for this are not clear but, as has been shown for nontypable *Haemophilus influenzae*[18, 19] and the pneumococcus, otitis-prone children may fail to develop the normal immune response to these pathogens. In adults, chronic obstructive pulmonary disease is the most consistently reported underlying illness associated with *M. catarrhalis* respiratory infection.[20] In adults with respiratory infections, underlying immunoglobulin deficiency is an interesting, though quantitatively less important, risk factor for *M. catarrhalis* infection; this association has been reported several times, and the clinical course appears more severe than in patients with chronic lung disease.[21–25] Cases reported in association with acquired immunodeficiency disease[26] may represent the indirect effect of human immunodeficiency virus infection on B-cell function.

Soto-Hernandez and colleagues looked for phenotypic differences between 27 isolates of *M. catarrhalis* from patients colonized with the organism, from patients with pneumonia, and from patients with tracheobronchitis.[27] Eighteen of 27 strains were serum-resistant, a lower percentage than previously described by Chapman and colleagues.[28] Isolates from patients with pneumonia tended to have higher minimal inhibitory concentrations (MICs) with ampicillin. A study by Jordan and colleagues showed that disease-causing isolates of *M. catarrhalis* were more likely to be serum-resistant (43%) than colonizing (13%) strains, but bacteremic strains were no more serum-resistant than pneumonia-causing strains.[29] The mechanism of complement resistance seems to involve binding or inactivation of one of the terminal complement components or intermediates involved in the membrane attack complex; this resistance is abolished by trypsin treatment, suggesting that complement resistance is mediated by an *M. catarrhalis*–associated protein.[30]

The various phenotypic differences described by different authors (hemagglutination, beta-lactamase production, serum sensitivity) need to be correlated with the antigenic differences between outer membrane proteins described by Murphy and Loeb[14, 17] and the differences defined by restriction endonuclease methods described by Patterson and colleagues[31] to see if virulence is related to particular strains of the organism. At present it would seem that the ability of the organism to cause disease is both host- and microbe-related.

EPIDEMIOLOGY

Natural Reservoir and Colonization

Several studies have established that *M. catarrhalis* colonizes the nasopharynx of up to 7.4% of adults and 50%

of children.[32] Vaneechoutte and colleagues recovered this organism in 49.9% of saliva specimens of children aged 3–12 years.[33] Faden and colleagues evaluated a large cohort of infants, following them prospectively from birth to 2 years of age.[34] Of the 120 children evaluated at 13 routine visits, 66% were colonized by 1 year and 77.5% by 2 years. During visits for otitis media, the colonization rate increased to 63% compared with a rate of 27% during routine visits. Otitis-prone children were colonized on 44.4% of all visits compared with 16.7% of children who did not have otitis media. The study demonstrated that children tended to acquire and eliminate a number of different strains, and that intrafamilial spread of the same strain of *M. catarrhalis* was frequent. The study of Fadden and colleagues seemed to confirm previous observations from their group[35] and others[36, 37] that there was a relationship between the frequency of colonization and the development of otitis media, as well as a positive relationship between organisms recovered simultaneously in the nasopharynx and middle ear.

A seasonality in adult lower respiratory infection with *M. catarrhalis* is demonstrable,[38–41] with more infections occurring in the winter months.

Transmission

Restriction endonuclease typing has been applied to *M. catarrhalis.* Patterson and colleagues used three restriction enzymes in a study of a hospital outbreak of *M. catarrhalis* infection.[31] Seven isolates (from five patients and two staff members) appeared to be of the same clone, whereas four other isolates displayed different patterns. In a study of 14 other *M. catarrhalis* strains (not associated with the outbreak) it was noted that there were 12 different patterns.[31]

Murphy studied the outer membrane proteins (OMPs) of 50 strains of *M. catarrhalis* from different sources and noted a high degree of similarity in OMP patterns,[42] a somewhat surprising observation because OMPs of other gram-negatives organisms, both enteric organisms and *H. influenzae,* show more obvious differences in molecular weight.[14, 17, 42, 43] This work suggests that it will be possible to develop a serotyping system based on antigenic differences in LOSs of strains of *M. catarrhalis.* The conserved nature of the LOS raises the prospect of using the LOS molecule as a vaccine.[42, 43]

Other promising methods to study outbreaks include the API ZYM research kit, which suggests that most clinical isolates fall into three common patterns of enzyme production.[44] Sodium dodecyl sulfate polyacrylamide gel electrophoresis of whole-cell protein, together with immunoblotting with normal serum and restriction endonuclease analysis using the Taq 1 enzyme, was applied by Morgan and colleagues to 38 isolates in a suspected nosocomial outbreak[45]; the results, as with other studies of nosocomial outbreaks, suggested that several distinct strains were involved and that the combination of the three techniques described was sufficiently reproducible and discriminatory to constitute suitable investigative tools.

IMMUNITY

Patients with disorders of antibody production appear to be more susceptible to *M. catarrhalis* infection.[21] This suggests that immunity to *M. catarrhalis* is acquired during childhood and most adults have considerable protective immunity. Therefore, there has been considerable interest in antibody responses to *M. catarrhalis*. Additionally, demonstration of a rise in specific antibody against *M. catarrhalis* after putative infection is proof the organism is a significant pathogen and not a colonizer, and the test could potentially have diagnostic utility.

Various methods have been used to investigate antibody responses to *M. catarrhalis* in patients infected with the organism. Using complement-fixing technique, Brorson and Malmvall demonstrated complement-fixing antibodies in 25 of 97 patients with maxillary sinusitis and also in 1 of 20 healthy persons.[46] Using an immunodiffusion method, Eliasson found that 69% of 90 human serums had precipitating antibodies to a hot acid extract of *M. catarrhalis*.[47] In a study of children with otitis media caused by *M. catarrhalis* in which an enzyme immunoassay (EIA) was used (the whole organism serving as antigen), immunoglobulin G (IgG) and A (IgA) antibodies were found in the serums, and an increase in antibody titer was demonstrated when acute and convalescent serums were compared.[48] Chapman and colleagues used a bactericidal assay in patients with *M. catarrhalis* pneumonia or tracheobronchitis and found that 32% of acute-phase serums and 90% of convalescent-phase serums showed increasing bactericidal activity against *M. catarrhalis*.[28] Black and Wilson, studying patients with acute exacerbations of bronchitis, reported that convalescent serums had significantly higher titers than acute serums, which in turn had higher titers than serums from healthy controls.[49] Chi and colleagues, using an EIA with a hot acid–extracted protein antigen of *M. catarrhalis* (the P-protein), found acute-phase titers to be increased in patients with *M. catarrhalis* pneumonia or bronchitis when compared with healthy controls; convalescent serums showed increased antibody titers in 46% of pneumonia patients and 50% of tracheobronchitis patients.[50] Goldblatt and colleagues, using a whole-cell enzyme-linked immunosorbent assay (ELISA), showed that antibody to *M. catarrhalis* was first detectable around 4 years of age and was demonstrable in all healthy adults.[51] Their subsequent work has suggested that the recognition of antigen appears to be subclass-restricted to IgG3, and that antibodies directed against whole organisms and against OMPs may not be strain-specific.[52] Faden and colleagues studied the systemic and local antibody responses to *M. catarrhalis* in 14 children with otitis media; their data seemed to suggest that young children develop a local antibody response to *M. catarrhalis* in the middle ear during otitis media, but that they fail to develop systemic antibody in a uniform manner.[53]

Animal studies of *M. catarrhalis* pneumonia have shown that this organism elicits a striking neutrophil response in the murine lung, one that far exceeds that generated by other commensals[54]; McCracken's group in Dallas has identified a large conserved protein on the surface of *M. catarrhalis* that is a target for protective antibodies in a murine model; antibodies to this protein could be demonstrated in convalescent human serum but not acute-phase serum, indicating that strains growing in vivo express this molecule.[55]

The consensus of studies of immunity is that roughly half of all patients develop an antibody response after *M.* *catarrhalis* infection and that it is a weak immunologic stimulant. Since the initiation, frequency, and duration of nasopharyngeal colonization with *M. catarrhalis* is greater with this organism than with other potential middle ear pathogens, it is possible that a form of systemic tolerance to this organism develops. It appears unlikely from these studies that antibody testing will be of diagnostic value, since baseline antibody levels are present in healthy controls and a rise in convalescent titers does not occur consistently.

PATHOGEN IN EAR, NOSE, AND THROAT INFECTION

The clinical syndromes of otitis media, sinusitis, and mastoiditis are discussed in detail in subsequent chapters. The clinical picture of infection caused by *M. catarrhalis* and producing these syndromes is not unique and cannot be distinguished on clinical grounds. The syndrome of purulent tracheitis caused by this organism is confined to children[56–58] and may occur in a normal host.[59] For a review of lower respiratory infections the reader is referred to the reviews by Verghese and others.[1, 20, 38]

TREATMENT

From 80% to 90% of strains of *M. catarrhalis* produce beta-lactamase.[60] There is evidence that beta-lactamase production is a recent event in the history of this organism, and that older strains were penicillin-sensitive.[61, 62] Beta-lactamase production in *M. catarrhalis* was first noted in 1977 in Sweden, France, and England.[63–65]

The beta-lactamases of *M. catarrhalis* are termed BRO-1 and BRO-2; BRO-1 is found in approximately 90% of beta-lactamase producing strains of *M. catarrhalis*.[60, 66] The BRO enzymes are relatively weak enzymes, perhaps because they are strongly cell-associated.[67] Although they have a broad spectrum, they have their greatest effect against penicillin and ampicillin (a 256-fold increase in MICs) and less against the cephalosporins. Curiously, cefaclor is hydrolyzed by BRO-1 at a much higher rate than the older cephalosporin-like cephaloridine. Numerous studies have looked at the susceptibility of *M. catarrhalis* to common oral beta-lactam and non–beta-lactam agents.[68–73] Beta-lactamase–producing strains of *M. catarrhalis* are not necessarily labeled ampicillin-resistant by clinical microbiology laboratories.[60] Clinical evidence suggests that all beta-lactamase–producing strains of *M. catarrhalis* be considered resistant to penicillin and ampicillin regardless of their MIC.[60] Susceptibility testing of *M. catarrhalis* is both medium- and inoculum-dependent (as it is for *H. influenzae*). Tetracycline resistance was first reported in 1983 among isolates in Sweden; by 1988, rates of resistance of 15% and 43% were being reported from the Netherlands and China, and in that year tetracycline-resistant isolates, as well as erythromycin-resistant isolates, were reported in the United States.[74–76]

Beta-lactamase–producing strains are inhibited by ampicillin-clavulanic acid (MIC90 of 0.125 μg/mL), cefixime (MIC90 of 0.5 μg/mL), cefuroxime (MIC90 of 2.0 μg/mL), and cefaclor (MIC90 of 2.0 μg/mL), though the ability of the BRO-1 enzyme to break down cefaclor is noted above. Non–beta-lactam agents also show good activity against *M. catarrhalis*. Typical MIC90s (in micrograms per milliliter) for some commonly used agents are tetracycline, 0.5; trimethoprim-sulfamethoxazole, 0.25; ciprofloxacin, 0.015, and erythromycin, 0.25.

SUMMARY

M. catarrhalis is part of the normal oral flora and an important cause of otitis media in children. Organisms producing disease tend to colonize the oropharynx first; many different strains are responsible for clinical disease. Antigenicity seems to reside in the outer membrane protein, which is antigenically relatively conserved. The organism is most often beta-lactamase–producing; tetracycline and erythromycin resistance occurs sporadically.

References

1. Verghese A, Berk SL: *Moraxella (Branhamella) catarrhalis.* Infect Dis Clin North Am 1991; 5: 523–538.
2. Berk SL: From *Micrococcus* to *Moraxella*: The reemergence of *Branhamella catarrhalis.* Arch Intern Med 1990; 150: 2254–2257.
3. Gordon JE: The gram-negative cocci in colds and influenza. J Infect Dis 1921; 29: 462–494.
4. Osler W: The Principles and Practice of Medicine. Classics of Medicine Series. Birmingham, Alabama: Gryphon, 1978, p 512.
5. Cushing H: The life of Sir William Osler, vol 2. Oxford: Clarendon Press, 1952, p 672.
6. Catlin BW: *Branhamella catarrhalis*: An organism gaining respect as a pathogen. Clin Microbiol Rev 1990; 3: 293–320.
7. Catlin BW: Transfer of the organism named *Neisseria catarrhalis* to *Branhamella* gen. nov. Int J Syst Bacteriol 1970; 20: 155–159.
8. Bovre K: Family VIII. *Neisseriaceae* Prévot 1933, 119. In: Krieg NR, Holt JG (eds): Bergey's Manual of Systematic Bacteriology, vol. 1. Baltimore: Williams & Wilkins, 1984, pp 288–290.
9. Bovre K: Genus II. *Moraxella* Lwoff 1939, 173 emend. Henriksen and Bovre 1968, 391. In: Krieg NR, Holt JG (eds): Bergey's Manual of Systematic Bacteriology, vol. 1. Baltimore: Williams & Wilkins, 1984, pp 296–303.
10. Doern GV: *Branhamella catarrhalis*: Phenotypic characteristics. Am J Med 1990; 88(5A): 33S–35S.
11. Shurin PA, Marchant CD, Kim CH, et al.: Emergence of beta-lactamase-producing strains of *Branhamella catarrhalis* as important agents of acute otitis media. Pediatr Infect Dis J 1983; 2: 34–38.
12. Louie M, Ongsansoy EG, Forward KR: Rapid identification of *Branhamella catarrhalis*: A comparison of five rapid methods. Diagn Microbiol Infect Dis 1990; 13(3): 205–208.
13. Marrs CF, Weir S: Pili (fimbriae) of *Branhamella* species. Am J Med 1990; 88(5A): 36S–40S.
14. Murphy TF: The surface of *Branhamella catarrhalis*: A systematic approach to the surface antigens of an emerging pathogen. Pediatr Infect Dis J 1989; 8(suppl): S75–S77.
15. Wistreich GA, Baker RF: The presence of fimbriae (pili) in three species of *Neisseria.* J Gen Microbiol 1971; 65: 167–173.
16. Hellio R, Guibourdenche M, Collatz E, et al.: The envelope structure of *Branhamella catarrhalis* as studied by transmission electron microscopy. Ann Inst Pasteur Microbiol 1988; 139: 515–525.
17. Murphy TF, Loeb MR: Isolation of the outer membrane of *Branhamella catarrhalis.* Microb Pathog 1989; 6: 159–174.
18. Prellner K, Christensen P, Hoevlius B, Rosen C: Nasopharyngeal carriage of bacteria in otitis-prone and non-otitis-prone children in day centres. Acta Otolaryngol (Stockh) 1984; 98: 343–350.
19. Yamanaka N, Faden H: Antibody response to outer membrane protein of nontypable *H. influenzae* in otitis-prone children. J Pediatr 1993; 122: 212–218.
20. Hager H, Verghese A, Alvarez S, et al.: *Branhamella catarrhalis* respiratory infections. Rev Infect Dis 1987; 9: 1140–1149.
21. Karnad A, Alvarez S, Berk SL: *Branhamella catarrhalis* pneumonia in patients with immunoglobulin abnormalities. South Med J 1986; 79: 1360–1362.
22. Diamond LA, Lorber B: *Branhamella catarrhalis* pneumonia and immunoglobulin abnormalities: A new association. Am Rev Respir Dis 1984; 129: 876–878.
23. Srinivasan G, Raff MJ, Templeton WC, et al.: *Branhamella catarrhalis* pneumonia. Report of two cases and review of the literature. Am Rev Respir Dis 1981; 123: 553–555.
24. Cox PM Jr, Colloff E: *Neisseria catarrhalis* empyema in an immunodeficient host. Am Rev Respir Dis 1979; 120: 471–472.
25. McNeely DJ, Kitchens CS, Kluge RM: Fatal *Neisseria (Branhamella) catarrhalis* pneumonia in an immunodeficient host. Am Rev Respir Dis 1976; 114: 399–402.
26. Wong VK, Ross LA: *Branhamella catarrhalis* septicemia in an infant with AIDS. Scand J Infect Dis 1988; 20: 559–560.
27. Soto-Hernandez JL, Holtsclaw-Berk S, Harvill LM, et al.: Phenotypic characteristics of *Branhamella catarrhalis* strains. J Clin Microbiol 1989; 27: 903–908.
28. Chapman AJ, Musher DM, Jonsson S, et al.: Development of bactericidal antibody during *Branhamella catarrhalis* infection. J Infect Dis 1985; 151: 878–882.
29. Jordan KL, Berk SH, Berk SL: A comparison of serum bactericidal activity and phenotypic characteristics of bacteremic, pneumonia-causing strains, and colonizing strains of *Branhamella catarrhalis.* Am J Med; 1990; 88(5A): 28S–32S.
30. Verduin C, Jansze M, Hol C, et al.: Differences in complement activation between complement-resistant and complement-sensitive *Moraxella (Branhamella) catarrhalis* strains occur at the level of membrane attack complex formation. Infect Immun 1994; 62: 589–595.
31. Patterson JE, Patterson TF, Farrel P, et al: Evaluation of restriction endonuclease analysis as an epidemiologic typing system for *Branhamella catarrhalis.* J Clin Microbiol 1989; 27: 944–946.
32. Calder MA, Croughan MJ, McLeod DT, et al: The incidence and antibiotic susceptibility of *Branhamella catarrhalis* in respiratory infections. Drugs 1986; 31(suppl 3): 11–16.
33. Vaneechoutte M, Verschraegen G, Claeys G, et al.: Selective medium for *Branhamella catarrhalis* with acetazolamide as a specific inhibitor of *Neisseria* spp. J Clin Microbiol 1988; 26: 2544–2548.
34. Faden H, Yasuaki H, Hong J, et al.: Epidemiology of *Moraxella catarrhalis* in children during the first 2 years of life: Relationship to otitis media. J Infec Dis 1994; 169: 1312–1317.
35. Faden H, Stenievich J, Brodsky L, Bernstein J, Ogra PL: Changes in nasopharyngeal flora during otitis media of childhood. Pediatr Infec Dis J 1990; 9: 623–626.
36. Schwartz R, Rodriguez WJ, Mann R, et al.: The nasopharyngeal culture in acute otitis media: A reappraisal of its usefulness. JAMA 1979; 241: 2170–2173.
37. Dickinson DP, Loos BG, Dryja DM, Berstein JM: Restriction fragment mapping of *Branhamella catarrhalis*: A new tool for studying the epidemiology of this middle ear pathogen. J Infect Dis 1988; 158: 205–208.
38. Sarubbi FA, Myers JW, Williams JJ, et al.: Respiratory infections caused by *Branhamella catarrhalis.* Selected epidemiologic features. Am J Med 1990; 88(5A): 9S–14S.
39. McLeod DT, Ahmad F, Power JT, et al.: Bronchopulmonary infection due to *Branhamella catarrhalis.* Br Med J 1983; 287: 1446–1447.
40. Pollard JA, Wallace RJ Jr, Nash DR, et al.: Incidence of *Branhamella catarrhalis* in the sputa of patients with chronic lung disease. Drugs 1986; 31(suppl 3): 103–108.
41. McLeod DT, Ahmad F, Capewell S, et al.: Increase in bronchopulmonary infection due to *Branhamella catarrhalis.* Br Med J 1986; 292: 1103–1105.
42. Murphy TF: Studies of the outer membrane proteins of *Branhamella catarrhalis.* Am J Med 1990; 88(5A): 41S–45S.
43. Murphy TF, Bartos LC: Surface-exposed and antigenically conserved determinants of outer membrane proteins of *Branhamella catarrhalis.* Infect Immun 1989; 57: 2938–2941.
44. Peiris V, Heald J: Rapid method for differentiating strains of *Branhamella catarrhalis.* J Clin Pathol 1992; 45: 532–533.
45. Morgan M, McKenzie H, Enright M, et al.: Use of molecular methods to characterize *Moraxella catarrhalis* strains in a suspected outbreak of

nosocomial infection. Eur J Clin Microbiol Infect Dis 1992; 11: 305–312.

46. Brorson JE, Malmvall BE: *Branhamella catarrhalis* and other bacteria in the nasopharynx of children with longstanding cough. Scand J Infect Dis 1981; 13: 111–113.

47. Eliasson I: A protein antigen characteristic of *Branhamella catarrhalis.* Acta Pathol Microbiol Scand B 1980; 88: 281–286.

48. Leinonen M, Luotonen J, Herva E, et al.: Preliminary serologic evidence for a pathogenic role of *Branhamella catarrhalis.* J Infect Dis 1981; 144: 570–574.

49. Black AJ, Wilson TS: Immunoglobulin G (IgG) serological response to *Branhamella catarrhalis* in patients with acute bronchopulmonary infections. J Clin Pathol 1988; 41: 329–333.

50. Chi DS, Verghese A, Moore C, et al.: Antibody response to P-protein in patients with *Branhamella catarrhalis* infections. Am J Med 1990; 88(5A): 25S–27S.

51. Goldblatt D, Seymour ND, Levinsky RJ, et al.: An enzyme-linked immunosorbent assay for the determination of human IgG subclass antibodies directed against *Branhamella catarrhalis.* J Immunol Methods 1990; 128: 219–225.

52. Goldblatt D, Turner MW, Levinsky RJ: *Branhamella catarrhalis*: Antigenic determinants and the development of the IgG subclass response in childhood. J Infect Dis 1990; 162: 1128–1135.

53. Faden H, Hong J, Murphy T: Immune response to outer membrane antigens of *Moraxella catarrhalis* in children and otitis media. Infect Immun 1992; 60: 3824–3829.

54. Verghese A, Berro E, Berro J, et al.: Pulmonary clearance and phagocytic cell response in a murine model of *Branhamella catarrhalis* infection. J Infect Dis 1990; 162: 1189–1192.

55. Helminen M, Maciver I, Latimer J, et al.: A large, antigenically conserved protein on the surface of *Moraxella catarrhalis* is a target for protective antibodies. J Infect Dis 1994; 170: 867–872.

56. Ernst TN, Philp M: Bacterial tracheitis caused by *Branhamella catarrhalis.* Pediatr Infect Dis J 1987; 6: 574.

57. Wong VK, Mason WH: *Branhamella catarrhalis* as a cause of bacterial tracheitis. Pediatr Infect Dis J 1987; 6: 945–946.

58. Alligood GA, Kenny JF: Tracheitis and supraglottis associated with *Branhamella catarrhalis* and respiratory syncytial virus. Pediatr Infect Dis J 1989; 8: 190–191.

59. Singh RP, Marwaha RK: Fulminant *Branhamella catarrhalis* tracheitis. Ann Trop Paediatr 1990; 10: 221–222.

60. Wallace RJ Jr, Nash DR, Steingrube VA: Antibiotic susceptibilities and drug resistance in *Moraxella (Branhamella) catarrhalis.* Am J Med 1990; 88(5A): 46S–50S.

61. Baumann P, Doudoroff M, Stanier RY: Study of the *Moraxella* group: I. Genus *Moraxella* and the *Neisseria catarrhalis* group. J Bacteriol 1968; 95: 58–73.

62. Reyn A: Family I. *Neisseriaceae* Prevot 1933. In: Buchanan RE, Gibbons NE (eds): Bergey's Manual of Determinative Bacteriology, 8th ed. Baltimore: Williams & Wilkins Co, 1974, pp 427–423, 442–443.

63. Percival A, Corkill JE, Rowlands J, et al.: Pathogenicity of and beta-lactamase production by *Branhamella (Neisseria) catarrhalis.* Lancet 1977; 2: 1175.

64. Philippon A, Riou JY, Guibourdenche M, et al.: Detection, distribution and inhibition of *Branhamella catarrhalis* β-lactamases. Drugs 1986; 31(suppl 3): 64–69.

65. Malmvall BE, Brorsson JE, Johnsson J: In vitro sensitivity to pencillin V and beta lactamase production of *Branhamella catarrhalis.* J Antimicrob Chemother 1977; 3: 374–375.

66. Wallace RJ Jr, Steingrube VA, Nash DR, et al.: BRO β-lactamases of *Branhamella catarrhalis,* and *Moraxella* subgenus *Moraxella,* including evidence for chromosomal β-lactamase transfer by conjugation in *B. catarrhalis, M. nonliquefaciens,* and *M. lacunata.* Antimicrob Agents Chemother 1989; 33: 1845–1854.

67. Farmer T, Reading C: β-Lactamases of *Branhamella catarrhalis* and their inhibition by clavulanic acid. Antimicrob Agents Chemother 1982; 21: 506–508.

68. Sweeney KG, Verghese A, Needham CA: In vitro susceptibilities of isolates from patients with *Branhamella catarrhalis* pneumonia compared with those of colonizing strains. Antimicrob Agents Chemother 1985; 27: 499–502.

69. Alvarez S, Jones M, Holtsclaw-Berk S, et al.: In vitro susceptibilities and beta-lactamase production of 53 clinical isolates of *Branhamella catarrhalis.* Antimicrob Agents Chemother 1985; 27: 646–647.

70. Doern GV, Jones RN: Antimicrobial susceptibility testing of *Haemophilus influenzae, Branhamella catarrhalis,* and *Neisseria gonorrhoeae.* Antimicrob Agents Chemother, 1988; 32: 1747–1753.

71. Doern GV, Tubert T: Detection of β-lactamase activity among clinical isolates of *Branhamella catarrhalis* with six different β-lactamase assays. J Clin Microbiol 1987; 25: 1380–1383.

72. Doern GV, Tubert T: Effect of inoculum size on results of macrotube broth dilution susceptibility tests with *Branhamella catarrhalis.* J Clin Microbiol 1987; 25: 1576–1578.

73. Doern GV, Tubert T: In vitro activities of 39 antimicrobial agents for *Branhamella catarrhalis* and comparison of results with different quantitative susceptibility test methods. Antimicrob Agents Chemother 1988; 32: 259–261.

74. Kallings I: Sensitivity of *Branhamella catarrhalis* to oral antibiotics. Drugs 1986; 31(suppl 3): 17–22.

75. Davies BI, Maesen FP: The epidemiology of respiratory tract pathogens in southern Netherlands. Eur Respir J 1988; 1: 415–420.

76. Brown BA, Wallace RJ Jr, Flanagan CW, et al.: Tetracycline and erythromycin resistance among clinical isolates of *Branhamella catarrhalis.* Antimicrob Agents Chemother 1989; 33: 1631–1633.

CHAPTER TWENTY-ONE

Aldona L. Baltch
Raymond P. Smith

Pseudomonas aeruginosa and Aerobic Gram-Negative Bacilli

▼

Pseudomonas aeruginosa and other facultative and aerobic gram-negative bacilli are known to be pathogens or colonizers in ear, nose, and throat (ENT) infections. More common serious infections are those seen with *P. aeruginosa*. This chapter includes a discussion about these microorganisms, their pathogenetic factors, and a brief description of the infections they may cause. For more detailed descriptions of specific infections including these as well as other pathogens, the reader is referred to specific chapters of the book. The recent epidemiology of nosocomial ENT infections is given at the end of this chapter.

PSEUDOMONAS AERUGINOSA

P. aeruginosa is a ubiquitous organism, most capable of surviving in moist environments in nature as well as in hospitals.[1] It survives in exopolysaccharide slime layers, releasing planktonic forms from microcolonies.[2] A rare organism as a cause of infections in patients at the turn of the 20th century, during the past 40 years, *P. aeruginosa* has become one of the most significant and feared causes of infection in hospitalized patients. Although the overall rate of *P. aeruginosa* infections shows a minor decline since 1985, *P. aeruginosa* remains the fourth most commonly isolated pathogen in U.S. hospitals.[3]

P. aeruginosa infections continue to be most common in patients with neutropenia, intravascular monitoring devices, thermal injury, organ transplantation, or instrumentation of the genitourinary or respiratory tracts. A common preceding history of these patients includes immunosuppressive therapy and previous use of antimicrobial agents. Preceded by colonization with *P. aeruginosa,* these patients frequently develop infections with this organism. The mortality rate from serious *P. aeruginosa* infections remains high, as seen in bacteremia, in which mortality still reaches 30% to 60%.[4, 5]

Pseudomonas aeruginosa—The Microorganism

Of the many species of *Pseudomonas* described in Bergey's manual, only several are significant pathogens for humans. *P. aeruginosa* is the most common one. *Pseudomonas mallei* (*Burkholderia mallei*) and *Pseudomonas pseudomallei* (*Burkholderia pseudomallei*) are rarely observed causing disease in the Western world, whereas *Pseudomonas cepacia* (*Burkholderia cepacia*) and *Pseudomonas maltophilia* (*Stenotrophomonas maltophilia*) are opportunistic pathogens observed in patients with cystic fibrosis or hospitalized patients with decreased host defenses.

P. aeruginosa is a non–spore-forming, gram-negative slender rod. It is 1–5 μm in length and 0.5–1 μm in width. Figure 21–1 depicts the glycocalix surrounding the organism. *P. aeruginosa* usually has a single polar flagellum and multiple pili. It is motile, is aerobic, and requires oxygen for

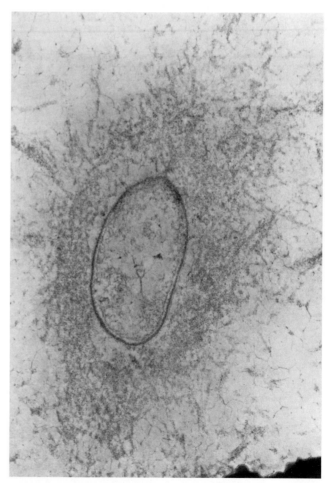

Figure 21–1. Electron micrograph of a section of ruthenium red-stained glycocalix of *Pseudomonas aeruginosa*. (From Doggett RG [ed]: *Pseudomonas aeruginosa*: Clinical Manifestations of Infection and Current Therapy. New York: Academic Press, 1979.)

the production of its toxins. In 1882 Géssard identified *P. aeruginosa* from wounds of patients showing "blue pus."[6]

P. aeruginosa is an opportunist. It can be a pathogen for humans, animals, insects, and plants. Because its growth requirements are simple, it can use inorganic carbon sources for proliferation. Selective media containing cetyltrimethylammonium bromide (cetrimide) may assist the laboratory in the isolation of *P. aeruginosa*, especially the nonpigmented forms. Although a number of colonial types may be observed on agar, the usually characteristic pigmentation and fruity odor of aminoacetophenone are well known to the microbiologist. Mucoid colonies frequently observed in patients with cystic fibrosis are usually nonpigmented. *P. aeruginosa* is the only bacterial species known to produce a pigment, called pyocyanin. This is a water-soluble, blue, nonfluorescent phenazine pigment that is soluble in chloroform. Magnesium, potassium, glycerol, and iron increase the production of this pigment. A yellow-green, also water-soluble fluorescent pigment that is insoluble in chloroform, is called pyoverdin. Iron-deficient media stimulate its production. Intense green fluorescence is observed when culture plates are observed under an ultraviolet light (wavelength ~245 nm). Various other pigment combinations are also seen, i.e., pyorubin (red) or pyomelin (brown to black). Salts of fatty acids released by autolysis from crystals cause the iridescent patches with a metallic sheen on culture plates.

P. aeruginosa is indophenol oxidase–positive, and it does not ferment glucose or other carbohydrates in media with high nitrogen content. It characteristically grows at 42 °C. Other fluorescent members of *Pseudomonas*, i.e., *Pseudomonas fluorescens, Pseudomonas putida,* will not grow at this temperature. In contrast, these organisms grow at 4 °C, whereas *P. aeruginosa* may not.[7] Resistance or the acquisition of resistance to various antimicrobial agents is well known to the clinician interested in *P. aeruginosa.* This resistance may be related to enzyme production (beta-lactamases), a permeability barrier, inadequate transport of antimicrobials, and other reasons.

Pathogenesis of *P. aeruginosa* Infections

The interaction of the host with *P. aeruginosa* is a complex process that includes adherence, replication and persistence, and tissue injury.[8] As well pointed out by Woods and Vasil,[8] the number and types of *P. aeruginosa* virulence factors are truly surprising. Historically, early descriptions of serious disseminated *P. aeruginosa* infections usually concerned children, and the infections were marked by diarrhea and cutaneous manifestations.[9] In 1894, Williams and Cameron described an enterotoxin from *P. aeruginosa.*[10] In the past 30 years, severe disseminated *P. aeruginosa* infections have usually occurred in adults and have rarely been accompanied by gastrointestinal or cutaneous manifestations such as ecthyma gangrenosum.[11] *P. aeruginosa* infections today are usually nosocomial in origin and occur in immunocompromised hosts such as those with malignancies, neutropenia, burns, and transplants, and in intensive care unit (ICU) patients receiving prolonged multiple antibiotic therapy. In *P. aeruginosa* infections of ENT patients, both nosocomial infections (sinusitis in intubated patients in the ICU) and community-acquired infections (malignant external otitis; sinusitis in cystic fibrosis patients) are described.

Table 21–1 lists the cell wall–associated factors and exoproducts (virulence factors) that may be released from *P. aeruginosa* in both localized and systemic infections.

Table 21–1. PATHOGENIC FACTORS OF *Pseudomonas aeruginosa*

Adhesins
Flagella
Siderophores, iron-binding proteins (pyochelin, pyoverdin)
Mucoexopolysaccharide, alginate
Lipopolysaccharide (LPS, endotoxin)
Exotoxin A
Exoenzyme S
Cytotoxin
Phospholipase C (heat-labile hemolysin, nonhemolytic phospholipase C)
Heat-stable hemolysin
Proteases (lasA, lasB, alkaline protease)
Others: pyocyanin, phytotoxic factor, hydrocyanic acid

Adhesins

The currently known *P. aeruginosa* adhesion to cells occurs through pili and nonpilus adhesion.[12, 13] The bacteria bind to mucosal surfaces that are not covered by fibronectin.[14] Antibodies to pili (polyclonal and monoclonal) inhibit this interaction, which is usually irreversible.[15] Three gangliosides have been identified as possible receptors.[16] Nonpilus adhesins and exoenzyme S (ADP-ribosyl transferase exoproduct) may also contribute to the adhesive properties of *P. aeruginosa* to epithelial cells.[17]

Flagella

The motility and persistence of *P. aeruginosa* may depend on its usually polar flagella. A mutant aflagellar strain demonstrated decreased virulence in an animal model.[18] The motility of *P. aeruginosa* may be an important factor in the spread of infection.[19]

Siderophores, Iron-Binding Proteins

Pyochelin and pyoverdin are *P. aeruginosa* siderophores (iron chelators) that allow survival of the organism in environments with poor iron resources.[20] They are complex organic compounds. It has been demonstrated that the outer membrane protein of *P. aeruginosa* may serve as a receptor for pyochelin.[21] Thus, *P. aeruginosa* is capable of overcoming the host defenses that have iron in forms of lactoferrin or transferrin; by secreting siderophores, the bacteria can have the available iron chelated and can use it for their own function and growth. Furthermore, one of the *P. aeruginosa* toxins, exotoxin A, is produced in greater quantities when *P. aeruginosa* is grown in iron-deficient medium.[22]

Mucoexopolysaccharides (Slime, Alginate)

Two high-molecular-weight polysaccharides (slime and alginate) are produced by *P. aeruginosa.*[23, 24] These polysaccharides, which are loosely bound to the bacterial surface, can interfere with the phagocytosis of *P. aeruginosa* (Fig. 21–1).[25, 26] The development of mucoid strains with large quantities of alginate are noted in cystic fibrosis patients with pulmonary infections.[27] These mucoid colonies revert to nonmucoid ones on laboratory media. Recently, Woods and colleagues demonstrated the conversion of a nonmucoid phenotype to a mucoid one in vivo.[28]

ADP-Ribosyl Transferases (Exotoxin A and Exoenzyme S)

Exotoxin A. Exotoxin A is an ADP-ribosyl transferase toxin of *P. aeruginosa.*[29] It is produced by about 95% of the strains.[30] Its mode of action is similar to that of diphtheria toxin, and it includes inhibition of protein synthesis by a nicotinamide adenine dinucleotide (NAD) dependent adenosine diphosphate (ADP) ribosylation of elongation factor 2. Exotoxin A–deficient mutants are less pathogenic.[31] Antibody to exotoxin A protects the experimental animal. Like staphylococcal enterotoxins, exotoxin A has been classified as a "superantigen," capable of inducing the production of interleukin-1 and acting as a T-cell mitogen.[32] These cytokines may further promote the detrimental effects of *P. aeruginosa* exoproducts on the already-immunocompromised hosts. Although previously published work indicated that antibody to exotoxin A was associated with better survival in *P. aeruginosa* bacteremia,[33] more recent studies were unable to demonstrate similar observations.[34] High antibody levels to lipopolysaccharide (LPS) were associated with better survival of patients in both studies.

Exoenzyme S. Exoenzyme S is the second ADP-ribosyl transferase toxin of *P. aeruginosa.*[35] Rather than ADP-ribosylating elongation factor 2, however, it modifies various eukaryotic cell proteins including the cytoskeletal protein of these cells. When immunologic techniques are used, exoenzyme S appears to be produced by 90% of the strains, but direct evidence for toxin production has been demonstrated by 40% of *P. aeruginosa* isolates.[36] Mutants unable to produce exoenzyme S appear to be less pathogenic to experimental animals.[37]

Cytotoxin

Cytotoxin is a tissue injury–causing toxin of *P. aeruginosa.*[38] It is localized in the periplasmic space of the bacterium and, like staphylococcal alpha toxin, it causes pore formation in most eukaryotic cell membranes.[39, 40] Cytotoxin can decrease granulocyte function, but it has no effect on serum or complement.[41] Furthermore, it is known to cause leukotriene B$_4$ (LTB$_4$) generation, which is abolished by specific arachidonic acid inhibitors.[42] A cytotoxin-deficient mutant was less pathogenic for leukopenic mice.[43] Protection by antibody to cytotoxin was clearly demonstrated in this animal model. Better survival of bacteremic patients with high levels of antibody to cytotoxin has been demonstrated.[34] As with other *P. aeruginosa* virulence factors, high serum antibody concentrations are observed in cystic fibrosis patients.[44] By immunologic techniques, all *P. aeruginosa* isolates tested in one study were cytotoxin-positive.[45] The prevalence of the cytotoxin gene, however, has been difficult to demonstrate in these strains. The possibility that cytotoxin gene heterogeneity may exist is currently under investigation. The finding that the cytotoxin gene in the PA158 strain of *P. aeruginosa* is carried on a temperate bacteriophage may also indicate a reason for the differences in the production of cytotoxin by different *P. aeruginosa* strains.[46]

Endotoxin (Lipopolysaccharide)

As a gram-negative organism, *P. aeruginosa* possesses endotoxin, or lipopolysaccharides, as a part of the bacterial cell wall. It has three components: O-specific polymeric side chains, core oligosaccharide, and lipid A. Although toxic LPS properties are related to lipid A, the O-antigen is both strain-specific and species-specific. LPS causes the production of cytokines, including tumor necrosis factor α (TNF-α), which can lead to the clinical presentation of septic shock.[47] Antibody to LPS is known to opsonize bacteria and increase the phagocytic properties of phagocytes. *P. aeruginosa* LPS has as yet been studied inadequately.[48–50] *P. aeruginosa* LPS has cellular, biologic, and molecular activities similar to those of LPS of many other gram-negative organisms. However, biochemically *P. aeruginosa* LPS is more heterogeneous than the LPS of *Salmonella*. Differences have been observed in the lipid A protein and the concentration of phosphorus in the LPS molecule of *P. aeruginosa*. Some investigators have questioned the potency of *P. aeruginosa* LPS, because its LD$_{50}$ (50% lethal dose) varies from 20 to 450 μg.[51] The possibility that the pathogenicity of *P. aeruginosa* LPS is increased in the presence of exotoxin A has recently been suggested.[22] Antibody to LPS of *P. aeruginosa* is both serotype-dependent and protective. Thus, although similarities do exist in the various LPS effects of *P. aeruginosa* and those of LPS of other gram-negative bacteria (pyrogenicity, immunogenicity, macrophage activation, complement activation, production of Shwartzman reaction), a number of differences in the characterization and activities of *P. aeruginosa* LPS from those of other gram-negative organisms have been recognized.

Hemolysins

Two hemolysins are produced by *P. aeruginosa*. The heat-labile hemolysin, phospholipase C, acts on lung surfactant.[52] It may also be responsible for the induction of alginate production. *P. aeruginosa* isolates from blood cultures and urinary tract isolates are greater producers of this enzyme.[53] Phospholipase C is produced by all *P. aeruginosa* isolates studied to date. Antibody production against this enzyme occurs in humans.[54] Phospholipase C can cause severe inflammation, increased vascular permeability, dermal necrosis, platelet aggregation, adverse effects on macrophages, and death.[55] The inflammatory reaction due to this enzyme may be a result of the activation of arachidonic acid. Deletion of the phospholipase C gene causes loss of virulence.[56]

The heat-stable glycolipid hemolysin has an adverse effect on cilial motion and can emulsify phosphatides present in eukaryotic cell membranes.[57] Another phospholipase with no known hemolytic action on human or sheep erythrocytes has been described.[58]

Proteases

P. aeruginosa produces three proteases: alkaline protease, lysine-specific protease, and elastase. These enzymes cause hemorrhage and necrosis; degrade mucins; inhibit chemotaxis, bactericidal activities of phagocytes, and lymphocyte proliferation; and cleave interleukin-2.[59–61] Approximately 90% of *P. aeruginosa* are protease producers. Two gene-encoded proteins of *P. aeruginosa* protease have activity on elastin. LasA can "nick" elastin, and lasB allows better access to the elastin itself.[62] In addition to the degradation of elastin, elastase degrades immunoglobulins, complement, basement membranes, human collagen, laminin, and human α1 protease inhibitor. By its effect on the fifth component of complement (C_5), elastase causes the production of C_{5a}, a substance causing the attraction of polymorphonuclear leukocytes, and thus contributing to the inflammation caused by *P. aeruginosa*.[63] Alkaline protease, lysine-specific protease, and elastase may all work in concert. Their local effects on lung and skin may be especially important. However, antibody concentrations to protease or elastase in *P. aeruginosa* bacteremia do not correlate with patient survival.[34]

Specific Ear, Nose, and Throat Infections Caused by *Pseudomonas aeruginosa*

Serious *P. aeruginosa* infections most commonly occur in hospitalized patients who are immunocompromised and/or seriously ill in ICUs. However, ENT infections due to *P. aeruginosa* are commonly community-acquired. Special reference must be given to malignant external otitis, perichondritis, simple external otitis, and chronic otitis media with otorrhea.[64] Other serious *P. aeruginosa* infections are those related to sinuses, especially maxillary sinuses, in intubated patients or those with nasogastric tubes in ICUs.[65] Patients with cystic fibrosis may have sinusitis in addition to pulmonary infections.[66] Only a brief description and treatment of these entities is provided in this chapter. The reader is referred to Chapters 35, 36, 38, and 41 for details of these infections.

Ear Infections

Malignant External Otitis. This infection was originally described in 1959 as osteomyelitis of the temporal bone,[67] but the term *malignant otitis externa* was used by Chandler in 1968.[68] This disease is rare in children, and it usually occurs in immunocompromised patients, i.e., elderly diabetic patients.[64, 69] Microangiopathy, trauma, and colonization of the external ear canal, in some cases after aural canal irrigation with unsterile water, are possible predisposing factors to this serious infection. These patients present with severe pain, otorrhea, and the presence of granulation tissue in the ear canal, but they usually have an intact tympanic membrane. Cranial nerve paralysis can occur. Brain abscess, meningitis, and dural sinus thrombosis are ominous complications. Although other microorganisms may be found in the otorrheic fluid, *P. aeruginosa* is virtually always there. Isolation of the organism and appropriate antimicrobial susceptibility studies should be performed. Any involvement of the bone must be determined by computed tomography (CT) scans, and in some cases by magnetic resonance imaging (MRI).[69, 70] Historically, the treatment of this disease entity was surgical, but currently proper antibiotic administration has altered the need for drastic surgery. Indeed, the use of fluoroquinolones, i.e., the currently available ciprofloxacin, has been quite successful.[71] The use of proper beta-lactams with aminoglycosides should be considered for patients infected with quinolone-resistant *P. aeruginosa* or in those with other serious complications listed above. The use of hyperbaric oxygen is currently being evaluated.[72]

Simple External Otitis. Isolation of *P. aeruginosa* from acute external otitis fluid is common and occurs in 49% of patients with external otitis.[73] Prolonged exposure to water is notorious in most of these cases. This infection is painful. The ear canal may be occluded because of swelling, and there may be cervical adenopathy. Treatment is usually directed to cleansing of the ear canal and placement of a "wick" containing 2% acetic acid with hydrocortisone for at least 48 hours. Topical antipseudomonal agents are also used. Although antistaphylococcal agents are frequently prescribed, careful follow-up of the patient who is not improving should direct the clinician to obtain a culture and to consider systemic antipseudomonal antibiotics.

Auricular Perichondritis. This infection has been described after ear piercing.[74, 75] Perichondritis occurs also in patients with burns, after resection of the auricle, or as a complication of malignant external otitis.[76] Pain, redness, and swelling of the ear can be associated with systemic symptoms. Cultures and sensitivity studies are indicated. The use of appropriate antipseudomonal antibiotics usually causes a resolution of the infection; if untreated, auricular chondritis can lead to severe disfigurement of the ear.

Chronic Otitis Media with Otorrhea. This *P. aeruginosa* infection is most common in children. It likely is associated with an immature or underdeveloped eustachian tube.[77] Otorrhea and a tympanic membrane perforation are seen in the clinical presentation. Because otitis media is rarely caused by *P. aeruginosa*, chronic otitis media with tympanic membrane perforation is most commonly related to previous colonization of the external ear canal with *P. aeruginosa*.[78] Although some patients are cured with effective antipseudmonal antibiotics, many relapse and may require mastoidectomy or other surgical procedures. Many of these patients have a history of middle ear infections and tympanic membrane perforation with poor healing. Because this disease entity requires the exclusion of a cholesteatoma, a CT scan and an audiologic evaluation of the patient's hearing may be in order. The treatment of chronic otitis media with otorrhea remains a dilemma. In the presence of otorrhea, chronic tympanic membrane perforation and an edematous external ear canal, most clinicians carefully culture the fluid and treat the patient with an appropriate oral antipseudomonal antibiotic. Should this approach fail, systemic antipseudomonal therapy and possibly surgery may be indicated.

Sinuses

Recently, *P. aeruginosa* sinusitis has been identified as an important acute ENT infection in ICU patients who are intubated or have nasogastric tubes.[65] Fever, leukocytosis, and fluid, usually in the maxillary sinus, have been recognized in such patients. The tube should be removed and appropriate systemic antipseudomonal antibiotics given. The occasional need for surgical drainage should be recognized.

Maxillary or even pansinusitis due to *P. aeruginosa* is known to occur in patients with acquired immunodeficiency syndrome (AIDS).[79–82] In these patients, infections of the sinuses are very difficult to treat, but early recognition and proper antibiotic and surgical attention may be helpful to the patient. In a trauma unit, sinusitis in patients with facial injuries is an important nosocomial *P. aeruginosa* infection. In one study, of the 32 patients with facial injuries and sinusitis, 11 were associated with *P. aeruginosa*.[83]

P. aeruginosa has been recognized as a pathogen in 1%–5% of chronic sinusitis patients.[84] Bone involvement should be determined by CT and/or MRI studies. The presence of *P. aeruginosa* in chronic sinusitis should be approached aggressively with both medical (proper antipseudomonal antibiotics) and surgical therapy. Chronic sinusitis with *P. aeruginosa* as the pathogen has also been recognized in patients with cystic fibrosis.[66, 85]

Throat

The presence of *P. aeruginosa* in the throat is usually related to colonization of the airway or acquisition of this organism in a nosocomial setting, especially while undergoing antimicrobial therapy for an infection elsewhere in the body. In one study, 3% of the patients had *P. aeruginosa* in the throat on admission.[86] Acquisition of the organism in the gastrointestinal (GI) tract usually occurs within 4–5 weeks after admission, and it is observed in at least 11% of the patients.[86] Attention should be given to such patients, especially if they are neutropenic, because of possible invasion of this organism from the GI tract into the systemic circulation. Prevention of colonization is most important, because treatment is usually ineffective.[87] Therefore, foods such as lettuce, tomatoes, or fresh fruit should be eliminated from the diets of such patients.

Wound Infections

P. aeruginosa can occur as a colonizer or a pathogen in patients who have undergone extensive surgical procedures of the throat, sinuses, nose, or ears. The epidemiology of nosocomial ENT infections is discussed at the end of this chapter. Because *P. aeruginosa* can be an aggressive pathogen, once the diagnosis of a soft tissue infection is made, therapy with an appropriate beta-lactam antimicrobial plus an aminoglycoside, with proper attention to surgical débridement, should be used.

Other *Pseudomonas, Burkholderia* and *Stenotrophomonas* Infections

Based on ribosomal RNA homology, a reclassification of the genus *Pseudomonas* has been described.[88] These changes and new names have been published, but some of them have not yet been confirmed by the International Committee on Nomenclature. The *Pseudomonas* genus now includes *Pseu-*

domonas aeruginosa, Pseudomonas fluorescens, Pseudomonas putida, Pseudomonas stutzeri, Pseudomonas alcaligenes, Pseudomonas pseudoalkaligenes, Pseudomonas species strain CDC Group 1, *Pseudomonas diminuta,* and *Pseudomonas vesicularis.* Other species are now in the genus *Burkholderia.* They are *Burkholderia pseudomallei, Burkholderia mallei, Burkholderia cepacia, Burkholderia gladioli,* and *Burkholderia picketti. Pseudomonas maltophilia,* later called *Xanthomonas maltophilia,* is now named *Stenotrophomonas maltophilia.*

Most of these organisms thrive in moist environments, including water and soil, but they can also be pathogens causing systemic or organ infections, as seen especially in patients with cystic fibrosis and in bone marrow transplant units. It is important for the clinician to be aware of these organisms, because of their marked difference in antimicrobial susceptibilities when compared with *P. aeruginosa.* Proper knowledge of the antimicrobial susceptibility patterns for these microbes is essential for the treatment of such nosocomial (sporadic or epidemic) and community-acquired *Pseudomonas, Burkholderia,* or *Stenotrophomonas* infections.

Therapy of *Pseudomonas aeruginosa* Infections

Antimicrobial Therapy

A number of beta-lactam drugs including cephalosporins, penicillins and carbapenems, aminoglycosides, and quinolones have been used successfully for therapy of *P. aeruginosa* infections (Table 21–2). In treating patients with serious *P. aeruginosa* infections, one has to choose effective therapy, frequently in combinations, without delay, even within hours. If the infection is nosocomial, appropriate review of the

Table 21–2. BETA-LACTAM, AMINOGLYCOSIDE, AND FLUOROQUINOLONE ANTIBACTERIAL AGENTS FOR TREATMENT OF *Pseudomonas aeruginosa* INFECTIONS

Penicillins	Aminoglycosides
Piperacillin	Tobramycin
Azlocillin	Amikacin
Mezlocillin	Gentamicin
Ticarcillin	Netilmicin
Carbenicillin	Isepamicin†
Cephalosporins	**Fluoroquinolones**
Ceftazidime	Ciprofloxacin
Cefepime*	Sparfloxacin*
Cefpirome*	Levofloxacin*
Cefsulodin†	
FK037*	
Monobactams	
Aztreonam	
Carbapenems	
Imipenem	
Meropenem*	
Biapenem*	

*Investigational
†Not available in the United States.

particular susceptibilities of the *P. aeruginosa* isolates in the hospital is essential, because of increasing resistance to antibacterial agents. The clinical data for monotherapy are inadequate, and therefore in most serious *P. aeruginosa* infections, a beta-lactam plus aminoglycoside combination is recommended.[89] The efficacy of the addition of rifampin to this combination is still in question and needs to be evaluated further in both clinical and experimental studies.[90, 91] Carbapenems, singly or in combination with aminoglycosides, are generally used in specific cases where resistance to antipseudomonal penicillins or cephalosporins is observed.[92] Although the significance of in vitro demonstration of synergy between the beta-lactams and aminoglycosides is still in question, few if any clinicians would choose monotherapy in serious *P. aeruginosa* infections. More recently, the use of fluoroquinolones, especially ciprofloxacin, has made a considerable impact in the therapy of malignant external otitis.[69, 71] Unfortunately, its wide general use has resulted in increasing numbers of strains resistant to this and other quinolones. The use of combinations of quinolones and beta-lactams or aminoglycosides has not been adequately evaluated to date. Therapy for serious *P. aeruginosa* infections should be prolonged (weeks) with careful follow-up for possible recurrence in ENT and other infections.

Immunotherapy and Immunoprophylaxis

Vaccines and polyclonal and monoclonal antibodies are being evaluated for the prevention and treatment of *P. aeruginosa* infections. Although the use of specific *P. aeruginosa* exoproduct antibody appears to be effective and protective in experimental animals, such studies are limited in humans. To date, antibody to LPS, cytotoxin, and toxin A correlates with better patient survival in *P. aeruginosa* bacteremia.[33, 34] Hyperimmune intravenous gamma globulin from subjects previously immunized with *P. aeruginosa* O (LPS)/toxin A antigens (O-PS-toxin A) and *Klebsiella* capsular polysaccharide vaccine is currently being studied in ICU patients.[93] Studies are continuing on the effectiveness of immunoglobulins prepared from screened plasma units of subjects demonstrating high concentrations of *P. aeruginosa* antibody to Fisher immunotypes 1, 2, 4, and 6.[94, 95] The use of monoclonal antibodies to mucoid exopolysaccharide, outer membrane proteins, flagella, core polysaccharide of LPS, O-antigen, and others is under study in animal models. Early vaccine studies based on *P. aeruginosa* LPS were associated with considerable side effects. Other vaccines including the 16-valent *P. aeruginosa* vaccine (PEV-1) were evaluated in animals and humans.[96] Currently an octavalent vaccine is being studied.[97] Other vaccines to various exoproducts of *P. aeruginosa*, pili, ribosomes, and outer membrane proteins are under investigation. The E5 murine monoclonal antibody evaluation in patients with gram-negative sepsis, including *P. aeruginosa*, is still under study.[98] Cytokines, including TNF-α, have been only minimally studied in *P. aeruginosa* infections.[99]

Thus, therapy of serious *P. aeruginosa* infections is complex. The prevention of colonization and infection remain most essential for both hospitalized and community patients. A multifactorial approach outlined in this chapter may be of importance in reducing and controlling *P. aeruginosa* infections.

FACULTATIVE AND AEROBIC GRAM-NEGATIVE BACTERIA

Gram-negative bacteria cause a variety of community-acquired and nosocomial ENT infections. The purpose of this section is to briefly review the medically important microbiology of important or unusual gram-negative bacteria other than *P. aeruginosa* in ENT infections and briefly describe the presentation and diagnosis of ENT infections caused by unusual facultative or aerobic gram-negative bacteria.

Microbiology and Virulence

Gram-negative bacteria are described morphologically by selected biochemical reactions and according to growth and nutrient requirements. Bacteria described as *aerobic* grow in an environment containing modest amounts of oxygen and high reduction-oxidation potential. *Facultative* gram-negative bacteria grow well in either aerobic or *anaerobic* environments.[100] This is important in ENT infections, because many chronic or nosocomial infections are the result of mixed infections and predisposing conditions that promote the growth of aerobic, facultative, and strictly anaerobic organisms (see Chapter 22).

The structural differences between gram-negative bacteria and gram-positive bacteria can be described briefly: gram-negative bacteria have a "thinner" cell wall, differing in peptidoglycan composition from that of gram-positive bacteria, and have a unique outer membrane (external to the cell wall) composed of lipopolysaccharide, outer membrane proteins, and pili or fimbriae, which can be attachment factors to mucosae.[101] Like gram-positive organisms associated with ENT infections (e.g., *Streptococcus pneumoniae*), gram-negative bacteria can also have a carbohydrate capsule external to the outer "membrane." The single most important virulence factor for most gram-negative bacteria is outer membrane LPS.[102] Endotoxin activity resides in LPS, which is released during bacterial growth. Endotoxin is a critical first messenger in the initiation of inflammatory responses, primarily by stimulating cells to synthesize and release the proinflammatory cytokines TNF-α, interleukin-1, interleukin-6, and interleukin-8.[102] Endotoxin also induces the lipoxygenase pathway of arachidonic acid metabolism in host cell membranes, causing the production of LTB_4, a potent chemotactic factor for polymorphonuclear leukocytes.[102] The resulting intense local inflammatory response is especially important in such ENT infections as otitis and sinusitis, in which closed spaces lined by mucosa are the sites of infection. Gram-negative bacteria may also produce a variety of toxins (as illustrated by *P. aeruginosa* earlier in this chapter); factors that allow the invasion of cells, such as that seen in *Shigella*; or factors that prevent phagocytosis or intracellular killing by phagocytes, as with *Legionella*. Examples of gram-negative bacteria found in ENT infections are seen in Tables 21–3 and 21–4. These are not comprehensive lists of all gram-negative bacteria.

Growth requirements for gram-negative bacteria vary tremendously. Appropriate conditions for bacterial isolation are listed in Tables 21–3 and 21–4 as well as in the text. It is always important to inform the microbiology and surgical

Table 21–3. MICROBIOLOGIC FEATURES OF SOME FACULTATIVE GRAM-NEGATIVE BACTERIA IMPORTANT IN OTOLARYNGOLOGIC INFECTIONS

Microorganism	Characteristics and Virulence Factors	Relevance to ENT Infection	Culture Needs
Enterobacteriaceae	Facultative	Almost never primary or sole pathogens	Blood agar, MacConkey's agar
Escherichia coli	Capsule, endotoxin, hemolysins	Chronic sinusitis, otitis Nosocomial sinusitis, otitis	Blood agar, MacConkey's agar
Klebsiella pneumoniae and *Klebsiella oxytoca*	Capsule, endotoxin (recognized as airway pathogens)	Chronic sinusitis, otitis Nosocomial sinusitis, otitis	Blood agar, MacConkey's agar
Klebsiella rhinoscleromatis	Capsule	Cause of scleroma	Blood agar, MacConkey's agar
Klebsiella ozaenae	No known factors	Cause of ozena (atrophic rhinitis)	Blood agar, MacConkey's agar
Enterobacter, Serratia, Citrobacter species (spp.)	Endotoxin	Nosocomial sinusitis, otitis (intubated patients)	Blood agar, MacConkey's agar
Proteus spp.	Endotoxin, motility	Chronic otitis externa, media (as part of polymicrobial infection)	Blood agar, MacConkey's agar
Yersinia pestis	Endotoxin, intracellular invasion	Plague: cervical bubo	Blood agar, MacConkey's agar
Yersinia enterocolitica	Intracellular invasion	Acute or chronic sinusitis	Blood agar, MacConkey's agar
Vibrionaceae	Facultative		
Vibrio parahaemolyticus *Vibrio vulnificus* *Vibrio alginolyticus*	Saltwater	Otitis externa, media	Thiocitrate bile salts agar
Pasteurellaceae	Facultative		
Pasteurella multocida	Endotoxin, capsule	Sinusitis, otitis (rare)	Blood agar, MacConkey's agar
Haemophilus influenzae	Capsule, outer membrane proteins, lipo-oligosaccharide	Epiglottitis, sinusitis, otitis	Chocolate agar, high CO_2 levels
Haemophilus spp.	Outer membrane proteins	Sinusitis, otitis	Chocolate agar

ENT, ear, nose, and throat.

pathology laboratories of the diagnosis under consideration when specimens are submitted.

Facultative Gram-Negative Bacilli

Enterobacteriaceae

The Enterobacteriaceae are an extremely varied group of facultative, glucose-fermenting, oxidase-negative, small-to-plump gram-negative bacteria, usually found in the GI tract.[103] In ENT infections, the Enterobacteriaceae are usually opportunistic pathogens. Most Enterobacteriaceae are found in small numbers in chronic infection (otitis, sinusitis, mastoiditis) along with other more common bacterial causes of ENT infection[104–111] and appear to follow tissue injury from other infections, trauma, alteration of normal clearance mechanisms, or extreme impairment of immune defenses. Although Enterobacteriaceae possess unique mechanisms for attachment to GI and urinary mucosae, they generally lack tropism for the mucosa of the upper respiratory tract. Enterobacteriaceae probably contribute to ENT disease primarily by releasing endotoxin, a structural component of the external cell envelope.[101] Some genera produce cytotoxic enzymes, hemolysins, and preoteolytic enzymes, but the role of these products in pathogenesis is very poorly understood in comparison to that seen with *P. aeruginosa*.

Enterobacteriaceae are found with differing frequency as causes of nosocomial sinusitis and otitis, well-recognized problems in adult and pediatric patients with indwelling endotracheal or nasogastric tubes.[112] Sepsis occurs in severe

Table 21–4. MICROBIOLOGIC FEATURES OF SOME AEROBIC GRAM-NEGATIVE BACTERIA IMPORTANT IN OTOLARYNGOLOGIC INFECTIONS

Organisms	Characteristics and Virulence Factors	Relevance to ENT Infection	Culture Needs
Francisella tularensis	Cell wall, capsule	Tularemia with oropharyngeal and cervical involvement	Cysteine-enriched media; buffered charcoal yeast extract agar
Legionella species (spp)	Intracellular survival and growth	Occasional sinusitis (nosocomial)	Buffered charcoal yeast extract agar
Neisseriaceae			
Neisseria meningitidis	Endotoxin, capsule, outer membrane proteins	Nasopharyngitis, sepsis from pharynx	Chocolate agar
Neisseria gonorrhoeae	Pili, outer membrane proteins	"Culture negative" pharyngitis	Thayer-Martin medium
Neisseria spp.	Unknown	Otitis, sinusitis	Chocolate agar
Moraxella spp.	Adhesin proteins	Otitis, sinusitis, conjunctivitis	Blood, chocolate agars
Acinetobacter spp.	Endotoxin, capsule	Nosocomial sinusitis	Blood, chocolate, MacConkey's agars
Kingella spp.	Endotoxin	Sinusitis	Chocolate, enriched liquid media (blood culture media)
Bordetella spp.	Filamentous hemagglutinin, adenylate cyclase toxin, endotoxin, tracheal cytotoxin	Pertussis syndrome; *rare* focal (sinus) infection	Supplemented Bordet-Gengou medium (innoculate *immediately* after taking nasopharyngeal specimen on alginate swab)

ENT, ear, nose, and throat

cases,[112] and antimicrobial-resistant bacteria, such as *Enterobacter, Serratia,* and *Citrobacter* species, are frequently found.[112, 113]

A small number of Enterobacteriaceae, such as *Klebsiella rhinoscleromatis,* appear to cause primary disease of the upper respiratory tract and are treated in detail.

Escherichia coli, Klebsiella pneumoniae, Klebsiella oxytoca. These are found in a small (<20%) fraction of otitis media cases in ill newborns[111] and in as many as 5%–10% of cases of chronic otitis media[104–111] and chronic sinusitis.[84, 104–111]

***Enterobacter, Serratia, Citrobacter* Species.** These are almost exclusively found in nosocomial sinusitis or otitis, or in the soft tissues related to invasive procedures. Antimicrobial resistance is frequent, and most infections are polymicrobial.[112, 113]

***Proteus* Species.** These organisms are frequently found in both cutaneous infections, such as chronic otitis externa or pustular disease of the external nose,[106] and chronic otitis media. In chronic otitis media and sinusitis cases, *Proteus* species are often part of the flora of intracranial extension such as brain abscess.[114]

Klebsiella rhinoscleromatis. *K. rhinoscleromatis* is a facultative diplobacillus. The only known source or reservoir of the organism is humans, and *K. rhinoscleromatis* is the cause of scleroma of the upper and lower respiratory mucosae (*rhinoscleroma*).

Microbial Pathogenesis. Little is known about adhesive or virulence determinants of *K. rhinoscleromatis,* and host factors may be extremely important in the disease process. *K. rhinoscleromatis* invades the respiratory mucosa at junctions between squamous and ciliated epithelium.[115] This is especially noted in the presence of iron-deficiency states.[115] When isolated from human tissue or respiratory secretions, *K. rhinoscleromatis* is invariably heavily *encapsulated,* with the immunologically unique somatic and capsular antigen combination O2K3.[115] It is thought that the capsule both limits

phagocytosis and, in unknown ways, inhibits some aspect of phagocytic killing by tissue macrophages.[115] Intracellular killing is minimal, and a granulomatous inflammatory mass forms, a process analogous to that of many diseases in which intracellular persistence of bacteria leads to chronic, but ineffective, cellular inflammation of tissues.

Host factors in patients with scleroma include diminished numbers of CD4 lymphocytes and a decreased response of helper T cells to interleukin-2.[115] Of great interest is a recent report of two European patients with moderately advanced infection with human immunodeficiency virus who developed classic rhinoscleroma after visits to endemic areas.[116] Given the relative rarity of rhinoscleroma, even two cases suggest T-cell deficiency as an important risk factor.

Epidemiology. Areas of endemicity (>80% of cases) include Eastern and Central Europe; Latin America including Mexico; South America; Africa; India; and Indonesia.[115] Person-to-person transmission is the only known means of spread. Scleroma is rare in the United States, but changing immigration patterns demand that U.S. physicians be aware of the disease.[115]

Clinical Manifestations. *K. rhinoscleromatis* initiates an indolent (many months to years) process, characterized by fetid discharge, crusting, granulomatous mass, and cicatrization, by growing in histiocytes of the tissue of the airway. Masses can occur at any site in the upper respiratory tract. The nose is most common (>90%, rhinoscleroma), followed by the pharynx (pharyngoscleroma, 15%–40%), the tracheobroncial tree (15%), the larynx (laryngoscleroma, 2%–3%), and the paranasal sinuses (2%–25%) (Fig. 21–2).[115, 117, 118]

Diagnosis and Treatment. Differential diagnosis includes all the "necrotizing midline" syndromes, including leprosy and rare cases of late syphilis. Cultures of secretions are positive in at least 60% of cases, and biopsies in 80%. Immunoperoxidase staining is sensitive and highly specific because of the uniqueness of the capsular antigen.[115] Pathologic examination at the early (precicatrization) stages of the

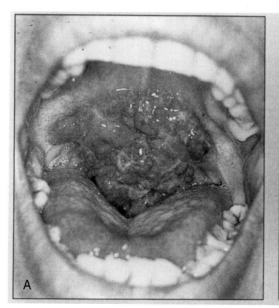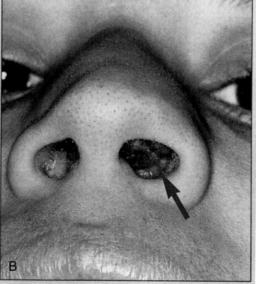

Figure 21–2. Pharyngeal *(A)* and nasal *(B)* scleroma caused by *Klebsiella rhinoscleromatis* in a young male. Note the invasive mass of the palate and the obstructing mass of the naris *(arrow).* (From Fred HL: Case in point: Rhinoscleroma. Hosp Pract [Off Ed] 1994; 29: 20.)

disease shows bacteria-laden histiocytes (Mikulicz's cells) and Russell's bodies, allowing frozen section diagnosis.[119]

Therapy is usually medical and surgical, with caution to treat with antimicrobials before definitive surgery to prevent dissemination to the head and neck. Streptomycin and systemic or topical rifampin have been used extensively.[115] Recent experience with orally administered fluoroquinolones[120, 121] has been favorable. Prolonged therapy (>3–6 months) along with ablative and corrective surgery is needed.[115, 120–122]

Klebsiella ozaenae. *K. ozaenae* is an occasional isolate from the respiratory tract, blood stream, and other sites.[123] Isolation of *K. ozaenae* from the nasal mucosa is associated with squamous metaplasia and other chronic sinonasal diseases. Interestingly, spread of *K. ozaenae* from the nose to other sites (meningitis, etc.) is frequently associated with preexisting nasal mucosal diseases, such as metaplasia, midline granuloma, or leprosy.[123, 124] Virulence factors of *K. ozaenae* are not known. *K. ozaenae* is apparently the cause of ozena, an infectious form of atrophic rhinitis seen in underdeveloped countries, especially in South Asia or in developed countries with crowded living conditions.

Yersinia pestis. This small, coccobacillary nonmotile member of the genus *Yersinia* is the cause of plague. It is a facultatively intracellular pathogen and grows readily on routine laboratory media. The organism has several distinct virulence determinants that allow it to proliferate in mammalian cells.[125] Expression of virulence is controlled by the environmental calcium concentration. The external F-1 antigen may inhibit phagocytosis.[125] In the United States, plague is usually seen in the Southwest and results from the bites of fleas of infected animals. *Y. pestis* proliferates and spreads to regional nodes, which rapidly swell and cause pain. Fifty percent of patients are bacteremic, and death is frequent in untreated patients. Aspiration of swollen nodes (bubos), culture, and fluorescent stain of the contents are important diagnostic tests. Throat cultures are frequently positive.

Yersinia enterocolitica. *Y. enterocolitica* is a motile organism and is most frequently a GI pathogen. It is occasionally seen as a cause of sinus infection in Northern Europe and Japan.[126] Airway infection is presumed to be the result of ingestion of contaminated food or drink.[126] The laboratory can readily isolate and identify the organism.

Other Enterobacteriaceae. Organisms such as *Salmonella*, *Edwardsiella*, and *Hafnia* are occasionally seen as causes of sepsis in the newborn as a result of contamination from the mother's GI tract at birth. Isolation from nares and ear canals suggests an ENT source for the infections.[127]

Vibrionaceae

The vibrios (*Vibrio parahaemolyticus*, *Vibrio vulnificus*, *Vibrio alginolyticus*) are facultative, small gram-negative bacteria that differ from the Enterobacteriaceae in that they are oxidase-positive. They are found in saltwater and are usually causes of enteritis but have recently been reported as pathogens in otitis externa and otitis media among patients swimming in saltwater.[128] A history of exposure to saltwater should prompt a request to the laboratory to use thiocitrate bile salts medium for the detection of vibrios from drainage in affected ears.

Pasteurellaceae

Pasteurella multocida. *Pasteurella* organisms are small, nonmotile facultative bacilli. A large carbohydrate capsule is the major virulence factor. Of this genus, *Pasteurella multocida* is an occasional cause of acute and chronic infection of the paranasal sinuses. Most human infections are associated with contact with animals, primarily domestic cats and dogs.[129, 130] Diagnosis is readily made by standard culture methods.

***Haemophilus influenzae* (see Chapter 19) and Other *Haemophilus* Species.** Haemophilus species (*Haemophilus parainfluenzae*, *Haemophilus aphrophilus*, *Haemophilus paraphrophilus*, *Haemophilus haemolyticus*, *Haemophilus parahaemolyticus*) are small, facultative coccobacilli that are highly pleomorphic in gram-stained specimens. Fastidious nutrient requirements can make identification in mixed cultures difficult, but clinical laboratories generally use media to detect *Haemophilus* in appropriate airway specimens. Protoporphyrins and NAD are two factors that are variably required for aerobic growth by different species. Virulence factors of *Haemophilus* include carbohydrate capsules (antiphagocytic, types a–f), lipo-oligosaccharide (analogous to LPS of Enterobacteriaceae), and outer membrane proteins.[131, 132] *All* the *Haemophilus* species are found in acute or chronic ENT infections.

Aerobic Gram-Negative Bacilli

Francisella tularensis

F. tularensis is the cause of tularemia, a serious infection of the skin, respiratory tract, lymphatic tissue, and occasionally other organs. ENT presentations of tularemia are common and extremely difficult to diagnose.[133–135]

Microbiology. *F. tularensis* is a small, aerobic, somewhat pleomorphic gram-negative coccobacillus. The cell wall of *F. tularensis* is high in fatty acids compared with those of similar organisms,[135] and this, along with a lipid-rich capsule, may be an important virulence factor.[135, 136] The LPS of *F. tularensis* seems to have less endotoxin activity than that of members of the Enterobacteriaceae,[135] so virulence is more likely related to the external cell envelope (cell wall and capsule). The infectious inoculum varies from strain to strain but can be as low as 50–100 organisms.[135]

Epidemiology. *F. tularensis* strains are found primarily in the northern latitudes in the United States, Europe, and Asia. The most important animal reservoirs and vectors are rodents and lagomorphs (rabbits). *F. tularensis* can be transmitted to humans by infected animal secretions, but the most important means of transmission of *F. tularensis* to humans in the United States are ticks and flies. *F. tularensis* can also survive harsh environmental conditions, including water. Ingestion of *F. tularensis* also leads to tularemia. Of all strains worldwide, biogroup A is the most virulent and is the predominant strain found in the United States. There are many differences among strains of *F. tularensis* in their preference and virulence for animal hosts, as well as severity of disease in humans. Epidemiologic factors of *F. tularensis* infection, then, include occupational exposure (trappers, hunters), exposure to ticks or biting flies, and mucosal contamination by *F. tularensis* from water or wild game.

Clinical Presentations. The ENT manifestations of *F. tularensis* infection depend on the mode of infection: vector bite, mucosal contact (oropharyngeal or conjunctival), and primary lymphadenitis.[133–135] Disease caused by vector bites (or other cutaneous inoculation) presents with the formation of a rapidly growing inflamed cutaneous papule that appears with or follows the development of regional adenopathy. The papule ulcerates, leaving a tender ulcer. About 11% of all tularemia presents with cervical or occipital adenopathy in association with a mild to severe systemic illness characterized by fever (>101 °F), malaise, headache, and sore throat. Ulcers are usually found on the head and neck in children,[133] who acquire insect-borne tularemia more commonly. Thus, the ENT physician might become involved with a case of tularemia because of severe systemic illness and cervical or occipital adenopathy.

Pharyngeal tularemia results from the ingestion of virulent *F. tularensis*. Mucosal ulcers are seen anywhere in the oropharynx, but the frequency is unknown. The predominant findings are severe throat pain, exudative pharyngitis, and tonsillitis, reflecting the lymphatic tropism of *F. tularensis*. Exudates can be severe enough to mimic the pseudomembrane of diphtheria.[133]

A third ENT presentation is primary lymphadenitis, usually cervical or occipital, as part of an acute or prolonged systemic illness.[133–135]

The most common complication of tularemia, and one of the most useful diagnostic signs, is the rapid progression to suppurative adenitis with deep abscess formation. This can occur even after partial treatment and can persist for long periods.[135] Pneumonia, sepsis, meningitis, and a wide variety of skin rashes, including erythema nodosum occur as well.

Diagnosis. *F. tularensis* has very specialized nutritional requirements in the laboratory, and the diagnosis can be missed if cultures are not properly performed. Appropriate cultures include blood, pharyngeal exudate, and lymph node aspirates. Serologic studies (enzyme-linked immunosorbent assay, microagglutination) are very useful, but only after 2 weeks of illness, so acute diagnosis is based on history and appropriate microbiologic testing. The laboratory needs to be informed of the suspected diagnosis in order to use appropriate media (cysteine-enriched blood agar, thioglycolate, Thayer-Martin medium, buffered charcoal yeast extract [*Legionella*] agar) and to protect laboratory workers against exposure.

Treatment of all forms of tularemia except central nervous system infection is usually with streptomycin or gentamicin.[133–136]

Legionellaceae

Legionella species are aerobic, weakly catalase-positive, unencapsulated gram-negative coccobacilli. *Legionella* species are nutritionally fastidious, and special media are required. *Legionella* species produce a variety of extracellular enzymes, but their role in pathogenesis is unknown. *Legionella* species survive and replicate in human mononuclear phagocytes. *Legionella* species were found to be the cause of pneumonia in 30% of surgical patients with head and neck

cancer.[137] *Legionella pneumophila* is occasionally found as a cause of sinusitis in conditions in which mucociliary clearance or cell-mediated immunity are impaired. Potable water appears to be the primary source of *Legionella,* and wound infections are seen when tap water is used for irrigation. Clinical suspicion should be directed at *L. pneumophila* when "culture-negative" purulent sinusitis occurs in the nosocomial setting or in a patient with an impaired cell-mediated immunity.[138] The standard medium for isolation is buffered charcoal yeast extract agar.[139]

Neisseriaceae

Moraxella. *Moraxella catarrhalis* is the most important member of this genus (see Chapter 20). *Moraxella* are strictly aerobic, oxidase-positive nonmotile gram-negative diplococci. Differentiation from *Neisseria* and other *Moraxella* is complex, but several rapid biochemical tests allow rapid presumptive identification.[140] *M. catarrhalis* organisms sometimes appear as diplobacilli in poorly stained clinical specimens, but generally resemble *Neisseria* species. *M. catarrhalis* can be a saprophyte or a pathogen of the upper and lower respiratory tracts. The mechanisms by which *M. catarrhalis* causes disease in the airway are not well understood. Adherence to mucosa at all levels of the respiratory tract is critical in the disease process, and protein adhesins are most important.[140] Differentiation between *Moraxella* and nonpathogenic *Neisseria* should always be performed in light of the high (>80%) frequency of penicillin resistance in *Moraxella.*[140, 141]

***Neisseria meningitidis* and Other *Neisseria*.** The *Neisseria* are gram-negative diplococci in clinical specimens. The organisms are primarily aerobic, but some are facultative. *Neisseria* are nonmotile, utilize glucose to differing degrees, and are somewhat fastidious in transportation and growth requirements. The major virulence determinants of the pathogenic *Neisseria* are the external polysaccharide capsules, outer membrane proteins, and LPS.[142]

The *Neisseria* species potentially pathogenic for the respiratory tissues of humans include *Neisseria gonorrhoeae, Neisseria meningitidis, Neisseria sicca, Neisseria subflava, Neisseria flavescens, Neisseria mucosa, Neisseria lactamica, Neisseria weaveri,* and *Neisseria cinerea.*[143]

Neisseria meningitidis. There are nine capsular serotypes (A, B, C, D, X, Y, Z, W-135, 29E) of *N. meningitidis*. A, B, and C account for most serious disease of humans. Capsules are antiphagocytic, many strains produce proteases that cleave mucosal immunoglobulin A, and *N. meningitidis* is rich in lipopolysaccharide. Organisms are carried on the pharyngeal mucosa and may cause a mild nasopharyngitis. Meningitis and septicemia occur as a result of bacteremia. Otitis and sinusitis are occasional sources of *N. meningitidis* by culture.

Neisseria gonorrhoeae. This organism is a major cause of sexually transmitted mucosal disease and ophthalmia neonatorum. Although *N. gonorrhoeae* infection of the pharyngeal mucosa is usually asymptomatic, it is an occasional cause of relapsing symptomatic pharyngitis,[144] with "negative" routine cultures. Taking an appropriate sexual history and using appropriate culture media (Thayer-Martin media) readily allow diagnosis.

Other *Neisseria* Species. Some of these species are *normal* commensals of the airway but are occasionally isolated from infections of the sinuses, ears, and epiglottis.

Acinetobacter and *Kingella*. *Acinetobacter* comprises 17 species of small, pleomorphic organisms. They are catalase-positive and are able to utilize a wide variety of nutrients. Their pathogenic mechanisms are not known. They are usually pathogens in cases of nosocomial sinusitis and can be highly antibiotic-resistant.

Kingella. *Kingella* organisms are small coccobacillary members of the family Neisseriaceae. They are occasionally seen in ENT infections because they are able to persist on respiratory mucosa and, in compromised hosts, invade tissue. Epiglottitis has been reported in compromised hosts.[140]

Bordetella Species

The *Bordetella* are *minute* gram-negative coccobacilli. Their primary importance in airway infection in humans is *pertussis*, a complex toxin-mediated disease (see Chapter 49). All four species of *Bordetella* (*Bordetella pertussis, Bordetella parapertussis, Bordetella bronchiseptica, Bordetella avium*) are aerobic, have pili that facilitate attachment, and produce a variety of toxins that both are immunomodulating and affect tissue function.

Structural elements that are pathogenic include a variant LPS with very potent endotoxin activity.[145]

B. bronchiseptica is a common cause of the economically important atrophic rhinitis of piglets,[145, 146] but it is rarely a cause of focal ENT infection in humans.[147] The true frequency of infection in humans due to *B. bronchiseptica* is not known, and it is not clear when the clinician should request cultures for the organism using Bordet-Gengou medium.[148]

Other Gram-Negative Bacteria (*Actinobacillus, Cardiobacterium, Eikenella* Species)

These small, heterogeneous facultative bacteria are common components of polymicrobial infections related to dental sources and can also be found in chronic infections of the middle ear and paranasal sinuses.[149] *Eikenella* is an important pathogen in relation to human bites[148] and has been reported as a cause of invasive orbital infection emanating from a chronically infected paranasal sinus.[150, 151]

Mycobacterium leprae

M. leprae is the cause of leprosy, a disease with many ENT manifestations (see Chapter 23). It is briefly discussed here because it is a part of the differential diagnosis of chronic nasopharyngeal processes, including rhinoscleroma and syphilis.

M. leprae is a gram-variable, acid-fast member of the family *Mycobacteriaceae*. *M. leprae* is an obligate intracellular organism, with lipid-rich external cell layers. Growth is very slow in animals, and the doubling time averages about 14 days.[152] It cannot be grown in the clinical laboratory, so clinical diagnosis must be supplemented by acid-fast stains of biopsied tissue. Because of low temperature requirements for replication, *M. leprae* thrives in the upper respiratory tract of humans.[152]

The ENT manifestations of leprosy are primarily found in the nasal mucosa (obstruction due to thickening), with destruction of the cartilage. In Mexican patients, diffuse dermal thickening of the perinasal and forehead skin may be present. Leprosy is endemic in Asia, Latin America, Africa, and the Pacific. Transmission is by intimate contact; thus ethnic, geographic, and social histories are required for diagnosis. Biopsies of the skin and affected airway mucosa are the best diagnostic tests. An acid-fast stain of biopsied tissue should be requested. The treatment of infection due to *M. leprae* is complicated by poor compliance and drug resistance (see Chapter 12). However, dapsone once daily with rifampin monthly for several years frequently results in resolution of leprosy in which few bacilli (*paucibacillary* infection) are found. For heavier infection (*multibacillary*), daily rifampin and dapsone with or without clofazimine can be used.[153] Response begins in weeks to months, and therapy can be lifelong.

Spirochaeteceae: *Treponema pallidum*

No discussion of gram-negative bacilli causing infections of the ears, nose, and throat is complete without a mention of *Treponema pallidum*, the cause of syphilis. *T. pallidum* is a coiled, almost helical, highly motile organism that is structurally similar to more common gram-negative bacilli. In addition to an LPS component of the outer membrane, *T. pallidum* also has an additional phospholipid envelope that shields many surface proteins from immune surveillance. Virulence factors are poorly understood, but adherence to skin structures is critical in pathogenesis. The organism can be maintained briefly but not cultured in the clinical laboratory.[154]

The clinical settings in which a microbiologic diagnosis of syphilis must be made include congenital syphilis, with mucocutaneous, cartilage, and bony abnormalities of the nasal and oral structures (osteochondritis, snuffles, mucous patches); primary syphilis, with a chancre of the skin or mucous membranes, from contact with another infected lesion; secondary syphilis, with a split papule of the nasal fold, mucous patches, diffuse adenopathy; tertiary syphilis, with a perforated nasal septum, destructive mass of cartilage of the nose, larynx, pharynx, and palate (*gumma*, late benign syphilis). The differential diagnosis includes neoplasm, mycobacterial infection, scleroma, and midline necrosis syndromes.

Diagnosis is by clinical suspicion, the use of nontreponemal (rapid plasma reagin, venereal disease research laboratories) and treponemal (fluorescent treponemal antibody–absorption) serologic tests, dark-field examination of "wet" lesions in congenital, primary, and secondary disease; and serologic examination and biopsies in tertiary syphilis.[155]

EPIDEMIOLOGY OF NOSOCOMIAL EAR, NOSE, AND THROAT INFECTIONS DUE TO *P. aeruginosa* AND OTHER GRAM-NEGATIVE AEROBIC OR FACULTATIVE BACILLI

Pseudomonas aeruginosa

During the past 40 years, *P. aeruginosa* infections have become frequent as nosocomial infections in immunocom-

Table 21–5. NOSOCOMIAL INFECTIONS OF HOSPITALIZED PATIENTS IN U.S. HOSPITALS

Site of Infection	Frequency	Percent
Ear	468	0.2
Sinuses	883	0.5
Upper respiratory tract	1,147	0.6
Mouth	2,258	1.2
Blood stream	24,842	12.8
Pneumonia	30,818	15.9
Surgical sites	31,127	16.0
Urinary tract	65,778	33.9
Other	36,812	19.0

NNIS (National Nosocomial Infections Surveillance) data, Centers for Disease Control and Prevention, Atlanta, Georgia, 1986–July 1995.

promised or debilitated hosts.[3] No more than 3% of human adults carry this organism in the GI tract on admission to the hospital.[86] Once *P. aeruginosa* establishes itself in the respiratory tract or the ear as a colonizer, it may be difficult to eradicate it. Data from the National Nosocomial Infections Surveillance (NNIS) system (1985–1991) indicate that *Escherichia coli* was the most commonly isolated pathogen in hospitals (13.9%), whereas *P. aeruginosa* was the 4th overall pathogen and the 2nd most common gram-negative pathogen (10.1%) in nosocomial infections in the United States.[3] In this study, the overall *P. aeruginosa* infection rate was 4.0 cases per 1000 discharges. Urinary tract infections, pneumonia, surgical site infections, and bacteremia were described most frequently (35%, 15%, 16%, and 12%, respectively). It should be noted that in ICUs, *P. aeruginosa* was the most commonly isolated pathogen in pulmonary infections (17.5%) and the 3rd most common isolate in surgical site infections (10.9%). Higher *P. aeruginosa* infection rates were observed in large teaching hospitals (4.9 cases per 1000 discharges) compared with small hospitals (2.6 cases per 1000 discharges). Overall, however, from 1985 to 1991 there has been a trend to a decrease in *P. aeruginosa* infections and an increase in gram-positive infections and those with

Candida albicans. Less than one infection with *P. aeruginosa* per 1000 discharges was reported for surgical site infections during this time period.

Analysis of the most recent data from the NNIS system (personal communication, R. Gaynes, M.D., Centers for Disease Control and Prevention, Atlanta, Georgia) includes the most recent information concerning nosocomial ENT infections. Criteria for diagnosis of infection were given previously.[156] Table 21–5 shows that nosocomial ENT infections are infrequent; they represent 2.5% of the total infections reported. Tables 21–6 and 21–7 provide the distribution of the microorganisms in nosocomial ear and sinus infections. Gram-negative bacteria were detected in 42.9% of ear and 50.7% of sinus infections. *P. aeruginosa* was the most commonly detected gram-negative organism in the ear infections (18.5% of total isolates) and the second in sinus infections (11.7% of total isolates). Table 21–8 indicates that of the 4539 nosocomial ENT infections (ear, sinus, upper respiratory tract, and mouth), only 27.87% were related to surgical procedures. Great concern has been expressed by many clinicians and laboratory investigators about the increasing resistance of *P. aeruginosa* to potent antibacterial agents, including beta-lactams, carbapenems, aminoglycosides, and fluoroquinolones. Table 21–9 shows the resistance rates of *P. aeruginosa* isolates from nosocomial ENT infections from 1986 to July 1995. High resistance rates (4.7%–15.9%) are reported for the four antipseudomonal antimicrobials listed.

To control the spread and outbreaks of *P. aeruginosa* infections in hospitals, one must understand the various reservoirs of *P. aeruginosa,* i.e., environmental sources, medical equipment, food, medication, fluids, and disinfectants.[3] Person-to-person transmission by hand contact is not uncommon. Recognition of the problem, specific features of the organism regarding antibiotic-susceptibility patterns, serotyping, pyocine-typing, and phage-typing, and more recently molecular-typing techniques (pulsed-field gel electrophoresis) are important methods used to recognize an outbreak. Asepsis, isolation precautions, environmental control, and meticulous hand washing are important in the prevention and control of *P. aeruginosa* infections.

Table 21–6. PATHOGENS ASSOCIATED WITH NOSOCOMIAL EAR INFECTIONS

Gram-Negative Pathogens	Percent	Gram-Positive Pathogens	Percent
Pseudomonas aeruginosa	18.5	*Staphylococcus* coagulase negative	20.9
Enterobacter species (spp.)	4.9	*Staphylococcus aureus*	12.0
Escherichia coli	3.3	*Enterococcus*	6.2
Klebsiella pneumoniae	3.1	Other gram-positive aerobes	4.9
Proteus mirabilis	2.9	*Candida albicans*	2.9
Citrobacter spp.	2.0	*Aspergillus* spp.	1.8
Acinetobacter spp.	1.8	*Streptococcus pneumoniae*	1.8
Haemophilus influenzae	1.6	Other *Streptococcus* spp.	1.6
Other nonenteric organisms	1.1	Other fungi	1.6
Other enteric organisms	0.9	Group B *Streptococcus*	0.9
Other *Klebsiella* spp.	0.4	Other *Candida* spp.	0.9
Other *Proteus* spp.	0.4	Gram-positive anaerobes	0.4
Serratia marcescens	0.4	Group D *Streptococcus*	0.4
Other *Pseudomonas* spp.	0.2	Group A *Streptococcus*	0.2
Other *Serratia* spp.	0.2	Other *Staphylococcus* spp.	0.2
Other	1.2	Other	0.4
	42.9		57.1

NNIS data, Centers for Disease Control and Prevention, Atlanta, Georgia, 1986–July 1995.

Table 21–7. PATHOGENS ASSOCIATED WITH NOSOCOMIAL SINUS INFECTIONS

Gram-Negative Pathogens	Percent	Gram-Positive Pathogens	Percent
Enterobacter species (spp.)	11.9	*Staphylococcus aureus*	16.5
Pseudomonas aeruginosa	11.7	*Staphylococcus* coagulase negative	7.2
Klebsiella pneumoniae	4.2	Other *Streptococcus* spp.	6.0
Escherichia coli	4.0	*Candida albicans*	5.8
Acinetobacter spp.	3.0	*Enterococcus*	5.0
Other nonenteric aerobes	2.7	Other fungi	1.7
Proteus mirabilis	2.4	*Aspergillus* spp.	1.6
Haemophilus influenzae	2.3	Other gram-positive aerobes	1.1
Serratia marcescens	1.8	Other *Candida* spp.	1.0
Other *Klebsiella* spp.	1.4	Gram-positive mixed bacteria	0.5
Citrobacter spp.	1.2	Gram-positive anaerobes	0.4
Gram-negative anaerobes	0.9	Group B *Streptococcus*	0.3
Other nonenteric aerobes	0.7	*Torulopsis* spp.	0.2
Other *Pseudomonas*	0.4	Group A *Streptococcus*	0.2
Gram-negative mixed bacteria	0.3	Group D *Streptococcus*	0.2
Other *Proteus* spp.	0.3	Other *Staphylococcus* spp.	0.1
Other *Serratia* spp.	0.2	Other	1.5
Other *Bacteroides* spp.	0.2		
Bacteroides fragilis	0.1		
Other	1.0		
	50.7		49.3

NNIS data, Centers for Disease Control and Prevention, Atlanta, Georgia, 1986–July 1995.

Although *P. aeruginosa* infections are most commonly nosocomial, there has been a trend for *P. aeruginosa* to be a cause of community-acquired infections as well. Although ENT infections, i.e., *P. aeruginosa* infections related to the ear (malignant otitis media), are most commonly observed as community-acquired infections, even the number of serious systemic infections, i.e., bacteremia, have increased in number as infections acquired in the community.[157] Serious respiratory tract and sinus infections in cystic fibrosis patients or in patients with AIDS continue to be mostly acquired in the community.

Other Gram-Negative Aerobic or Facultative Bacilli

ENT infection due to facultative and aerobic gram-negative bacilli other than *H. influenzae* and *Moraxella* species is most commonly nosocomial in origin. Gram-negative bacilli, primarily Enterobacteriaceae, occur infrequently in acute community-acquired otitis media and sinusitis, and slightly more commonly as part of a mixed flora in community-acquired chronic sinusitis and otitis media.

Gram-negative facultative and aerobic bacilli other than *P. aeruginosa* are common causes of nosocomial infections of the lung, urinary tract, blood stream and surgical site.[3] From the reporting period 1985–1991, the NNIS system reported that *E. coli, Enterobacter,* and *Klebsiella* species accounted for 33.5%, 23.3%, 5.2%, and 10.5% of nosocomial infections of the urinary tract, lung, blood stream and surgical site, respectively, in critical care patients.[3] In patients with nosocomial infections outside the critical care units, *E. coli, Klebsiella,* and *Proteus* species were found in 39.5% of urinary tract infections. For lung, blood stream, and surgical site infections, facultative and aerobic bacilli other than *P. aeruginosa* were found at rates similar to those seen in critical care patients.

In nosocomial ENT infections, however, members of the Enterobacteriaceae and *Acinetobacter* species are found commonly. Tables 21–6 and 21–7 show the distribution of causative microorganisms in nosocomial ear and sinus infections. *Enterobacter* species and *P. aeruginosa* are de-

Table 21–8. NUMBER OF NOSOCOMIAL EAR, NOSE, AND THROAT INFECTIONS RELATED TO SURGICAL PROCEDURES

Site of Infection	Infections Related to Surgery	Infections Unrelated to Surgery	Total
Ear	85	358	443
Sinuses	322	524	846
Upper respiratory tract	318	765	1083
Oral	540	1627	2167
Total	1265 (27.87%)	3274 (72.13%)	4539

NNIS data, Centers for Disease Control and Prevention, Atlanta, Georgia, 1986–July 1995.

Table 21–9. PERCENTAGE OF NOSOCOMIAL ANTIBIOTIC-RESISTANT *Pseudomonas aeruginosa* ISOLATES FROM EAR, NOSE, AND THROAT INFECTIONS

Antibiotic	Number Tested	Percent Resistant
Imipenem	113	15.9
Aztreonam	115	15.7
Ceftazidime	187	15.0
Ciprofloxacin	169	4.7
Total	747	

NNIS data, Centers for Disease Control and Prevention, Atlanta, Georgia, 1986–July 1995.

tected in 11.9% and 11.7% of total isolates reported in sinus infections. Other gram-negative infections account for 27.1% of total infections reported. In nosocomial ear infections, however, gram-negative pathogens other than *P. aeruginosa* account for 24.4% of total pathogens, compared with 18.5% for *P. aeruginosa*. The frequency of isolation of *Enterobacter* species and *Acinetobacter* species is of special concern because of antimicrobial resistance and difficult therapeutic challenges.

Control of nosocomial infection due to gram-negative bacilli depends heavily on the appropriate use of barrier precautions for contaminated secretions and judicious use of antimicrobial agents. In ENT surgery, airway secretions can be copious, and normal oropharyngeal flora will promptly be dominated by gram-negative bacilli from the patient's own gastrointestinal tract. Antimicrobial resistance can be induced during therapy, especially with *Enterobacter* species, and resistant organisms can also be acquired from other patients if barrier precautions and hand washing are not carefully performed by personnel.

References

1. Doggett RG: Microbiology of *Pseudomonas aeruginosa*. In: Doggett RG (ed): *Pseudomonas aeruginosa*: Clinical Manifestations of Infection and Current Therapy. New York: Academic Press, 1979, pp 1–7.
2. Ward KH, Olson ME, Lam K, Costerton JW: Mechanism of persistent infection with peritoneal implants. J Med Microbiol 1992; 36: 406–413.
3. Beck-Sagué CM, Banerjee SN, Jarvis WR: Epidemiology and control of *Pseudomonas aeruginosa* in U.S. hospitals. In: Baltch AL, Smith RP (eds): *Pseudomonas aeruginosa* Infections and Treatment. New York, Marcel Dekker, 1994, pp 51–71.
4. Baltch AL, Griffin PE: *Pseudomonas aeruginosa* bacteremia: Clinical study of 75 patients. Am J Med Sci 1977; 274: 119–129.
5. Hilf M, Yu VL, Sharp J, et al.: Antibiotic therapy for *Pseudomonas aeruginosa* bacteremia: Outcome correlations in a prospective study of 200 patients. Am J Med 1989; 87: 540–546.
6. Géssard C: Sür le colorations bleue des lignes à pansements. C R Hebdom Seances Acad Sci D 1882; 94: 536–538.
7. Zwadyk P: *Pseudomonas*. In: Joklick WK, Willett H, Amos DR, Wilfert CM (eds): Zinsser Microbiology, 20th ed. Norwalk, Connecticut: Appleton & Lange, 1992, pp 576–583.
8. Woods DE, Vasil ML: Pathogenesis of *Pseudomonas aeruginosa* infections. In: Baltch AL, Smith RP (eds): *Pseudomonas aeruginosa* Infections and Treatment. New York: Marcel Dekker, 1994, pp 21–50.
9. Fraenkel E: Weitere Untersuchungen über de Menschenpathogenität des *Bacillus pyocyaneus*. Z Hyg Infect 1917; 84: 369–424.
10. Williams EP, Cameron BA: Upon general infection by *Bacillus pyocyaneus* in children. J Pathol Bacteriol 1897; 3: 344–351.
11. Bodey GP, Bolivar R, Fainstein V, Jadeja L: Infections caused by *Pseudomonas aeruginosa*. Rev Infect Dis 1983; 5: 279–301.
12. Woods DE, Straus DC, Johanson WG Jr, et al.: Role of pili in adherence of *Pseudomonas aeruginosa* to mammalian buccal epithelial cells. Infect Immun 1980; 29: 1146–1151.
13. Ramphal R, Koo L, Ishimoto KS, et al.: Adhesion of *Pseudomonas aeruginosa* pili-deficient mutants to mucin. Infect Immun 1991; 59: 1307–1311.
14. Woods DE, Straus DC, Johanson WG Jr, Bass JA: Role of fibronectin in the prevention and adherence of *Pseudomonas aeruginosa* to buccal cells. J Infect Dis 1981; 143: 784–790.
15. Doig P, Sastry PA, Hodges RS, et al.: Inhibition of pilus-mediated adhesion of *Pseudomonas aeruginosa* to human buccal epithelial cells by monoclonal antibodies directed against pili. Infect Immun 1990; 58: 124–130.
16. Baker NR, Hanson GC, Leffler H, et al.: Glycosphingolipid receptors for *Pseudomonas aeruginosa*. Infect Immun 1990; 58: 2361–2366.
17. Baker NR, Minor V, Deal C, et al.: *Pseudomonas aeruginosa* exoenzyme S is an adhesin. Infect Immun 1991; 59: 2859–2863.
18. Montie TC, Doyle-Huntzinger D, Craven RC, Holder IA: Loss of virulence associated with absence of flagellum in an isogenic mutant of *Pseudomonas aeruginosa* in the burned mouse model. Infect Immun 1982; 38: 1296–1298.
19. Drake D, Montie T: Flagella, motility and invasive virulence of *Pseudomonas aeruginosa*. J Gen Microbiol 1988; 134: 43–52.
20. Weinberg ED: Iron and infection. Microbiol Rev 1978; 42: 45–66.
21. Sokol PA, Woods DE: Demonstration of an iron-siderophore-binding protein in the outer membrane of *Pseudomonas aeruginosa*. Infect Immun 1983; 40: 665–669.
22. Hirakata Y, Furuya N, Takeda K, et al.: In vivo production of exotoxin A and its role in endogenous *Pseudomonas aeruginosa* septicemia in mice. Infect Immun 1993; 61: 2468–2473.
23. Liu PV: Extracellular toxins of *Pseudomonas aeruginosa*. J Infect Dis 1974; 130: S94–S99.
24. Pier GB, Sidberry HF, Zolyomi S, Sadoff JC: Isolation and characterization of a high-molecular-weight polysaccharide from the slime of *Pseudomonas aeruginosa*. Infect Immun 1978; 22: 908–918.
25. Oliver AM, Weir DM: Inhibition of bacterial binding to mouse macrophages by *Pseudomonas aeruginosa* alginate. J Clin Lab Immunol 1983; 10: 221–224.
26. Eftekhar F, Speert DP: Alginase treatment of mucoid *Pseudomonas aeruginosa* enhances phagocytosis by human monocyte derived macrophages. Infect Immun 1988; 56: 2788–2793.
27. Evans LR, Linker A: Production and characterization of the slime polysaccharide of *Pseudomonas aeruginosa*. J Bacteriol 1973; 116: 915–924.
28. Woods DE, Sokol PA, Bryan LE, et al.: In vivo regulation of virulence in *Pseudomonas aeruginosa* associated with genetic rearrangement. J Infect Dis 1991; 163: 143–149.
29. Iglewski BH, Liu PV, Kabat D: Mechanisms of action of *Pseudomonas aeruginosa* exotoxin A: Adenosine diphosphate-ribolysation of mammalian elongation factor 2 in vitro and in vivo. Infect Immun 1977; 15: 138–144.
30. Bjorn MJ, Vasil ML, Sadoff JC, Iglewski BH: Incidence of exotoxin production of *Pseudomonas aeruginosa* species. Infect Immun 1977; 16: 362–366.
31. Woods DE, Cryz SJ, Friedman RL, Iglewski BH: Contribution of toxin A and elastase to virulence of *Pseudomonas aeruginosa* in chronic lung infection in rats. Infect Immun 1982; 36: 1223–1228.
32. Misfeldt ML: Microbial "superantigens." Infect Immun 1990; 58: 2409–2413.
33. Pollack M, Young LS: Protective activity of antibody to exotoxin A and lipopolysaccharide at the onset of *Pseudomonas aeruginosa* septicemia. J Clin Invest 1979; 63: 276–286.
34. Baltch AL, Smith RP, Franke M, et al.: Survival and serum antibody concentration to cytotoxin, exotoxin A, lipopolysaccharide, protease and elastase in patients with *Pseudomonas aeruginosa* bacteremia. Clin Infect Dis (in press).
35. Iglewski BH, Sadoff JC, Bjorn MJ, Maxwell ES: *Pseudomonas aeruginosa* exoenzyme S: An adenosine diphosphate ribosyltransferase distinct from toxin A. Proc Natl Acad Sci USA 1978; 75: 3211–3215.
36. Sokol PA, Iglewski BH, Hager TA, et al.: Production of exoenzyme S by clinical isolates of *Pseudomonas aeruginosa*. Infect Immun 1981; 34: 147–153.
37. Woods DE, Sokol PA: Use of transposon mutants to assess the role of exoenzyme S in chronic pulmonary disease due to *Pseudomonas aeruginosa*. Eur J Clin Microbiol 1985; 4: 163–169.
38. Sharmann W: Purification and characterization of leucocidin from *Pseudomonas aeruginosa*. J Gen Microbiol 1976; 93: 292–302.
39. Kluftinger JL, Lutz F, Hancock REW: *Pseudomonas aeruginosa* cytotoxin: Periplasmic localization and inhibition of macrophages. Infect Immun 1989; 57: 882–886.
40. Bishop MB, Baltch AL, Hill A, et al.: The effect of *Pseudomonas aeruginosa* cytotoxin and toxin A on human polymorphonuclear leukocytes. J Med Microbiol 1987; 24: 315–324.
41. Baltch AL, Hammer MC, Smith RP, et al.: Effects of *Pseudomonas aeruginosa* cytotoxin on human serum and granulocytes and their microbicidal, phagocytic and chemotactic functions. Infect Immun 1985; 48: 498–506.
42. Baltch AL, Franke M, Tanaka Y, et al.: Generation of leukotriene B$_4$ (LTB$_4$) by *Pseudomonas aeruginosa* cytotoxin. Abstr Ann Meet Am Soc Microbiol B-287:73, 1991.

43. Bopp L, Baltch AL, Hammer MC, et al.: Isolation and characterization of a transposon-induced cytotoxin-deficient mutant of *Pseudomonas aeruginosa*. Toxicon 1994; 32: 27–34.

44. Baltch AL, Winnie G, Smith RP: Serum antibody concentration of *Pseudomonas aeruginosa* cytotoxin and toxin A in cystic fibrosis patients. Abstr Ann Meet Am Soc Microbiol E-119:147, 1989.

45. Baltch AL, Obrig TG, Smith RP, et al.: Production of cytotoxin by clinical strains of *Pseudomonas aeruginosa*. Can J Microbiol 1987; 33: 104–111.

46. Hayashi T, Baba T, Hatsumoto H, Terawaki Y: Phage-conversion of cytotoxin production in *Pseudomonas aeruginosa*. Mol Microbiol 1990; 4: 1703–1709.

47. Hess DG, Tracey KJ, Fong Y, et al.: Cytokine appearance in human endotoxemia and primate bacteremia. Surg Gynecol Obstet 1988; 166: 147–153.

48. Pitt TL: Lipopolysaccharide and virulence of *Pseudomonas aeruginosa*. Antibiot Chemother 1989; 42: 1–7.

49. Wilkinson SG, Galbraith L: Studies of lipopolysaccharides from *Pseudomonas aeruginosa*. Eur J Biochem 1975; 52: 331–343.

50. Kropinski AM, Jewell B, Kuzio J, et al.: Structure and functions of *Pseudomonas aeruginosa* lipopolysaccharide. Antibiot Chemother 1985; 36: 58–73.

51. Kropinski AM, Kuzio J, Angus BL, Hancock REW: Chemical and chromatographic analysis of lipopolysaccharide from an antibiotic supersusceptible mutant of *Pseudomonas aeruginosa*. Antimicrob Agents Chemother 1982; 21: 310–319.

52. Berka RM, Vasil ML: Phospholipase C (heat-labile hemolysin) of *Pseudomonas aeruginosa*: Purification and preliminary characterization. J Bacteriol 1982; 152: 239–245.

53. Baltch AL, Griffin PE, Hammer M: *Pseudomonas aeruginosa* bacteremia: Relationship of bacterial enzyme production and pyocine types with clinical prognosis in 100 patients. J Lab Clin Med 1979; 93: 600–606.

54. Berka RM, Gray GL, Vasil ML: Studies of phospholipase C (heat-labile hemolysin) in *Pseudomonas aeruginosa*. Infect Immun 1981; 34: 1071–1074.

55. Vasil ML, Graham LM, Ostroff RM, et al.: Phospholipase C: Molecular biology and contribution to the pathogenesis of *Pseudomonas aeruginosa*. Antibiot Chemother 1991; 44: 34–47.

56. Ostroff RM, Wretlind B, Vasil ML: Mutation in the hemolytic phospholipase C operon results in decreased virulence of *Pseudomonas aeruginosa* PA01 grown under phosphate limiting conditions. Infect Immun 1989; 57: 1369–1373.

57. Hingley ST, Hastie AT, Kueppers F, et al.: Effect of ciliastatic factors from *Pseudomonas aeruginosa* on rabbit respiratory cilia. Infect Immun 1986; 51: 254–262.

58. Ostroff RM, Vasil ML: Identification of a new phospholipase C activity by analysis of an insertional mutation in the hemolytic phospholipase C structural gene of *Pseudomonas aeruginosa*. J Bacteriol 1987; 169: 4597–4601.

59. Nicas T, Iglewski BH: The contribution of exoproducts to virulence of *Pseudomonas aeruginosa*. Can J Microbiol 1985; 31: 387–392.

60. Kharazmi A, Döring G, Hoiby N, Valerus NH: Interaction of *Pseudomonas aeruginosa* alkaline protease and elastase with human polymorphonuclear leukocytes in vitro. Infect Immun 1984; 43: 161–165.

61. Theander TG, Kharazmi A, Pederson BK, et al.: Inhibition of human lymphocyte proliferation and cleavage of interleukin 2 by *Pseudomonas aeruginosa* proteases. Infect Immun 1988; 56: 1673–1677.

62. Peters JE, Galloway DR: Purification and characterization of an active fragment of the LasA protein from *Pseudomonas aeruginosa*: Enhancement of elastase activity. J Bacteriol 1990; 172: 2236–2240.

63. Schultz DR, Miller KD: Elastase of *Pseudomonas aeruginosa* activation of complement components and complement-derived chemotactic and phagocytic factors. Infect Immun 1974; 10: 128–135.

64. Rubin Grandis J, Yu VL: *Pseudomonas aeruginosa* infections of the ear. In: Baltch AL, Smith RP (eds): *Pseudomonas aeruginosa* Infections and Treatment. New York, Marcel Dekker, 1994, pp 401–419.

65. Koltai PJ, Maisel BO, Goldstein JC: *Pseudomonas aeruginosa* in chronic maxillary sinusitis. Laryngoscope 1985; 95: 34–37.

66. Davidson TM, Murphy C, Mitchel M, et al.: Management of chronic sinusitis in cystic fibrosis. Laryngoscope 1995; 105: 354–358.

67. Meltzer PE, Kelemen G: Pyocyaneus osteomyelitis of the temporal bone, mandible and zygoma. Laryngoscope 1959; 69: 1300–1316.

68. Chandler JR: Malignant external otitis. Laryngoscope 1968; 78: 1257–1294.

69. Rubin J, Yu VL: Malignant external otitis: Insights into pathogenesis, clinical manifestations, diagnosis and therapy. Am J Med 1988; 85: 391–398.

70. Gold S, Som PM, Lawson W, et al.: Radiographic findings in progressive necrotizing "malignant" external otitis. Laryngoscope 1984; 94: 363–366.

71. Sade J, Lang R, Goshen S, Kitzes-Cohen R: Ciprofloxacin treatment of malignant external otitis. Am J Med 1989; 87(suppl 5A): 138S–141S.

72. Davis JC, Gates GA, Lerner C, et al.: Adjuvant hyperbaric oxygen in malignant external otitis. Arch Otolaryngol Head Neck Surg 1992; 118: 89–93.

73. Cassisi N, Cohn A, Davidson T, Witten BR: Diffuse external otitis: Clinical and microbiologic findings in the course of a multicenter study on a new otic solution. Ann Otol Rhinol Laryngol 1977; 86(Suppl 38): 1–16.

74. Cossette JE: High ear-piercing-perichrondreal abscess. Otolaryng Head Neck Surg 1993; 107: 967–968.

75. Turkeltaub SH, Habal MB: Acute *Pseudomonas* chondritis as a sequel to ear piercing. Ann Plast Surg 1990; 24: 279–282.

76. Dowling JA, Foley FD, Montcrief JA: Chondritis of the burned ear. Plast Reconstr Surg 1968; 42: 115–122.

77. Antonelli PJ, Juhn SK, Chap TL, Giebink GS: Acute otitis media increases middle ear susceptibility to nasal infection of *Pseudomonas aeruginosa*. Otolaryng Head Neck Surg 1994; 110: 115–121.

78. Kenna MA, Bluestone CD, Reilly JS, Lusk RP: Medical management of chronic suppurative otitis media with cholesteatoma in children. Laryngoscope 1986; 96: 146–151.

79. O'Donnell JG, Sorbello AF, Condeluci DV, Barnish MJ: Sinusitis due to *Pseudomonas aeruginosa* in patients with human immunodeficiency virus infection. Clin Infect Dis 1993; 16: 404–406.

80. Rubin J, Honigberg R: Sinusitis in patients with acquired immunodeficiency syndrome. Ear Nose Throat J 1990; 69: 460–463.

81. Grant A, von Schoenberg M, Grant HR, Miller RF: Paranasal sinus disease in HIV antibody positive patients. Genitourin Med J 1993; 69: 208–212.

82. Farr RW, Ramadan HH: Report of *Pseudomonas aeruginosa* sinusitis in a patient with AIDS. W V Med J 1993; 89: 284–285.

83. Caplan ES, Hoyt NJ: Nosocomial sinusitis. JAMA 1982; 247: 639–641.

84. Karma P, Jokippi L, Sipila P, et al.: Bacteria in chronic maxillary sinusitis. Arch Otolaryngol 1979; 105: 386–390.

85. Moss RB, King VV: Management of sinusitis in cystic fibrosis by endoscopic surgery and serial antimicrobial lavage. Arch Otolaryngol Head Neck Surg 1995; 121: 566–572.

86. Murthy SK, Baltch AL, Smith RP, et al.: Oropharyngeal and fecal carriage of *Pseudomonas aeruginosa* in hospital patients. J Clin Microbiol 1989; 27: 35–40.

87. Levinson ME: Factors influencing colonization of the gastrointestinal tract with *Pseudomonas aeruginosa*. In: Young VM (ed): *Pseudomonas aeruginosa*: Ecologic aspects and patient colonization. New York: Raven Press, 1977, pp 97–109.

88. Gilligan PH: *Pseudomonas* and *Burkholderia*. In: Murray PR, Baron EJ, Pfaller MA, et al. (eds): Manual of Clinical Microbiology. Washington, DC: ASM Press, 1994, pp 509–519.

89. Baltch AL, Smith RP: Combinations of antibiotics against *Pseudomonas aeruginosa*. Am J Med 1985; 79(suppl 1A): 8–16.

90. Valdes J, Baltch AL, Franke MA, et al.: Comparative therapy with cefpirome alone and in combination with rifampin and for gentamicin against a disseminated *Pseudomonas aeruginosa* infection in leukopenic mice. J Infect Dis 1990; 162: 1112–1117.

91. Korvick JA, Peacock JE, Murder RR, et al.: Addition of rifampin to combination therapy of *Pseudomonas* bacteremia. Prospective trial using the Zelen protocol. Antimicrob Agents Chemother 1992; 36: 620–625.

92. Craig WA, Ebert SC: Antimicrobial therapy in *Pseudomonas aeruginosa* infections. In: Baltch AL, Smith RP (eds): *Pseudomonas aeruginosa* Infections and Treatment. New York: Marcel Dekker, 1994, pp 441–517.

93. Cryz SJ Jr, Fürer E, Sadoff JC, et al.: Production and characterization of a hyperimmune intravenous immunoglobulin against *Pseudomonas aeruginosa* and *Klebsiella* species. J Infect Dis 1991; 163: 1055–1061.

94. Böhn D: Experiences with a *Pseudomonas* immunoglobulin in ventilated patients with *Pseudomonas* pneumonia in a surgical intensive care station. Infection 1987; 15(suppl 2): S64–S66.

95. Pilz G, Class I, Boekstegers P, et al.: *Pseudomonas* immunoglobulin therapy in patients with *Pseudomonas* sepsis and septic shock. Antibiot Chemother 1991; 44: 120–135.

96. Miller JM, Pilsbury JF, Jones RJ, et al.: A new polyvalent *Pseudomonas* vaccine. Med Microbiol 1977; 10: 19–27.

97. Cryz SJ Jr, Fürer E, Que JU, et al.: Clinical evaluation of an octavalent *Pseudomonas aeruginosa* conjugate vaccine in plasma donors and in bone marrow transplants and cystic fibrosis patients. Antibiot Chemother 1991; 44: 157–162.

98. Greenman RL, Schein RM, Martin MA, et al.: A controlled clinical trial of E5 murine monoclonal IgM antibody to endotoxin in the treatment of gram-negative sepsis. JAMA 1991; 266: 1097–1102.

99. Louie A: Cytokines and endotoxin in the pathogenesis of systemic *Pseudomonas aeruginosa* infection. In: Baltch AL, Smith RP (eds): *Pseudomonas aeruginosa* Infections and Treatment. New York: Marcel Dekker, 1994, pp 547–585.

100. Bacterial growth, nutrition and control. In: Volk WA, Benjamin DC, Kadner RJ, Parsons TJ (eds): Essentials of Medical Microbiology. Philadelphia; JP Lippincott Co, 1991, pp 257–263.

101. Nicas TI, Eisenstein BI: Introduction to bacterial diseases. In: Mandell GL, Bennett JE, Dolin R (eds): Principles and Practice of Infectious Diseases. New York: Churchill Livingstone, 1995, pp 1753–1754.

102. Tramont E, Hoover DL: General or non-specific host defense mechanisms. In: Mandell GL, Bennett JE, Dolin R (eds): Principles and Practice of Infectious Diseases. New York: Churchill Livingstone, 1995, pp 30–34.

103. Farmer JJ III, Kelly MT: Enterobacteriaceae. In: Balows A, Hausler WJ Jr, Herrmann KL, et al. (eds): Manual of Clinical Microbiology. St Louis: CV Mosby, 1987, pp 289–328.

104. Brook I, Finegold SM: Bacteriology of chronic otitis media. JAMA 1979; 241: 487–488.

105. Erkan M, Aslan T, Sevuk E, Guney E: Bacteriology of chronic suppurative otitis media. Ann Otol Rhinol Laryngol 1994; 103: 771–774.

106. Hussain MA, Ali EM, Ahmed HS: Otitis media in Sudanese children: Presentation and bacteriology. East Afr Med J 1991; 68: 679–685.

107. Kenna MA: Treatment of chronic suppurative otitis media. Otolaryngol Clin North Am 1994; 27: 457–472.

108. Orbello PW Jr, Park RI, Belcher LJ, et al.: Microbiology of chronic sinusitis in children. Arch Otolaryngol Head Neck Surg 1991; 117: 980–983.

109. Van Cauwenberge PB, Vander-Mijnsbrugge AM, Ingels KJ: The microbiology of acute and chronic sinusitis and otitis media: A review. Eur Arch Otorhinolaryngol 1993; 250(suppl 1): S3–S6.

110. Wald ER: Sinusitis in infants and children. Ann Otol Rhinol Laryngol 1992; 101: 37–41.

111. Burton DM, Seid DB, Kearns DB, Pransky SM: Neonatal otitis media: An update. Arch Otolaryngol Head Neck Surg 1993; 119: 672–675.

112. Rouby JJ, Laurent P, Gosnach M, et al.: Risk factors and clinical relevance of nosocomial maxillary sinusitis in the critically ill. Am J Respir Crit Care Med 1994; 150: 776–783.

113. Holzapfel L, Chevret S, Madinier G, et al.: Influence of long-term oro- or nasotracheal intubation on nosocomial maxillary sinusitis and pneumonia: Results of a prospective, randomized, clinical trial. Crit Care Med 1993; 21: 1132–1138.

114. Pit S, Jamal F, Cheah FK: Microbiology of cerebral abscess: A four-year study in Malaysia. J Trop Med Hygiene 1993; 96: 191–196.

115. Andraca R, Edson RS, Kern EB: Rhinoscleroma: A growing concern in the United States? Mayo Clinic experiences. Mayo Clin Proc 1993; 68: 1151–1157.

116. Paul C, Pialoux G, Dupont B, et al.: Infection due to *Klebsiella rhinoscleromatis* in two patients infected with human immunodeficiency virus. Clin Infect Dis 1993; 16: 441–442.

117. Busch RF: Rhinoscleroma occurring with airway obstruction. Otolaryngol Head Neck Surg 1993; 109: 933–936.

118. Lenis A, Ruff T, Diaz JA, Ghandour EG: Rhinoscleroma. South Med J 1988; 81: 1580–1582.

119. Dharan M, Nactigal D, Rosen G: Intraoperative demonstration of Mikulicz cells in nasal scleroma. A case report. Acta Cytol 1993; 37: 732–734.

120. Perkins BA, Hamill RJ, Musher DM, O'Hara C: In vitro activities of streptomycin and 11 oral antimicrobial agents against clinical isolates of *Klebsiella rhinoscleromatis*. Antimicrob Agents Chemother 1992; 36: 1785–1787.

121. Trautman M, Held T, Ruhnke M, Schnoy N: A case of rhinoscleroma cured with ciprofloxacin. Infection 1993; 21: 403–406.

122. Borgsein J, Sada E, Cortes R: Ciprofloxacin for rhinoscleroma and ozena. Lancet 1993; 342: 122.

123. Tang LM, Chen ST: *Klebsiella ozaenae* meningitis: Report of two cases and review of the literature. Infection 1994; 22: 58–61.

124. Zohar Y, Talmi YP, Strauss M, et al.: Ozena revisited. J Otolaryngol 1990; 19: 345–349.

125. Butler T: *Yersinia* species, including plague. In: Mandell GL, Bennett JE, Dolin R (eds): Principles and Practice of Infectious Diseases. New York: Churchill Livingstone, 1995, pp 2071–2074.

126. Fenwick SG: Pharyngitis and infections with *Yersinia enterocolitica*. N Z Med J 1992; 105: 112.

127. Eavey RD: Abnormalities in the neonatal ear: Otoscopic observations, histologic observations, and a model for contamination of the middle ear by cellular contents of amniotic fluid. Laryngoscope 1993; 103: 1–31.

128. Hornstrup MK, Gahrn-Hansen B: Extraintestinal infections caused by *Vibrio parahaemolyticus* and *Vibrio alginolyticus* in a Danish county, 1987–1992. Scand J Infect Dis 1993; 25: 735–740.

129. Arashima Y, Kumasaka K, Okuyama K, et al.: The first report of human chronic sinusitis by *Pasteurella multocida* subsp. *multocida* in Japan. Kansenshogaku Zasshi 1992; 66: 232–235.

130. Nakano H, Sekitani T, Ogata Y, et al.: Paranasal sinusitis due to *Pasteurella multocida*. Nippon Jibiinkoka Gakkai Kaiho 1993; 96: 192–196.

131. Kilian M: *Haemophilus*. In: Ballows A, Hausler WJ Jr, Herrmann KL, et al. (eds): Manual of Clinical Microbiology, 5th ed. Washington, DC: American Society for Microbiology, 1991, pp 463–470.

132. Wilson R, Moxon ER: Molecular mechanisms of *Haemophilus influenzae* pathogenicity in the respiratory tract. In: Donachie W, Griffiths E, Stephen J (eds): Bacterial Infections of Respiratory and Gastrointestinal Mucosae. Washington, DC: IRL Press, 1988; 24: 29–38.

133. Jacobs RF, Condrey YM, Yamauchi T: Tularemia in adults and children: A changing presentation. Pediatrics 1985; 76: 818–822.

134. Luotonen J, Syrjälä H, Jokinen K, et al.: Tularemia in otolaryngologic practice. An analysis of 127 cases. Arch Otolaryngol Head Neck Surg 1986; 112: 77–80.

135. Nordahl SH, Hoel T, Scheel O, Olofsson J: Tularemia: A differential diagnosis in oto-rhinolaryngology J Laryngol Otol 1993; 107: 127–129.

136. Tärnvik A: Nature of protective immunity to *Francisella tularensis*. Rev Infect Dis 1989; 11: 440–450.

137. Johnson JT, Yu VL, Best MG, et al.: Nosocomial legionellosis in surgical patients with head and neck cancer: Implications for epidemiological reservoir and mode of transmission. Lancet 1985; 2: 298–300.

138. Lowry PW, Tompkins LS: Nosocomial legionellosis: A review of pulmonary and extrapulmonary syndromes. Am J Infect Control 1993; 21: 21–27.

139. Vickers RM, Ying YC, Yu VL, et al.: Prospective evaluation of laboratory diagnostic methods for *Legionella* in culture-confirmed patients (Abstract). Am Soc Microbiol 1994; c17.

140. Graham DR, Band JD, Thornsberry C, et al.: Infections caused by *Moraxella catarrhalis*, *Moraxella urethralis*, *Moraxella*-like groups M-5 and M-6, and *Kingella kingae* in the United States, 1953–1980. Rev Infect Dis 1990; 12: 423–431.

141. Kowalski RP, Harwick JC: Incidence of *Moraxella* conjunctival infection. Am J Ophthalmol 1986; 101: 437.

142. Verheul AFM, Snippe H, Poolman JT: Meningococcal lipopolysaccharides: Virulence factor and potential vaccine component. Microbiol Rev 1993; 57: 34–49.

143. Boslego JW, Tramont E: *Neisseria meningitidis*. In: Gorbach SL, Bartlett JG, Blacklow NR (eds): Infectious Diseases. Philadelphia: WB Saunders Co, 1992, pp 1452–1456.

144. Wiesner PJ, Tronca E, Bonin P, et al.: Clinical spectrum of pharyngeal gonococcal infection. N Engl J Med 1973; 288: 181–185.

145. Weiss AA, Hewlett EL: Virulence factors of *Bordetella pertussis*. Annu Rev Microbiol 1986; 40: 661.

146. Gueirard P, Guiso N: Virulence of *Bordetella bronchiseptica*: Role of adenylate cyclase hemolysin. Infect Immun 1993; 61: 4072–4078.

147. Yamaguchi M, Matsui Y, Tanaka E, et al.: A case of sino-bronchial syndrome with repeatedly detected *Bordetella bronchiseptica* from sputum. Nippon Naika Gakkai Zasshi 1992; 81: 1105–1107.

148. Woolfrey BF, Moody JA: Human infections associated with *Bordetella bronchiseptica*. Clin Microbiol Rev 1991; 4: 243–255.

149. McGowan JE Jr, Steinberg JP: Other gram-negative bacilli. In: Mandell GL, Bennett JE, Dolin R (eds): Principles and Practice of Infectious Diseases. New York: Churchill Livingstone, 1995, pp 2107–2012.

150. Hemady R, Zimmerman A, Katzen BW, Karesh JW: Orbital cellulitis caused by *Eikenella corrodens* (see comments). Am J Ophthalmol 1992; 114: 584–588.

151. Perez-Diaz L, de Pablos M, Michaus ML, et al.: Periorbital abscess and paranasal sinusitis caused by *Eikenella corrodens* (letter). Enferm Infecc Microbiol Clin 1993; 11: 344–345.

152. Rees RJW: The microbiology of leprosy. In: Hastings RC (ed): Leprosy. Edinburgh: Churchill Livingstone, 1985, pp 186–190.

153. Gelber RH: Leprosy (Hansen's disease). In: Mandell GL, Bennett JE, Dolin R (eds): Principles and Practice of Infectious Diseases. New York: Churchill Livingstone, 1995, pp 2245–2249.

154. Musher DM: The biology of *Treponema pallidum*. In: Holmes K, Mardh P, Sparling F, et al. (eds): Sexually Transmitted Diseases. New York: McGraw-Hill, 1990, pp 205–206.

155. Kampmeier RH: Late benign syphilis. In: Holmes K, Mardh P, Sparling F, et al.: Sexually Transmitted Diseases. New York: McGraw-Hill, 1990, pp 251–262.

156. Garner JS, Jarvis WR, Emori TG, et al.: CDC definitions for nosocomial infections, 1988. Am J Infect Control 1988; 16: 128–140.

157. Baltch AL: *Pseudomonas aeruginosa* bacteremia. In: Baltch AL, Smith RP (eds): *Pseudomonas aeruginosa* Infections and Treatment. New York: Marcel Dekker, 1994, pp 73–128.

Itzhak Brook

CHAPTER TWENTY-TWO

Oropharyngeal Anaerobes

▼

MICROBIOLOGY

Before the advent of anaerobic microbiology, the bacteria of the oropharynx were thought to consist mainly of facultative organisms such as *Staphylococcus aureus* and *Streptococcus pyogenes*. With the entry of anaerobic bacteriologic methodology into the clinical microbiology laboratory, anaerobic bacteria have been shown to be major pathogens of ear, nose, and throat infections.

Description of Pathogens

The anaerobic bacteria that predominate in head and neck infection are of oral flora origin.[1–3] They include the pigmented *Prevotella* and *Porphyromonas* species (previously called *Bacteroides melaninogenicus* group), which include *Prevotella melaninogenicus, Prevotella intermedius, Prevotella oralis, Prevotella oris, Prevotella buccae,* and *Porphyromonas asaccharolyticus; Fusobacterium* species, which include *Fusobacterium nucleatum* and *Fusobacterium necrophorum; Bacteroides ureolyticus* (all are anaerobic gram-negative bacilli) and *Peptostreptococcus* species.[1, 2] These organisms are a potential source of a variety of chronic infections such as otitis; sinusitis; aspiration pneumonia; empyema; and lung, oropharynx, and dental abscesses.[1, 2] Most infections involving anaerobic bacteria are polymicrobial and include multiple anaerobic as well as aerobic bacteria, and the number of isolates varies between two and seven per site.[1, 2]

Microbial Characteristics

Anaerobic bacteria do not grow on solid media in the presence of room air (10% carbon dioxide and 18% oxygen), whereas facultative anaerobic bacteria grow in both the presence and the absence of air. Microaerophilic bacteria grow poorly or not at all aerobically but grow better under 10% carbon dioxide or anaerobically. Anaerobes can be divided into strict anaerobes that are unable to grow in the presence of >0.5% oxygen or moderate anaerobes that are capable of growing at between 2% and 8% oxygen.[1] Anaerobes generally do not possess catalase, but some clinical isolates can produce superoxide dismutase that can protect them from oxygen.

Virulence Factors

Anaerobes contribute to the severity of infection through their synergy with their aerobic counterparts and with each other.[4] Anaerobes take longer to become virulent. This is because some of the major virulence factors of certain anaerobic species (i.e., the production of a capsule) are expressed only after the infection has become chronic.[5]

Many of the anaerobes involved in ear, nose, and throat infections possess a number of virulence factors. Encapsulation of gram-negative anaerobic bacilli (*Bacteroides, Fusobacterium, Prevotella,* and *Porphyromonas* species) and *Peptostreptococcus* species has been found to be higher when they are isolated from patients with tonsillitis[6] and head and neck abscesses,[7] as compared with their rate of encapsulation when they are part of the normal oral flora. *Fusobacterium* species are capable of producing lipopolysaccharides, neutrophil cytotoxic substances, leukotoxins, and deoxyribonuclease, all associated with virulence.[8] Inhibition of chemotaxis and production of tissue-destroying toxins have been observed for *F. nucleatum, P. asaccharolytica,* and *Porphyromonas gingivalis.* Pigmented *Prevotella* and *Porphyromonas* organisms can degrade serum proteins,[8] and *P. gingivalis* and *F. nucleatum* have enhanced adherence to oral epithelial cells. Other virulence factors include coagulation promotion and spreading factors.[8]

An indirect pathogenic role of anaerobes is their ability to produce the enzyme beta-lactamase. Beta-lactamase-producing bacteria can be involved directly in the infection and protect not only themselves but also other penicillin-susceptible organisms from the activity of penicillins. This can occur when the enzyme beta-lactamase is secreted into the infected tissue or abscess fluid in sufficient quantities to degrade the beta-lactam ring of penicillin before it can kill the susceptible bacteria.[9] In vitro studies have demonstrated protection of penicillin-susceptible aerobic and anaerobic bacteria from penicillin by beta-lactamase-producing bacteria (i.e., protection of group A streptococci by *S. aureus* or *Bacteroides* species.) In vivo studies using animal models of abscess or pneumonia showed survival of group A beta hemolytic *Streptococcus* (GABHS) or *Prevotella* species due to the presence of beta-lactamase-producing *Bacteroides, Prevotella,* or *Fusobacterium* organisms.[9] Beta-lactamase-producing bacteria can be recovered from more than half of respiratory tract infections.[2] The predominant anaerobic beta-lactamase-producing bacteria are pigmented *Prevotella* and *Porphyromonas, Bacteroides,* and *Fusobacterium* species; they have been isolated from recurrently inflamed tonsils,[9] chronic otitis,[10] sinusitis,[11] and abscesses of the head and neck.[2] Up to 50% of these organisms can produce beta-lactamase.[12] "Free" beta-lactamase has been detected within the core of inflamed tonsils and aspirates of acute and chronic ear and sinus infections.[2]

The high incidence of recovery of beta-lactamase–producing bacteria in upper respiratory tract infections may be due to the selection of these organisms after antimicrobial therapy with beta-lactam antibiotics. The emergence of penicillin-resistant flora can occur after only a short course of penicillin, and these organisms can spread to other individuals.[13]

EPIDEMIOLOGY

Natural Reservoirs

Most human mucosal and epithelial surfaces including the oropharynx are colonized with aerobic and anaerobic microorganisms that are referred to as the *normal* or *indigenous* flora.[3] The organisms that prevail in one body system predictably belong to certain major bacterial species. These sets of bacterial flora remain stable throughout life. The relative and total number of each type of organism, however, can be affected by factors such as age, diet, anatomic variations, illness, hospitalization, and antimicrobial therapy.

The microflora of the oral cavity are complex and contain many kinds of aerobic and facultative and obligate anaerobes. The establishment of the normal oral flora is initiated at birth. Certain organisms such as lactobacilli and anaerobic streptococci reach high numbers within a few days after birth. *Actinomyces, Fusobacterium,* and *Nocardia* species are acquired by the age of 6 months. Thereafter, *Prevotella, Porphyromonas, Bacteroides, Leptotrichia, Propionibacterium,* and Candida species are also established as part of the oral flora.

Anaerobic bacteria are present in large numbers in both the mouth and the oropharynx, particularly in patients with poor dental hygiene, caries, or periodontal disease. Anaerobic bacteria can adhere to tooth surfaces and contribute, through the elaboration of metabolic products, to caries and periodontal disease that can range from gingivitis to periodontitis.[1, 2] Anaerobic bacteria outnumber the aerobic counterpart in a ratio of 10:1 to 100:1. The number of anaerobic strains, however, varies between locations within the oropharynx. The distribution of organisms within the oral cavity seems to be a function of their ability to adhere to the oral mucous membrane surfaces. The differences in numbers of the anaerobic microflora probably occur because of the considerable variation in the oxygen concentration in parts of the oral cavity. The periodontal pockets are the most anaerobic area in the oral cavity. The maxillary and mandibular buccal folds contain less oxygen than the tongue surfaces. The buccal folds are more anaerobic than the gingival sulcus. The ratio of anaerobic bacteria to aerobic bacteria in saliva is approximately 10:1, and the total number of anaerobic bacteria is 1.1×10^8/mL.

Links to Humans

Anaerobes are especially important in the chronic form of many otolaryngologic infections, but proper techniques for anaerobic transportation, cultivation, and identification are necessary for consistent isolation. Anaerobes have been isolated from acute[14] and chronic[10, 15] otitis media,

cholesteatoma,[16, 17] mastoiditis,[18] tonsillar and retropharyngeal abscesses,[19] recurrent tonsillitis,[9] suppurative thyroiditis,[20] parotitis,[21] chronic sinusitis,[11] cervical lymphadenitis,[22] wound infection after head and neck surgery,[23] deep neck infection,[24] and dental infection[25] (Table 22–1).

COLONIZATION, TRANSMISSION, PATHOGENESIS, IMMUNOLOGY

Many otolaryngologic infections evolve over several stages (Fig. 22–1). The initial infection is often viral, and this compromises local immunity, allows adherence of bacterial pathogens to damaged mucous membranes, and causes edema and swelling. The aerobic bacterial components of the oropharyngeal flora become the first pathogens. Aerobic and facultative anaerobic bacteria are not susceptible to oxygen and are therefore generally more immediately virulent than their anaerobic counterparts. However, as the infection progresses, oxygen is consumed by the aerobic bacteria, the pH is lowered, and the developing edema decreases the blood flow to the area, thereby generating conditions more ideal for anaerobes. As the infection becomes protracted and chronic, anaerobic bacteria become predominant. Polymicrobial aerobic-anaerobic bacterial flora are recovered during this state; mixed infection allows synergistic virulent relationships between aerobic and anaerobic bacteria.[4]

PATHOGENS IN EAR, NOSE, AND THROAT INFECTIONS

Pharynx, Tonsil, and Adenoid

Indirect evidence is mounting that anaerobes are involved in both acute and chronic tonsillitis. The evidence is mainly derived from studies of complications of anaerobic tonsillitis (i.e., bacteremia, abscesses). Anaerobic bacteria play a major role in complications of tonsillitis. The organisms associated with the infection are *Fusobacterium* species, gram-negative anaerobic bacilli, and *Peptostreptococcus* species. Polymicrobial aerobic and anaerobic flora predominate in peritonsillar and retropharyngeal abscesses, where the number of isolates is between 1 and 12 (average 5 anaerobes or 2 aerobes).[1, 2, 19] These organisms can be isolated from 25% of suppurative cervical lymph nodes and are mostly associated with the presence of dental or tonsillar infections.[22] Anaerobic organisms have been associated with thrombophlebitis of the internal jugular veins, which often causes postanginal sepsis.[1]

The pathogenic role of anaerobes in the acute inflammatory process in the tonsils is also supported by several clinical observations: their recovery in tonsillar or retropharyngeal abscesses in many cases without any aerobic bacteria,[19] the isolation of anaerobes from tonsils in Vincent's angina,[1] the recovery of encapsulated pigmented *Prevotella* and *Porphyromonas* species in acutely inflamed tonsils,[6] the isolation of anaerobes from the core of recurrently inflamed non-GABHS tonsils,[26] and the response to antibiotics in patients with non-GABHS tonsillitis.[27, 28] Furthermore, im-

Table 22–1. AEROBIC AND ANAEROBIC BACTERIA ISOLATED IN UPPER RESPIRATORY TRACT INFECTIONS

Type of Infection	Aerobic and Facultative Organisms	Anaerobic Organism
Otitis media: acute	*Streptococcus pneumoniae* *Haemophilus influenzae** *Moraxella catarrhalis**	*Peptostreptococcus* spp.
Otitis media: chronic, and mastoiditis	*Staphylococcus aureus** *Escherichia coli** *Klebsiella pneumoniae** *Pseudomonas aeruginosa** *Peptostreptococcus* spp.	Pigmented *Prevotella* and *Porphyromonas* spp.* *Bacteroides* spp.* *Fusobacterium* spp.*
Peritonsillar and retropharyngeal abscess	*Streptococcus pyogenes* *S. aureus** *S. pneumoniae*	*Fusobacterium* spp.* Pigmented *Prevotella* and *Porphyromonas* spp.* *Peptostreptococcus* spp.
Recurrent tonsillitis	*S. pyogenes* *H. influenzae** *S. aureus**	*Fusobacterium* spp.*
Suppurative thyroiditis	*S. pyogenes* *S. aureus**	Pigmented *Prevotella* and *Porphyromonas* spp.* *Peptostreptococcus* spp.
Sinusitis: acute	*H. influenzae** *S. pneumoniae* *M. catarrhalis**	*Peptostreptococcus* spp.
Sinusitis: chronic	*S. aureus** *S. pneumoniae* *H. influenzae**	*Bacteroides fragilis* group* Pigmented *Prevotella* and *Porphyromonas* spp.* *Peptostreptococcus* spp.
Cervical lymphadenitis	*S. aureus** *Mycobacterium* spp.	Pigmented *Prevotella* and *Porphyromonas* spp.* *Peptostreptococcus* spp.
Postoperative infection disrupting oral mucosa	*Staphylococcus* spp.* Enterobacteriaceae* *Staphylococcus* spp.*	*Fusobacterium* spp.* *Bacteroides* spp.* Pigmented *Prevotella* and *Porphyromonas* spp.* *Peptostreptococcus* spp.
Deep neck species	*Streptococcus* spp. *Staphylococcus* spp.*	*Bacteroides* spp.* *Fusobacterium* spp.* *Peptostreptococcus* spp.
Odontogenic complications	*Streptococcus* spp. *Staphylococcus* spp.*	Pigmented *Prevotella* and *Porphyromonas* spp.* *Peptostreptococcus* spp.
Oropharyngeal: Vincent's angina and necrotizing ulcerative gingivitis	*Streptococcus* spp. *Staphylococcus* spp.*	*Fusobacterium necrophorum** Spirochetes

*Organisms that have the potential of producing beta-lactamase.

mune response against *P. intermedia* can be detected in patients with non-GABHS tonsillitis[29]; an immune response can also be detected against *P. intermedia* and *F. nucleatum* in patients who recovered from peritonsillar cellulitis or abscesses[30] and infectious mononucleosis.[31]

Metronidazole therapy also alleviated the symptoms of tonsillar hypertrophy and shortened the duration of fever in patients with infectious mononucleosis.[27] Since metronidazole has no antiviral or aerobic antibacterial efficacy,[1] suppression of the oral anaerobic flora may contribute to dimin-

Figure 22–1. Interactions between organisms in respiratory infections.

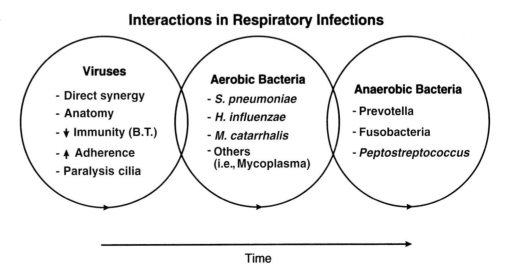

Interactions in Respiratory Infections

ishing the inflammatory process induced by the Epstein-Barr virus. This is supported by the increased recovery of *P. intermedia* and *F. nucleatum* during the acute phases of infectious mononucleosis.[32]

GABHS, *Staph. aureus,* and viruses are generally associated with tonsillar and peritonsillar infections. However, anaerobes also have been isolated from the cores of tonsils of children with recurrent GABHS[33] and non-GABHS tonsillitis[26] and peritonsillar and retropharyngeal[19] abscesses. The number of isolates per tonsil varied between 3 and 11. Beta-lactamase-producing strains of pigmented *Prevotella* and *Porphyromonas* species, *Bacteroides fragilis, Fusobacterium* species, and *S. aureus* were isolated from the tonsils of more than 75% of children with recurrent GABHS tonsillitis[9, 33, 34] and from 40% of children with non-GABHS tonsillitis.[26] Similar organisms were recovered from patients with adenoiditis and adenoid hypertrophy.[35]

Recurrent pharyngotonsillitis and failure to eradicate the GABHS with penicillin can be a serious clinical problem. One explanation for penicillin failure is that repeated administrations result in selection of beta-lactamase-producing bacteria.[9] The recovery of these bacteria in more than three quarters of the patients with recurrent GABHS tonsillitis,[9, 33, 34] the ability to measure beta-lactamase activity in the core of these tonsils,[36] and the response of patients to antimicrobials effective against beta-lactamase-producing bacteria (i.e., clindamycin or amoxicillin plus clavulanic acid[9, 37, 38] support the role of these aerobic as well as anaerobic organisms in the inability of penicillin to eradicate GABHS tonsillitis.

Ear Infection

Whenever adequate aerobic techniques have been employed, substantial numbers of anaerobic bacteria have been recovered from patients with acute, serous, and chronic otitis media.[1, 2, 10, 12, 14, 15]

Acute Otitis Media

Anaerobes, mainly *Peptostreptococcus* species and *Propionibacterium acnes* were isolated from about 25% of ear aspirates of acute otitis media. Anaerobic bacteria were isolated in about 50% of the patients in conjunction with aerobic and facultative bacteria.[14] However, since the external ear canal was not sterilized before the aspiration of specimens, the possibility of contamination by normal bacterial flora of the ear canal exists. Since the anaerobic bacteria recovered in acute otitis media are susceptible to antimicrobials commonly used to treat acute otitis media, the recovery of anaerobes does not require a change in the recommended empiric antimicrobial therapy for this infection. However, more studies are needed to elucidate the role of anaerobes in acute otitis media.

Serous Otitis Media

Anaerobes were isolated in 23 of 57 (41%) of the patients with serous otitis media.[39] Anaerobes were recovered as the only isolate in 17% of the culture-positive specimens, and in an additional 26% they were found mixed with aerobes

and facultative organisms. The predominant anaerobes were *Peptostreptococcus* species and pigmented *Prevotella* and *Prophyromonas* species. The role of microorganisms in the pathogenesis of serous otitis media is not yet defined, however. Since organisms can be recovered in about 50% of serous otitis media aspirates, antimicrobial agents are often administered to patients in an attempt to eradicate these bacteria. The presence of bacteria, many of which produce beta-lactamase, raises the question whether antibiotics also effective against these bacteria should be used in the treatment of serous otitis media. Controlled studies of therapy may clarify the role of anaerobic bacteria in the pathogenesis of the inflammatory process in serous otitis media.

Chronic Suppurative Otitis Media

The high number of cultures showing no bacterial growth in some studies of chronic suppurative otitis media may be attributed to the use of inappropriate microbiologic methods for the recovery of anaerobes.[1] Several studies reported the recovery of anaerobes in about 50% of the patients with chronic suppurative otitis media[1, 2, 10, 15] and those with cholesteatoma.[16, 17] The variability in the rate of isolation of anaerobes in these studies may be attributed to differences in the geographic locations of the studies and to laboratory methodologies. The predominant anaerobes recovered in these studies were *Peptostreptococcus*; pigmented *Prevotella* and *Porphyromonas*; and *Fusobacterium* species. Many of these organisms can produce beta-lactamase and might have contributed to the high failure rate of beta-lactam antibiotics in the therapy of this infection. Anaerobic bacteria were recovered, mixed with other anaerobic or aerobic bacteria, and the number of isolates ranged between 2 and 6 per specimen. Anaerobes were isolated from 23 of 24 (96%) specimens of chronic mastoiditis[18] and from most patients with intracranial abscesses that complicate chronic suppurative otitis media.[1, 2]

Anaerobic bacteria are often recovered from infected cholesteatomas.[16, 17] Cholesteatoma that often accompanies chronic suppurative otitis media can enhance the absorption of bone. The production of organic acids by anaerobic bacteria may promote the process of bone destruction.[17] Since cholesteatoma associated with chronic suppurative otitis media contains bacteria similar to those recovered from chronically infected ears,[16] the cholesteatoma may serve as a nidus of the chronic infection.

Sinus Infection

Infections of sinuses do not occur if proper aeration and drainage are maintained. However, disease may develop when allergy, viral infection, or anatomic obstruction occurs, preventing normal drainage. In the first stages of infection, the most common pathogens are similar to those recovered in acute otitis media: *S. pneumoniae, H. influenzae,* and *Moraxella catarrhalis.* Anaerobic organisms become involved as the infection becomes chronic and the levels of tissue oxygen decline.[40] Although anaerobes are generally isolated from only about 10% of patients with acute sinusitis, they can be isolated from up to 67% of patients with chronic infection.[1, 2] The predominant anaerobes are pigmented *Prevotella* and *Porphyromonas; Fusobacterium*; and *Peptostreptococcus.*[1, 2] An average of three anaerobes per sinus aspirate were recovered in children and adults with chronic sinusitis.[11]

Sinus infection may spread via anastomosing veins or contiguously to the central nervous system. Intracranial complications include orbital cellulitis,[41] meningitis, cavernous sinus thrombosis, and epidural, subdural, and brain abscesses.[1, 2]

Dental Infections

All odonotogenic infections involve anaerobic bacteria (see Chapter 55). These include pulpitis, periapical or dental abscess, and perimandibular space infections. Infections can originate in the dental structures or in the surrounding soft tissues. Root canal infection can progress to a periapical abscess, which may involve the surrounding alveolar bone.[1, 2] The organisms isolated from these infections are *Prevotella, Porphyromonas, Fusobacterium,* and *Peptostreptococcus* species, microaerophilic streptococci and *Streptococcus salivarius.*[25]

Gingival crevice and gum infections that include gingivitis, periodontitis, and pyorrhea generally involve anaerobic bacteria.[42] Vincent's angina (or trench mouth) is a distinct form of ulcerative gingivitis; the causative organisms include *Fusobacterium* species and anaerobic spirochetes, although definitive studies using anaerobic microbiologic methods remain to be performed.

Deep Neck Infection

Deep neck infections generally follow oral, dental, and pharyngeal infections and are usually polymicrobial, involving the anaerobic organisms that caused the primary infections. The predominant pathogens are *Peptostreptococcus, Fusobacterium* species, and anaerobic gram-negative bacilli.[24, 43] These infections are potentially life-threatening, because of their ability to compromise the airways, involve the vascular system, and extend to vital structures. Although the administration of antimicrobials with proper coverage against anaerobes is essential, surgical drainage and débridement are crucial in the management of deep neck infections.

Miscellaneous

Parotitis

Of all the salivary glands, the parotid gland is most commonly affected by an inflammatory process. Predisposing factors include dehydration, malnutrition, oral neoplasms, immunosuppression, sialolithiasis, and medications that diminish salivation. Viral parotitis can be caused by paramyxovirus (mumps), Epstein-Barr virus, coxsackievirus, human immunodeficiency virus, and influenza A and parainfluenza viruses. Acute suppurative parotitis is generally caused by *S. aureus, Streptococcus* species, and, rarely, aerobic gram-

negative bacteria. Anaerobic bacteria, mostly *Peptostreptococcus, Bacteroides,* and pigmented *Prevotella* and *Porphyromonas* species, have also been recognized as an important cause of this infection.[21] Empiric antibiotic therapy should be directed against both aerobic and anaerobic bacteria. Surgical drainage may be indicated when pus has formed.

Cervical Lymphadenitis

Cervical lymphadenitis is characterized by an inflammation of one or more lymph nodes in the neck (see Chapter 57). The anterior cervical, the submandibular, or the posterior cervical nodes are the most prevalent sites of infection. The most common causes in children are viruses. The organisms that cause acute unilateral infection associated with facial trauma or impetigo are *S. aureus* and *S. pyogenes.* Cat scratch and mycobacterial infections are important in chronic infections. Anaerobic bacteria have been isolated in about 25% of the infections, often in pure culture[22]; the predominate anaerobes were *Fusobacterium* and *Peptostreptococcus* species. The recovery of anaerobes was often associated with a primary dental, periodontal, or tonsillar infection.

Thyroiditis

Anaerobic bacteria such as anaerobic gram-negative bacilli and *Peptostreptococcus* species have been identified as causative agents in thyroiditis.[1, 2, 20] *Eikenella corrodens* and *Actinomyces* species have also been reported. Since methodologies for the recovery of anaerobic bacteria were not uniformly used in all past reports, the true role of these organisms is unknown.

Infected Cysts

Thyroglossal duct cysts, cystic hygromas, branchial cleft cysts, laryngoceles, and dermoid cysts can become inflamed and cause local infection.[2] The organisms that can cause secondary infection of these cysts can originate from either the skin or the oropharynx. Blockage of these cysts predisposes to infection by preventing the evacuation of their contents. *S. aureus* and *S. pyogenes* are the predominant aerobic isolates, whereas pigmented *Prevotella* and *Porphyromonas* species and *Peptostreptococcus* species[44] are the predominant anaerobes.

Infection After Head and Neck Surgery

Wound infection frequently occurs after head and neck surgery, especially after surgery for malignant tumors. The occurrence of these infections is related to the exposure of the surgical site to the oropharyngeal flora and the fact that the surgical site is compromised because of the decreased blood supply and the presence of necrotic tissues. Postsurgical head and neck wounds are generally infected by polymicrobial aerobic and anaerobic flora; the average number of isolates varies from one to nine (average six).[23] The most frequently recovered isolates are *Peptostreptococcus* species, *Staph. aureus,* anaerobic gram-negative bacill (i.e., *Bacteroides* species), *Fusobacterium* species, and enteric gram-negative rods. The presence of polymicrobial flora in postsurgical wounds after head and neck cancer surgery warrants the use of antimicrobial agents that are effective against these organisms in the prophylaxis and therapy of this infection.[45]

LABORATORY DIAGNOSIS

Anaerobic infections present special methodologic problems not encountered in other types of bacterial infections. Recovery of anaerobes is often suboptimal for a number of reasons. The clinical specimen may not be placed in anaerobic conditions for transport to the laboratory. The specimen may be contaminated by normal flora. Many laboratories are not equipped to identify anaerobes accurately.[1, 2] Finally, anaerobes require a longer time for isolation than aerobes.

Specimens must be obtained free of contamination, excluding saprophytic organisms or normal flora so that culture results can be interpreted correctly (Table 22–2). Because indigenous anaerobes often are present on the surfaces of skin and mucous membranes in large numbers, even minimal contamination of a specimen with the normal flora can give misleading results. On this basis, specimens can be designated according to their acceptability for anaerobic culture to either the acceptable or unacceptable category. Materials that are appropriate for anaerobic cultures should be obtained with a technique that bypasses the normal flora. Unacceptable specimens include coughed sputum, bronchoscopy aspirates, gingival and throat swabs, feces, and gastric aspirates. However, selective media may be used to detect only a possible pathogen, such as *Clostridium difficile,* in stool obtained from a patient with colitis.

Acceptable specimens include blood specimens; aspirates of body fluids (pleural, pericardial, cerebrospinal, and joint fluids); abscess contents; deep aspirates of wounds; and specimens collected by special techniques, such as transtracheal aspirates or direct lung puncture (see Table 22–2). Direct needle aspiration probably is the best method of obtaining a culture, whereas the use of swabs is much less desirable. Specimens obtained from sites that are normally sterile may be collected after thorough skin decontamination.[2]

Table 22–2. METHODS FOR COLLECTION OF ANAEROBIC BACTERIAL SPECIMENS FROM EAR, NOSE, AND THROAT INFECTIONS

Infection Site	Methods
Abscess or body cavity	Aspiration by syringe and needle (after incision: syringe, or swab [less desirable]).
Tissue or bone	Surgical specimen using tissue biopsy or curet.
Sinuses	Aspiration after decontamination, or surgical specimen.
Ear	Tympanocentesis after decontamination of ear canal; in perforation: cleanse ear canal and aspirate through perforation.
Lung	Transtracheal aspiration or lung puncture.
Pleura	Thoracentesis.

Specimen Transportation

The specimens should be placed into an anaerobic transporter as soon as possible after their collection. Aspirates of liquid specimens or tissues are always preferred to swabs. Several systems for the collection of all three culture forms are commercially available. These transport media are very helpful in preserving anaerobes until the time of inoculation.

Liquid specimens may be inoculated into a commercially available anaerobic transport vial, which is devoid of oxygen and sometimes contains an indicator. A plastic or glass syringe and needle also may be used for transport. After the specimen is collected and all air bubbles are expelled from the syringe and needle, the needle tip should be inserted into a sterile rubber stopper. Because air gradually diffuses through the wall of a plastic syringe, no more than 30 minutes should elapse before the specimen is processed. This inexpensive transport device for liquid specimens is especially useful in the hospital situation.[46]

Swabs may be placed into the sterilized tubes containing carbon dioxide or prereduced anaerobically sterile Carey and Blair semisolid media. A preferred method is to use a swab that has been placed in a prereduced anaerobic tube. Tissue specimens can be transported anaerobically in an anaerobic jar or in a Petri dish placed in a sealed plastic bag that can be rendered anaerobic by use of a catalyzer.

Laboratory Diagnosis

Laboratory diagnosis begins with the examination of a Gram-stained smear of the specimen. The types of organisms present suggest appropriate initial therapy and serve as a quality control on the final culture results. The laboratory should be able to recover all the morphologic types in the approximate ratio in which they are seen on Gram's stain. The techniques for cultivation of anaerobes should provide optimal anaerobic conditions throughout processing. Detailed procedures can be found in microbiology manuals.[46, 47]

Antimicrobial Susceptibility Testing

The susceptibility of anaerobic bacteria to antimicrobial agents has become less predictable. Resistance to several antimicrobial agents especially by anaerobic gram-negative bacilli and *Fusobacterium* species has increased over the past decade.[2] It is important, therefore, to perform susceptibility testing for anaerobes recovered from sterile body sites or those that are clinically important and have variable susceptibilities.

Screening of anaerobic gram-negative bacilli isolates (particularly *Prevotella, Bacteroides,* and *Fusobacterium* species) for beta-lactamase activity may be helpful. This can provide information regarding their penicillin susceptibility. However, occasional bacterial strains may resist beta-lactam antibiotics through other mechanisms.

Routine susceptibility testing of all anaerobic isolates is extremely time-consuming and in many cases unnecessary. Susceptibility testing should be limited to anaerobes isolated from blood cultures, bone, central nervous system, and serious otolaryngologic infections, as well as to anaerobic bacteria isolated in pure culture from properly collected specimens. Antibiotics tested should include penicillin, a broad-spectrum penicillin, a penicillin plus a beta-lactamase inhibitor, clindamycin, chloramphenicol, a second-generation cephalosporin (e.g., cefoxitin), metronidazole, and a carbapenem (e.g., imipenem).

TREATMENT

The recovery from an anaerobic infection depends on prompt and proper management. The strategy for therapy of anaerobic infections consists of surgical drainage of pus, débridement of any necrotic tissue, and appropriate antimicrobial therapy. Certain types of adjunctive therapy such as hyperbaric oxygen may also be useful. Antimicrobial therapy is in many patients the only form of therapy required, whereas in others it is an important adjunct to a surgical approach.

Since anaerobic bacteria are generally recovered mixed with aerobic organisms, selection of proper therapy becomes more complicated. In the treatment of mixed infection the choice of the appropriate antimicrobial agents should provide for adequate coverage of most of the pathogens.

Antimicrobial Drugs

Penicillins. Penicillin G is the drug of choice when the infecting strains are susceptible to this drug. However, as more species of anaerobic gram-negative bacilli have become resistant to penicillin, its use in head and neck infections has declined. Strains that are resistant to penicillins are all *B. fragilis* group and over half of *Prevotella, Porphyromonas,* and *Fusobacterium* species. However, penicillin is active against most *Actinomyces, Peptostreptococcus,* and *Propionibacterium* species and microaerophilic streptococci. Ampicillin and amoxicillin generally are equally active to penicillin, but the semisynthetic penicillins are less active than the parent compound. Methicillin, nafcillin, and the isoxazolyl penicillins have unpredictable activity and frequently are inferior to penicillin G against anaerobes. A beta-lactamase inhibitor (e.g., clavulanic acid) is combined with a penicillin (e.g., amoxicillin) for an oral preparation or with ticarcillin, ampicillin, or piperacillin for parenteral use. Most aerobic gram-negative bacilli are also susceptible to these agents.

Carbapenems. Carbapenems (imipenem-cilastatin and meropenem) are effective against a wide variety of aerobic and anaerobic gram-positive and gram-negative organisms. They possess excellent activity against beta-lactamase-producing anaerobic gram-negative bacilli and are an effective single agent for the therapy of mixed aerobic-anaerobic infection.

Cephalosporins. The antimicrobial spectrum of the first-generation cephalosporins against anaerobes is similar to that of penicillin G, although they are less active on a weight basis. Similar to what is seen with penicillin G, most strains of *B. fragilis* group and many of the *Prevotella* and *Fusobacterium* species are resistant to cephalosporins as a result of cephalosporinase production. Some of the second-generation

cephalosporins (cefoxitin and to a lesser degree cefotetan) are resistant to this enzyme and are therefore effective against most of the *B. fragilis* group as well as other anaerobic gram-negative bacilli. The third-generation cephalosporins (e.g., cefotaxime, ceftriaxone, ceftazidime) are only effective against about 50% of anaerobic gram-negative bacilli.

Chloramphenicol. Although it is a bacteriostatic drug, chloramphenicol is one of the most active antimicrobial drugs against anaerobes, and resistance to this drug is rare. Even though several failures to eradicate anaerobic infections, including bacteremia, with chloramphenicol have been reported,[1] this drug has been used for over 25 years for the treatment of anaerobic infections. It is regarded as a good choice for treatment of serious anaerobic infections when the nature and susceptibility of the infecting organisms are unknown. Because of its good penetration through the blood-brain barrier, it is used in infections of the central nervous system.

Clindamycin. Clindamycin has a broad range of activity against anaerobic organisms and has proved its efficacy in clinical trials. Approximately 95% of the isolated anaerobic bacteria are susceptible to easily achievable levels of clindamycin. *B. fragilis* as well as other anaerobic gram-negative bacilli are generally sensitive to levels below 3 μg/mL. There are, however, reports of resistant strains associated with clinical infections, although these are uncommon. Clindamycin is frequently used in combination with aminoglycosides or other agents effective against Enterobacteriaceae for the treatment of mixed aerobic-anaerobic infections.

Metronidazole. This drug shows excellent bactericidal activity against most obligate anaerobic bacteria, such as *B. fragilis* group, other species of anaerobic gram-negative bacilli, and *Fusobacterium* and *Clostridium* species. Occasional strains of anaerobic gram-positive cocci and nonsporulating gram-positive bacilli are highly resistant. Microaerophilic streptococci, *P. acnes,* and *Actinomyces* species are almost uniformly resistant. Aerobic and facultative anaerobes are usually highly resistant. More than 90% of obligate anaerobes are susceptible to less than 2 μg/mL metronidazole.

Because of its lack of activity against aerobic bacteria, additional antimicrobial agents effective against these organisms should be administered whenever they are also present. The use of metronidazole seems advantageous in central nervous system infections because of its excellent penetration across the blood-brain barrier.

Tetracyclines. Tetracycline has currently limited usefulness because of the development of resistance by virtually all types of anaerobes. The tetracycline analogues doxycycline and minocycline are more active than the parent compound.

Vancomycin. Vancomycin is effective against all gram-positive anaerobes but is inactive against gram-negative anaerobic bacteria. Little clinical experience exists for the treatment of anaerobic bacteria using vancomycin.

References

1. Finegold SM: Anaerobic Bacteria in Human Disease. New York: Academy Press, 1977.

2. Brook I: Pediatric Anaerobic Infection, Diagnosis and Management, 2nd ed. Philadelphia, Mosby, 1989.

3. Rosebury T: Microorganisms Indigenous to Man. New York: McGraw-Hill, 1962.

4. Brook I: Enhancement of growth of aerobic and facultative bacteria in mixed infections with *Bacteroides* sp. Infect Immun 1985; 50: 929–931.

5. Brook I, Myhal LA, Dorsey HC: Encapsulation and pilus formation of *Bacteroides* sp. J Infect 1991; 25: 251–257.

6. Brook I, Gober AE: *Bacteroides melaninogenicus,* its recovery from tonsils of children with acute tonsillitis. Arch Otolaryngol 1983; 109: 818–820.

7. Brook I: Recovery of encapsulated anaerobic bacteria from orofacial abscesses. J Med Microbiol 1986; 22: 171–176.

8. Hofstad T: Virulence determinants in non spore-forming anaerobic bacteria. Scand J Infect Dis 1989; 62(suppl): 15–24.

9. Brook I: The role of beta-lactamase-producing bacteria in the persistence of streptococcal tonsillar infection. Rev Infect Dis 1984; 6: 601–607.

10. Brook I: Prevalence of beta-lactamase-producing bacteria in chronic suppurative otitis media. Am J Dis Child 1985; 139: 280–284.

11. Brook I, Thompson DH, Frazier EH: Microbiology and management of chronic maxillary sinusitis. Arch Otolaryngol Head Neck Surg 1994; 120: 1317–1320.

12. Brook I: Beta-lactamase-producing bacteria in head and neck infection. Laryngoscope 1988; 98: 428–433.

13. Brook I, Gober AE: Emergence of beta-lactamase-producing aerobic and anaerobic bacteria in the oropharynx of children following penicillin chemotherapy. Clin Pediatr 1984; 23: 338–341.

14. Brook I, Anthony BV, Finegold SM: Aerobic and anaerobic bacteriology of acute otitis media in children. J Pediatr 1978; 92: 13–15.

15. Sweeney G, Picozzi GL, Browning GG: A quantitative study of aerobic and anaerobic bacteria in chronic suppurative otitis media. J Infect 1982; 5: 47–55.

16. Brook I: Aerobic and anaerobic bacteriology of cholesteatoma. Laryngoscope 1981; 91: 250–255.

17. Iino Y, Hoshimi E, Tomioko S, et al: Organic acids and anaerobic microorganisms in the contents of the cholesteatoma sac. Ann Otol Rhinol Laryngol 1983; 92: 91–94.

18. Brook I: Aerobic and anaerobic bacteriology of chronic mastoiditis in children. Am J Dis Child 1981; 135: 478–479.

19. Brook I, Frazier EH, Thompson DH: Aerobic and anaerobic microbiology of peritonsillar abscess. Laryngoscope 1991; 101: 289–292.

20. Bussman YC, Wong ML, Bell MJ, et al.: Suppurative thyroiditis with gas formation due to mixed anaerobic infection. J Pediatr 1977; 90: 321–322.

21. Brook I: Aerobic and anaerobic microbiology of acute suppurative parotitis. Laryngoscope 1991; 101: 170–172.

22. Brook I: Aerobic and anaerobic bacteriology of cervical adenitis in children. Clin Pediatr 1980; 19: 693–696.

23. Brook I, Hirokawa, R: Post surgical wound infection after head and neck cancer surgery. Ann Otol Rhinol Laryngol 1989; 98: 323–325.

24. Chow AW, Roser SM, Brady FA: Orofacial odontogenic infections. Ann Intern Med 1978; 88: 392–402.

25. Brook I, Frazier EH, Gher ME: Aerobic and anaerobic microbiology of periodontal abscess. Oral Microbiol Imm 1991; 6: 123–125.

26. Brook I, Yocum P: Comparison of the microbiology of group A strepto-coccal and non-group A streptococcal tonsillitis. Ann Otol Rhinol Larngol 1988; 97: 243–246.

27. Helstrom SA, Mandl PA, Ripa T: Treatment of infectious mononucleosis with metronidazole. Scand J Infec Dis 1978; 10: 7–9.

28. Putto A: Febrile exudative tonsillitis: Viral or streptococcal. Pediatrics 1987; 80: 6–12.

29. Brook I, Foote PA Jr, Slots J, Jackson W: Immune response to *Prevotella intermedia* in patients with recurrent non-streptococcal tonsillitis. Ann Otol Rhinol Laryngol 1993; 102: 113–116.

30. Brook I, Foote PA, Slots J: Immune response to *Fusobacterium nucleatum* and *Prevotella intermedia* in patients with peritonsillar cellulitis and abscess. Clin Infect Dis 1995; 20: S220–S221.

31. Brook I, de Leyva F: Immune response to *Fusobacterium nucleatum* and *Prevotella intermedia* in patients with infectious mononucleosis. J Med Microbiol 1996; 131–134.

32. Brook I, de Leyva F: Microbiology of tonsillar surfaces in infectious mononucleosis. Arch Pediatr Adolesc Med 1994; 148: 171–173.

33. Brook I, Yocum P, Friedman EM: Aerobic and anaerobic bacteria in tonsils of children with recurrent tonsillitis. Ann Otol Rhinol Laryngol 1981; 90: 261–263.

34. Tuner K, Nord CE: Beta-lactamase-producing microorganisms in recurrent tonsillitis. Scand J Infect Dis 1983; 39(suppl): 83–85.

35. Brook I: Aerobic and anaerobic bacteriology of adenoids in children: A comparison between patients with chronic adenotonsillitis and adenoid hypertrophy. Laryngoscope 1981; 91: 377–382.

36. Brook I, Yocum P: Quantitative measurement of beta-lactamase level in tonsils of children with recurrent tonsillitis. Acta Otolaryngol Scand 1984; 98: 556–559.

37. Kaplan EL, Johnson OR: Eradication of group A streptococci from treatment failure of the upper respiratory tract by amoxicillin with clavulanate after oral penicillin. J Pediatr 1988; 113: 400–403.

38. Brook I, Hirokawa R: Treatment of patients with a history of recurrent tonsillitis due to group A beta-hemolytic streptococci. Clin Pediatr 1985; 24: 331–336.

39. Brook I, Yocum P, Shah K, et al: Aerobic and anaerobic bacteriological features of serous otitis media in children. Am J Otolaryngol 1983; 4: 389–392.

40. Carenfelt C, Lundberg C: Purulent and non-purulent maxillary sinus secretions with respect to pO_2, pCO_2 and pH. Acta Otolaryngol 1977; 84: 138–143.

41. Brook I, Friedman EM, Rodriguez WJ, Contoni G: Complications of sinusitis in children. Pediatrics 1980; 66: 568–572.

42. Loeshe WJ, Syed SA, Laughon BE, Stoll J: The bacteriology of acute necrotizing ulcerative gingivitis. J Periodontal 1981; 53: 223–230.

43. Bartlett JG, Gorbach SL: Anaerobic infections of the head and neck. Otolaryngol Clin North Am 1976; 9: 655–678.

44. Brook I: Microbiology of infected epidermal cysts. Arch Dermatol 1989; 125: 1658–1661.

45. Johnson JT, Yu VL, Myers RN, Wagner RL: Assessment of the need for gram negative bacterial coverage on antibiotic prophylaxis for oncological head and neck surgery. J Infect Dis 1987; 155: 331–333.

46. Summanen P, Baron EJ, Citron DM, et al.: Wadsworth Anaerobic Bacteriology Manual, 5th ed. Belmont, California: Star Publishing Co, 1993.

47. Murray PR, Baron EJ, Pfaller MA, et al.: Manual of Clinical Microbiology, 5th ed. Washington, D.C.: American Society for Microbiology, 1995.

Irmgard Behlau
Thomas M. Daniel

Mycobacterial Diseases: Tuberculosis, Leprosy, and Other Mycobacterial Infections

TUBERCULOSIS

The Lord shall unite thee with a consumption, and with a fever, and with an inflammation . . . and they shall pursue thee until thou perish.

DEUTERONOMY 28:22

Description

Tuberculosis is the oldest documented infectious disease, and it continues to be an important global health problem today. During the Industrial Revolution, tuberculosis was known as "the White Plague" and caused up to one fourth of adult deaths in Western Europe. It reached epidemic proportions in the United States in the 19th century, with an annual death rate of nearly 1% of the population in some cities. As living conditions in these countries began to improve, the prevalence of tuberculosis declined. Yet it remains a major cause of death in overpopulated and poorer countries.

On the basis of bacteriologic features and DNA homology, the *Mycobacterium tuberculosis* complex is a member of the family Mycobacteriaceae, order Actinomycetales, and consists of *M. tuberculosis, Mycobacterium bovis, Mycobacterium africanum* (a rare cause of human tuberculosis in Africa), and *Mycobacterium ulcerans* (cutaneous disease seen in Africa and Australia). *M. tuberculosis* is by far the primary cause of tuberculosis, with *M. bovis* accounting for less than 1% of the tuberculosis cases in the United States. Therefore, tuberculosis caused by *M. tuberculosis*, the tubercle bacillus, is the focus of this section unless noted otherwise.

M. tuberculosis is an obligate aerobe, non–spore-forming, nonmotile slender, and slightly bent and beaded rod. Owing to its high lipid content (25%), heat or detergents are required for staining, and mycobacteria characteristically resist destaining by acid-alcohol treatment and thus are referred to as acid-fast bacilli. *M. tuberculosis* grows slowly (doubling time 20–24 hours). On solid media (Löwenstein-Jensen or Middlebrook 7H10) incubated at 37° C, buff-colored, dry, and wrinkled-appearing colonies are visible in 3–6 weeks.

Epidemiology

M. tuberculosis infects 1.7 billion people, a third of the world's population. About eight million cases occur annu-

ally, with three million deaths per year. In poorer countries, tuberculosis accounts for 6% of infant deaths, nearly 20% of adult deaths, and 26% of avoidable deaths.[1]

In the United States, there was a steady decline in the number of tuberculosis cases since national reporting began in 1953, reaching a low in 1985 (22,201 cases). Then, from the mid-1980s through 1992, there was a transient increase in new cases; fortunately from 1993 through 1995, the number of tuberculosis cases reported in the United States has resumed its previous decline.[2] This transient increase in tuberculosis cases has been attributed to the following factors: (1) increased immigration from countries where tuberculosis is endemic; (2) the increased susceptibility to tuberculosis by persons infected with human immunodeficiency virus (HIV); (3) worsening social conditions in urban areas with interrelated factors of poverty, overcrowding, homelessness, and illicit drug use; and (4) neglect of tuberculosis control programs. A resurgence of tuberculosis is cause enough for concern, but the new outbreaks have a frightening difference from earlier outbreaks of the disease. In some locations, notably including New York City, many of the bacteria now causing new cases of tuberculosis are resistant to one or more of the drugs used to treat *M. tuberculosis*. Because the fatality rate of treating multidrug-resistant tuberculosis is approximately 20% despite treatment with second-line drugs,[3] this form of disease has set off a panic, especially among health-care workers caring for these patients. In HIV-infected persons, the fatality rate from multidrug-resistant tuberculosis approaches 100%.

In impoverished countries, tuberculosis continues to be a major cause of death, and its incidence shows no signs of decline. In some countries, the estimated annual incidence of tuberculosis is equivalent to that seen during the White Plague era in Western Europe and North America (400 cases per 100,000 population). The global AIDS epidemic has resulted in unprecedented increases in tuberculosis incidence in such areas as sub-Saharan Africa, where tuberculosis is the single most important cause of morbidity and mortality.

Reservoir, Transmission, Pathogenesis, Virulence Factors, and Immunity

Humans are the only reservoir for *M. tuberculosis*, despite its ability to infect other primates. Although now a rare cause of tuberculosis in countries that routinely pasteurize milk, *M. bovis* infection due to ingestion of contaminated milk from infected cows had been a major problem, especially in children.

Transmission of *M. tuberculosis* is from person to person via the respiratory route. The efficiency of transmission depends on the presence of lung cavitation that harbors a higher concentration of organisms, the expulsive force of a cough or sneeze, and the presence of liquefaction necrosis that has a lower viscosity. People in close contact with patients who are "smear-positive" have 25%–80% chance of becoming infected, depending on their length and closeness of exposure and the state of the infected patient.[4,5] Yet, the rate of infection for contacts of "smear-negative, culture-positive" patients (5%) is the same as in their community.[6] Transmission by fomites is rare. Infection can occur by dermal inoculation of bacilli.

Almost all tuberculosis infections are due to inhalation of small-particle aerosols (<10 μm) from pulmonary secretions by patients with active pulmonary tuberculosis. These tiny-droplet nuclei are inhaled (evading the mucociliary mechanisms of the lower respiratory tract), are deposited in the terminal bronchioles and alveoli, and begin to replicate. Because of greater air flow to the lower and mid-lung fields, bacilli tend to be deposited in these regions. The tubercle bacilli implanted into the terminal air spaces are ingested by macrophages lining the alveoli. The mycobacteria multiply within these phagocytes and eventually destroy them.

Within tissue macrophages, mycobacteria evade host microbicidal killing by virtue of specific virulence factors, many of which remain unknown. Factors that may contribute to *M. tuberculosis* survival within the macrophage are the following: (1) its ability to prevent acidification of the phagosome, which is a vacuole that forms around the bacilli (phagocyte), and inhibition of phagolysosomal fusion, thereby avoiding cellular hydrolytic lysosomal enzymes; (2) the ability of phenolic glycolipids that are abundant in the cell wall to scavenge, and thus detoxify, oxygen radicals; and (3) production of factors by the bacteria that interfere with macrophage activation.

After a short period of replication (about 14–21 days), unimpeded growth in the lungs is associated with lympho-hematogenous spread to the hilar nodes and extrapulmonary sites. This dissemination is usually silent and is accompanied almost simultaneously by the onset of delayed-type hypersensitivity. Most infected persons develop cell-mediated immunity in 4–6 weeks, and subsequently tuberculous foci become infiltrated by blood mononuclear cells. Activated T lymphocytes generate cytokines (interferon-γ, tumor necrosis factor-α, interleukin-2) that enable the tissue macrophages and the newly arrived blood monocytes to destroy mycobacteria. A tubercle is formed with a caseous, necrotic center consisting of dead and live bacilli and cellular debris surrounded by granulation tissue containing lymphocytes and macrophages. Activated macrophages (epithelioid cells, histiocytes) may fuse into Langhans's giant cells. Whether this lesion progresses or regresses depends on the ability of activated macrophages to further ingest and destroy the pathogen. In 90%–95% of infected persons, immune mechanisms halt tuberculous infection. Small caseous foci are dissolved and replaced by fibrous tissue. Larger foci (>5

mm) develop fibrous capsules, which may calcify with time. These larger foci may be reactivated years later if the host's immune response is compromised. In both reactivation tuberculosis and progressive primary infection, the mycobacterial load within the caseous center increases. Tumor necrosis factor and procoagulant factors lead to thrombosis of blood vessels, ischemia, and necrosis. Release of reactive oxygen metabolites, proteinases, and lipases hydrolyzes and liquefies the caseum. Finally, adjacent bronchioles become necrotic, and cavity formation occurs.

Morbidity and mortality rates from tuberculosis are greater at the extremes of age. The risk of developing disease after infection of an otherwise normal host with *M. tuberculosis* is about 3%–5% during the first year and persists at a lower incidence for life, declining to less than 0.1% per year in adults with normal chest radiographs. However, young adults, especially females, have a greatly increased risk of both reactivation of dormant lesions and of progressive disease following primary infection.[7] Positive tuberculin reactors with pulmonary scars, however, have an 0.8% per year risk of developing disease. Factors that are associated with increased risk of clinical tuberculosis are cancer, immunosuppressive therapy, HIV infection, alcoholism, silicosis, diabetes mellitus, malnutrition, gastrectomy, and chronic renal insufficiency.

Clinical Manifestations

Tuberculosis infection is usually divided into pulmonary tuberculosis and tuberculosis affecting all other organ systems (extrapulmonary). In the United States in immunocompetent hosts, pulmonary tuberculosis accounts for 82% of infections, and extrapulmonary tuberculosis accounts for 18%[8] (Table 23–1). In the HIV population, extrapulmonary tuberculosis may account for up to one half of infections, and one third of patients present with both extrapulmonary and pulmonary tuberculosis[9] (see Table 23–1).

Table 23–1. TUBERCULOSIS CASES BY ANATOMIC SITE: UNITED STATES

Site	Frequency (%)	
	HIV Negative*	HIV Positive†
Pulmonary Only	82.0	43.2
Lymphatic	5.1	32.4
Pleural	4.6	10.8
Genitourinary	2.2	9.5
Bone/Joint	1.7	4.1
Miliary/Hematogenous	1.4	21.6
Central Nervous System	0.9	2.7
Other	2.1	10.8

*National data reviewed by Bloch AB, Reider HL, Kelly GD, et al: The epidemiology of tuberculosis in the United States: implications for diagnosis and treatment. Clin Chest Med 1989; 10: 297–313.

†Combined data (n = 74) from two series reported by Chaison RE, Schecter GE, Theuer CP, et al.: Tuberculosis in patients with the acquired immunodeficiency syndrome: Clinical features, response to therapy, and survival. Am Rev Respir Dis 1987; 136: 570–574; and Modilevsky T, Sattler FR, Barnes PF: Mycobacterial disease in patients with human immunodeficiency virus infection. Arch Intern Med 1989; 149: 2201–2205. Total exceeds 100% because many patients had disease in more than one site.

Pulmonary Tuberculosis

Primary Tuberculosis Infection. After inhalation, *M. tuberculosis* replicates in the middle and/or lower lobes. A nonspecific pneumonitis with hilar lymph node enlargement is common.

Reactivation Tuberculosis. In persons previously infected with *M. tuberculosis*, reactivation of latent foci may occur. Host factors that attenuate the cellular immune response favor reactivation. The most common site of reactivation is in the apices of the lungs. There is a wide spectrum of disease ranging from minimal infiltrates to pneumonia or progressive nodular pulmonary lesions with central caseating necrosis to liquefaction necrosis and resultant cavitation, scarring, and fibrosis with prominent constitutional and respiratory symptoms. Fatigue, weight loss, low-grade fever, and drenching night sweats are common systemic manifestations, and cough productive of scant, blood-tinged sputum is a common respiratory manifestation. Rales over the upper lung fields, at times heard only after coughing, and dullness to percussion may be present with extensive apical disease, and amphoric breath sounds may be present with extensive cavitation.

Exogenous Reinfection. Immunity following primary tuberculous infection usually offers nearly complete protection from disease due to exogenous reinfection. However, disease due to exogenous reinfection certainly occurs on some occasions. It is most often seen in situations of high exposure and in patients with acquired immunodeficiency syndrome (AIDS), whose protective immune mechanisms are severely compromised.

Differential Diagnosis. Pulmonary tuberculosis must be differentiated from (1) carcinoma of the lung, (2) other granulomatous processes such as sarcoidosis, (3) fungal infections such as histoplasmosis, coccidioidomycosis, blastomycosis, and cryptococcosis, (4) bacterial lung abscesses, and (5) infection by other mycobacteria such as *Mycobacterium kansasii* and the *Mycobacterium avium-intracellulare-scrofulaceum* (MAIS) complex. In immigrants from southeast Asia, infection with *Pseudomonas pseudomallei* (melioidosis) should be considered. In the evaluation of carcinoma of the lung, screening for tuberculosis by skin testing should always be done, the two processes may occur simultaneously.

Extrapulmonary Tuberculosis

The incidence of extrapulmonary tuberculosis is much greater in the immunocompromised host, especially in patients with AIDS. Diagnosis of extrapulmonary tuberculosis is often difficult because symptoms and signs are nonspecific, the number of organisms that cause disease is low compared with that of pulmonary tuberculosis, and biopsy is often required to make the diagnosis.

Tuberculous Lymphadenitis. Tuberculous lymphadenitis is the most frequent manifestation of extrapulmonary tuberculosis (see Table 23–1).[8]

In localized lymph node disease, single anatomic loci of lymph nodes are diseased and represent the major organ system involved. The most common sites involved are the cervical lymph nodes (scrofula) or the retroperitoneal nodes.

In addition, bilateral or unilateral hilar adenopathy can develop without obvious parenchymal disease. When cervical lymph node disease is present, breakdown and drainage can occur with either minimal or no constitutional symptoms.

Generalized lymph node involvement represents a disease process between the phase of complete containment of primary infection and miliary disease. Constitutional symptoms such as fever and weight loss may prompt the initial impression of a lymphoreticular neoplastic process.

Lymph node involvement due to drainage of an infected organ is a more common cause of lymph node infection than primary lymph node disease. Hilar adenopathy resulting from a pulmonary infection is an example.

Tuberculous Pleuritis. Pleurisy with effusion is the second most common manifestation of extrapulmonary tuberculosis. This syndrome follows shortly after primary infection and is due to a breakdown of tuberculous granulomas into the pleural space, with an outpouring of fluid and cellular material into this space. The onset of tuberculous pleurisy tends to be more abrupt; low-grade fever accompanied by a "heaviness" of the chest and pleuritic pain are common manifestations. Cough and sputum production are usually minimal or absent. Needle biopsy of the parietal pleura may reveal granulomas. Untreated, tuberculous pleurisy temporarily remits with a period of quiescence, but active pulmonary tuberculosis eventually develops in at least two thirds of patients.

Genitourinary. Renal tuberculosis, usually spread by hematogenous seeding, presents as sterile pyuria and microscopic hematuria. Complications include cavitation and scarring of the renal parenchyma, and if tubular spread to the ureters and bladder occurs, possible ureteral strictures may form. Diagnosis is by multiple large-volume cultures of morning urine samples.

Genital infection, rarely, may also result from sexual transmission and is usually insidious. In females, it may remain asymptomatic, and chronic salpingitis may result in sterility. In males, it most commonly presents as nontender, nodular induration of the prostate or the epididymis. Biopsy is required for diagnosis.

Skeletal Tuberculosis. Tuberculosis has a predilection for large weight-bearing structures such as the lower thoracic spine (Pott's disease) and weight-bearing joints (hips and knees). It results either from hematogenous seeding of the spine or from the pleural space via lymphatic channels to the paravertebral lymph nodes. Patients often present with pain. If the disease progresses, spinal cord compression from collapse of vertebral bodies may result in paraplegia. Paravertebral abscess formation may also occur and extend along fascial planes. Diagnosis may be attempted by needle biopsy, but often open biopsy is required. Other skeletal manifestations of tuberculosis include synovitis and arthritis.

Miliary Tuberculosis. Acute miliary tuberculosis can occur shortly after the primary infection when the infection is not contained, and there is early massive dissemination of the bacilli. The onset tends to be abrupt with prominent constitutional and respiratory symptoms. Yet, between episodes of fever the patient may feel well. More commonly, miliary tuberculosis is due to reactivation disease. Patients have an indolent and insidious onset, low-grade bacteremia, and absent focal symptoms. Typical findings on chest radiographs are soft, uniformly distributed, fine millet seed–like nodules; of note, radiologic findings tend to lag about 1 month behind clinical symptoms and signs. Laboratory manifestations of disease include cholestatic liver dysfunction, leukopenia, thrombocytopenia, sterile pyuria, and chronic meningitis. Pathognomonic yellow-white choroidal tubercles may be seen on fundoscopy late in the disease. The diagnosis can be difficult and expectorated sputum often is negative. Bone marrow biopsies are positive in two thirds of patients. Tuberculin skin test anergy is common and should not deter consideration of the diagnosis. Miliary tuberculosis should be considered in the differential diagnosis of fever of unknown etiology. Without treatment, prognosis is often death; with treatment, the prognosis is guarded.

Central Nervous System. Central nervous system tuberculosis may result from seeding of the leptomeninges during primary infection (most often in children) or from reactivation of latent meningeal foci (in adults). Meningeal tuberculosis patients present with headache and possibly a stiff neck or photophobia. Owing to the predilection for basilar distribution, cranial nerve signs such as sixth nerve paresis are common findings. Tuberculosis may also present as an isolated tuberculoma of the cortex or meninges, causing localized neurologic signs or focal seizures. The cerebrospinal fluid demonstrates lymphocytosis and a high protein and low glucose concentration. Diagnosis is difficult, requiring at least three samples of cerebrospinal fluid for staining and culture of concentrated fluids.

Gastrointestinal. Gastrointestinal tuberculosis is usually a sequela of extensive cavitary pulmonary disease with contamination of the gastrointestinal tract by swallowed organisms. Postgastrectomy patients are more susceptible because stomach acid usually destroys the bacilli.

Tuberculous peritonitis results from hematogenous seeding of the peritoneum or from an abdominal lymphatic or genitourinary organ source. Onset is usually insidious and an exudative effusion develops. Diagnosis is difficult, requiring repeated large volume paracentesis; peritoneal biopsy may be needed.

Tuberculous Pericarditis. This manifestation most commonly occurs from drainage of an infected lymph node into the pericardium. It also may occur from an extension of tuberculous pleuritis into the pericardium or from hematogenous spread. Patients present with fever, pericardial pain, and a friction rub. Complications include cardiac tamponade and constrictive pericarditis. A pericardial biopsy may be required for diagnosis.

Ocular Tuberculosis. Chorioretinitis and uveitis are the most common manifestations. The diagnosis is difficult to establish and may be helped by an exposure history, positive tuberculin skin test result, and abnormal chest radiograph. Tuberculosis cannot be distinguished on clinical examination from sarcoidosis or systemic mycoses. Choroidal tubercles may be present in miliary disease, and their recognition is crucial in this diagnosis.

Tuberculosis and AIDS

HIV-infected patients have a special risk of acquiring primary tuberculosis and reactivation of previously acquired infections. Tuberculosis represents a major cause of morbidity and mortality in HIV-infected patients. Extrapulmonary manifestations of tuberculosis are seen in nearly one half of AIDS patients, with tuberculous lymphadenitis predominant.[9] Diagnosis of tuberculosis in AIDS patients, as in other severely immunocompromised patients, deserves special attention. Often the manifestations of disease are atypical because of the lack of an appropriate immune response. Tuberculin skin test responses are depressed owing to severe CD4 T-cell depletion. Nearly one half of AIDS patients have atypical radiographic findings of the chest, such as diffuse fine infiltrates, pneumonic infiltrates, hilar adenopathy, perihilar infiltrates, pleural effusions, and even normal chest radiographs in the presence of sputum-positive tuberculosis.

Specific Manifestations of the Ear, Nose, and Throat

Cervical Lymphadenitis. Tuberculous lymphadentitis of the cervical lymph nodes (scrofula) (Fig. 23–1) is a disease that was recognized in antiquity. European monarchs claimed the power to heal scrofula with their touch. Clovis of France, who included the touching of persons with scrofula in his coronation ceremony in 496 A.D. may have been the first ruler to touch scrofulous persons, and for many generations his descendants claimed to have inherited his healing power. Scrofula became known as "the king's evil." Louis XIV is said to have touched 2500 persons. At the beginning of

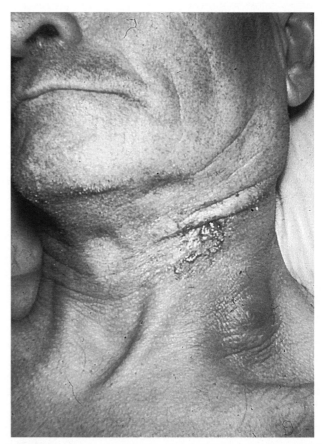

Figure 23–1. Patient with tuberculous lymphadenitis of the right cervical lymph node (scrofula). (Courtesy of H. Provine, BS)

the seventeenth century, Shakespeare described touching for scrofula in Macbeth, Act IV, Scene 3:

> . . . . strangely visited people,
> All swoln and ulcerous, pitiful to the eye,
> The mere despair of surgery, he cures;
> Hanging a golden stamp about their necks,
> Put on with holy prayers.

Samuel Johnson was touched by Queen Anne, the last British monarch to practice touching regularly. Johnson was disfigured by the scars left by his scrofula, which later required surgical drainage.

Scrofula is usually indolent, and its relatively benign course may have contributed to the success claimed for the royal touch. It accounts for two thirds of tuberculous adenitis. Five percent of all scrofula patients have associated active pulmonary tuberculosis,[10] and 15% have radiographic evidence consistent with previous pulmonary tuberculosis. Any of the cervical nodes may be involved, but the anterior triangle of the neck (Fig. 23–2) is the most frequent site of disease. One third of patients have bilateral disease.[11] Early in the disease process, tuberculous nodes are rubbery and nontender. With disease progression, they become firm and matted. Infrequently, abscess formation and chronic draining fistulas may develop.

Diagnosis is commonly established by biopsy. Bi-

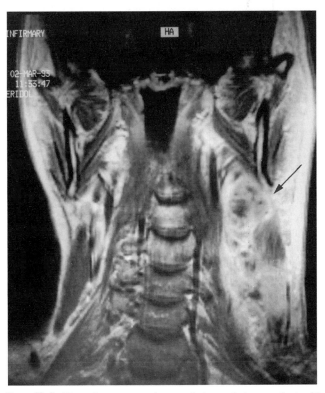

Figure 23–2. Magnetic resonance image of the neck in a patient with tuberculous lymphadenitis. Sagittal view of large tuberculous necrotic cavities in the left neck from the level of the angle of the mandible (arrow) inferiorly to the level of the inferior thyroid cartilage. There are enlarged nodes and inflammatory tissue that extends inferiorly to the level of the lower neck. (Courtesy of R. Fabian, MD, A. S. Baker, MD, and D. Kim, MD)

opsy specimens should be submitted for Ziehl-Neelsen stain (Fig. 23–3), routine and mycobacterial cultures, and histopathologic examination. Approximately 20% of cases are culture-positive and histopathology-negative. An increasingly popular approach to diagnosing tuberculous cervical lymphadenitis is fine needle aspiration for cytology,[11, 12] which has a reported sensitivity of approximately 75%. Concerns regarding this approach are that a negative fine needle aspirate must be followed up by excisional biopsy in 25% of cases and that inadequate material may be obtained for culture and subsequent sensitivity tests. Antimycobacterial treatment must always be instituted at or preferably before the time of surgery. This important point deserves emphasis. Failure to provide adequate chemotherapy at the time of surgical manipulation may lead to postoperative fistulas in the surgical wound site and to hematogenous dissemination with subsequent miliary disease. Liquefaction necrosis in the nodes of nonsurgical cases may require biweekly drainage by a large-bore needle.

In younger children, most cases of scrofula are caused by nontuberculous mycobacteria such as the MAIS complex, *M. kansasii*, and *Mycobacterium malmoense*. The clinical presentation is similar to that of tuberculous adenitis, often with a single, nontender node that may progress to necrosis and fistula formation. Diagnosis is by biopsy. There are unique histologic features that may suggest an atypical mycobacterial infection, such as ill-defined nonpalisading granulomas, irregular or serpiginous granulomas, and lack of caseation.[10] However, definitive diagnosis depends on culture. Culture identification of the offending organism is also important in directing therapy because nontuberculous mycobacterial disease requires the use of different drugs than those used for tuberculosis. Spontaneous resolution of limited disease may occur after puberty (which may also have contributed to the success of the royal touch). In limited atypical mycobacterial infections, excision of the node is the only treatment required. In cases of nodal rupture or more widespread disease, specific chemotherapy is required.

The most important differential diagnosis of tuberculous lymphadenitis is Hodgkin's disease, which can present with cervical lymphadenopathy and constitutional symptoms of fever, weight loss, and night sweats similar to those of tuberculosis.

Laryngeal Tuberculosis. At the turn of the century, tuberculosis was the most common condition to affect the larynx, and one fourth to one half of patients with pulmonary tuberculosis had laryngeal involvement. Nicolo Paganini had laryngeal tuberculosis. As his death approached, he continued to play the violin, but his voice was so hoarse he was unable to announce the names of the works he performed. Today, laryngeal tuberculosis accounts for less than 1% of all cases of tuberculosis.[13] Tuberculosis of the larynx was seen with advanced pulmonary disease and resulted from seeding of the mucosal surfaces during expectoration in bed-bound patients. Recent studies suggest that lymphatic and hematogenous dissemination are more common modes of spread, and cavitary pulmonary disease is seen in only a minority of patients (15%).[14] In contrast to the symptoms at the turn of the century, the anterior larynx is affected twice as frequently as the posterior larynx.[15]

Dysphonia is the principal presenting symptom. Other

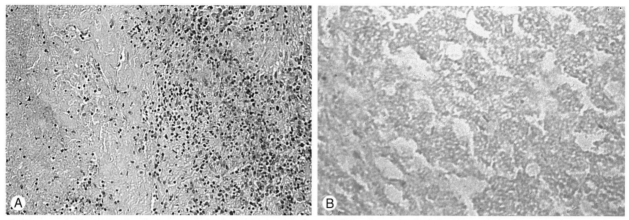

Figure 23–3. *A* and *B*, Necrotizing granulomatous lymphadenitis (cervical node) with focal giant cell formation (×16) with acid fast bacilli (×100). (Courtesy of Massachusetts General Hospital, Pathology Dept., Boston, Mass.)

manifestations include cough, weight loss, fever, dyspnea, dysphagia, laryngeal stridor, and hemoptysis.[14] The complaint of dysphagia may be out of proportion to the extent of pathologic problems seen on laryngeal examination.[16] Findings on laryngoscopy are noteworthy for the varied appearance of tuberculous laryngitis. The disease ranges from an infiltrative laryngitis with mucosal hypertrophy to granulomatous nodules to fibrosis. Ulceration appears to be much less common than in the past. The most common sites affected are the vocal folds, ventricular bands, supraglottis, aryepiglottic folds, arytenoids, posterior commissure, and subglottis (Fig. 23–4)[14, 15] Stridor may be due to granulations occluding the supraglottis or to stenosis and fibrosis of the larynx, which may necessitate tracheostomy.[14, 17] Tuberculous laryngitis is among the most infectious of all forms of tuberculosis.

Because of the varied appearance of tuberculous laryngitis, biopsy is essential. As pulmonary involvement accompanies laryngeal tuberculosis in 90% of cases, radiographic

examination of the chest should be done first. Common radiographic findings include bilateral, poorly defined, nodular shadows involving predominantly the upper and middle zones and occasionally the lower zones. Cavitation (15%) is seen less frequently than in the past, and a miliary pattern (15%) may also be seen.[14] Sputum microscopy test results are positive in about three fourths of patients with laryngeal tuberculosis.[15, 16] Tuberculous laryngitis responds rapidly to chemotherapy and has a favorable prognosis with treatment. The differential diagnoses are carcinoma of the larynx and chronic laryngitis; both can be easily excluded by biopsy.[16, 18, 19]

Pharyngeal Tuberculosis. At the turn of the century, 1.4% of all adenoids and 6.5% of all tonsils that were removed from asymptomatic patients were infected by tubercle bacilli. Tonsillar tuberculosis, usually due to *M. bovis* infection from contaminated cow's milk, was seen in more than one third of patients (children) with cervical lymphadenitis at the beginning of the century,[20, 21] in contrast, it is rarely seen today. This clearly reflected the high incidence of tuberculosis and the paucity of symptoms and signs often associated with pharyngeal tuberculosis. Infection of the pharynx is usually slowly progressive and presents with chronic nodular irregularities of mucosal surfaces. Rarely, a more acute form is seen, which presents with small pink nodules with yellow "apple-jelly" centers. These nodules eventually coalesce, forming areas of raised bosselated epithelium covered by a mucinous secretion.

Nasopharyngeal tuberculosis is usually due to a primary infection. It is accompanied by cervical lymphadenopathy 70% of the time; cervical lymphadenopathy may also be the only feature in 50% of cases.[22] Mahindra and colleagues[23] reported that one fourth of children with tuberculous cervical lymphadenopathy had tuberculous infection of the adenoids. Other associated manifestations include nasal obstruction and nasal discharge. Only 30% of patients have any manifestations of systemic disease, with transitory low-grade fever and malaise uncommon. Because of tubercle formation occurring deep within the adenoid tissue, examination usually reveals only hypertrophic but normal-appearing adenoids. Radiographic evidence of lung involvement is seen in only 20% of cases, and hilar involvement is seen more frequently (up to 50%).[23]

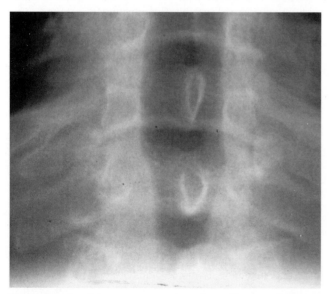

Figure 23–4. Coned-down anteroposterior radiographic view of the neck with slight asymmetric prominence of the left subglottic airway in a patient with laryngeal tuberculosis. (Reprinted by permission of Schafer DF: Case 34–1994: laryngeal tuberculosis. N Engl J Med 1994; 331: 728–734, Massachusetts Medical Society.)

Diagnosis is by biopsy. Acid-fast bacilli (AFB) are seen in only a small percentage of specimens submitted for direct examination. Antimycobacterial treatment should produce a rapid response. Differential diagnosis includes other granulomatous processes and carcinoma.

Aural Tuberculosis. At the turn of the century, 2% of all suppurative otitis media in Scottish children was due to tuberculosis, mostly *M. bovis*.[24] The incidence was directly correlated with *M. bovis* infection from unpasteurized milk in bottle-fed children, and the infection affected over 50% of 1-year-olds and 25% of 2-year-olds with suppurative otitis media. Nearly all of these children had associated lymphadenopathy, half had facial palsy, and 20% had labyrinthine infection.

Currently, primary aural tuberculosis (Fig. 23–5) is extremely rare; it has been reported in the literature fewer than 10 times since 1960.[25, 26] The spread of bacilli, mainly *M. bovis*, is to the middle ear via the eustachian tube, and no other focus of infection can be found.[25a] More commonly, tubercle bacilli may spread to the middle ear via a hematogenous or lymphatic route or directly via the eustachian tube from a primary focus in an adjacent organ. Patients often present with a painless ear that is chronically draining, unresponsive to antibiotics, and, if the diagnosis is delayed, hearing loss. The tympanic membrane in aural tuberculosis initially becomes thickened, and an effusion develops that produces a conductive hearing loss. Tubercles may develop on the tympanic membrane, producing multiple perforations that may coalesce to form a central or total perforation. Sensorineural hearing loss may occur if the labyrinth becomes involved.[27] Findings on otoscopy include painless otorrhea, tympanic membrane perforations, and pale granulation tissue that may extend into the ear canal. Many patients have associated mastoid swelling. Bony sequestra may be seen. Facial palsy (20%)[25a, 28] and labyrinth destruction with sensorineural hearing loss[26] may complicate this disease. Lymphadenopathy of the high jugular nodes may occur. Meningitis and intracranial complications, if they are present, are secondary to hematogenous spread rather than a result of direct spread, as the dura typically forms an effective barrier to disease extension.[29–31] As of yet, there has been no reported increased incidence of aural tuberculosis in HIV-infected persons.[31a]

Microscopy of the aural discharge has a sensitivity of 73%, and culture of middle ear mucosa has a sensitivity of 96%.[28] Therefore, if the initial screening is normal, surgical biopsy is required. Because 50% of patients have associated pulmonary involvement, radiographic examination of the chest should be performed. Aural tuberculosis is best treated with conservative antituberculosis therapy, which should be instituted as quickly as possible to avoid its major sequela, profound hearing loss.[25a, 32] Surgical intervention may be indicated for a subperiosteal abscess, fistula formation, labyrinthitis, progressive disease due to resistant organisms or atypical mycobacteria, and intracranial extension.[33] Aural tuberculosis should be considered in the differential diagnosis of chronic middle ear discharge, which includes Wegener's granulomatosis, sarcoidosis, and fungal and nocardial infections.

Oral Tuberculosis. Even at the turn of the century when tuberculosis was much more common in industrialized Western countries, oral tuberculosis was very uncommon;[34, 35] currently, it is extremely rare. It was seen most often secondary to pulmonary tuberculosis. Primary infection had been seen with oral contamination by ingestion of *M. bovis*[36] and associated with poor oral hygiene or mucosal damage, including dental extraction. The most common sites affected are the gum, tongue, palate, and floor of the mouth. It presents as a painless, nonhealing ulcer with associated regional lymphadenopathy. Biopsy with culture must be obtained. Histopathologic examination and microscopy and culture may sometimes be unrevealing, however, because of the paucity of organisms and limited inflammation present. In high-risk patients with supporting evidence from a reactive tuberculin skin test and chest radiograph, repeat biopsies may need to be attempted. The differential diagnosis of oral

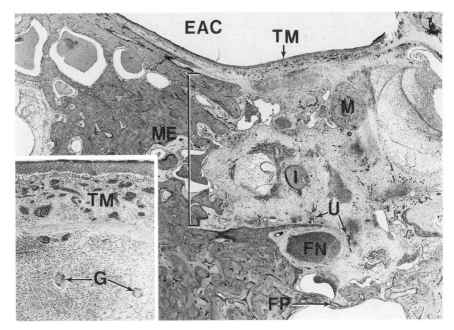

Figure 23–5. Histologic section through the middle-ear space in a patient with acute tuberculous otitis media and mastoiditis. The middle ear (ME) is filled with granulation tissue. The lining of the middle-ear space is ulcerated (U), and there is early resorption of bone. The tympanic membrane (TM, inset: higher power view of area bracketed in main photomicrograph) is markedly thickened by infiltration with inflammatory cells and multinucleated giant cells (G). EAC = external ear canal; FN = facial nerve; FP = footplate of stapes; I = incus; M = malleus. Original magnification, ×9 (inset, ×70). (From Skolnik, PR, Nadol, JB, Baker, AS: Tuberculosis of the middle ear: Review of the literature with an instructive case report. Rev Infect Dis 1986; 8: 403–410. Published by the University of Chicago.)

tuberculosis includes carcinoma, syphilis, sarcoidosis, and deep fungal infections.

Nasal Tuberculosis. Nasal disease is another rare manifestation of tuberculosis. As in the early 1900s, women appear to be affected twice as often as men.[37, 38] Nasal tuberculosis often reflects primary disease. It is painless and may present with symptoms of chronic rhinitis and nasal obstruction. It has few, if any, associated systemic systems. Early, there is a pale nasal mucosa with tiny, nonblanching "apple-jelly" nodules. With progression of disease, the mucosa becomes more granular, the nodules coalesce, and the nasal septum may perforate, leaving a pale and irregular mucosal border. The bony septum tends not to perforate. Diagnosis is by biopsy. It is important to examine the biopsy material carefully by both AFB stain and culture because tubercle bacilli are so few and are therefore difficult to detect. Culture definitively distinguishes this from other mycobacterial diseases, including *Mycobacterium leprae*. Treatment is conservative with antimycobacterial agents. Differential diagnosis includes not only other mycobacterial diseases but also chronic granulomatous diseases such as Wegener's granulomatosis[39] and carcinoma.

Tuberculosis of the Salivary Glands. Tuberculosis of the salivary glands is the rarest otolaryngologic manifestation. It may present as a chronic encapsulation of the gland or a more acute and diffuse inflammatory process. In order of frequency, the glands most commonly affected are the parotid gland, submandibular gland, and sublingual gland. It is believed that the salivary glands are infected by lymphatic drainage from an adjacent site. For parotid gland tuberculosis, the pharynx or tonsils are believed to be infected first, with infection of the intraparotid lymph nodes via the lymphatic channels, or infection may arise from the parotid duct. Patients are often asymptomatic, with pain only in the late stages, and facial palsy is rare. Tuberculosis of the salivary glands is often without radiologic evidence of pulmonary infection. Fine needle aspiration for AFB stain, culture, and cytology may be attempted, but if test results are negative, then surgical biopsy is needed. Conservative antimycobacterial therapy is recommended. Surgery is rarely needed. The differential diagnosis is carcinoma, from which it is clinically indistinguishable.

Cervical Spine Tuberculosis. The cervical spine is affected in less than one fifth of adult patients with Pott's disease of the spine, which typically affects the T10 segment. In children, spinal disease is more common and can affect the cervical spine more frequently. Often the presenting symptom is pain with resultant neck stiffness. With disease progression, cervical nerve roots are involved and pain is referred down the arms. Infection of the cervical spine is by hematogenous spread, and there may be concurrent radiographic evidence of pulmonary disease. Cervical spine tuberculosis often presents as a retropharyngeal abscess, less commonly behind the sternomastoid, and it can even appear as a parotid mass.[40] Computed tomography scan and magnetic resonance imaging demonstrate bony destruction, and definitive diagnosis can often be made by needle aspiration of a retropharyngeal abscess. If this procedure is nondiagnostic, then surgical biopsies must be obtained. Treatment is medical if diagnosed relatively early. Surgery is indicated for large abscesses, neurologic deficits, and spinal instability.

Prognosis is good if neurologic deficits are early and minimal, but with more advanced deficits, full recovery may not occur even with chemotherapy and surgical decompression. The differential diagnosis is usually metastatic carcinoma to the spine.

Diagnosis

Unlike other opportunistic infections, tuberculosis is highly contagious by aerosolization for even healthy individuals. Therefore, appropriate care and adherence to infection control procedures should be undertaken when obtaining secretions and biopsy material for examination and cultures. In most cases, these precautions include wearing gowns, high-efficiency filtration masks, gloves, and goggles to protect the eyes. A well-ventilated room is especially important when performing laryngoscopy or bronchoscopy. In one well-documented outbreak, the risk of infection for those attending a bronchoscopy in a poorly ventilated intensive care unit alcove was 75 times that for the nursing personnel caring for the patient.[41]

Laboratory

Despite suspicion of mycobacterial infection, definitive diagnosis is made only by observing AFB on staining or culture from secretions, fluids, or tissue from the sites of disease. Often only a few tubercle bacilli, which are slender, curved, and often beaded rods in pairs, are seen on typical smears. Many laboratories use a fluorochrome stain, with phenolic auramine or auramine-rhodamine, and counterstain with potassium permanganate in the initial staining procedure. This enhances the sensitivity of picking up fluorescent orange-yellow bacteria against a dark background. If this initial screen produces a positive result, staining by the more labor-intensive Ziehl-Neelsen technique and scanning under $\times 100$ magnification must be done. Cultures, which are the most sensitive, should always be obtained prior to instituting therapy and as a part of any biopsy procedure. Cultures also allow mycobacterial speciation and drug sensitivities, the latter, with the increasing isolation of multidrug-resistant organisms, being increasingly important. Commonly, cultures on Lowenstein-Jensen slants take 4–8 weeks. Newer methods in clinical mycobacteriology are developing that will allow for rapid diagnosis of infection with mycobacterial species. The BACTEC H60 system is being incorporated into many larger, urban, and more modern mycobacteriology laboratories. This system employs a ^{14}C-labeled substrate medium, which is highly specific for mycobacteria, that can alert the clinician in about 7–14 days to possible infection. Other techniques still in the experimental phase include polymerase chain reaction amplification using *M. tuberculosis*-specific primers, enzyme-linked immunosorbent assay (ELISA) techniques based on the recognition of serum immunoglobulin (Ig) IgG antibody to selected mycobacterial antigens and, in some reference laboratories, high-performance chromatographic techniques based on identifying mycobacteria by their specific cell wall components.

Evaluation by histologic examination for AFB is less sensitive, more difficult, and more time-consuming than culture and may be unrewarding. Histology is useful as evidence of the underlying granulomatous process and for its ability to rule out concurrent diseases such as carcinoma.

Clinical laboratory test results tend to be normal or very nonspecific in the diagnosis of tuberculosis. If abnormal, they may represent more extensive disease or an underlying host disease process. A mild peripheral blood monocytosis, elevated erythrocyte sedimentation rate, and an anemia may be present. Depending on the manifestation of tuberculosis, specific organ abnormalities may be seen.

Classic patterns on chest radiographs of primary tuberculosis reveal mediastinal lymphadenopathy with a small area of pneumonitis, often in the lower or mid-lung field. Reactivation tuberculosis typically presents as a patchy or nodular infiltrate in the apical posterior segment of the upper lobes or the superior segments of the lower lobes (subapical). With more advanced reactivation disease, cavitation supervenes in these areas. Fibrotic scarring, volume loss in the involved lobes, and upward retraction may occur. In extrapulmonary tuberculosis, there may be evidence of a concurrent pulmonary infection or evidence of a healed and calcified primary lesion either in the periphery or in the hilar lesion suggestive of tuberculosis.

Tuberculin Skin Test

The tuberculin skin test is the standard method for identifying persons previously infected with *M. tuberculosis*. Intracutaneous administration of five tuberculin units of tuberculin purified protein derivative (Mantoux's test) is superior to the multiple puncture method (tine test), although the latter is often used to screen persons at low risk in physicians' offices. The tuberculin skin test is applied to the volar aspect of the forearm, and the response is read by measuring the transverse diameter of induration (not erythema) by gentle palpation at 48–72 hours.

Cross-reactions are due to infection with mycobacteria other than *M. tuberculosis* and vaccination with bacille Calmette-Guérin. In general, the larger the induration the greater the probability of infection with *M. tuberculosis*. In most low-risk populations, using 15-mm induration as the cutoff point best identifies infection with *M. tuberculosis*.[42] However, in persons who recently have had close contact with a patient with tuberculosis, persons whose chest radiographs are consistent with tuberculosis, and persons who are profoundly immunosuppressed (such as HIV-infected patients), who are likely to show blunted responses to the organism, a reaction larger than 5 mm should be considered positive. Reactions greater than 10 mm are positive in patients at increased risk of tuberculosis. Waning of skin test reactivity can occur with advancing age, at a rate of 5% per year. Reactivity can be accentuated by repeated testing (booster effect) and can be confused with a true, new skin test conversion. False-negative tuberculin reactions are associated with cellular immune hyporesponsiveness. Concurrent viral infections (HIV, measles, varicella virus), lymphoreticular malignancies, malnutrition, sarcoidosis, immunosuppressive drugs, chronic renal failure, and overwhelming illness of any kind are in this category. Approximately half of patients with miliary (disseminated) disease and 25% of those with pulmonary tuberculosis have a negative skin test result.[43] Despite its limitations, tuberculin skin testing may be useful both to assist in the diagnosis of suspected cases of tuberculosis and to identify persons who may need preventive therapy. Even in the presence of a positive reaction to control antigens such as mumps, a negative tuberculin skin test result does not exclude the diagnosis of tuberculosis.

Treatment

Medical

Prompt institution of effective therapy remains the key to preventing spread of tuberculosis in the population. Once sputum smears become negative in response to treatment, the patient can be considered noninfectious. Hospitalized patients receiving treatment for newly diagnosed tuberculosis are usually considered noninfectious after 14 days of therapy, provided the number of AFB seen on sputum smears declines.

Specific chemotherapeutic regimens for treatment of both pulmonary and extrapulmonary tuberculosis, prophylaxis, and prevention are discussed in Chapter 12.

Surgical

In general, since the advent of available chemotherapeutic agents in the 1950s, medical treatment is preferred for the management of all forms of tuberculosis. Special instances of surgical intervention have been discussed in relation to each specific clinical manifestation.

Prognosis

In general, with rapid diagnosis and treatment of both pulmonary and extrapulmonary tuberculosis with effective chemotherapeutic agents, prognosis is good. The exceptions to this are miliary tuberculosis, multidrug-resistant tuberculosis, and tuberculosis in an immunocompromised host. In advanced tuberculosis, the damage tuberculosis and the host immune response have inflicted on a particular organ may not be reversible.

OTHER MYCOBACTERIA

Mycobacteria other than tuberculosis and leprosy represent a heterogeneous group. They have been referred to as nontuberculous mycobacteria, atypical mycobacteria, mycobacteria other than tuberculosis, and other mycobacteria. We use the least erroneous name, "other mycobacteria," and attempt to refer to the individual species name whenever possible.

Other mycobacteria were recognized as saprophytes or pathogens for various nonprimate animal species. Only since the 1950s have other mycobacteria been increasingly recognized as able to cause human disease. Currently 2%–10% of all mycobacterial infections in the United States are due to these other mycobacteria, with a higher incidence observed in patients with malignancy or in an immunocompromised state, especially with AIDS. The difficulty is to determine whether the isolation of these other mycobacteria is clinically significant. We discuss only those that have the greatest impact on human disease and are most likely to be encountered by the otolaryngologist.

Mycobacterium avium-intracellulare Complex

M. avium was first identified in 1890 as the avian tubercle bacillus, the cause of tuberculosis of chickens and sporadic cases of pulmonary infections in chicken farmers. In the 1950s a series of patients with pulmonary disease was reported to be infected with what was called the Battey bacillus, later named *M. intracellulare.*

M. intracellulare has been found to be almost indistinguishable by routine laboratory criteria from *M. avium.* This has prompted a name change to *M. avium-intracellulare* (MAI) complex. MAI is nonchromogenic bacillus. With acid-fast staining, it usually appears short and coccobacillary, although early in culture, long, thin bacilli may be seen. Staining is usually uniform without beading or banding. Growth for MAI is moderate for mycobacteria at 10–21 days at 37° C. MAI colonies are smooth, sometimes with "asteroid" margins, either opaque and domed or transparent and flat, and become more yellow with age, independent of light.

MAI is ubiquitous in the environment and appears to be endemic in the southeastern United States. The number of MAI infections has increased over the last two decades, and in 1980 only *M. tuberculosis* was recovered with greater frequency than MAI.[44] The greatest upsurge in MAI infections during the past decade has been in patients with end-stage AIDS, to the point that in some settings MAI is more frequently recovered than *M. tuberculosis.*

MAI is of low pathogenicity and, until recently, was considered a colonizer that rarely caused disease. Aerosols are an important mode of acquisition of respiratory disease. In immunocompetent patients with underlying lung disease or in immunosuppressed patients, MAI can colonize the tracheobronchial tree, preexisting areas of bronchiectasis, or old scarred and fibrosed cavities. It is presumed that MAI gains access due to a disruption of normal mucociliary clearance or factors that retard clearance such as excess mucus production, abnormally tenacious secretions, or anatomic abnormalities. In the case of silicosis, there may also be an element of macrophage dysfunction that potentiates invasive disease. Possible water-associated disease has also been reported for MAI. This may be due to some traumatic break in the skin in a susceptible host. The massive involvement of the gastrointestinal tract seen in disseminated disease also suggests the possibility of an oral route of infection from contaminated water. Despite a potentially high organism burden (up to 10^6 bacteria/mL of blood and 10^{10} bacteria/g of tissue), the cellular inflammatory response is typically minimal. In addition, patients with disseminated or multifocal MAI disease tend to be immunodeficient, and disseminated MAI has been reported in up to 50% of patients with end-stage AIDS.[45]

In general, *M. avium* strains seem more virulent for humans than *M. intracellulare.* Enhanced virulence has also been associated with plasmids. Interestingly, half of clinical isolates and only 5% of soil isolates contain plasmids.[46]

Strains of MAI may be associated with a wide spectrum of mycobacterial disease, including pulmonary disease, childhood lymphadenitis, and opportunistic disseminated infection in patients who have diminished cellular immunity, especially AIDS.

Pulmonary infection due to MAI usually occurs in association with preexisting lung disease—silicosis, chronic bronchitis, emphysema, healed tuberculosis, and bronchiectasis—and in elderly women. Early manifestations are often minimal and include a nonproductive cough and mild malaise. Then a productive cough, hemoptysis, and nonpleuritic chest pain develop with onset of systemic manifestations that may include malaise, fever, chills, and night sweats. As the disease progresses, dyspnea, weight loss, and a more persistent fever occur. Without treatment, disease is usually progressive.

Extrapulmonary disease for MAI may be either localized or disseminated. In general, localized disease may occur as a result of direct inoculation, from contamination of the oropharynx as in cervical lymphadenitis, or contiguous spread. Patients with single-site extrapulmonary MAI generally do not have obvious deficits of immunity. Cutaneous, soft tissue, and skeletal infections; genitourinary tract involvement; meningitis; gastrointestinal ulcers; pericarditis; and otomastoiditis have been reported.

Disseminated and multifocal extrapulmonary MAI disease occurs most commonly in immunocompromised hosts, especially AIDS patients.[47] Those with disseminated disease have an even more pronounced deficit in immunity. Disseminated MAI infection is diagnosed in 50% of AIDS patients at autopsy. The most important risk factor is a CD4 count less than 100 cells/μL of blood. Clinical findings associated with disseminated MAI include fever, sweats, malaise, wasting, diffuse peripheral and central lymphadenitis, infiltrative hepatosplenomegaly, refractory diarrhea, and anemia or pancytopenia secondary to massive infiltration of the bone marrow.

M. scrofulaceum

M. scrofulaceum was initially isolated in 1956. Its name derived from its recognition as a cause of scrofula in preschool children. Its incidence in the United States appears to be declining, and that may be why cervical lymphadenitis in children seems to be due to MAI infection more frequently than *M. scrofulaceum* infection. The portal of entry is believed to be the oral cavity. *M. scrofulaceum* has been isolated from soil, water, raw milk, and oysters. *M. scrofulaceum* is able to form a light-yellow to deep-orange pigment even in the dark (scotochromogenic). *M. scrofulaceum* forms a typically smooth, buttery, and globoid colony 10–28 days at temperatures ranging from 25°–37° C.

The most common manifestation of infection is cervical lymphadenitis, predominantly in children 1–5 years of age. The disease is usually unilateral, involving a single node or cluster in the submandibular area. This is in contrast to *M. tuberculosis*, which more frequently involves the tonsillar, cervical, and supraclavicular nodes. Involvement of lymph nodes of the head and extremities is infrequent. Children are usually healthy and free of constitutional symptoms, and pain is either minimal or absent. Infection may first be noticed when the node ruptures but, at times, fibrosis and calcification may have already developed. Uncommonly, progressive pulmonary disease, bone and soft tissue disease, conjunctivitis, meningitis, and hepatitis have been reported. Disseminated disease is rare and is usually associated with serious underlying immunosuppressive defects.

M. kansasii

The "yellow bacillus" was initially isolated in 1953. It is the second most common cause of pulmonary disease due to other mycobacteria. On acid-fast smear, it characteristically appears longer, thinner, and more beaded than *M. tuberculosis* and MAI. It has prominent transverse banding (cross-barred). Most strains are photochromogenic (development of beta-carotene crystals on exposure to light) and grow by 21 days on solid media.

M. kansasii has been isolated infrequently from water, milk supplies, and swine. Its natural reservoir is unknown. No person-to-person transmission has been documented. It has geographic preferences that include the central and southern United States, England, Wales, and Japan. Chronic obstructive lung disease and pneumoconiosis predispose to infection. Miners, welders, sandblasters, and painters are at highest risk. Owing to the infrequency of *M. kansasii* in the environment, recovery of this organism is more likely to indicate invasive disease.

Chronic pulmonary disease is the most common manifestation of *M. kansasii* infection. Patients may present with a chronic, sparsely productive cough; mild fever; malaise; and nonpleuritic chest pain resembling an indolent pneumonia. Extensive unilateral upper zone disease is common, but is generally milder than tuberculosis or MAI with less fibronodular and confluent shadowing. Multiple thin-walled cavities with minimal inflammatory reaction, scarring, and endobronchial spread are typically seen on chest radiographs.

In some geographic areas, *M. kansasii* is a major cause of cervical lymphadenitis in children. Disseminated disease has been recognized recently but only rarely with far-advanced disease or in immunocompromised hosts such as patients with leukemia and other malignancies, patients undergoing bone marrow and renal transplantation, and patients with AIDS.[48]

M. marinum

M. marinum was identified in 1926 as a cause of saltwater fish disease. On acid-fast smears, this bacillus appears relatively long with frequent cross-barring. This photochromogen grows optimally at 30°–32° C (unable to grow at 37° C), and colonies appear in 7–14 days.

Natural reservoirs are water and aquatic organisms. It is common along the Gulf Coast of the United States. Human infections are usually associated with some aquatic activity. Cutaneous disease occurs as a result of trauma, often minor,

to skin in contaminated, nonchlorinated fresh or salty water. It enters through abraded skin and may form a nodule, which can spread along lymphatics, cause verrucous lesions, or ulcerate. Pathologically early granulomatous lesions show collections of polymorphonuclear cells surrounded by histiocytes. Older lesions consist of lymphocytes, epithelioid cells, and occasional Langhans's giant cells, usually without caseation (the so-called "swimming pool" or "fish tank granuloma"). Its inability to grow at 37° C explains its limitation to superficial, cooler body tissues.

The skin lesions that are the most common manifestation may be of two types. The less common presentation is sporotrichosis-like, in which the primary area of inoculation develops into an abscess, with secondary spread of nodules along the lymphatics. The more typical presentation is after a 2–3-week incubation, and a single, small, tender subcutaneous papulonodule develops, usually involving the elbow, knee, toe, or finger ("swimming pool granuloma"). It may progress, acquiring a blue-purple hue, suppurate, and ulcerate. Infections of tendon sheath, bone, and synovium have been described in association with penetrating injuries. One case of sclerokeratitis has been reported.[49] Dissemination is rare but has been reported in both apparently immunocompetent and immunocompromised hosts.

M. xenopi

M. xenopi was originally thought to be an infrequent and relatively benign cause of disease. Despite being a scotochromogen, it is classified with the nonchromogens because of antigenic similarities to MAI. It grows optimally at 42°–43° C. Colonies are smooth and on cornmeal agar have filamentous extension. Acid-fast–stained specimens reveal long, filamentous rods that are tapered at both ends and arranged in palisades.

Despite being first isolated from a toad, *Xenopus laevis*, birds are the natural reservoir of *M. xenopi*. Geographic preferences include Ontario and the United States, southeast England, Scandinavia, and Australia. It has been isolated from hot- and cold-water sources. Clusters of nosocomial pulmonary infections have occurred in association with contaminated hot-water generators.

It infrequently causes pulmonary disease, and then usually in patients with underlying lung disease or predisposing conditions (alcoholism, malignancy, or diabetes mellitus). Pulmonary infections resemble tuberculosis with multinodular densities, often showing cavitary formation (in more than 90% of cases) and fibrosis. Extrapulmonary disease is rare. *M. xenopi* has been isolated from human tonsils.[50] Prosthetic joint, sinus tract, epididymis, osseous, and lymph node infections have also been reported. Reports of disseminated disease are becoming more common, notably in AIDS patients. It is noteworthy for resistance to many chemotherapeutic agents and occurrence of relapses.

M. malmoense

M. malmoense was first isolated in 1954 and identified in 1977 as a cause of chronic pulmonary disease that resembled tuberculosis in Sweden. Since then more than 180 cases have been reported, mostly from Europe and occasionally from the United States. It may be underreported because some strains take much longer to grow (8–12 weeks) than the amount of time most laboratories hold their specimens. In contrast to other mycobacteria, which are endemic in nature, *M. malmoense* has been isolated only from human sources and captured wild armadillos in Louisiana, never from an inanimate object. On acid-fast smears, the organism appears coccoid or as short bacilli without crossbands.

Typically, patients present with a chronic pulmonary infection that resembles tuberculosis and MAI, in the setting of preexisting lung disease such as pneumoconiosis. Extrapulmonary manifestations of disease are much less common. The most frequent extrapulmonary infection is cervical adenitis, which occurs almost exclusively in children. Unilateral cervical lymphadenitis presenting as an abscess is the most frequent appearance, with constitutional symptoms rare. Mediastinal lymphadenitis, tenosynovitis, and cutaneous lesions have also been reported. Disseminated disease is rare, and in all cases reported, patients have had a severe underlying immunodeficiency, either AIDS or leukemia.[51]

M. szulgai

M. szulgai was first described in 1972. It is an uncommon pathogen producing primarily pulmonary disease similar to *M. tuberculosis*. It has an RNA sequence that is more than 99% homologous to that of *M. malmoense*. The chief characteristic of this organism is that at 37° C it is a scotochromogen, and at 25° C it is a photochromogen. It requires about 2–4 weeks for growth. It has been isolated from snails and tropical fish. It can also be confused with more common tap-water contaminants, but it is not an environmental contaminant.

Most patients develop chronic pulmonary disease similar to that caused by the other mycobacteria. Most of the clinical isolates have been associated with clinical disease; therefore, if isolated, *M. szulgai* has a higher likelihood of causing disease than the other mycobacteria. Two thirds of the 30 reported cases involved pulmonary disease similar to that caused by *M. tuberculosis*. Other infections have involved the skin and soft tissue, bone and joints, cervical lymph nodes,[52] and even dissemination.

M. haemophilum

M. haemophilum was first described in 1978 in Israel when it was isolated from a skin abscess of an immunosuppressed patient with Hodgkin's disease. It is unique among mycobacteria in its absolute requirement for iron in the form of hemin (factor X) or ferric ammonium citrate in vitro. The main presentation of *M. haemophilum* infection is in immunocompromised persons, including AIDS, lymphoma, leukemia, and transplant patients. Most cases have involved skin and soft tissue infection. One or multiple painful chronic nodules develop, often on the extremities. They may develop into an abscess with draining purulent material and may also ulcerate. Other sites of involvement have included the lungs, bone, synovial tissue, and submandibular lymph nodes.[53]

Rapid Growers
(*M. chelonae* and *M. fortuitum*)

M. fortuitum and *M. chelonae* account for more than 95% of the reported infections due to rapid growers. Rare infections have been reported with other fast growers such as *M. smegmatis*, *M. thermoresistibile*, and *M. flavescens*. They are usually regarded as nonpathogenic commensals or environmental contaminants. Under the right host conditions, all other mycobacteria can and many have been reported to cause pulmonary or extrapulmonary disease in humans.

Acid-fast–stained bacilli often appear pleomorphic, ranging from long filamentous forms to short, thick rods. At times, they appear beaded or swollen, and nonstaining ovoid bodies may be seen at one end. Nonpigmented colonies grow rapidly in 3–7 days at 25°–40° C on both mycobacterial and routine bacteriologic media. They may be confused with diphtheroids. Unlike other mycobacteria, they may not stain with auramine-rhodamine used in fluorescence microscopy, and sodium hydroxide (commonly used in specimen decontamination in mycobacteriology laboratories) is toxic to these microorganisms.

These organisms are ubiquitous in nature and can be readily recovered from soil, dust, and water. They can be found in moist areas in hospitals, contaminated biologicals, aquariums, domestic animals, and marine life. Because they are highly resistant to antibiotics, antiseptics, and disinfectants, rapid growers are important nosocomial pathogens. Contamination of equipment, solutions, or water in the hospital setting may lead to small in-hospital pseudoepidemics. Most human infections are acquired by inoculation during accidental trauma, surgery, or injection. Pulmonary infection may be acquired hematogenously or by aspiration. There is no evidence for person-to-person transmission. These organisms are geographically widespread but are most frequently isolated in the southeastern United States.

Infections of the skin and soft tissue are the most common form of disease. Six weeks to 6 months after initial inoculation, subcutaneous erythematous nodules develop. They either form into well-circumscribed abscesses or form an almost confluent mass of cellulitis with multiple draining fistulas. The drainage is often a cloudy serous fluid. With pressure, thick, white necrotic material can often be expressed from within the lesion. In general, the nodules progress slowly, with chronic inflammation, ulceration, sinus tract formation, and exudates that resemble sporotrichosis. Systemic symptoms are absent.

Pulmonary infections due to *M. chelonae* and *M. fortuitum* occur most frequently in patients with underlying lung disease, such as cystic fibrosis, old tuberculosis, or in patients receiving immunosuppressive therapy, but in contrast to other mycobacteria they are often seen in patients without underlying disease. Bronchopulmonary infections usually occur following aspiration, especially of lipoidal material.[54] The lung infection due to *M. fortuitum-chelonae* is indistinguishable from that due to other mycobacteria;[55] although cavitation tends to be less frequent than in other mycobacterial lung infections. Clinical exacerbations occur for years, but the course remains progressive.

Other clinical syndromes associated with these fast growers include lymphadenitis; ocular infections; suppurative arthritis; osteomyelitis; endocarditis; meningitis; peritonitis due to indwelling peritoneal catheters; chronic urinary tract infections; bacteremia related to indwelling intravenous catheters; and otitis media associated with tympanotomy tubes or intraoral or facial infection. Disseminated disease is rare; it usually occurs in immunocompromised persons and is associated with a high mortality rate.

Specific Manifestations of the Ears, Nose, and Throat

Cervical Lymphadenitis. At the turn of the century when mycobacterial infections were prevalent, *M. tuberculosis* complex was almost exclusively the cause of mycobacterial lymphadenitis. With the decline in tuberculosis in industrialized countries, infections due to other mycobacteria have been identified and recognized as an important cause of cervical lymphadenitis in recent years. *M. tuberculosis* is still the most common cause of cervical lymphadenitis in adults, whereas the other mycobacteria are the most common cause of cervical adenitis in children.[56] When *M. scrofulaceum* was initially described, it was the most common other mycobacterium that caused cervical lymphadenitis. Yet, reports in the last couple of decades have reported that MAI is by far the most common pathogen.[56, 57] These differences probably reflect geographic differences but may also reflect the changing epidemiology of cervical lymphadenitis. In general, other mycobacterial cervical lymphadenitis seems most prevalent in the southeastern United States, with *M. kansasii* having a preference in the urban midwest and southwest[58] and *M. avium-intracellulare* in the rural southeast[59] and Massachusetts.[60] *M. scrofulaceum* is not as geographically defined.

The clinical presentation of other mycobacterial cervical lymphadenitis is indistinguishable from *M. tuberculosis*, except that concurrent pulmonary infection is much less frequent.

Aural. Infections of the ear due to other mycobacteria have rarely been reported and have always been sporadic. There have been two cases due to MAI[61, 62] and two cases due to *M. fortuitum*.[63, 64] The source of infection in these cases was not identified. In 1988 there was an epidemic of 17 cases of otitis media caused by *M. chelonae* from a single otolaryngology practice. These patients presented similarly to patients with tuberculous otitis media with a painless chronic otorrhea with exuberant granulation tissue. But unlike aural tuberculosis, these infections occurred by direct ear inoculation rather than by secondary spread to the middle ear from a pulmonary source. Of note, the lack of an intact tympanic membrane was an important risk factor; *M. chelonae* was cultured only from ears with a tympanotomy tube in place or perforation of the tympanic membrane. These infections were due to not using a high-level disinfection or sterilization of ear, nose, and throat instruments between examinations of patients to prevent transmission of this organism.[65] These infections were also very difficult to eradi-

cate and often required surgical intervention along with multiple antimycobacterial therapy.

Laryngeal. A case has been described of an infected tracheal tube site with *M. chelonae* presumptively following inoculation from contaminated water in a humidifier spray (A. S. Baker, personal communication, 1995).

In general, infections of the larynx, pharynx, or nose by other mycobacteria have been rarely reported and are usually due to direct inoculation of previously damaged tissues or occur in an immunocompromised host.

Diagnosis

The same techniques for making the diagnosis of other mycobacteria hold true for *M. tuberculosis*. Definitive diagnosis requires visualizing acid-fast organisms on staining or culture from secretions, fluid, or tissue from the sites of disease. However, unlike tuberculosis, in which isolation of a single colony of *M. tuberculosis* is always clinically significant, the other mycobacterial species may colonize body surfaces or secretions without causing disease. In addition, because other mycobacteria are often ubiquitous in soil, water, and dust, they are frequent contaminants of clinical specimens. Thus, the differentiation among contamination, colonization, and disease must be made.

The following general guidelines have been adopted[66, 67] and may be helpful in establishing the diagnosis of a true infection by other mycobacteria:

1. The organism is isolated multiple times from the same body site or from different body sites. The site of isolation is also crucial; in the absence of environmental contamination, isolation of the organism from a normally sterile tissue or fluid is significant.
2. The organism is grown from a single specimen on several different media; growing multiple colonies of the organism on each culture medium is preferable.
3. The organism is detected in smears or in histologic sections.
4. The presence of a clinical illness and/or histopathologic process is consistent with a mycobacterial etiology, and other reasonable causes for disease have been excluded.
5. There is a response, either clinically and/or histopathologically, to appropriate antimycobacterial therapy.
6. The organism is eliminated from clinical specimens as the patient's condition improves.

If the organism is rare, it is important to report how it was identified by stating the results of the specific biochemical tests used, preferably with confirmation by a reference laboratory. Often it is important not only to distinguish the organism from other bacteria but also from other mycobacteria, because the necessary medical and surgical therapy may differ. Skin testing with purified protein derivatives from various species of other mycobacteria is not useful owing to a lack of adequately standardized antigens and cross-reactivity due to shared antigens leading to poor specificity of the presently available reagents. The diagnosis of disseminated infection is made by isolation of organisms from the blood, bone marrow, or liver tissues.

Treatment

Medical

Therapy for atypical mycobacteria must be individualized. In general, these mycobacteria are very resistant to standard antituberculosis agents, although *M. kansasii*, *M. szulgai*, and *M. marinum* are more susceptible to these agents than the other species. Documented pulmonary infections may require multiple-drug regimens. Consultation is advisable in these and other infections in which disease is documented and therapy is being considered.

Surgical

Localized disease (e.g., a single lymph node or skin nodule) can often be treated by surgical excision alone. Again, consultation is advised to assess whether systemic involvement is present and whether combination surgical-medical therapy is indicated.

LEPROSY

Description

M. leprae, the etiologic agent of leprosy (Hansen's disease), has been known since the late nineteenth century as the cause of a chronic granulomatous infection of the skin, mucous membranes, and peripheral nerves. It has been responsible for millions of infections worldwide.

M. leprae is an acid-fast bacillus indistinguishable morphologically from other mycobacteria. It is an obligate intracellular parasite that may remain viable outside the body for several days. It cannot be cultivated in artificial media or tissue culture, so it is propagated in armadillos and in the footpads of mice. The bacillus multiplies exceedingly slowly, with an optimal doubling time of 11–13 days.

Epidemiology

Humans and nine-banded armadillos are its only known hosts in nature. The number of leprosy cases decreased from approximately 12 million in 1982 to 6 million in 1991.[68] However, caution regarding disease eradication is suggested by a similar optimism for the eradication of tuberculosis being recently shattered, the worldwide incidence of new cases has yet to decline, and most of the current leprosy patients reside in areas with poor medical infrastructures for delivery of effective therapy. Leprosy is endemic to Asia, Africa, the islands of the Pacific, and Latin America. Within the United States, most cases have been reported in areas with a warm climate, including California, Texas, Louisiana, Hawaii, Florida, and Puerto Rico. However, the vast majority of infections in the United States were acquired abroad. In endemic areas, household contacts of lepromatous cases have attack rates of 6%–13%.[69]

Colonization, Transmission, Pathogenesis, and Immunity

Like the *M. tuberculosis* complex, *M. leprae* is transmissible from person to person. Traditionally, entry of bacilli via the skin was considered important, but there have been only occasional case reports of direct skin inoculation. The respiratory tract, specifically via nasal droplet transmission, may be the primary mode of infection. A patient with lepromatous leprosy may discharge up to 10^9 organisms from a sneeze, cough, or speaking.[70] The nasal turbinates are encountered early in infection; their cool, moist environment favors growth; and transmission is enhanced by abraded mucosa. The incubation period is frequently 3–5 years but may range from 6 months to decades.

Its pathogenicity and ability to survive in the host are poorly understood. The best-characterized possible virulence factor is phenolic glycolipid-1 (PGL-1), a prominent surface lipid specific for *M. leprae*. PGL can mediate phagocytosis of the bacterium into the macrophage and also helps protect the bacterium from oxidative killing by chemically scavenging hydroxyl radicals and superoxide anions.

Owing to skin-test positivity to *M. leprae*–specific PGL-1 and lepromin (whole, killed *M. leprae*), it is believed that only about 10% of individuals who become infected develop disease. *M. leprae* itself is not toxic to its host cell, and the manifestations of disease are the result of the host immune response to the organism. The clinical spectrum of disease depends on the extent of cell-mediated immunity expressed toward *M. leprae*. High levels of cell-mediated immunity and delayed hypersensitivity effectively control bacillary replication and lead to the formation of organized epithelioid cell granulomas producing the tuberculoid form of disease, whereas absence of cell-mediated immunity (anergy) results in lepromatous leprosy with resultant abundant bacilli within inactivated macrophages. Between these two poles, there is a spectrum of disease with moderate cell-mediated immunity (borderline tuberculoid), borderline, and minimal cell-mediated response (borderline lepromatous). *M. leprae* is a systemic infection due to hematogenous spread of bacilli, which accounts for its invasion of skin and nerves.

The defect in cell-mediated immunity seen in lepromatous patients is extremely specific. These patients do not suffer increased morbidity following infection by other pathogens associated with defects in cellular immunity (such as viruses, protozoa, or fungi), nor do these patients have an increased risk for neoplasia. Patients with lepromatous leprosy do have an increased number of circulating CD8 lymphocytes that can be specifically activated by *M. leprae* antigens.

Clinical Manifestations

The clinical presentation varies a great deal, depending on the host immune response, and is predictive of disease complications. Clinical manifestations are largely confined to the skin, upper respiratory system, testes, and peripheral nerves. Most of the serious sequelae are a result of *M. leprae* having a unique tropism for peripheral nerves. In the full tuberculoid (TT) and borderline tuberculoid (BT) disease, there are one

Figure 23–6. Patient with lepromatous leprosy. *A,* Classic leonine facies with thickening of the supraciliary ridge and absent eyebrows due to diffuse infiltration of the dermis. *B,* Punch biopsy from the border of a hypopigmented area of the trunk revealing abundant acid-fast bacilli (×100). *C,* Near total opacification of the left cornea with scarring and diffuse edema and a rubeotic iris. (Courtesy of N.A. Hynes, MD, M. Raizman, MD, and A. S. Baker, MD.) *D,* Avascular punctate keratitis of the superior temporal quadrant of the right eye with an elevated iris lesion (leproma) at the 9 o'clock position and mild nuclear sclerosis. (From Carus NH, Raizman MB, Williams DL, Baker AS: Relapse of *Mycobacterium leprae* infection with ocular manifestations. Clin Infect Dis 1995; 20: 776–780. Published by the University of Chicago.)

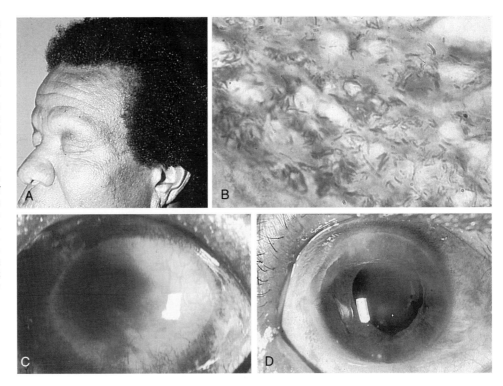

or a few large, well-demarcated hypopigmented macules, often elevated with erythematous borders. The lesions are often hairless, without sweat glands, and anesthetic. Large asymmetric peripheral nerves near the lesions may be swollen. Uncommonly, patients may have a large and functionally impaired nerve trunk without skin lesions as the sole manifestation (neural leprosy). Tuberculoid leprosy does not result in upper respiratory signs and symptoms. In borderline leprosy (BB), skin lesions are more numerous and appear poorly defined. The bacilli are more frequently demonstrated on biopsy, most often in the nerves. This stage is often less stable than either the tuberculoid or lepromatous forms, and patients normally progress to either the tuberculoid or lepromatous forms. The most severe forms of leprosy are the borderline lepromatous (BL) and full lepromatous (LL) forms. The replication of the organism is poorly contained, and patients often have diffuse disease. Systemic involvement is common, with the organism found in many organs of the body. Even in the most advanced cases, destructive lesions are limited to areas of the body that are several degrees cooler than 37° C, including the skin, peripheral nerves, anterior portions of the eyes, upper respiratory passages above the larynx, ears, testes, and the hands and feet.

Skin lesions are of many variable types, including macules, papules, nodules, or plaques and a thickened dermis. Thickening of the facial skin results in leonine facies. Also, there is often a loss of the lateral eyebrows (madarosis) from diffuse infiltration of the dermis (Fig. 23–6A). Owing to the massive infiltration with bacilli (Fig. 23–6B) in lepromatous patients, the upper respiratory tract, particularly the nasal mucosa, is affected. Patients may complain of chronic nasal congestion due to atrophic rhinitis and epitaxis. If left untreated, this process can extend to the nasal cartilage, leading to septal collapse and the classic "saddle nose" deformity

(Fig. 23–7). Peripheral neuropathy in lepromatous patients is often generalized, symmetric, and associated with distal anesthesia of the hands and feet. In untreated lepromatous patients, a high level continuous bacteremia is very common, and organisms can often be seen in stained smears of peripheral blood "buffy" coats.

Ocular complications are the result of primary infection of the eye as well as secondary damage because of neural involvement. The eye is involved in approximately 50%–90% of patients with leprosy, with blindness occurring in about 5%. The ciliary body is often involved and may present with signs 25–30 years after the initial onset. Infection of the eye (Fig. 23–6C and D) may result in prominent corneal nerves, conjunctivitis, superficial punctate keratitis, scleral nodules, and chronic uveitis. Seventh nerve involve-

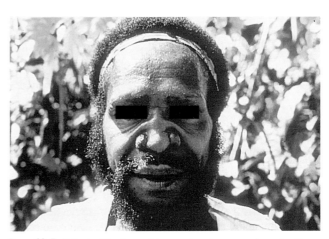

Figure 23–7. Patient with advanced lepromatous leprosy and nasal collapse. (Courtesy of H. Provine, BS)

ment or the ophthalmic division of the trigeminal nerves is not uncommon. Leprosy patients deserve an ocular examination every 5 years.

The differential diagnosis of the skin lesions includes sarcoidosis, lupus vulgaris, lupus erythematosus, dermal leishmaniasis, and yaws. The differential diagnosis of the peripheral neuropathy includes nutritional, HIV-induced, and other neurologic disorders. The combination of a chronic skin disease and peripheral neuropathy in a patient from an endemic area should suggest leprosy.

Diagnosis

The diagnosis of leprosy is primarily clinical and presumptive. One relies on the clinical symptom complex, epidemiologic history, and the correlation of typical histopathologic lesions with the presence of acid-fast organisms in the skin biopsy specimen. An elliptic excision biopsy, 12–15 mm, is preferred and should include central and peripheral areas of the lesion and should be deep enough to remove subcutaneous tissues en bloc. In tuberculoid leprosy the number of bacilli may be sparse, whereas in lepromatous leprosy numerous bacilli may be found. In addition, bacilli may also be found in the discharge from the mouth and the nose. Biopsy specimens should always be stained with both hematoxylin and eosin stain and an acid-fast stain (preferably Fite's), because *M. leprae* may not be acid-fast when stained with the more typical mycobacterial Ziehl-Neelsen staining procedure. PCR-based techniques are being explored to significantly decrease the time to definitive diagnosis and have the potential to be used to monitor the adequacy of therapy.[71]

M. leprae fails to grow on conventional mycobacteriologic culture media. In general, the organism cannot be grown in vitro at this time, and inoculation of armadillos or the footpads of mice is required.

Skin tests and serologic tests are not yet widely available. Most promising is a serologic test based on detection of antibody to the *M. leprae*–specific PGL-1. The level of antibody response correlates with bacillary load. Therefore, in lepromatous patients this assay has a sensitivity of more than 95%, and in tuberculoid leprosy it is 30% sensitive. It is 100% specific, so it may be useful in confirming a diagnosis or as an epidemiologic tool.

Treatment

Medical

Treatment is primarily medical. See Chapter 12 for recommended agents and doses.

Surgical Therapy

Surgical indications are primarily orthopedic or ophthalmic. Patients with permanent disability require specialized treatment by physical therapists and surgeons. Surgical ophthalmic therapy is directed toward the ocular deformity to repair lid function and provide corneal protection. Nasal collapse (Fig. 23–7), though not as common in the postantibiotic era,

still affects some patients. Nasal reconstruction surgery can largely ameliorate the cosmetic defect, making the appearance of affected patients socially acceptable. Similar cosmetic surgery on the ears may also be beneficial.

References

1. Bloom BR, Murray JL: Tuberculosis: Commentary on reemergent killer. Science 1992; 257: 1055–1064.
2. Anonymous: Tuberculosis Morbidity: United States, 1994. MMWR CDC Surveill Summ 1995; 44: 387–395.
3. Goble M, Iseman MD, Madsen RN-C, et al.: Treatment of 171 patients with pulmonary tuberculosis resistant to isoniazid and rifampin. N Engl J Med 1993; 328: 527–532.
4. Stead WW: Tuberculosis among the elderly person: An outbreak in a nursing home. Ann Intern Med 1981; 94: 606.
5. Honk VH, Kent DC, Baker JH: The Byrd study: In-depth analysis of a microoutbreak of tuberculosis in a closed environment. Arch Environ Health 1968; 16: 1968.
6. Stylbo K: Recent advances in epidemiological research in tuberculosis. Adv Tuberc Res 1980; 20: 1.
7. Zeidberg LD, Gass RS, Dillon A, et al.: The Williamson County tuberculosis study: A twenty-four year epidemiologic study. Am Rev Respir Dis 1963; 87: 1–88.
8. Bloch A, Reider M, Kelly G, et al.: Clin Chest Med 1989; 10: 297.
9. Small PM, Schecter GF, Goodman PC, et al.: Treatment of tuberculosis in patients with advanced human immunodeficiency virus infection. N Engl J Med 1991; 324: 289.
10. Dandapat M, Mishra B, Dash SP, Kar PK: Peripheral lymph node tuberculosis: A review of 80 cases. Br J Surg 1986; 77: 911–912.
11. Lee K, Tami T, Lalwani AK, Schecter G: Contemporary management of cervical tuberculosis. Laryngoscope 1992; 102: 60–64.
12. Lau SK, Wei WI, Hsu C, Engzell UC: Efficacy of fine-needle aspiration cytology in the diagnosis of tuberculous cervical lymphadenopathy. J Laryngol Otol 1990; 104: 24–27.
13. Galietti F, Giorgis GE, Oliaro A, et al.: Tuberculosis of the larynx. Panminerva Med 1989; 31: 134–136.
14. Soda A, Rubio H, Salazar M: Tuberculosis of the larynx: Clinical aspects of 19 patients. Laryngoscope 1989; 99: 1147–1150.
15. Bailey CM, Windle-Taylor PC: Tuberculous laryngitis. Laryngoscope 1981; 91: 93–100.
16. Hunter AM, Millar JW, Wightman AJA, Horne NW: The changing pattern of laryngeal tuberculosis. J Laryngol Otol 1981; 95: 393–398.
17. Gertler R, Ramages L: Tuberculous laryngitis: A one-year harvest. J Laryngol Otol 1985; 99: 1119–1125.
18. Bull TR: Tuberculosis of the larynx. BMJ 1966; 2: 991–992.
19. Chodosh P, Willis W: Tuberculosis of the upper respiratory tract. Larngoscope 1970; 80: 679–696.
20. Mitchell A: Report on the infection of children with bovine tubercle bacillus. BMJ 1914; 200: 125–133.
21. Fordyce A, Carmichael E: Nasopharyngeal and cervical glandular tuberculosis in children. Lancet 1914; 260: 23–26.
22. Waldron J, van Hasselt C, Skinner D, Arnold M: Tuberculosis of the nasopharynx: Clinicopathological features. Clin Otolaryngol 1992; 17: 57–59.
23. Mahindra S, Malik G, Sohail M: Primary tuberculosis of the adenoids. Acta Otolaryngol (Stockh) 1981; 92: 173–180.
24. Turner L, Fraser JS: Tuberculosis of the middle-ear cleft in children: A clinical and pathological study. J Laryngol Rhinol Otol 1915; 30: 209–247.
25. Ozcelik T, Ataman M, Gedikoglu G: An unusual presentation: Primary tuberculosis of the middle ear cleft. Tuber Lung Dis 1995; 76: 178–179.
25a. Windle-Taylor PC, Bailey CM: Tuberculosis otitis media: A series of 22 patients. Laryngoscope 1980; 90: 1039–1044.
26. Skolnik PR, Nadol JB Jr, Baker AS: Tuberculosis of the middle ear: Review of the literature with an instructive case report. Rev Infect Dis 1986; 8: 403–410.
27. Davidson S, Creter D, Leventon G, Katznelson D: Tuberculosis of the middle ear in an infant. Arch Otolaryngol Head Neck Surg 1989; 115: 876–877.
28. Ramages MB, Gertler R: Aural tuberculosis: A series of 25 patients. J Laryngol Otol 1985; 99: 1073–1080.

29. Proctor B, Lindsay JR: Tuberculosis of the ear. Arch Otolaryngol 1942; 35: 221–249.

30. Harbert F, Riordan D: Tuberculosis of the middle ear. Laryngoscope 1964; 74: 198–204.

31. Birrell JF: Aural tuberculosis in children. Proc R Soc Med 1973; 66: 331–338.

31a. Gettler, JF, Casarona J: Tuberculous otitis media in an HIV-infected patient. Infect Dis Clin Prac 1995; 4: 68–69.

32. MacAdam AM, Rubio T: Tuberculous otomastoiditis in children. Am J Dis Child 1977; 131: 152–156.

33. Ma K, Tang P, Chan KW: Aural tuberculosis. Am J Otol 1990; 11: 174–177.

34. Bryant JC: Oral tuberculosis. Am Rev Tuberc 1939; 39: 738–744.

35. Douglass BE, Foss EL: Tuberculosis of the tongue. Mayo Clin Proc 1957; 32: 374–376.

36. Miller FJW: Recognition of primary tuberculous infection of skin and mucosae. Lancet 1953; 1: 5–9.

37. Thompson SC: Diseases of the Nose and Throat, 2nd ed. Cassell & Co., Ltd, 1919: 632–654.

38. Gentric A, Garre M: Nasal tuberculosis: two cases in elderly patients. Clin Infect Dis 1992; 15: 176–177.

39. Harrison A, Knight R: Tuberculosis of the nasopharynx misdiagnosed as Wegener's granulomatosis. Thorax 1986; 41: 219–220.

40. Dilkes M, McGilligan J, Chapman J: A rare presentation of tuberculosis of the cervical spine. J Laryngol Otol 1991; 105: 786–787.

41. Catanzaro A: Nosocomial tuberculosis. Am Rev Respir Dis 1982; 125: 559–562.

42. Society AT: The tuberculin skin test. Am Rev Respir Dis 1981; 124: 356.

43. Nash DR, Douglass JE: Anergy in active pulmonary tuberculosis. Chest 1980; 77: 32.

44. Good RC, Silcos VA, Kilburn JO, Plikaytis BD: Isolation of nontuberculous mycobacteria in the United States. J Infect Dis 1982; 146: 829–833.

45. Welch K, Finkbeiner W, Alpers CE, et al.: Autopsy findings in the acquired immune deficiency syndrome (AIDS). JAMA 1984; 252: 1152–1159.

46. Meissner PS, Palkinham JOI: Plasmid DNA profiles as epidemiological markers for clinical and environmental isolates of *M. avium, M. intracellulare,* and *M. scrofulaceum.* J Infect Dis 1986; 153: 325.

47. Greene JB, Sidhu GS, Lewin S, et al.: *Mycobacterium avium-intracellulare:* A cause of disseminated life-threatening infection in homosexuals and drug abusers. Ann Intern Med 1982; 97: 539–546.

48. Sherer R, Sable R, Sonnenberg M: Disseminated infection with *Mycobacterium kansasii* in the acquired immunodeficiency syndrome. Ann Intern Med 1986; 105: 710.

49. Schonherr U, Naumann GOH, Lang GK, et al.: Sclerokeratitis caused by *Mycobacterium marinum.* Am J Ophthalmol 1989; 238: 607.

50. Stewart CJ, Dixon JMS, Curtis BA: Isolation of mycobacteria from tonsils, nasopharyngeal secretions, and lymph nodes in East Anglia. Tubercle 1970; 51: 178–83.

51. Zaugg M, Salfinger M, Opravil M, Luthy R: Extrapulmonary and disseminated infections due to *Mycobacterium malmoense:* Case report and review. Clin Infect Dis 1993; 16: 549–549.

52. Dylewski JS, Zackon HM, Latour AH, et al.: *Mycobacterium szulgai:* An unusual pathogen. Rev Infect Dis 1987; 9: 578–80.

53. Dawson DJ, Blacklock ZM, Kaane DW: *Mycobacterium haemophilum* causing lymphadenitis in an otherwise healthy child. Med J Austr 1981; 2: 289–290.

54. Sanders WEJ: Lung infection caused by rapidly growing mycobacteria. J Respir Dis 1982; 3: 30–38.

55. Griffith DE, Wallace RJ: Pulmonary disease due to rapidly growing mycobacteria. Semin Respir Med 1988; 9: 505.

56. Lai KK, Stottmeier KD, Sherman IH, McCabe WR: Mycobacterial cervical lymphadenopathy. JAMA 1984; 25: 1286–1288.

57. Schaad UB, Votteler TP, McCracken GH, Nelson JD. Management of atypical mycobacterial lymphadenitis in childhood: a review based on 380 cases. J Pediatr 1979; 95: 356.

58. Black BG, Chapman JS. Cervical adenitis in children due to human and unclassified mycobacteria. Pediatrics 1964; 33: 887–893.

59. Morimoto MG, Rothrock AG, Stottmeier KD: Isolation of acid-fast organisms from surgical specimens. J Clin Microbiol 1979; 10: 589–600.

60. Smith DH, Doherty RA, DeLemos RA: Unclassified mycobacterial infection and disease in children residing in Massachusetts. J Pediatr 1965; 67: 759–767.

61. Kinsella JP, Grossman M, Black S: Otomastoiditis caused by *Mycobacterium avium-intracellulare.* Pediatr Infect Dis J 1986; 5: 704–706.

62. Wardrop PA, Pillsbury HCI: *Mycobacterium avium* acute mastoiditis. Arch Otolaryngol 1984; 110: 686–687.

63. Austin WK, Lockey MW: *Mycobacterium fortuitum* mastoiditis. Arch Otolaryngol 1976; 102: 558–560.

64. Neitch SM, Sydnor JB, Schleupner CJ: *Mycobacterium fortuitum* as a cause of mastoiditis and wound infection. Arch Otolaryngol 1982; 108: 11–14.

65. Lowry PW, Jarvis WR, Oberle AD, et al: *Mycobacterium chelonae* causing otitis media in an ear-nose-and-throat practice. N Engl J Med 1988; 319: 978–982.

66. Wallace RJ Jr, O'Brien R, Glassroth J, et al.: Diagnosis and treatment of disease caused by nontuberculous mycobacteria. Am Rev Respir Dis 1990; 142: 940–53.

67. Weinberger M, Berg SL, Feuerstein IM, Pizzo PA, et al.: Disseminated infection with *Mycobacterium gordonae:* Report of a case and critical review of the literature. Clin Infect Dis 1992; 14: 1229–1239.

68. Noordeen SK: A look at world leprosy. Lepr Rev 1991; 62: 72–86.

69. Rao PSS, Karat ABA, Kaliaperumal VG, et al.: Transmission of leprosy within households. Int J Lepr 1975; 43: 45.

70. Shepard CC: The nasal excretion of *Mycobacterium leprae* in leprosy. Int J Lepr 1966; 30: 10.

71. Carus NH, Raizman MB, Williams DL, Baker AS: Relapse of *Mycobacterium leprae* infection with ocular manifestations. Clin Infect Dis 1995; 20: 776–780.

CHAPTER TWENTY-FOUR

Michael C. Bach

Nocardia

▼

Nocardiosis is caused by an aerobic actinomycete; Eppinger first described the infection in humans in 1890 after Nocard described bovine farcy in cattle in 1888.[1] It is a suppurative necrotizing infection usually acquired by the respiratory route, although infection by inoculation from contaminated soil does occur.

MICROBIOLOGY

Nocardia has a very characteristic morphologic appearance on Gram's stain. It is seen as delicate branching beaded gram-positive filaments (Fig. 24–1).[2] These may occasionally break up during preparation of the stain and may be seen as small rod forms resembling diphtheroids. With the Kinyoun's stain, using 1% sulfuric acid instead of the usual acid alcohol decolorizer used for tuberculosis identification, the organism is acid-fast.

Nocardia grows on most culture media; however, it is a slow grower. Colonies usually begin to be seen at 48–72 hours, and most cultures plates are usually discarded before this time. Occasionally growth may take up to 10–14 days. This is an important issue in terms of isolation of the organism since the laboratory should be notified of the suspicion of *Nocardia* so that plates can be held for longer periods of time.

There are a number of species of *Nocardia*. The most important is the *Nocardia asteroides* complex, which comprises *N. asteroides, Nocardia farcinica,* and *Nocardia nova*.[3, 4] These three are currently differentiated on the basis of antimicrobial susceptibility patterns and some growth and chemical characteristics. *Nocardia brasiliensis* is much less common and is usually seen as an inoculation disease although disseminated infections can occur. *Nocardia otitidis-caviarum* is also much rarer and can also cause systemic disease. A few cases caused by *Nocardia transvalensis* have also been reported.[5] *Actinomyces,* the cause of actinomycosis, resembles *Nocardia* on smear. It more commonly results in the appearance of yellow "sulfur" granules in exudate from the infected area; however, this may be seen with *Nocardia* as well. *Nocardia* is aerobic, whereas *Actinomyces* is a strict anaerobe.

HISTOLOGY

Although polymorphonuclear leukocytes predominate in the tissues infected with *Nocardia,* the predominant cell controlling the spread of this organism is the activated T cell, thus explaining the correlation of defects in cell-mediated immunity and nocardiosis.[2] The infection is a necrotizing

process with cavitation found especially in tissues such as the lung and brain. The organism is not visualized on routine hematoxylin and eosin staining or periodic acid–Schiff but may be well seen with the Brown-Brenn stain and methenamine silver stain.

EPIDEMIOLOGY

The most common method of entry of *Nocardia* is by inhalation into the respiratory tract. It can then disseminate to multiple organs via the blood stream. The brain is a favored site, as is the kidney. The organism may be found in soil, and after traumatic inoculation it can either cause a localized infection or spread by lymphatics and result in a sporotrichoid-type lesion. Although *Nocardia* may be cultured from respiratory secretions as a commensal, its isolation usually implies disease, and it should be evaluated seriously as a potential pathogen.

EAR, NOSE, AND THROAT INFECTIONS

There have been very few cases of *Nocardia* related to infections of the ear, nose, and throat (Table 24–1). Isolated case reports document mastoiditis with spread locally to the temporal lobe[6] or as a tonsillar infection unresponsive to the usual antibacterial agents.[7] It has been found as a rare cause of sinusitis[8] and as a cervicofacial infection in children[9] and adults.[10] *Nocardia* has been isolated from a vallecular cyst,[11] as well as from the parotid gland, middle ear effusion, and pharyngeal ulcers.[12]

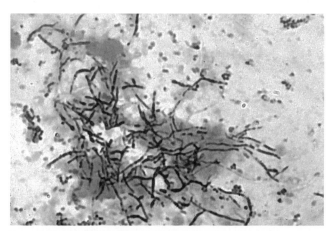

Figure 24–1. Photomicrograph of a Gram's stain of exudate showing branching filaments of *Nocardia* (×1000).

Table 24–1. *NOCARDIA* AND EAR, NOSE, AND THROAT INFECTION

Age	Underlying Disease	Site of Infection	Diagnosis	Treatment	Outcome	First Author
10	None	Mastoid Brain	Mastoiditis Brain abscess	Surgery TMP-SMX	Cured	Cox[6]
22	None	Tonsil	Peritonsillar abscess	Surgery TMP-SMX	Cured	Adair[7]
39	None	Maxillary sinus	Maxillary sinusitis	Surgery Sulfadiazine	Cured	Katz[8]
2	None	Facial pustule	Pustule	Surgery TMP-SMX	Cured	Lampe[9]
5	None	Cheek pustule Cervical node	Pustule and lymphadenitis	TMP-SMX	Cured	Lampe[9]
3	None	Nasal pustule	Pustule	TMP-SMX	Cured	Lampe[9]
33	HIV	Submandibular space	Dental abscess Submandibular abscess	Surgery TMP-SMX	Cured	Seidel[10]
55	None	Vallecula	Vallecular abscess	Surgery	Cured	Burton[11]

TMP-SMX, trimethoprim-sulfamethoxazole; HIV, human immunodeficiency virus.

DIAGNOSIS

Although this organism can cause disease in normal hosts, it is the presence of a defect in cell-mediated immunity that often raises the possibility of the organism. Infection unresponsive to usually effective antibiotics, the presence of necrosis and suppuration, and concomitant pulmonary or intracerebral processes should at least engender a suspicion of *Nocardia*. It should also be considered as a potential pathogen in pyogenic lesions with sterile routine cultures. It may be grown from the blood and certainly from the affected site. Gram's stain of a smear from the infected area is the most helpful diagnostic clue; if this shows the typical morphology of this organism, it should immediately prompt the laboratory to look for this slow-growing pathogen in culture. There are no reliable serologic tests at the present time.

TREATMENT

Sulfonamides, now often in the form of trimethoprim-sulfamethoxazole, are the backbone of therapy (Table 24–2).[13] Patients require a long course of therapy, in the range of 4–6 months, depending on the site, immune status of the patient, and severity of infection. If sulfonamides are used alone, then one generally tries to achieve blood levels of 10%–15

Table 24–2. THERAPY OF *NOCARDIA*

Antibiotic	Species	Dose
Sulfamethoxazole	Most	2 g twice daily
TMP-SMX*	Most	1–2 DS twice daily†
Minocycline	Most	100–200 mg twice daily
Amikacin	Most	7.5 mg/kg every 12h
Imipenem-cilastatin	Most‡	250–500 mg every 8h
Ceftriaxone	Many‡	1 g every 24h
Cefotaxime	Many‡	1 g every 8h

*Trimethoprim-sulfamethoxazole.
†1 DS (double-strength tablet) contains 160 mg trimethoprim and 800 mg sulfamethoxazole.
‡*Nocardia farcinica* is often resistant.

mg% 2 hours after a dose. The usual drug used in this situation is sulfamethoxazole 2 g twice daily. Trimethoprim-sulfamethoxazole is used in doses of one to two double-strength tablets twice daily.

In the sulfonamide-allergic patient or patients who do not seem to be responding to sulfonamides, minocycline has excellent activity and is usually given in a dose of 100–200 mg twice daily depending on patient tolerance.[14] In patients with disseminated or bulky disease or who are immunosuppressed and often critically ill, amikacin, often in combination with imipenem-cilastatin or a third-generation cephalosporin (ceftriaxone or cefotaxime), is very effective.[15] Antimicrobial susceptibility testing by a reference laboratory should be requested for any significant isolate of *Nocardia* since this testing takes time, is often very laboratory-dependent, and may be critical in patients who fail to respond to initial therapy.

N. farcinica is highly resistant to most antibiotics but seems to be very susceptible to amikacin. *N. asteroides* is usually sensitive to amikacin, imipenem-cilastatin, and the third-generation cephalosporins. Where significant pus formation is present, surgical drainage is often necessary along with antimicrobial therapy.

Nocardia often occurs in conjunction with or is followed by other opportunistic pathogens. If a patient is not responding to standard therapy and the organism is susceptible to the agents being used, consideration should be given to reaspiration or rebiopsy to be sure another pathogen is not present.

References

1. McNeil MM, Brown JM: The medically important aerobic actinomycetes: Epidemiology and microbiology. Clin Microbiol Rev 1994; 7: 357.
2. Beeman BL, Beeman L: *Nocardia* Species: Host–parasite relationships. Clin Microbiol Rev 1994; 7: 213.
3. Wallace RJ Jr, Tsukamura M, Brown BA, et al.: Cefotaxime-resistant *Nocardia asteroides* strains are isolates of the controversial species *Nocardia farcinica*. J Clin Microbiol 1990; 28: 2726.
4. Wallace RJ Jr, Brown BA, Tsukamura M, et al.: Clinical and laboratory features of *Nocardia nova*. J Clin Microbiol 1991; 29: 2407.
5. McNeil MM, Brown JM, Georghiou PR, et al.: Infections due to *Nocardia transvalensis*. Clin Infect Dis 1992; 15: 453–463.

6. Cox F, Hall JE, Ballenger CE, et al.: *Nocardia asteroides* brain abscess following mastoidectomy. Pediatr Neurol 1986; 2: 183–184.

7. Adair JC, Amber IJ, Johnston JM: Peritonsillar abscess caused by *Nocardia asteroides*. J Clin Microbiol 1987; 25; 2214–2215.

8. Katz P, Fauci AS: *Nocardia asteroides* sinusitis. JAMA 1987; 238: 2397–2398.

9. Lampe RM, Baker CJ, Septimus EJ, et al.: Cervicofacial nocardiosis in children. J Pediatr 1981; 99: 593–595.

10. Seidel JF, Younce DC, Hupp JR, et al.: Cervicofacial nocardiosis: Report of case. J Oral Maxillofac Surg 1994; 52: 188–191.

11. Burton DM, Burgess LPA: Nocardiosis of the upper aerodigestive tract. Ear Nose Throat J 1990; 69: 350–353.

12. Young LS, Armstrong D, Blevins A, et al.: *Nocardia asteroides* infection complicating neoplastic disease. Am J Med 1971; 50: 356–367.

13. Wallace RJ, Steele LC, Sumter G, et al.: Antimicrobial susceptibility patterns of *Nocardia asteroides*. Antimicrob Agents Chemother 1988; 32: 1776–1779.

14. Bach MC, Gold O, Finland M: Activity of minocycline against *Nocardia asteroides*: Comparison with tetracycline and agar-dilution and standard disc-diffusion tests and with sulfadiazine in an experimental infection of mice. J Lab Clin Med 1973; 81: 787–793.

15. Gombert ME: Antimicrobial management of *Nocardia asteroides* infection. Infect Med 1994; 11: 448–452.

▼ *Fungi*

M. Hong Nguyen
Alan M. Sugar

CHAPTER TWENTY-FIVE

Aspergillus

▼

HISTORY

The name *Aspergillus* was coined by Micheli, a priest and botanist, in 1729 to describe the microscopic structure of an organism that resembles an aspergillum, a device used in churches to sprinkle holy water. The first human disease was reported by Sluyter in 1847.[1] Virchow in 1856 described four autopsy-proven cases of *Aspergillus* infection in patients with chronic lung disease.[1] An increased interest in *Aspergillus* came in the latter part of the nineteenth century, when a link between allergic disease caused by *Aspergillus* and occupational exposures such as those of wig cleaners or pigeon feeders was made.[2] In the mid–twentieth century, more clinical syndromes associated with *Aspergillus* were described, such as pulmonary aspergilloma, allergic bronchopulmonary aspergillosis, and invasive aspergillosis.[1]

PATHOGEN

There are more than 150 *Aspergillus* species, of which *Aspergillus fumigatus* and *Aspergillus flavus* are the species most often implicated in human infection. Identification of *Aspergillus* species is based on the differences in the morphologic characteristics, including color and shape of conidial head, numbers of phialides, shape of vesicles, markings and color of conidiophores, and shape of Hülle cells.[2]

EPIDEMIOLOGY

Aspergillus is ubiquitous in nature with no geographic distinction and is found in soil, food products, and decomposing organic material. The primary mode of *Aspergillus* acquisition is via inhalation of spores. Cases of hypersensitivity pneumonitis in individuals exposed to compost piles, decomposing haystacks, and moldy oats; of invasive aspergillosis in oncologic or bone marrow transplant patients exposed to *Aspergillus* spores during hospital construction or renovation; and of allergic bronchopulmonary aspergillosis and invasive aspergillosis secondary to smoking marijuana contaminated with *Aspergillus*[3] have been reported.

Aspergillus spores in the hospital environment can also gain access to susceptible hosts via burn wounds or during surgery (open heart, organ transplant, and cataract surgeries), or via direct inoculation, as in cases of *Aspergillus* endophthalmitis and endocarditis in intravenous drug users.

HOST DEFENSE

Aspergillus species are opportunistic pathogens. Alveolar macrophages provide the first-line protection against *Aspergillus* by phagocytizing the spores. Neutrophils are active against the mycelial form of *Aspergillus* found in infected tissue.[4] Either line of defense is able to protect against uncontrolled proliferation of *Aspergillus*, although neutrophils are relatively more important than macrophages in host defense.[4]

The most significant risk factor for *Aspergillus* infection is the presence and duration of granulocytopenia; the risk of *Aspergillus* infection increases tremendously after 4 weeks of granulocytopenia.[5] High-dose corticosteroid therapy also predisposes patients to aspergillosis by impairing both macrophage and granulocyte functions. Other risk factors include receipt of cytotoxic or immunosuppressive drugs; hematologic malignancy, especially leukemia; acute rejection of bone marrow transplant or solid organ transplant; and the use of antibacterial agents.

DIAGNOSIS

The diagnosis of invasive aspergillosis requires the demonstration of hyphae within tissue and the growth of fungus from tissue. The presence of *Aspergillus* on a smear or culture does not necessarily indicate invasive infection, since the organism may colonize some sites. The presence of septate dichotomous branching hyphae is not specific for *Aspergillus* infection, whereas other organisms such as *Fusarium* or *Pseudallescheria* and other molds can have a similar morphologic appearance on histopathologic examination.

Serologic testing for the diagnosis of invasive aspergillosis has not proved useful. Tests for circulating antigen detection still are research tools and are not generally clinically available.

ASPERGILLUS EAR, NOSE, AND THROAT INFECTION

Otitis Externa

Although *Aspergillus* isolated from an ear canal usually represents a saprophyte rather than a pathogen, *Aspergillus* infection of the external ear and auricle (otitis externa) can occur. Indeed, *Aspergillus* is the most common cause of fungal otitis externa (or otomycosis), with *Aspergillus niger* and *A. fumigatus* accounting for 54% and 25%, respectively, of the 171 cases of fungal otitis in one study.[6] *Aspergillus* otitis externa occurs more commonly in warm and humid climates. Patients with open-cavity mastoidectomy and those who wear a hearing aid with an occlusive ear mold are at higher risk.

The symptoms of *Aspergillus* otitis externa are indistinguishable from those of otitis externa due to bacteria. However, pain is often the predominant symptom of otitis externa with a bacterial cause, and pruritus is the predominant symptom in otomycosis.[6] On physical examination, inflammation with hyperemia, edema, and narrowing of the ear canal are invariably seen. In addition, granulomatous myringitis with granulation tissue of the middle ear is often present.[6] A wet, blotting paper–like mass (comprising mycelial mat and exfoliated epithelial scales) can also be visualized. A black mass of moldy growth in the external ear is characteristic of fungal otitis.

Thorough cleaning and débridement are the mainstay of management of *Aspergillus* otitis externa. Antifungal agents have been used in conjunction with surgical débridement. Topical flucytosine, nystatin ointment, clotrimazole or boric acid powder, and clotrimazole (Lotrimin) drops have all been shown to be effective. Systemic antifungal agents are indicated for refractory cases.

Malignant Otitis Externa

Although *Aspergillus* otitis externa is common, malignant otitis externa caused by *Aspergillus* is extremely rare. As of 1994, only 13 cases have been reported in the English literature,[7] and of those, 7 were immunocompromised, 2 had diabetes mellitus, and 2 had chronic ear disease; 2 patients had no underlying diseases. *A. fumigatus* and *A. flavus* were the etiologic agents. The disease is characterized by an insidious progressive course. The signs and symptoms are indistinguishable from those of malignant otitis externa caused by *Pseudomonas aeruginosa*. Since *Aspergillus* can be commensal within the external ear, the diagnosis requires the demonstration of branching septate hyphae within tissue of the external canal in addition to a positive culture for *Aspergillus* species. Multiple histologic sections are often necessary to identify the presence of fungal hyphae.[7] Ther-

apy entails the combination of aggressive surgical débridement and antifungal agents; amphotericin B (with a total dose of 1.5–2 g) has been the standard antifungal agent used. Cure with itraconazole after a course of amphotericin B (total dose of 800–1050 mg) (two cases), or after failure with amphotericin B (one case) has been reported.[7, 8] The role of liposomal amphotericin B formulations is being evaluated and likely will be useful.

Sinusitis

Aspergillus is the most common cause of fungal sinusitis. *Aspergillus* sinusitis can be classified into four different forms: (1) acute fulminant form, frequently involves immunocompromised hosts and is associated with a high mortality; (2) indolent, noninvasive form that, on some occasions, can become locally invasive; (3) aspergilloma (fungus ball); and (4) allergic, which frequently affects atopic patients (Table 25–1).[9] For further details, see Chapter 43.

Tracheobronchitis

Aspergillus tracheobronchitis is a rare clinical entity. In a review of histologically proven cases of *Aspergillus* at the National Institutes of Health between 1953 and 1960, only 5 of the 98 patients had isolated involvement of the bronchial or tracheal wall.[1] Three major patterns of *Aspergillus* tracheobronchitis have been described: allergic, saprophytic, and invasive (Table 25–2).[10, 11]

A compromised host immune system is the most important predisposing factor for *Aspergillus* tracheobronchitis. Although most cases have been reported in patients with malignancy; prolonged neutropenia; or receipt of chemotherapy, corticosteroids, or broad-spectrum antibiotics, there have been increasing reports of *Aspergillus* tracheobronchitis in human immunodeficiency virus (HIV)–infected patients[11, 12] and in patients with lung or heart-lung transplants.[12, 14] In HIV-infected patients, the spectrum of disease ranges from focal mucoid impaction to pseudomembrane formation with mucosal ulceration to tissue invasion. In lung or heart-lung transplant recipients, the infection is mostly confined to the transplanted lung; the common finding is ulcerative tracheobronchitis. Although neutropenia; the administration of corticosteroid or broad spectrum of antibiotics; diabetes mellitus; underlying pulmonary or hepatic diseases; and intravenous

Table 25–1. CHARACTERISTICS, THERAPY, AND OUTCOME ACCORDING TO TYPE OF *ASPERGILLUS* SINUSITUS

Type	Underlying Disease	Onset of Disease	Sinus Involved	Pathologic Characteristics	Therapy	Prognosis
Aspergilloma	None	Chronic	Single	Minimal inflammation	Curettage	Good
Allergic	Atopy or asthma; nasal polyp	Chronic	Multiple	Mucin ball plug	Débridement, ? steroid, ± antifungal*	Good
Indolent	None	Chronic	Single	Chronic inflammation Localized disease	Débridement ± antifungal*	Good
Fulminant	Immunocompromised	Acute	Multiple	Destructive invasive	Débridement and antifungal	Poor

*Antifungal agent is indicated if there is tissue invasion.

Table 25–2. *ASPERGILLUS* **TRACHEOBRONCHITIS**

Classification	Presentation	Bronchoscopic Findings	Pathologic Findings
Allergic			
Allergic bronchopulmonary aspergillosis	Wheezes; cough; production of fungal casts or plugs; patchy lung infiltrates, central bronchiectasis; eosinophilia	Mucoid impaction of bronchi, Charcot-Leyden crystals	Bronchi with mucus, Curschmann's spirals, eosinophils, and inflammatory cells
Bronchocentric granulomatosis	Cough, wheezing, dyspnea, chest pain	Segmental bronchial obstruction by "cheesy" materials	Granulomas with necrotic areas
Saprophytic			
Mucoid impaction	Fever, cough, dyspnea, chest pain, hemoptysis, upper respiratory infection	Mucoid impaction of bronchi, upper lobe involvement	Thin, fibrotic bronchial walls containing atrophied cartilage and mucous glands; eosinophils and chronic inflammatory cells
Obstructive bronchial aspergillosis	Fever, cough, dyspnea, chest pain, hemoptysis, production of fungal casts	Fungal cast impaction of bronchi, lower-lobe involvement	(Not available)
Invasive			
Tracheobronchitis	Wheezes, dyspnea, cough	Mild inflammation of tracheobronchial tree	Acute, chronic inflammation, noninvasive hyphae present
Ulcerative bronchitis	Wheezes, dyspnea, cough	Focal bronchial ulcerations; hyphae invading cartilage and surrounding tissues	Ulcerative necrosis
Pseudomembranous tracheobronchitis	Severe dyspnea	Extensive pseudomembrane, hemorrhagic necrotic mucosa surrounding the trachea and necrotic materials	Extensive necrosis membrane consisting of inflammatory cells and mycelia

Adapted from Kramer MR, Denning DW, Marshall SE, et al: Ulcerative tracheobronchitis after lung transplantation: A new form of invasive aspergillosis. Am Rev Respir Dis 1991; 144: 552–556.

drug use are risk factors for *Aspergillus* infection in HIV-infected patients, the use of immunosuppressive therapy; a decrease in the cough reflex; impairment of mucociliary function; and an immunologic reaction between graft and host in the lung are risk factors in lung transplant recipients.[13]

Local damage to the airway, either from prolonged mechanical ventilatory support, neoplastic infiltration, or severe bacterial tracheobronchitis can also predispose to *Aspergillus* tracheal colonization with subsequent invasion.[14]

The diagnosis of *Aspergillus* tracheobronchitis is easily overlooked. If the diagnosis is not made early, *Aspergillus* tracheobronchitis can progress to local invasion, dissemination, airway obstruction, and death. Thus, mucous plugs or necrotic debris obtained during bronchoscopy should be submitted for histopathologic examination and fungal culture, especially when the patients are immunocompromised. Although itraconazole has been effective in the treatment of *Aspergillus* tracheobronchitis, relapse after the discontinuation of this agent has been documented.[13] Amphotericin B with or without aggressive surgical resection is indicated for refractory cases.

Laryngitis

Aspergillus laryngitis is rare and often occurs in immunocompetent hosts.[15, 16] To date, several cases have been attributed to the occupational exposure to *Aspergillus* that leads to colonization with subsequent invasion.[15, 16] Progressive hoarseness is the most common presenting symptom. Indirect laryngoscopy reveals an ulcerative lesion, the histopathologic examination of which shows superficial involvement of hyphae with mucosal necrosis. Pseudoepitheliomatous hyperplasia simulating squamous cell carcinoma of the larynx has also been reported.[16] *Aspergillus* laryngitis has a good prognosis. Cure has been documented with local excision of the lesion and amphotericin B therapy. Itraconazole would also be expected to be satisfactory for adjunctive medical therapy.

Other Entities

Aspergillus epiglottitis is extremely rare and occurs predominantly in immunocompromised hosts.[1, 17] The clinical picture is indistinguishable from that of bacterially caused epiglottitis; however, a suggestive clue to this diagnosis is the presence of a necrotic epiglottis.[17] Although rare, this diagnosis should be entertained in immunocompromised patients who complain of sore throat or dysphagia, or who present with signs of airway obstruction, especially when these symptoms do not respond to antibacterial agents.

Aspergillus infection of the oropharynx with involvement of the tongue and soft palate has been rarely reported.[1] These lesions were mostly necrotic ulcers that can extend locally to involve the hypopharynx and epiglottis. In one study, all patients with oropharyngeal aspergillosis were symptomatic, with complaints of intense local pain, oral bleeding, and odynophagia.[1]

References

1. Young RC, Bennett JE, Vogel CL, et al.: Aspergillosis: The spectrum of the disease in 98 Patients. Medicine 1970; 49: 147–173.
2. Kwon-Chung KJ, Bennett JE (eds): Aspergillosis. In: Medical Mycology. Malvern, PA, Lea & Febiger, 1992, pp 201–247.
3. Kagen SL: *Aspergillus*: An inhalable contaminant of marijuana. N Engl J Med 1981; 304: 483–484.
4. Schaffner A, Douglas H, Braude A: Selective protection against conidia by mononuclear and against mycelia by polymorphonuclear phagocytes in resistance to *Aspergillus*. J Clin Invest 1982; 69: 617–631.
5. Gerson SL, Talbot GH, Hurwitz S, et al.: Prolonged granulocytopenia: The major risk factor for invasive pulmonary aspergillosis in patients with acute leukemia. Ann Intern Med 1984; 100: 345.
6. Paulose KO, Khalifa SA, Shenoy P, Sharma RK: Mycotic infection of ear (otomycosis): A prospective study. J Laryngol Otol 1989; 103: 30–35.
7. Gordon G, Giddins NA: Invasive otitis externa due to *Aspergillus* species: Case report and review. Clin Infect Dis 1994; 19: 866–870.
8. Phillips P, Bryce G, Shepherd J, Mintz D: Invasive external otitis caused by *Aspergillus*. Rev Infect Dis 1990; 12: 277–281.
9. Blitzer A, Lawson W: Fungal infections of the nose and paranasal sinuses: Part 1. Otolaryngol Clin North Am 1993; 26: 1007–1035.
10. Katzenstein AL, Liebow AA, Friedman PJ: Bronchocentric granulomatosis, mucoid impaction, and hypersensitivity reactions to fungi. Am Rev Respir Dis 1975; 3: 497–537.
11. Denning DW, Follansbee SE, Scolaro M, et al.: Pulmonary aspergillosis in the acquired immunodeficiency syndrome. N Engl J Med 1991; 324: 654–662.
12. Kemper CA, Hostetler JS, Follansbee SE, et al.: Ulcerative and plaque-like tracheobronchitis due to infection with *Aspergillus* in patients with AIDS. Clin Infect Dis 1993; 17: 344–352.
13. Biggs VJ, Dummer S, Holsinger FC, et al.: Successful treatment of invasive bronchial aspergillosis after single-lung transplantation. Clin Infect Dis 1994; 18: 123–124.
14. Clarke A, Skelton J, Fraser RS: Fungal tracheobronchitis: Report of 9 cases and review of literature. Medicine 1991; 70: 1–14.
15. Rao PB: Aspergillosis of larynx. J Laryngol Otol 1974; 88: 377–379.
16. Kheir SM, Flint A, Moss JA: Primary aspergillosis of the larynx simulating carcinoma. Hum Pathol 1983; 14: 184–186.
17. Bolivar R, Gomez LG, Luna M, et al.: *Aspergillus* epiglottitis. Cancer 1983; 51: 367–370.

Alan M. Sugar

CHAPTER TWENTY-SIX

Mucormycosis

▼

Mucormycosis is one of the more uncommon fungal infections, but because the disease is usually rapidly progressive and ultimately fatal without appropriate treatment, it needs to be recognized early so that life-saving therapy can be instituted. In contrast to mycotic diseases such as candidiasis and aspergillosis, which are caused by fungi classified in only one genus (e.g., *Candida* or *Aspergillus*), mucormycosis is caused by any 1 of at least 10 different genera (Table 26–1). Of most importance to the physician, however, is that the disease caused by each of these different fungi is similar and characterized by vascular invasion, tissue infarction, and tissue necrosis.

Mucormycosis has also been known by different names. For example, the designation *phycomycosis* is no longer tenable, since the classification of the organisms has relegated the name Phycomycetes obsolete. Some prefer to refer to mucormycosis as zygomycosis, after the class name of the fungi. However, some members of the Zygomycetes, the Entomophthorales, cause a distinctly different disease, primarily in tropical climates, so the term *zygomycosis* is unnecessarily confusing to those in medicine. Since mucormycosis is widely recognized in clinical medicine as a distinct clinical syndrome, it seems to be the preferable term by which to refer to this disease. A more detailed discussion of the intricacies of taxonomy and nomenclature can be found in other specialty sources.[1, 2]

PATHOGENS

The agents of mucormycosis are ubiquitous in the environment. The fungi grow as molds in the environment and in tissue. Thus, the pathogenic Mucorales do not have a yeast form. The hyphae as seen in tissue are characteristic in appearance and are virtually pathognomonic when visualized under the microscope (Fig. 26–1). Characteristically, the hyphae of the fungi causing mucormycosis are large in diameter (10–20 μm) and nonseptate, with branches occurring at right angles to the main filament (see Fig. 26–1). This contrasts with the thinner, septate hyphae that branch at acute angles of *Aspergillus, Fusarium,* and other molds.

There is nothing distinctive about the fluffy colonies that grow on agar in the microbiology laboratory. Growth is usually rapid, with visible colonies present on agar within 2–5 days. Identification of the genus is usually within the grasp of most microbiology laboratories, but for a species identification or the name of a less common member of the Mucorales, the help of a reference laboratory may be required. The precise identification of these fungi is desirable, since questions of epidemiology and drug susceptibility may hinge on knowing as much as possible about a patient's isolate.

EPIDEMIOLOGY

There is no geographic prevalance of these fungi, and they typically grow well on decaying matter. Spores presumably become airborne and are inhaled into the respiratory tract, especially the nasal sinuses and the lungs. Should spores come to rest on medical devices, such as adhesive tape, the spores can be implanted directly onto the skin with the resulting development of primary cutaneous mucormycosis. Similarly, direct implantation of the spores is well described in cases of trauma, especially motor vehicle accidents. This last scenario is less important for the otolaryngologist, since this type of mucormycosis is typically seen on the torso and extremities. However, with appropriate trauma to the head and neck, mucormycosis in these areas would be expected to occur, and the same principles concerning diagnosis and management would hold as for the disease in other areas of the body.

COLONIZATION, TRANSMISSION, PATHOGENESIS, AND IMMUNITY

People are presumably exposed to the spores of the Mucorales in the air daily. The rarity of the disease attests to the low virulence of this group of microorganisms. Mucormycosis involving the head and neck and lungs is thought to be acquired from the inhalation of spores present in the environment and circulating in the ambient air. Person-to-person spread does not occur, and the disease is not contagious. Thus, no special infection-control precautions need be instituted when caring for patients with mucormycosis.

Once landing in the sinuses of the upper airway or in the pulmonary alveoli, the spores must be able to germinate, despite encountering cell-mediated and humoral host defenses. In the normal animal, inoculation with *Rhizopus* spores into the lungs elicits no discernible illness.[3] Examination of the lungs of these animals reveals ungerminated

Table 26–1. MUCORMYCOSIS—ETIOLOGIC AGENTS

Absidia	*Mortierella*
Mucor	*Saksenaea*
Rhizomucor	*Apophysomyces*
Cunninghamella	*Cokeromyces*

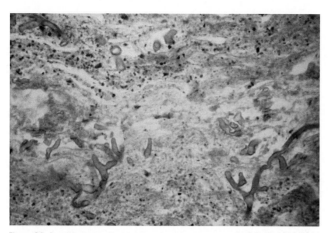

Figure 26–1. Histologic picture of mucormycosis. Nonseptate hyphae characterize mucormycosis. Biopsy may be the best means to make the diagnosis of patients with invasive mucormycosis.

spores.[4–6] Once removed from the lungs, however, these spores are capable of germination and the formation of viable hyphae. Thus, the intact animal possesses a growth-inhibitory mechanism but is apparently unable to actually kill the spore form of the fungus. If these same *Rhizopus*-inoculated animals are rendered diabetic, with streptozotocin, for example, the spores begin to germinate within the lungs and the animals develop fatal mucormycosis. The basic mechanisms underlying this reversal of normal host defenses are not well understood. It is clear that hyperglycemia or acidosis per se is not sufficient to impair the innate host defense mechanisms. In vitro incubation of pulmonary alveolar macrophages in acidic and/or hyperglycemic conditions is not sufficient in abrogating inherent macrophage fungistatic activity.[6, 7]

Recently, laboratory evidence for the role of iron in the pathogenesis of mucormycosis has been delineated, in response to the observation that there is an increased frequency of mucormycosis in patients who are receiving deferoxamine.[8] In the laboratory, in the presence of serum and iron-loaded deferoxamine (feroxamine), the growth of *Rhizopus* is enhanced more than that of *Aspergillus* or *Candida*.[8] It is quite remarkable that the normal growth-inhibitory effect of serum is abrogated by iron and deferoxamine. Presumably, the deferoxamine is functioning as a siderophore, making the iron available to the fungus and thus encouraging its growth.

Although much remains to be learned concerning the mechanisms of host defenses against the fungi causing mucormycosis, it is apparent that neutrophils are an important line of defense and that other innate defenses such as natural killer cells and circulating humoral factors may play some role. The paucity of cases of mucormycosis in acquired immunodeficiency disease (AIDS)[9, 10] reflects the relative roles of neutrophils compared with lymphocytes and macrophages in preventing the growth of the Mucorales in the human body.

PATHOGEN IN EAR, NOSE, AND THROAT

Mucormycosis is typically classified into six different syndromes, all of which share the same basic pathologic pro-

cesses. Rhinocerebral mucormycosis is perhaps the most common manifestation and certainly the most important for the otolaryngologist. Central nervous system, pulmonary, gastrointestinal, and cutaneous are other well-defined presentations of mucormycosis. The sixth grouping is that of miscellaneous cases, involving isolated involvement of certain target organs, such as trachea, kidney, heart, or bone (Fig. 26–2).[11–16]

Occasionally, mucormycosis can present as an isolated lesion of the central nervous system, with the typical appearance and behavior of a brain abscess.[17] Despite appropriate evaluation, the sinuses and the remainder of the respiratory tract are normal, without evidence of signs of infection. Most of these patients are intravenous drug users. Presumably, fungus-contaminated drug is injected into the blood stream and the organism comes to rest in the brain.

LABORATORY DIAGNOSIS

Careful examination of tissue obtained by biopsy is the key to success in making the correct diagnosis. Since other illnesses and other fungi can produce symptoms and signs compatible with mucormycosis, presumptive identification of the fungus by microscopic examination of tissue or by identifying the organism once a mold grows in the microbiology laboratory from suitably obtained specimens is critical to proper management of the patient. Simple swabs of an abnormal area are not sufficient to make a definitive diagnosis, since fungi can typically grow on mucosal surfaces without causing disease. The demonstration of tissue invasion by hyphae is the only sure diagnostic method.

Although hyphae can be seen on routine hematoxylin and eosin stained tissue sections, special stains with periodic acid–Schiff (PAS) or Gomori methenamine silver (GMS) are useful adjunctive tools. PAS stains the fungus red, and GMS or other silver staining methods stain the organism black, against a greenish background. Such demonstration of tissue invasion by hyphae establishes the diagnosis of mucormycosis.

The hyphae of the Mucorales are often seen penetrating

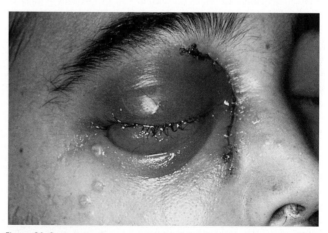

Figure 26–2. Patient demonstrates orbital involvement by mucor. Eyelid edema erythema and paralysis are the hallmarks. The incision between the nose and eye indicates recent surgery.

into blood vessels, thus explaining the clinical manifestations of infarction and necrosis of involved tissue. The inflammatory response typically consists of infiltration with neutrophils and a generalized vasculitis involving both arteries and veins. Tissue obtained from patients with more chronic disease often has a mononuclear cellular infiltrate, and occasional giant cells may be seen.

TREATMENT

The most successful outcomes result from the combination of early diagnosis, correction of underlying predisposing causes, aggressive surgical débridement, and appropriate antifungal therapy. Once the diagnosis is made, a multidisciplinary approach is critical to ensure the best result. Surgical removal of dead and dying tissue is critical. A common strategy of piecemeal, daily débridement of the infected area is not recommended, since the end result is often as disfiguring, or more so, than an initial large-scale débridement. Because of the location of vital structures including major blood vessels, nerves, and the brain, such surgery is often fraught with technical difficulties, but infarcted and devitalized tissue must be removed. In general, patients in whom less was done in the operating room have a poorer prognosis than patients who receive aggressive surgical débridement during the initial stages of treatment (Figs. 26–3 and 26–4).

Medical therapy is less problematic, since only amphotericin B has been shown to be effective in treating mucormycosis. The Mucorales are relatively more resistant to amphotericin B, so higher doses than usual need to be employed, at least in the earliest stages of therapy. Thus amphotericin B 1–1.5 mg/kg/day should be administered to patients very quickly once the decision is made to start such therapy. The patient should be sodium-replete and well hydrated. Several good sources concerning the administration of amphotericin B are in the recent medical literature.[18–20]

The duration of therapy has to be based on how the infection is responding to treatment, as well as how severe the toxicity of amphotericin B is. At doses of less than 2–3 g of amphotericin B, most of the renal toxicity is reversible,

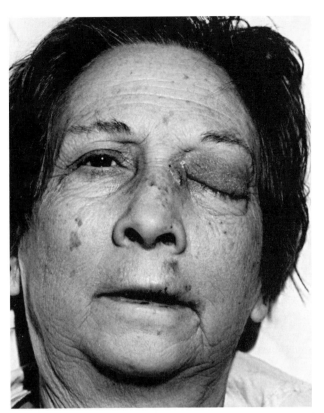

Figure 26–4. Patient underwent surgery to remove invasive mucormycosis involving the ethmoid sinus. Paralysis of the eyelid and residual discoloration of the surrounding skin are apparent.

but as higher doses are administered, some degree of permanent renal impairment should be expected. In an attempt to decrease the acute and chronic side effects of amphotericin B, several different liposomal formulations of amphotericin B (amphotericin B lipid complex [ABLC], unilamellar amphotericin B, [AmBisome], amphotericin B colloidal dispersion [ABCD]) have been introduced into clinical study.[21–23] The toxicity of these preparations is thought to be less than those associated with the usual formulation of amphotericin B, but the efficacy of these preparations, especially compared with that of amphotericin B, is not yet clear. Anecdotal reports do suggest that some patients who have not responded to amphotericin B have responded to one or another liposomal amphotericin B therapies.[22, 24] Given the uncontrolled nature of these observations, it is not clear how to assess the relative roles of amphotericin B and liposomal amphotericins. Consultation with an infectious disease physician familiar with mucormycosis and the treatment options is encouraged.

Hyperbaric oxygen has been used with some success in the treatment of the various mucormycosis syndromes.[25–28] Given the problems with reporting bias and the difficulties in performing appropriately controlled clinical trials, it is difficult to completely evaluate the role of this adjunctive measure in the treatment of patients with mucormycosis. Nevertheless, if facilities for the administration of hyperbaric oxygen are available and there are no contraindications to its use, the use of hyperbaric oxygen can be considered on a case-by-case basis.

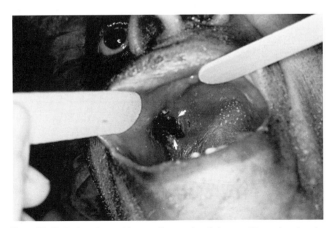

Figure 26–3. Patient has evidence of necrosis of the maxillary alveolus due to invasive mucormycosis.

Presently, there are no methods for the prevention of mucormycosis. Since the spores are ubiquitous and easily airborne, there seems to be little that can be done to prevent exposure to these organisms. On the other hand, supportive care during periods of intense immunosuppression, such as chemotherapy for malignancies, and tight control of blood sugar levels in diabetic patients, should result in minimizing the risk of invasive mucormycosis.

References

1. Kwon-Chung KJ, Bennett JE: Medical Mycology. Philadelphia: Lea & Febiger, 1992.
2. Sugar AM: Agents of mucormycosis and related species. In: Mandell GL, Bennett JE, Dolin R (eds): Principles and Practice of Infectious Diseases, 4th ed. New York: Churchill Livingstone, 1995, pp 2311–2321.
3. Waldorf AR, Halde C, Vedros NA: Murine model of pulmonary mucormycosis in cortisone treated mice. Sabouraudia 1982; 20: 217–224.
4. Schaffner A, Davis CE, Schaffner T, et al.: In vitro susceptibility of fungi to killing by neutrophil granulocytes discriminates between primary pathogenicity and opportunism. J Clin Invest 1986; 78: 511–524.
5. Waldorf AR, Peter L, Polak AM: Mucormycotic infection in mice following prolonged incubation of spores in vivo and the role of spore agglutinating antibodies on spore germination. Sabouraudia 1984; 22: 101–108.
6. Waldorf AR, Ruderman N, Diamond RD: Specific susceptibility to mucormycosis in murine diabetes and bronchoalveolar macrophage defense against *Rhizopus*. J Clin Invest 1984; 74: 150–160.
7. Waldorf AR, Levitz SM, Diamond RD: In vivo bronchoalveolar macrophage defense *Rhizopus oryzae* and *Aspergillus fumigatus*. J Infect Dis 1984; 150: 752–760.
8. Boelaert JR, de Locht M, Van Custem J, et al.: Mucormycosis during deferoxamine therapy is a siderophore-mediated infection. In vitro and in vivo animal studies. J Clin Invest 1993; 91: 1979–1986.
9. Blatt SP, Lucey DR, DeHoff D, Zellmer RB: Rhinocerebral zygomycosis in a patient with AIDS. J Infect Dis 1991; 164: 215–216.
10. Sanchez MR, Pongewilson I, Moy JA, et al.: Zygomycosis and HIV infection. J Am Acad Dermatol 1994; 30(suppl 5, pt 2): 904–908.
11. Brown OE, Finn R: Mucormycosis of the mandible. J Oral Maxillofac Surg 1984; 44: 132–136.
12. Clarke A, Skelton J, Fraser RS: Fungal tracheobronchitis. Report of 9 cases and review of the literature. Medicine 1991; 70: 1–14.
13. Davila R, Moser SA, Grosso LE: Renal mucormycosis: A case report and review of the literature. J Urol 1991; 145: 1242–1244.
14. Eisenberg L, Wood T, Boles R: Mucormycosis. Laryngoscope 1977; 87: 347–356.
15. Gussen R, Canalis RF: Mucormycosis of the temporal bone. Ann Otol Rhinol Laryngol 1982; 91: 27–32.
16. Schwartz JRL, Nagle NG, Elkins RC, et al.: Mucormycosis of the trachea. An unusual cause of acute upper airway obstruction. Chest 1982; 81: 653–654.
17. Siddiqi SU, Freedman JD: Isolated central nervous system mucormycosis. South Med J 1994; 87: 997–1000.
18. Bennett JE: Treatment of cryptococcal, candidal and coccidioidal meningitis. In: Remington JS, Swartz MN (eds): Current Clinical Topics in Infectious Diseases, vol 2. New York: McGraw-Hill Book Co, 1980, pp 54–67.
19. Gallis HA, Drew RH, Pickard WW: Amphotericin B: 30 years of clinical experience. Rev Infect Dis 1990; 12: 308–329.
20. Khoo SH, Bond J, Denning DW: Administering amphotericin B–A practical approach. J Antimicrob Chemother 1994; 33: 203–213.
21. Demarie S, Janknegt R, Bakkerwoudenberg IAJM: Clinical use of liposomal and lipid-complexed amphotericin B. J Antimicrob Chemother 1994; 33: 907–916.
22. Fisher EW, Toma A, Fisher PH, Cheeseman AD: Rhinocerebral mucormycosis: Use of liposomal amphotericin B. J Laryngol Otol 1991; 105: 575–577.
23. Leake HA, Appleyard MN, Hartley JPR: Successful treatment of resistant crytococcal meningitis with amphotericin B lipid emulsion after nephrotoxicity with conventional intravenous amphotericin B. J Infect 1994; 28: 319–322.
24. Lim KKT, Potts MJ, Warnock DW, et al.: Another case report of rhinocerebral mucormycosis treated with liposomal amphotericin B. Clinical Infect Dis 1994; 18: 653–654.
25. De la Paz MA, Patrinely MA, Marines HM, et al.: Adjunctive hyperbaric oxygen in the treatment of bilateral cerebro-rhino-orbital mucormycosis. Am J Ophthalmol 1992; 114: 208–211.
26. Ferguson BJ, Mitchell TG, Moon R, et al.: Adjunctive hyperbaric oxygen for treatment of rhinocerebral mucormycosis. Rev Infect Dis 1988; 10: 551–559.
27. Fisher EW, Toma A, Fisher PH, Chessman AD: Rhinocerebral mucormycosis: Use of liposomal amphotericin B. J Laryngol Otol 1991; 105: 575–577.
28. Munckhof W, Jones R, Tosolini FA, et al.: Cure of *Rhizopus* sinusitis in a liver transplant recipient with liposomal amphotericin B. Clin Infect Dis 1993; 16: 183.

Paul L. Williams

CHAPTER TWENTY-SEVEN

Coccidioidomycosis

▼

HISTORY

Posada, an Argentine pathologist, was the first to describe disseminated coccidioidomycosis in 1894. The etiologic agent *Coccidioides immitis* was first identified at Stanford by Rixford and Gilchrist in 1896 but was originally thought to be a protozoan. The genus *Coccidioides* was so named because of its resemblance to the protozoan *Coccidia*. *Immitis* means "not mild" in Latin. *C. immitis* was characterized as a fungus in 1900 by Ophüls and Moffitt. Ophüls was successful in delineating its life cycle and identified the lung as the portal of entry for infection. Although coccidioidomycosis was originally thought to be a fatal infection, by the mid 1930s, Dickson and Gifford were able to demonstrate that the usual presentation was a self-limited pulmonary infection. They coined the term valley fever, which referred to the central valley of California where most infections appeared to occur. Later Smith went on to characterize disseminated coccidioidomycosis and pointed out the increased risk of disseminated disease developing in nonwhites, particularly blacks and Filipinos. He was responsible for developing the first useful skin test reagent (coccidioidin) and the first useful serologic test for coccidioidomycosis using the complement-fixation technique.[1, 2]

DESCRIPTION OF THE PATHOGEN

C. immitis lives in the soil as a mold characterized by elongated structures called hyphae that contain septated bodies called arthroconidia, which resemble barrels. Arthroconidia (also called arthrospores) are approximately 5 μm in diameter and can be easily disarticulated from each other and become aerosolized. Intertwined branching hyphae are referred to as mycelium, and this is how the fungus appears in culture media. Arthrospores become naturally aerosolized by wind currents or mechanically aerosolized by means of machinery engaged in excavation or agricultural pursuits. Once arthrospores are inhaled into the lungs, a biologic transformation occurs (hence the term dimorphic) in which the arthroconidia "round up" into structures termed spherules. Immature spherules are 10 μm in diameter. They divide internally by mitotic division, producing endospores, which are between 2 and 5 μm in diameter. Mature spherules containing hundreds of endospores can reach 80–100 μm in diameter. When they mature sufficiently, they rupture, releasing hundreds of endospores into surrounding tissues. Each endospore can, in turn, become an individual spherule, again capable of maturing as described above. This then represents a tremendous multiplication potential of the organism, stress-

ing the reserves of even the most resilient immune response. When cultured from sputum or other infected biologic tissues or secretions at 25 °C, the organisms in this spherule-endospore phase transform back into the mycelial phase within 3–7 days (Fig. 27–1). Typical mycelia on culture media appear white to whitish-gray and "membranous," reflecting the mycelium phase. Colonies later develop aerial structures or hyphae that can be easily identified microscopically. These structures are extremely infectious, and it is necessary to advise microbiology personnel that valley fever is being considered, so that appropriate protection can be enforced using protected biohazard hoods.[2–4]

ECOLOGY AND EPIDEMIOLOGY

C. immitis is a fungus endemic to several Central and South American countries in addition to the southwestern portion of the United States, in regions termed the lower Sonoran life zone (Fig. 27–2). This arid environment is characterized by sandy, alkaline soil and sporadic rainfall generally limited to winter and early spring that enhances the growth of the fungus in the soil. In the United States, *C. immitis* is concentrated in the southern San Joaquin Valley (central valley) of California, notably in Kern and Tulare counties. The organism is spottily distributed in the endemic area and lives in an altitude range of from sea level to 3000 feet. The organism is found most abundantly 1 to 2 in. under the soil surface.[5]

It has been estimated that 100,000 cases of coccidioidomycosis occur annually in the United States.[6] The number of cases deriving from Mexico and Central and South America is unknown. Most cases occur during the summertime or early fall, when the soil is maximally dry, allowing easy disruption and aerosolization of the soil and resultant disarticulation of arthroconidia. Vocational and advocational pursuits associated with soil disruption set the stage for an increased risk of acquisition. However, a history of unusual dust exposure is not always obtained, and certainly simply residing in the endemic area constitutes a risk factor.[5] The skin test conversation rate approximates 1.5%–4% per year in the endemic area as documented by skin test conversation test studies in the 1960s and 1970s.[7, 8] Dust storms appear to represent a particular risk to immunologically naive individuals, and one of the great epidemics of coccidioidomycosis in this century was due to a dust storm that occurred in the southern San Joaquin Valley in 1977. This dust storm was associated with a 20-fold increase in the number of cases ordinarily reported.[9] A recent earthquake in the Los Angeles area (Northridge, California) was associated with

Saprobic phase   Parasitic phase

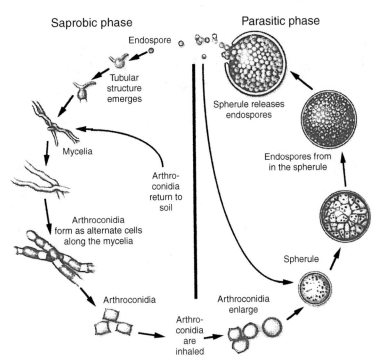

Figure 27–1. The life cycle of *C. immitis*. (Courtesy of H. B. Levine, Ph.D.)

an outbreak of coccidioidomycosis associated with dust generated from the earthquake.[10] Another epidemic of coccidioidomycosis in this century occurred from 1991 to 1994 in the central valley of California and accounted for over 10,000 reported cases.[11] In comparison, 1500 cases would ordinarily have occurred. This epidemic was thought to be due to an increase in rain in the winter, which enhanced the growth of the fungus in the soil. Other contributory factors included a rapid influx of immunologically naive immigrants to the area and numerous construction projects associated with such growth. The cost of caring for individuals so infected in Kern County alone approximated $50 million.[13]

Coccidioidomycosis is a classic example of a "traveler's disease," and there have been many cases reported of individuals sojourning briefly in the endemic area, returning to

their native states or countries, and 2–3 weeks later developing symptomatic pulmonary coccidioidomycosis.[12]

ACQUISITION AND GENERAL NATURE OF INFECTION IN THE HUMAN HOST

Coccidioidomycosis is not a contagious disease and is almost always acquired from the inadvertent inhalation of invisible arthroconidia from contaminated dust. Ten or fewer arthroconidia may be all that are necessary to be inhaled in order to establish pulmonary infection.[5] Sixty percent of infections are asymptomatic, recognizable only by skin testing or serologic studies. Forty percent of infections are symptomatic and are generally associated with pulmonary symptoms that can include fever, night sweats, profound fatigue, cough, exertional dyspnea, and occasional hemoptysis or pleurisy. Most patients experience these symptoms for 3 to 6 weeks and recover without apparent ill effects, becoming "naturally immunized." Roentgenographic studies on these individuals may demonstrate unilateral or bilateral pulmonary infiltrates, hilar adenopathy, and nodules that may later cavitate and grow, posing a threat of pyopneumothorax.[14] Rarely, acute primary disease can be overwhelming and present with life-threatening miliary pneumonia and sepsis syndrome.[15, 16]

Chronic pulmonary coccidioidomycosis can develop in a minority of patients and be roentgenographically indistinguishable from tuberculosis.[17]

Disseminated coccidioidomycosis occurs when spherules or endospores pass from the lung hematogenously to involve virtually any body organ. Disseminated coccidioidomycosis is usually symptomatic, but occasionally it can be silent, particularly when it involves the liver, spleen, kidney, or eye. There have been a few reported cases of cardiac involvement and gastrointestinal tract involvement.[2, 18] Dis-

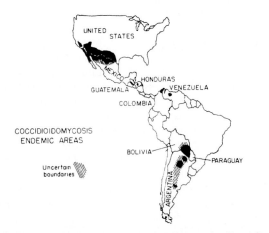

Figure 27–2. The endemic regions of coccidioidomycosis. (From Stevens DA (ed): Coccidioidomycosis, A Text. New York: Plenum Book Company, 1980.)

semination is thought to occur in approximately 1 of 100 cases of infection in whites and as often as 1 in 10 in blacks and perhaps more often in Filipinos,[5] presumably secondary to factors having to do with a selective immunologic incompetency termed *selective anergy.*[19] Recent epidemiologic studies associated with the 1991–1994 epidemic in California indicate that there is a 5% overall risk of dissemination.[10] Other associations characterized by an increased risk of potentially fatal primary or disseminated coccidioidomycosis include patients with acquired immunodeficiency syndrome; individuals receiving cytotoxic or immunosuppressive therapy for neoplastic and immunologically mediated disorders; pregnant women, particularly in the final trimester of pregnancy; and young children or infants. Males are also more likely to disseminate than are females.[2, 5, 7]

Rarely, primary cutaneous disease can occur because of direct inoculation of *C. immitis* into the skin by direct puncture from contaminated objects (i.e., infected thorns or contaminated needles).[2] Sexual transmission has been suggested in individuals with genitourinary dissemination, but additional confirmatory studies will be necessary before this potential risk can be clarified.[20] Nosocomial transmission has occurred when unsuspecting orthopedic personnel opened an infected cast in a patient having undergone surgery for bone and joint coccidioidomycosis.[21]

PATHOLOGY

During the initial phase of tissue infection, the body's immunologic response involves the recruitment of polymorphonuclear cells and macrophages. Over days to weeks, there gradually develops a mononuclear migration (T lymphocytes and macrophages) to the site of infection, supplanting the polymorphonuclear response and thereby producing granulomatous inflammation often with multinucleated giant cells (Fig. 27–3). Later, central necrosis (caseation necrosis) and fibrotic reactions occur. Spherules are often found in the center of these granulomatous reactions. The histopathologic identification of spherules within biologic tissue is pathognomonic of active infection and never represents contamination. Organisms that can be demonstrated by routine hema-

toxylin and eosin stain are often better appreciated with the use of Gomori methenamine silver stain, which demonstrates the organism as black contrasting with a green background. The identification of *C. immitis* can often be enhanced by cytocentrifugation or digestion centrifugation techniques, using fluorescent antibody techniques or fluorescent dye (Calcofluor).[2, 22, 23]

IMMUNOLOGIC RESPONSE TO *C. IMMITIS* INFECTION

Although leukocyte activation and migration to the site of *C. immitis* infection is well documented, the overall immunologic impact of this response does not appear to be pivotal to the control of infection. The principal controlling arm of the immune response in humans is the cellular immune response. This is characterized by the activation and recruitment of T lymphocytes, particularly those associated with the type I CD4 (helper T cell) characteristic.[24–27] A favorable T-cell response is verifiable by the findings of a positive skin test to coccidioidal antigen (usual test strength coccidioidin [Spherulin]). A positive skin test generally means immunologic competency. Conversely, a depressed or absent response in the setting of disseminated coccidioidomycosis denotes a poor prognosis for recovery, and generally about 60% of patients with disseminated coccidioidomycosis have a negative skin test reaction. Many times these individuals demonstrate a *selective anergic state,* whereby they are skin test–negative to coccidioidal antigen but retain delayed dermal hypersensitivity to other recall antigens. This dichotomy may be explained by an *antigen excess* situation in which there is a large fungal "load" involved in the infectious process in addition to inhibitory factors produced by the fungus itself, which can impair cellular immunity.

DIAGNOSIS

The establishment of *C. immitis* as the etiologic agent involved in infection is accomplished by histopathologic iden-

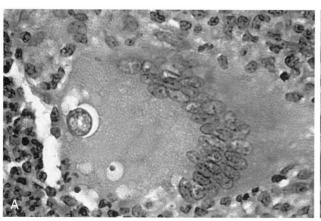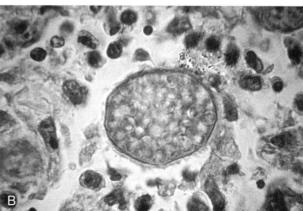

Figure 27–3. *A*, The histopathologic appearance of *C. immitis* in a skin biopsy from a lesion involving the external ear. ×400 hematoxylin and eosin stain. Multinucleated giant cell with an engulfed coccidioidal spherule; surrounding mononuclear and polymorphonuclear response. *B*, ×1000 Giemsa's stain demonstrating a mature coccidioidal spherule containing endospores from a skin biopsy with surrounding mononuclear inflammation.

tification or culture of the organism in biologic tissues or secretions.

The culture of *C. immitis* from biologic tissues or fluids is accomplished generally quite easily on routine bacteriologic media or mycologic media such as Sabouraud's medium at 35–37 °C. Growth can be enhanced in a 5%–10% CO_2 environment. *C. immitis* resistance to cycloheximide may be useful in differentiating this fungus from other fungi that can appear macroscopically similar on culture media. Growth usually occurs within 3–5 days, and colonies may appear white to gray and appear membranous. Definitive microbiologic identification cannot be made by microscopic identification of mycelium on culture plates alone. Definitive identification requires either the identification of the parasitic form by inoculation of colonies into animals or by using special tests that measure extracellular coccidioidal antigens produced by the growing fungus on culture media (DNA probe test).[23]

Serologic diagnosis can be accomplished by the identification of immunoglobulin M (IgM) antibodies, which are generally produced in the first 2–4 weeks of acute infection or by the subsequent identification of IgG antibodies, which are generally produced 4–6 weeks after initial infection and may last for months even in self-limited infections. IgM antibody usually fades by 2–6 months in self-limited infection but in chronic infections may persist indefinitely along with an IgG antibody. In progressive disseminated coccidioidomycosis, one sees increasing production of IgG antibody, resulting in high titers. Conversely, during clinical improvement, falling IgG antibody levels are generally observed (Fig. 27–4). Falsely positive serologic tests for coccidioidomycosis are rare.

The tube precipitin assay is both sensitive and reasonably specific for detecting IgM. IgM can also be detected in a very sensitive and specific manner using an immunodiffusion test, and sensitivity can be further enhanced by concentration of serum. The most useful and reliable test for the detection of IgG antibody is the complement fixation test, which has the advantage of excellent sensitivity and specificity but also provides prognostic information. A complement fixation titer of greater than 1:4 reflects recent or current infection, whereas titers in excess of 1:16 are consistent with disseminated disease. An immunodiffusion test for IgG antibody is available and is both sensitive and specific but appears not to measure the exact antibody that is measured by the complement fixation testing and therefore does not generally have the same useful prognostic implications.[8] A number of antigen detection systems are currently under investigation but are not available clinically.

EXTRAPULMONARY DISSEMINATED COCCIDIOIDOMYCOSIS

The most common sites of disseminated coccidioidomycosis include skin and soft tissue, bone and joint, and meninges.[2, 7, 18, 28] Very commonly multiple organs are involved concomitantly, and the investigating physician must evaluate for other sites of involvement at the time of initial diagnosis of disseminated coccidioidomycosis at any site.

C. IMMITIS INFECTION OF THE TISSUES OF THE HEAD AND NECK

Frauenfelder and Schwartz reported that *C. immitis* infection of the soft tissues of the head and neck occurred in 7% of 240 patients with disseminated coccidioidomycosis in a study done at the University of Arizona.[29] These authors did not specify whether these lesions were cutaneous or subcutaneous, or represented adenitis. Eight additional patients had evidence of osteomyelitis with lytic destruction of bone involving the parietal, maxillary, and mandibular bones. These areas of bone involvement were contiguous oftentimes to areas of soft tissue involvement (abscesses, sinus tracts, etc.). Only one of their patients had soft tissue involvement alone. Of the 17 patients reported to have head and neck involvement, 16 were nonwhite.

Coccidioidal infections of the tissues of the upper airway including larynx and trachea have been reported but appear relatively uncommon. When they occur, these infections can be life-threatening, leading to airway compromise.

Deep soft tissue abscesses of the throat and pharynx with or without lymphadenitis have also been reported but appear relatively uncommon. Often there is a concomitant osteomyelitis of the cervical vertebral bodies with the development of prevertebral and posterior pharyngeal abscesses. These can grow, enlarge, and subsequently compromise either the upper airway or the gastrointestinal tract.

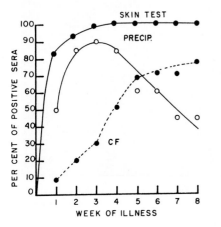
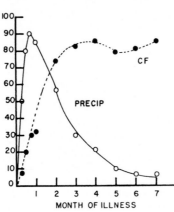

Figure 27–4. Temporal sequence of precipitin antibody (predominantly IgM antibody) and complement fixation antibody (predominantly IgG antibody) and skin test reactivity in patients with primary nondisseminated coccidioidomycosis. (From Stevens DA [ed]: Coccidioidomycosis, A text. New York: Plenum Book Company, 1980, p 106.)

There are no published data on the frequency of lymphadenitis of the head or neck, but it is the author's impression that cervical adenitis is the most common manifestation of disseminated coccidioidomycosis involving the head and neck. Supraclavicular coccidioidal adenitis often represents the initial manifestation of dissemination from the original pulmonary site of infection. Unfortunately, in many reports in the literature, the descriptions of the nature of subcutaneous abscesses or masses involving the head and the neck are merely descriptive and lack histopathologic analysis.

A knowledge of travel history to the endemic area is critical for the inclusion of disseminated coccidioidomycosis within the differential diagnosis of patients presenting with inflammatory processes involving the head and neck. The simple question "Where have you been in the last year?" may be the most important question asked by the consulting ear, nose, and throat specialist. The second most important question would be "Have you ever had a serious lung infection or other serious infections including fungal infections?" Obviously a history of past pulmonary coccidioidomycosis or previous disseminated coccidioidomycosis to another body site would be a significant clue directing further investigation.

Osteomyelitis

Osteomyelitis is one of the most common forms of disseminated coccidioidomycosis, and *C. immitis* can infect multiple bone sites concomitantly (40% of the cases). The vertebral column and the skull appear to be particularly common sites of involvement.[29] The interested reader is referred to several excellent reviews on this subject.[30, 31] Roentgenographically, these lesions appear lytic and well demarcated, having the appearance of either a uniloculated or a multiloculated abscess. Periosteal new bone formation is uncommon. Sclerosis with cortical thickening appears to be a late finding. Definitive diagnosis requires a bone biopsy. The presumptive diagnosis when bone biopsy is not feasible is suggested by a positive coccidioidal serologic response and/or evidence of disseminated disease to another body organ. Although vertebral lesions occur more commonly in the thoracic and lumbar regions of the spine, cervical involvement leading to spine destabilization and occasionally to prevertebral abscesses has been reported. Oftentimes, multiple sites of spine involvement are present concomitantly. The intervertebral disc is generally spared. Sinus tracts are common and are derived from deep bone involvement and/or prevertebral abscesses. Occasionally such areas of involvement can compromise the upper airway. Winter and colleagues reported 12 cases of disseminated coccidioidomycosis involving the spine, including 4 patients with cervical spine involvement.[32] All these patients were nonwhite and all were male. All received intravenous amphotericin B. Two of the four underwent fusion. Two underwent débridement with irrigation. Three survived. These authors recommend the following conditions under which surgical intervention including incision and drainage and evacuation of all necrotic tissue is necessary:

1. All patients with clinical or roentgenographic evidence

suggesting the presence of a large coccidioidal abscess contiguous with the site of spinal involvement that compromises either the upper airway or gastrointestinal tract or causes progressive local or systemic symptoms

2. All patients with impending instability of the spine (fusion necessary also)

Henley-Cohn and colleagues reported four patients with acute airway obstruction developing secondary to deep neck coccidioidal abscesses contiguous with cervical vertebral osteomyelitis.[33] It is noteworthy that the two patients who underwent complete débridement responded best to therapy. The importance of complete débridement has been stressed by Winter and colleagues.[32] Discitis and gibbous deformity of the spine resembling tuberculosis have been uncommonly reported (McGahan and colleagues).[34]

Cutaneous Involvement

A complete review of cutaneous disseminated coccidioidomycosis is beyond the scope of this chapter. Jacobs has tabulated the various appearances of disseminated cutaneous coccidioidomycosis (Table 27–1).[35] A representative example of how disseminated coccidioidomycosis can appear is shown in Figure 27–5. Disseminated cutaneous coccidioidomycosis requires therapeutic intervention even though the extent of cutaneous involvement may be minimal, as there may be other occult sites of disseminated disease present concomitantly.

Coccidioidal Involvement of the Soft Tissues of the Head and Neck (Subcutaneous Involvement Including Adenitis)

Dissemination to "soft tissues" is common.[12] Forbus has also described subcutaneous coccidioidal tissue involvement as being common in cases of disseminated disease and describes the gross appearance to be that of a suppurative granulomatous mass with associated regional inflammation often resulting in draining sinus tracts commonly associated with deeper areas of involvement such as osteomyelitis (Fig. 27–6).[28] Kafka and Catanzaro have reviewed the pediatric literature on disseminated coccidioidomycosis and reported 14 cases of extrapulmonary disseminated disease.[36] Six of

Table 27–1. LESIONS OF SECONDARY (DISSEMINATED) CUTANEOUS COCCIDIOIDOMYCOSIS

I. Papules	III. Granulomatous lesions
A. Solitary	A. Nodular
B. Multiple	B. Fungating
1. Grouped	C. Ulcerative
a. Plaquelike	D. Scarring
b. Verrucous	IV. Subcutaneous abscesses
2. Miliary	A. Ulcerating
II. Pustules	B. Sinusal
A. Furuncular	
B. Vegetating	

From Jacobs PH: Cutaneous coccidioidomycosis. In: Stevens DA (ed): Coccidioidomycosis, A Text. New York: Plenum Book Company, 1980, p 215.

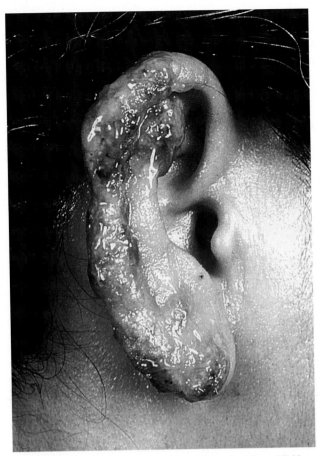

Figure 27–5. Filipino female with documented disseminated coccidioidomycosis involving the external ear.

their patients presented with soft tissue abscesses involving the head, face, or neck. In three instances, adjacent areas of bone involvement were roentgenographically verified. One patient presented with bilateral cervical adenitis. All patients were nonwhite. These authors suggest that neck abscesses probably represented coccidioidal adenitis in that the location of the subcutaneous abscess was consistent with such an association. Unfortunately, no histopathologic studies were performed to verify this. Sinus tract formation was often associated with subcutaneous abscesses or masses, and oftentimes there appeared to be an area of osteomyelitis nearby. Four of the patients received intravenous amphotericin B, and all responded. One patient with axillary and cervical adenitis was unable to tolerate amphotericin B but nonetheless spontaneously improved. This patient did demonstrate a positive skin test reaction to coccidioidal antigen. The majority of patients presented with disseminated disease, which occurred within 6 months of primary pulmonary infection. However, these authors point out that as long as 2–5 years can elapse from the time of initial pulmonary involvement to the time of dissemination. They point out that subcutaneous abscesses can occur anywhere in the body and can appear in solitary fashion or can present with multiple areas of involvement. Kafka and Catanzaro underscore the importance of surgical débridement of both bone and subcutaneous tissues for best therapeutic results.

DeClercq and Chole describe a 62-year-old man with

a large, painful coccidioidal retropharyngeal abscess with evidence of concomitant C3 osteomyelitis.[37] Surgical treatment involved placement of a tracheostomy and transoral aspiration of 30 cc of purulent material and subsequent débridement of the C3 vertebral body and C2–C4 disc spaces with ultimate fusion of C2–C4.

Laryngeal and Tracheal Involvement

Coccidioidal involvement of the larynx and trachea is less common than cutaneous and subcutaneous sites of infection and, when present, is commonly associated with respiratory compromise (Table 27–2). Of the 14 patients described, 9 had biopsy-proven areas of tracheal or laryngeal disseminated coccidioidomycosis. In five patients, the diagnosis was inferred on the basis of other data (shown). The ages of the patients ranged from 4½ months to 45 years. The majority (9) were male. Nonwhites outnumbered whites (7 versus 3). The majority of the patients (6) presented with acute respiratory embarrassment of less than 1 month's duration, whereas in four instances symptoms were of greater than 1 month's duration. When specified, 30% of the patients had evidence of cervical adenitis. Of 12 patients for whom data were provided, 5 had other sites of disseminated disease, including cervical osteomyelitis in 2 instances. Concomitant pulmonary involvement was present in the majority of patients (9) and provided a clue as to the diagnosis. The majority of patients presented with acute airway compromise and required either a tracheostomy or intubation. Skin test data were provided in only nine instances, and in four patients a positive coccidioidal skin test was documented. In nine instances in which antifungal treatment was given, a favorable outcome was documented in seven patients, with two patients "status pending." All patients resided in the area of endemicity. Surprisingly, there was only 1 instance of a patient with an immunocompromising condition (nephrotic syndrome).

Miscellaneous Sites of Ear, Nose, and Throat Infection

A Russian case of coccidioidal infection of the maxillary sinus, palate, and pharynx resembling Wegener's granuloma-

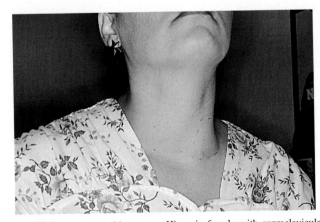

Figure 27–6. A 23-year-old pregnant Hispanic female with supraclavicular mass representing initial focus of disseminated coccidioidomycosis.

Table 27–2. REPORTED CASES OF TRACHEAL-LARYNGEAL COCCIDIOIDOMYCOSIS

Reference	Gross Appearance and/or Biopsy	Age	Sex	Race	Nature and Duration of Symptoms Before Diagnosis or Therapy	Presence of Regional Adenopathy	Other Sites of Dissemination	Concomitant Pulmonary Involvement	Presence of Airway Complications	Require Tracheostomy Intubation	Skin Test Status	Comp Fix Titer	Therapy	Outcome	Hx Resident Endemic Area	Other Immunocompromising Conditions
Boyle, et al.[38]	Diffuse supraglottic edema with near total compromise of the airway. Bx lymph node: caseating granuloma, multinucleated giant cells and/or spherules	40 yr	F	W	Hoarseness × 6 wk Temp to 38.3 °C, night sweats, dry cough, fatigue	Yes	No	No	No	No	NS	1:32	Fluconazole	Pending	Yes	No
Mumma[39]	Invasive granulomatous lesion of the epiglottis. Bx: positive coccidioidal granuloma.	37 yr	M	B	Pharyngitis × 5 mo, dysphagia or odynophagia, hoarseness, weight loss, hemoptysis × 2 wk	Yes	No	No	No	No	Negative	1:32	NS	NS	Yes	No
Singh et al.[40]	Fungating granuloma with ulcer involving vestibule with endolaryngeal thickening, excoriation, edema. Tumor mass obstructing rima glottidis. Bx trachea: positive C. immitis.	34 yr	M	B	Weight loss and cough × 3 mo, hoarseness, dysphagia × 1 mo	Yes	Skin, bone	Yes	Yes	Yes	Negative	NS	No (pre-ampB era)	NS	Yes	No
Platt[41]	Irregular mass aryepiglottic area involving vocal cords. Bx: positive spherules.	45 yr	M	NS	Fever, malaise, hemoptysis, weight loss, dyspnea, hoarseness × 1 yr	No	No	Yes	No	No	Positive	1:256	IV ampB IV miconazole	NS	Yes	No
Ward et al.[42]	Granulomatous appearance post commissure, false cords, and aryepiglottic folds.	20 yr	F	NS	NS	NS	Meninges	NS	NS	NS	NS	NS	NS	NS	NS	NS
Ward et al.[42]	Obstructive granuloma of trachea.	19 mo	F	NS	NS	NS	NS	Yes	Yes	NS	NS	Positive titer	NS	NS	NS	NS
Ward et al.[42]	Granular lesion of anterior commissure and subglottic fold, subglottic stenosis. Bx: positive spherules.	4 1/2 mo	M	H	Wheezing and cough × 3 mo	NS	NS	Yes	Yes	Yes	Negative	1:32	IV ampB	Improved	Yes	No

Table continued on following page

Table 27–2. REPORTED CASES OF TRACHEAL-LARYNGEAL COCCIDIOIDOMYCOSIS *(Continued)*

Reference	Gross Appearance and/or Biopsy	Age	Sex	Race	Nature and Duration of Symptoms Before Diagnosis or Therapy	Presence of Regional Adenopathy	Other Sites of Dissemination	Concomitant Pulmonary Involvement	Presence of Airway Complications	Require Tracheostomy Intubation	Skin Test Status	Comp Fix Titer	Therapy	Outcome	Hx Resident Endemic Area	Other Immuno-compromising Conditions
Gardner et al.[43]	Friable subglottic mass. Bx: positive granulomas and spherules.	13 mo	M	W	Cough or stridor × 3 mo	No	No	No	Yes	Yes	Positive	1:8	IV ampB	Improved	Yes	No
Kafka and Catanzaro[36]	Laryngeal abscess.	8 yr	F	H	Respiratory distress × 1 wk; cough, poor weight gain × 2 yr	NS	Skin: cervical, inguinal, leg abscess	Yes	NS	NS	Negative	1:2048	IV ampB	Lost to f/u	NS	NS
Moskowitz et al.[44]	Large right paratracheal mass, endotracheal mass.	5 yr	M	H	Stridor or wheezing × 2 wk	NS	Yes, site NS	Yes	Yes	Yes	Positive	NS	IV ampB × 5 wk, miconazole × 2 wk	Improved	NS	NS
Benitz, et al.[45]	Irregular mass of granulation tissue below vocal cord on anterior laryngeal wall or edema. Bx: acute and chronic inflammation with granulomatous lymphadenitis. Spherules present.	5 yr	M	NS	Pleurisy, cough, fever, night sweats × 5 wk, wheezing or stridor × 1 wk	No	NS	Yes	Yes	Yes	Positive	1:8	IV ampB	Improved	NS	NS
Hajare and Gibson[46]	Epiglottic and subglottic edema. Polypoid granulomatous mass involving true and false vocal cords and anterior commissure. Bx: positive spherules.	2 1/2 yr	M	H	Respiratory distress or stridor × 2 day	No	No	No	Yes	Yes	NS	1:32	IV ampB × 4 wk, ketoconazole × 1 yr	Improved	Yes	Nephrotic syndrome requiring steroid Rx
Winter, et al.[47]	Granulomatous mass obstructing airway caused by penetrating paratracheal lymph node. Bx: coccidioidal granulomas.	2 1/2 yr	F	W	Cough, dyspnea with apneic episodes, fever × 3 day	NS	No	Yes	Yes	No (tracheostomy could not be done due to location of stenosis)	Positive	1:4	Surgical only (endobronchial débridement)	Improved	Yes	No
Oliver[48]	Fungating mass interarytenoidal area extending into ventricles; laryngeal ulcer.	34 yr	M	B	Cough, wheezing, dysphagia, weight loss × 4 mo	No	Skin, bone	No	Yes	Yes	Negative (positive PPD = selective anergy)	NS	No (pre-ampB era)	Pending	Yes	No

NS = not specified; W = White; H = Hispanic; B = Black; AmpB = amphotericin B; Comp Fix = complement fixation; Hx = history; Rx = treatment; Flu = fluconazole; PPD = purified protein derivative of tuberculin; Bx = biopsy.

tosis has been reported.[49] Although the English abstract summary of this case does not give demographic information on this patient, the patient apparently presented with purulent discharge from the nose and had headache, fever, and maxillary sinus and tooth pain. Surgical exploration revealed a defect in the maxillary sinus consistent with osteomyelitis; a coccidioidal mass was found in the lower nasal meatus; and an apparent area of palatal osteomyelitis was also present. The outcome and type of therapy used were not specified in the abstract.

Coccidioidal otitis media and otitis externa with involvement of the ossicles and mastoid sinus have been described in a 23-year-old Hispanic woman with systemic lupus erythematosus who presented with left ear pain.[50] These areas required surgical débridement and were treated with both intravenous and local amphotericin B irrigation. This patient also had a documented periauricular and cervical coccidioidal adenitis and developed a partial left facial nerve paralysis requiring surgical decompression. Coccidioidal otitis media requiring tympanoplasty and drainage has also been described in a 43-year-old white man who responded to applications of amphotericin B ointment topically and a short course of intravenous amphotericin B.[50]

THERAPY

Amphotericin B has been the "gold standard" since it became available for intravenous therapy in 1957. Amphotericin B acts by disrupting the normal architecture of the fungal cell membrane, producing damage to the integrity of the cell membrane and subsequently allowing leakage of important intracellular substances, thereby leading to inhibition of growth. Amphotericin B is a notoriously toxic agent requiring intravenous administration and frequent monitoring for toxicity by laboratory testing. It is currently reserved for the treatment of life-threatening coccidioidomycosis given the availability of several oral agents including ketoconazole (an imidazole) and several triazole compounds (itraconazole and fluconazole), all of which have been shown to be effective in the treatment of disseminated coccidioidomycosis. Fluconazole is also available for intravenous delivery. All these agents work by inhibiting the synthesis of ergosterol, the major sterol of the fungal cell membrane. This leads to destabilization of the cell wall, loss of important intracellular substances, and subsequent inhibition of growth. Both amphotericin B and the oral azoles appear to be inhibitory (fungistatic) rather than fungicidal against *C. immitis.* No comparative studies of amphotericin B versus these agents have ever been undertaken nor are they likely to be undertaken. However, a randomized double-blind study comparing the efficacy and toxicity of itraconazole versus fluconazole in the treatment of nonmeningeal disseminated disease or chronic pulmonary disease is in progress. Results may be available by 1997. Itraconazole requires the presence of food and low gastric pH for optimal absorption, whereas fluconazole does not.[51]

Amphotericin lipid complex agents have been used in the treatment of disseminated coccidioidomycosis and are potentially less toxic than amphotericin B with comparable efficacy, but published experience with these agents in the treatment of disseminated coccidioidomycosis is limited.[7]

The treatment of coccidioidomycosis can be complex and problematic. In such circumstances, an infectious disease consultation is recommended.

References

1. Deresinski SC: History of coccidioidomycosis: "Dust to dust." In: Stevens DA (ed): Coccidioidomycosis, A Text. New York: Plenum Book Company, 1980, pp 1–20.
2. Stevens DA: *Coccidioides immitis.* Principles and practice of infectious diseases. In: Mandell GL, Douglas RG, Bennett JE (eds): New York: Churchill Livingstone, 1980, pp 2008–2016.
3. Huppert M, Sun SH: Overview of mycology, and the mycology of *Coccidioides immitis.* In: Stevens DA (ed): Coccidioidomycosis, A Text. New York: Plenum Book Company, 1980, pp 21–40.
4. Cole GT, Kirkland TN: Conidia of *Coccidioides immitis,* their significance in disease initiation. In: Cole GT, Hoch HC (eds): The Fungal Spores and Disease Initiation in Plants and Animals. New York: Plenum Press, 1991, pp 405–443.
5. Pappagianis D: Epidemiology of coccidioidomycosis. Curr Top Med Mycol 1988; 2: 199–238.
6. Dickson EC, Gifford MA: *Coccidioides* infection (coccidioidomycosis): II. The primary type of infection. Arch Intern Med 1938; 62: 853–871.
7. Galgiani JN: Coccidioidomycosis. West J Med 1993; 159: 153–171.
8. Drips WD, Smith CE: Epidemiology of coccidioidomycosis. JAMA 1964; 1909: 136–138.
9. Einstein HE, Johnson RH: Coccidioidomycosis: New aspects of epidemiology and therapy. Clin Infect Dis 1993; 16: 349–356.
10. Schneider E, Hajjeh R, Spiegel R, Gunn R, et al.: A coccidioidomycosis outbreak following the Northridge earthquake, Ventura County, California, Jan–Mar 1994. Abstract 13. In: Proceedings of the 5th International Conference on Coccidioidomycosis, Stanford University Aug 24–27, 1994. National Foundation for Infectious Disease. In press 1995.
11. Einstein HE: The great epidemic of the early 1990's. Abstract 9 presented at the Centennial Conference on *Coccidioides immitis.* In: Proceedings of the 5th International Conference on Coccidioidomycosis, Stanford University, August 24–27, 1994. National Foundation for Infectious Disease. In press 1995.
12. Drutz DJ, Catanzaro A: Coccidioidomycosis: Part I. Am Rev Respir Dis 1978; 117: 559–585.
13. Caldwell J, Welch G, Johnson R, Einstein H: The economic impact of coccidioidomycosis in Kern County, California. Abstract 11 presented at the Centennial Conference on *Coccidioides immitis.* In: Proceedings of the 5th International Conference on Coccidioidomycosis, Stanford University, August 24–27, 1994. National Foundation for Infectious Disease. In press 1995.
14. Catanzaro A, Drutz DJ: Pulmonary coccidioidomycosis. In: Stevens DA (ed): Coccidioidomycosis, A Text. New York; Plenum Book Company, 1980, pp 135–145.
15. Lopez AM, Williams PL, Ampel NM: Acute pulmonary coccidioidomycosis mimicking bacterial pneumonia and septic shock. Am J Med 1993; 95: 236–239.
16. Arsura E, Ismail Y, Abraham J, Billinghausen P, et al.: Cytokine response in septic shock syndrome secondary to disseminated coccidioidomycosis. Abstract 35 presented at the Centennial Conference on *Coccidioides immitis.* In: Proceedings of the 5th International Conference on Coccidioidomycosis, Stanford University, August 24–27, 1994. National Foundation for Infectious Disease. In press 1995.
17. Catanzaro A, Drutz DJ: Pulmonary coccidioidomycosis. In: Stevens DA (ed): Coccidioidomycosis, A Text. New York: Plenum Book Company, 1980, pp 147–161.
18. Stevens DA: Coccidioidomycosis. N Engl J Med 1995; 332: 1077–1082.
19. Cox RA, Vivas JR, Gross R, et al.: In vivo and in vitro cell mediated responses in coccidioidomycosis. Am Rev Respir Dis 1976; 114: 937–943.
20. Perez J, Abraham J: Coccidioidomycosis: A new sexually transmitted disease. Abstract 27 presented at the Centennial Conference on *Coccidioides immitis.* In: Proceedings of the 5th International Conference on

Coccidioidomycosis, Stanford University, August 24–27, 1994. National Foundation for Infectious Disease. In press 1995.

21. Eckmann BH, Schaefer GL, Huppert M: Bedside interhuman transmission of coccidioidomycosis via growth on fomites: An epidemic involving 6 persons. Am Rev Respir Dis 1964; 89: 175–185.

22. Ampel NM, Widen MA, Galgiani JN: Coccidioidomycosis: Clinical update. Rev Infect Dis 1989; 11: 897–911.

23. McClenny N, Widen MA, Sutton JA: Detection methods for *Coccidioides immitis* in the clinical lab. Abstract 4 presented at the Centennial Conference on *Coccidioides immitis*. In: Proceedings of the 5th International Conference on Coccidioidomycosis, Stanford University, August 24–27, 1994. National Foundation for Infectious Disease. In press 1995.

24. Mosmann JR, Coffman RL: TH1 and TH2 cells: Different patterns of lymphokine secretion lead to different functional properties. Annu Rev Immunol 1989; 7: 145–173.

25. Cox RA: Coccidioidomycosis. In: Murphy JW (ed): Fungal Infections and Immune Responses. New York: Plenum Press, 1993, pp 173–211.

26. Heinzel FP: Th1 and Th2 cells in the cure and pathogenesis of infectious diseases. Curr Opin Infect Dis 1995; 8: 151–155.

27. Cole GT, Kirkland TN: Conidia of *Coccidioides immitis*, their significance in disease initiation. In: Cole GT, Hoch HC (eds): The Fungal Spore and Disease Initiation in Plants and Animals. New York: Plenum Press, 1991, pp 403–443.

28. Forbus WD: Coccidioidomycosis: A study of 95 cases of the disseminated type with special reference to the pathogenesis of the disease. Mil Surg 1946; 654–713.

29. Frauenfelder D, Schwartz AW: Coccidioidomycosis involving head and neck. Plast Reconstr Surg 1967; 39(6): 549–553.

30. Iger M: Coccidioidal osteomyelitis. In: Ajello L (ed): Coccidioidomycosis: Current Clinical and Diagnostic Status. Miami: Symposium Specialist Medical Books, 1977, pp 165–190.

31. Deresinski SC: Coccidioidomycosis of bone and joints. In: Stevens DA (ed): Coccidioidomycosis, A Text. New York: Plenum Book Company, 1980, pp 195–211.

32. Winter WG, Larson RK, Zettas JP, Libtke RI: Coccidioidal spondylitis. J Bone Joint Surg Am 1978; 60-A(2): 240–244.

33. Henley-Cohn J, Boles R, Weisberger E, Ballantyne J: Upper airway obstruction due to coccidioidomycosis. Laryngoscope 1979; 89: 355–366.

34. McGahan JP, Graves DS, Palmer PE: Coccidioidal spondylitis. Radiology 1980; 136: 5–9.

35. Jacobs PH: Cutaneous coccidioidomycosis. In: Stevens DA (ed): Coccidioidomycosis, A Text. New York: Plenum Book Company, 1980, pp 213–224.

36. Kafka JA, Catanzaro A: Disseminated coccidioidomycosis in children. J Pediatr 1981; 98(3): 355–361.

37. DeClercq LD, Chole RA: Retropharyngeal abscess in the adult. Otolaryngol Head Neck Surg 1980; 88: 684–689.

38. Boyle JO, Coulthard SW, Mandel RM: Laryngeal involvement in disseminated coccidioidomycosis. Arch Otolaryngol Head Neck Surg 1991; 117: 433–438.

39. Mumma CS: Coccidioidomycosis of the epiglottis. Arch Otolaryngol Head Neck Surg 1953; 58: 306–309.

40. Singh H, Yast CJ, Gladney JH: Coccidioidomycosis with endolaryngeal involvement. Arch Otolaryngol 1956; 3: 244–247.

41. Platt MA: Laryngeal coccidioidomycosis. JAMA 1977; 237(12): 1234–1235.

42. Ward PH, Morledge D, Berci G, Schwartz H: Coccidioidomycosis of the larynx in infants and adults. Ann Otol Rhinol Laryngol 1977; 86: 655–660.

43. Gardner S, Seilheimer D, Catlin F, et al.: Subglottic coccidioidomycosis presenting with persistent stridor. Pediatrics 1980; 66(4): 623–625.

44. Moskowitz PS, Sue JY, Gooding CA: Tracheal coccidioidomycosis causing upper airway obstruction in children. AJR Am J Roentgenol 1982; 139: 596–600.

45. Benitz WE, Bradley JS, Fee WE, Loomis JC: Upper airway obstruction due to laryngeal coccidioidomycosis in a 5-year-old child. Am J Otolaryngol 1983; 4(5): 367–370.

46. Hajare S, Gibson FB: Laryngeal coccidioidomycosis causing airway obstruction. Pediatr Infect Dis J 1989; 8(1): 54–55.

47. Winter B, Villaveces J, Spector M: Coccidioidomycosis accompanied by acute tracheal obstruction in a child. JAMA 1966; 195(2): 1101–1104.

48. Oliver EA: Coccidioidomycosis with cutaneous involvement. AMA Arch Dermatol Syphil 1954; 70: 537–538.

49. Arievich AM, Zabrokritskaia DM: Vestnik Otorinolaringologii 1970; 32(3): 60–64.

50. Harvey RP, Pappigianis D, Cochran J, Stevens DA: Otomycosis due to coccidioidomycosis. Arch Intern Med 1978; 138: 1434–1435.

51. Sugar AM: Fluconazole and itraconazole, current status and prospects for anti-fungal therapy. In: Remington JS, Swartz MN (eds): Current Clinical Topics in Infectious Diseases. Cambridge: Blackwell Scientific Publications, 1993, pp 74–98.

M. Hong Nguyen
Alan M. Sugar

CHAPTER TWENTY-EIGHT

Candida

▼

HISTORY

Oral thrush, a common manifestation of *Candida* infection, was recognized by Hippocrates in the fourth century B.C. Although the "thrush fungus" was isolated much earlier than 1846, the association of this fungus and the oral lesion was not made until 1846, when Berg reproduced thrush in healthy babies by inoculating them with the thrush materials.[1] Over the next century, at least 100 names were given to this fungus, of which *Monilia albicans* (*albicans*, from Latin meaning "to whiten") remained favored for several decades. Berkhout, in 1923, reclassified this organism to the genus *Candida* (from Latin meaning "white," given the white morphology of the organism on agar plates).

Shortly after the identification of the fungus, the association between *Candida* infection and serious debilitating disease was recognized. The first documentation of invasive disease was reported by Zenker, who described a case of cerebral candidiasis.[1] The introduction of antibacterial agents in the 1940s precipitated a wide spectrum of infection caused by *Candida albicans*, including endophthalmitis, endocarditis, osteomyelitis, and peritonitis. Furthermore, since the mid-1970s, with advances in medical-surgical technology, therapeutic interventions such as chemotherapy and transplantation, and an increase in immunocompromised patients, *C. albicans* has emerged as an important nosocomial pathogen. In addition, over the past several years, there has been an increase in the incidence of infection caused by other *Candida* species, such as *Candida glabrata, Candida tropicalis, Candida parapsilosis*, and *Candida krusei*.[2]

DESCRIPTION OF THE PATHOGEN

Candida species are fungi that reproduce by budding, most growing as yeasts. *C. albicans*, however, is dimorphic and can grow either as a yeastlike form or as a hyphal form. *Candida* grows well on agar plates and forms smooth, white to cream-colored colonies. The organism stains Gram-positive.

The genus *Candida* comprises close to 200 species, among which *C. albicans, C. tropicalis, C. glabrata (Torulopsis glabrata), C. parapsilosis, C. krusei, Candida guilliermondii*, and *Candida lusitaniae* are medically important species. *C. albicans* can be reliably differentiated from other *Candida* species by its ability to form germ tubes in serum or albumin-containing media, and chlamydospores on corn meal polysorbate-80 agar. The differentiation between the non-*albicans Candida* species is based mainly on biochemical tests (e.g., carbohydrate assimilation and fermentation, ni-trate usage, urease production) and enzymatic reactions. The commercially available packages (such as API 20C [Analytab Products, Plainview, New York] or Vitek [BioMerieux Vitek, Hazelwood, Missouri]) have facilitated the identification of yeasts in the clinical laboratory.

EPIDEMIOLOGY

Candida species are ubiquitous in nature. They can be isolated from the environment, including water, soil, air, plants, and animal manure. *Candida* species are normal commensals of the gastrointestinal and genital tract of humans and can also be found in the oropharynx, in sputum, or on skin.

Although the source of candidiasis is frequently endogenous, direct transmission of *Candida* from humans to humans (such as the acquisition of thrush in newborns via the maternal birth canal, balanitis in men via sexual contact with candidal vaginitis) can also occur. In addition, nosocomial spread of *Candida* has been reported, probably by transmission through the hands of health-care workers.

LABORATORY DIAGNOSIS

Candida is a frequent colonizer of humans, especially hospitalized patients; therefore, the diagnosis of invasive candidiasis requires the isolation of fungus on culture and detection of either yeast forms, pseudohyphae, or hyphae within tissue. These morphologic forms can be observed microscopically using potassium hydroxide wet mount; Calcofluor stain can assist in the detection of these organisms by binding to chitin in the cell wall and causing the fungus to brightly fluoresce. *Candida* species can also be visualized by hematoxylin and eosin or Giemsa's stains, although methenamine silver or periodic acid–Schiff stain facilitates the detection of *Candida* on clinical samples.

Lysis-centrifugation blood cultures (Isolator, E.I. du Pont de Nemours, Wilmington, Delaware) are more effective than the biphasic blood cultures in recovering *Candida* species from blood. However, culture of blood is not a sensitive means to diagnose invasive candidiasis. In one study of disseminated candidiasis, candidemia was detected in only 50% of these cases.[3]

Positive culture for *Candida* at a normally sterile site is the "gold standard" for the diagnosis of candidiasis. However, although most *Candida* species can be recovered within 48 hours of incubation, a few *Candida* species such as *C. guilliermondii* and *C. glabrata* require a longer incubation time for growth. Therefore, laboratory personnel should be alert for cases in which *Candida* or other fungi are clinically suspected so that the cultures can be held for 2–3 weeks.

Detection of antibodies or *Candida* antigens has not been particularly useful, but refinements in the detection of certain *Candida* metabolites may become clinically useful in the future.

HOST DEFENSE

Intact skin and mucous membranes are important factors in the host defense against *Candida* infection. Once candidal invasion occurs, polymorphonuclear cells provide a major host defense; myeloperoxidase, hydrogen peroxide, and superoxide anion are major mechanisms for intracellular killing of these organisms.[4]

Lymphocytes appear to be the primary host defense against mucocutaneous candidiasis. Patients with T-cell defects, including chronic mucocutaneous candidiasis, thymic dysplasia, or acquired immunodeficiency syndrome (AIDS), are at high risk for oropharyngeal candidiasis. The role of macrophages, humoral factors, and complement in the defense against *Candida* remains to be elucidated.

The risk factors for deep-seated candidiasis include diabetes mellitus; prolonged administration of antibacterial agents; abdominal surgery; severe burns; intravenous drug use; the presence of intravenous catheters; immunosuppression such as bone marrow or organ transplantation; malignancy; neutropenia; and the administration of corticosteroids or chemotherapeutic or other cytotoxic agents.

EAR, NOSE, AND THROAT CLINICAL SYNDROMES

Oral Candidiasis

Candida can cause a variety of oral infections, of which thrush and denture stomatitis are the most common. Lehner classified the candidal oral lesions into five clinical entities:[5]

1. *Acute pseudomembranous candidiasis* (or thrush). This is characterized by discrete white plaques resembling "a membrane of lard"[6] on the buccal mucosa, tongue, and throat. These plaques, upon scraping, yield a raw, erythematous, and painful surface.

Thrush is uncommon in healthy patients and occurs mainly in patients recently receiving antibacterial agents or inhaled corticosteroids, and in immunocompromised patients (e.g., patients with malignancy; neutropenia; receipt of systemic corticosteroid or chemotherapeutic agents; or AIDS). In AIDS patients, the appearance of thrush is a marker for the progression of human immunodeficiency virus disease. Thrush usually appears as the CD4 counts fall to below 200/mm^3. Thrush can also affect infants, who can acquire *Candida* either from the maternal birth canal, a health-care worker's hands, or objects such as pacifiers.[6]

The diagnosis of thrush is frequently made based on its appearance in the oral cavity. Scrapings of the oral lesions for potassium hydroxide smear, Gram's stain, or culture can be confirmatory. Because *Candida* can be a normal inhabit-

ant of the mouth, the sole presence of this organism on the oral culture does not fulfill the diagnosis of thrush.

Azole agents (ketoconazole, fluconazole, itraconazole) are highly effective against thrush and have proved to be superior to clotrimazole troches. However, cases of thrush refractory to these agents have been reported. The therapeutic failure of these cases has been attributed to the development of antifungal resistance (especially to azole agents) in some cases, and to the defect in host defenses in others. The problem of oral thrush refractory to antifungal therapy is most often seen in patients with advanced AIDS (CD4 counts <50/mm^3), especially when they had received long-term, low-dose fluconazole therapy. Itraconazole, amphotericin B, or the addition of flucytosine to these agents has been successful in some cases of refractory oral candidiasis.

2. *Chronic atrophic candidiasis* (or denture stomatitis). This is characterized by chronic inflammation of the portion of the palate that comes into contact with the denture plates. The lesion often begins as a local focus of hyperemia, which then progresses to generalized hyperemia and swelling, and if untreated, can lead to granular papillary hyperplasia. This condition is rarely symptomatic, except when it progresses to involve the corner of the mouth (angular cheilitis, see below). The therapy requires topical antifungals or antiseptics, denture disinfection with agents such as chlorhexidine, and discontinuing the use of dentures.

3. *Angular cheilitis* (or perleche). This is characterized by erythema, inflammation and fissure at the corner of the mouth. This condition is frequently associated with denture stomatitis. It is not exclusively caused by *Candida*, but also by bacteria such as *Staphylococcus aureus*. Iron or vitamin deficiencies appear to predispose patients to angular cheilitis.

4. *Chronic hyperplastic candidiasis* (or *Candida* leukoplakia). This is characterized by raised, white patches which firmly adhere to the buccal mucosa, lips and tongue. *Candida* leukoplakia should be separated from oral leukoplakia due to other etiologies such as cigarette smoking and premalignant changes. Most cases of *Candida* leukoplakia respond to topical or systemic antifungal therapy; for refractory cases, surgical resection is required.

5. *Acute atrophic candidiasis* (or midline glossitis). This is characterized by erythema and loss of papillae at the center of the tongue. It is still controversial as to whether this lesion is truly due to *Candida*.

Other Clinical Entities

With the exception of thrush, *Candida* infections of the ear, nose, and throat are uncommon. However, the recognition of these infections is important, since therapy is available and early diagnosis might alter the disease course, improve outcome, and prevent further candidal invasion or dissemination.

1. *Candida laryngitis* is a rare manifestation of candidal infection. It has been reported in all sex and age groups. The vocal cord is the most common site of involvement.[7] The predisposing factors include: newborn, diabetes mellitus, endotracheal intubation, chronic mucocutaneous candidiasis, the use of systemic or inhaled corticosteroids, malignancy, and severe burn.[7] The most common presentation is hoarseness in adults, and respiratory stridor and distress in neonates.[8] The spectrum of the disease ranges from minor infection in severely debilitated patients to life threatening respiratory distress.[7] *Candida* laryngitis can also provide a focus for subsequent development of disseminated candidiasis.

The diagnosis relies on indirect laryngoscopy with culture and biopsy of the involved tissue. Laryngeal ulcers with coexisting pseudomembrane formation are often visualized on the laryngoscopy.

The disease often responds to topical antifungal agents; however, in immunocompromised hosts, systemic antifungal agents should be considered; amphotericin B or an azole agent, especially fluconazole, should be used depending on the patient's underlying condition. Early recognition and therapy of this disease may minimize complications such as laryngeal scarring, improve morbidity, and help to prevent systemic dissemination.

2. *Candida epiglottitis* can occur as an isolated, locally invasive infection, or as part of a disseminated disease.[9] The earliest presentation is laryngeal stridor followed by dysphagia, refractory pharyngitis, and odynophagia.[9] Few cases of rapidly progressive sore throat followed by an obstructive airway have also been reported.[9] The diagnosis is by indirect laryngoscopy with culture sent from swab and biopsy material. Intravenous amphotericin B should be considered in patients with sustained neutropenia.

3. *Candida sinusitis* is a rare cause of sinusitis in both immunocompetent and immunocompromised hosts.[10] *Candida* sinusitis often runs a more benign clinical course than other types of fungal sinusitis (e.g., *Mucor* or *Aspergillus* sinusitis) with less local inva-sion. The prognosis is good with local debridement and antifungal therapy.

References

1. Kwon-Chung KJ, Bennett JE: Candidiasis. In: Medical Mycology. Malvern, Pennsylvania: Lea & Febiger, 1992, pp 280–336.
2. Nguyen MH, Peacock JE Jr, Tanner DC, et al.: The changing face of candidemia: Emergence of the non-*C. albicus* species and antifungal resistance. Am J Med 1996, in press.
3. Hart PD, Russell E Jr., Remington JS: The compromised host infection–deep fungal infection. J Infect Dis 1969; 120: 169–191.
4. Edwards JE Jr: *Candida* species. In: Mandell GL, Bennett JE, Dolin R (eds): Principles and Practice of Infectious Disease. Edinburgh: Churchill Livingstone, 1995, p 1943.
5. Lehner T: Oral candidosis. Dent Practit 1967; 17: 209–216.
6. Odds FC: *Candida* and Candidosis. A Review and Bibliography, 2nd ed. London: Balliere Tindall, 1988.
7. Tashjian LS, Peacock JE Jr: Laryngeal candidiasis. Report of seven cases and review of the literature. Arch Otolaryngol 1984; 110: 806–809.
8. Jacobs RF, Yasuda K, Smith AL, et al.: Laryngeal candidiasis presenting as respiratory stridor. Pediatrics 1972; 69: 234–236.
9. Walsh TJ, Gray WC: *Candida* epiglottitis in immunocompromised patients. Chest 1987; 91(4): 482–485.
10. Dooley DP, McAllister K: Candidal sinusitis and diabetic ketoacidosis. A brief report. Arch Intern Med 1989; 149: 962–964.

Luciano Z. Goldani
Alan M. Sugar

CHAPTER TWENTY-NINE

Dimorphic and Miscellaneous Fungi

▼

The fungi discussed in this chapter include the dimorphic pathogens and some miscellaneous fungi that, although rare, may be encountered in a busy otolaryngologic practice. The term *dimorphic* refers to the growth of the fungi in two morphologic forms, mold and yeastlike. The mold form typically grows in the environment and consists of multinucleate threadlike masses called *hyphae* or *mycelia*. Mycelia reproduce by the formation of spores or conidia, which are thought to be the infective form of the organism. Once at the elevated temperature of the human body, these fungi undergo a transition to a yeastlike form and reproduce by either budding or endosporulation (in the case of *Coccidioides immitis*). It is the characteristic microscopic appearance of the yeastlike forms of the dimorphic fungi that allows a definitive diagnosis before culture results are available.

BLASTOMYCOSIS

Mycology

Blastomyces dermatitidis, the causative agent of blastomycosis, is a thermally dimorphic fungus producing mycelia with 2–10 μm, round to oval or pear-shaped conidia at 25 °C, and broad-based budding yeasts with thick refractile walls varying in size from 8 to 15 μm up to 30 μm in diameter at 37° C (Fig. 29–1).[1] Like *Histoplasma capsulatum*, *B. dermatitidis* is an ascomycete and has a teleomorphic form, *Ajellomyces dermatitidis*. Growth of *B. dermatitidis* is favored by soil containing organism matter, acid pH, and moisture.[1]

Epidemiology

The organism may be found in microfoci enriched with animal excreta. The presence of decaying organic material appears to be required to support the sustained growth of *B. dermatitidis* in soil.[1]

Endemic and sporadic cases account for the majority of cases of blastomycosis, but a few epidemics of infection from point sources have also been described. Despite underreporting, it is clear that most cases of blastomycosis occur in the states surrounding the Mississippi and Ohio rivers and in the southeastern United States, with the greatest numbers (in descending order) in Kentucky, Arkansas, Mississippi, North Carolina, Tennessee, Louisiana, Illinois, and Wisconsin.[1]

Pathogenesis

Blastomycosis is acquired by inhalation of the conidia that are thought to be found in the soil. At body temperature, conidia are converted to their yeast form, which may disseminate from the lungs via hematogenous and lymphatic routes throughout the body, causing a wide spectrum of clinical manifestations.[2]

Neutrophils are recruited first to sites of infection, but lymphocytes arrive later, leading to pyogranuloma formation. Cellular immune responses, as measured by in vitro reactivity of circulating lymphocytes of *B. dermatitidis*, may be demonstrated in immunocompetent patients.[1]

Clinical Manifestations

The most common initial symptoms of blastomycosis are related to pulmonary disease or systemic symptoms. Constitutional symptoms include weight loss, fever, malaise, fatigue, and other nonspecific complaints but offer little diagnostic help. The most common feature of blastomycosis is a pulmonary infiltrate.[2] The majority of patients have either an alveolar or a masslike infiltrate. The primary pulmonary disease can present with acute pneumonia-like symptoms of fever, night sweats, purulent cough, weight loss, and chest pain. Chronic pneumonia with symptoms that usually last 2 to 6 months is also seen in patients with blastomycosis. These patients may be misdiagnosed as having a malignancy or tuberculosis. Some patients with pulmonary infiltrates may have no pulmonary symptoms. Physical examination may reveal skin lesions, which are classically painless, nodular, or papular initially but may later enlarge to form large abscesses or ulcers if left untreated. This is the most common extrapulmonary site of blastomycosis and is seen in up to 80% of cases of extrapulmonary blastomycosis. The cutaneous lesions have often been mistaken for keratoacanthoma, squamous cell carcinoma, pyodermal infection, syphilis, and tuberculosis.

Blastomycosis, a systemic illness, has also been reported to involve, in particular, bone, and also genitourinary tract, liver, heart, adrenal glands, and several sites in the extracranial head and neck region.[3]

Head and Neck Involvement. Head and neck manifestations of blastomycosis are summarized in Table 29–1. Like other complications in blastomycosis, lung or skin involvement is almost always associated with these manifestations.

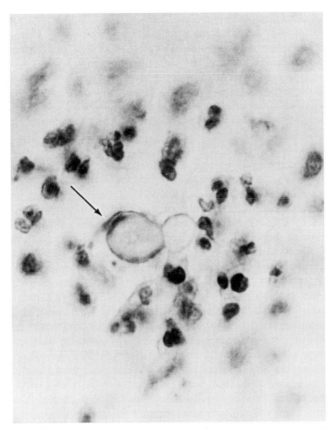

Figure 29–1. Gomori methenamine silver stain showing the organism *B. dermatitidis* (arrow) with the broadbased bud and double-contoured walls.

In the majority of the cases, otolaryngologic consultation was reserved for laryngeal disease or nasal involvement, although some patients with skin lesions might seek otolaryngologic consultations. In a retrospective study of 123 patients with blastomycosis, Reder and Neel described 23 patients with head and neck involvement.[4] Of these 23 patients, 16 (69.6%) had blastomycotic lesions of the skin of the head and neck, 5 (21.7%) had lesions of the larynx, and 2 (8.7%) had lesions involving the nose. Of all the patients, 4.7% had laryngeal involvement as a presenting site.

Oropharyngeal and Intranasal Involvement. The oral and nasal cavities have been described as presenting sites of blastomycosis. It is often difficult to distinguish the oral lesions from those of actinomycosis.[5, 6] Nasal involvement

Table 29–1. HEAD AND NECK INVOLVEMENT IN BLASTOMYCOSIS

Site	Percentage
Skin	50–75
Oral cavity	10–30
Larynx	5–10
Lymph nodes	5–10
Thyroid	2
Nasal cavity	<1
Ear	<1
Paranasal sinuses	<1

Data from Blastomycosis I. A review of 198 collected cases in Veterans Administration hospitals. Am Rev Respir Dis 1964; 89: 659–672.

occurs near the vestibule or alar rim, and mucosal lesions are uncommon. Lesions in the mouth and nasal and oropharyngeal area in blastomycosis are not found with the same frequency as the lesions seen in disseminated histoplasmosis. One exception is laryngeal involvement. The larynx has been reported to be the next most common presenting site in the head and neck region. Witorsch and Utz suggested that the larynx is infected as a result of hematogenous dissemination from a pulmonary focus rather than as a result of direct primary inoculation, because almost all patients with laryngeal blastomycosis have evidence of the disease at other sites.[3] Biopsy of the larynx reveals histologic features similar to those in the skin. The laryngeal lesions have been confused clinically with well-differentiated squamous cell carcinoma, resulting in radical surgical excision.

Although only rarely reported, lesions of the nasal mucous membrane occur singly and in association with oral mucosal lesions. Their gross and microscopic appearance is quite similar to that of the oral lesions. In a study by Witorsch and Utz, the nasal lesions were mucocutaneous, as they were continuous with lesions of the nasal skin.[3] However, Gerwin and Myer have reported a 38-year-old woman without mucosal or skin lesions who was complaining of an intranasal mass and intermittent periods of bleeding for 4 months.[7] The mass was biopsied, and culture of the intranasal mass grew *B. dermatitidis*.

Extensive Bone, Epidural, and Middle Ear Involvement. Angtuaco and colleagues reported two patients with extensive nasopharyngeal and temporal bone involvement with extension from disseminated disease to the entire middle ear, base of the skull, and epidural space.[8] These cases would be categorized as deep infiltrating lesions, and the major diagnostic consideration would be malignant neoplasms, such as primarily squamous cell carcinomas of either the lymphoepitheliomatous or transitional cell type, rhabdomyosarcoma, adenocarcinoma, adenoid cystic carcinoma, lymphoma, sarcoma, and metastatic disease.

Sinus Involvement. Reports of parasinus involvement have been limited. Several series of patients with blastomycosis failed to reveal evidence of sinus involvement. Greer reported one case of blastomycosis involving the maxillary sinus that was successfully treated with amphotericin B.[9] Istorico and colleagues reported two patients with nasopharyngeal masses due to *B. dermatitidis* that were found by radiologic scans to involve the paranasal sinus.[10] In another report, Day and Stucker described a woman with a right upper lobe pneumonia due to *B. dermatitidis*.[11] Several months later, after a long period of noncompliance with her medication, she presented with nasal airway obstruction, facial pain, and a nodule near her medial canthus. A right nasoantral window and Caldwell-Luc procedure were performed (Fig. 29–2), and the biopsy specimen of the right maxillary sinus revealed *B. dermatitidis*.

Otitis Media with Head and Neck Masses. A nasopharyngeal mass with bony destruction, middle ear opacification, and central nervous system involvement due to *B. dermatitidis* has been reported in two patients with disseminated blastomycosis.[10] Both patients presented with fever, headache, and ear pain and were treated initially with antibiotics for bacterial otitis media. Initial evaluation suggested neoplastic diseases, but biopsy of the mass confirmed *B.*

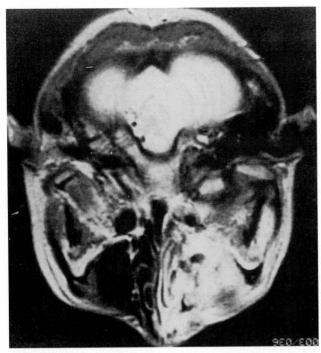

Figure 29–2. Axial gadolinium-enhanced magnetic resonance imaging scan showing extensive involvement of the right maxillary sinus and soft tissue overlying the front wall sinus.

dermatitidis in both patients. Therefore, fungal infection due to *B. dermatitidis* should be considered as a cause of mass lesions and otitis media in patients from areas in which blastomycosis is endemic.

Central Nervous System. Central nervous system involvement by *B. dermatitidis* was estimated by Parker and colleagues to constitute 2.5% of all cerebral mycoses.[12] Intracerebral involvement results from either hematogenous spread in disseminated disease or contiguous spread from the sinuses or from a primary focus in the nasopharynx. The predominate intracerebral lesions are noncaseating granulomas and on brain computed tomography (CT) scans appear as nodular enhancing lesions that may be confused with tumoral lesions. Acute and chronic meningitis may be a predominant manifestation. Cerebrospinal fluid cultures or smears, biopsy specimens, and correlative data aid in the accurate diagnosis of blastomycosis.

Blastomycosis in Special Hosts. Blastomycosis in children 16 years of age or younger have been reported in only 3.5% of 376 reported cases.[1] Clinical manifestations were similar in both adults and children, with the exception of epididymitis or prostatitis, which were not reported in children.

Blastomycosis is an uncommon infection among immunocompromised patients, including patients with acquired immunodeficiency syndrome (AIDS).[13] The scarcity of reported cases of blastomycosis in patients with AIDS is consistent with observations of a similarly low incidence of blastomycosis among bone marrow and solid transplant recipients.

In a review of 15 patients with AIDS who developed blastomycosis, disseminated disease was described in 8 patients (53.3%).[13] Curiously, oropharyngeal involvement was

not identified. However, 5 patients (33.3%) had cerebral or meningeal blastomycosis.

The definitive diagnosis of blastomycosis was established by culture in 14 patients (93%), and a presumptive diagnosis was made on the basis of the typical morphologic appearance of the organism in an additional patient.

Diagnosis

The diagnosis of blastomycosis is made by identification of the fungus in tissue or exudate followed by culture. Unlike the situation with some organisms, *B. dermatitidis* is easy to detect in both smears and cultures. Colonization or contamination with the fungus in tissue does not occur as it occurs with members of the genus *Aspergillus* and *Candida*. In addition to examinations of sputum, skin, and mucosal lesion scrapings by wet preparations with potassium hydroxide, and histopathologic section, cytologic preparations are useful for dependable diagnosis. The relative ease of diagnosis in many cases by direct smear or culture should be appreciated, because other diagnostic techniques are not as reliable as they are for other infections. Clinically available tests include complement fixation antibodies, enzyme immunoassay antibodies, and immunodiffusion precipitin bands. As a rule, serologic tests for blastomycosis lack sensitivity and specificity. With blastomycosis, these assays have been useful as tools for epidemiologic assessments.

It is important to emphasize the complementary role of CT and magnetic resonance imaging (MRI) in diagnosing lesions involving the sinuses, bone, middle ear, and central nervous system aside from their detection of soft-tissue masses. Early lesions may be better visualized by MRI, whereas calcification and bony destruction may be better seen on CT scans.

The distinction between blastomycosis and paracoccidioidomycosis or coccidioidomycosis in histopathologic section is usually easy in experienced hands but may be so difficult that only culture can resolve the question. Fortunately, the endemic regions of blastomycosis have almost no overlap with those of the other two mycoses.

Treatment

The presence of pleural disease or any extrapulmonary infection during the course of illness requires antifungal treatment. Amphotericin B is effective in the treatment of blastomycosis.[14] Intravenous amphotericin B in a dosage of 2.0 g resulted in cure without relapse in up to 97% of patients.

Ketoconazole has in vitro activity against *B. dermatitidis* comparable to that of amphotericin B; however, it has fewer toxic effects. The initial trial from the NIH Mycoses Study Group was not optimistic, however.[14a] Of 16 patients with blastomycosis, 7 were cured, 4 were considered to have been treatment failures, and 5 had relapses of infection. Other clinical trials of ketoconazole have shown that with adequate doses (400–800 mg taken orally each day for at least 6 months) blastomycosis was cured in 89% of patients.[15]

Newer imidazole and triazole antifungal agents are being developed. Itraconazole, a triazole antifungal agent given orally has recently been investigated in clinical trials. Its major advantage over ketoconazole is that it has a lower degree of toxicity, especially in regard to endocrinopathies associated with ketoconazole therapy. Itraconazole has been shown to have efficacy in blastomycosis (200–400 mg daily for at least 6 months). Experience with fluconazole is more limited, but preliminary evidence suggests that at doses up to 400 mg/day, it is less effective than itraconazole.

In the very ill or immunocompromised patient, amphotericin B remains the treatment of choice, but after improvement, a switch to ketoconazole or itraconazole may be appropriate.

HISTOPLASMOSIS

Mycology

Histoplasma capsulatum var. *capsulatum* is an ascomycete of the family Arthrodermataceae. It grows as a mold in the soil and on appropriate culture media at temperatures of less than 35 °C. Hyphae bear tuberculate macroconidia that are 8–14 μm in diameter and smaller microconidia (2–5 μm) that are the infectious form of the organism.[16] At temperatures above 35 °C and in human tissues, *H. capsulatum* grows as a yeast measuring 2–4 μm in diameter. The sexual state is known as *Emmonsiella capsulata*, although some believe that the correct taxonomic placement is in the genus *Ajellomyces*, as a second species, *Ajellomyces capsulata*.

Pathogenesis

Infection with *H. capsulatum* develops when microconidia or hyphal elements are inhaled and convert into yeasts in the lungs or when organisms in old foci of infection reactivate during immunosuppression.[17]

T-cell immunity plays the key role in determining the outcome of infection with *H. capsulatum*. These T cells activate macrophages, enhancing their fungicidal capabilities. Individuals with impaired T-cell immunity fail to control infection with *H. capsulatum*. Exposure to heavy inocula may also overcome these immune mechanisms. Because exposure to *H. capsulatum* is common in endemic areas, reinfection occurs frequently. Illnesses tend to be milder and shorter in recurrent cases. Contrasted to exogenous reinfection, endogenous reactivation of latent infection is probably rare in histoplasmosis.[17]

Epidemiology

H. capsulatum is found primarily in microfoci containing large amounts of rotted guano where starlings, pigeons, and grackles have roosted or bats have inhabited. Although such exposures can be identified in most small outbreaks, a history of exposure cannot be elicited in most *H. capsulatum* infections. Several large urban outbreaks occurred without recognizable exposure.[18]

In the United States, most cases have occurred within regions recognized to be endemic for histoplasmosis, especially along the Ohio and Mississippi River valleys.

Clinical Manifestations

Pulmonary Histoplasmosis. Only 1% of persons develop symptomatic illness after exposure to low-inoculum exposure, whereas 50%–100% develop symptoms with heavy exposure. Acute self-limited illnesses constitute the majority of symptomatic cases. About 1 in 2000 infected individuals develops progressive or cavitary infection. About 80% of symptomatic patients initially present with flulike, acute pulmonary diseases. Symptoms include fever (90%–100%), chills (90%–100%), headache (90%), thigh pain (39%), myalgia (90%), anorexia (85%), nonproductive cough (50%–95%), and retrosternal or pleuritic chest pain (60%–85%).[16] Chronic pulmonary histoplasmosis is characterized by chronic pulmonary symptoms and apical lung lesions that progress with inflammation, cavitation, and fibrosis. Mediastinal fibrosis and fibrosing mediastinitis are unusual clinical presentations of histoplasmosis.[16]

Disseminated Histoplasmosis. Disseminated histoplasmosis, which includes a progressive clinical illness with evidence of extrapulmonary spread of infection, occurs in 1 of 2000–5000 acute infections. About half the patients are receiving immunosuppressive therapy or suffer illnesses that depress cellular immunity, such as lymphoma, lymphocytic leukemia, hyposplenic disorders, or AIDS.[19] Old age also predisposes to dissemination. Most patients present with fever, fatigue, and weight loss of 1–2 months in duration. Although this clinical presentation may be rapidly fatal, a subacute presentation over 1–3 months is characteristic. Respiratory complaints of cough or dyspnea occur in half the patients. Other common findings include hepatosplenomegaly and lymphadenopathy. Less commonly, patients present with a sepsis syndrome, meningitis, or gastrointestinal involvement. Renal failure may also complicate this disease.[19]

A variety of skin lesions such as erythematous, diffuse maculopapules, pustules, folliculitis, plaques, or nodules occur in about 10% of cases with disseminated presentation.

Oropharyngeal and Laryngeal Involvement in Disseminated Histoplasmosis. The granulomatous lesions of disseminated histoplasmosis may be found in any site of the upper respiratory tract.[20, 21] From 40% to 75% of adults and 18% of children with progressive disseminated histoplasmosis have oropharyngeal involvement.[22] Goodwin and Des Prez found that 66% of those with chronic disseminated disease demonstrated oropharyngeal ulcers, and 24% had laryngeal lesions.[23] Smith and Utz, in a prospective study in 1972, demonstrated that only 15% of patients studied manifested isolated laryngeal disease, but 42% manifested orolaryngeal disease as part of disseminated histoplasmosis.[24] Mucous membrane lesions can occur in acute dissemination but are more common in more indolent cases. The usual sites are gums, tonsillar pillars, tongue, buccal mucosa, lip, and palate.[25, 26] Patients usually present with only one mucous membrane lesion. Progression is indolent, accompanied by ulceration. A distinct, heaped-up margin is characteristic, as is induration, even to the point of feeling hard or tumorlike. Local oropharyngeal and laryngeal involvement may be the only sign of disseminated infection.[27] The medical literature describes numerous instances in which laryngeal symptoms led to the diagnosis of histoplasmosis. In 1950, Roberts and Forman first described two cases of laryngeal histoplasmosis.[27] In another report, Hutchinson described a case in which disease was apparently limited not only to the larynx but more specifically to the right vocal fold (Fig. 29–3).[28] Firm, painful ulcers with heaped up edges, involving the tongue, buccal mucosa, pharynx, and larynx, are characteristic in this form of the disease. The lesions resemble tuberculosis and malignancy, which are the important differential diagnoses. The common presenting manifestations are sore throat, hoarseness, gingival ulceration, dysphagia, and occasionally stridor. On visualization, the laryngeal mucosa may appear pearly white and edematous or inflamed and ulcerative.

Occasionally, histoplasmosis involving the mandible has been described, as part of disseminated disease.[29]

Diagnosis

The diagnosis is made by taking a swab specimen from the center of an ulcer for microscopy and culture. Special stains (e.g., Gomori methenamine silver and periodic acid–Schiff–Gridly stains) usually demonstrate numerous macrophages containing yeast forms. Microscopically, the lesions of histoplasmosis may resemble tuberculoid granulomas with central caseation necrosis, giant cells, lymphocytes, plasma cells, and large numbers of macrophages, making it extremely difficult to distinguish histoplasmosis from tuberculosis. A high index of suspicion for histoplasmosis must be maintained, as the organism is not easily demonstrable on hematoxylin and eosin stain.

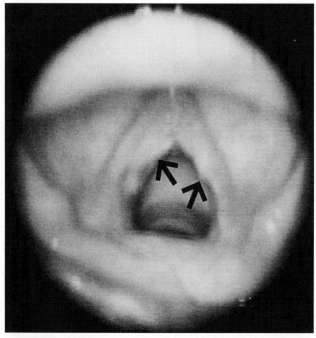

Figure 29–3. Appearance of the vocal fold masses *(arrows)* due to *H. capsulatum.*

H. capsulatum has been isolated in culture from blood, bone marrow, respiratory secretions, or localized skin lesions in >85% of cases of disseminated histoplasmosis. Growth on fungal media is relatively slow, requiring incubation for 4–5 days to several weeks. Definitive identification requires conversion of the mold to the yeast form, demonstration of specific reactivity with anti–*H. capsulatum* antiserums, or reactivity with nucleic acid probes.

The detection of antigen in body fluids permits the rapid diagnosis of disseminated histoplasmosis, such as seen in patients with AIDS. Antigen testing is performed by radio-immunoassay or enzyme immunoassay, using polyclonal antibodies to *H. capsulatum*. The specificity of antigen detection has been greater than 98%. Tests for antigen may be negative in 5%–10% of cases, mostly in those with mild clinical manifestations or localized sites of dissemination. Cross-reactions have occurred in patients with coccidioidomycosis, paracoccidioidomycosis, and blastomycosis.

Serologic tests are less sensitive than cultures or antigen detection in patients with disseminated histoplasmosis.

Treatment

Antifungal treatment is reserved for the more severe forms of histoplasmosis, such as disseminated histoplasmosis. The mortality rate of untreated disseminated histoplasmosis is >80%. With amphotericin B treatment, the mortality is between 7% and 23%, establishing the effectiveness of therapy.[30] Clinical improvement usually occurs within 1 week of treatment, although some patients may require 2 weeks. Relapsing infection, occurring in 5%–23% of treated cases, is more frequent in patients receiving less than 30 mg/kg of amphotericin B, supporting a total dose of at least 35 mg/kg, and at least 2 g in adults weighing less than 60 kg. Disseminated histoplasmosis relapses predictably (>90%) in patients with AIDS, which should be excluded if no other cause for relapse can be identified. Furthermore, because cure is unachievable, no basis exists for giving a large total dose in the initial treatment course of amphotericin B. A reasonable approach would be to give 1.0–1.5 g of amphotericin B over a 6–8 week period of induction therapy, followed by indefinite maintenance therapy with ketoconazole (400 mg daily), itraconazole (200 mg/day) or amphotericin B (50–100 mg weekly).

Ketoconazole is highly active in vitro against *H. capsulatum*: 90% of strains are inhibited by 0.1 μg/mL. Ketoconazole is effective treatment in nonimmunocompromised patients, with response rates of 70%–100%. However, ketoconazole is not an acceptable treatment for histoplasmosis in immunocompromised patients.[31]

Itraconazole given in doses of 200 mg 3 times daily for 3 days and then twice daily for 12 weeks is highly effective for patients with mild histoplasmosis, inducing remission in 85% of cases.[32] However, treatment failures occur in patients with moderately severe disease. The response to itraconazole was slower than the response to amphotericin B,[32] supporting the regimen of initial treatment with amphotericin B for patients with moderately severe or severe clinical manifestations. Interactions with drugs that reduce the absorption of itraconazole (H₂ antagonists and omeprazole) or accelerate its metabolism (rifampin, rifabutin, phenytoin, carbamazepine, and barbiturates) must be recognized before this treatment option is selected.

The role of fluconazole in induction therapy is under investigation in a prospective trial with an 800-mg daily dose.

PARACOCCIDIOIDOMYCOSIS

Mycology

Paracoccidioidomycosis is the most prevalent systemic mycosis in Latin America.[33] Its etiologic agent, *Paracoccidioides brasiliensis*, is a thermally dimorphic fungus only known in its asexual state.

The fungus grows as a yeast form in host tissues and in the laboratory when incubated at 37 °C; growth becomes apparent after 10–15 days of incubation from a single mother cell. In the yeast phase, the colonies are soft, wrinkled, cream-colored and composed of yeast cells of different sizes (4–30 μm), usually oval to elongated with multiple budding cells. Yeast cells have a well-defined thick refractile cell wall and a cytoplasm that contains lipid droplets. The mycelial form grows after 20–30 days of incubation at room temperature. Colonies are white, small, and irregular, covered by short aerial mycelia that often adhere to the agar, breaking its surface. Microscopically, the hyphae are thin and septate, and in usual laboratory media, sparse chlamydospores are the only additional structures seen. Culture and histologic diagnosis rely upon the most characteristic feature of the yeast form, which is the "pilot's wheel" appearance, i.e, a mother cell surrounded by multiple peripheral daughter cells.[34]

Epidemiology

The estimated number of infected individuals in the entire area of endemicity, where approximately 90 million people live, is close to 10 million. The disease is restricted to South and Central America and distributed heterogeneously throughout Latin America. Areas of high endemicity are located next to areas of very low incidence. The highest number of cases have been reported from Brazil, Colombia, and Venezuela.[35] Sporadic cases of paracoccidioidomycosis have been described in the United States. The majority of patients were immigrants from endemic areas of Central and South America, and reactivation of latent disease was the most probable mechanism for developing the disease.

Pathogenesis

Although the microniche of *P. brasiliensis* in nature is still unknown, it has been accepted that the fungus lives in soil, where it grows in the mycelial form. Conidia produced by the mycelium on simple natural media are a size compatible with aerial dispersion. Disease is acquired by inhaling conidia, which cause local pulmonary infection often followed by extrapulmonary dissemination.[36] Although neutrophils participate in the early inflammatory response to *P. brasiliensis*, the predominant tissue reaction is granulomatous.[37] The predominance of CD4 T lymphocytes in granulomas from patients with paracoccidioidomycosis provides clues to possible roles for T-cell subsets in immunoregulation. Depression of the cell-mediated immune response is a common finding in paracoccidioidomycosis and correlates strongly with the acute progressive form of the disease. It has been hypothesized that impaired cell-mediated responses in paracoccidioidomycosis are caused by the infection itself and that they contribute to the success of the pathogen. *P. brasiliensis*–induced impairment of cell-mediated immune responses is known to be reversible after successful antifungal therapy.

In an immunocompetent host, fungal growth is halted and the interaction ends with no apparent damage to the host (subclinical infection). If the host-fungus balance is upset by immunosuppression or other unknown causes, then infection progresses and gives rise to full-blown disease.[38]

Reactivation of latent disease seems to be the mode of acquisition of paracoccidioidomycosis in patients with AIDS. Because of the lack of cellular immunity, patients with AIDS experience severe progressive forms of paracoccidioidomycosis.

Clinical Manifestations

A wide spectrum of clinical manifestations is seen in patients with paracoccidioidomycosis, ranging from an indolent (chronic) form to a rapidly progressive disseminated disease (acute or subacute form). The chronic form usually affects adults older than 30 years of age, the clinical course is prolonged (frequently exceeding 6 months), and almost always the patient reveals pulmonary and mucosal involvement.[38] Lymph node enlargement can also be observed but is not a dominant finding. The acute form of paracoccidioidomycosis usually affects children, adolescents, and young adults. The clinical course is characterized by short duration, usually 1–2 months, with clinical manifestations compatible with involvement of the reticuloendothelial system, i.e., lymphadenopathy, hepatomegaly, and splenomegaly. Mucosal and pulmonary involvement are unusual.

Oropharyngolaryngeal Involvement. Oropharyngolaryngeal manifestations may be the first presentation and are fairly common.[39] Because of its frequency, early investigators postulated that the fungus would initially invade the oropharyngeal mucosa and then disseminate through the body by the lymphatic route. Concomitant pulmonary involvement is detectable in most of the cases as part of the chronic form of paracoccidioidomycosis. In a study of 343 patients with paracoccidioidomycosis, lesions involving the oral cavity were seen in 275 cases (80.1%), larynx in 41 (11.9%), pharynx in 24 (6.9%), and nasal mucosa in 3 (0.87%).[40] Lesions involving more than one site were seen in 91 cases (26%). Adenopathy with mucosal lesions were seen in 37 cases (10%).

Oral lesions are generally multiple in 85% of the cases, usually involving the gingiva or alveolar mucosa, followed by palate, lips, buccal mucosa, and, rarely, the tongue (Figs. 29–4 and 29–5). These lesions are generally silent, but

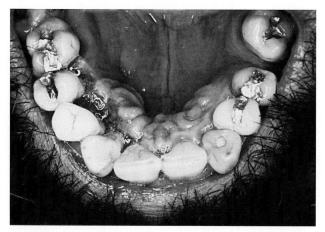

Figure 29–4. Oral mucosa involvement by *P. brasiliensis*. Note the mulberry-like infiltrative lesions of the gums behind the incisors and bicuspids.

when tooth extractions and surgical manipulation take place, exacerbation and dissemination of the infection to the other sites of the oral mucosa and lymph nodes become apparent.

Oropharyngolaryngeal lesions were first referred to as ulcerative mulberry-like (moriforme) stomatitis, thus defined because of the similarity of the ulcerative infiltrating process to the fine granulations of the mulberry fruit.[39] These lesions are located in the gums, mouth floor, lips, cheeks, soft palate, uvula, and pillars and are accompanied by abundant salivation and a painful reaction to mastication and swallowing. Oropharyngeal ulcerated lesions characterized by ulceration with a granular, rough, and irregular bottom are also seen in patients with paracoccidioidomycosis. Hypertrophic lesions predominate in the lips and cheeks and are characterized by an increase in a densely cellular infiltration of tissues.[41]

Another form occasionally seen is occult paracoccidioidic tonsillitis, which is characterized by gross features that give no indication of a mycotic lesion. The tonsils acquire a firm consistency and peritonsillar adherence occurs. Satellite

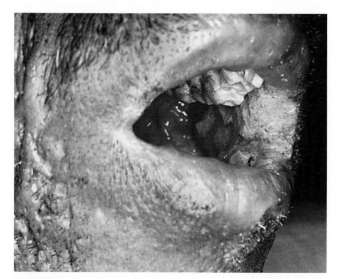

Figure 29–5. Oral mucosa involvement by *P. brasiliensis*. Note the thickened, infiltrated, white plaque on buccal mucosa.

adenopathy is frequently observed. Hoarseness, odynophagia, dysphagia, sore throat, dyspnea, and a "husky voice" are frequent clinical manifestations.[41]

Differential diagnosis of oropharyngeal lesions include tegumentary leishmaniasis, tuberculosis, syphilis, and neoplasms.

Lymph Node Involvement. Lymphadenopathy may be the major complaint, as is generally the case in children, adolescents, and young adults who exhibit the acute or subacute form of paracoccidioidomycosis. In patients with the chronic form, lymphadenopathy may be present, although it is not a major complaint and is frequently related to the presence of respiratory and mucocutaneous lesions.

The most common site of lymph node involvement is the cephalic segment, followed by the supraclavicular and axillary segments. In the cephalic segment, the submandibular and anteroposterior cervical lymph nodes are the most common areas of involvement. Abdominal lymphatic involvement, particularly the mesenteric lymph nodes, is also seen in some patients, and may be accompanied by malabsorption syndrome.

Patients with the nonsuppurative inflammatory type of adenopathy present with lymph nodes that are usually painless, noncoalescent, and without redness or heat. In the suppurative type, lymph nodes present fluctuation or a fistula, regardless of size.

Diagnosis

Paracoccidioidomycosis should be considered in patients with mucosal lesions, lymphadenopathy, and pulmonary involvement who have lived in or visited endemic areas of Central and South America.[35] Chest x-ray examination is important to assess lung involvement. Diagnosis is usually made by direct microscopic examination on potassium hydroxide preparation and culture of a clinical specimen, most commonly in sites such as skin, mucosa, and lymph node aspirates.[34] Oropharyngeal lesions, because of their frequency and easy access to the lesions, permit the collection of material for mycologic examination (Table 29–2).

By direct microscopy, *P. brasiliensis* is easily identified by its pilot wheel appearance, a mother cell surrounded by multiple buds. The organism grows on conventional Sabouraud or brain-heart infusion medium. Yeast forms usually take 10–14 days to grow at 37 °C. Anti–*P. brasiliensis* antibodies can be measured by different methods such as

Table 29–2. OROPHARYNGEAL AND CERVICAL LYMPH NODE INVOLVEMENT IN 471 PATIENTS WITH PARACOCCIDIOIDOMYCOSIS

Site	No. of Patients	Percentage
Oral cavity	275	58.8
Larynx	41	8.7
Pharynx	24	5.1
Nasal fossae	3	0.6
Cervical lymph nodes (adenopathy)	18	3.8
Cervical lymph nodes (adenopathy) plus oropharynx	19	4.0
Multiple sites	91	19.5
Total	471	100

counter-immunoelectrophoresis (CIE) and enzyme-linked immunosorbent assay. This is an option for the cases in which neither microscopy nor culture are positive. Immuno-compromised patients such as patients with AIDS are known to have a high rate of false-negative serologic results. Recently, a *P. brasiliensis* antigen assay detected circulating antigens in patients with paracoccidioidomycosis and AIDS and could be a promising diagnostic tool in this setting. Moreover, a polymerase chain reaction assay that can detect small amounts of *P. brasiliensis* DNA has recently been developed in our laboratory. This is another tool that might aid in diagnosis of paracoccidioidomycosis in immunocompromised patients, such as those with AIDS.

Treatment

Treatment of paracoccidioidomycosis in immunocompetent patients involves an initial phase of treatment with antifungal agents effective against *P. brasiliensis*, which include sulfonamide derivatives, sulfonamide-trimethoprim combination, amphotericin B, or azole derivatives, and a maintenance treatment for up to 1–2 years.[42]

Sulfonamide derivatives such as sulfadiazine are the oldest and the least efficient drugs against *P. brasiliensis*. Trimethoprim-sulfamethoxazole has proved to be very effective in the initial treatment of paracoccidioidomycosis at a dose of 800 mg/160 mg twice daily for 6 months, followed by a prolonged maintenance treatment with a daily half-dose of sulfadoxine (500 mg twice weekly) for up to 1 year after serologic tests become negative.

Amphotericin B is the most effective drug available for the treatment of paracoccidioidomycosis. Because of its toxicities, amphotericin B is indicated for severe cases or cases resistant to other drugs. Treatment should aim for a target dose of approximately 1.0 mg/kg body weight. The drug can be given on alternate days, and the total dose need not exceed 30 mg/kg. Maintenance treatment for months or years is generally necessary in order to effect a true cure.

The azole compounds are very effective in the treatment of paracoccidioidomycosis. Ketoconazole is generally recommended at a daily dose of 400 mg for 3 months, followed by a daily dose of 200 mg for 3 months. Itraconazole and fluconazole are also active against *P. brasiliensis*. Recent studies have shown that itraconazole is more effective than fluconazole for treatment of paracoccidioidomycosis. Clinical cure was obtained in 99% of the patients treated with a 100-mg/day dose of itraconazole for 6 months. Clinical experience with fluconazole is still restricted, and it may be a promising antifungal agent to treat central nervous involvement of paracoccidioidomycosis.[42]

MISCELLANEOUS FUNGI

Rhinosporidiosis

Rhinosporidiosis is a chronic granulomatous disease characterized by the formation of polypoid masses of inflamed mucous membranes, leading to indolent growth of a friable, soft, red-to-purple, vascular, lobulated polyp.[43] Tiny white dots may be seen underneath the epithelia, giving a characteristic strawberry-like surface. The etiologic agent is *Rhinosporidium seeberi*, an endosporulating organism believed by most microbiologists to be a fungus. The definite mode of transmission is unknown, but trauma is believed to be essential for disease development.

Oropharyngeal Involvement

Mucous membranes of the head and neck, such as those of the lachrymal sac, epiglottis, uvula, tongue, larynx, palate, tonsil, trachea, ethmoid sinus, or maxillary sinus are occasionally affected by *R. seeberi*. Rhinosporidial lesions of the tonsil, palate, or uvula are commonly sessile, resembling granulomas.[44] Hoarseness invariably accompanies laryngeal lesions.[45] Infection usually involves the nose with unilateral nasal obstruction by sessile granulomatous masses in 69.9% of the cases. Symptoms may be present for many years. In most of the cases, no systemic symptoms accompany rhinosporidiosis of the mucous membranes. Bacterial sinusitis may be precipitated by a paranasal sinus ostium. A thin, mucoid nasal discharge, sometimes with blood tingling, is often noted. Pain and frank epistaxis are uncommon, although nasal itching may occur.[46] Polypoid masses are sometimes visualized in the oropharynx or posterior nasopharynx.

Ocular involvement is the second most common site, responsible for 15.5% of the cases. The palpebral conjunctiva is the site most often involved, with the bulbar conjunctiva, corneal limbus, lachrymal caruncle, and canthus less often involved.[47]

Skin lesions have been rare, but have usually been found in association with nearby lesions of the nose and conjunctiva. However, multiple skin lesions are even rarer, indicating either multiple sites of inoculation or hematogenous dissemination.

Diagnosis

Since *R. seeberi* has not been successfully cultured in the laboratory, diagnosis relies on histopathologic analysis of the excised specimen or microscopic examination of nasal discharge or paranasal sinus irrigation fluid. Special stains are not usually necessary. The sporangia and the extruded spores confirm the diagnosis.[46] The sporangia from *R. seeberi* should not be confused with the spherules of *C. immitis*, which have smaller and thinner walls than the sporangia of *R. seeberi*. Furthermore, the sporangium of *R. seeberi* stains with mucicarmine, unlike *C. immitis*. The characteristic red-to-purple polypoid appearance of the lesion is also very helpful in diagnosis. Examination of the polyp may reveal the superficial location of the sporangia, which can be seen as small white dots with the naked eye.

Treatment

Spontaneous disappearance of the lesions is unusual. Surgical excision has been the only successful therapy. The optimal procedure is obtained by excision at the base of the polyp. In a series of 255 cases, lesions recurred in 27 patients after surgical removal.[44]

Phaeohyphomycosis

Ajello and colleagues proposed the term *phaeohyphomycosis* to cover all infections of a cutaneous, subcutaneous, and systemic nature caused by Hyphomycetes (*Alternaria, Anthopsis, Aureobasidium, Bipolaris, Cladosporium, Curvularia, Dactylaria, Exophiala, Exerohilium, Fonsecaea, Hormonema, Lecythophora, Mycocentrospora, Nigrospora, Oidiodendron, Phialemonium, Phialophora, Ramichloridium, Sarcinomyces, Scytalidium, Taeniolella, Tetraploa, Ulocladium*), Ascomycetes (*Arnium, Chaetomium*), and Coelomycetes (*Coniothyrium, Hendersonula, Phoma*), fungi that develop in the host tissues in the form of dark-walled dematiaceous septate mycelial or hyphal elements.[48] Such fungi produce a wide variety of clinical syndromes in humans including mycetoma, chromoblastomycosis, tinea nigra, black piedra, keratitis, and onychomycosis.[48]

Paranasal Sinus Involvement

New cases of sinusitis due to dematiaceous fungi, such as *Drechslera biseptata, Bipolaris spicifera, B. australiensis, B. hawaiiensis, Exserohilum rostratum, E. mcginnisii, Curvularia lunata, Alternaria* species, and *Cladosporium trichoides* have been reported in the medical literature.[49, 50]

Phaeohyphomycotic sinusitis is an indolent disease that may remain confined to the sinus cavity or may spread to contiguous structures over months and years. Clinical findings include allergic rhinitis-like symptoms, nasal polyps, postnasal drip, recurrent bacterial sinusitis, or intermittent sinus pain. Commonly a large mass has filled one or more of the paranasal sinuses, rather than just thickening of the mucosa.[51] Systemic complaints, such as fever and malaise, are rarely seen. Although leukocytosis is not a common feature, up to 20% of eosinophilia may be present. The ethmoid and maxillary sinuses are the most common sinuses involved. On CT scan, the thin lateral wall between the ethmoid and the orbit, the lamina papyracea, may be bowed laterally. Sometimes this may be visible as exophthalmos or broadening of the nasal bridge. Less commonly, the inferior wall of the ethmoid bows downward and medially into the nasal cavity. The sphenoid sinus is involved in a late stage and the frontal sinus usually spared.

Surgical findings include a thick, tenacious, inspissated, dark mucus likened to "rubber cement." Generally bony walls are thinned but intact. Species of *Alternaria* have caused necrotic lesions of the nasal septum in patients with acute leukemia or AIDS.

Differential diagnosis includes chronic allergic rhinitis with sinusitis and carcinoma of the sinus.

Diagnosis

Diagnosis relies on biopsy and histopathologic analysis of the specimen. Special stains are required to see the hyphae in deep tissue, though hyphae within the sinus mucosa are often visible with hematoxylin and eosin staining. Hyphae are usually yellowish-brown, regular-to-moniliform hyaline with or without budding cells, septate, occasionally branched, and 2–4 μm in diameter. Hyphae may be sparse or massive. In some cases, pigment on the hyphal wall may be too faint to be detected.

Material from surgical drainage or excision is cultured on Sabouraud agar, malt extract agar, or potato dextrose agar and incubated at both 30 and 37 °C for 10–20 days. Colonies of phaeohyphomycotic agents vary from yeastlike to woolly, depending on the species, but they are all deeply pigmented, gray, dark olive gray, dark brown, or nearly black.

Treatment

Surgical procedures, such as ethmoidectomy or the Caldwell-Luc procedure, have excellent results. However, symptoms may return in weeks or months, and sometimes five or more surgical procedures are needed, particularly if the surgeon does not aggressively clean out the affected area. A follow-up with CT scan or MRI should be done after surgery to define the postsurgical anatomy.

In the absence of surgery, it is not certain if any other treatment has any impact on the disease. Intravenous amphotericin B, oral ketoconazole, and oral itraconazole have all been advocated, but the appropriate dosage and duration of therapy are unknown. Itraconazole appears to be the most promising drug.[52]

Basidiomycosis

There are 16,000 species recognized within the phylum Basidiomycota, and they are widely distributed in nature. Only a few members of Basidiomycetes have been associated with human infection such as endocarditis, pneumonia, and sinusitis.[53]

Oropharyngeal, Sinus, and Neurologic Involvement

Sinus involvement by *Schizophyllum commune* has been described in the medical literature. Restrepo and colleagues have reported a 4-month-old child without any evidence of immunologic abnormality or illness who developed ulceration and perforation of the palate.[54] Further work-up revealed evidence of ocular, orbit, maxillary sinus, and base-of-the-brain involvement. Biopsy of the palate ulcer revealed a chronic inflammatory process in which submucosa had been penetrated by hyphae with walls of various degrees. Initial therapy with amphotericin B seemed to have resulted in a favorable outcome. Unfortunately, the patient lost follow-up after leaving the hospital. Presumed maxillary sinusitis by *S. commune* has been described in three other patients.[55, 56] Sinus contents removed by surgery consisted of necrotic debris and purulent material mixed with bacteria and thick-walled hyphae, branched with occasional clamp connections. Although severe acute and subacute inflammation was seen in the mucosal sections, no actual invasion of hyphae into the sinus mucosa was detected in two cases. One of these three patients had AIDS.

Fusariosis

Fusarium species, which are soil saprophytes with a worldwide distribution, have increasingly been reported from colonizing and disseminated infection in patients with severe underlying diseases.[57] *Fusarium* species most often reported from human infection have been *Fusarium solani, Fusarium oxysporum*, and *Fusarium moniliforme*.[57, 58]

The incidence of *Fusarium* species causing human infections, especially invasive disease in the compromised host, has been increasing. Infection due to *Fusarium* may be localized or hematogenously disseminated.

Disseminated Disease

The disseminated cases to date have occurred in patients with a hematopoietic malignant disorder except for three patients who were receiving corticosteroid therapy, three who were severely neutropenic from either aplastic anemia or from treatment from neuroblastoma, and a burn patient. Clinical manifestations in those patients included fever and myalgia, followed in 66% of cases by skin lesions.[59] These lesions, which resemble ecthyma gangrenosum in appearance and on histopathologic study, tend to be multiple and located on the extremities. Each lesion begins with focal pain and macular or papular erythema. The portal of entry into the body has been obscure, although an indwelling intravascular catheter was implicated in five cases. Patients who have fusariosis at a site of probable inoculation only infrequently develop disseminated infection. Blood cultures were positive in 59% of disseminated cases.

Oronasopharynx and Sinus Involvement in Disseminated Fusariosis

Involvement of the orbit and the oral, nasal, sinus, and lung tracts is relatively common in patients with disseminated fusariosis. In a review article, 9 of 29 patients (31%) with disseminated fusariosis described in the medical literature revealed sinus and oronasopharyngeal involvement.[57]

Clinical manifestations such as severe maxillary sinusitis, mucosal ulcerations, and tracheobronchitis extending from the base of the tongue through the larynx have been described in these patients. Sinus and mucosa biopsy with culture were important diagnostic tools to establish the involvement of these organs by *Fusarium* species. However, skin involvement with multiple necrotic lesions was detected in the majority of these patients, and skin biopsy with culture led to the diagnosis in most of the cases. Infection in other organ sites, including the central nervous system, gastrointestinal tract, and kidney, was less frequently documented.

Despite the high frequency of antemortem detection and institution of one or more antifungal therapies with high-dose amphotericin B alone or plus 5-fluorocytosine in 23 patients with disseminated fusariosis, only 5 (22%) had resolution of the fusariosis.

Localized Fusariosis

Fusarium species have caused infections in the immunocompetent human host, but they have usually been limited to superficial sites such as the nail plate or have been a superinfecting agent of deep skin ulcers, third-degree burns, or surgical wounds. Less commonly, these organisms have been documented as etiologic agents in localized tissue infections such as keratomycosis; endophthalmitis; peritonitis; paronychia; post-traumatic lesions of the bone, joint, or skin; brain abscess; and invasive nasal infection.

Invasive Nasal Infection

Valenstein and Schell have described a diabetic woman who presented with a 3-week history of fever, malaise, and fatigue.[60] Physical examination revealed a black 1×1.5 cm eschar located in the posterior portion of her left middle turbinate. The infection simulated early rhinocerebral mucormycosis clinically. However, the excisional biopsy of the lesion revealed hyphae that were readily identified in hematoxylin and eosin and periodic acid–Schiff stained sections of paraffin-embedded tissue. Culture of the lesion grew *F. oxysporum*. The patient eventually was found to have adenocarcinoma of the sigmoid colon.

An important feature of this novel pattern of *Fusarium* infection is the potential for clinical and histologic confusion with early rhinocerebral mucormycosis, which might lead to unnecessary nasal and sinus exploration.

Penicilliosis marneffei

Because members of the genus *Penicillium* are abundant in the environment, *Penicillium* species are among the most common laboratory contaminants. When a common *Penicillium* is isolated from a patient, a diagnosis of penicilliosis can be confirmed only through examining tissue sections for the presence of the fungus.[61]

Among numerous species of the genus *Penicillium*, *Penicillium marneffei* is the only species known to be a primary pathogen of humans, with at least 30 reports in the medical literature. This species is unique among the members of *Penicillium* by having thermal dimorphism, and it is geographically restricted to Southeast Asia and part of the Far East.[62] *P. marneffei* infection affects either immunocompetent or immunocompromised hosts, such as patients with AIDS or Hodgkin's disease and those receiving corticosteroid.[63]

The clinical manifestations of penicilliosis marneffei have included fever, weight loss, anemia, and gradual progression to death unless treated. Although cases with localized disease have been reported, disseminated progressive penicilliosis is the most common form of the disease. The course of the illness ranges from 1 month to 3 years. Lymph nodes, lungs, liver, and skin are the organs most commonly involved.

Nasopharyngeal involvement by *P. marneffei* was described in a patient with nasopharyngeal carcinoma. The organism was seen but not cultured in necrotic tissue at the site of the nasopharyngeal carcinoma.[64]

Microscopic examination of histopathologic sections stained with Gomori methenamine silver or periodic acid–Schiff shows yeastlike cells with cross-walls and confirms the diagnosis. Microscopically, the fungi when in histiocytes closely resemble *H. capsulatum*. To culture *P. marneffei*, clinical samples can be inoculated onto Sabouraud agar slants with antibacterial antibiotics and incubated at 25 and 37 °C to demonstrate thermal dimorphism.

Amphotericin B appears to be the drug of choice for

penicilliosis marneffei, especially for those patients who are critically ill. The organism appears to be susceptible to flucytosine, and some patients have responded to the combination of flucytosine and amphotericin B. Itraconazole may offer an oral alternative to amphotericin B.[65] Deaths early during therapy indicated the need for prompt diagnosis.

References

1. Bradsher RW: Blastomycosis. Infect Dis Clin North Am 1988; 2: 877–898.

2. Sarosi GA, Davies SF: Blastomycosis. Am Rev Respir Dis 1979; 120: 911–938.

3. Witorsch P, Utz JP: North American blastomycosis: A study of 40 patients. Medicine 1968; 47: 169–200.

4. Reder PA, Neel B: Blastomycosis in otolaryngology: Review of a large series. Laryngoscope 1993; 103: 53–58.

5. Rose HD, Gingrass DJ: Localized oral blastomycosis mimicking actinomycosis. Oral Surg 1982; 54: 12–14.

6. Scully C, Paes de Almeida O: Oral manifestations of the systemic mycosis. J Oral Pathol Med 1992; 21: 289–294.

7. Gerwin JM, Myer CM III: Intranasal blastomycosis. Am J Otolaryngol 1981; 2: 267–273.

8. Angtuaco EEC, Angtuaco EJC, Glasier CM, Benitez WI: Nasopharyngeal and temporal bone blastomycosis: CT and MR findings. Am J Neurol Radiol 1991; 12: 725–728.

9. Greer AE: North American blastomycosis of a nasal sinus: Report of a case. Dis Chest 1960; 38: 454–458.

10. Istorico LJ, Sanders M, Jacobs RF, et al.: Otitis media due to blastomycosis: Report of two cases. Clin Infect Dis 1992; 14: 355–358.

11. Day TA, Stucker FJ: Blastomycosis of paranasal sinuses. Otolaryngol Head Neck Surg 1994; 110: 437–440.

12. Parker JC, McClaskey JJ, Lee RS: The emergence of candidosis. The postmortem cerebral mycosis. Am J Clin Pathol 1978; 70: 31–36.

13. Papas PG, Pottage JC, Powderly WG, et al.: Blastomycosis in patients with the acquired immunodeficiency syndrome. Ann Intern Med 1992; 116: 853–857.

14. Abernathy RS: Amphotericin therapy of North American blastomycosis. Antimicrob Agents Chemother 1967; 3: 208–211.

14a. Dismukes WE, Stamm AM, Graybill JR, et al.: Treatment of systemic mycoses with ketoconazole: Emphasis on toxicity and clinical response in 52 patients. Ann Intern Med 1983; 98: 13–20.

15. National Institute of Allergy and Infectious Diseases Mycoses Study Group: Treatment of blastomycosis and histoplasmosis with ketoconazole: Results of a prospective, randomized clinical trial. Ann Intern Med 1985; 103: 861–872.

16. Wheat LJ: Systemic fungal infections: diagnosis and treatment. I. Histoplasmosis. Infect Dis Clin North Am 1988; 2: 841–859.

17. Deepe GS Jr, Bullock WE: Histoplasmosis: Granulomatous inflammatory response. In: Gallin JI, Goldstein IM, Snyderman R (eds): Inflammation: Basic Principles and Clinical Correlates. New York: Raven Press, pp 733–749.

18. Grayston JT, Fuscolon ML: The occurrence of histoplasmosis in epidemics: Epidemiological studies. Am J Public Health 1953; 43: 665–676.

19. Wheat LJ: Endemic mycosis in AIDS. Clin Microbiol Rev 1995; 8: 146–159.

20. Bennett DE: Histoplasmosis of the oral cavity and larynx. Arch Intern Med 1980; 59: 1–33.

21. Calcaterra TC: Orolaryngeal histoplasmosis. Laryngoscope 1970; 80: 111–120.

22. Pillsbury HC III, Sasaki CT: Granulomatous disease of the larynx. Otolaryngol Clin North Am 1982; 15: 539–551.

23. Goodwin RA, Des Prez RM: Histoplasmosis. Am Rev Respir Dis 1978; 157: 929–956.

24. Smith JW, Utz JP: Progressive disseminated histoplasmosis: A prospective study of 26 patients. Ann Intern Med 1972; 75: 557–565.

25. Scully C, Almeida OP: Orofacial manifestations of the systemic mycosis. J Oral Pathol Med 1992; 21: 289–294.

26. Rajah V, Essa A: Histoplasmosis of the oral cavity, oropharynx and larynx. J Laryngol Otol 1993; 107: 58–61.

27. Roberts SE, Forman FS: Histoplasmosis. A deficiency disease: Report of two cases with laryngeal involvement. Ann Oral Rhinol Laryngol 1950; 59: 809–822.

28. Hutchinson HE: Laryngeal histoplasmosis simulating carcinoma. J Pathol Bacteriol 1952; 64: 309–319.

29. Dobleman TJ, Scher N, Goldman M, Doot S: Invasive histoplasmosis of the mandible. Head Neck 1989; 11: 81–84.

30. Sarosi GA, Davies SF: Gastrointestinal involvement in histoplasmosis. Pract Gastroenterol 1984; 8: 19–31.

31. Dismukes WE, Cloud G, Bowles C, et al.: Treatment of blastomycosis and histoplasmosis with ketoconazole. Ann Intern Med 1985; 103: 861–872.

32. Wheat LJ, Hafwer RE, Ritchie M, Schneider D: Itraconazole is effective treatment for histoplasmosis in AIDS: Prospective multicenter noncomparative trial. Abstract 1206. In: Program and Abstracts of the 32nd Interscience Conference on Antimicrobial Agents and Chemotherapy. Washington, DC: American Society for Microbiology, p 312.

33. Restrepo A: The ecology of *Paracoccidioides brasiliensis*: A puzzle still unsolved. J Med Vet Mycol 1985; 23: 323–334.

34. Bethlem NM, Lemle A, Bethlem E, Wanke B: Paracoccidioidomycosis. Semin Respir Med 1991; 12: 81–86.

35. Greer DL, Restrepo A: La epidemiologia de la paracoccidioidomycosis. Bol Sanit Panam 1977; 83: 428–445.

36. Franco M, Mendes RP, Moscardi-Bacchi, Montenegro MR: Paracoccidioidomycosis. Baillieres's Clin Trop Med Commun Dis 1989; 4: 185–220.

37. Motta I, Pupo JA: Granulomatose paracoccidiodica ("Blastomycose brasileira"): I. Estudo anatomo-clinico das lesões cutâneas. II. Estudo clínico das blastomycoses tegumentares. An Fac Med São Paulo 1936; 12: 407–423.

38. Giraldo RA, Restrepo F, Gutierrez M, et al.: Pathogenesis of paracoccidioidomycosis: A model based on the study of 46 patients. Mycopathologia 1976; 58: 63–70.

39. Paiva LJ, Lacaz CS: Oropharyngolaryngeal lesions. In: Franco M, Lacaz C, Restrepo-Moreno A, Del Negro G (eds): Paracoccidioidomycosis. Boca Raton, Florida: CRC Press, 1994, p 267.

40. Rapoport A, Santos IC, Sobrinho JA, et al.: Importancia da blastomicose sul americana (B.S.A.) no diagnostico diferencial com as neoplasias malignas de cabeca e pescoco. Rev Bras Cir Cab Pesc 1974; 1: 13–33.

41. Sposto MR, Mendes-Gianni MJ, Moraes RA, et al.: Paracoccidioidomycosis manifesting as oral lesions: Clinical, cytological and serological investigation. J Oral Pathol Med 1994; 23: 83–87.

42. Mendes RP, Negroni R, Arechavala A: Treatment and control of cure. In: Franco M, Lacaz CS, Restrepo-Moreno A, Del Negro G (eds): Paracoccidioidomycosis. Boca Raton, Florida: CRC Press, 1994, p 373.

43. Fortin R, Meisels A: Rhinosporidiosis. Acta Cytol 1974; 18: 169–173.

44. Satyanarayana C: Rhinosporidiosis with a record of 255 cases. Acta Otolaryngol 1960; 51: 348–366.

45. Pillai OSR: Rhinosporidiosis of the larynx. J Laryngol Otol 1974; 88: 277–280.

46. Prins LC, Tnage RA, Dingemans KP: Rhinosporidiosis in the Netherlands. ORL J Otorhinolaryngol Relat Spec 1983; 45: 237–244.

47. Neumayr TG: Bilateral rhinosporidiosis of the conjunctiva. Arch Ophthalmol 1964; 71: 379–381.

48. Ajello L, Georg LK, Steigbigel RT, Wang CJ: A case of phaeohyphomycosis caused by a new species of *Phialophora*. Mycologia 1974; 66: 490–498.

49. Bartynski JM, McCaffrey TV, Frigas E: Allergic fungal sinusitis secondary to dematiaceous fungi: *Curvularia lunata* and *Alternaria*. Otolaryngol Head Neck Surg 1990; 103: 32–39.

50. Frenkel L, Kuhls TL, Nitta K, et al.: Recurrent bipolaris sinusitis following surgical and antifungal therapy. Pediatr Infect Dis J 1987; 6: 1130–1132.

51. Aviv JE, Lawson W, Bottone EJ, et al.: Multiple intracranial mucoceles associated with phaeohyphomycosis of the paranasal sinuses. Arch Otolaryngol Head Neck Surg 1990; 116: 1210–1213.

52. Sharkey PK, Graybill JR, Rinaldi MG, et al.: Itraconazole treatment of phaeohyphomycosis. J Am Acad Dermatol 1990; 23: 577–586.

53. Greer DL: Basidiomycetes as agents of human infections: A review. Mycopathologia 1979; 65: 133–139.

54. Restrepo A, Greer DL, Robledo M: Ulceration of the palate caused by a basidiomycete *Schizophyllum commune*. Sabouraudia 1973; 11: 201–204.

55. Kern ME, Uecker FA: Maxillary sinus infection caused by the homobasidiomycetous fungus *Schizophyllum commune*. J Clin Microbiol 1986; 23: 1001–1005.

56. Rosenthal J, Katz R, DuBois DB, et al.: Chronic maxillary sinusitis associated with the mushroom *Schizophyllum commune* in a patient with AIDS. Clin Infect Dis 1992; 14: 46–48.

57. Anaisse E, Kantarijian H, Jones P: Fungal infection caused by *Fusarium* in cancer patients. Am J Clin Oncol 1987; 10: 86–87.

58. Collins MS, Rinaldi MG: Cutaneous infection in man caused by *Fusarium moniliforme*. Sabouradia 1977; 15: 151–160.

59. Merz WG, Karp JE, Hoagland M, et al.: Diagnosis and successful treatment of fusariosis in the compromised host. J Infect Dis 1988; 158: 1046–1055.

60. Valenstein P, Schell MS: Primary intranasal *Fusarium* infection. Arch Pathol Lab Med 1986; 110: 751–754.

61. DiSalvo AF, Fickling AM, Ajello L: Infection caused by *Penicillium marneffei*. Am J Clin Pathol 1973; 60: 259–263.

62. Capponi M, Sureau P, Segretain G: Penicilliose de *Rhizomys sinensis*. Bull Soc Pathol Exot 1956; 49: 418–421.

63. Deng ZL, Conner DH: Progressive disseminated penicilliosis caused by *Penicillium marneffei*: Report of eight cases and differentiation of the causative organism from *Histoplasma capsulatum*. Am J Clin Pathol 1985; 84: 323–327.

64. Piehl MR, Kaplan RL, Harber MH: Disseminated penicilliosis in a patient with acquired immunodeficiency syndrome. Arch Pathol Lab Med 1988; 112: 1262–1264.

65. Hilmarsdottir I, Meynard JL, Rogeaux O, et al.: Disseminated *Penicillium marneffei* infection associated with human immunodeficiency virus: A report of two cases and a review of 35 published cases. J Acquir Immune Defic Synd 1993; 6: 466–471.

Ann R. Falsey
Caroline Breese Hall

C H A P T E R   T H I R T Y

Viruses

▼

Viruses are a diverse group of pathogens responsible for a large percentage of all acute infectious diseases. This chapter reviews those agents causing syndromes likely to be encountered by the otolaryngologist. Upper respiratory infections (URIs) are an important cause of human disease by virtue of their frequency and associated disability. The average preschool child experiences 6–10 colds per year, and the average adult has 2–4 colds per year. Women in the child-bearing ages of 20–30 years have the highest rates of URIs in adults.[1] Colds account for 17% of acute illness visits to health-care providers, and an average of two drugs are recommended per patient visit.[2, 3] In addition to enormous amounts of money spent on over-the-counter medications, URIs are a major cause of school and work absenteeism. Viruses are the major cause of acute respiratory infections that include the common cold, pharyngitis, laryngitis, and bronchitis. The supply of viruses that infect the respiratory tract is abundant; thus, even if immunity to one is good, there is a nearly endless number of viruses and subtypes. Direct viral invasion or secondary bacterial infection may result in the complications of otitis media, sinusitis, and pneumonia (Fig. 30–1). The common respiratory viruses are reviewed with attention to specific clinical syndromes, diagnosis, and treatment if available (Table 30–1). In addition, several members of the herpesvirus family including Epstein-Barr virus (EBV), herpes simplex virus (HSV), and varicella-zoster virus (VZV), all of which cause diseases affecting the ears, nose, and throat, are discussed. Lastly, viral causes of parotitis and mumps are considered.

RESPIRATORY VIRUSES

Rhinovirus

Rhinoviruses are single-stranded RNA viruses belonging to the picornavirus family and are the major cause of the common cold.[4] Approximately 70%–80% of rhinovirus infections are symptomatic. Illness is typically self-limited and characterized by nasal congestion, sneezing, mild sore throat, and cough.[1] Viremia is not observed, and this may be because the virus does not replicate well at 37 °C. Minimal damage is caused by direct viral invasion of the epithelium.[5] Rather, symptoms are due to the release of inflammatory mediators, such as bradykinin and lysyl bradykinin, which cause vascular engorgement, influx of neutrophils, and pro-

duction of mucus.[6] These events may lead to changes in resident bacterial flora and predispose to secondary bacterial infection.[7]

Complications of rhinovirus infections occur in a minority of cases because of impairment of drainage of the paranasal sinuses and middle ear. Otitis media occurs in approximately 2% of common colds.[8] Experimental rhinovirus infection in adults has been shown to cause marked changes in eustachian tube function and middle ear pressure lasting as long as 10 days.[9] In addition, viral infection of the middle ear may help explain antibiotic failure in children with acute otitis media.[10] Presumed bacterial sinusitis complicates common colds in approximately 0.5% of cases.[8] However, involvement of the paranasal sinuses in colds is common. In a recent study of 31 early cold sufferers who were examined by computed tomography (CT), more than 80% had abnormalities of their ethmoid and/or maxillary sinuses, and over one third had abnormal frontal or sphenoid sinuses.[11]

The treatment of rhinovirus infections is currently symptomatic. Short courses of experimental treatment with intranasal interferon-α2 provide modest benefits, while long-term prophylaxis with interferon has been hampered by unacceptable side effects.[5] Diagnosis of secondary bacterial infection of the sinuses and middle ear is a difficult clinical problem that is discussed in other chapters. These conditions require appropriate antimicrobial treatment.

Coronaviruses

Coronaviruses are a group of RNA viruses belonging to the family Coronaviridae, first recognized in 1965 as an agent causing the common cold.[4] Two of these strains, 229E and OC43, have been shown to be a major cause of URIs in children and adults, implicated in approximately 10%–20% of cases.[12] Colds associated with coronavirus are generally mild and characterized by nasal congestion and sore throat, but the virus occasionally causes lower respiratory symptoms in young children.[13] Diagnosis is difficult to make since the organism is not easily isolated and serologic tests are generally not available except in research settings.

Influenza Viruses

Influenza viruses are single-stranded RNA viruses belonging to the family Orthomyxoviridae. Three types of influenza

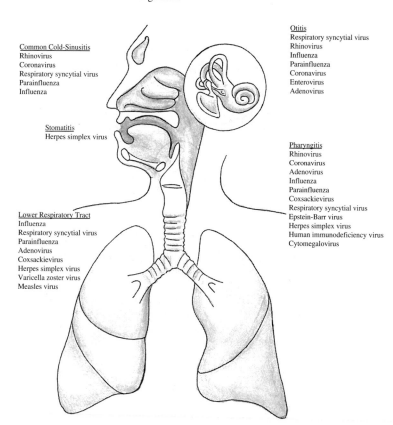

<u>Common Cold-Sinusitis</u>
Rhinovirus
Coronavirus
Respiratory syncytial virus
Parainfluenza
Influenza

<u>Stomatitis</u>
Herpes simplex virus

<u>Lower Respiratory Tract</u>
Influenza
Respiratory syncytial virus
Parainfluenza
Adenovirus
Coxsackievirus
Herpes simplex virus
Varicella zoster virus
Measles virus

<u>Otitis</u>
Respiratory syncytial virus
Rhinovirus
Influenza
Parainfluenza
Coronavirus
Enterovirus
Adenovirus

<u>Pharyngitis</u>
Rhinovirus
Coronavirus
Adenovirus
Influenza
Parainfluenza
Coxsackievirus
Respiratory syncytial virus
Epstein-Barr virus
Herpes simplex virus
Human immunodeficiency virus
Cytomegalovirus

Figure 30–1. Viruses that infect the respiratory tract shown by anatomic location. RSV (respiratory syncytial virus), HSV (herpes simplex virus), VZV (varicella-zoster virus), EBV (Epstein-Barr virus), HIV (human immunodeficiency virus), and CMV (cytomegalovirus).

Table 30–1. RESPIRATORY VIRUSES

Virus	Subgroups	Primary Transmission	Incubation (Days)	Season	Syndrome	Diagnosis	Antiviral
Rhinovirus	>100	Fomites	2–3	All year Peak: fall–spring	URI	Culture (NP/NW)	None
Coronavirus	≥5	Unknown	1–2	Winter–spring	URI Bronchitis	Research only	None
Influenza	A, B, C	Aerosol	2	Winter	Flulike illness Pneumonia	Culture (NP/NW) Serologic test Rapid antigen	Amantadine Rimantadine Ribavirin
Respiratory syncytial virus	A, B	Large-droplet, fomites	3–5	Winter	URI Bronchiolitis Pneumonia	Culture (NP/NW) Serologic test Rapid antigen	Ribavirin
Parainfluenza	1, 2, 3	Large-droplet, fomites	1–4	Fall–early winter Spring	Croup Bronchiolitis Pneumonia	Culture (NW/NP) Serologic test	None
	4a, 4b			All year	URI		
Adenovirus	47	Fecal–oral Large-droplets, fomites	2–14	All year	URI, LRI Pharyngitis Pharyngo-conjunctival fever	Culture (NP/NW, stool conjunctiva)	None
Enteroviruses	67	Fecal–oral	3–7	Summer	URI, LRI Febrile illnesses Herpangina Hand-foot-and-mouth	Culture (NP/NW vesicles, stool)	None

NP/NW, nasopharyngeal swab or wash; URI, upper respiratory infection; LRI, lower respiratory infection.

virus have been identified: A, B, and C with subtypes and strains within the types. Influenza C likely represents another genus and causes only mild illness. Influenza pandemics occur at irregular intervals and are caused by a major change in either of the two surface proteins, the hemagglutinin (H) and the neuraminidase (N). The current circulating subtypes are H3N2 and H1N1. All three types of influenza may be present during the same season, although dominance may vary. Influenza A predominates most years with influenza B becoming dominant every 2–4 years.[4]

Influenza is most efficiently transmitted through inhalation of small aerosols.[14] After entering the body, the virus multiples in the ciliated columnar epithelium of the upper and lower respiratory tract, causing cell necrosis and sloughing.[15] There is considerable variation in the severity of illness caused by influenza infection, which is influenced by age, general health, and previous immune status. Typical influenza is characterized by the abrupt onset of fever, headache, myalgias, sore throat, and a nonproductive cough. A clear nasal discharge is common, but nasal obstruction is uncommon. The pharynx may be hyperemic, but exudate is rarely present.[16] Complications of influenza include primary viral pneumonia as well as secondary bacterial pneumonia.[17] In children an interstitial pneumonia that cannot be differentiated from other types of viral pneumonia is common. Additionally, influenza viruses have also been implicated as a cause of otitis media in children.[18] Eighty percent of adults challenged with influenza A virus developed eustachian tube dysfunction, and 20% developed otitis with effusion.[19]

Generally, uncomplicated influenza in healthy persons does not require therapy. Amantadine and rimantadine are both licensed in the United States for the treatment and prevention of influenza A. Neither has activity against influenza B. Both drugs, when administered early in illness, have been shown to shorten illness and reduce symptoms.[20] The dosage of amantadine for young healthy persons is 200 mg orally initially, then 100 mg orally twice daily thereafter. The dosage must be reduced in elderly persons and those with renal impairment. Unfortunately, central nervous system (CNS) side effects and drug resistance limit the usefulness of these drugs. Ribavirin is a nucleoside analogue that demonstrates antiviral activity against both influenza A and B; however, clinical efficacy of this drug for the treatment of influenza has not been clearly established.[20]

Respiratory Syncytial Virus

Respiratory syncytial virus (RSV) is a single-stranded RNA virus belonging to the Paramyxoviridae family. RSV is recognized worldwide as the most important cause of serious respiratory infections in young children and causes yearly epidemics of disease in temperate climates.[21] By the age of 2 years most people are infected; however, immunity is incomplete and reinfections occur throughout life.[22] Generally, reinfection in older children and healthy young adults causes a URI.[23]

Both upper and lower respiratory tract diseases are attributable to RSV. Signs of infection include fever, nasal congestion, pharyngitis, and otitis media.[24] In a 14-year longitudinal study of respiratory illnesses in children, one third of RSV infections were associated with acute otitis media.[25] RSV has also been recovered from middle ear effusions of children with otitis, supporting its direct role in the pathogenesis of otitis media.[26] Involvement of the lower respiratory tract occurs most frequently with young children with primary infection and may be manifested as croup, bronchitis, bronchiolitis, or pneumonia. Nonspecific symptoms, such as lethargy and poor feeding, may be seen in infants.[24] Ribavirin has been shown to be clinically effective in reducing the severity of illness in infants infected with RSV.[27] Ribavirin therapy is indicated for the treatment of hospitalized infants at high risk for serious disease or immunocompromised hosts with documented RSV infection.[24]

Parainfluenza Viruses

Parainfluenza viruses are single-stranded RNA viruses belonging to the paramyxovirus family. Parainfluenza viruses are a very common cause of respiratory illness in humans; however, the epidemiology and specific syndromes vary with age and virus serotype.[4] Illness rates with parainfluenza are highest in children under 4 years of age so that by 5 years of age, approximately 75% of the population has been infected.[28] Parainfluenza virus types 1 and 2 are the leading cause of croup, have a peak incidence at the ages of 2–6 years, and occur in fall–early winter epidemics. Parainfluenza 1 tends to occur in odd-numbered years, whereas parainfluenza 2 is less predictable.[29] Parainfluenza 3 causes approximately 40% of its infections in the first 12 months of life. Peaks of activity are seen in the spring or summer in North America. Bronchiolitis and pneumonia are the most common clinical syndromes. Parainfluenza 4 is not commonly identified and causes mild URIs and asymptomatic infections.[1, 30]

In addition to lower respiratory tract infection, parainfluenza viruses may cause pharyngitis, conjunctivitis, and otitis media. In a study involving 363 children, parainfluenza virus was detected in the nasopharyngeal secretions of 4% of children with acute otitis media.[31] Reinfection with parainfluenza viruses occurs throughout life, with illness generally manifesting as a mild URI.

Adenoviruses

The adenoviruses were discovered in 1953 by Rowe and colleagues when the organism was isolated from degenerating adenoidal tissue.[32] These viruses are double-stranded DNA viruses and belong to the family Adenoviridae. Adenovirus infections are ubiquitous, and primary infection usually takes place in the first few years of life. This group of viruses causes the widest variety of illnesses of all the respiratory viruses. Approximately 50% of adenovirus infections are symptomatic.[33] Of symptomatic infections, nearly 60%–80% involve the respiratory tract, with the remaining 40% associated with CNS, urinary tract, gastrointestinal, and undifferentiated febrile illnesses.[34]

When adenovirus infection causes respiratory disease in children, it usually takes the form of coryza, pharyngitis, or bronchiolitis.[35] Adenovirus pharyngitis may be indistinguishable from group A streptococcal disease.[36] Adenovirus type 4 has been associated with epidemics of acute respiratory illness in military recruits, in whom up to one fifth require hospitalization.[37] Pharyngoconjunctival fever is a common illness seen by physicians at summer camps and is characterized by the acute onset of conjunctivitis, pharyngitis, rhinitis, and cervical adenitis. Adenovirus type 3 is the usual agent, and contaminated swimming water has been implicated as the source of disease in outbreaks.[38]

No specific treatment for adenovirus infection is available. Recently, ganciclovir has been evaluated as a possible treatment for severe adenovirus infections, and results show some promise.[39] Live vaccine for adenovirus types 4 and 7 has been used successfully in military populations but is not recommended for use in the general population.

VIRUSES CAUSING OROPHARYNGEAL DISEASE

Enteroviruses

The genus *Enterovirus* is one of four genera belonging to the Picornaviridae family. The enteroviruses are RNA viruses consisting of five different groups and a total of 67 different agents: group A coxsackieviruses, group B coxsackieviruses, echoviruses, polioviruses, and the newer enteroviruses, types 68–71.[40] Although these agents share certain biologic characteristics, individual agents cause widely varied clinical manifestations. More than 50% of the infections are asymptomatic. Most of the reported cases occur in young children (56% <10 years and 26% <1 year of age). Infections are most common in the summer and may result in URIs, pneumonia, exanthems, nonspecific fevers, and neurologic symptoms.[41–43]

Herpangina is a syndrome characterized by a vesicular enanthem of the soft palate and fauces accompanied by fever, sore throat, and painful swallowing.[44] Children between the ages of 3 and 10 years are most commonly affected. Coxsackieviruses from group A (1–10, 16, 22) are the most common agents, but occasionally echoviruses and coxsackievirus B have been implicated. Characteristic findings are 6–12 punctate macules on the soft palate, which then ulcerate in 24–48 hours. A nodular variant has been described in which tiny nodules packed with lymphocytes appear in the same distribution but do not ulcerate.[45] Patients generally do not appear very ill and recover in 2–7 days. Herpangina can be confused with herpes simplex stomatitis but can be distinguished by the lack of anterior mouth involvement and systemic toxicity.[44]

Hand-foot-and-mouth disease is a syndrome most commonly caused by coxsackievirus A16 and is characterized by vesicular stomatitis and exanthem. Children are most commonly affected and present with fevers of 38–39 °C and vesicles on the buccal mucosa and tongue. Cutaneous lesions are seen in approximately 75% of cases. The classic rash is found on the hands and feet (both palmar and extensor surfaces), as well as the genitalia and buttocks.[46]

Human Immunodeficiency Virus

The acquired immunodeficiency syndrome (AIDS), which was first recognized in 1981, is caused by infection with a retrovirus, human immunodeficiency virus (HIV) 1 and, to a lesser extent, HIV-2. Exposure to HIV may be followed by an acute febrile illness 1–8 weeks later, at the time of seroconversion. This primary infection syndrome may take the form of a mononucleosis-like illness or acute encephalopathy. Febrile pharyngitis is a characteristic of primary HIV infection. Marked pharyngeal erythema has been described, as well as mucosal ulceration but no exudate. In some cases lymphadenopathy and a nonpruritic maculopapular rash on the upper body may develop.[47] More advanced HIV infection has been associated with a number of other conditions affecting the head and neck: parotid gland enlargement, chronic serous otitis, facial nerve palsies, and hypertrophy of nasopharyngeal lymphatic tissues.[48]

Epstein-Barr Virus

EBV is a double-stranded DNA virus in the Herpesviridae family and the cause of heterophile-positive infectious mononucleosis. The virus is worldwide in distribution and does not appear to be seasonal.[49] The initial route of infection is through the nasopharyngeal epithelial cells and lymphoid tissues of the throat. During a 3–7 week incubation period, viral replication and dissemination occur throughout the lymphoreticular system.[50] EBV, like other herpesviruses, establishes latent infection. Salivary tissues are the recognized repository of EBV, and virus can be periodically detected in the oral secretions of normal persons. Shedding is sustained for months after infection and gradually diminishes over time.[51] Epidemiologic data suggest that EBV is an agent of low contagiousness and that infection of susceptible individuals requires intimate contact and the exchange of saliva.[52, 53]

The classic syndrome of mononucleosis is defined as fever, pharyngitis, and adenopathy, with prominent constitutional symptoms. Gastrointestinal complaints such as nausea, abdominal pain, and vomiting are noted in 5%–12% of cases and may be due in part to hepatitis and splenomegaly. Pharyngitis associated with EBV may be severe, and exudates are observed in roughly 30% of cases. Hyperplasia of the pharyngeal lymphatic tissue is usually visible during the second week of illness. A palatal enanthem, which consists of sharply circumscribed red spots 0.3–1.0 mm in diameter, distributed symmetrically at the junction of the hard and soft palates and lasting about 4–5 days, has also been described. Periorbital edema has been reported in up to one third of cases.[49–53] Diffuse lymphadenopathy is common but usually is most prominent in the posterior cervical chain. Nodes are freely movable and only mildly tender to palpation. EBV infection is generally a self-limited illness lasting 2 or 3 weeks.

Although most patients recover uneventfully, a variety of complications including hemolytic anemia, splenic rupture, myocarditis, and encephalitis are reported.[50] Airway obstruction from grossly enlarged tonsils is a rare, but potentially fatal complication of infectious mononucleosis.[54, 55] Burkitt's lymphoma, nasopharyngeal carcinoma, and lymphoproliferative diseases in recipients of organ transplants have been associated with EBV infection.[49] Replicating EBV has also been found in the epithelial cells of oral hairy leukoplakia, an exophytic growth of epithelial cells on the tongue and buccal mucosa of AIDS patients.[56]

Diagnosis of EBV infection is made by the combination of the appropriate clinical picture, the presence of absolute lymphocytosis with atypical lymphocytes, and the presence of heterophile antibodies (agglutinins directed against surface antigens on sheep, bovine, or horse red blood cells). In the 2nd or 3rd week of illness, approximately 85%–90% of patients develop these immunoglobulin M (IgM) antibodies, which usually disappear in 3–6 months.[49] False-positive heterophile tests are rare; however, young children may have a false-negative heterophile antibody. EBV-specific IgM and IgG can also be measured and are almost always present at the onset of symptoms.

Patients with uncomplicated infectious mononucleosis usually require only symptomatic therapy. The exudative tonsillopharyngitis often leads to bacterial throat cultures in which group A hemolytic streptococci can be recovered in 3%–30% of patients.[57] Colonization versus infection is impossible to distinguish clinically. Ampicillin or amoxicillin should be avoided, since these agents frequently cause rash in patients with infectious mononucleosis. Several antiviral agents, such as acyclovir, ganciclovir, zidovudine, or foscarnet show in vitro activity against EBV; however, these agents have not demonstrated clinical benefit.[49, 58]

The use of corticosteroids in the routine management of acute mononucleosis is controversial. The cumulative results of several small controlled studies suggest that the use of corticosteroids hastens resolution of fever and sore throat but overall provides no significant or reproducible benefit. Therefore, the routine use of steroids cannot be recommended.[50] However, corticosteroids are indicated in severe exudative tonsillitis, or pharyngeal or laryngeal edema, *when* there is impending airway obstruction. In these cases, a short course of prednisone, 40–60 mg/day, can be given for 7–10 days with a rapid taper once clinical response is noted.[54, 55]

Herpes Simplex Virus

HSVs are double-stranded DNA viruses that are members of the Herpesviridae family. There are two major antigenic types: HSV-1 and HSV-2. Although HSV-1 is most commonly associated with oral-facial lesions and HSV-2 with genital lesions, each virus may infect either region.[59] HSV infections are common, worldwide, and without seasonality. Seroprevalence depends on the HSV type and population studied. Approximately 40% of young adults in the United States have antibody to HSV-1.[60]

Direct contact with infected oral secretions is the principal mode of HSV-1 spread. Asymptomatic salivary excretion has been reported in approximately 6% of adults and children. Infection may be transmitted by asymptomatic salivary excretions as well as from contact with active lesions. However, the titer from active lesions is 100–1000-fold higher than from asymptomatic subjects.[59] On entry into the skin or mucous membranes, HSV replicates locally in the epidermis and dermis. After primary infection, HSV may become latent within sensory nerve ganglions with reactivated virus spreading along peripheral nerve pathways.[61]

Gingivostomatitis and pharyngitis are the most frequent manifestations of primary HSV-1 infection, and recurrent herpes labialis is the most common manifestation of HSV-1 reactivation. In primary infection when the host lacks immunity, systemic signs and symptoms of fever and malaise are common. Primary HSV gingivostomatitis is most frequently seen in children. Vesicles develop on the soft palate, buccal mucosa, tongue, and floor of the mouth, with lesions commonly extending to the lips and chin. Children may appear toxic and become dehydrated from poor oral intake. The disease generally runs its course in 10–14 days. In college-age persons, primary HSV has been isolated in 6%–11% of students presenting with sore throats.[62, 63] Exudates or ulcerative lesions were noted on the posterior pharynx or tonsillar pillars. Lesions were also noted on the lips, gingiva, and buccal mucosa in some cases. Clinical differentiation from bacterial pharyngitis may be difficult.

Recurrent oral herpes is frequently preceded by prodromal symptoms of tingling or itching for 6–48 hours before the onset of vesicles. Vesicles are typically at the border of the outer lip and usually most painful in the first 24 hours. Crusting of the ulcer occurs within 48 hours, with gradual resolution in 8–10 days.[64, 65] The mean monthly recurrence of oral-labial HSV-1 is approximately 0.12 per month, and of HSV-2, 0.001 per month.[66]

HSV infection in immunosuppressed patients may involve deep mucosal and cutaneous layers causing necrosis and bleeding. Infection can evolve into esophagitis, tracheobronchitis, or pneumonia, or can disseminate. Patients with atopic eczema are also at risk of developing severe oral-facial HSV infections (eczema herpeticum), which may rapidly involve extensive areas of skin and occasionally disseminate.[59]

Specific diagnosis of HSV infection by viral isolation is available in most laboratories. Vesicles contain the highest titers of virus in the first 24–48 hours, when they can be unroofed or aspirated and fluid obtained for culture. Viral growth is usually detectable in 24–48 hours.[61] Rapid diagnosis of HSV can be made by scraping cells from suspect lesions and preparing a Giemsa or Wright stain. The presence of multinucleated giant cells indicates infection with a herpesvirus.

Several antiviral agents are available for the treatment of HSV; they include vidarabine, acyclovir, and foscarnet. Acyclovir is the most widely used compound and is available in three formulations: topical 5% ointment and oral and intravenous preparations. The use of topical acyclovir for oral HSV is not effective.[67] Oral acyclovir has been effective at reducing symptoms during initial episodes of genital herpes but has not been studied in primary oral-facial episodes. It is reasonable to consider therapy with oral acyclovir in severe primary cases. Oral acyclovir has a slight clinical benefit in recurrent herpes labialis only if initiated very early (during prodrome) and cannot be recommended as a routine treatment. Frequently, recurrent herpes labialis or ultraviolet radiation–induced herpes labialis can be suppressed with daily oral acyclovir, 200 mg given five times daily; however, it is generally not warranted in the immunocompetent host. In the immunocompromised host, acyclovir is useful for both treatment and suppression of mucocutaneous HSV lesions. For the treatment of acute episodes, intravenous acyclovir 5 mg/kg/day, or oral acyclovir 200–400 mg five times daily, can reduce viral shedding, local symptoms, and the time to heal.[67] Treatment is also indicated for extensive eczema herpeticum.[59] Foscarnet is a new antiviral that is effective for the treatment of acyclovir-resistant HSV.

Varicella-Zoster Virus

VZV is a double-stranded DNA virus belonging to the Herpesviridae family. VZV is the cause of two human diseases: varicella (chickenpox) and herpes zoster (shingles). Varicella reflects primary infection, and zoster represents reactivation of latent virus. In the United States 90% of people are infected with chickenpox virus before the age of 15 years.[68] Herpes zoster can occur at any age but primarily affects elderly persons and those who are immunocompromised.[69] Herpes zoster is characterized by a unilateral vesicular erruption with a dermatomal distribution. Thoracic and lumbar dermatomes are most commonly involved.

Herpes zoster oticus, also known as Ramsay Hunt syndrome, is caused by reactivation of VZV from the geniculate ganglion. Ramsay Hunt syndrome is characterized by ipsilateral facial paralysis and herpetic lesions on the tympanic membrane, external auditory canal, pharynx, and pinna. Patients may have loss of taste and salivation as well as hearing loss, hyperacusis, tinnitus, and vertigo. The pathogenesis of Ramsay Hunt syndrome is felt to be inflammation of both the seventh nerve nucleus and the peripheral nerve.[70]

Management is aimed at protecting the eye and preventing permanent nerve damage resulting in irreversible facial paralysis and deafness. Prognosis for complete recovery of seventh cranial nerve function is less favorable in Ramsay Hunt syndrome when compared with Bell's palsy.[70] Recommendations for treatment are based on small uncontrolled studies. Some authorities recommend corticosteroids at a dose of 60 mg of prednisone in divided doses for 6 days with a taper over the next week if the patient is stable. If pain or paralysis progresses the dose should be maintained at 60 mg for an additional 5–7 days.[70, 71] Acyclovir appears to be beneficial; however, its use has been reported only in small series of patients. Outcomes of treated patients were better when compared with those of historical controls.[72, 73] Intravenous acyclovir at 5 mg/kg/day or oral acyclovir at 800 mg five times daily should be considered.

Mumps

Mumps virus is a RNA virus and a member of the Paramyxoviridae family. Mumps is endemic throughout the world with peak activity from January to May.[30] Epidemic parotitis is caused by mumps virus; however, since the introduction of the live attenuated vaccine in 1967, the pattern of the disease has changed. Other viral agents associated with parotitis include coxsackievirus A, EBV, influenza A, parainfluenza viruses, and lymphocytic choriomeningitis virus.[74–77] The incubation period is from 2 to 4 weeks. Symptoms of mumps include malaise, headache, and earache, which are followed by fever and parotid swelling. Stensen's duct is erythematous and edematous. Parotid swelling is usually bilateral but may be unilateral in 25% of cases. Inflammation may also occur in other salivary glands, occasionally causing swelling of the tongue. Mumps infection has also been associated with meningoencephalitis, orchitis, and pancreatitis.

A definitive diagnosis of mumps infection can be made by isolation of the virus from saliva up to 9 days after the onset of symptoms. Virus can also be cultured from urine and cerebrospinal fluid.[30] Diagnosis can be made retrospectively by serologic examination. Therapy for viral parotitis is supportive. Antipyretics, analgesics, and warm or cold packs may be helpful for discomfort.

References

1. Gwaltney JM, Hendley JO, Simon G, Jordan WS: Rhinovirus infections in an industrial population: II. Characteristics of illness and antibody response. JAMA 1967; 202: 494–550.
2. National Center for Health Statistics: Current Estimates from the National Health Interview Survey, United States, 1985. Vital and Health Statistics, Series 10. Washington, D.C.: Public Health Services, 1986, p 160.
3. Cypress BK: Medication therapy for office visits for selected diagnoses. In: National Center for Health Statistics: The National Ambulatory Medical Care Survey, United States 1980. Vital and Health Statistics Series 13, No. 71, Washington, D.C.: Public Health Service.
4. Anderson LJ, Patriarca PA, Hierholzer JC, Noble GR: Viral respiratory illnesses. Med Clin North Am 1983; 67: 1009–1031.
5. Sperber SJ, Hayden FG: Minireview. Chemotherapy of rhinovirus colds. Antimicrob Agents Chemother 1988; 321: 409–419.
6. Proud D, Reynolds CJ, Lecapra S, et al.: Nasal provocation with bradykinin induces symptoms of rhinitis and sore throat. Am Rev Respir Dis 1988; 137: 613–616.
7. Ramirez-Ronda CH, Fuxench-Lopez Z, Naverez M: Increased pharyngeal colonization during viral illness. Arch Intern Med 1982; 141: 1599–1603.
8. Gwaltney JM: Rhinoviruses. In: Mandell GL, Bennett JE, Dolan R (eds): Principles and Practice of Infectious Diseases, 4th ed. New York: Churchill Livingstone, 1995, pp 1656–1663.
9. McBride TP, Doyle WJ, Hayden FG, Gwaltney JM: Alterations of the eustachian tube, middle ear and nose in rhinovirus infection. Arch Otolaryngol Head Neck Surg 1989; 115: 1054–1059.
10. Sung BS, Chonmaitree T, Broemeling LD, et al.: Association of rhinovirus infection with poor bacteriologic outcome of bacterial viral otitis media. Clin Infect Dis 1993; 17: 38–42.
11. Gwaltney JM, Phillips CD, Miller RD, Riker DK: Computed tomographic study of the common cold. N Engl J Med 1994; 330: 25–30.
12. Hendley OJ, Fishburne HB, Gwaltney JM: Coronavirus infections in working adults: Eight year study with 229E and OC43. Am Rev Respir Dis 1972; 105: 805–811.
13. Flowers DI, Clarke JR, Valman HB, MacNaughton MR: Epidemiology of coronavirus respiratory infections. Arch Dis Child 1983; 50: 500–503.
14. Alford RH, Kasel JA, Gerome PJ, et al.: Human influenza resulting from aerosol inhalation. Proc Soc Exp Biol Med 1966; 122: 800–804.
15. Harmon MW, Kendal AP: Influenza viruses. In: Schmidt NJ, Emmons RW (eds): Diagnosis Procedures for Viral, Rickettsial and Chlamydial Infections, 6th ed. Washington, DC: American Public Health Association, 1989, pp 631–668.
16. Betts RF: Influenza virus. In: Mandell GL, Bennett JE, Dolin R (eds): Principles and Practice of Infectious Diseases, 4th ed. New York: Churchill Livingstone, 1991, pp 1546–1567.
17. Louria BD, Blumenfield HL, Ellis JT, et al.: Studies on influenza in the pandemic of 1957–1958: II. Pulmonary complications of influenza. J Clin Invest 1959; 38: 213–265.
18. Chonmaitree T: Viral otitis media. Pediatr Ann 1990; 19: 522–532.
19. Doyle WJ, Buchman CA, Skoner DP, et al.: Nasal and otologic effects of experimental influenza A virus infection. Ann Otol Rhinol Laryngol 1994; 103: 59–69.
20. Douglas RG: Prophylaxis and treatment of influenza. N Engl J Med 1990; 322: 443–449.
21. Brandt CD, Kim HW, Arrobio J, et al.: Epidemiology of respiratory

syncytial virus infection in Washington DC: II. Composite analysis of eleven consecutive yearly epidemics. Am J Epidemiol 1973; 98: 355–364.

22. Henderson FW, Collier AM, Clyde WA Jr, Denny FW: Respiratory syncytial virus infections, reinfections and immunity: A prospective, longitudinal study in young children. N Engl J Med 1979; 30: 530–534.

23. Johnson KM, Bloom HH, Mufson MA, Chanock RM: Natural reinfection of adults by respiratory syncytial virus—possible relation to mild upper respiratory diseases. N Engl J Med 1962; 267: 68–71.

24. Hall CB, McCarthy CA: Respiratory syncytial virus. In: Mandell GL, Bennett JE, Dolin R (eds): Principles and Practice of Infectious Diseases, 4th ed. New York: Churchill Livingstone, 1995, pp 1501–1519.

25. Henderson FW, Collier AM, Sanyal MA, et al.: A longitudinal study of respiratory syncytial virus and bacteria in the etiology of acute otitis media with effusion. N Engl J Med 1982; 30: 1377–1383.

26. Klein JO, Teele DW: Isolation of viruses and mycoplasmas from middle ear effusions: A review. Ann Otol Rhinol Laryngol 1976; 85(S5): 140–141.

27. Hall CB, McBride JT, Walsh EE, et al.: Aerosolized ribavirin treatment of infants with respiratory syncytial virus infection: A randomized double-blind study. N Engl J Med 1983; 308: 1443–1447.

28. Monto AS, Sullivan KM: Acute respiratory illness in the community. Frequency of illness and agents involved. Epidemiol Infect 1993; 110: 145–160.

29. Knott AM, Long C, Hall CB: Parainfluenza viral infections in pediatric outpatients; seasonal patterns and clinical characteristics. Pediatr Infect Dis 1994; 13: 269–273.

30. Mufson MA: Parainfluenza viruses, mumps virus and Newcastle disease virus. In: Schmitt NJ, Emmons RW (eds): Diagnostic Procedures for Viral, Rickettsial and Chlamydial Infections, 6th ed. Washington, D.C.: American Public Health Association: 1989, pp 669–692.

31. Arola M, Roustkanen O, Ziegler T, et al.: Clinical role of respiratory virus infection in acute otitis media. Pediatrics 1990; 86: 848–855.

32. Rowe WP, Huebner RJ, Gillmore LK, et al.: Isolation of a cytopathogenic agent from human adenoids undergoing spontaneous degeneration in tissue culture. Proc Soc Exp Biol Med 1953; 84: 570–573.

33. Piedra PA: Epidemiology and clinical manifestations of adenovirus infection in children. Contemp Pediatr 1994; 11: 15.

34. Schmitz H, Wigand R, Heinrich W: Worldwide epidemiology of human adenovirus infections. Am J Epidemiol 1983; 117: 455–456.

35. Angella JJ, Connor JD: Neonatal infection caused by adenovirus type 7. J Pediatr 1968; 73: 474–478.

36. Glezen WP, Clyde WA, Senior RJ, et al.: Streptococci, mycoplasmas and viruses associated with acute pharyngitis. JAMA 1967; 202: 119–124.

37. McNamara MJ, Pierce WE, Crawford YE, Miller LF: Patterns of adenovirus infections in the respiratory diseases of naval recruits. Am Rev Respir Dis 1962; 86: 485–497.

38. Sobel G, Aronson B, Aronson S, et al.: Pharyngo-conjunctival fever. Am J Dis Child 1956; 92: 596.

39. Wregitt TG, Gray JJ, Ward KN, et al.: Disseminated adenovitis infection after liver transplantation and its possible treatment with ganciclovir. J Infect 1989; 19: 88–89.

40. Moore M: Enteroviral disease in the United States, 1970–79. J Infect Dis 1982; 146: 103–108.

41. Grandien M, Forsgren M, Ehrnst A: Enteroviruses and reoviruses. In: Schmidt NJ, Emmons RW (eds): Diagnostic Procedures for Viral, Rickettsial and Chlamydial Infections, 6th ed. Washington, D.C.: American Public Health Association, 1989, pp 513–578.

42. Hable KA, O'Connell EJ, Herrmann EC: Group B coxsackieviruses as respiratory pathogens. Mayo Clin Proc 1970; 45: 170–176.

43. Cherry JD: Enteroviruses: Polioviruses (poliomyelitis) enteroviruses, coxsackieviruses, echoviruses, and enteroviruses. In: Feigin RD, Cherry JD (eds): Textbook of Pediatric Infectious Diseases, 3rd ed. Philadelphia: WB Saunders Co, 1992, pp 1705–1753.

44. Modlin JF: Coxsackieviruses, echoviruses and newer enteroviruses. In: Mandell GL, Bennett JE, Dolin R (eds): Principles and Practice of Infectious Diseases, 4th ed. New York: Churchill Livingstone, 1995, pp 1620–1636.

45. Steigman AJ, Lipton MM, Braspennic H: Acute lymphonodular pharyngitis: A newly described condition due to coxsackie A virus. J Pediatr 1962; 61: 331–336.

46. Miller GD: Hand-foot-and-mouth disease. JAMA 1968; 203: 827–830.

47. Valle SL: Febrile pharyngitis as the primary sign of HIV infection in a cluster of cases linked by sexual contact. Scand J Infect Dis 1987; 19: 13–17.

48. Lindstrom C, Pincus R, Leavitt EB, Urbina MC: Otologic neurologic manifestations of HIV-related disease. Otolaryngol Head Neck Surg 1993; 108:680–687.

49. Andiman WA: Epstein-Barr Virus. In: Schmidt NJ, Emmons RW (eds): Diagnostic Procedures for Viral, Rickettsial and Chlamydial Infections, 6th ed. Washington, DC: American Public Health Association, 1989, pp 407–452.

50. Strauss SE, Cohen JI, Tosato G, Meier J: Epstein-Barr virus infections: Biology, pathogenesis and management. Ann Intern Med 1993; 118: 45–58.

51. Neiderman JC, Miller G, Pearson HA, et al.: Infectious mononucleosis: Epstein-Barr virus shedding in saliva and the oropharynx. N Engl J Med 1976; 294: 1355–1359.

52. Sawyer RN, Evans AS, Niederman JC, McCollum RW: Prospective studies of a group of Yale University freshmen: I. Occurrence of infectious mononucleosis. J Infect Dis 1971; 123: 263–270.

53. Hoagland RS: Infectious Mononucleosis. New York; Grune & Stratten, 1967.

54. Schumacher HR, Jacobson WA, Bemill CR: Treatment of infectious mononucleosis. Ann Intern Med 1963; 58: 217–228.

55. Brandtonbrener A, Epstein A, Wu S, Phair J: Corticosteroid therapy in Epstein-Barr virus infection. Effect on lymphocyte class, subset, and response to early antigen. Arch Intern Med 1986; 146: 337–379.

56. Greenspan JS, Greenspan D, Lennett ET, et al.: Replication of Epstein-Barr virus within the epithelial cells of oral hairy leukoplakia, an AIDS-associated lesion. N Engl J Med 1985; 313: 1564–1571.

57. Bennike T: Penicillin treatment of infectious mononucleosis: Comparison of effects in ninety-nine patients with and in sixty-seven patients without penicillin therapy. Arch Intern Med 1951; 87: 181–189.

58. Anderson J, Britton S, Ernberg I, et al.: Effect of acyclovir on infectious mononucleosis: A double-blind, placebo-controlled study. J Infect Dis 1986; 153: 283–290.

59. Corey L, Spear PG: Infections with herpes simplex virus. N Engl J Med 1986; 314: 686–691.

60. Wentworth BB, Alexander ER: Seroepidemiology of infections due to members of the herpes virus group. Am J Epidemiol 1971; 94: 496–507.

61. Hirsch MS: Herpes simplex virus. In: Mandell GL, Bennett JE, Dolin R (eds): Principles and Practice of Infectious Diseases, 4th ed. New York: Churchill Livingstone, 1995, pp 1336–1345.

62. Glezen WP, Fernald GW, Lohr JA: Acute respiratory disease of university students with special reference to the etiologic role of herpes virus hominis. Am J Epidemiol 1975; 101: 111–121.

63. McMillan JA, Weiner LB, Higgins AM, Lamparella VJ: Pharyngitis associated with herpes-simplex virus in college students. Pediatr Infect Dis J 1993; 12: 280–284.

64. Young SK, Rose NH, Buchanan RA: A clinical study for the control of facial mucocutaneous herpes virus infections: I. Characterization of natural history in a professional school population. Oral Surg 1978; 41: 498–507.

65. Spruance S, Overall JC, Kein ER, et al.: The natural history of recurrent herpes simplex labialis. Implications for antiviral therapy. N Engl J Med 1977; 297: 69–75.

66. Lafferty WE, Coombs RW, Benedetti J, et al.: Recurrence after oral and genital herpes simplex virus infection. N Engl J Med 1987; 316: 1444–1449.

67. Whitely RJ, Grann JW: Acyclovir: A decade later. N Engl J Med 1992; 327: 782–789.

68. Strauss S, Ostrove JM, Inchaupe G, et al.: Varicella-zoster virus infections: Biology, natural history, treatment and prevention. Ann Intern Med 1988; 108: 221–237.

69. Bucci FA, Schwartz RA: Neurologic complications of herpes zoster. Am Fam Pract 1988; 37: 185–192.

70. Crabtree JA: Herpes zoster oticus and facial paralysis. Otolaryngol Clin North Am 1974; 7: 369–373.

71. Robillard RB, Hilsinger RL, Adour KK: Ramsay Hunt facial paralysis: Clinical analyses of 185 patients. Otolaryngol Head Neck Surg 1986; 95: 292–297.

72. Uri N, Meyer W, Greenberg E, Kitzes-Cohen R: Herpes zoster oticus: Treatment with acyclovir. Ann Otol Rhinol Laryngol 1992; 101: 161–162.

73. Adour KK: Otological complications of herpes zoster. Ann Neurol 1994; 35: S62–S64.

74. Brook I: The swollen neck: Cervical lymphadenitis, parotitis, thyroiditis, and infected cysts. Infect Dis Clin North Am 1988; 2: 221–237.

75. Zollar LM, Mufson MA: Acute parotitis associated with parainfluenza-3 virus infection. Am J Dis Child 1970; 199: 147–148.

76. Brill SJ, Gilggillan RF: Acute parotitis associated with influenza A: A report of twelve cases. N Engl J Med 1977; 296: 1391–1392.

77. Lewis JM, Utz JP: Orchitis, parotitis and meningoencephalitis due to lymphocytic choriomeningitis virus. N Engl J Med 1961; 265: 776–780.

Chien Liu

CHAPTER THIRTY-ONE

Mycoplasma pneumoniae

▼

HISTORY

In the 1930s, in adolescents and young adults a number of cases of benign pneumonitis clinically quite distinct from the "typical" pneumococcal pneumonia occurred. Reimann classified this disease as a new clinical entity.[1] This illness accounted for a significant morbidity in combat troops during World War II, and the U.S. Army Surgeon General officially adopted the diagnosis "primary atypical pneumonia, etiology unknown" for military patients.[2] Peterson and colleagues reported the development of cold agglutinins in many of these patients, and this was helpful in the diagnosis of primary atypical pneumonia.[3] In 1944 Eaton and colleagues isolated a filtrable agent from sputum specimens and lung suspensions of patients with the diagnosis of primary atypical pneumonia, and this agent was thought to be a virus.[4] Subsequently, by applying the immunofluorescent staining technique, Liu confirmed Eaton's studies and developed a specific serologic test for the diagnosis of primary atypical pneumonia.[5, 6] In 1962, Chanock, Hayflick, and Barile succeeded in cultivating the agent in cell-free media and demonstrated it to be a cell wall–deficient organism.[7] The term *Mycoplasma pneumoniae* was adopted in 1963 (Table 31–1).[8]

MICROBIOLOGY

Mycoplasmas are a group of the smallest free-living organisms lacking a cell wall. They require complex media containing beef heart infusion supplemented with serum, yeast, DNA, and RNA for growth. *M. pneumoniae* grows slowly aerobically and anaerobically on the surface of agar, forming "mulberry-like" colonies without a "fried egg" appearance. Microscopically, detectable colonies usually take 6–12 days to appear. *M. pneumoniae* causes rapid and complete beta hemolysis of guinea pig erythrocytes by means of hydrogen peroxide production; hemadsorbs erythrocytes onto its colonies; ferments glucose; and reduces tetrazolium and methylene blue under aerobic conditions.[9] The virulence factors of *M. pneumoniae* have not been extensively studied. However, it possesses a membrane-associated 169-kD protein, called P1, which is known to mediate the adherence of *M. pneumoniae* to host cells, a step necessary for initiating infection. Persons infected with *M. pneumoniae* produce a vigorous antibody response against this adhesin.[10] Antigens of mycoplasma species may act as immunomodulators by their interactions with lymphocytes and act as T-lymphocyte mitogens. They are able to activate cytotoxic T cells in vitro and also appear to induce polyclonal B-cell activation.

EPIDEMIOLOGY

Infections associated with *M. pneumoniae* are found worldwide. There is no seasonal preponderance for sporadic cases, but the peak incidence appears to be in the cooler months of the year and may be cyclic. Infections are seen more commonly in children of school age and in young adults. The proportion of pneumonia with *M. pneumoniae* as causal agent is greatest among the 15–19 year olds.[11] The incidence of respiratory infections without evidence of pneumonia may be 10–20 times as high. Among cases of community-acquired pneumonia, *M. pneumoniae* stands only second to pneumococcus as the etiologic agent and is estimated to be responsible for 15%–20% of cases.[12, 13] Humans are the only natural hosts; no animal reservoir has been identified.

COLONIZATION, PATHOGENESIS, AND IMMUNITY

M. pneumoniae is not part of the regular resident flora of the human respiratory tract. Its spread is likely by droplet

Table 31–1. EVENTS ASSOCIATED WITH ESTABLISHING *MYCOPLASMA PNEUMONIAE* AS THE CAUSE OF PRIMARY ATYPICAL PNEUMONIA

Year	Events	Reference
1938	Reimann described atypical pneumonia in young adults.	Reimann[1]
1942	U.S. Army Surgeon General's Office adopted diagnosis "primary atypical pneumonia, etiology unknown."	U.S. Army Surgeon General[2]
1943	Cold agglutinin was used for diagnosis of primary atypical pneumonia (PAP).	Peterson et al.[3]
1944	Eaton and colleagues isolated filtrable agent from sputum and lung specimens collected from PAP patients.	Eaton et al.[4]
1957	Liu detected growth of Eaton agent in chick embryo tracheal cells and developed specific serologic diagnostic test for PAP.	Liu,[5] Liu et al.[6]
1962	Chanock and colleagues succeeded in culturing Eaton agent in artificial media and found it to be a cell wall–deficient organism.	Chanock et al.[7]
1963	Name *Mycoplasma pneumoniae* was adopted for etiologic agent of PAP.	Chanock et al.[8]

infection from close contacts such as in families or among military recruits living in barracks. Transmission appears to occur during the acute stage of the infection.

After gaining access to the human host, *M. pneumoniae* grows extracellularly as filamentous forms that adhere to epithelial cells of the respiratory tract by specialized structures at one end of the microorganism. It is usually not invasive and multiplies on the respiratory epithelium without infiltrating into the cells or tissues. Few autopsy reports on mycoplasma pneumonia are available. Parker and colleagues reported studies on fatal cases of primary atypical pneumonia seen at the Boston City Hospital in 1942 and 1943; these studies showed that the cut surfaces of the lungs displayed a characteristic miliary nodular appearance.[14] Microscopically, these nodules consisted of a mononuclear type of alveolar exudate, an interstitial infiltration composed predominantly of plasma cells, and swollen alveolar lining cells. In organ tissue culture studies, *M. pneumoniae* produces ciliary inactivation and eventually destroys the cells of the mucosa.[15] The mechanism is not entirely clear but appears to involve the ability of *M. pneumoniae* to attach to the neuraminic acid receptors and to generate hydrogen peroxide to elicit the damage.

M. pneumoniae infection induces humoral antibody response and local accumulation of both immunoglobulin G (IgG) and IgA antibodies, leading to recovery. In persons exposed to naturally occurring disease as well in human volunteer challenge experiments, resistance to reinfection is present.[16] However, the duration of immunity is unknown, as second episodes of pneumonia have been documented.[17]

CLINICAL MANIFESTATIONS

M. pneumoniae is a respiratory pathogen. Pneumonia remains the most recognizable and major clinical manifestation, although other systems can also be involved.[18]

Pneumonia

The incubation period is generally 2–3 weeks. Onset is usually insidious with fever and cough. Sore throat, nasal congestion, and coryza are reported in about half the patients. Chills, but not rigors, and malaise are common. In the early stage, the cough is usually nonproductive or yields a small amount of mucoid sputum. Pleuritic chest pain and hemoptysis are rare. On physical examination, the patient often does not appear severely ill. Findings in the lungs are usually not very striking. Moist rales are commonly heard, but egobronchophony and bronchial breathing are uncommon. Chest x-ray films may show bronchopneumonia involving one or more lobes, radiating from the hilar region toward the periphery. The lower lobes are involved more frequently. Often the roentgenographic findings and the physical findings do not coincide. Small amounts of pleural effusion may be detectable in 5%–25% of patients with *M. pneumoniae* pneumonia, particularly if a lateral decubitus roentgenograph is taken.

Laboratory examinations are not particularly remarkable. The hemogram is usually normal, with mild leukocytosis

seen in occasional patients. No characteristic renal or hepatic functional abnormalities are present. A rise in cold agglutinin titers may be seen in approximately 50%–60% of patients.[6] This usually develops during the 2nd and 4th weeks of illness and disappears in 6–8 weeks.

Even without specific treatment, defervescence with falling of fever gradually to normal temperature occurs by lysis in 8–10 days. However, roentgenographic clearance of the lungs may take 2–3 weeks. In treated cases, the defervescence and pneumonic clearance may be hastened by 2–3 days.[19]

Infections Related to Ears, Nose, and Throat

In human volunteer studies with experimentally induced *M. pneumoniae* infections, Rifkind and colleagues reported a high incidence of ear involvement in which 12 of 27 seronegative volunteers developed myringitis.[20] The myringitis varied from mild edema of the tympanic membrane to a severe inflammatory reaction, with two patients showing vesicles on the tympanic membrane (bullous myringitis). In naturally occurring *M. pneumoniae* infections, both bullous myringitis and middle ear effusions have been reported.[21, 22] Sobeslavsky and colleagues reported the isolation of *M. pneumoniae* from three children with otitis media; two of the isolations were from throat swabs, and the other was from middle ear fluid.[22] Two reviews on the etiologic role of *M. pneumoniae* in bullous myringitis and middle ear effusion have concluded that it rarely causes such infections naturally.[23, 24] Rhinitis has been reported as a major manifestation of *M. pneumoniae* infection in children younger than 1 year of age.[25] Epidemiologic studies of *M. pneumoniae* infection in families have shown that upper respiratory syndromes and tracheobronchitis are the most common manifestations.[21, 26] However, it would be impossible to distinguish these nonpulmonary respiratory *M. pneumoniae* infections from those with other causes based on clinical grounds alone.

Involvement of Other Organ Systems

Almost every organ system has been reported to be involved in *M. pneumoniae* infections. The incidence of nonrespiratory involvements is low. However, some of these infections can be quite severe with high morbidity and deaths. Stevens-Johnson syndrome with erythematous vesicles and bullae involving the skin and mucous membranes has been described as a nonpulmonary manifestation in mycoplasmal pneumonia.[27] Patients with high cold agglutinin antibody titers may develop hemolytic anemia, paroxysmal cold hemoglobinuria, Raynaud's syndrome, and disseminated intravascular coagulopathy.[28] Cardiac involvement with pericarditis and myocarditis associated with *M. pneumoniae* infection has been documented.[29, 30] Complications involving the central nervous system in *M. pneumoniae* infections have been estimated to occur in 0.1% of infected patients. Aseptic meningitis, meningoencephalitis, cerebral ataxia, transverse myelitis, and Guillain-Barré syndrome have been described. There appeared to be no correlation between the severity of the respiratory symptoms or the cold agglutinin antibody titers and the development of neurologic complications.[31, 32]

Laboratory Diagnosis

It is difficult if not impossible to make a definitive diagnosis of *M. pneumoniae* infection based on clinical grounds alone. Isolation of the organism is feasible, yet the fastidious and slow growth renders this procedure impractical. Determination of the cold agglutinin titer, although not entirely specific and present in only about 60% of patients with *M. pneumoniae* pneumonia, is useful because it is generally available in all routine hospital laboratories. A titer of 1:64 or greater suggests a current or recent infection. A complement-fixation (CF) test is also widely available and relatively specific as a serologic procedure to diagnose *M. pneumoniae* infections. It is more useful in epidemiologic studies and as a means to confirm a retrospective diagnosis. CF antibodies do not rise until 2–4 weeks in *M. pneumoniae* infections and may persist for many months afterward. An enzyme immunoassay to detect serum IgM and IgG antibodies against *M. pneumoniae* has been developed.[33–35] Detection of both serum immunoglobulins is desirable because adults may show only an IgG antibody response against *M. pneumoniae* infections.[34] Among patients with positive CF antibodies against *M. pneumoniae*, the enzyme immunoassay test has a sensitivity of 98% and a specificity of 99%.[33] However, IgM antibodies generally do not become positive until 1 week after infection, and the test is therefore not very helpful for establishing an early diagnosis to initiate specific antimicrobial therapy.

Detection of *M. pneumoniae* antigens in sputum specimens can be accomplished by enzyme immunoassay as well as by DNA probes (Gen-Probe).[36, 37] Although both methods are highly specific, one study comparing these two techniques showed that the antigen-capture indirect enzyme immunoassay was more sensitive than Gen-Probe, 91% versus 22%, respectively.[38] Two Gen-Probe studies, one from Canada[39] and the other from Japan,[40] both using the commercial kits manufactured by Gen-Probe Corp., San Diego, California, showed a sensitivity of 89% and 76.7% and a specificity of 89% and 91.7%, respectively. In another comparative study on throat washings from *M. pneumoniae*–infected patients, the sensitivity and specificity were considerably less.[41] The manufacturer of the diagnostic kits recommends that throat swabs be used for assay. Polymerase chain reaction (PCR) has been used to detect *M. pneumoniae*. The DNA from different *M. pneumoniae* strains can be detected by PCR, whereas the DNA from other mycoplasma species does not cross-react with that of *M. pneumoniae*.[42, 43] When throat swab samples from hamsters experimentally infected with *M. pneumoniae* were tested, PCR was more sensitive and reliable than conventional culture techniques. In artificially seeded human bronchoalveolar lavages, PCR was shown to detect 10^2–10^3 organisms (Table 31–2).[42]

Treatment

Many patients with *M. pneumoniae*, including those with pneumonia, recover spontaneously without specific therapy. However, appropriate antibiotic treatment improves the patients' well-being and lessens the duration of the illness. Beta-lactam antibiotics are not effective because *M. pneumoniae* is a cell wall–deficient bacterium. Tetracyclines, macrolides, and quinolones are effective.[44] Clinical experiences have shown no significant differences between tetracyclines and erythromycin, although tetracyclines are contraindicated for use in children. The newer macrolides, clarithromycin and azithromycin, are effective and better-tolerated and can be dosed once or twice daily.[45, 46] The cost of these new macrolides is many times more than that of erythromycin and tetracyclines. The quinolones, ciprofloxacin and lomefloxacin, have a minimal inhibitory concentration (MIC) 1000-fold more potent than the MIC of erythromycin against *M. pneumoniae*.[47, 48] Again, they are more expensive and are not for use in children. Since the contribution of *M. pneumoniae* in causing otitis and myringitis is probably small, management of the ear infections should follow the routine antimicrobial therapy regimens for bacterial infections rather than those of *M. pneumoniae* infections.[49]

Table 31–2. LABORATORY DIAGNOSTIC TESTS FOR *M. PNEUMONIAE* INFECTIONS

Test	Sensitivity/Specificity	Comments
Culture of organisms	+ +/+ + +	Slow and fastidious growth; not generally available in routine hospital laboratories.
Serologic techniques		
Cold agglutinins	+/+ +	Generally available in hospital laboratories; only 60%–70% of *M. pneumoniae* patients show positive results.
Complement fixation	+ +/+ +	Antibody develops after 1 week of infection, and may persist for years; good for epidemiologic and retrospective diagnosis.
IgM-IgG determinations	+ +/+ + +	IgM level rises at 7–10 days of infection; specificity good; still not sufficiently sensitive to guide early initiation of specific therapy.
Antigen detection		
Antigen-capture immunoassay	+ + +/+ + +	Both assays showed excellent specificity against a range of mycoplasma species with only *M. pneumoniae* and *Mycoplasma genitalium* reacting.
cDNA probe	+ + +/+ + +	Diagnostic Gen-Probe kits are available commercially to help in establishing early diagnosis.
PCR	+ + +/+ + +	Probably most sensitive and specific if performed properly; not generally available except in research laboratories.

cDNA = complementary DNA, PCR = polymerase chain reaction.

References

1. Reimann HA: An acute infection of the respiratory tract with atypical pneumonia. JAMA 1938; 111: 2377.
2. US Army Surgeon General's Office: Official statement. Primary atypical pneumonia, etiology unknown. War Med 1942; 2: 330.
3. Peterson CL, Ham TH, Finland M: Cold agglutinins (autohemagglutinins) in primary atypical pneumonia. Science 1943; 97: 167.
4. Eaton MD, Meiklejohn G, Van Herick W: Studies on the etiology of primary atypical pneumonia; a filterable agent transmissible to cotton rats, hamsters, and chick embryos. J Exp Med 1944; 79: 649.
5. Liu C: Studies on primary pneumonia: I. Localization, isolation and cultivation of a virus in chick embryos. J Exp Med 1957; 106: 455.
6. Liu C, Eaton MD, Heyl JT: Studies on primary atypical pneumonia: II. Observations concerning the development and immunological characteristics of antibody in patients. J Exp Med 1959; 109: 545.
7. Chanock RM, Hayflick L, Barile MP: Growth on an artificial medium of an agent associated with atypical pneumonia and its identification as a PPLO. Proc Natl Acad Sci USA 1962; 48: 41.
8. Chanock RM, Dienes L, Eaton MD, et al.: *Mycoplasma pneumoniae*: Proposed nomenclature for primary atypical pneumonia organism (Eaton agent). Science 1963; 140: 662
9. Mycoplasma and ureaplasmas. In: Koneman EW, Allen SD, Janda WM, et al. (eds): Color Atlas and Text of Diagnostic Microbiology, 4th ed. Philadelphia: JB Lippincott Co, 1992, p 675.
10. Jacobs E, Pilatschek A, Kleinman B, et al.: Use of adherence protein of *Mycoplasma pneumoniae* as antigen for enzyme-linked immunosorbent assay (ELISA). Isr J Med 1987; 23: 709.
11. Foy HM, Kenny GE, McMahan R, et al.: *Mycoplasma pneumoniae* pneumonia in an urban area: Five years of surveillance. JAMA 1970; 214: 1665.
12. Foy HM, Kenny GE, Cooney MK, et al.: Long term epidemiology of infection with *Mycoplasma pneumoniae*. J Infect Dis 1979; 139: 681.
13. Community-acquired pneumonia in adults in British hospitals in 1982–83: A survey of aetiology, mortality, prognostic factors, and outcome. From the Research Committee of the British Thoracic Society and the Public Health Laboratory Service. Q J Med 1986; 62: 195.
14. Parker F Jr, Jollife LS, Finland M: Primary atypical pneumonia: Report of 8 cases with autopsies. Arch Pathol 1947; 44: 581.
15. Carson JL, Collier AM, Hu SS: Ultrastructural observations on cellular and subcellular aspects of experimental *Mycoplasma pneumoniae* disease. Infect Immun 1980; 29: 1117.
16. Foy HM, Kenny GE, Cooney MK, et al.: Naturally acquired immunity to pneumonia due to *Mycoplasma pneumoniae*. J Infect Dis 1983; 147: 967.
17. Foy HM, Kenny GE, Sefi R, et al.: Second attacks of pneumonia due to *Mycoplasma pneumoniae*. J Infect Dis 1977; 135: 673.
18. Baum SG: *Mycoplasma pneumoniae* and atypical pneumonia. In: Mandell GL, Bennett JE, Dolin R (eds): Principles and Practice of Infectious Diseases, 4th ed. New York: Churchill Livingstone, 1995, p 1701.
19. McIntosh JC, Gutierrez HH: Myoplasmal infections: Epidemiology, immunology, diagnostic techniques, and therapeutic strategies. Immunol Allergy Clin North Am 1993; 13: 43.
20. Rifkind D, Chanock R, Kravetz HM, et al.: Ear involvement (myringitis) and primary atypical pneumonia following inoculation of volunteers with Eaton agent. Am Rev Respir Dis 1962; 85: 7479.
21. Foy HM, Grayston JT, Kenny GE, et al.: Epidemiology of *Mycoplasma pneumoniae* infection in families. JAMA 1966; 197: 859.
22. Sobeslavsky O, Syrucek L, Bruckova M, et al.: The etiological role of *Mycoplasma pneumoniae* in otitis media in children. Pediatrics 1965; 35: 652.
23. Roberts DB: The etiology of bullous myringitis and the role of mycoplasmas in ear disease: A review. Pediatrics 1980; 65: 761.
24. Klein JO, Teele DW: Isolation of viruses and mycoplasmas from middle ear effusions: A review. Ann Otol Rhinol Laryngol 1976; 85: 140.
25. Mok JY, Waugh PR, Simpson H: *Mycoplasma pneumoniae* infection: A follow-up study of 50 children with respiratory illness. Arch Dis Child 1979; 54: 506.
26. Balassanian N, Robbins FC: *Mycoplasma pneumoniae* infection in families. N Engl J Med 1967; 277: 719.
27. Levy M, Shear NH: *Mycoplasma pneumoniae* infections and Stevens-Johnson syndrome. Clin Pediatr 1991; 30: 42.
28. Jacobson LB, Longstrech GF, Edgington TS: Clinical and immunologic features of transient cold agglutinin hemolytic anemia. Am J Med 1973; 554: 514.
29. Sands MJ, Satz JE, Soloff LA: Pericarditis and perimyocarditis associated with active *Mycoplasma pneumoniae* infection. Ann Intern Med 1977; 86: 544.
30. Karjalainen J: A loud third heart sound and asymptomatic myocarditis during *Mycoplasma pneumoniae* infection. Eur Heart J 1990; 11: 960.
31. Koskiniemi M: CNS manifestations associated with *Mycoplasma pneumoniae* infections: Summary of cases at the University of Helsinki and review. Clin Infect Dis 1993; 1(suppl): S52.
32. Mills RW, Schoolfield L: Acute transverse myelitis associated with *Mycoplasma pneumoniae* infection: A case report and review of the literature. Pediatr Infect Dis J 1992; 11: 228.
33. Uldum SA, Jensen JS, Sondergard-Anderson J, et al.: Enzyme immunoassay for detection of immunoglobulin M (IgM) and IgG antibodies to *Mycoplasma pneumoniae*. J Clin Microbiol 1992; 30: 1198.
34. Sillis M: The limitations of IgM assays in the serological diagnosis of *Mycoplasma pneumoniae* infections. J Med Microbiol 1990; 33: 253.
35. Vikerfors T, Brodin G, Grandien M, et al.: Detection of specific IgM for the diagnosis of *M. pneumoniae* infections: A clinical evaluation. Scand J Infect Dis 1988; 20: 601.
36. Kok TW, Varkanis G, Marmion BP, et al.: Laboratory diagnosis of *Mycoplasma pneumoniae* infection: 1. Direct detection of antigen in respiratory exudates by enzyme immunoassay. Epidemiol Infect 1988; 101: 669.
37. Tilton RC, Dias F, Kidd H, et al.: DNA probe versus culture for detection of *Mycoplasma pneumoniae* in clinical specimens. Diagn Microbiol Infect Dis 1988; 10: 109.
38. Harris R, Marmion BP, Varkanis G, et al.: Laboratory diagnosis of *Mycoplasma pneumoniae* infection: Comparison of methods for the direct detection of specific antigen or nucleic acid sequences in respiratory exudates. Epidemiol Infect 1988; 101: 685.
39. Dular R, Kajioka R, Kasatiya S: Comparison of Gen-Probe commercial kit and culture technique for the diagnosis of *Mycoplasma pneumoniae* infection. J Clin Microbiol 1988; 26: 1068.
40. Hata D, Fumiyuki K, Mochizuki Y, et al.: Evaluation of DNA probe test for rapid diagnosis of *Mycoplasma pneumoniae* infections. J Pediatr 1990; 116: 273.
41. Kleemola MSR, Karalaninen JE, Raty RKH: Rapid diagnosis of *Mycoplasma pneumoniae* infection: Clinical evaluation of a commercial probe test. J Infect Dis 1990; 162: 70.
42. Bernet C, Garret M, de Barbeyrac B, et al.: Detection of *Mycoplasma pneumoniae* by using the polymerase chain reaction. J Clin Microbiol 1989; 27: 2492.
43. Kai M, Yamanouchi I, Kamiya S, et al.: Rapid diagnostic method for *Mycoplasma pneumoniae* by polymerase chain reaction. Nippon Rinsho 1992; 50(suppl): 433.
44. McCormack WM: Susceptibility of mycoplasmas to antimicrobial agents: Clinical implications. Clin Infect Dis 1993; 1(suppl): S200.
45. Schonwald S, Gunjaca M, Kolacny-Babic L, et al.: Comparison of azithromycin and erythromycin in the treatment of atypical pneumonias. J Antimicrob Chemother 1990; 25: 123.
46. Rylander M, Hollander H: In vitro comparison of the activity of doxycycline, tetracycline, erythromycin and a new macrolide, CP 62993, against *Mycoplasma pneumoniae, Mycoplasma hominis* and *Ureaplasma urealyticum*. Scand J Infec Dis 1988; 53(suppl): 12.
47. Waiters KB, Casell GH, Canupp KC, et al.: In vitro susceptibilities of mycoplasmas and ureaplasmas to new macrolides and aryl-fluoroquinolones. Antimicrob Agents Chemother 1988; 32: 1500.
48. Casell GH, Waiters KB, Pate MS, et al.: Comparative susceptibility of *Mycoplasma pneumoniae* to erythromycin, ciprofloxacin and lomefloxacin. Diagn Microbiol Infect Dis 1989; 12: 433.
49. Canafax DM, Giebink GS: Antimicrobial treatment of acute otitis media. Ann Otol Rhinol Laryngol 1994; 163(suppl): 11.

Margaret R. Hammerschlag

CHAPTER THIRTY-TWO

Chlamydia

▼

DESCRIPTION

The genus *Chlamydia* is a group of obligate intracellular parasites that have a unique developmental cycle with morphologically distinct infectious and reproductive forms. All members of the genus have a gram-negative envelope without peptidoglycan, share a genus-specific lipopolysaccharide antigen, and use host adenosine triphosphate (ATP) for the synthesis of chlamydial protein. The genus now contains four species: *Chlamydia trachomatis, Chlamydia pneumoniae* (TWAR strain), *Chlamydia psittaci* and *Chlamydia pecorum.*

Members of the genus are distinguished by a unique developmental cycle involving an infectious, metabolically inactive extracellular form (elementary body) and a noninfectious metabolically active intracellular form (reticulate body). The elementary bodies, which are 200–400 μm in diameter, attach to the host cell and are taken into the cell by endocytosis that is not dependent on the microtubule system. The elementary body remains within a membrane-lined phagosome; fusion with the host cell liposomes does not occur. The elementary bodies differentiate into reticulate bodies, which then undergo binary fusion, forming the characteristic intracytoplasmic inclusions. After approximately 36 hours, the reticulate bodies condense back into elementary bodies, and infectivity increases. At about 48 hours, release of mature elementary bodies may occur by cytolysis or by a process of exocytosis of individual elementary bodies. Cell division is also unaffected during infection. Thus, one daughter cell may contain an inclusion, the other can remain uninfected. This is probably the biologic basis for prolonged subclinical infection, which is a hallmark of human chlamydial infection.

C. trachomatis is divided into two biovars with 15 serovars. The first isolates of *C. pneumoniae* were serendipitously obtained during trachoma studies in the 1960s.[1] TW-183 was isolated from the eye of a child with suspected trachoma in Taiwan, and IOL-207 was isolated from the eye of a child with trachoma in Teheran. Subsequently, serologic studies of an outbreak of mild pneumonia among schoolchildren in rural Finland in the late 1970s suggested that an organism related to TW-183 was the cause.[2] After the recovery of a similar isolate from the respiratory tract of a college student with pneumonia in Seattle, Grayston and colleagues applied the designation TWAR after their first two isolates, TW-183 and AR-39.[1] On the basis of inclusion morphology and staining characteristics in cell culture, TWAR was initially considered a *C. psittaci* strain. Subsequent analyses, however, have demonstrated that this organism is distinct from both *C. psittaci* and *C. trachomatis* (Table 32–1). Initial

ultrastructural studies demonstrated that the elementary bodies of *C. pneumoniae* have a pear-shaped appearance caused by a loose periplasmic membrane, whereas the elementary bodies of *C. trachomatis* and *C. psittaci* are round. However, ultrastructural studies of IOL-207 and other strains of *C. pneumoniae* revealed round elementary bodies similar in appearance to those of the other two chlamydial species.[3] Restriction endonuclease pattern analysis and nucleic acid hybridization studies suggest a high degree (>95%) of genetic relatedness among the *C. pneumoniae* isolates examined so far.[4]

EPIDEMIOLOGY

The natural reservoir of *C. trachomatis* and *C. pneumoniae* appears to be only humans. *C. psittaci* infects practically every mammalian and avian species. Infection in humans occurs primarily after avian exposure. *C. pecorum* has recently speciated off from *C. psittaci* and infects cows and sheep. Human infection has not been reported so far. No animal or avian vector has been identified for *C. pneumoniae.*

Table 32–1. CHARACTERISTICS OF CHLAMYDIA

Feature	Chlamydia pneumoniae	Chlamydia trachomatis	Chlamydia psittaci
Number of serovars	1	15	At least 4 avian serovars
Percentage of DNA homology to *C. pneumoniae*	94–100	<5	<10
Plasmid	No	Yes	Yes (rarely no)
Contains glycogen	No	Yes	No
Resistant to sulfonamides	Yes	No	Yes
Morphology of elementary body	Round, pear-shaped	Round	Round
Natural host	Humans	Humans	Birds, mammals
Population	All ages	Infants; sexually active adults	Poultry workers, veterinarians, bird fanciers
Mode of transmission	Aerosol: person to person	Vertical: mother to infant	Aerosol: animal to person
Respiratory diseases	Pneumonia, bronchitis, pharyngitis, sinusitis, otitis media	Pneumonia in infants	Pneumonia

COLONIZATION, TRANSMISSION, PATHOGENESIS, AND IMMUNITY

C. trachomatis is a sexually transmitted pathogen. Respiratory infection is essentially limited to infants who acquire the infection vertically from an infected mother during parturition. The prevalence of *C. trachomatis* infection in pregnant women ranges from 2% to more than 30% depending on the population. More than 75% of women with endocervical chlamydial infection are asymptomatic. The infant can be infected at one or more anatomic sites, including the conjunctiva, nasopharynx, rectum, and vagina. The nasopharynx is the most frequent site. Approximately 20%–50% of infants born to infected women become infected. The most frequent clinical manifestation is conjunctivitis. The majority of respiratory infections are asymptomatic. *C. pneumoniae* appears to be transmitted person to person via infected aerosol droplets.[5] *C. pneumoniae* can remain viable on plastic (Formica) countertops for 30 hours and can survive small-particle aerosolization.[6, 7] Spread within families and enclosed populations such as military recruits has been well described.[1, 8]

Like *C. trachomatis*, *C. pneumoniae* is also capable of causing subclinical infection. Approximately 2%–5% of subjectively healthy, asymptomatic adults and children can have *C. pneumoniae* isolated from the nasopharynx.[9, 10]

C. psittaci is primarily transmitted through aerosolized fecal material from birds and other animals. Many birds and animals can also be subclinically infected. Person-to-person transmission is rare. As human infections due to *C. trachomatis* and *C. pneumoniae* are rarely fatal, there are limited data on pathogenesis; such data that exist are associated with trachoma and female genital infection with *C. trachomatis*.

C. pneumoniae has been demonstrated to have a marked ciliastatic effect on human ciliated bronchial epithelial cells in vitro.[11] Decreases in ciliary motility leading to impairment of mucociliary clearance might be an important facilitating factor in *C. pneumoniae* respiratory infections. This effect may also facilitate coinfection with other pathogens. Several recent studies have found that as many as 20% of patients with *C. pneumoniae*–associated pneumonia are infected with other pathogens, especially *Mycoplasma pneumoniae* and *Streptococcus pneumoniae*.[12] It has not been established that *C. pneumoniae* has a direct toxic effect on respiratory cells in humans as described for *M. pneumoniae*. However, as it is an intracellular parasite, one can assume that some cellular damage does occur.

Little is also known about immunity to chlamydial infections in humans. Limited data suggest that local or mucosal immunity is important. Preliminary studies of *C. pneumoniae* and reactive airway disease suggest that bronchospasm in infected patients may be mediated by immunoglobulin E (IgE).[10] Since chlamydiae are obligate intracellular parasites, we consider an individual to be subclinically infected rather than colonized.

PATHOGENS IN EAR, NOSE, AND THROAT
Epidemiology of the Organism

C. trachomatis is primarily a sexually transmitted pathogen. Approximately 20%–50% of infants born to infected women become infected in the nasopharynx; however, less than

25% of those infants with nasopharyngeal infection develop pneumonia. This nasopharyngeal infection may persist for at least 3 years after birth. The association of *C. trachomatis* with other respiratory infections is tenuous. There is one specific situation in which *C. trachomatis* can cause pneumonia in older children and adults: immunosuppression. There have been several well-documented cases of pneumonia due to *C. trachomatis* in patients with leukemia, bone marrow transplant recipients, and acquired immunodeficiency syndrome (AIDS) patients. These adults had none of the characteristic findings of infantile *C. trachomatis* pneumonia.

C. pneumoniae appears to be a frequent respiratory pathogen affecting all age groups. Recent epidemiologic studies have found *C. pneumoniae* infection in 10%–20% of children and adults with community-acquired pneumonia and bronchitis.[1, 12–14]

Specific Ear, Nose, and Throat Diseases

Of the three chlamydial species known to cause disease in humans, *C. pneumoniae* is the only species that causes infections that are of importance to the ear, nose, and throat practitioner.

Otitis Media

Isolation of a chlamydial species, *C. trachomatis*, from middle ear fluid was first reported by Tipple and colleagues.[15] The organism was isolated from the middle ear aspirates of 3 of 11 infants with chlamydial pneumonia. These infants were all younger than 3 months of age and had typical infantile chlamydial pneumonia and what was described as "serous" otitis media. This may not imply a causal relationship, as the middle ear is contiguous with the nasopharynx and the organism is present in the mucosa of the nasopharynx. Infants with chlamydial pneumonia have a significant degree of nasal congestion, which can lead to eustachian tube dysfunction; thus the presence of serous otitis media may not be directly attributable to the presence of *C. trachomatis* in middle ear fluid. However, subsequent studies that have examined middle ear fluids from older infants and children with acute and chronic otitis media have not found convincing evidence of *C. trachomatis* as an etiologic agent of otitis. Four studies have examined middle ear fluids from a total of 337 children ranging in age from 5 months through 12 years.[16–19] *C. trachomatis* was isolated from ear fluids of 5 of these children enrolled in two of the studies.[17, 18] Chang and colleagues isolated *C. trachomatis* from ear aspirates of 3 of 26 (11.5%) children with acute and persistent otitis media; however, the age of only one of these children, 10 months, was given.[17] The culture method used was iododeoxyuridine-treated McCoy's cells with iodine staining, which would be species-specific for *C. trachomatis*. In the second study, Dawson and colleagues isolated presumptive *C. trachomatis* from two ear aspirates from 217 Australian aboriginal children with chronic otitis media.[18] The positive children were 4 and 8 years of age. They used McCoy's cells but confirmed the isolates with a genus-specific monoclonal antibody; thus, it is possible that both isolates may have actually been *C. pneumoniae*. Considering that perinatally acquired nasopharyngeal *C. trachomatis* infections may persist for at least 2 years, it is possible that the organism may be isolated from middle ear fluids beyond early infancy.[20] However, a causal relationship has not been established. *C. pneumoniae* is a more likely candidate as a cause of otitis media in older children and adults.

Ogawa and colleagues isolated *C. pneumoniae* from 6 of 43 patients with otitis media with effusion.[21] Four of the positive patients were adults, 36–59 years of age, with chronic otitis. The remaining two patients were children, 5 and 7 years of age, also with a history of recurrent and chronic otitis media. Both girls had a history of cough, rhinorrhea, and fever. Preliminary results of a study of children with acute otitis in the United States indicated isolation of *C. pneumoniae* by culture from the middle ear fluids of 7 of 88 (7.9%) children.[22] The children ranged in age from 5 months to 12 years. One of the positive children was 8 months of age. He presented with acute otitis media and a flulike illness with a fever of 103.2° F. *C. pneumoniae* was the only organism isolated from his ear fluid. *C. pneumoniae* was isolated from the nasopharynx of two of the children, both of whom had negative ear fluid cultures.

Sinusitis

Clinical symptoms compatible with sinusitis, usually maxillary, have been reported to occur frequently in patients with respiratory infection due to *C. pneumoniae*.[1, 23] However, there are no studies that have conclusively demonstrated a causal relationship. Hashigucci and colleagues reported the isolation of *C. pneumoniae* from a maxillary sinus aspirate of a 47-year-old man with clinical and radiographic evidence of sinusitis.[24] The patient initially presented with a complaint of 3 days of stuffy nose and purulent nasal discharge. He did not respond to treatment with clindamycin and returned with a complaint of facial pain and headache. He responded to treatment with 10 days of roxithromycin (a 14-membered-ring macrolide antibiotic not available in the United States).

Pharyngitis and Tonsillitis

In 1983, Komaroff and colleagues reported serologic evidence that *C. trachomatis* might be responsible for 20% of pharyngitis in adults.[25] However, subsequent studies using culture failed to isolate the organism from children and adults with pharyngitis.[26, 27] *C. trachomatis* has been isolated in the pharynx of both heterosexual and homosexual men and women and appears to be associated with sexual practices.[28, 29] These patients were asymptomatic. It does appear that the serologic evidence reported by Komaroff was probably due to *C. pneumoniae*. Sore throat and hoarseness are prominent clinical complaints in patients with *C. pneumoniae*–associated pneumonia and bronchitis.[1, 13, 23] These findings also were significantly more frequent with *C. pneumoniae* infection than in patients with *M. pneumoniae* or viral infection.[1, 13] Pharyngitis can also be the primary presentation of *C. pneumoniae* infection; most are individual case reports, and limited data are available from controlled studies in which culture has been done. Grayston and colleagues found that less than 1% of patients with pharyngitis who did not develop lower respiratory tract involvement had *C. pneumoniae* infection.[1] However, *C. pneumoniae* can also be isolated from the nasopharynx of 2%–5% of asympto-

matic adults and children.[5, 10] A later study by Huovinen and colleagues found serologic evidence of *C. pneumoniae* infection in 9 of 106 (8.5%) adult patients with pharyngitis.[30] However, recent data suggest that the criteria for serologic diagnosis of *C. pneumoniae* infection may not be very specific. Hyman and colleagues[9] found that 19 of 101 (19%) asymptomatic, subjectively healthy, culture and polymerase chain reaction (PCR) negative adults fulfilled the serologic criteria for acute *C. pneumoniae* infection, i.e., the IgM titer was ≥1:16, the IgG titer was ≥1:512. *C. pneumoniae* may have a role in pharyngitis but awaits definitive studies to confirm any etiologic role.

LABORATORY DIAGNOSIS

The definitive diagnostic method for *C. trachomatis* or *C. pneumoniae* infection in any respiratory tract specimen remains cell culture. Culture of *C. trachomatis* is fairly well standardized and widely available. Most laboratories use cycloheximide-treated McCoy's cells. A major problem with chlamydial culture in general is maintaining the cold chain. Specimens must be refrigerated and if not cultured within 48 hours, frozen at −80° C. Culture of *C. trachomatis* takes 48–72 hours. Culture of *C. pneumoniae* is more difficult and not widely available. The cell lines of choice are HEp-2 and HL cells.[31] Culture confirmation should be performed by fluorescent antibody staining with species-specific monoclonal antibodies. Although there are numerous nonculture methods available for the detection of *C. trachomatis*, including direct fluorescent antibody (DFA) tests, enzyme immunoassays (EIAs), DNA hybridization, and PCR assays, all are approved primarily for genital sites in adults. DFAs and EIAs have approval for nasopharyngeal specimens from infants with suspected *C. trachomatis* pneumonia; however, the performance with respiratory specimens can be extremely variable, with sensitivities as low as 30% compared with culture.[32, 33] Nonculture tests have not been evaluated nor should they be used with throat, sinus, or other respiratory specimens.

All the currently available EIAs use polyclonal and/or genus-specific monoclonal antibodies and thus can detect *C. pneumoniae*. However, they are very insensitive compared with culture. PCR and related DNA-amplification tests will be the methods of choice in the future. Preliminary studies look very promising, and kits are currently being developed commercially.[34]

Since *C. pneumoniae* was initially very difficult to isolate by culture, Grayston proposed a set of criteria for serologic diagnosis using a modification of the microimmunofluorescence (MIF) test developed for *C. trachomatis*.[1] For acute infection, the patient should have a fourfold rise in the IgG titer or a single IgM titer of ≥1:16 or IgG titer of ≥1:512. Past or preexisting infection is defined as an IgG titer ≥1:16 and <1:512. However, as previously stated, as many as 19% of healthy, uninfected adults may meet the criteria for acute infection.[5] In children, the opposite occurs. Two studies that identified 54 children with community-acquired pneumonia and asthma who were culture-positive for *C. pneumoniae* found that only 12 (22%) had serologic evidence of acute infection and 40 (74%) had no detectable antibody by MIF even after 2 or more months of follow-up.[10, 12] As many *C.*

pneumoniae infections are chronic, a fourfold rise in IgG titer may be difficult to demonstrate.

The definitive diagnosis of *C. pneumoniae* infection remains identification of the organism by culture, PCR, or related test.

TREATMENT

Chlamydial species are susceptible to tetracyclines, macrolides, and quinolones. *C. pneumoniae* and *C. psittaci* are resistant to sulfonamides. To date, there have also been few published data describing the response of *C. pneumoniae* to antimicrobial therapy.[14] Most of the treatment studies of pneumonia caused by *C. pneumoniae* published so far have relied entirely on diagnosis by serologic tests; thus, microbiologic efficacy could not be assessed. Anecdotal reports have suggested that prolonged courses, up to 3 weeks, of either tetracyclines or erythromycin may be needed to eradicate *C. pneumoniae* from the nasopharynx of adults with flulike illness and pharyngitis.[23] Recent results of a multicenter study comparing erythromycin suspension to clarithromycin suspension, for 10 days, in children 3–12 years of age with radiographically proven pneumonia found both drugs to be equally efficacious, eradicating the organism in 86% and 79% of the children, respectively.[12] Preliminary data examining azithromycin in adults with pneumonia and bronchitis found an eradication rate of 75%.[14]

Based on these limited data, we can suggest the following regimens for respiratory infection due to *C. pneumoniae*: in adults, doxycycline 100 mg, twice daily for 14–21 days; tetracycline 250 mg four times daily for 14–21 days; or azithromycin, 1.5 g over 5 days (some patients may need to be retreated); for children, erythromycin suspension 50 mg/kg/day for 10–14 days, or clarithromycin suspension, 15 mg/kg/day in two doses for 10 days.

References

1. Grayston JT, Campbell LA, Kuo CC, et al.: A new respiratory tract pathogen: *Chlamydia pneumoniae* strain TWAR. J Infect Dis 1990; 161: 618.
2. Saikku P, Wang SP, Kleemola M, et al.: An epidemic of mild pneumonia due to an unusual strain of *Chlamydia psittaci*. J Infect Dis 1985; 151: 832.
3. Carter MW, Al-Mahdawi SAH, Giles IG, et al.: Nucleotide sequence and taxonomic value of the major outer membrane protein gene of *Chlamydia pneumoniae* 10L-207. J Gen Microbiol 1991; 137: 465.
4. Campbell LA, Kuo CC, Grayston JT: Characterization of the new *Chlamydia* agent, TWAR, as a unique organism by restriction endonuclease analysis and DNA-DNA hybridization. J Clin Microbiol 1987; 25: 1911.
5. Hyman CL, Augenbraun MH, Roblin PM, et al.: Asymptomatic respiratory tract infection with *Chlamydia pneumoniae* TWAR. J Clin Microbiol 1991; 29: 2082.
6. Falsey AR, Walsh EE: Transmission of *Chlamydia pneumoniae*. J Infect Dis 1993; 168: 493.
7. Theunissen HJH, Lemmens-deen Toom NA, Burggraaf A, et al.: Influence of temperature and relative humidity on the survival of *Chlamydia pneumoniae* in aerosols. Appl Environ Microbiol 1993; 59: 2589.
8. Yamazaki T, Nakada N, Sakurai N, et al.: Transmission of *Chlamydia pneumoniae* in young children. J Infect Dis 1990; 162: 1390.
9. Hyman CL, Roblin PM, Gaydos CA, et al.: Prevalence of asymptomatic nasopharyngeal carriage of *Chlamydia pneumoniae* in subjectively healthy adults: Assessment by polymerase chain reaction–enzyme immunoassay and culture. Clin Infect Dis 1995; 20: 1174.
10. Emre U, Roblin PM, Gelling M, et al.: The association of *Chlamydia pneumoniae* infection and reactive airway disease in children. Arch Pediatr Adolesc Med 1994; 148: 727.
11. Shemer-Avni Y, Lieberman D: *Chlamydia pneumoniae*—Induced ciliostasis in ciliated bronchial epithelial cells. J Infect Dis 1995; 171: 1274.
12. Block S, Hedrick J, Hammerschlag MR, et al.: *Mycoplasma pneumoniae* and *Chlamydia pneumoniae* in pediatric community-acquired pneumonia: Comparative efficacy and safety of clarithromycin vs erythromycin ethylsuccinate. Pediatr Infect Dis 1995; 14: 471.
13. Grayston JT, Aldous MB, Easton A, et al.: Evidence that *Chlamydia pneumoniae* causes pneumonia and bronchitis. J Infect Dis 1993; 168: 1231.
14. Hammerschlag MR: Antimicrobial susceptibility and therapy of infections caused by *Chlamydia pneumoniae*. Antimicrob Agents Chemother 1994; 38: 1873.
15. Tipple MA, Beem MO, Saxon EM: Clinical characteristics of the afebrile pneumonia associated with *Chlamydia trachomatis* infection in infants. Pediatrics 1979; 63: 192.
16. Hammerschlag MR, Hammerschlag PE, Alexander ER: The role of *Chlamydia trachomatis* in middle ear effusions in children. Pediatrics 1980; 66: 615.
17. Chang MJ, Rodriguez WJ, Mohla C: *Chlamydia trachomatis* in otitis media in children. Pediatr Infect Dis 1982; 1: 95.
18. Dawson VM, Coelen RJ, Murphy S, et al.: Microbiology of chronic otitis media with effusion among Australian aboriginal children. Role of *Chlamydia trachomatis*. Aust J Exp Biol Med Sci 1985; 63: 99.
19. Blackston ML, Lovchik JC, Gray WC: Presence of *Chlamydia trachomatis* in tympanocentesis fluid assessed by immunofluorescence microscopy and cell culture. Otolaryngol Head Neck Surg 1989; 100: 348.
20. Bell TA, Stamm WE, Wang SP, et al.: Chronic *Chlamydia trachomatis* infections in infants. JAMA; 267: 400.
21. Ogawa H, Hashiguchi K, Kazuyama Y: Recovery of *Chlamydia pneumoniae* in six patients with otitis media with effusion. J Laryngol Otol 1992; 106: 490.
22. Block S, Hedrick J, Hammerschlag MR: Unpublished data.
23. Hammerschlag MR, Chirgwin K, Roblin PM, et al.: Persistent infection with *Chlamydia pneumoniae* following acute respiratory illness. Clin Infect Dis 1992; 14: 178.
24. Hashigucci K, Ogawa H, Suzuki T, et al.: Isolation of *Chlamydia pneumoniae* from the maxillary sinus of a patient with purulent sinusitis. Clin Infect Dis 1992; 15: 570.
25. Komaroff AL, Aronson MD, Pass TM, et al.: Serologic evidence of chlamydial and mycoplasmal pharyngitis in adults. Science 1983; 222: 927.
26. Gerber MA, Ryan RW, Tilton RC, et al.: Role of *Chlamydia trachomatis* in acute pharyngitis in young adults. J Clin Microbiol 1984; 20: 993.
27. Huss H, Jungkind D, Amodio P, et al.: Frequency of *Chlamydia trachomatis* as the cause of pharyngitis. J Clin Microbiol 1985; 22: 858.
28. Jones RB, Rabinovitch RA, Katz BP, et al.: *Chlamydia trachomatis* in the pharynx and rectum of heterosexual patients at risk for genital infection. Ann Intern Med 1985; 102: 757.
29. McMillan A, Sommerville RG, McKie PM: Chlamydial infection in homosexual men: Frequency of isolation of *Chlamydia trachomatis* from the urethra, ano-rectum and pharynx. Br J Vener Dis 1981; 57: 47.
30. Huovinen P, Lahtonen R, Ziegler T, et al.: Pharyngitis in adults: The presence and coexistence of viruses and bacterial organisms. Ann Intern Med 1989; 110: 612.
31. Roblin PM, Dumornay W, Hammerschlag MR: Use of HEp-2 cells for improved isolation and passage of *Chlamydial pneumoniae*. J Clin Microbiol 1992; 30: 1968.
32. Roblin PM, Hammerschlag MR, Cummings C, et al.: Comparison of two rapid microscopic methods and culture for detection of *Chlamydia trachomatis* in ocular and nasopharyngeal specimens from infants. J Clin Microbiol 1989; 27: 968.
33. Hammerschlag MR, Roblin PM, Gelling M, et al.: Comparison of two enzyme immunoassays to culture for the diagnosis of chlamydial conjunctivitis and respiratory infection in infants. J Clin Microbiol 1990; 28: 1725.
34. Gaydos CA, Roblin PM, Hammerschlag, et al.: Diagnostic utility of PCR-enzyme immunoassay, culture and serology for detection of *Chlamydia pneumoniae* in symptomatic and asymptomatic patients. J Clin Microbiol 1994; 32: 903.

SYNDROMES

▼ *Ear Infections*

▼ *Sinus Infections*

▼ *Throat Infections*

▼ *Miscellaneous Syndromes and Infections*

Charles D. Bluestone

CHAPTER THIRTY-THREE

Otitis Media

▼

Otitis media is the most common disease diagnosed by clinicians in the United States and is prevalent throughout the world. It affects all ages, both sexes, and all races. It is the most common diagnosis made by physicians in the United States.[1] Although relatively infrequent in adults, these infections primarily affect infants and young children and to a lesser degree, older children and teenagers. It is estimated that over $5 billion is spent annually to provide health care to patients with middle ear infections in the United States.[2] Of the estimated 120 million prescriptions written for oral antimicrobial agents each year in the United States, more than one fourth are for the treatment of otitis media, the most common middle ear infection. Myringotomy with the insertion of a tympanostomy tube is the most common minor surgical procedure performed in children for which a general anesthetic is required, and tonsillectomy and adenoidectomy are still the most common major surgical procedures performed in children; many of them are for the prevention of otitis media. Otitis media is, indeed, a major health problem.

CLINICAL DESCRIPTION AND DIAGNOSIS

The clinician should be familiar with the clinical description of the various types of otitis media and the diagnostic characteristics of each type. In addition to the medical history, the pneumatic otoscope is an invaluable diagnostic aid that should be used in all age groups.[3] Tympanometry is helpful in confirming the presence or absence of a middle ear effusion.[4] Audiometry is not diagnostic of middle ear effusion but can be beneficial in the decision-making process in managing the individual patient.

The rapid, brief onset of signs and symptoms of infection in the middle ear generally is termed acute otitis media. Synonyms such as acute suppurative or purulent otitis media are acceptable. One or more of the following symptoms are present: otalgia (or pulling of the ear in the young infant), fever, or irritability of recent onset. The tympanic membrane is full or bulging, is opaque, and has limited mobility or none to pneumatic otoscopy, all of which are indicative of a middle ear effusion. The acute onset of ear pain, fever, and a purulent discharge (otorrhea) through a perforation of the tympanic membrane (or tympanostomy tube) would also be evidence of acute otitis media.

When the diagnosis of acute otitis media is in doubt or when determination of the etiologic agent is desirable,

aspiration of the middle ear should be performed by the clinician; if the clinician is not skilled in this procedure, the patient can be referred to an otolaryngologist.[5] Today, with the emergence of resistant bacterial organisms causing otitis media, such as beta-lactamase–producing *Haemophilus influenzae* and *Moraxella catarrhalis*, and the more recent troublesome rise in penicillin- and multidrug-resistant pneumococcus,[6, 7] tympanocentesis is an evermore important diagnostic procedure. Indications for tympanocentesis (or myringotomy) include the following:

1. Otitis media in patients who have severe otalgia, are seriously ill, or appear toxic
2. Unsatisfactory response to antimicrobial therapy
3. Onset of otitis media in a child who is receiving appropriate and adequate antimicrobial therapy
4. Otitis media associated with a confirmed or potential suppurative complication
5. Otitis media in a newborn infant, a sick neonate, or an immunologically deficient patient, any of whom might harbor an unusual organism[5]

Unfortunately, nasopharyngeal cultures do not accurately identify the causative organism in children with acute otitis media.

After an episode of acute otitis media, the middle ear may have an effusion that remains for weeks to months; this has been termed persistent middle ear effusion. The signs and symptoms associated with a persistent middle ear effusion are usually the same as those of an otitis media with effusion, which are described below.

Otitis media with effusion is a relatively asymptomatic middle ear effusion, which has many synonyms, such as secretory, nonsuppurative, or serous otitis media. Pneumatic otoscopy frequently reveals either a retracted or a concave tympanic membrane, the mobility of which is limited or absent. However, fullness or even bulging may be visualized. In addition, an air-fluid level or bubbles, or both, may be observed through a translucent tympanic membrane. The duration (not the severity) of the effusion can be classified as acute (less than 3 weeks), subacute (3 weeks to 3 months), or chronic (longer than 3 months). The most important distinction between this type of disease and acute otitis media is that the signs and symptoms of acute infection (e.g., otalgia, fever) are lacking in otitis media with effusion, but hearing loss is usually present in both conditions.

Chronic suppurative otitis media is a stage of ear disease in which there is chronic infection of the middle ear and mastoid, and in which a "central" perforation of the tympanic membrane (or a patent tympanostomy tube) and discharge (otorrhea) are present. The infection is a sequela of acute otitis media, most frequently when there is a preexisting defect in the tympanic membrane, such as a perforation, or a tympanostomy tube in place. Mastoiditis is invariably a part of the pathologic process. The condition has been called chronic otitis media, but this term can be confused with chronic otitis media with effusion, which is not characterized by perforation. It is also called chronic suppurative otitis media and mastoiditis, chronic purulent otitis media, and chronic otomastoiditis. The most descriptive term is chronic otitis media with perforation, discharge, and mastoiditis, but this is not common usage. When a cholesteatoma is also present, the term chronic suppurative otitis media with cholesteatoma is used; however, an acquired aural cholesteatoma does not have to be associated with chronic suppurative otitis media.

EPIDEMIOLOGY

The National Center for Health Statistics recently reported that the diagnosis of otitis media has increased from about 10 million in 1975 to almost 25 million in 1990;[1] most likely, even more patients have the diagnosis today. As reported by the center, the annual visit rate for children younger than 2 years of age statistically increased by 224% during the period of the study, and significant increases occurred in older children until the age of 10 years, but not as dramatically; there was no significant increase in the diagnosis in children who were older than 10 years of age and in adults (Fig. 33–1). In Boston, a survey of about 17,000 office visits during the first year of life revealed that acute otitis media was the diagnosis in approximately one third of visits for illness and one fifth of all office visits.[8] Several studies in the United States and Scandinavia have reported that almost 90% of children have had at least one bout of otitis media by the time they reach their 5th birthday.

Persistent middle ear effusion for weeks to months after the onset of acute otitis media was frequent in Boston children:[9] 70% of children still had effusion at 2 weeks, 40% had effusion at 1 month, 20% at 2 months, and 10% at 3 months. Similar results of persistent middle ear effusion after an episode of acute otitis media have been noted in recent studies from other centers, except for the study by Kaleida and colleagues.[10] They included in their study recurrent acute otitis media, which occurred in 50% of subjects during the following 3 months, and the point prevalence of middle ear effusion ranged between 40% at 30 days and 23% at 90 days after the onset of the initial attack. The conclusion from these studies is that persistent middle ear effusion that frequently follows an attack of acute otitis media usually clears without further treatment.[4]

Otitis media with effusion is also commonly present in infants and children, especially those who attend a daycare center. In Pittsburgh, approximately 50% of children 2–6 years of age observed monthly over a 2-year period in a daycare center had one or more episodes, which were usually associated with an upper respiratory tract infection; however, the study also revealed that two thirds of the episodes spontaneously cleared within a month.[11] In a similar study of 126 school children 5–12 years of age, the incidence of otitis media with effusion was found to be much lower in children 6 years of age and older.[12] In many children, the duration of effusion may be as short as 1 or several days. Thus, relatively asymptomatic otitis media with effusion is relatively frequent in healthy children but usually resolves without

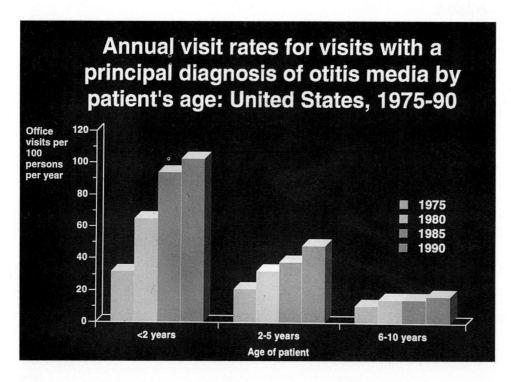

Figure 33–1. Office visits with the principal diagnosis of otitis media in the United States. (From Shappert SM: Office visits for otitis media: United States, 1975–1990. Vital and Health Statistics of the Centers for Disease Control 1992; 214: 1–18.)

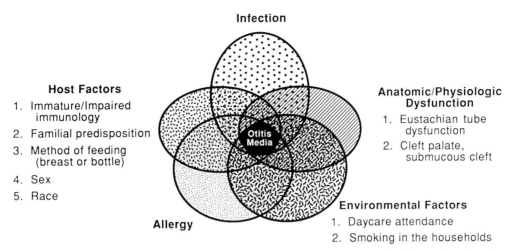

Figure 33–2. Factors related to the etiology and pathogenesis of otitis media. (From Bluestone CD, Klein JO: Otitis media atelectasis and eustachian tube dysfunction. In Bluestone CD, Stool SE, Kenna MA (eds): Pediatric Otolaryngology, 3rd ed. Philadelphia: WB Saunders Co., 1996, p 412.

medical or surgical intervention, and the incidence decreases after the age of 5 years. Past studies reported that black children had a lower incidence of middle ear disease than white children, but a recent study from Pittsburgh, in which both black and white infants were prospectively followed from birth to 2 years of age, found no difference in the incidence of either acute otitis media or otitis media with effusion.[13] Otitis media with effusion is also common in adults. In a recent report from Israel, during a 3-year period, 167 adults had the disease diagnosed, and the most common association was paranasal sinusitis.[14]

ETIOLOGY AND PATHOGENESIS

The pathogenesis of otitis media is multifactorial and includes factors such as infection (viral and bacterial); anatomic factors, such as eustachian tube dysfunction; host factors, such as young age or immature or impaired immunologic status; the presence of upper respiratory allergy; familial predisposition; the presence of older siblings in the household; male sex; race (e.g., Native Americans, Australian Aborigines); the method of feeding (bottle versus breast); and environmental factors, such as daycare attendance and passive smoking (Fig. 33–2). The increase in daycare attendance in the age group during the same period is the most likely cause of the dramatic rise. In the daycare environment, infants and young children develop frequent upper respiratory tract infections that commonly result in otitis media, since their eustachian tubes are functionally and structurally immature and they have immature immune systems.

Dysfunction of the eustachian tube appears to be the most important factor in the pathogenesis of middle ear disease in all age groups. This hypothesis was first suggested more than 100 years ago by Politzer.[15] However, later studies suggested that otitis media was a disease primarily of the middle ear mucous membrane and was caused by infection or allergic reactions in this tissue, rather than by dysfunction of the eustachian tube.[16, 17] But more recent studies conducted at the Children's Hospital of Pittsburgh, which involved humans as well as animals, have shown that the "*hydrops*

ex vacuo" theory as originally proposed by Adam Politzer over a century ago is most likely the primary pathogenic mechanism in many patients; dysfunction of the eustachian tube also promotes viruses and bacteria to enter the middle ear, which results in otitis media.[18–23]

ANATOMY AND PHYSIOLOGY OF EUSTACHIAN TUBE

The eustachian tube is part of a system of contiguous organs including the nose, palate, nasopharynx, middle ear, and mastoid air cells (Fig. 33–3). The eustachian tube, in reality, is not a tube but also an organ consisting of a lumen with its mucosa, cartilage, surrounding soft tissue, peritubal muscles (i.e., tensor veli palatini, levator veli palatini, salpingopharyngeus, and tensor tympani), and superior bony support, the sphenoid sulcus. The eustachian tube has at least three physiologic functions with respect to the middle ear: (1) *pressure regulation* of the middle ear to equilibrate gas

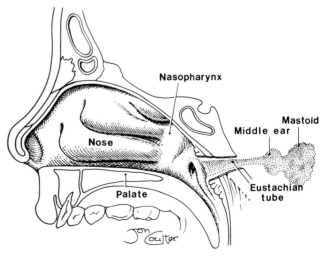

Figure 33–3. Eustachian tube is part of a system made up of the organs at either end of the tube.

pressure in the middle ear with atmospheric pressure; (2) *protection* from nasopharyngeal sound pressure and secretions; and (3) *clearance* of secretions produced within the middle ear into the nasopharynx (see Fig. 33–2). A basic understanding of these physiologic functions is helpful in comprehending the role of the eustachian tube in the pathogenesis of middle ear disease.

Pressure Regulation of Middle Ear (Ventilatory Function)

The most important function of the eustachian tube is regulation of pressure within the middle ear, since hearing is optimal when the middle ear gas pressure is relatively the same as the air pressure in the external auditory canal, i.e., tympanic membrane and middle ear compliance is physiologic. In ideal tubal function, intermittent active opening of the eustachian tube, due only to contraction of the tensor veli palatini muscle during swallowing, maintains nearly ambient pressures in the middle ear.[19, 24–26] Opening of the eustachian tube permits gas exchange and equalization of pressures between the environment and the middle ear. Under physiologic conditions the fluctuations in ambient pressure are bidirectional (i.e., either to or from the middle ear), relatively small in magnitude, and not readily appreciated.[27] These fluctuations reflect the rise and fall in barometric pressures associated with changing weather conditions and elevation, or both. However, the changes in middle ear pressure show mass directionality, can achieve appreciable magnitudes, and can result in pathologic changes. A major reason for these conditions is that the middle ear is a relatively rigid (i.e., noncollapsible) gas pocket, which is surrounded by mucous membrane, in which gases are exchanged between the middle ear space and the mucosa. Differential pressure exceeds 54 mm Hg between the middle ear space at atmospheric pressure and the microcirculation in the mucous membrane. This represents a diffusion-driven gradient from the middle ear cavity to the mucosa that can produce an underpressure (relative to ambient pressure) in the middle ear of more than 600 mm H_2O during equilibration.

Normal eustachian tube function was studied in Sweden using a pressure chamber in which children who were considered to be otologically normal were evaluated.[28] Eustachian tube function was evaluated in 53 children and compared with function in 55 adults, all of whom had intact tympanic membranes and who were apparently otologically healthy. The study revealed that 35.8% of the children could not equilibrate applied negative intratympanic pressure by swallowing, whereas only 5% of the adults were unable to perform this function. Children from 3 to 6 years of age had worse function than those aged 7–12 years. In this study and a subsequent one conducted by the same research group, children who had tympanometric evidence of negative pressure within the middle ear had poor eustachian tube function.[29] The conclusion from these studies is that even in apparently otologically normal children, eustachian tube function is not as good as in adults, and this is related to the higher incidence of middle ear disease in children.

Since infants have inefficient active tubal opening, then how do they physiologically regulate middle ear gas pressure? One possible explanation is that they inflate their middle ear during crying. Evidence that this occurs is the finding of positive middle ear pressures on tympanograms when infants who have no middle ear effusion are crying; also, a bulging tympanic membrane can be seen when pneumatic otoscopy is performed. Perhaps this is the compensatory mechanism used by infants during descent when they are passengers in airplanes. Even though pressure regulation of the middle ear is the most important of the functions of the eustachian tube, the protective and clearance functions are also important in maintaining the physiologic state.

Protective Function

In the physiologic state, the eustachian tube protects the middle ear because of the tube's anatomic structure, which depends also on an intact middle ear and mastoid so that a middle ear and mastoid gas pocket or cushion is present. The protective function has been assessed only by radiographic techniques,[18, 30, 31] which were modifications of a tubal patency test described by Wittenborg and Neuhauser.[32] In these studies radiopaque material was instilled into the nose and nasopharynx of children who had otitis media and compared with the material in those who were otologically normal. In the physiologic state, contrast material entered the nasopharyngeal end of the eustachian tube during swallowing activity but did not enter the middle ear. By contrast, the dye did reflux into the middle ear in some patients who had middle ear disease, especially during closed-nose swallowing. At rest, the normal eustachian tube is collapsed and the tubal lumen is closed, thus preventing liquid from entering the nasopharyngeal end of the tube. During swallowing, when the proximal end (i.e., cartilaginous portion) opens, liquid can enter this part of the tube but does not gain entrance into the middle ear, due to the narrow midportion of the tube, the isthmus. The entire eustachian tube–middle ear system is similar in this function to a flask with a long, narrow neck in which the mouth of the flask represents the nasopharyngeal end; the narrow neck, the isthmus; and the bulbous portion, the middle ear and mastoid air cell system.[5, 18]

Clearance Function

The clearance function of the eustachian tube is also important in maintaining the physiologic state of the middle ear. Clearance of secretions from the middle ear is provided by the mucociliary system of the eustachian tube and some areas of the middle ear mucous membrane. Also involved in the clearance of middle ear secretions is the pumping action of the eustachian tube during closing. The clearance function has been studied by instilling radiopaque material into the middle ear of children whose tympanic membranes were not intact, or when the material entered the middle ear (intact tympanic membrane) from the nasopharynx,[18, 31] and following insertion of foreign material into the middle ear in animal models.[33, 34] Such material flows toward the middle ear portion of the eustachian tube and out the tube. This movement is related to ciliary activity that occurs in the eustachian tube and parts of the middle ear; these ciliated cells in the middle ear are increasingly more active as their location becomes more distal to the opening of the eustachian tube.[35] In a series of elegant experiments by Honjo and colleagues, the eustachian tube was shown to pump liquid out of the middle ear in both animal models and humans.[36, 37]

Surface Tension Factors

Surface tension factors that could be involved with normal eustachian tube function have been identified by several investigators. Birken and Brookler isolated surface tension–lowering substances from washings of eustachian tubes of dogs.[38] They postulated that these substances could act to enhance eustachian tube functions, like surfactant in the lung. Rapport and colleagues described a similar substance and demonstrated the effect of washing out the eustachian tube on the opening pressure in the experimental animal;[39] others also have demonstrated a surfactant-like phospholipid in the middle ear and eustachian tube of animals and humans.[40–42] In a recent study in gerbils, Fornadley and Burns produced middle ear effusions by injecting killed *Streptococcus pneumoniae* into the middle ear through the tympanic membrane, which increased the opening pressure of the eustachian tube.[43] When the investigators introduced exogenous surfactant, the opening pressure dropped. From these studies, it is apparent that the clearance function of the eustachian tube–middle ear system is important in maintaining a healthy middle ear. Because otitis media is so common in humans, efficient removal of middle ear effusions must depend, to a large extent, on these functions.

DYSFUNCTION OF EUSTACHIAN TUBE

Abnormal function of the eustachian tube that can cause otitis media and related conditions can be due to (1) impairment of the pressure regulation function of the tube, (2) loss of the protective function of the eustachian tube–middle ear, and (3) impairment of clearance function of the tube and middle ear. Pathologic changes in other parts of the system, such as nasal obstruction or palatal dysfunction, may also adversely influence eustachian tube–middle ear function.

Impairment of Pressure Regulation (Functional Obstruction)

Impairment of the regulation of pressure within the middle ear can be caused by either: (1) anatomic obstruction or (2) failure of the opening mechanism (i.e., functional obstruction) of the eustachian tube.

Anatomic Obstruction of Eustachian Tube

Anatomic (i.e., "mechanical") obstruction of the tube can be either intraluminal, periluminal, or peritubal. Obstruction of the lumen or within the periluminal tissues (i.e., intrinsic obstruction) can be due to inflammation secondary to infection,[21, 44, 45] or allergy.[46] Obstruction within the bony portion (i.e., middle ear end) of the tube is usually due to acute or chronic inflammation of the mucosal lining, which may also be associated with polyps or a cholesteatoma. Total obstruction may be present at the middle ear end of the tube. Stenosis of the eustachian tube has also been diagnosed but is a rare finding. Peritubal obstruction (i.e., extrinsic obstruction) could be the result of compression caused by a tumor or possibly an adenoid mass.[31, 47]

Failure of Opening Mechanism of Eustachian Tube

Failure of the opening mechanism may be due either to persistent collapse of the eustachian tube caused by increased tubal compliance (i.e., lack of stiffness, or "floppy"), to an inefficient active opening mechanism, or both. This has also been termed functional obstruction of the eustachian tube—the tube is not anatomically (i.e., mechanically) obstructed, but it is functionally obstructed—which was first described by Bluestone in infants with unrepaired palatal clefts who had chronic otitis media with effusion.[30] Failure of the opening mechanism of the eustachian tube is common in infants and younger children without cleft palate or history of middle ear disease,[29, 48] but is more common in those children with middle ear disease.[18, 49–51]

A possible explanation for the opening failure of the tube in infants and young children may be related to the cartilage support, since the length of eustachian tube cartilage is less in infants than in older children and adults,[52] and the cell density of the cartilage decreases with advancing age,[53] which could affect the stiffness of the tubal cartilage in the infant and young child. If the tubal cartilage lacks stiffness, then the lumen may not open in response to contraction of the tensor veli palatini muscle. Also, the density of elastin in the cartilage is less in the infant,[54] and Ostmann's fat pad is less in volume in the infant than in the adult, but the width is similar between the two age groups.[55]

Inefficient active opening of the eustachian tube is another possible reason that could be related to the marked age differences in the craniofacial base. The angle of the tube in the child is different from that of the adult. In the adult, the tube is approximately 45° related to the horizontal plane, but in infants this inclination is only 10°.[56] This difference in the angle has been thought by some to be related to possible clearance problems in children, but this hypothesis has not been confirmed. It is more likely that the difference in angulation has an effect on the function of the active opening mechanism (i.e., tensor veli palatini muscle contraction). Swarts and Rood found that the angular relationship between the tensor veli palatini muscle and the cartilage varies in the infant but is relatively stable in the adult.[57]

Loss of Protective Function

The middle ear may not be protected from unwanted nasopharyngeal secretions when (1) the eustachian tube has abnormal patency, (2) the tube is relatively short, (3) abnormal gas pressure develops at either end of the tube, or (4) there is a nonintact middle ear and mastoid, e.g., perforation of the tympanic membrane, which results in a loss of the middle ear gas pocket or cushion.

Abnormal Patency of Eustachian Tube

The eustachian tube is open even at rest (i.e., patulous tube) in extreme cases of abnormal patency of the eustachian tube. Lesser degrees of abnormal patency result in a semipatulous eustachian tube that is closed at rest but has low resistance in comparison with the normal tube. Increased patency of the tube may be due to abnormal tube geometry or to a decrease in the peritubal pressure, such as occurs after weight loss or possibly as a result of periluminal factors. Since the eustachian tube has been found to be highly compliant in infants and young children, this increase in distensibility of the tube may result in abnormal patency, especially when there is high nasopharyngeal pressure. But, in teenagers and adults the patulous tube has been found to be too stiff, compared with the normally compliant tube.[58] A patulous eustachian tube usually permits gas to flow readily from the nasopharynx into the middle ear, which thus effectively regulates middle ear pressure; however, unwanted secretions from the nasopharynx can more readily gain access, i.e., reflux, to the middle ear when the tube is abnormally patent. Certain special populations have been found to have patulous or semipatulous eustachian tubes, such as Native Americans,[59] and patients who have Down's syndrome and middle ear disease.[60]

The Short Eustachian Tube

Most likely, the most important difference in the anatomy of the eustachian tube between infants and young children, and older children and adults, is the length of the tube; the tube is shorter in children younger than 7 years of age (Table 33–1).[61] Young children with a cleft palate have eustachian tubes that are statistically shorter than those in age-matched controls younger than 6 years of age; also the tube is shorter in children with Down's syndrome.[61]

The shorter the tube, the more likely secretions can reflux into the middle ear. An analogy can be made to the length of the urethra: females of all ages have more urinary tract infections than males because the urethra is shorter in the female. This may be one explanation for the frequent occurrence of troublesome otorrhea in infants and young children, especially those who have a cleft palate, or have Down's syndrome, when the tympanic membrane is not intact.

Abnormal Gas Pressures

If high negative pressure develops in the middle ear, secondary to obstruction of the eustachian tube, because of either anatomic obstruction or failure of active opening, or both, aspiration of nasopharyngeal secretions into the middle ear may result in middle ear disease. At the other end of the

Table 33–1. DEVELOPMENTAL DIFFERENCES BETWEEN ANATOMY OF EUSTACHIAN TUBE IN INFANTS AND ADULTS

Anatomic Features of Tube	Compared with Adult Tube, Infant Tube is	Reference
Length of tube	Shorter	Sadler-Kimes et al., 1989
Angle of tube to horizontal plane (degrees)	10 versus 45	Proctor, 1967[56]
Angle of TVP to cartilage	Variable versus stable	Swarts and Rood, 1993[57]
Cartilage cell density	Greater	Yamaguchi et al., 1990[53]
Elastin at hinge portion of cartilage	Less	Matsune et al., 1993[54]
Ostmann's fat pad	Relatively wider	Aoki et al., 1994[55]

From Bluestone CD, Klein JO: Otitis media, atelectasis, and eustachian tube dysfunction. In: Bluestone CD, Stool SE, Kenna MA (eds): Pediatric Otolaryngology, 3rd ed. Philadelphia: WB Saunders Co, 1996.
TVP = Tensor veli palatini muscle.

system, high positive nasopharyngeal pressures can result in insufflation of secretions into the middle ear, which may occur during blowing the nose, during crying in the infant, or when nasal obstruction is present. Swallowing when the nose is obstructed (owing to inflammation or enlarged adenoids) results in an initial positive nasopharyngeal air pressure followed by a negative-pressure phase. When the tube is pliant, positive nasopharyngeal pressure might insufflate infected secretions into the middle ear, especially when the middle ear has a high negative pressure; with negative nasopharyngeal pressure, such a tube could be prevented from opening and could be further obstructed functionally, which has been referred to as Toynbee's phenomenon.[48, 62, 63] Rapid alterations in ambient pressures, which can occur during swimming and diving, during airplane flying, and when patients receive hypobaric pressure treatments, may also result in aspiration or insufflation of nasopharyngeal secretions.

Nonintact Middle Ear–Mastoid Air Cells

When the anatomy of the eustachian tube is normal, nasopharyngeal secretions are prevented from entering the middle ear, but this protection is also due to the "cushion" (or "pocket") of gas that is within the intact middle ear and mastoid–air cell system. When a perforation of the tympanic membrane is present, or in the extreme condition, when a radical mastoidectomy is present (the eardrum is absent, and the middle ear, mastoid, and ear canal communicate, forming a single cavity), the gas pocket is lost, which may allow secretions from the nasopharynx to reflux into the middle ear.[18, 49]

Impairment of Clearance Function

Clearance of normal and unwanted secretions from the middle ear into the nasopharynx can be affected by several conditions that can occur in the eustachian tube and middle ear. Ohashi and colleagues demonstrated in studies conducted in guinea pigs that bacteria, their toxins, and irradiation can impair ciliary function.[64] Also, Park and associates[65] demonstrated that influenza A virus alters the ciliary activity and dye transport function in the eustachian tube of the chinchilla. Most investigators consider impairment of the clearance function to be related to failure to resolve middle ear effusions as opposed to being the primary cause of the disease.[66] However, patients who have ciliary dysmotility in their upper respiratory tract mucous membrane have been observed to have chronic middle ear effusions.[67] Also, tubal pumping action is most likely ineffective when the opening mechanism is inadequate, and this function has been demonstrated to be impaired when negative pressure was present within the middle ear.[68, 69]

Role of Allergy in Eustachian Tube Function

Allergy may affect the eustachian tube and middle ear and cause otitis media by one or more of the following possible mechanisms: (1) middle ear mucosa functioning as a "shock (target) organ,"[70–72] (2) inflammatory swelling of the mucosa of the eustachian tube,[46] (3) inflammatory obstruction of the nose, i.e., "Toynbee's phenomenon", or (4) aspiration of bacteria-laden allergic nasopharyngeal secretions into the middle ear cavity.[49] Another possible mechanism has been proposed by Doyle.[73] This hypothesis is based on the possible increase in circulating anti-inflammatory mediators as the result of local allergic reactions in the mucosa of the nose or stomach, which in turn could alter the middle ear mucosal permeability and result in altered gas exchange. Studies at the Children's Hospital of Pittsburgh involving adult volunteers have shown there is an effect on eustachian tube function when there are changes in the nose. Table 33–2 shows the summary of these studies that demonstrated a relationship among intranasal challenge with allergens, virus, and mediators in volunteers who did and did not have allergic rhinitis, and the effect on nasal and eustachian tube function.[20, 21, 46, 74–79] It seems reasonable that children with signs and symptoms of upper respiratory allergy may have otitis media as a result of the allergic condition. Most likely, however, these children also have a preexisting dysfunction of the eustachian tube. However, some investigators have

Table 33–2. EFFECT OF NASAL CHALLENGE ON NASAL AND EUSTACHIAN TUBE FUNCTION: STUDIES AT CHILDREN'S HOSPITAL OF PITTSBURGH

Nasal Provocation	Nasal Function		Eustachian Tube Function	
	Normal	*Allergic*	*Normal*	*Allergic*
Allergens (pollens, mite)	No	Yes	No	Yes
Virus (rhinovirus, influenza A)	Yes	Yes	Yes	Yes
Mediators				
Histamine	Yes	Yes	No	Yes
Prostaglandin D$_2$	Yes	Yes	No	Yes
Methacholine	Yes	Yes	No	No

Yes = adverse effect, no = little effect. Studies at Children's Hospital of Pittsburgh.

concluded that allergy is not the cause of the middle ear disease but plays a role in the persistence of effusion.[66]

Cleft Palate and Eustachian Tube Function

Virtually all infants with an unrepaired cleft palate have middle ear effusions.[80, 81] Palate repair appears to improve middle ear status, but middle ear disease nonetheless often continues or recurs even after palate repair.[82] Studies suggest failure of the opening mechanism in infants with an unrepaired cleft palate.[30, 83, 84] Histopathologic temporal bone studies have confirmed that the eustachian tube of cleft palate patients is not anatomically obstructed, which would give credence to failure of the opening mechanism, i.e., functional as opposed to anatomic obstruction, as the underlying defect. The other anatomic findings, such as the abnormal cartilage and lumen, abnormal insertion ratio of the tensor veli palatini muscle into the cartilage, deficient attachment of the tensor veli palatini muscle into the lateral lamina of the cartilage, and deficient elastin at the hinge portion of the cartilage,[85–89] most likely explain the functional obstruction identified by radiographic and manometric eustachian tube function tests. Also, animals in which the palate had been surgically split develop otitis media with effusion.[84, 90, 91] From these studies in humans and animals, it appears that the high incidence of otitis media in children with cleft palate is related to failure of the opening mechanism and may also be related to the deficient length of the eustachian tube. If infants with an intact palate are able to inflate their middle ears during crying, as a physiologic compensatory mechanism for their ineffective active tubal opening, then infants with an unrepaired cleft palate have an additional handicap.

Other Causes of Eustachian Tube Dysfunction

Abnormal function of the eustachian tube has also been reported to be associated with deviation of the nasal septum;[92, 93] trauma induced by nasogastric and nasal endotracheal tubes;[94, 95] trauma to the palate, pterygoid bone, or tensor veli palatini muscle; injury to the trigeminal nerve or, more specifically, to the mandibular branch of this nerve;[96] and trauma associated with surgical procedures, such as palatal or maxillary resection for tumor.[97] Neoplastic disease, either benign or malignant, that invades the palate, pterygoid bone, or tensor veli palatini muscle can cause otitis media,[98] as a result of failure of the opening mechanism of the tube.[97, 99, 100]

EUSTACHIAN TUBE IN THE PATHOGENESIS OF OTITIS MEDIA

Acute Otitis Media

Acute otitis media most likely develops in the following sequence: the patient has an antecedent event (usually an upper respiratory viral infection) that results in congestion of the respiratory mucosa of the upper respiratory tract, including the nasopharynx and eustachian tube; congestion of the mucosa in the eustachian tube results in obstruction of the tube; negative middle ear pressure develops and, if prolonged, is followed by "aspiration" of potential pathogens (viruses and bacteria) from the nasopharynx into the middle ear. Since the eustachian tube is obstructed, an effusion due to the infection accumulates in the middle ear; microbial pathogens proliferate in the secretions, resulting in a suppurative and symptomatic otitis media. In a recent study conducted by Buchman and colleagues, this cascade of events was reproduced in 27 adult volunteers in whom influenza A virus was inoculated into the nose.[101] All subjects developed a nasal infection, 16 (59%) subsequently developed high negative middle ear effusion, and in one subject, an acute otitis media was present; the middle ear aspirate revealed the virus and *S. pneumoniae*.

In children with recurrent episodes of acute otitis media or otitis media with effusion, an anatomic or physiologic abnormality of the eustachian tube appears to be an important, if not the most important, factor. The child with such an underlying abnormality of the eustachian tube may be subject to recurrent episodes of acute otitis media. The pathogenesis of recurrent acute otitis media in 50 otitis-prone children (defined as greater than 11 episodes of acute otitis media) was studied in Sweden by Stenstrom and colleagues.[50] Employing the pressure chamber to test eustachian tube function, they found the otitis-prone children to have significantly poorer active tubal function than 49 normal (control) children who had no history of acute otitis media. This finding indicates that the pathogenesis of recurrent acute otitis media is the result of functional, as opposed to mechanical, obstruction of the eustachian tube. However, it is likely that infants and young children who have short, floppy eustachian tubes can reflux or insufflate nasopharyngeal secretions into the middle ear during a viral upper respiratory tract infection. Another possible mechanism is progressive ascending infection from the nasopharynx into the mucosa of the eustachian tube, which most likely occurs when there is an indwelling obstructing foreign object in the nasopharynx, such as a nasogastric or nasotracheal tube in place.

Otitis Media with Effusion

The acute onset of otitis media with effusion, although a relatively asymptomatic condition in children, most likely has a similar sequence of events as described above for acute otitis media, since bacteria can be isolated from middle ear effusions of patients with otitis media with effusion,[102, 103] but prolonged negative pressure within the middle ear can cause a sterile middle ear effusion. Otitis media with effusion has been produced in the monkey animal model after excision of,[104] and injection of botulinum toxin into,[19, 105] the tensor veli palatini muscle, which resulted in an opening failure of the eustachian tube, middle ear underpressures, and effusion. These experiments confirm the hydrops ex vacuo theory of the pathogenesis of middle ear effusion, which postulates that in the absence of eustachian tube

opening, the gas exchange from the middle ear into the microcirculation of the mucous membrane causes a middle ear underpressure, followed by transudation of effusion. Alper and associates were also able to produce middle ear effusion in the monkey shortly after inducing middle ear negative pressure by flushing the middle ear with CO_2.[105] Because tubal opening is possible in a middle ear with an effusion, aspiration of nasopharyngeal secretions might occur, thus creating the clinical condition in which otitis media with effusion and recurrent acute bacterial otitis media with effusion occur together. The most dramatic example of the "ex vacuo" cause of acute middle ear effusion is after barotrauma, e.g., descent during scuba diving or airplane flying.

In two elegant studies by McBride and colleagues[45] and Buchman and colleagues[21] that involved adult volunteers, nasal challenge with rhinovirus resulted in eustachian tube obstruction and negative middle ear pressure, and in two subjects middle ear effusion developed. The two individuals who had a middle ear effusion had negative middle ear pressure before the challenge. None of the subjects who had normal middle ear pressure before the challenge developed an effusion, which would indicate that a viral infection will result in a middle ear effusion if the patient has a preexisting dysfunction of the eustachian tube.[21] Doyle and colleagues also demonstrated that intranasal challenge of influenza A virus in 33 healthy adult volunteers resulted in eustachian tube obstruction and negative middle ear pressure, and in 5 of 21 infected subjects, middle ear effusion developed.[20] Most likely, influenza A virus is more virulent than rhinovirus. Periods of upper respiratory tract infection may then result in atelectasis of the tympanic membrane–middle ear (i.e., high negative middle ear pressure), sterile otitis media with effusion, or acute bacterial otitis media.

In a study of eustachian tube function in 163 ears of Japanese children and adults who had otitis media with effusion and chronic otitis media, Iwano and colleagues found impaired active opening function of the tube in children and adults.[51] They concluded the tube was functionally obstructed; however, "organic" (i.e., mechanical or anatomic) obstruction was considered also to be involved in the pathogenesis in adults.

Persistent Middle Ear Effusion

The pathogenesis of persistent middle ear effusion after the initial stage of a viral or bacterial infection in the middle ear, or after transudation of effusion when high negative pressure is within the middle ear, is probably similar. There is stimulation of cytokines, such as interleukin-1, interleukin-2, interleukin-6, tumor necrosis factor, and interferon-γ, from inflammatory cells of the middle ear mucous membrane,[106–111] followed by two pathways of inflammation: (1) upregulation of submucosal receptors, primarily selectins and integrins that trap into the mucosa lymphocytes, which also produce cytokines and inflammatory mediators; and (2) stimulation of inflammatory mediators, such as leukotrienes, prostaglandins, thromboxane, prostacyclin, and platelet-activating factor,[112–118] which in turn can promote fluid leakage from the mucous membrane. At this stage there is probably an increase in blood flow within the mucous membrane, because of engorgement of blood vessels and angioneogenesis, which then results in further negative pressure within the middle ear because of an increase in perfusion of N_2 into the microcirculation of the mucosa.[27] In addition, the effusion that is produced is "trapped" in the middle ear because of the anatomy of the system, i.e., a closed space in which there is a narrow outlet, the eustachian tube. Also, the mucociliary system and the pumping action of tubal opening and closing is most likely impaired. Thus, persistent middle ear effusion results.

Eustachian Tube Dysfunction

Dysfunction of the eustachian tube can be due to either tubal obstruction or a patulous tube and result in signs and symptoms referable to the ear, despite the lack of a middle ear effusion. Obstruction of the tube can cause middle ear negative pressure, retraction of the tympanic membrane, hearing loss, and, in its severe form, atelectasis of the middle ear, i.e., loss of the middle ear space. Obstruction can be due to inflammation or failure of the opening mechanism and can be acute or chronic, but evidently infrequent periodic tubal opening occurs to prevent the accumulation of an effusion. A patulous tube can cause patients to complain of autophony and hearing their own breathing in the ear, since the eustachian tube is open at rest, i.e., in the absence of swallowing activity. Both conditions have been documented during the last trimester of pregnancy.[119] Eustachian tube obstruction is not uncommon in girls during puberty; this may be related to hormonal changes, but the underlying cause of this problem has not been reported.

Chronic Suppurative Otitis Media

Chronic suppurative otitis media (without cholesteatoma) is the chronic stage that follows an attack of acute otitis media in which a perforation of the tympanic membrane, or tympanostomy tube, is present, followed by continuous discharge. From our studies of the pathogenesis of chronic suppurative otitis media,[120, 121] it appears that the sequence of events may be in one of two ways: When the tympanic membrane is not intact, bacteria from the nasopharynx can gain access to the middle ear due to reflux of nasopharyngeal secretions, especially when there is inflammation (secondary to infection or possibly allergy) of the nose, nasopharynx, or paranasal sinuses through the eustachian tube, since the middle ear "gas cushion" is lost. In most instances, these bacteria are initially the same as those isolated when acute otitis occurs behind an intact tympanic membrane, such as *S. pneumoniae* and *H. influenzae*, and when acute otorrhea develops when tympanostomy tubes are in place.[122] After the acute otorrhea, *Pseudomonas aeruginosa*, *Staphylococcus aureus*, and other organisms from the external ear canal enter the middle ear through the nonintact tympanic membrane, which results in the chronic infection. The second common way in which chronic otitis media occurs is by contamination of the middle ear cleft from organisms (e.g., *P. aeruginosa*) that are present in water that enters through the nonintact eardrum during bathing and swimming.

MICROBIOLOGY

The bacteria causing acute otitis media in children have remained relatively constant for the past decades, but only recently has there been a report describing the bacteria causing this infection in adults in the United States.[123] Figure 33–4 shows that these organisms in the two populations are the same. *S. pneumoniae* was the predominant pathogen cultured from aspirates of children who had acute otitis media during decade of the 1980s; however, this rate significantly increased from 29% in 1980 to 44% in 1989.[102] *H. influenzae* was the second most common pathogen isolated

Figure 33–4. Comparison of bacterial etiology of acute otitis media between children and adults. (From Bluestone CD, Stephenson JS, Martin LM: Ten-year review of otitis media pathogens. Pediatr Infect Dis J 1992; 11: 7–11; and Celin SE, Bluestone CD, Stephenson J, et al.: Bacteriology of acute otitis media in adults. JAMA 1991; 266: 2249–2252, Copyright 1991, American Medical Association.)

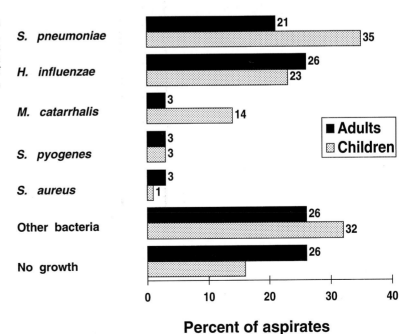

Percent of aspirates

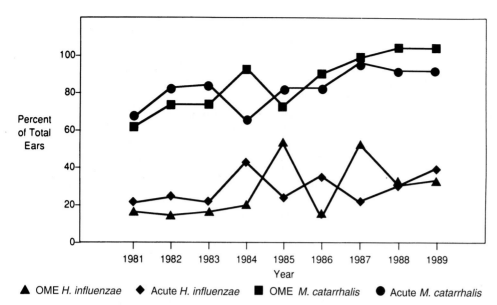

Figure 33–5. Percent beta-lactamase–producing *H. influenzae* and *M. catarrhalis* in acute otitis media and otitis media with effusion (OME). 1981–1989. (From Bluestone CD, Stephenson JS, Martin LM: Ten-year review of otitis media pathogens. Pediatr Infect Dis J 1992; 11(8 Suppl): 7–11.)

▲ OME *H. influenzae*   ◆ Acute *H. influenzae*   ■ OME *M. catarrhalis*   ● Acute *M. catarrhalis*

in acute ear infections in children. In adults, these two bacteria were also the most commonly isolated.[123] Before 1980, the incidence of *M. catarrhalis* was less than 10%, but it is now present in 14% of acute effusions in children; only 3% of middle ear aspirates obtained from adults had this bacterium. Group A beta-hemolytic streptococcus and *S. aureus* also cause this infection in both children and adults, but not as frequently as pneumococcus and *H. influenzae*. Respiratory viruses have been cultured from as many as 19% of acute effusions.[124] Anaerobic bacteria are infrequently cultured from middle ear aspirates of children.

The percentage of *H. influenzae* (primarily nontypable in otitis media) that are beta-lactamase–producing in children is now more than 30% in the Pittsburgh area (Fig. 33–5). This percentage increased during the 1980s, as did the rate of beta-lactamase–producing *M. catarrhalis*. Currently, most, if not all, strains of *M. catarrhalis* isolated from children's middle ears produce beta-lactamase. In the study of adults, 22.5% of *H. influenzae* produced beta-lactamase and both isolates of *M. catarrhalis* were beta-lactamase–producing. Overall, 9% of the adults had beta-lactamase–producing organisms.

The rate of isolation of penicillin-resistant *S. pneumoniae* from the middle ear is increasing in the United States.[6, 7] Mason and colleagues reported that the middle ear was the most common site in which resistant pneumococcus was isolated at their children's hospital in Houston.[125] Reichler and colleagues reported a high rate of nasopharyngeal carriage of resistant pneumococcus in children attending a day-care center in Ohio;[126] this was attributed to the use of antimicrobial treatment and prophylaxis for otitis media. Figure 33–6 shows that the rate of these resistant organisms has increased at the Children's Hospital of Pittsburgh from 12% in 1988 to 31% in 1994.

With the relatively recent emergence of resistant bacterial organisms causing otitis media, such as beta-lactamase–producing *H. influenzae* and *M. catarrhalis*, and the more recent troublesome rise in penicillin-resistant—as well as multidrug-resistant—pneumococcus, tympanocentesis should

be considered in patients who are seriously ill or appear toxic, or in those children and adults who fail to improve rapidly on appropriate and adequate antimicrobial therapy.[5] The change in the incidence of these pathogens and the increasing emergence of beta-lactamase–producing organisms has an important impact on the management of acute otitis media today.

In the past, otitis media with effusion was assumed to be sterile, since several reports described unsuccessful attempts to culture bacteria; however, later studies identified bacteria by means of smears and cultures in a small percentage of middle ear effusions. In a study of 4589 middle ear aspirates from ears with chronic otitis media with effusion from our center during the 1980s, about two thirds had bacteria isolated; of the one third that were considered to be pathogens, the most common bacteria were *H. influenzae*, *M. catarrhalis*, and *S. pneumoniae*, which are the common pathogens

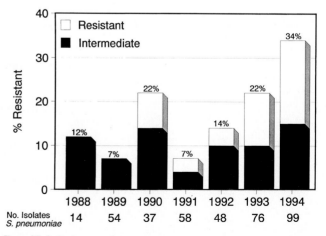

| No. Isolates *S. pneumoniae* | 14 | 54 | 37 | 58 | 48 | 76 | 99 |

Figure 33–6. Resistance of *S. pneumoniae* to penicillin G from middle ear aspirates: Children's Hospital of Pittsburgh. Breakpoint for susceptibility for penicillin <0.1 μg/mL. Isolates tested by broth microdilution using Mueller-Hinton medium containing 2% lysed sheep blood. (Courtesy R. Wadowsky, Children's Hospital of Pittsburgh, unpublished data.)

found in middle ear aspirates from children with acute otitis media.[102] In addition, *Staphylococcus epidermidis* was cultured from many middle ears when it was not cultured from the external canal of the same ear. (A culture preceded sterilization and tympanocentesis.) Beta-lactamase activity was similar to that reported for isolates from ears with acute otitis media.

Post and colleagues found that 77.3% of middle ear effusions had evidence of the three major organisms (i.e., *H. influenzae, M. catarrhalis*, and *S. pneumoniae*) by polymerase chain reaction, whereas only 28.9% of the aspirates were culture-positive (Fig. 33–7).[103] The investigators postulated that bacteria may have a larger role in the inflammatory process than previously believed.

Unfortunately, information concerning the microbiology of otitis media with effusion that occurs in adults is not available.

Chronic suppurative otitis media develops from a chronic bacterial infection; however, the bacteria that caused the initial episode of acute otitis media with perforation and otorrhea may not be those that are isolated from the chronic discharge when there is chronic infection in the middle ear and mastoid. In fact, Mandel and associates reported that infants and young children who had the acute onset of otorrhea through a tympanostomy tube usually had the common organisms that cause acute otitis media when the tympanic membrane is intact, whereas, in older children, especially in the summer, the predominant organism was frequently *Pseudomonas*, presumably due to contamination of the middle ear during swimming.[122] Thus, the antimicrobial therapy recommended for acute otitis media may not be effective for most cases of chronic suppurative otitis media. The microbiology of chronic suppurative otitis media without cholesteatoma in children has been reported by Kenna Bluestone, and colleagues.[120] From the 51 ear cultures obtained from 36 children, 23 microbiologic species were isolated. One organism was isolated from 18 ears, two from 20 ears, three from 3 ears, four from 4 ears, and five from 2

ears. The most common bacterial species isolated was *P. aeruginosa*, which was present in 34 ears (67%) and was the only isolate in 16 ears (31%). Of the 15 children who had bilateral otorrhea, 11 (73%) had the same organism(s) identified in both middle ears: seven children had *P. aeruginosa* isolated, four had *S. aureus*, and one each had *S. epidermidis, Candida albicans*, and diphtheroids.

The bacteriology of chronic suppurative otitis media with cholesteatoma in children and adults has been reported. The most common aerobic microbiologic organisms isolated were *P. aeruginosa* and *S. aureus*, and the most frequent anaerobic organisms were *Bacteroides, Peptostreptococcus*, and *Peptococcus* species. It is important to make the distinction between chronic suppurative otitis media with and without cholesteatoma, since tympanomastoid surgery is indicated when cholesteatoma is present, whereas medical management may be effective when it is not.

MANAGEMENT

Acute Otitis Media

Some clinicians question the need for antimicrobial therapy in patients who have acute otitis media; however, most experts in the United States today agree that acute otitis media should be actively treated with an antimicrobial agent.[127] A large clinical trial by Kaleida and colleagues found that children who had "severe" acute otitis media and who had been randomized to receive myringotomy without antibiotic had statistically more initial treatment failures than those who received an antimicrobial agent, with or without the adjunctive use of a myringotomy.[128] As part of that trial, another group of children who had "nonsevere" acute otitis media were randomized to either antibiotic or placebo, and those in the placebo group also had more treatment failures, as well as more time with middle ear effusion, compared with those in the antibiotic group.

Another reason to administer antimicrobials when acute otitis media is diagnosed is that the rate of suppurative complications has decreased in the antibiotic era. Withholding antibiotics today will most likely result in an increase in complications. Indeed, Hoppe and colleagues reported that the rate of acute mastoiditis has statistically increased recently in their children's hospital in Germany, which they attribute in some cases to withholding antimicrobial agents.[129]

The drug currently recommended for initial empiric therapy of acute otitis media is amoxicillin, since it is active both in vitro and in vivo against most strains of *S. pneumoniae* and *H. influenzae*, and it is relatively inexpensive in the United States.[130] If the patient is allergic to the penicillins, a combination of erythromycin and sulfisoxazole, or one of the new macrolides, azithromycin or clarithromycin, is advocated; as an alternative, one of the newer cephalosporins could be used, if the patient does not have hypersensitivity to these agents and does not have an immediate hypersensitivity reaction to the penicillins. If beta-lactamase–producing *H. influenzae* or *M. catarrhalis* is isolated by tympanocentesis or from otorrhea fluid—in which case amoxicillin would not be appropriate—then the choices also would be these

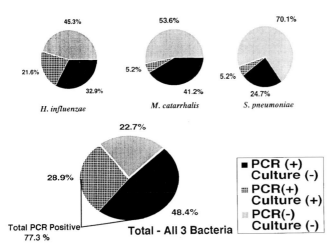

Figure 33–7. Comparison of culture and polymerase chain reaction results from 97 middle ear effusions from children with otitis media with effusion analyzed for *H. influenzae, M. catarrhalis*, and *S. pneumoniae*. (Adapted from Post JC, Preston RA, Aul JJ, et al: Molecular analysis of bacterial pathogens in otitis media with effusion. JAMA 1995; 273: 1598–1604, Copyright 1995, American Medical Association.)

antimicrobials or amoxicillin-clavulanate. Currently, there are six cephalosporins that are effective for treatment of acute otitis media: the second-generation agents, cefaclor, loracarbef, cefuroxime axetil, and cefprozil, and the third-generation drugs, cefpodoxime and cefixime. Trimethoprim-sulfamethoxazole would also be an appropriate alternative. The clinical efficacy of these antimicrobial agents is summarized in Table 33–3. Even though no data are available on the efficacy of these antimicrobial agents for treatment of adults with acute otitis media, the recommendations discussed above should be applied to adults as well, since the causative organisms are similar in adults and children. Thus, empiric use of such agents as the tetracyclines, penicillin V, erythromycin, or cephalexin is not recommended as monotherapy. The quinolones, such as ciprofloxacin, are not indicated in children younger than 17 years of age, and the efficacy of these antimicrobial agents has not been reported in adults with acute otitis media.

When a penicillin-resistant pneumococcus is isolated from the middle ear, from otorrhea or by tympanocentesis, the agent should be selected according to the results of the susceptibility testing. Many antibiotics have been suggested, such as clindamycin, rifampin, erythromycin, clarithromycin, cefuroxime-axetil, cefprozil, and cefpodoxime, but at this time there is no oral agent that has been demonstrated to be effective against this frequently multidrug-resistant bacterium in clinical trials; parenteral vancomycin is the drug of choice today when the patient is seriously ill and toxic.

Most cases of acute bacterial otitis media improve significantly within 48–72 hours when appropriate antimicrobial therapy is administered; if signs and symptoms of infection progress despite antimicrobial therapy, the patient should be reevaluated within 24 hours, since a suppurative complication may have developed or a concurrent serious infection (e.g., an infant may have meningitis). Persistent or recurrent pain or fever, or both, during treatment would signal the need for tympanocentesis and myringotomy (for Gram's stain, culture, and susceptibility testing), selection of another antimicrobial agent, or both. Selection of an antibiotic at

this stage would depend on the results of the culture and susceptibility testing. If amoxicillin was initially administered, then one of the alternative antimicrobial agents recommended above would be reasonable as empiric therapy until the results of the culture are available, or if culture was not obtained.

Most patients should probably be reexamined at the end of the course of antibiotic therapy (i.e., after 10–14 days), when about half will have persistent effusion. The presence of effusion after a 10-day trial of an antimicrobial agent is common in infants and children and is usually asymptomatic, but myringotomy can be helpful in older patients if even relatively mild symptoms are present, such as fullness in the ear, hearing loss, tinnitus, or vertigo. Mandel and colleagues recently conducted a clinical trial in children, in which 20-day therapy was compared with the traditional 10-day course.[131] They recommend having children who are asymptomatic return for their first follow-up visit in 4 weeks, since further treatment with antimicrobial therapy immediately after a 10-day treatment in the trial provided no long-term advantage. Patients who still have any signs or symptoms of acute infection should be reevaluated during or at the end of the initial course of treatment, since further evaluation and therapy may be indicated.

When an asymptomatic middle ear effusion persists after the initial 10-day antimicrobial therapy for acute otitis media, further treatment also may be indicated, but as described above most of these effusions will spontaneously resolve without further therapy. Factors that would be important in deciding to treat or not to treat this stage of the disease are similar to those described later in the section on otitis media with effusion.

Persistent Middle Ear Effusion

If the middle ear effusion persists after the initial 10-day antimicrobial therapy, one or more of the following treatment

Table 33–3. EFFICACY OF ORAL ANTIMICROBIAL AGENTS MEDIA*

Antimicrobial Agent	Streptococcus pneumoniae (35%)†	Haemophilus influenzae (23%) Beta-lactamase		Moraxella catarrhalis (14%) Beta-lactamase		Streptococcus pyogenes (3%)	Staphylococcus aureus (1%) Beta-lactamase	
		Neg (66%)	Pos (34%)	Neg (10%)	Pos (90%)		Neg (50%)	Pos (50%)
Amoxicillin	+	+	−	+	−	+	+	−
Amoxicillin-clavulanate	+	+	+	+	+	+	+	+
Cefaclor	+	+	±	+	±	+	+	+
Loracarbef	+	+	+	+	+	+	+	+
Cefuroxime axetil	+	+	+	+	+	+	+	+
Cefprozil	+	+	+	+	+	+	+	+
Cefixime	+	+	+	+	+	+	−	−
Ceftibutin	+	+	+	+	+	+	−	−
Cefpodoxime	+	+	+	+	+	+	+	+
Clarithromycin	+	+	+	+	+	+	+	+
Azithromycin‡	+	+	+	+	+	+	+	+
Erythromycin-sulfisoxazole								
Trimethoprim-sulfamethoxazole	+	+	+	+	+	−	+	+

*Based on available data from clinical trials and laboratory studies.
†Percentage of bacteria found in middle ear aspirates of acute otitis media (Pittsburgh Otitis Media Research Center).
‡Not available in liquid formulation.
 + = effective or susceptible; − = not effective or not susceptible; ± = marginally effective or marginally susceptible; neg = negative, pos = positive.

options have been advocated to hasten the resolution of the effusion during the next, *subacute*, phase:

1. Another 10-day course of therapy with the same antimicrobial agent that was used initially, since the optimal duration of antibiotic treatment for acute otitis media has not been defined

2. If amoxicillin was given initially, a course of an alternative antimicrobial agent that is effective against resistant organisms

3. A topical or systemic nasal decongestant or systemic antihistamine, or a combination of these drugs

4. Administration of systemic corticosteroids

5. Eustachian tube–middle ear inflation employing the method of Valsalva or Politzer

Despite the use of these treatment options by their advocates, none of these commonly employed methods has been shown to be effective in randomized, controlled trials of children with subacute middle ear effusions. As described above, the trial by Mandel and colleagues found no long-term advantage in retreating asymptomatic children with an antimicrobial agent at this stage.[131] Also, two additional Pittsburgh studies that involved more than 1000 infants and children demonstrated a lack of efficacy of a combination of an oral decongestant and antihistamine, with and without amoxicillin, in eliminating persistent middle ear effusion, although these studies did not test the efficacy of this combination in patients older than 12 years, or in those children who had documented nasal allergy.[132] With our current understanding of this stage of otitis media, clinicians do not have to treat patients who have asymptomatic (except for hearing loss) persistent middle ear effusion still present after 2 weeks, since most patients will be effusion-free at the end of 3 or 4 months without further treatment.[10] However, the patient should be reexamined during this period to determine if the effusion has persisted for 3 months or longer, at which point the effusion is chronic and should be treated as described later in the section on otitis media with effusion. Also, some patients may benefit from further treatment at an earlier time; this is also described below.

Recurrent Acute Otitis Media

If attacks of acute otitis media are frequent and close together, prevention is desirable. Several avenues of investigation are open: a search for respiratory allergy may prove fruitful; roentgenograms (or imaging) of the paranasal sinuses may reveal sinusitis; immunologic studies may be of value in the infant and young child if other organs are involved (i.e., the lung), but if the patient is 5 or 6 years of age or older, an evaluation of immune function might be helpful even if recurrent or chronic ear disease is the only apparent problem, and a more complete evaluation of the head and neck may uncover a tumor, especially in adolescents and adults. If none of the above conditions are present, then one or more of the popular methods of prevention may be attempted. For infants and children who have frequent episodes of acute otitis media, without evidence of chronic middle ear effusion, the most common nonsurgical and surgical methods currently employed for prevention are (1) che-

moprophylaxis with an antimicrobial agent or agents, (2) myringotomy with insertion of a tympanostomy tube, (3) adenoidectomy, and (4) pneumococcal vaccine in children who are 18–24 months of age or older.

Antimicrobial prophylaxis for the prevention of recurrent acute otitis media has been demonstrated to be effective.[133] For the child who has repeated episodes of otitis media, it seems reasonable to recommend amoxicillin 20 mg/kg in one dose (given at bedtime).[134] If the child is allergic to the penicillins, a daily dose of sulfisoxazole 50 mg/kg may be substituted. This prophylactic regimen should be continued during the respiratory season.

Patients receiving antimicrobial prophylaxis should be examined at frequent and regular intervals (every 6–8 weeks) to be certain that inapparent middle ear effusion, which might become chronic, does not occur. It is important to stress that prolonged antimicrobial prophylaxis is inappropriate if long-standing chronic middle ear effusion is present. When this occurs, the patient should be managed as described below.

Myringotomy and tympanostomy tube placement should be considered for patients who are prophylaxis failures, since this operation has been shown to be effective, compared with nonsurgical controls, for the prevention of recurrent acute otitis media in otitis-prone infants. A clinical trial reported by Casselbrant and colleagues has shown that both amoxicillin prophylaxis and myringotomy and tympanostomy tube insertion were more effective than placebo in reducing the rate of recurrent acute otitis media;[134] for those children who fail prophylaxis, tubes were then suggested as an alternative. Today, with the emergence of resistant bacteria, myringotomy and tube insertion may be a reasonable alternative to antimicrobial prophylaxis.[135] Adenoidectomy, with or without tonsillectomy, is frequently advocated for the prevention of recurrent acute otitis media, but only one randomized, controlled study has been reported that has shown the efficacy of adenoidectomy, albeit limited, for this condition. Paradise and colleagues did demonstrate a significant difference in the attack rate of acute otitis media in children who had been randomized to receive adenoidectomy compared with those who did not receive this operation; all subjects in this clinical trial had at least one myringotomy and tympanostomy tube insertion before random assignment.[136] As a note of caution, however, adenoidectomy in infants should only be recommended selectively (such as in those who also have severe nasal obstruction due to obstructive adenoids), since the operation carries some degree of increased risk in this age group.

Currently, when infants and children have frequently recurrent acute otitis media, the decision should be between administering an antibiotic in a prophylactic dose or myringotomy and insertion of a tympanostomy tube, and in selected patients, adenoidectomy. Although not effective in infants, the administration of the currently available pneumococcal vaccine is recommended for older children.

Otitis Media with Effusion

Otitis media with effusion in most children resolves without active treatment in 2 or 3 months, but treatment may be indicated in some children, because there are possible complications and sequelae associated with this condition. Since hearing loss of some degree usually accompanies a middle ear effusion, treatment may be warranted when long-standing hearing loss is present. Although the significance of this hearing loss is still uncertain, such a loss may impair cognitive and language function and result in disturbances in psychosocial adjustment. Important factors that should be considered when deciding to treat (and which treatment) or not to treat are listed in Table 33–4.

As with a patient who has had recurrent acute otitis media, before a nonsurgical or surgical method of management of patients with frequently recurrent or chronic effusions is initiated, a thorough search for an underlying cause should be attempted, as described above when patients have recurrent acute otitis media.

If active treatment is elected, there are only a few options that have been shown to be effective. Even though a combination of an oral decongestant and an antihistamine was thought to be effective—and widely used—in the past, two Pittsburgh studies that involved over 1000 infants and children failed to demonstrate their efficacy in eliminating middle ear effusion, although these studies did not test the efficacy of this combination in patients older than 12 years, or in children who had documented nasal allergy.[132, 138] The efficacy of systemic corticosteroid therapy for treatment of otitis media with effusion has been tested in clinical trials, most of which showed some benefit.[139] Yet, some clinicians consider the risks of corticosteroid therapy for otitis media with effusion in children to outweigh its possible benefits.[4] Clinical trials have not yet been reported that have tested the efficacy of topical nasal treatment, immunotherapy, and control of allergy in children who have nasal allergy and middle-ear disease. Nevertheless, this method of management seems reasonable in children who have frequently recurrent or chronic otitis media with effusion and evidence of upper respiratory allergy. Inflation of the eustachian tube–middle ear using Politzer's method or Valsalva's maneuver has been advocated for more than a century for this condition. However, a randomized, controlled trial by Chan and Bluestone found a lack of efficacy of middle ear inflation for chronic otitis media with effusion, and therefore it is not recommended in children;[140] efficacy in adults remains uncertain. Inflation may be effective for all age groups for the management of middle ear effusion that follows barotrauma (e.g., after air travel or scuba diving).

Of all the medical treatments that have been advocated, a trial of an antimicrobial agent would appear to be most appropriate in those children who have not received an antibiotic recently. Because bacteria similar to those found in acute otitis media have been isolated from a significant proportion of middle ear aspirates in children with chronic otitis media with effusion, the antibiotic chosen for treatment should be the same as that recommended for children who have acute otitis media. As in acute otitis media, amoxicillin is a reasonable choice for treating otitis media with effusion, since a recently reported study by Mandel and associates demonstrated its efficacy, albeit limited, in the 518 infants and children with otitis media with effusion who participated in the study.[132] Other antimicrobial agents have also been recommended, but none have been reported to be more effective than amoxicillin at this time. Although no trial has been reported in which the efficacy of a longer than 10-day course of amoxicillin has been tested for otitis media with effusion, it is possible that longer therapy is more effective than shorter therapy. At this time, however, prolonging antimicrobial treatment for longer than 2–4 weeks would appear to be excessive and is not recommended. A metaanalysis of the effect of antimicrobial agents in the treatment of otitis media with effusion reported by Rosenfeld and Post confirmed their efficacy.[141] Two other more recent metaanalyses also verified their short-term effect, but as expected, there was no long-term efficacy.[4, 133] Other strategies, such as antimicrobial prophylaxis or surgery, are required for long-term control, since the disease is frequently recurrent because of repeated exposure to upper respiratory tract infections.

If nonsurgical methods of management fail and the effusion is chronic, surgical intervention should be considered, and referral of the patient to an otolaryngologist is appropriate. In 109 Pittsburgh children with chronic otitis media with effusion that was unresponsive to amoxicillin, and who were followed monthly for 3 years, myringotomy and tympanostomy tube insertion was shown to be more effective than myringotomy without tube insertion or no surgery.[142] The outcome of this study was confirmed in a more recently reported clinical trial conducted by the same group, which was similar in design to the first one and involved 111 subjects.[143]

The current indications for insertion of tympanostomy tubes in children are listed in Table 33–5.[135] These indications are derived from clinical trials, as well as a long experience with otitis media in children, in which the occurrence is vastly more common than in adults. Unfortunately, there are no similar published clinical trials that have been conducted in adults, but the clinician can use the outcomes of the studies in children as a guide to treating adults. However, there are some important differences, such as the usual intolerance of adults when even relatively asymptomatic middle-ear effusion of short duration is present, and the feasibility of performing myringotomy, with and without

Table 33–4. FACTORS IN DECIDING TO TREAT OTITIS MEDIA WITH EFFUSION

1. Degree and duration of associated conductive hearing loss
2. Age: young infants are unable to communicate about their symptoms and may have suppurative disease
3. Associated acute purulent upper respiratory tract infection
4. Concurrent permanent conductive or sensorineural hearing loss
5. Presence of speech or language delay associated with effusion and hearing loss
6. Dysequilibrium, vertigo, or tinnitus
7. Alterations of tympanic membrane, such as severe atelectasis, especially a deep retraction pocket
8. Middle ear changes, such as adhesive otitis or ossicular involvement
9. Previous surgery for otitis media, e.g., tympanostomy tube placement or adenoidectomy
10. Frequency: when episodes recur frequently, such as in 6 of preceding 12 months
11. Persistence: effusion that persists for 3 months or longer, i.e., chronic otitis media with effusion

Adapted from Bluestone CD, Klein JO: Clinical practice guideline on otitis media: Strengths and weaknesses. Otolaryngol Head Neck Surg 1995; 112: 507–511.

Table 33–5. INDICATIONS FOR TYMPANOSTOMY TUBE INSERTION

1. Chronic otitis media with effusion unresponsive to medical management 3 or more months bilateral, or 6 or more months unilateral; earlier when significant hearing loss (e.g., >25 dB), speech or language delay, severe retraction pocket, disequilibrium or vertigo, or tinnitus is present
2. Recurrent episodes of middle ear effusion not meeting criteria for chronic disease, but cumulative duration excessive (e.g., 6 of 12 months)
3. Recurrent acute otitis media, especially when antimicrobial prophylaxis fails to reduce frequency, severity, and duration of attacks; minimal frequency three or more episodes in 6 months, or four or more in 12 months, with one recent
4. Eustachian tube dysfunction (with or without effusion), when persistent, recurrent signs and symptoms (e.g., hearing loss [usually fluctuating], disequilibrium or vertigo, tinnitus, or a severe retraction pocket) not relieved by medical treatment are present
5. Tympanoplasty when eustachian tube function is poor (e.g., surgery for cholesteatoma)
6. Suppurative complication present or suspected

Adapted from Bluestone CD, Klein JO, Gates GA: "Appropriateness" of tympanostomy tubes. Setting the record straight. Arch Otolaryngol Head Neck Surg 1994; 120: 1051–1053, Copyright 1994, American Medical Association.

tympanostomy tube insertion, using local anesthesia in teenagers and adults. Thus, surgical intervention should be considered at a much earlier stage in the natural history of acute otitis media, persistent middle ear effusion, recurrent acute otitis media, and otitis media with effusion in older patients.

Adenoidectomy, in conjunction with myringotomy and tympanostomy tube insertion or myringotomy alone, can benefit some children. Table 33–6 shows the design and outcomes of the clinical trials conducted in the United States and Great Britain. Even though some of the earlier studies failed to show a consistent advantage of the operation, the more recent randomized clinical trials reported by Maw,[149] Gates and colleagues,[150] and Paradise and associates[136] did show efficacy of adenoidectomy. Because the effectiveness of adenoidectomy for chronic otitis media with effusion is apparently unrelated to adenoid size,[151] the selection of children who might benefit from adenoidectomy at present must be based on the potential benefits weighed against the costs and potential risks. For children who have recurrent or chronic otitis media with effusion and who have had one or more myringotomy and tympanostomy tube operations in

the past, adenoidectomy is a reasonable option. The presence of upper airway obstruction (due to obstructive adenoids), recurrent acute or chronic adenoiditis, or both conditions would also be more compelling indications to consider adenoidectomy.

Chronic Suppurative Otitis Media

Today, medical management of chronic suppurative otitis media without cholesteatoma is directed toward eliminating the infection from the middle ear and mastoid. Since the bacteria most frequently cultured are gram-negative, antimicrobial agents should be selected to be effective against these organisms. A suspension that contains polymyxin B, neomycin, and hydrocortisone (Cortisporin), or one that has neomycin, polymyxin E, and hydrocortisone (Coly-Mycin), has been advocated, but owing to concern about the potential ototoxicity of these agents, caution is advised. In children, orally administered antibiotics are usually not effective unless an organism that will be susceptible, such as *S. aureus*, is seen on Gram's stain or is cultured from the discharge. Oral antibiotics are also effective against the organisms that commonly cause acute otitis media, such as pneumococcus and *H. influenzae*; however, ciprofloxacin, an oral antimicrobial agent with activity against most of the organisms that cause chronic suppurative disease, may be effective, although randomized clinical trials demonstrating efficacy for this infection have not been reported. However, treatment of adults who have chronic suppurative otitis media with the quinolones when the causative organism is *Pseudomonas* seems reasonable.

When topical antibiotic medication is elected, the patient should return to the outpatient facility daily so that the discharge can be aspirated thoroughly. Frequently, the discharge resolves rapidly with this type of treatment, within a week or two. Also, if ototopical agents are used, patients (and parents) should be informed of the potential for ototoxicity. As an alternative, we hospitalize the children and administer a parenteral beta-lactam antipseudomonal drug, such as ticarcillin. The middle ear is aspirated daily. In most children, the middle ear is free of discharge within 7–10 days, and the signs of otitis media are greatly improved or absent.

Table 33–6. CLINICAL TRIALS OF ADENOIDECTOMY FOR OTITIS MEDIA

First Author	No. of Subjects	Random Arms	Age Range (yr)	Otitis Media Outcome
McKee[144] (1st trial)	413	T&A versus no surgery	2–15	Reduction 1st year, but not 2nd year
McKee[145]	200	T&A versus A	2–15	No difference between T&A versus A
Mawson[146]	404	T&A versus no surgery	<16	No difference
Roydhouse[147] (1st trial)	379	T&A versus no surgery	<13	Reduction in 1st year, but less reduction in 2nd year
	173	T&A versus no surgery and control		
Roydhouse[148] (2nd trial)	100	A-M&T versus M&T	3.7–14	No reduction observed
Maw[149]	103	T&A versus A versus no surgery	2–12	Significant reduction for 1 year; T&A = A
Gates[150]	578	M versus M&T versus A-M versus A-M&T	4–8	Significant reduction in A&M, and A&M&T versus M&T, and M for 2 years
Paradise[136]	99 random (114 nonrandom)	A versus no surgery	1–15	Significant reduction for 2 years

T&A = tonsillectomy and adenoidectomy; A = adenoidectomy; M = myringotomy; M&T = myringotomy and tube.

If the discharge fails to respond to intensive medical therapy, surgery on the middle ear and mastoid is indicated. Kenna and colleagues[120] reported on a study of 36 pediatric patients with chronic suppurative otitis media, all of whom received parenteral antimicrobial therapy and daily otic toilet, 32 (89%) experienced resolution of their initial infection with medical therapy alone; 4 children required tympanomastoidectomy. In a follow-up of that study, 51 of the original 66 were evaluated for their long-term outcomes.[121] Of these 51 children, 40 (78%) had resolution of their initial or recurrent infection after medical treatment, and 11 (22%) had to have mastoid surgery eventually. Failure was associated with older children and as early recurrence. Even though similar large-scale clinical trials of parenteral antimicrobial therapy have not been reported in adults, this management option also seems reasonable before performing mastoid surgery in this age group. When the infection can be eliminated by the methods described above, recurrence can usually be prevented by one of the following measures: prophylactic antimicrobial therapy; removal of the tympanostomy tube; or surgical repair of the tympanic membrane defect. The choice depends on the age of the patient and the function of the eustachian tube.[5]

If chronic suppurative otitis media is present with cholesteatoma, tympanomastoid surgery is indicated. Preoperative antimicrobial therapy, and possibly perioperative prophylaxis, may be helpful in reducing postoperative infection and should promote better healing.

References

1. Shappert SM: Office visits for otitis media: United States, 1975–90. From Vital and Health Statistics of the Centers for Disease Control. Published in National Center for Health Statistics, 1992; 214: 1–18.
2. Gates GA: Cost effectiveness considerations in otitis media treatment. Sixth International Symposium on Recent Advances in Otitis Media. Fort Lauderdale, Florida, June 4–8, 1995.
3. Bluestone CD, Klein JO: Otitis Media in Infants and Children, 2nd ed. Philadelphia: WB Saunders Co, 1995.
4. Stool SE, Berg AO, Carney CJ, et al.: Otitis Media with Effusion in Young Children. Clinical Practice Guideline No. 12. AHCPR Pub No 94–0622. Rockville, Maryland: Agency for Health Care Policy and Research, Public Health Service, US Department of Health and Human Services, July 1994.
5. Bluestone CD, Klein JO: Otitis media, atelectasis, and eustachian tube dysfunction. In: Bluestone CD, Stool SE, Kenna MA (eds): Pediatric Otolaryngology, 3rd ed. Philadelphia: WB Saunders Co, 1996, pp 388–582.
6. Spika JS, Facklam RR, Plikaytis BD, Oxtoby MJ: Antimicrobial resistance of Streptococcus pneumoniae in the United States, 1979–1987. J Infect Dis 1991; 163: 1273–1278.
7. Welby PL, Keller DS, Cromien JL, et al.: Resistance to penicillin and no-beta-lactam antibiotics of Streptococcus pneumoniae at a children's hospital. Pediatr Infect Dis J 1994; 13: 281–287.
8. Teele DW, Klein JO, Rosner B, et al.: Middle ear disease and the practice of pediatrics. Burden during the first five years of life. JAMA 1983; 249: 1026–1029.
9. Teele DW, Klein JO, Rosner BA, The Greater Boston Otitis Media Study Group: Epidemiology of otitis media during the first seven years of life in children in Greater Boston: A prospective, cohort study. J Infect Dis 1989; 160: 83–99.
10. Kaleida PH, Bluestone CD, Rockette HE, et al.: Amoxicillin-clavulanate potassium compared with cefaclor for acute otitis media in infants and children. Pediatr Infect Dis J 1987; 6: 265–271.
11. Casselbrant ML, Brostoff LM, Cantekin EI, et al.: Otitis media with effusion in preschool children. Laryngoscope 1985; 95: 428–436.
12. Casselbrant ML, Brostoff LM, Cantekin EI, et al.: Otitis media in children in the United States. In: Sade J (ed): Proceedings of the International Conference on Acute and Secretory Otitis Media. Amsterdam: Kugler Publications, 1986, pp 161–164.
13. Casselbrant ML, Mandel EM, Kurs-Lasky M, et al.: Otitis media in a population of black American and white American infants, 0–2 years of age. Int J Pediatr Otorhinolaryngol 1995; 33: 1–16.
14. Finkelstein Y, Ophir D, Talmi YP, et al.: Adult-onset otitis media with effusion. Arch Otolaryngol Head Neck Surg 1994; 120: 517–527.
15. Politzer A: Ueber die willkurlichen Bewegungen des Trommelfells. Weiner Med Halle Nr 1862; 18: 103.
16. Zollner R: Anatomie, Physiologie und Klinik der Ohrtrompete. Berlin: Springer-Verlag, 1942.
17. Sade J: Pathology and pathogenesis of serous otitis media. Arch Otolaryngol 1966; 84: 297–305.
18. Bluestone CD, Paradise JL, Beery QC: Physiology of the eustachian tube in the pathogenesis and management of middle ear effusions. Laryngoscope 1972; 82: 1654–1670.
19. Casselbrant ML, Cantekin EI, Dirkmaat DC, et al.: Experimental paralysis of tensor veli palatini muscle. Acta Otolaryngol (Stockh) 1988; 106: 178–185.
20. Doyle WJ, Skoner DP, Hayden F, et al.: Nasal and otologic effects of experimental influenza A virus infection. Ann Otol Rhinol Laryngol 1994; 103: 59–69.
21. Buchman CA, Doyle WJ, Skoner D, et al.: Otologic manifestations of experimental rhinovirus infection. Laryngoscope 1994; 104: 1295–1299.
22. Alper CM, Tabari R, Seroky JT, Doyle WJ: Magnetic resonance imaging of the development of middle-ear effusion secondary to experimental paralysis of tensor veli palatini muscle. Otolaryngol Head Neck Surg 1994; 111: 122.
23. Swarts JD, Alper CM, Seroky JT, et al.: In vivo observation with magnetic resonance imaging of middle ear effusion in response to experimental underpressures. Ann Otol Rhinol Laryngol 1995; 104: 522–528.
24. Cantekin EI, Doyle WJ, Reichert TJ, et al.: Dilation of the eustachian tube by electrical stimulation of the mandibular nerve. Ann Otol Rhinol Laryngol 1979; 88: 40–51.
25. Honjo I, Okazaki N, Kumazawa T: Experimental study of the eustachian tube function with regard to its related muscles. Acta Otolaryngol (Stockh) 1979; 87: 84.
26. Rich AR: The innervation of the tensor veli palatini and levator veli palatini muscles. Bull Johns Hopkins Hosp 1920; 31: 305.
27. Doyle WJ, Seroky JT: Middle ear gas exchange in rhesus monkeys. Ann Otol Rhinol Laryngol 1994; 103: 636–645.
28. Bylander A: Comparison of eustachian tube function in children and adults with normal ears. Ann Otol Rhinol Laryngol 1980; 89: 20–24.
29. Bylander A, Tjernstrom O, Ivarsson A: Pressure opening and closing functions of the eustachian tube by inflation and deflation in children and adults with normal ears. Acta Otolaryngol (Stockh) 1983; 96: 255–268.
30. Bluestone CD: Eustachian tube obstruction in the infant with cleft palate. Ann Otol Rhinol Laryngol 1971; 80: 1–30.
31. Bluestone CD, Wittel RA, Paradise JL, Felder H: Eustachian tube function as related to adenoidectomy for otitis media. Trans Am Acad Ophthalmol Otolaryngol 1972; 76: 1325–1339.
32. Wittenborg MH, Neuhauser EB: Simple roentgenographic demonstration of eustachian tubes and abnormalities. Am J Roentgenol Radium Ther Nucl Med 1963; 89: 1194.
33. Albiin N, Hellstrom S, Stenfors LE: Clearance of effusion material from the attic space— an experimental study in the rat. Int J Pediatr Otorhinolaryngol 1983; 5: 1–10.
34. Stenfors LE, Hellstrom S, Albiin N: Middle ear clearance. Ann Otol Rhinol Laryngol 1985; 94 (suppl 120): 30–31.
35. Ohashi Y, Nakai Y, Koshimo H, Esaki Y: Ciliary activity in the in vitro tubotympanum. Arch Otorhinolaryngol 1986; 243: 317–319.
36. Honjo I, Okazaki N, Nozoe T, et al.: Experimental study of the pumping function of the eustachian tube. Acta Otolaryngol (Stockh) 1981; 91: 85–89.
37. Honjo I, Hayashi M, Ito S, Takahashi H: Pumping and clearance function of the eustachian tube. Am J Otolaryngol 1985; 6: 241–244.
38. Birken EA, Brookler KH: Surface tension lowering substance of the canine eustachian tube. Ann Otol Rhinol Laryngol 1972; 81: 268–271.
39. Rapport PN, Lim DJ, Weiss HS: Surface-active agent in eustachian tube function. Arch Otolaryngol 1975; 101: 305–311.

40. Hagan WE: Surface tension lowering substance in eustachian tube function. Laryngoscope 1977; 87: 1033–1045.

41. White P: Effect of exogenous surfactant on eustachian tube function in the rat. Am J Otolaryngol 1989; 10: 301–304.

42. Karchev T, Watanabe N, Fujiyoshi T, et al.: Surfactant-producing epithelium in the dorsal part of the cartilaginous eustachian tube of mice. Acta Otolaryngol (Stockh) 1994; 114: 64–69.

43. Fornadley JA, Burns JK: The effect of surfactant on eustachian tube function in a gerbil model of otitis media with effusion. Otolaryngol Head Neck Surg 1994; 110: 110–114.

44. Bluestone CD, Cantekin EI, Beery QC: Effect of inflammation on the ventilatory function of the eustachian tube. Laryngoscope 1977; 87: 493–507.

45. McBride TP, Doyle WJ, Hayden FG, Gwaltney JM: Alterations of the eustachian tube, middle ear, and nose in rhinovirus infection. Arch Otolaryngol 1989; 115: 1054–1059.

46. Friedman RA, Doyle WJ, Casselbrant ML, et al.: Immunologic-mediated eustachian tube obstruction: A double-blind crossover study. J Allergy Clin Immunol 1983; 71: 442–447.

47. Bluestone CD, Cantekin EI, Beery QC: Certain effects of adenoidectomy on eustachian tube ventilatory function. Laryngoscope 1975; 85: 113–127.

48. Bluestone CD, Beery QC, Andrus WS: Mechanics of the eustachian tube as it influences susceptibility to and persistence of middle ear effusions in children. Ann Otol Rhinol Laryngol 1974; 83: 27–34.

49. Bluestone CD, Cantekin EI, Beery QC, Stool SE: Function of the eustachian tube related to surgical management of acquired aural cholesteatoma in children. Laryngoscope 1978; 88: 1155–1163.

50. Stenstrom C, Bylander-Groth A, Ingvarsson L: Eustachian tube function in otitis-prone and healthy children. Int J Pediatr Otorhinolaryngol 1991; 21: 127–138.

51. Iwano T, Hamada E, Kinoshita T, et al.: Passive opening pressure of the eustachian tube. In: Lim DJ, Bluestone CD, Klein JO, et al. (eds): Recent Advances in Otitis Media. Proceedings of the Fifth International Symposium. Burlington, Ontario: Decker Periodicals, 1993, pp 76–78.

52. Siegel MI, Sadler-Kimes D, Todhunter JS: Eustachian tube cartilage shape as a factor in the epidemiology of otitis media. In: Lim DJ, Bluestone CD, Klein JO, Nelson JD (eds): Recent Advances in Otitis Media. Proceedings of the Fourth International Symposium. Philadelphia: BC Decker, 1988, pp 114–117.

53. Yamaguchi N, Sando I, Hashida Y, et al.: Histologic study of eustachian tube cartilage with and without congenital anomalies: A preliminary study. Ann Otol Rhinol Laryngol 1990; 99: 984–987.

54. Matsune S, Sando I, Takahashi H: Comparative study of elastic at the hinge portion of eustachian tube cartilage in normal and cleft palate individuals. In: Lim DJ, Bluestone CD, Klein JO, et al. (eds): Recent Advances in Otitis Media. Proceedings of the Fifth International Symposium. Burlington, Ontario: Decker Periodicals, 1993, pp 4–6.

55. Aoki H, Sando I, Takahashi H: Anatomic relationships between Ostmann's fatty tissue and eustachian tube. Ann Otol Rhinol Laryngol 1994; 103: 211–214.

56. Proctor B: Embryology and anatomy of the eustachian tube. Arch Otolaryngol 1967; 86: 503–514.

57. Swarts JD, Rood SR: Preliminary analysis of the morphometry of the infant eustachian tube. In: Lim DJ, Bluestone CD, Klein JO, et al. (eds): Recent Advances in Otitis Media. Proceedings of the Fifth International Symposium. Burlington, Ontario: Decker Periodicals, 1993, pp 111–113.

58. Sakakihara J, Honjo I, Fujita A, et al.: Compliance of the patulous eustachian tube. Ann Otol Rhinol Laryngol 1993; 102: 110–112.

59. Beery QC, Doyle WJ, Cantekin EI, et al.: Eustachian tube function in an American Indian population. Ann Otol Rhinol Laryngol 1980; 89: 28–33.

60. White BL, Doyle WJ, Bluestone CD: Eustachian tube function in infants and children with Down's syndrome. In: Lim DJ, Bluestone CD, Klein JO, Nelson JD (eds): Recent Advances in Otitis Media with Effusion. Proceedings of the Third International Symposium. Philadelphia: BC Decker, 1984, pp 62–66.

61. Sadler-Kimes D, Siegel MI, Todhunter JS: Age-related morphologic differences in the components of the eustachian tube/middle ear system. Ann Otol Rhinol Laryngol 1989; 98: 854–858.

62. Jorgensen F, Holmquist J: Toynbee phenomenon and middle ear disease. Am J Otolaryngol 1984; 5: 291–294.

63. Thompson AC, Crowther JA: Effect of nasal packing on eustachian tube function. J Laryngol Otol 1991; 105 (7): 539–540.

64. Ohashi Y, Nakai Y, Furuya H, et al.: Mucociliary diseases of the middle ear during experimental otitis media with effusion induced by bacterial endotoxin. Ann Otol Rhinol Laryngol 1989; 98: 479–484.

65. Park K, Bakaletz LO, Coticchia JM, Lim DJ: Effect of influenza A virus on ciliary activity and dye transport function in the chinchilla eustachian tube. Ann Otol Rhinol Laryngol 1993; 102: 551–558.

66. Mogi G, Kawauchi H, Kurono Y: Tubal dysfunction or infection? Role of bacterial infection and immune response. In: Mogi G (ed): Recent Advances in Otitis Media. Proceedings of the Second Extraordinary International Symposium on Recent Advances in Otitis Media. New York: Kugler Publications, 1993, pp 73–77.

67. Shikowitz MJ, Ilardi CF, Gero M: Immotile cilia syndrome associated with otitis media with effusion: A case report. In: Lim DJ, Bluestone CD, Klein JO, Nelson JD (eds): Recent Advances in Otitis Media. Proceedings of the Fourth International Symposium. Philadelphia: BC Decker, 1988, pp 304–307.

68. Nozoe T, Okazaki N, Koda Y, et al.: Fluid clearance of the eustachian tube. In: Lim DJ, Bluestone CD, Klein JO, Nelson JD (eds): Recent Advances in Otitis Media with Effusion. Proceedings of the Third International Symposium. Philadelphia: BC Decker, 1984, pp 66–68.

69. Takahashi H, Honjo I, Hayashi M, Fujita A: Clearance function of eustachian tube and negative middle ear pressure. Ann Otol Rhinol Laryngol 1992; 101: 759–762.

70. Miglets A: The experimental production of allergic middle ear effusions. Laryngoscope 1973; 83: 1355–1384.

71. Bernstein JM, Lee J, Conboy K, et al.: Further observations on the role of IgE-mediated hypersensitivity in recurrent otitis media with effusion. Otolaryngol Head Neck Surg 1985; 93: 611–615.

72. Bluestone CD: Eustachian tube function and allergy in otitis media. Pediatrics 1978; 61: 753–760.

73. Doyle WJ: Panel on etiology of otitis media with effusion: Role of allergy and tubal function. In: Mogi G (ed): Recent Advances in Otitis Media. Proceedings of the Second Extraordinary International Symposium on Recent Advances in Otitis Media. Amsterdam: Kugler Publications, 1994, pp 53–60.

74. Ackerman MN, Friedman RA, Doyle WJ, et al.: Antigen-induced eustachian tube obstruction: An intranasal provocative challenge test. J Allergy Clin Immunol 1984; 73: 604–609.

75. Doyle WJ, Friedman R, Fireman P, Bluestone CD: Eustachian tube obstruction after provocative nasal antigen challenge. Arch Otolaryngol 1984; 110: 508–511.

76. Skoner DP, Doyle WJ, Chamovitz AH, Fireman P: Eustachian tube obstruction after intranasal challenge with house dust mite. Arch Otolaryngol 1986; 112: 840–842.

77. Stillwagon PK, Doyle WJ, Fireman P: Effect of an antihistamine/decongestant on nasal and eustachian tube function following intranasal pollen challenge. Ann Allergy 1987; 58: 442–446.

78. Skoner DP, Doyle WJ, Fireman P: Eustachian tube obstruction (ETO) after histamine nasal provocation—a double-blind dose-response study. J Allergy Clin Immunol 1987; 79: 27–31.

79. Doyle WJ, Boehm S, Skoner DP: Physiologic responses to intranasal dose-response challenges with histamine, methacholine, bradykinin, and prostaglandin in adult volunteers with and without nasal allergy. J Allergy Clin Immunol 1990; 86: 924–935.

80. Stool SE, Randall P: Unexpected ear disease in infants with cleft palate. Cleft Palate J 1967; 4: 99–103.

81. Paradise JL, Bluestone CD, Felder H: The universality of otitis media in fifty infants with cleft palate. Pediatrics 1969; 44: 35–42.

82. Paradise JL, Bluestone CD: Early treatment of the universal otitis media of infants with cleft palate. Pediatrics 1974; 53: 48–54.

83. Bluestone CD, Wittel R, Paradise JL: Roentgenographic evaluation of eustachian tube function in infants with cleft and normal palates. Cleft Palate J 1972; 9: 93–100.

84. Doyle WJ, Cantekin EI, Bluestone CD: Eustachian tube function in cleft palate children. Ann Otol Rhinol Laryngol 1980; 89(suppl 68): 34–40.

85. Kitajiri M, Sando I, Hashida Y, Doyle WJ: Histopathology of otitis media in infants with cleft and high arched palates. In: Lim DJ, Bluestone CD, Klein JO, Nelson JD (eds): Recent Advances in Otitis Media with Effusion. Proceedings of the Third International Symposium. Philadelphia: BC Decker, 1984, pp 96–100.

86. Matsune S, Sando I, Takahashi H: Abnormalities of lateral cartilagi-

nous lamina and lumen of eustachian tube in cases of cleft palate. Ann Otol Rhino Laryngol 1991; 100: 909–913.

87. Matsune S, Sando I, Takahashi H: Insertion of the tensor veli palatini muscle into the eustachian tube cartilage in cleft palate cases. Ann Otol Rhinol Laryngol 1991; 100: 439–446.

88. Matsune S, Sando I, Takahashi H: Elastin at the hinge portion of the eustachian tube cartilage in specimens from normal subjects and those with cleft palate. Ann Otol Rhinol Laryngol 1992; 101: 163–167.

89. Shibahara Y, Sando I: Histopathologic study of eustachian tube in cleft palate patients. Ann Otol Rhinol Laryngol 1988; 97: 403–408.

90. Doyle WJ, Ingraham AS, Saad MM, Cantekin EI: A primate model of cleft palate and middle ear disease: Results of a one-year post cleft follow-up. In: Lim DJ, Bluestone CD, Klein JO, Nelson JD (eds): Recent Advances in Otitis Media with Effusion. Proceedings of the Third International Symposium. Philadelphia: BC Decker, 1984, pp 215–218.

91. Odoi H, Proud GO, Toledo PS: Effects of pterygoid hamulotomy upon eustachian tube function. Laryngoscope 1971; 81: 1242–1244.

92. McNicoll WD, Scanlon SG: Submucous resection. The treatment of choice in the nose-ear distress syndrome. J Laryngol Otol 1979; 93: 357–367.

93. McNicoll WD: Remediable eustachian tube dysfunction in diving recruits: Assessment, investigation, and management. Undersea Biomed Res 1982; 9: 37–43.

94. Tos M, Bonding P: Middle ear pressure during and after prolonged nasotracheal and/or nasogastric intubation. Acta Otolaryngol (Stockh) 1977; 83(3–4): 353–359.

95. Wake M, McCullough DE, Binnington JD: Effect of nasogastric tubes on eustachian tube function. J Laryngol Otol 1990; 104(1): 17–19.

96. Perlman HB: Observations on the eustachian tube. Arch Otolaryngol 1951; 53: 370.

97. Myers EN, Beery QC, Bluestone CD, et al.: Effect of certain head and neck tumors and their management on the ventilatory function of the eustachian tube. Ann Otol Rhinol Laryngol 1984; 93(suppl 114): 3–16.

98. Weiss MH, Liberatore LA, Kraus DH, Budnick AS: Otitis media with effusion in head and neck cancer patients. Laryngoscope 1994; 104: 5–7.

99. Takahara T, Sando I, Bluestone CD, Myers EN: Lymphoma invading the anterior eustachian tube: Temporal bone histopathology of functional tubal obstruction. Ann Otol Rhinol Laryngol 1986; 95: 101–105.

100. Yamaguchi N, Sando I, Hashida Y, et al.: Histopathologic study of otitis media in individuals with head and neck tumors. Ann Otol Rhinol Laryngol 1990; 99: 827–832.

101. Buchman CA, Doyle WJ, Skoner DP, et al.: Influenza A virus–induced acute otitis media. J Infect Dis 1995; 172: 1348–1351.

102. Bluestone CD, Stephenson JS, Martin LM: Ten-year review of otitis media pathogens. Pediatr Infect Dis J 1992; 11: S7–S11.

103. Post JC, Preston RA, Aul JJ, et al.: Molecular analysis of bacterial pathogens in otitis media with effusion. JAMA 1995; 273: 1598–1604.

104. Cantekin EI, Bluestone CD, Saez CA, et al.: Normal and abnormal middle ear ventilation. Ann Otol Rhinol Laryngol 1977; 86 (suppl 41): 1–15.

105. Alper CM, Tabari R, Seroky JT, Doyle WJ: Effects of dopamine, dobutamine and phentolamine on middle ear pressure and blood flow in cynomolgus monkeys. Acta Otolaryngol 1995; 115: 55–60.

106. Ophir D, Hahn T, Schattner A, et al.: Tumor necrosis factor in middle ear effusions. Arch Otolaryngol 1988; 114: 1256–1258.

107. Yellon RF, Leonard G, Marucha PT, et al.: Characterization of cytokines present in middle ear effusions. Laryngoscope 1991; 101: 165–169.

108. Yellon RF, Leonard G, Marucha P, et al.: Demonstration of interleukin 6 in middle ear effusions. Arch Otolaryngol 1992; 118: 745–748.

109. Yan SD, Huang CC: Tumor necrosis factor alpha in middle ear cholesteatoma and its effect on keratinocytes in vitro. Ann Otol Rhinol Laryngol 1991; 100: 157–161.

110. Juhn SK, Lees C, Amesara R, et al.: Role of cytokines in the pathogenesis of otitis media. In: Lim DJ, Bluestone CD, Klein JO, et al. (eds): Recent Advances in Otitis Media. Proceedings of the Fifth International Symposium. Burlington, Ontario: Decker Periodicals, 1993, pp 431–434.

111. Himi T, Suzuki T, Kadama H, et al.: Immunologic characteristics of cytokines in otitis media with effusion. Ann Otol Rhinol Laryngol 1992; 157: 21–25.

112. Bernstein JM, Okazaki T, Reisman RE: Prostaglandins in middle ear effusions. Arch Otolaryngol 1976; 102: 257–258.

113. Smith DM, Jung TTK, Juhn SK, et al.: Prostaglandins in experimental otitis media. Arch Otorhinolaryngol 1979; 225: 207–209.

114. Jung TTK, Linda L: Prostaglandins, leukotrienes, and other arachidonic acid metabolites in the pathogenesis of otitis media. Laryngoscope 1988; 98: 980–993.

115. Jung TTK, Park YM, Schlund D, et al.: Effect of prostaglandin, leukotriene and arachidonic acid on experimental otitis media with effusion in chinchillas. Ann Otol Rhinol Laryngol 1990; 99: 28–32.

116. Jung TTK: Arachidonic acid metabolites in otitis media pathogenesis. Ann Otol Rhino Laryngol 1988; 97: 14–18.

117. Nonomura N, Giebink GS, Zelterman D, et al.: Early biochemical events in pneumococcal otitis media: Arachidonic acid metabolites in middle ear fluid. Ann Otol Rhinol Laryngol 1991; 100: 385–388.

118. Rhee CK, Jung TTK, Miller S, Weeks D: Experimental otitis media with effusion induced by platelet activating factor. Ann Otol Rhinol Laryngol 1993; 102: 600–605.

119. Derkay CS, Bluestone CD, Thompson AR, Kardatske D: Otitis media in the pediatric intensive care unit: A prospective study. Otolaryngol Head Neck Surg 1989; 100: 292–299.

120. Kenna MA, Bluestone Cd, Reilly JS, Lusk RP: Medical management of chronic suppurative otitis media with cholesteatoma in children. Laryngoscope 1986; 96: 146–151.

121. Kenna MA, Rosane BA, Bluestone CD: Medical management of chronic suppurative otitis media without cholesteatoma in children—update 1992. Am J Otol 1993; 14: 469–473.

122. Mandel EM, Casselbrant ML, Kurs-Lasky M: Acute otorrhea: Bacteriology of a common complication of tympanostomy tubes. Ann Otol Rhinol Laryngol 1994; 103: 713–718.

123. Celin SE, Bluestone CD, Stephenson J, et al.: Bacteriology of acute otitis media in adults. JAMA 1991; 266: 2249–2252.

124. Chonmaitree T, Owen MJ, Howie VM: Respiratory viruses interfere with bacteriologic response to antibiotic in children with acute otitis media. J Infect Dis 1990; 162: 546–549.

125. Mason EO Jr, Kaplan SL, Lamberth LB, Tillman J: Increased rate of isolation of penicillin-resistant Streptococcus pneumoniae in a children's hospital and in vitro susceptibilities to antibiotics of potential therapeutic use. Antimicrob Agents Chemother 1992; 36: 1703–1707.

126. Reichler MR, Allphin AA, Breiman RF, et al.: The spread of multiple resistant Streptococcus pneumoniae at a day-care center in Ohio. J Infect Dis 1992; 166: 1346–1353.

127. Rosenfeld RM, Vertrees JE, Carr J, et al.: Clinical efficacy of antimicrobial drugs for acute otitis media: Metaanalysis of 5400 children from thirty-three randomized trials. J Pediatr 1994; 124: 355–367.

128. Kaleida PH, Casselbrant ML, Rockette HE, et al.: Amoxicillin or myringotomy or both for acute otitis media: Results of a randomized clinical trial. Pediatrics 1991; 87: 466–474.

129. Hoppe JE, Koster S, Bootz F, Niethammer D: Acute mastoiditis—relevant once again. Infection 1994; 22: 178–182.

130. Drugs for treatment of acute otitis media in children. Med Lett 1994; 36: 19.

131. Mandel EM, Casselbrant ML, Rockette HE, et al.: Efficacy of 20-versus 10-day antimicrobial treatment for acute otitis media. Pediatrics 1995; 96: 5–13.

132. Mandel EM, Rockette HE, Bluestone CD, et al.: Efficacy of amoxicillin with and without decongestant-antihistamine for otitis media with effusion in children. N Engl J Med 1987; 316: 432–437.

133. Williams RL, Chalmers TC, Stange KC, et al.: Use of antibiotics in preventing recurrent acute otitis media and in treating otitis media with effusion. JAMA 1993; 270: 1344–1351.

134. Casselbrant ML, Kaleida PH, Rockette HE, et al.: Efficacy of antimicrobial prophylaxis and of tympanostomy tube insertion for prevention of recurrent acute otitis media: Results of a randomized clinical trial. Pediatr Infect Dis 1992; 11: 278–286.

135. Bluestone CD, Klein JO, Gates GA: "Appropriateness" of tympanostomy tubes. Setting the record straight. Arch Otolaryngol Head Neck Surg 1994; 120: 1051–1053.

136. Paradise JL, Bluestone CD, Rogers KD, et al.: Efficacy of adenoidectomy for recurrent otitis media in children previously treated with tympanostomy-tube placement: Results of parallel randomized and nonrandomized trials. JAMA 1990; 263: 2066–2073.

137. Bluestone CD, Klein JO: Clinical practice guideline on otitis media

with effusion in young children: Strengths and weaknesses. Otolaryngol Head Neck Surg 1995; 112: 507–511.

138. Cantekin EI, Mandel EM, Bluestone CD, et al.: Lack of efficacy of a decongestant-antihistamine combination for otitis media with effusion ("secretory" otitis media) in children. N Engl J Med 1983; 308: 297–301.

139. Rosenfeld RM, Mandel EM, Bluestone CD: Systemic steroids for otitis media with effusion in children. Arch Otolaryngol Head Neck Surg 1991; 117: 984–989.

140. Chan KH, Bluestone CD: Lack of efficacy of middle-ear inflation: Treatment of otitis media with effusion in children. Otolaryngol Head Neck Surg 1989; 100: 317–323.

141. Rosenfeld RM, Post JC: Meta-analysis of antibiotics for the treatment of otitis media with effusion. Otolaryngol Head Neck Surg 1992; 106: 378–386.

142. Mandel EM, Rockette HE, Bluestone CD, et al.: Myringotomy with and without tympanostomy tubes for chronic otitis media with effusion. Arch Otolaryngol Head Neck Surg 1989; 115: 1217–1224.

143. Mandel EM, Rockette HE, Bluestone CD, et al.: Efficacy of myringotomy with and without tympanostomy tubes for chronic otitis media with effusion. Pediatr Infect Dis J 1992; 11: 270–277.

144. McKee WJE: A controlled study of the effects of tonsillectomy and adenoidectomy in children. Br J Prev Soc Med 1963; 17: 46–49.

145. McKee WJE: The part played by adenoidectomy in the combined operation of tonsillectomy with adenoidectomy: Second part of a controlled study in children. Br J Prev Soc Med 1963; 17: 133–140.

146. Mawson SR, Adlington R, Evans M: A controlled study evaluation of adenotonsillectomy in children. J Laryngol Otol 1967; 81: 777–790.

147. Roydhouse N: A controlled study of adenotonsillectomy. Arch Otolaryngol 1970; 92: 611–616.

148. Roydhouse N: Adenoidectomy for otitis media with effusion. Ann Otol Rhinol Laryngol 1980; 89 (suppl 68): 312–315.

149. Maw AR: Chronic otitis media with effusion (glue ear) and adenotonsillectomy: Prospective randomised controlled study. Br Med J 1983; 287: 1586–1588.

150. Gates GA, Avery CA, Prihoda TJ, Cooper JC Jr: Effectiveness of adenoidectomy and tympanostomy tubes in the treatment of chronic otitis media with effusion. N Engl J Med 1987; 317 (23): 1444–1451.

151. Gates GA, Avery CA, Prihoda TJ: Effect of adenoidectomy upon children with chronic otitis media with effusion. Laryngoscope 1988; 98: 58–63.

CHAPTER THIRTY-FOUR

Vincent N. Carrasco
Harold C. Pillsbury
Jonathan R. Workman

Mastoiditis

▼

Successful treatment of disease requires a full understanding of anatomy, normal physiology, and the pathophysiology of the disease process. This chapter begins with a description of normal ear anatomy and a discussion of the pathophysiology and epidemiology of infectious ear disease before progressing to the clinical aspects of diagnosis and treatment of mastoiditis.

ANATOMY

The middle ear cleft consists of the eustachian tube, middle ear, mastoid, and petrous portions of the temporal bone. It appears in the human fetus at 3 weeks of development as an outpouching of the first pharyngeal pouch known as the tubotympanic recess (Fig. 34–1). The distal part of the pouch expands into a budding sac at week 7, progressively pneumatizing to the middle ear and the epitympanum. The proximal part of the first pharyngeal pouch remains narrow and forms the eustachian tube by elongation and chondrification. During late fetal life, the tympanic cavity expands dorsally by vacuolization of the surrounding tissue to form the tympanic antrum. After birth, the bone of the developing mastoid process is invaded by tympanic cavity epithelium forming epithelial-lined air sacs. These pneumatized air sacs come in contact with the tympanic cavity through the mastoid antrum and continue to grow for as long as 19 years after birth.

The middle ear is lined with modified respiratory epithelium and is connected to the nasopharynx by the eustachian tube. The posterior wall of the tympanic cavity is the entrance to the mastoid antrum. It also houses the fossa incu-dis. The mastoid antrum is an air-filled sinus in the petrous portion of the temporal bone. The aditus ad antrum is an opening in the upper part of the anterior wall of the mastoid antrum. This opening leads anteriorly into the epitympanic recess. The middle ear is separated from the antrum not only by the ossicles but also by mucosal folds. Proctor[1] found that there are only two constant openings between the middle ear and the mastoid, the first between the tendon of the tensor tympani muscle and the stapes and the second between the short process of the incus and the stapedial tendon. Edema and inflammation can easily block these openings, causing poor aeration, development of an anaerobic environment, and potential sequestration of disease. This is an important concept when examining the pathophysiology of mastoid disease.

The medial wall of the antrum itself is related to the posterior semicircular canal. Posteriorly the antrum is closely related to the sigmoid sinus. The roof is the tegmen tympani with the middle cranial fossa above. The lateral wall is formed by the squamous portion of the temporal bone.

The mastoid air cells are a series of interconnecting cavities, lined by mucous membrane, with a flattened squamous nonciliated epithelium, continuous with that of the mastoid antrum and tympanic cavity.

PATHOPHYSIOLOGY

Acute pain of the ear, with continued strong fever, is to be dreaded, for there is danger that the man may become delirious and die.

HIPPOCRATES[2]

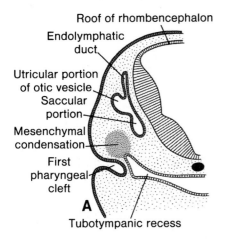

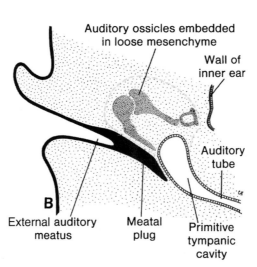

Figure 34–1. Demonstrates (A) the developing middle ear cleft and (B) auditory anatomy. (Courtesy of Sadler TW [ed]: Langman's Medical Embryology, 5th ed. Williams & Wilkins, Baltimore, 1985.)

Roof of rhombencephalon
Endolymphatic duct
Utricular portion of otic vesicle
Saccular portion
Mesenchymal condensation
First pharyngeal cleft
A
Tubotympanic recess

Auditory ossicles embedded in loose mesenchyme
Wall of inner ear
Auditory tube
B
External auditory meatus
Meatal plug
Primitive tympanic cavity

Today, armed with antimicrobial agents, diagnostic noninvasive imaging (such as computed tomography [CT] and magnetic resonance imaging [MRI]) and operative techniques to halt the progression of infection, the otolaryngologist is well equipped to avoid Hippocrates' prediction. Antibiotics have changed the course and outcome of acute otitis media and made acute mastoiditis infrequent.[3–6] Mastoiditis and its complications are therefore less common, but the sequelae of undiagnosed disease are still disastrous.

Mastoiditis typically begins as acute otitis media. *Acute, subacute,* or *chronic* otitis media and mastoiditis refer to the state of the mucosa in these pneumatized regions. The disease process progresses through the aditus ad antrum into the mastoid cavity. The clinical course of inflammatory diseases of the middle ear is therefore a continuum that begins as acute otitis media and progresses to infectious involvement of all pneumatized spaces of the temporal bone. Hawkins[7] defined mastoiditis as the presence of acute or subacute otitis media with posterior auricular swelling, erythema, tenderness, and a protruding ear with clouding of the ipisilateral mastoid air cells on CT scan. Glasscock and Shambaugh[8] describe acute suppurative otitis media by defining the progressive stages of the disease as follows.

Stage of Hyperemia

The mucoperiosteum of the middle ear spaces reacts to invading microorganisms by hyperemic swelling and closure of the eustachian tube. The hyperemic swelling extends to the antrum and pneumatic cells of the temporal bone. Earache and fever are common, with ear fullness and decrease in hearing also present. Treatment at this stage is antibiotics. Antihistamine-decongestants have not been shown to be efficacious in the treatment of otitis media.

Stage of Exudation

Hyperemia causes an outpouring of serum (from dilated permeable capillaries) containing fibrin, red blood cells, and polymorphonuclear leukocytes into the middle ear spaces. Increased pain and fever result, with a greater hearing loss, the loss of high-pitch frequencies greater than that of low. Treatment consists of antibiotics with and without myringotomy to relieve pain by releasing exudate under pressure.

Stage of Suppuration

Myringotomy or spontaneous perforation allows the ear to drain. At first, hemorrhagic secretions appear, followed by a mucopurulent discharge. The mucoperiosteum of the middle ear and air cells are thickened by new formation of capillaries and fibrous tissue. An infiltrate of lymphocytes, plasma cells, and polymorphonuclear leukocytes transforms the thick mucosal lining into granulation tissue. The infectious process is walled off in this manner, localizing it and promoting resolution. Severe pain is relieved by the release of pressure. Hearing loss continues in both low and high frequencies.

Stage of Coalescence or Surgical Mastoiditis

Progressive thickening of the hyperemic mucoperiostium begins to obstruct the free drainage of mucopurulent secretions. The epitympanum and the smaller periantral pneumatic cells close off the mastoid cavity that continues to secrete purulent material. Pus under pressure causes venous stasis, local acidosis, and decalcification of adjacent bone walls. Osteoclasts appear and dissolve the thin walls of the pneumatic cells. Separate pneumatic cells coalesce into larger cavities filled with purulent exudate and granulations. Spontaneous resolution occurs secondary to healing bone deposition underneath this exudate. Bony erosion also progresses in other portions of the temporal bone. At this stage intracranial and intratemporal complications are threatening to occur before spontaneous resolution.

The signs of coalescent mastoiditis include continued profuse purulent discharge from the ear for longer than 2 weeks, mastoid tenderness, and thickening of the periosteum. The ear protrudes from the side of the head, and a palpable mass is present posteriorly when the abscess approaches the surface. The posterosuperior wall of the osseous meatus sags because of periosteal thickening near the antrum. The tympanic membrane may protrude near the perforation because of obstruction of the perforation from the thickened tympanic mucosa. If the outer cortex perforates, a fluctuant subperiosteal abscess over the mastoid associated with the outward and downward displacement of the auricle results.

Treatment is to release purulence under pressure. A simple myringotomy is performed, and Gram's stain is done on the material, which is also cultured. Uncomplicated mastoiditis resolves with this regimen. If a subperiosteal abscess is found or another complication is suspected and confirmed by a CT scan, surgical drainage of the mastoid cavity is necessary. Incision and drainage with a cooldown period of the acute stage is advocated. This allows better visualization of surgical landmarks, thereby protecting vital structures. A decision about formal tympanomastoidectomy is made after resolution of the acute infection.

Stage of Complication

Extension of infection beyond the mucoperiosteal lining of the middle ear and pneumatic cells to an adjacent structure produces complications. This is discussed in greater detail later in the chapter.

Stage of Resolution

Cessation of the aural discharge occurs followed by closing of the central perforation. The exudate in the tympanum, antrum, and pneumatic cells is absorbed rapidly, and conductive hearing loss secondary to fluid resistance resolves. Mucoperiosteal thickening, which also causes an element of conductive hearing loss, resolves more slowly. The coalescent cavity fills with fibrous tissue and eventually ossifies. It is rare for acute suppurative otitis media to leave any permanent residue.

BACTERIOLOGY, ACUTE VERSUS CHRONIC MASTOIDITIS

Acute

The stages of mastoiditis represent a continuum beginning as middle ear disease extending to complications (Table 34–1). This way of looking at mastoiditis charts the progress of otitis media if left untreated or undertreated.

Acute mastoiditis ("classic" mastoiditis) was common before the antibiotic era, with patients quickly progressing. The classic presenting features, as described above, included retroauricular erythema, edema, and auricular displacement with occasional fluctuation behind the ear caused by a subperiosteal abscess. If a mastoidectomy was performed, pus and periostitis were encountered. Serious complications such as meningitis, cerebral abscess, thrombosis of the sigmoid sinus, Gradenigo's syndrome (petrous apicitis resulting in 6th-nerve palsy, diplopia, strabismus, lacrimation, and pain behind the eye [V1]), and Bezold's abscess (mastoiditis that progresses to subperiosteal abscess of the mastoid tip and presents as an abscess in the upper neck) were often found.

Organisms isolated from cases of mastoiditis can be expected to reflect the etiologic agents of middle ear infections. The most common cultures isolated from acute otitis media include *Streptococcus pneumoniae* (30%), *Haemophilus influenzae* (21%), *Branhamella catarrhalis* (12%), *Streptococcus pyogenes* (3%), *Staphylococcus aureus* (2%), other (20%), and no growth (20%).[9]

Results from large population centers, serving mainly indigent patients, show a high percentage of group A beta-hemolytic streptococci *(S. pyogenes)* isolated in cases of acute mastoiditis.[7, 10] Also seen are a large percentage of *S. aureus* in the isolates. This is in contrast to the other studies and may represent sampling error from the transcanal culture technique (Table 34–2).

Chronic Mastoiditis

Since the introduction of antibiotics "classic" mastoiditis has been replaced by a more chronic picture of "latent" (also described as *masked* or *acute-on-chronic*) mastoiditis. This condition is characterized by recurrent otitis media, treated with various antibiotics without preceding cultures.

Table 34–1. STAGES OF MASTOIDITIS

Acute suppurative otitis media	Bacterial meningitis in children
Streptococcus pneumoniae—most common	*Haemophilus influenzae*, type B
Haemophilus influenzae (nontypable)	*Streptococcus pneumoniae*
Moraxella (formerly *Branhamella*) catarrhalis (emerging common pathogen)	*Neisseria meningitidis*
Group A *Streptococcus*	Bacteremia from otitis media—in 3% of patients
Staphylococcus aureus (infrequent)	*Streptococcus pneumoniae*
Gram-negative bacilli (infrequent)	*Haemophilus influenzae* 4/50
	Salmonella 3/50
Cholesteatoma (intraoperative)	*Neisseria meningitidis* 2/50
Pseudomonas aeruginosa (most common aerobe)	*Staphylococcus aureus* 2/50
Bacteroides and *Peptococcus* (most common anaerobes) + *Peptostreptococcus*	Meningitis associated with acute otitis media
Propionibacterium acnes—most common anaerobe when only one organism found	High incidence of *Haemophilus influenzae*, type B
57% of cases grow 2–11 organisms (3 average)	*Haemophilus influenzae*
Foul-smelling ears grow 5–11 organisms, always anaerobes and aerobes	Nontypable *Haemophilus influenzae*
	Distinctly different from type B
Chronic otorrhea	A common cause of acute and chronic otitis media with effusion
Pseudomonas aeruginosa	Type B *Haemophilus influenzae*
Staphylococcus aureus	Causes: meningitis, cellulitis, epiglottitis, arthritis, septicemia, pneumonia
Other gram-negative organisms	Predominant in infants and young children under 5 years of age
Chronic otitis media with effusion, mastoiditis, chronic sinusitis, chronic tonsillitis	Effective vaccine given 18 months of age or younger
Haemophilus influenzae—most common	Bacteremia with type B 21.1-fold increased risk of meningitis compared with bacteremia with *S. pneumoniae*
Streptococcus pneumoniae	Rifampin good prophylaxis in at-risk contact
Branhamella catarrhalis	Anaerobes
Staphylococcus aureus	Play major roles in pathogenic synergism by protecting against host defenses, inactivating antibiotics, and creating suitable environment for other organisms
Bacteroides	Multiple anaerobes and facultative anaerobes colonize and act together
Acute mastoiditis	Anaerobes may persist, despite antibiotic treatment, in infected tissues
Streptococcus pneumonia—most common	Gram-negative anaerobes exert pathogenic activity via endotoxins that act via septic response–inducing mediators and may produce, or cause to be produced: beta-lactamase, leukocidin, proteases, collagenase, trypsin-like enzymes, dismutases, catalase, abscess-inducing capsular polysaccharides, lipases, heparinase, nucleases
Group A *Streptococcus*	
Staphylococcus epidermidis	
Haemophilus influenzae	
Anaerobes	
If perforation, canal culture not true pathogen in 25% of cases	
Intracranial abscesses (brain and subdural) of otogenic origin	
Streptococcus faecalis	
Proteus	
Bacteroides fragilis	

*Bacteria are listed in order of frequency.

Table 34–2. ORGANISMS ISOLATED FROM CASES OF ACUTE MASTOIDITIS

	Mathews[10]	Hawkins[7]	Rubin[38]	Rosen[20]
Aerobes				
Group A streptococci	15	9	3	2
S. pneumoniae	7	6	X*	3
S. aureus	6	6	5	1
Proteus mirabilis	4	X	4	X
S. viridans	1	X	X	1
P. vulgaris	1	X	X	X
Enterobacter	1	X	X	X
Anaerobes				
Bacteroides	4	1	1	X
Sterile cultures	9	X	9	9
Totals	49	22	22	16

*Variable not represented in this study.

The clinical history is long with incompletely controlled episodes of otitis media. The patient has neither protrusion of the pinna nor retroauricular edema and erythema. Mastoidectomy reveals granulation tissue in the mastoid cells in most cases, with pus and destruction of bone.

The otorrhea from an infected cholesteatoma is often malodorous because of frequent infection with anaerobic bacteria. The most common anaerobes include *Bacteroides, Peptococcus,* and *Peptostreptococcus* species and *Propionibacterium acnes.*[11] Uncomplicated chronic otorrhea characteristically cultures *Pseudomonas aeruginosa, S. aureus,* and a variety of other gram-negative organisms such as *Proteus* species, *Klebsiella* species, and *Escherichia coli.*[12] Brook[13] reported in a study of 24 patients with chronic mastoiditis that 290 (83%) had polymicrobial infections. The predominant isolates were anaerobic cocci, *Bacteroides* species, *P. aeruginosa,* and *S. aureus.*[13] Mathews and Oliver[10] reported *Proteus mirabilis, Bacteroides fragilis, Proteus* species, and *P. aeruginosa* (in order) as the most common chronic bacterial isolates. It should be noted that in 49% of cases, mixed cultures were isolated from chronic draining ears.

Masked Mastoiditis

The advent of antibiotics completely changed the course of mastoiditis and has created more subtle expressions of this disease. Masked mastoiditis is an indolent, smoldering temporal bone infection that has few clinical clues. It is a low-grade osteitis that is generally painless. The patient has a history of chronic ear infections that have been ineffectively treated with multiple courses of antibiotics. Classically the tympanic membrane is intact and the middle ear shows no sign of infection on otoscopic examination. The patient with masked mastoiditis progresses silently until a dramatic appearance of an infratemporal or intracranial complication makes its presence known.[14, 15]

The pathophysiology of masked mastoiditis is postulated as attic blockade in the face of resolved or static acute middle ear abnormality. Granulation tissue or cholesteatoma in the aditus ad antrum of the epitympanum seals off the mastoid air cells, preventing normal aeration of the mastoid.

As the oxygen tension and pH drop, an environment suitable for anaerobic pathogens, such as *Peptococcus* and *Bacteroides* species, develops. The group of high-risk patients who are at risk for the development of masked mastoiditis includes newborn infants, the immunosuppressed, chemotherapy- or steroid-treated patients, and diabetic or elderly patients.

Proper diagnosis is the first step in treatment. CT scan evaluation is done to rule out intra- or extracranial complications. Once the diagnosis has been made, the various complications are treated, a wide myringotomy, middle ear exploration, and mastoidectomy are then performed. Antibiotic coverage of anaerobic infection is continued until clinical and CT resolution of the patient's complication has occurred.

EPIDEMIOLOGY

Otitis media is a common health problem among infants and children in North America and throughout the world. In a study of Boston children observed from birth to 7 years of age, more than 90% of the children had at least one episode of acute otitis media, and approximately three quarters of the children had three or more episodes.[16] Children with early onset of otitis media are at high risk for recurrent otitis media and chronic otitis media as well as increased morbidity from associated complications. Boys may be at higher risk for otitis media than girls, and whites, American Indians, and Eskimos are at higher risk than blacks. Social class distribution data have been inconsistent. Congenital conditions such as cleft palate and Down's syndrome show that genetics may play a role in otitis media development, mainly through midface abnormalities associated with genetic syndromes. Environmental factors such as the season (winter and spring), exposure to passive smoking, and daycare attendance have been shown to increase otitis media prevalence. Breast-feeding appears to provide some protection.[17]

The development of acute mastoid osteitis as a complication of acute otitis media in the antibiotic era is rare. Before antibiotic agents, mastoiditis was the most common suppurative complication of acute otitis media and frequently resulted in death. The frequency of mastoidectomy for acute mastoiditis was 20% in 1938 and 2.8% in 1948, with an almost 90% reduction in the mortality rate during that period.[18] A study from Finland found that 29 cases of acute mastoiditis were reported during the period from 1956 to 1971.[19] A more recent study from Los Angeles, reports 54 cases of acute mastoiditis in children during the period from 1972 to 1982.[7] During the same 10-year period at Kaplan Hospital in Israel, 69 cases of acute mastoiditis were reported.[20]

During recent years a disturbing increased incidence of acute mastoiditis was observed at the University Children's Hospital, Tübingen, Germany (1975–1979: 1.4 patients per year; 1987–1992: 4.2 patients per year; p<.05). The authors attributed this increase to several factors. These included withholding antimicrobials for treatment of the preceding episode of otitis media; the use of suboptimal agents for therapy of otitis media (penicillin and erythromycin ethylsuccinate); and insufficient duration of treatment.[21]

Several reviews have shown the age range for acute mastoiditis to be from 2 months to 13–18 years of age. The majority of patients with coalescent mastoiditis are younger than 2 years of age, with a median age of 2–3 years. This age distribution parallels the prevalence of otitis media in younger populations.

The epidemiology of *extracranial and intracranial complications* of mastoiditis is detailed in the section on complications below. Briefly, the incidence of aural or extracranial complications is not well documented because of the rare occurrence of suppurative labyrinthitis, petrositis, and facial nerve paralysis.[22] Intracranial complications are more common and therefore better documented.[23–26] Before antibiotics, intracranial complications occurred in 2.3% of cases of acute or chronic middle ear infections. The introduction of antibiotics reduced this incidence to 0.15%. In both periods the majority of the complications were secondary to chronic suppuration. Patient age is an important consideration when examining the distribution of complications of otitis media. For example, approximately 75% of all cases of meningitis related to acute mastoiditis occur in patients younger than 10 years of age.

CLINICAL MANIFESTATION OF MASTOIDITIS

The clinical manifestations of mastoiditis are variable. They range from obvious retroauricular tenderness and protrusion of the pinna in acute mastoiditis to subtle ear pain behind an intact normal tympanic membrane in masked mastoiditis.

A complete past medical history is very important when evaluating a patient with suspected mastoiditis. It is especially important to obtain a detailed past history of any episode of acute otitis media before the presenting illness. Prior ear surgery should be noted; it is unusual in acute mastoiditis but common in chronic infections. Antimicrobial therapy before presentation, including specific antibiotic, dose, and duration, must be noted. It is crucial to assess the compliance and tolerance of antibiotic administration to uncover any undertreated acute otitis media. Included in the history should be a record of fever, loss of appetite, upper respiratory infection, otitis media, otalgia, otorrhea, retroauricular swelling, protrusion of the pinna, and retroauricular erythema. Physical signs of acute mastoiditis before admission were present in greater than 90% of patients in one study.[21]

Clinical findings during the initial examination in acute mastoiditis may include fever, cervical lymphadenopathy, rhinitis, abnormal tympanic membrane, retroauricular swelling, protrusion of the pinna, retroauricular erythema, and retroauricular tenderness. Retroauricular swelling is observed more often than protrusion of the pinna and retroauricular erythema. A thorough neurologic examination including a cranial nerve examination is critical at initial evaluation to assess for accompanying extracranial or intracranial complications. The signs and symptoms of these complications are discussed in the following section.

DIAGNOSIS: IMPORTANCE OF IMAGING

CT and MRI are the most important imaging modalities for evaluating the temporal bones and their associated intracranial structures.[27] Axial and coronal CT with magnified views are the "gold standard" radiologic examinations for inflammatory diseases of the temporal bone. Plain films and multidirectional tomography are obsolete and provide little additional information. Angiography is limited to detailed examination of vascular tumors or malformations in the temporal bone and vicinity. MR and CT angiography at present are excellent screening tools for vascular complications of mastoiditis where exquisite vessel detail is not essential for diagnosis.

Computed Tomography

CT is the best choice for evaluating infectious lesions involving the petromastoid complex[27] and is well suited for the evaluation of mastoiditis and its complications. CT is indicated in cases of acute otitis media when there is a clinical suggestion of coalescent mastoiditis[28, 29] or when there is evidence of its complications. Mafee and colleagues[30] found that CT proved valuable in the diagnosis and assessment of acute otomastoiditis, coalescent mastoiditis, and associated intratemporal, extracranial, and intracranial complications. In CT scans obtained for suspicion of coalescent mastoiditis, 8 of 14 showed no evidence of bone erosion and could be treated medically. The other 6 showed varied degrees of bony erosion, which was confirmed surgically.[30]

A CT scan should be performed when there is continued mucopurulent discharge from the middle ear, pain, and mastoid tenderness (the signs of coalescent mastoiditis as described above). The CT scan can be used to evaluate early bone destruction and aid the surgeon in the decision to proceed with medical treatment versus the need for mastoidectomy. The treatment algorithm for complications of mastoiditis is described below. The presence of cerebellar or meningeal signs and symptoms necessitates CT scanning of the head, with and without contrast material, to exclude intracranial and extracranial complications. Contrast-enhanced CT allows evaluation of the dural sinuses to rule out infectious thrombi. Otic hydrocephalus occurring with complete sinus thrombosis is a CT diagnosis.

We use high-resolution studies of the temporal bone. These are done in two projections using bone algorithms. Axial scanning with 1.0-mm-thick sections at 1-mm intervals clarifies the bony structures. The second projection is a coronal oblique, approximately 20 degrees less than a true coronal projection, with contiguous 1.0-mm-thick slices. Magnified images are then provided of the middle ear and mastoid alone. These images are of sufficient quality to visualize the stapes superstructure, round window, and sinus tympani.

Magnetic Resonance Imaging

MRI is significantly more sensitive for soft tissue abnormalities than is CT. It is the procedure of choice for evaluating the internal auditory canal, cerebellopontine angle, and cerebral parenchyma. It is also an important part of further evaluation for complications of mastoiditis initially diagnosed by CT. At present MRI offers no advantages over CT in the evaluation of mastoiditis.[31] New MRI sequences are under development to better evaluate the bony structures of the petrous bone. These techniques may one day surpass CT for evaluating the petrous bone, but at present CT remains the gold standard.[32] CT and MRI are complementary studies and should be obtained together when evaluating disease processes that require delineation of bone destruction and soft tissue extension. For example, both studies are important as part of the preoperative evaluation of glomus jugulare.

TREATMENT OF MASTOIDITIS

Patients presenting with uncomplicated acute mastoiditis should be initially treated with broad-spectrum intravenous antibiotics. A myringotomy incision with culture and Gram's stain of the effusion should be done before the start of antibiotic therapy. If gram-negative organisms are isolated from the ear, the antibiotic coverage is adjusted.

In chronic mastoiditis the predominant organisms are gram-negative bacilli. Augmented penicillins such as ampicillin plus sulbactam have good gram-negative aerobic and anaerobic coverage. If the culture isolates *Pseudomonas*, therapy is adjusted based on sensitivities. Ciprofloxacin can be used in adults with *Pseudomonas* isolates.

COMPLICATIONS

The natural history of mastoiditis has changed radically with the development of effective antimicrobial agents. Otitis media is treated early, preventing progression to more severe stages of disease. As a result, the complications of infectious ear disease that were once common are now rare. In the 5-year period immediately preceding the introduction of antibiotics, from 1928 to 1933, approximately 1 in 40 deaths in a large general hospital was caused by an intracranial complication of otitis media, with meningitis heading the list, sinus thrombosis second, and brain abscess last.[33] In a similar 5-year period from 1949 to 1954, only 1 in every 400 deaths was the result of ear disease, for a 10-fold reduction.

Kangsanarak and colleagues[15] reported 102 cases of intracranial and extracranial complications from 17,144 cases of suppurative otitis media. The prevalence of each complication was 0.24% and 0.45%, respectively. Facial paralysis, subperiosteal abscess, and labyrinthitis were the most common complications among the extracranial complication group, whereas meningitis and brain abscess were common in the intracranial complication group.[15]

Definition

A complication from suppuration in the pneumatized spaces of the temporal bone is defined as extension of inflammation beyond the confines of the lumen and its mucosa or products of that inflammation.[34] Complications occur from bone destruction secondary to enzymatic reabsorption or osteitis and inflammation of surrounding structures. This includes any portion of the surrounding bone, facial nerve, tympanic membrane, round window membrane, ossicles, adjacent blood vessels, or brain.

Otitis media, mastoiditis, and *petrositis* refer to mucosal inflammation and are not themselves considered complications of each other. Periosteal inflammation is not considered a complication of mastoiditis. Only when bone destruction occurs in these regions does a complication exist.

Classifications

Based on popular usage, complications of suppurative otitis media are classified into two categories. Complications of mastoiditis can be broken down into *aural, intratemporal,* or *extracranial,* and *intracranial* groups.[8, 35]

Aural or intratemporal or extracranial complications
  Mastoiditis with bone destruction
  Subperiosteal abscess
  Petrositis with bone destruction
  Facial paralysis
  Labyrinthitis (serous, suppurative, or chronic)
Intracranial complications
  Extradural abscess or granulation tissue in extradural
    space
  Lateral sinus thrombophlebitis or thrombosis
  Subdural abscess
  Meningitis
  Brain abscess
  Otitic hydrocephalus

Epidemiology

Studies analyzing intracranial complications have recently been performed by Gower and McGuirt,[23] Samuel and colleagues[25] and Kangsanarak and colleagues.[15] See Table 34–3. They report the most common intracranial complications are meningitis, brain abscess, and lateral sinus thrombosis. The most common extracranial complications from the study by Kangsanarak and colleagues include facial nerve paralysis, subperiosteal abscess, and labyrinthitis. All other complications were much less common. Kangsanarak and colleagues reported 77 patients with extracranial complications during a 7-year period (1983–1990). The frequencies of complications are as follows: facial nerve paralysis, 45; subperiosteal abscess, 31; labyrinthitis, 26; postauricular fistula or scar,

Table 34–3. PREVALENCE OF INTRACRANIAL COMPLICATIONS

	Gower[23] (n = 100)	Kangsanarak[15] (n = 43)	Samuel[25] (n = 224)
Meningitis	76	22	83
Brain abscess	6	18	53
Subdural effusion	5	X	X
Extradural abscess	X	7	49
Lateral sinus thrombosis	5	8	39
Otitic hydrocephalus	5	2	X
Subdural abscess	3	5	X

X, Variable not represented in this study.

14; coalescent mastoiditis, 11; pneumonia, 2; and pinna perichondritis, 1.

The age distribution in complications tends to follow fairly predictable patterns. For example, with the exception of meningitis in infants and young children, which may be associated with acute suppurative otitis media, all other complications tend to be associated with subacute or chronic middle ear infection.[35] Gower and McGuirt[23] found that 63 of 76 (83%) complications were secondary to acute otitis media and that meningitis was by far the number one complication; 56 of 63 (89%) occurred in children ≤10 years of age. Kangsanarak and colleagues[15] reported the opposite findings concerning acute versus chronic mastoiditis: 10 of 102 (10%) had complications secondary to acute otitis media, whereas 92 of 102 (90%) had complications secondary to chronic otitis media. Samuel[25] reported that 74% of all intracranial otogenic complications were in patients younger than 15 years of age.

Influencing Factors in the Development of Complications

The organisms involved have a significant influence on whether complications occur.[16] Nonperforated tympanic membrane–isolated organisms are usually single organism isolates and mimic the bacteria isolated from uncomplicated otitis media and mastoiditis. Isolates from perforated tympanic membranes are usually polymicrobial (5–11 different bacteria from one ear), resulting in a mixed infection of aerobes and anaereobes.[17]

Diagnosis of Mastoiditis Complications

Early signs and symptoms of neurootologic complications resulting from chronic suppurative otitis media are purulent malodorous drainage, headache, and deep ear pain.[18] Also reported are fever, lethargy, obtundation, retroorbital pain, emesis, blurred vision, sudden hearing loss, and vertigo. Signs and symptoms of this sort need careful investigation and represent masked subtle indicators of impending catastrophic sequelae.

Complications are also suspect when there is persistent acute or chronic otitis media with suppurative effusion or discharge accompanied by granulation tissue. Patients experiencing vestibular symptoms and increasing otalgia after initial cessation of long-standing discharge should also be evaluated.[18]

Management of Complications

The principles of the management of complications include (1) eradication of infection by antibiotics, (2) establishment of drainage, and (3) excision of infected tissue.

Complications involving bone destruction usually require mastoidectomy, parenteral antibiotics, and special management techniques specific for the complications involved.

Acute Coalescent Mastoiditis and Masked Mastoiditis, with or Without Subperiosteal Abscess

Myringotomy, or at least placement of a pressure equalization tube, is recommended as the initial treatment in less severe disease. When there is significant disease, such as systemic signs of toxicity and subperiosteal abscess, a canal wall-up mastoidectomy with a wide facial recess approach is performed. When disease is extensive and landmarks are not clearly definable, canal wall-down (modified radical mastoidectomy) is performed. If for some reason the disease is unresectable or there is cochlear invasion, radical mastoidectomy is performed. Ossicular reconstruction is reserved for a second-stage procedure in canal wall-up and modified radical mastoidectomy.

Chronic Mastoiditis

Treatment of chronic mastoiditis is the same as for chronic suppurative otitis media, with or without cholesteatoma—mastoidectomy for suppurative disease with inspection of the dura of the tegmen, the sigmoid sinus, and the facial nerve through thin bone. Reconstruction of the middle ear at the time of canal wall-up or wall-down mastoidectomy is controversial. If the disease is easily removed with reasonable confidence and the ear is not tremendously infected, ossicular reconstruction may be attempted. The patient and family are counseled regarding the philosophy of multiple staging so they understand the risks of a single-stage procedure and have realistic expectations.

Petrositis

Radical mastoidectomy or modified radical mastoidectomy are performed depending upon resectability. The five tracts to the petrous apex are opened as far as possible,[36] with the infracochlear route generally providing the deepest most direct drainage. If this does not resolve the infection a middle-fossa approach to exenterate the disease in the petrous apex may be necessary.

Labyrinthitis

Treatment in acute infection is myringotomy and antibiotics. In chronic infection, a tympanomastoidectomy (canal wall-up mastoidectomy) is performed. The ear is explored for fistulae. Lateral semicircular canal fistulae and cochlear fistulae are fixed with fascia at the time of mastoidectomy, but large fistulae may need a second operation after control of the acute process. Suppurative labyrinthitis quickly leads to meningitis. Treatment includes long-term parenteral antibiotics and in some cases surgical decompression of the labyrinth.

Facial Paralysis

For acute infection a myringotomy should be performed and the patient treated with intravenous antibiotics. We have found steroids useful in treating what is presumably swelling of the facial nerve in the bony facial nerve (fallopian) canal from inflammation. We generally observe the patient closely and do not perform acute mastoidectomy unless there are other significant complications. We have found that as soon as pressure is relieved and appropriate antibiotic therapy is instituted, facial paralysis resolves. In patients with complete facial paralysis, neurophysiologic testing is performed in order to gather objective data and provide a baseline for follow-up. The ear is rescanned using CT in 2–3 weeks for underlying abnormality, and mastoidectomy is performed at that time if appropriate.

In chronic infection, a mastoidectomy with exploration of the fallopian canal for invasive granulation tissue is indicated. Opening the sheath in the face of infection is contraindicated. If granulation tissue is found in the canal, then it should be opened along the length of involvement.

Extradural Granulation Tissue or Abscess

If abscess is found, canal wall-down mastoidectomy (modified radical) generally provides better drainage than intact canal wall procedures. Wide exposure of abnormal dura is indicated, and dural defects are defined and repaired using temporalis fascia and fibrin glue. Antibiotic therapy is an important part of treatment and should be based on culture results.

Dural Venous Thrombophlebitis

Complete mastoidectomy is performed for management of the extradural granulation tissue or pus. The sigmoid sinus is carefully exposed, and a small needle on a syringe is used to test the sinus for patency. If there is good blood flow, then eradication of disease in the middle ear and mastoid alone is adequate. If the sinus is thrombosed, the bone is removed from the sinus to the extent that tears can be controlled. A venotomy is performed and clot removed until free flow of blood is obtained. A completely solidified sinus with extension into the internal jugular vein and clinical signs of recurring sepsis may require ligation of the internal jugular vein in the neck.

Brain Abscess

The cerebral abscess should first be drained by the neurosurgeon, followed by the indicated ear surgery. Brain abscesses are usually not opened but drained under stereotactic guidance for culture and treated with antibiotics. Small abscesses that do not cause a mass effect are observed and treated nonsurgically with steroids and antibiotics alone. Rarely is an abscess in direct continuity with the ear and is not drained through the ear.

Otic Hydrocephalus

Patients can present with acute signs of increased intracranial pressure (ICP) or a more chronic process. The acutely ill patients require that the physician aggressively manage the mastoiditis, extradural granulations, and sigmoid sinus thrombophlebitis. The more chronic patients present with an indolent process that can include papilledema, visual abnormalities, cranial neuropathies (including sixth nerve palsy), and headache. Conservative management includes antibiotics, diuretics (carbonic anhydrase inhibitors to reduce ICP), visual monitoring by an ophthalmologist, and neurosurgical consultation for the ICP elevation. Occasionally, ventricular shunting is needed for control.

Subdural Abscess

Surgical control of mastoiditis, extradural granulations, or abscess, and sigmoid sinus thrombophlebitis, is necessary for recovery. The neurosurgical service performs a drainage procedure for the subdural abscess, and otologic procedures are performed as discussed above. Antibiotic therapy is aggressive and tailored to the organisms involved.

Meningitis

Meningitis is a complication of acute or chronic ear disease and is an emergency. Acute therapy is predominantly medical involving antibiotics with good central nervous system penetration. Myringotomy is performed to relieve pressure and provide drainage. More extensive surgical drainage is reserved for coalescent disease and abscess. The type of mastoid procedure is tailored to the nature of the disease encountered as discussed above.

Considerations for the Future

Inappropriate use of antibiotics eventually breeds resistant organisms. We have already seen the emergence of extremely aggressive strains of *Streptococcus*, and in-hospital strains of antibiotic-resistant *Staphylococcus* continue to proliferate. Cases involving human immunodeficiency virus, and the emergence of resistant strains of *Mycobacterium*, are becoming more common and require heightened clinical awareness on our part when dealing with patients with unusual presentations. These trends are anticipated to continue.

Three-dimensional surgical planning[37] will improve our preoperative planning for the treatment of ear disease. Minimally invasive surgical procedures may change our technical approaches to these problems, but the principles of disease management will generally remain the same.

CONCLUSION

Successful treatment of disease requires a full understanding of anatomy, normal physiology, and the pathophysiology of the disease process. Appropriate antibiotic therapy and aggressive surgical management, when necessary, will reduce complications and minimize the sequelae of infectious ear disease.

References

1. Proctor B: The development of the middle ear spaces and their surgical significance. J Laryngol Otol 1964; 78: 631.
2. Cawthorne T: The surgery of the temporal bone. J Laryngol Otol 1953; 67: 377.
3. Palva T, Pulkinen K. Mastoiditis: J Laryngol Otol 1959; 73: 573.
4. Mathews TJ: Acute and acute-on-chronic mastoiditis (a five-year experience at Groote Schuur Hospital). J Laryngol Otol 1988; 102(2): 115.

5. Palva T, Virtanen H, Makinen J: Acute and latent mastoiditis in children. J Laryngol Otol 1985; 99(2): 127.

6. Courville CB, Nielsen JM: Symposium: Intracranial complications of otitis media and mastoiditis in the antibiotic era. Laryngoscope 1955; 65: 31.

7. Hawkins D, Dru D, House J, Clark R: Acute mastoiditis in children: A review of 54 cases. Laryngoscope 1983; 93(May): 568.

8. Glasscock ME, Shambaugh G: Surgery of the Ear, 4th ed. Philadelphia: WB Saunders Co, 1990.

9. Bluestone CD, Lundgren K, Tos M, Takahara T: Frequency of bacteria isolated from middle ear effusions of children from the United States, Finland, Japan, and Denmark. Ann Otol Rhinol Laryngol 1990; 99(149): 42.

10. Mathews TJ, Oliver SP: Bacteriology of mastoiditis (a five-year experience at Groote Schuur Hospital). J Laryngol Otol 1988; 102(5): 397.

11. Harker LA, Koontz FP: The bacteriology of cholesteatomas. In: McCabe BF, Sade J, Abramson M (eds): Cholesteatoma: First International Conference. Birmingham, Alabama: Aesculapins Publishing, 1977, pp 264–267.

12. Fairbanks DNF: Antimicrobial Therapy in Otolaryngology—Head and Neck Surgery, 7th ed. Alexandria, Virginia: The American Academy of Otolaryngology—Head and Neck Surgery Foundation, 1994, p 74.

13. Brook I: Aerobic and anaerobic bacteriology of chronic mastoiditis in children. Am J Dis Child 1981; 135: 478.

14. Holt R, Gates G: Masked mastoiditis. Laryngoscope 1983; 93(8): 1034.

15. Kangsanarak J, Fooanant S, Ruckphaopunt K, et al.: Extracranial and intracranial complications of suppurative otitis media. Report of 102 cases. J Laryngol Otol 1993; 107(11): 999.

16. Klein J, Teele K, Resner B, et al.: Epidemiology of acute otitis media in Boston children from birth to seven years of age. In: Lim D, Bluestone C, Klein J, Nelson J (eds): Recent Advances in Otitis Media, vol 1, 1st ed. Philadelphia: BC Decker, 1988, p 14.

17. Daly K: Epidemiology of otitis media. Otol Clin North Am 1991; 24(4): 775.

18. Sorensen H: Antibiotics in suppurative otitis media. Otol Clin North Am 1977; 10: 45.

19. Juselius H, Kaltiokallio K: Complications of acute and chronic otitis media in the antibiotic era. Acta Otolaryngol (Stockh) 1972; 74: 445.

20. Rosen A, Ophir D, Marshak G: Acute mastoiditis: A review of 69 cases. Ann Otol Rhinol Laryngol 1986; 95(3, pt 1): 222.

21. Hoppe JE, Koster S, Bootz F, Niethammer D: Acute mastoiditis—Relevant once again. Infection 1994; 22(3): 178.

22. Neely J: Complications of suppurative otitis media: Part 1. Aural complications. Washington, D.C.: American Academy of Otolaryngology—Head and Neck Surgery Foundation, 1978, p 66. (Otol. CoCi, ed., self-instructional package vol. 78300).

23. Gower D, McGuirt WF: Intracranial complications of acute and chronic infectious ear disease: A problem still with us. Laryngoscope 1983; 93(August): 1028.

24. Ariza J, Casanova A, Fernandez VP, et al.: Etiological agent and primary source of infection in 42 cases of focal intracranial suppuration. J Clin Microbiol 1986; 24(5): 899.

25. Samuel J, Fernandes CM, Steinberg JL: Intracranial otogenic complications: A persisting problem. Laryngoscope 1986; 96(3): 272.

26. Samuel J, Fernandes CM: Lateral sinus thrombosis (a review of 45 cases). J Laryngol Otol 1987; 101(12): 1227.

27. Vignaud J, Jardin C, Rose L: The Ear: Diagnostic Imaging (CT Scanner, Tomography and Magnetic Resonance). New York: Masson Publishing, 1986.

28. Mafee M, Valvassori G, Dobben G: The role of radiology in surgery of the ear and skull base. Otol Clin North Am 1982; 15: 723.

29. Zizmor J, Noyek A: Inflammatory diseases of the temporal bone. Radiol Clin North Am 1974; 12: 491.

30. Mafee MF, Singleton EL, Valvassori GE, et al.: Acute otomastoiditis and its complications: Role of CT. Radiology 1985; 155(2): 391.

31. Latchaw R, Dreisbach J: Imaging the petrous bone and associated intracranial structures. In: Cummings C, Fredrickson J, Harker L, et al.: Otolaryngology Head and Neck Surgery, vol 4. St Louis: CV Mosby, 1994.

32. Brogan M, Chakeres D, Schmalbrock P: High resolution 3DFTMR imaging of the endolymphatic duct and soft tissues of the optic capsule. AJNR 1991; 12: 1.

33. Courville CB: Intracranial complications of otitis media and mastoiditis in the antibiotic era. Laryngoscope 1955; 65: 31.

34. Mawson SR: Diseases of the Ear, 3rd ed. Baltimore: Williams & Wilkins, 1974.

35. Neely JG: Intratemporal and intracranial complications of otitis media. In: Bailey BJ (ed): Head and Neck Surgery—Otolaryngology, vol 2. Philadelphia: JB Lippincott Co, 1993: 1607.

36. Fairbanks DNF: Antimicrobial Therapy in Otolaryngology—Head and Neck Surgery, 7th ed. Alexandria, Virginia: American Academy of Otolaryngology—Head and Neck Surgery Foundation, 1994, p 74.

37. Carrasco VN, Murkherji S, Soltys MS, et al.: A Realtime Interactive Three Dimensional Visualization System for Temporal Bone Surgical Planning. Key West, Florida: Southern Section of the Triologic Society, 1995.

Dennis I. Bojrab
Thomas E. Bruderly

CHAPTER THIRTY-FIVE

External Otitis

▼

Otitis externa is a broad term for a condition that includes inflammation and/or infection of the external auditory canal and auricle. This disease can range from mild inflammation and discomfort to a severe life-threatening disease. Otitis externa is one of the most common conditions seen in an otologic practice, affecting 3%–10% of the patient population.[1-3] The infection may be classified by location, cause, time course, and severity.

Otitis externa can be divided into six distinct subgroups: (1) acute diffuse (bacterial) (2) acute localized (circumscribed), (3) chronic, (4) eczematous, (5) fungal, and (6) necrotizing (malignant) (see Chapter 36). Identification and treatment of these various subgroups rely on a thorough understanding of the external auditory canal's anatomy and physiology along with the microbiology of the inciting organisms and pharmacotherapy to treat the offending pathogen.

NORMAL ANATOMY

Auricle (Pinna)

The external ear is composed of the auricle (pinna) and the external auditory canal. Both contain elastic cartilage derived from mesoderm and a small amount of subcutaneous tissue covered by skin with its adnexal appendages. The ear lobe is comprised of skin and fat but no cartilage. The auricle is derived from the hillocks of His—six hillocks, three from branchial arch one and three from branchial arch two.[4] During normal gestation, the cartilaginous hillocks merge to form the auricle along with selective growth of the mandible. The auricle arises from its original position near the lateral commissure of the mouth and migrates to the temporal area. The tragus and antitragus form a partial barrier lateral to the meatus of the external auditory canal. These structures act to focus and localize sound. The auricle normally rests at an angle of 30 degrees to the sagittal plane of the head. The auricle's growth parallels overall body growth until it reaches adult size at approximately age 9 years.

The auricle is composed of skin and elastic cartilage to form the tragus, anterior helical crus, concha, helix, antihelix, and antitragus (Fig. 35–1). The topography of the auricle is determined almost solely by the contour of its underlying cartilaginous frame. The flangelike auricle has a convex medial surface, which attaches to the head at its medial third; the lateral surface is concave. The major concavity of the lateral aspect of the pinna is the concha. Anteriorly, the tragus limits the concha as it extends over the orifice of the

external auditory canal. The concha is bounded by the antihelix and the anterior crus superiorly and posteriorly. The inferior extent of the concha is determined by the antitragus, which is separated from the antihelix posteriorly by the posterior auricular sulcus and from the tragus anteriorly by the intertragic notch and incisura. Anteroinferiorly, the crus of the helix is separated from the tragus by the anterior incisura. The helix and its furled edge sweep superiorly and posteriorly from the crus of the helix to the lobule.

The framework of the auricle, consisting of elastic cartilage, yields the contour of the external ear. This cartilage measures 0.5–2 mm in thickness. The structure of the auricle and the tragus functions to protect the middle and inner ear along with focusing and localizing sound. The auricle is attached to the cranium by skin, cartilage, and a complex of muscles and ligaments. There are three extrinsic ligaments and three extrinsic muscles; both sets are referred to as superior, anterior, and posterior. The superior ligament links the superior aspect of the bony external auditory canal to the spine of the cartilaginous helix; the anterior ligament connects the zygoma to the helix and tragus; and the posterior ligament attaches the eminence of the concha to the mastoid process. The three extrinsic muscles originate from the galea aponeurotica of the scalp. The superior auricular

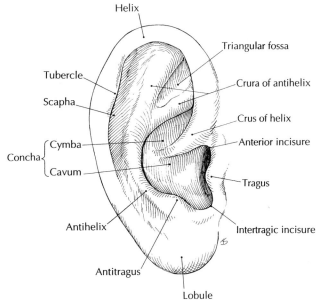

Figure 35–1. Anatomic illustration depicting the topographical features of the right auricle.

muscle inserts upon the eminence of the triangular fossa; the anterior auricular muscle inserts upon the spine of the helix; and the posterior auricular muscle inserts upon the eminence of the cavum concha.[3, 4]

The skin and subcutaneous tissue reproduce the irregular contour of the cartilaginous frame. The skin of the medial aspect is only loosely attached, whereas the skin on the lateral surface is snugly secured by subcutaneous areolar tissue. The usual skin adnexal structures are present, including sebaceous and sudoriferous (sweat) glands, and hair. The sebaceous glands are distributed both medially and laterally, especially in the regions of the concha and triangular fossa, where sudoriferous glands are sparse. A rudimentary type of hair is in abundance over the entire pinna. The hair of elderly males may be long and coarse, especially over the tragus and antitragus. The lobule, the inferior appendage of the pinna, is essentially a fibrofatty nodule with no known physiologic function.

External Auditory Canal

The external auditory canal is approximately 2.5 cm in length and serves as a channel for sound transmission to the middle ear (Fig. 35–2). It also functions to protect the middle and inner ear from foreign bodies and fluctuations in environmental conditions. The lateral third is cartilaginous and oriented in an upward and backward fashion. The medial two thirds of the external auditory canal are osseous and oriented in a downward and forward direction. Because of the different angulations of the fibrocartilaginous and osseous canal walls, the adult auricle must be pulled upward and posteriorly to achieve alignment during otoscopic examination. The anterior aspect of the fibrocartilaginous portion is pierced by two or three variably present vertical fissures known as the fissures of Santorini. These fissures are a

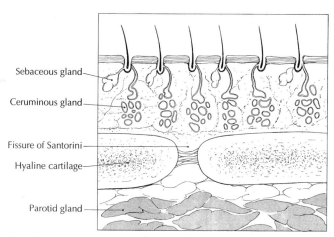

Figure 35–3. Cross-sectional microscopic view of the anterolateral wall in the fibrocartilaginous region of the external auditory canal featuring Santorini's fissure in close approximation to the parotid gland.

(labels: Sebaceous gland; Ceruminous gland; Fissure of Santorini; Hyaline cartilage; Parotid gland)

potential route for spread of infections or neoplasms between the external auditory canal and the parotid gland (Fig. 35–3).

The narrowest region of the external auditory canal is at the osseous and fibrocartilaginous junction. The inferior tympanic recess is a depression in the inferior and medial aspect of the osseous canal. The osseous canal is approximately 6 mm longer anteroinferiorly than posterosuperiorly because of the angulation of the tympanic membrane. This creates an acute angle between the tympanic membrane and the anteroinferior bony canal wall.

The skin of the osseous canal is thinner than that of the fibrocartilaginous portion, measuring approximately 0.2 mm in thickness, and is continuous with the epithelium of the tympanic membrane. The very thin dermal and subcutaneous layers have no glands or hair follicles. The skin of the fibrocartilaginous portion of the canal ranges from 0.5 to 1 mm in thickness with an epidermis of five layers (stratum corneum, stratum lucidum, stratum granulosum, stratum spinosum, and stratum basale) overlying true dermal and subcutaneous layers. This skin contains many hair follicles, sebaceous (lipid-producing) glands, and apocrine (ceruminous) glands. These three adnexal structures provide a protective function and are termed the apopilosebaceous unit (Fig. 35–4). The modified apocrine glands are found mainly on the superior and inferior walls of the canal. These apocrine glands are the ceruminous glands of the ear canal. They are located in the dermis and have three major components: (1) a coiled secretory portion, (2) a secretory duct within the dermis, and (3) a terminal funnel.[5] The lateral third of the fibrocartilaginous canal is replete with hair follicles, but they are less numerous in the medial aspect of the fibrocartilaginous portion. Arrector pili muscles are not found in association with hair follicles in any portion of the external auditory canal. Both sebaceous and modified apocrine glands develop from the outer root sheath of the hair follicles; hence, their numerical distribution follows a pattern similar to that of the hair follicles. An invagination of the epidermis forms the outer wall of the hair follicle, and the hair shaft forms the inner wall. The follicular canal is the space between these two structures. The alveoli of the sebaceous and apocrine glands empty into short, straight excre-

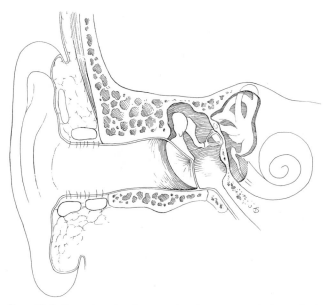

Figure 35–2. Coronal section demonstrating the osseous and fibrocartilaginous portions of a right ear canal.

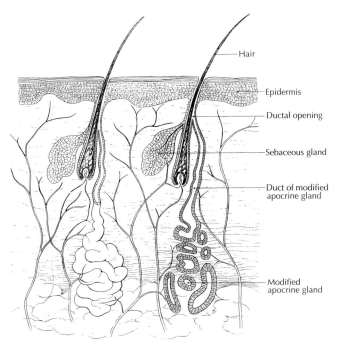

Hair

Epidermis

Ductal opening

Sebaceous gland

Duct of modified
apocrine gland

Modified
apocrine gland

Figure 35–4. Fibrocartilaginous portion of the external ear canal revealing the components of the apopilosebaceous unit.

tory ducts that drain into follicular canals. Obstruction of any part of the ductal system predisposes to infection.

The canal is normally a self-protecting and self-cleansing structure. The cerumen coat gradually works its way past the isthmus to the lateral part of the canal and sloughs externally. Instrumentation and excessive cleansing of the canal disturb this protective barrier and may lead to infection, either through the loss of cerumen or through direct tearing of the epithelial skin layer denuded of the protective cerumen, allowing access by offending microbes. The spread of infection to surrounding tissues may occur posterior to the cartilaginous canal, where lies dense connective tissue overlying the mastoid, or through the posterior bony canal, where several vessels penetrate the canal, especially along the tympanomastoid suture. Inferiorly, the canal is bound by the infratemporal fossa and base of skull. Infections extending through the floor of the canal may extend into these structures. Anterolaterally, the canal is bordered by the parotid gland and anteromedially by the temporomandibular joint. This anterolateral spread through the fissures of Santorini is a well-recognized pathway to this region.

The cerumen (ear wax) is the combination of secretions produced by the sebaceous and apocrine glands along with a variable component of desquamated epithelial cells. This combination forms an acidic coat to aid in preventing an infection of the external auditory canal. There are genetically and racially determined differences in the physical characteristics of cerumen. These differences vary the appearance and consistency of the cerumen and seem to be associated with the immunoglobulin and lysozyme content.[6–8]

The arterial supply to the auricle and the external auditory canal is the superficial temporal and the posterior auricular arteries, which are branches of the external carotid artery. Venous drainage from the external auditory canal and auricle

is by the superficial temporal vein to the retromandibular vein to the internal and external jugular veins, by the posterior auricular vein to the external jugular vein, and by the sigmoid sinus through the mastoid emissary vein.

Sensory innervation of the external auditory canal and auricle is supplied by cranial and cutaneous nerves. The cranial nerves are the auriculotemporal branch of the trigeminal, the sensory twigs of the facial, and the auricular branches of the glossopharyngeal and vagus nerves. The cutaneous branches are the greater auricular nerve and lesser occipital nerve emanating from the cervical plexus (C2–C3).

Lymphatic drainage is important in the spread of infections or neoplasms. The anterior drainage is through the fissures of Santorini to the preauricular, glenoid, and parotid regions, whereas the anterior superior region drains to the parotid and the superior deep cervical nodes. The inferior aspect drains to the infra-auricular nodal system located at the angle of the mandible. Drainage posteriorly is into the postauricular nodes and the superior deep cervical nodes.

ACUTE DIFFUSE OTITIS EXTERNA

Acute diffuse otitis externa (swimmer's ear) is an inflammatory and infectious process of the external auditory canal. *Staphylococcus epidermidis* and *Corynebacterium* species are the two most common organisms isolated in the external auditory canal of normal individuals, although *Pseudomonas aeruginosa* followed by *Staphylococcus aureus* are the most common pathogens cultured in acute diffuse otitis externa.[10–15] Other pathogens less commonly cultured are shown in Table 35–1, which lists the pathogenic organisms cultured in acute otitis externa and the appropriate antibiotic coverage for the offending organisms. The normal pH of the external auditory canal is mildly acidic, at a pH of 4–5.[9] The pathogenesis of acute diffuse otitis externa is a change in the normal environment and pH of the external auditory canal toward a more alkaline pH, which allows the growth of pathogenic bacteria. Factors involved in this process include an accumulation of moisture from a warm, humid climate; retention of water from swimming, bathing, snorkeling, and scuba diving; and the excessive removal of wax in the external auditory canal. Trauma from overzealous cleaning, scratching an itch with a foreign object, or even one's own fingernail can abrade and lacerate the canal, causing a defect in the canal skin and promoting otitis externa.[9, 16] These factors can lead to a rise in the pH of the external auditory canal from its normal acidic value to a neutral or alkaline environment in which bacteria can proliferate.

Acute diffuse otitis externa causes various signs and symptoms, depending on the severity and stage of the disease. Staging has been classified by Senturia[17] into preinflammatory and acute inflammatory stages, which are divided into mild, moderate, and severe.[17] The preinflammatory stage is defined by itching, edema, and the sensation of fullness. The acute inflammatory stage begins with increased itching, auricular tenderness, and pain penetrating the external auditory canal. Mild erythema and edema are appreciated in the patent external auditory canal. Exfoliation of skin along with a minimal amount of secretions can also be seen. The secretions during this stage are usually clear

Table 35–1. PATHOGENS CULTURED IN ACUTE OTITIS EXTERNA AND APPROPRIATE ANTIBIOTICS

Organisms	Quinolones		Miscellaneous Antibiotics					Aminoglycosides			Tetracyclines		Sulfonamides	
	Ciprofloxacin	Ofloxacin	Bacitracin	Chloramphenicol	Gramicidin	Polymyxin B	Polymyxin E (Colistin)	Neomycin	Gentamicin	Tobramycin	Tetracycline	Oxytetracycline	Sulfacetamide	Sulfisoxazole
Gram-positive														
Corynebacterium diphtheriae			•											
Staphylococcus species	•		•		•			•	•	•	•		•	•
Staphylococcus aureus	•	•	•					•	•	•	•		•	•
Staphylococcus epidermidis	•		•									•		
Streptococcus species			•	•							•	•	•	•
Streptococcus pneumoniae			•	•							•	•	•	•
Streptococcus pyogenes (group A beta-hemolytic)				•	•									
Gram-negative														
Bacteroides fragilis		•		•		•	•	•						
Citrobacter species	•	•				•	•	•	•		•	•		
Enterobacter aerogenes	•	•				•	•	•						
Enterobacter species	•	•				•	•	•						
Escherichia coli	•	•		•		•	•	•			•			
Haemophilus influenzae	•	•		•		•	•	•			•		•	•
Klebsiella pneumoniae	•	•				•	•	•				•	•	•
Klebsiella species	•	•				•	•	•	•			•	•	•
Proteus species	•	•				•	•	•					•	•
Pseudomonas aeruginosa	•	•				•	•		•	•			•	•

but can be cloudy (Figs. 35–5 to 35–10). The next stage of acute diffuse otitis externa is the moderate phase. During this phase, the itching, auricular tenderness, and pain in the external auditory canal are all intensified. The external auditory canal is still patent, but now the lumen is decreased owing to edema and debris of the thickened, irritated skin. Secretions now have an exudative content and are more profuse. These signs and symptoms continue to increase in severity until the severe stage of acute diffuse otitis externa is reached. At this stage, the pain is intolerable; there is even pain upon chewing, along with movement of soft tissue around the attachments of the ear. The lumen of the external auditory canal becomes more narrowed and can be obliterated by the increasing erythema and edema. The exudative content is a purulent greenish-yellow discharge (Figs. 35–11 and 35–12). The severe acute inflammatory stage of acute diffuse otitis externa is often associated with evidence of infection spread beyond the ear proper to surrounding soft tissues and regional lymph nodes.[8]

The diagnosis of acute otitis externa is not difficult. A thorough otologic history and examination reveal pertinent signs and symptoms for this diagnosis. The history almost

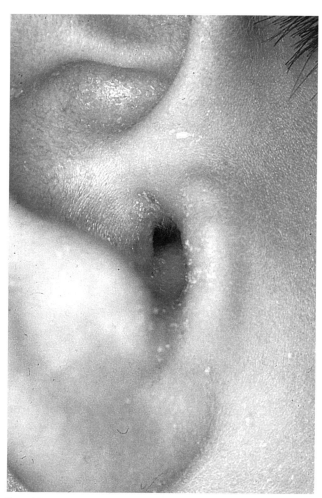

Figure 35–6. Mild acute diffuse otitis externa. A close-up view of Figure 35–5 revealing inflammation of the external auditory canal with circumferential yellow dried secretions.

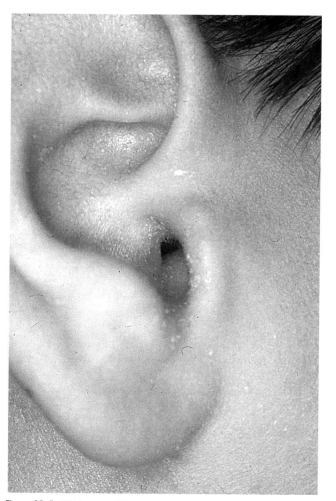

Figure 35–5. Mild acute diffuse otitis externa. A left ear demonstrating erythema and edema of the external auditory canal with yellow dried secretions around the meatus. A decrease in the size of the lumen is appreciated in the anterior inferior aspect of the canal wall.

always includes one of the previously mentioned inciting factors along with the symptoms of itching, tenderness, and pain.[18–20] This pain is exacerbated upon manipulation of the auricle and can even be present with chewing, i.e., movement of the temporomandibular joint. These common symptoms vary in intensity according to the severity of the disease. Other symptoms associated with acute otitis externa include hearing loss and a sensation of aural fullness and pressure.[21] These symptoms become more prominent as the external auditory canal lumen decreases in size. This decrease in the lumen's circumference allows for the accumulation of debris and secretions.[22] Common signs upon inspection and physical examination include an erythema and edema that can even include the tragus and concha.[23] Other observations are crusting and weeping secretions of the external auditory canal skin. On occasion, purulent otorrhea is appreciated. Palpation of the auricle and concha may yield intense pain. Two maneuvers that can be performed to elicit pain and tenderness are placing the examiner's index finger and thumb around the helix and pulling in a superoposterior direction and placing the examiner's index finger behind the ear lobule on the undersurface of the conchal bowl and applying pressure to the conchal bowl in a superior direction.

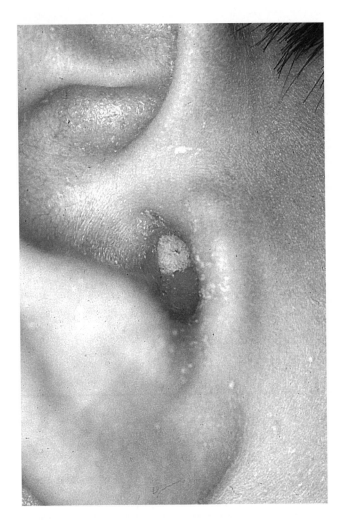

Figure 35–7. Mild acute diffuse otitis externa with placement of a Pope-otowick. Pope-otowick properly positioned in external auditory canal to facilitate the transport of medication.

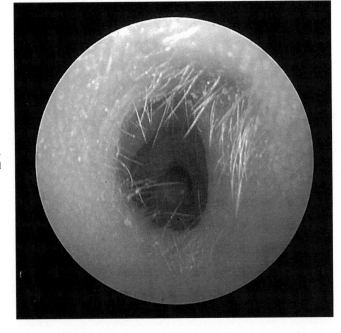

Figure 35–8. Mild acute diffuse otitis externa. This picture depicts the bony-cartilaginous junction. Erythema and edema of the bony canal are delineated from the less involved cartilaginous portion of the external auditory canal.

Figure 35–9. Mild acute diffuse otitis externa. A close-up view of Figure 35–8 reveals seropurulent secretions of the inferior aspect of the canal.

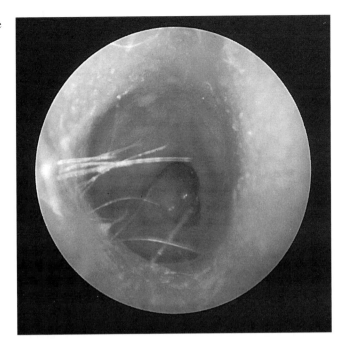

These two maneuvers are not well tolerated by patients with otitis externa. With advanced disease, fever and lymphadenopathy of the preauricular, postauricular, and anterior cervical regions can be appreciated.[24] With knowledge of the signs and symptoms, a good history, and otologic examination, the physician can make the diagnosis of acute otitis externa with confidence and begin empiric therapy.

Treatment

The treatment protocol for otitis externa employs basic fundamentals to resolve the infection and inflammation while promoting the restoration of the external auditory canal to its original healthy state. The first and most important step is a careful, thorough, and atraumatic cleaning of the external auditory canal with the aid of a microscope. Careful suctioning and débridement with the aid of picks and forceps under the microscope should allow for thorough cleansing of the ear canal. If the debris is thick, crusted, and difficult to remove, topical otic/ophthalmic drops or hydrogen peroxide can assist in débridement of the canal. The limiting factors in an adequate cleaning are patient tolerance and lumen size. The patient's already tender ear does not allow for much manipulation to facilitate cleaning; therefore, the patient must be informed that cooperation is needed to allow

Figure 35–10. Mild acute diffuse otitis externa. Treatment (see Figures 35–8 and 35–9) after the removal of the seropurulent secretions and the application of an antibiotic powder.

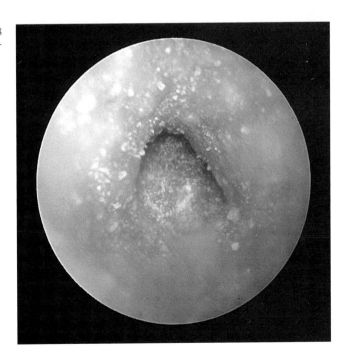

thorough cleaning. The size of the lumen decreases as the severity of the disease increases, hindering débridement of the canal. If the canal is near obliteration, cleaning by suctioning cannot be performed; a Pope-otowick or gauze strip can be placed in the external auditory canal. Care must be taken not to force the wick or strip too far into the canal, thus making its removal problematic or traumatizing the tympanic membrane. Once in place, the wick or strip is used as a conduit to facilitate the application of drops to the medial aspect of the external auditory canal. This wick can stay in place for 2–5 days with multiple daily application of drops to it. After removal of the wick, the canal is usually less obliterated, and cleaning can be performed. The frequency of cleaning varies according to the amounts of debris and secretions produced by the canal. If the production of secretions and debris is heavy, the ear should be cleaned every 1–2 days. Following the cleaning an acidic preparation (gentian violet, Merthiolate, or acetic acid) may be added in the office. However, if only a mild amount is being produced, then cleaning every 3–5 days is sufficient.

Adequate cleaning is necessary for the second step in the protocol: acidifying agents, topical antibiotic, and/or antifungal therapy. Table 35–2 lists the various topical agents. The preparations most commonly used for otitis externa are suspensions and solutions because of their ease of application. The pH range for the acidifying agents is 3.0–6.0, thus inhibiting the proliferation of the bacteria and fungi. The

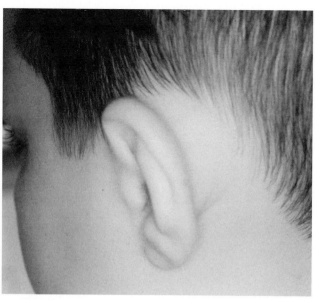

Figure 35–12. Moderate/severe acute diffuse otitis externa. A posterolateral view demonstrating erythema and edema of the postauricular region with lateralization of the ear.

major drawback to the use of the acidifying agents is patient noncompliance due to the burning and stinging upon application. Antibiotic preparations with and without steroids are available in both otic and ophthalmic solutions and suspensions. The otic preparations are more acidic than the ophthalmic preparations. Patients unable to tolerate the acidic otic drops may tolerate the more neutral ophthalmic drops. Ophthalmic drops also have a lower viscosity, allowing them to penetrate narrowed lumens with and without wicks to transport the medication.[21] Adverse effects of topical antibiotic preparations are antibiotic sensitivity and the possible overgrowth of resistant and opportunistic bacteria and fungi. Topical antifungal preparations range in pH from 4.5 to 8.0 and are usually well tolerated by the patient. The topical antibiotic and antifungal preparation can be used concomitantly if the disease is caused by both bacterial and fungal organisms. The dosage and duration of topical preparations should be three to four drops three to four times a day for 1–2 weeks.

Occasionally, oral antibiotics are indicated in the treatment of otitis externa. This is usually encountered in a severe case of otitis externa, caused most commonly by *P. aeruginosa* or *S. aureus*, which may cause a local cellulitis or lymphadenitis. Ten days of ciprofloxacin, at a usual dosage of 750 mg every 12 hours, or ofloxacin, at a usual dosage of 400 mg every 12 hours, or of an antistaphylococcal drug, such as dicloxacillin or cephalexin, at a usual dosage of 500 mg every 6 hours, can be used to treat severe cases of otitis externa.

The third component of the treatment of otitis externa is pain control. Pain is controlled systemically with nonsteroidal anti-inflammatory drugs (NSAIDs) or opioids and with steroid preparations applied topically. NSAIDs and opioid preparations are chosen according to the severity of the pain. Topical steroid-containing preparations decrease the inflammation and edema of the external auditory canal, resulting in less pain.

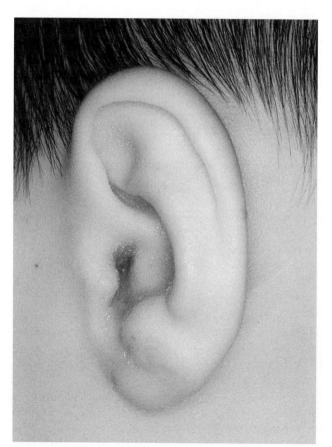

Figure 35–11. Moderate/severe acute diffuse otitis externa. Accumulation of exudative purulent discharge appreciated in an erythematous and edematous external auditory canal. Erythema is also noted in the postauricular region.

Table 35–2. TOPICAL MEDICATIONS FOR TREATMENT OF OTITIS EXTERNA[1]

Brand Name(s)	Antibiotic/Active Ingredients	Steroid	pH
Coly-Mycin S Otic Suspension	Neomycin sulfate 0.35%, colistin sulfate 0.3%, and thonzonium bromide 0.05%	Hydrocortisone 1%	5.0
Cortisporin Otic Solution	Neomycin sulfate 0.35% and polymyxin B sulfate 10,000 units	Hydrocortisone 1%	2.9–4
Cortisporin Otic Suspension			3.0–5.5
Pediotic Suspension			>4.1
Otobiotic Otic Solution	Polymyxin B sulfate 10,000 units	Hydrocortisone 0.5%	5.0–7.5
Pyocidin-Otic Solution			
Chloromycetin Otic Solution	Chloramphenicol 0.5%		4.0–8.0
Otic Domeboro Solution	Acetic acid 2%		4.5–6.0
VōSol Otic Solution	Acetic acid 2%		3.0
VōSol HC Otic Solution	Acetic acid 2%	Hydrocortisone 1%	3.0
Tridesilon Otic Solution	Acetic acid 2%	Desonide 0.05%	5.0–6.7
Gentian violet solution	Methylrosaniline chloride 1% and 2%		<6.1
Thimerosal solution	Merthiolate 1:1000		6.7
Castellani paint	Phenol 1.5%		2.8–3.7
Vasocidin Ophthalmic Solution	Sulfacetamide sodium 10%	Prednisolone acetate 0.25%	6.2–8.2
Metimyd Ophthalmic Suspension	Sulfacetamide sodium 10%	Prednisolone acetate 0.5%	5.0–6.0
Bleph-10 Ophthalmic Solution	Sulfacetamide sodium 10%		7.4
Gantrisin Ophthalmic Solution	Sulfisoxazole 4%		7.2–7.9
Tobradex Ophthalmic Suspension	Tobramycin 0.3%	Dexamethasone 0.1%	6.0–8.0
Tobrex Ophthalmic Solution	Tobramycin 0.3%		7.0–8.0
Garamycin Ophthalmic Solution	Gentamicin 0.3%		6.5–7.5
Chloromycetin Hydrocortisone[2]	Chloramphenicol 0.25%	Hydrocortisone 0.5%	7.1–7.5
Chloromycetin Ophthalmic Solution	Chloramphenicol 0.5%		7.0–7.5
Ciloxan Ophthalmic Solution	Ciprofloxacin hydrochloride 0.3%		3.5–5.5
Ocuflox Ophthalmic Solution	Ofloxacin 0.3%		6.0–6.8
Chibroxin Ophthalmic Solution	Norfloxacin 0.3%		5.2
Fungizone Lotion	Amphotericin B 3%		6.5–6.7
Nystatin Suspension	Nystatin 100,000 units/mL		—
Lotrisone Cream	Clotrimazole 1%	Betamethasone dipropionate 0.05%	5.0–7.0
Lotrimin	Clotrimazole 1%		
Solution			4.5–8.0
Lotion			—
Cream			5.0–7.0
Cresylate Solution	*m*-Cresyl acetate 25%		4.5
Decadron Solution		Dexamethasone 0.1%	7–8.5
Inflamase Forte Ophthalmic Solution		Prednisolone sodium acetate 1%	6.2–8.2
Pred Forte Ophthalmic Suspension		Prednisolone sodium acerate 1%	5.0–6.0
Elocon Lotion		Mometasone furoate 0.1%	4.5

[1]Not all of the drugs are approved by the U.S. Food and Drug Administration for otologic use. Caution should be used with the above preparations in the presence of tympanic membrane perforation.

[2]Discontinued by Parke-Davis in 1994.

Many cases of uncomplicated acute otitis externa may be managed with débridement and topical application of acidic and drying agents, such as 0.25% acetic acid, acetic acid and alcohol solutions, Merthiolate, and gentian violet. One may initially débride the external ear canal and paint the ear canal with Merthiolate or gentian violet and have the patient come back in 1–3 days, or one can débride the external ear canal, have the patient use acetic acid and alcohol solutions two times a day for 4–7 days, and then re-examine the patient.

ACUTE LOCALIZED OTITIS EXTERNA

Acute localized (circumscribed) otitis externa is also known as furunculosis. Acute localized otitis externa is a local infection of the outer superoposterior third of the external auditory canal. This infectious lesion can arise from single or multiple obstructed apopilosebaceous units. The pathogenesis is usually introduced by a traumatic incident to the apopilosebaceous unit that renders it dysfunctional. The pathogenic organism is usually *S. aureus*, although other

Staphylococcus and *Streptococcus* species have been cultured. The signs and symptoms of acute localized otitis externa include pain, itching, edema, erythema, decreased hearing if the edema occludes the canal, and pustules that may form an abscess. Diagnosis is by physical examination that yields evidence of a furuncle with pain and tenderness on auricular maneuvers. The presentation of the furuncle can vary, depending on the stage of the infection. The two different stages are composed of a superficial, pointing abscess, or a deep, diffuse, erythematous infection. Treatment of acute localized otitis externa depends on the stage of the infection. A deep diffuse infection is treated with local heat, oral opioid analgesics, and oral antibiotics. A superficial, pointing furuncle is treated by incision and drainage followed by topical and oral antibiotics along with oral analgesics.

CHRONIC OTITIS EXTERNA

Chronic otitis externa is a thickening of the external auditory canal skin caused by a persistent low-grade infection and inflammation. The signs and symptoms of chronic otitis externa include the most common symptom of itching along with mild discomfort, asteatosis (lack of cerumen), and dry hypertrophic skin lining the external auditory canal. This hypertrophic skin can vary in thickness, causing minimal stenosis to canal obliteration. The diagnosis of chronic otitis externa is by history and physical examination. The patient complains of an unrelenting pruritus with mild discomfort and flaking dry skin in the external auditory canal. Only upon manipulation of the external auditory canal and auricle is pain a complaint. Occasionally, a mucopurulent otorrhea is appreciated with excoriated skin predisposing the canal to an acute exacerbation (Fig. 35–13). The bacteriology of chronic otitis externa from culture reports varies from non-specific to normal flora of the external auditory canal. In chronic otitis externa, even normal flora can yield an unwarranted effect of dry hypertrophic skin in the external auditory canal. Frequently, patients have been on topical otic antibiotics and oral antibiotics for weeks to months prior to their referral to an otolaryngologist. Treatment of chronic otitis externa is to restore the external auditory canal skin to its original healthy state and to promote the reproduction of cerumen. This can be accomplished with otomicroscopic cleaning and débridement with application of an acidic and drying agent. This procedure may be performed weekly until the cerumen production returns. Application of topical antibiotic and steroid preparations after débridement must utilize a different topical regimen from that previously prescribed by the referring physician.

Rarely is surgical intervention deemed necessary to reverse the disease process if the preceding protocol is followed. The goal of surgery is to allow proper cleaning and observation of the external auditory canal and for more normal aeration (drying) to the ear canal. The surgical procedures performed for chronic otitis externa are to enlarge the width of the external auditory canal. Martin, Hirsch and Smelt[25] describe a conchal flap meatoplasty that was first performed by Hinds and Gray in the late 1950s. This technique enlarges the meatus by eliminating the sharp rim at the junction of the conchal bowl and the posterior canal wall cartilage along with thinning the skin and increasing the circumference of the external auditory canal. Paparella[26] describes a procedure that comprises removing all of the osseous and cartilaginous canal skin, widening the osseous canal with a bur, and enlarging the external opening to the meatus by excising a strip of skin and conchal cartilage and then applying a split-thickness skin graft.

ECZEMATOUS OTITIS EXTERNA

Eczematous otitis externa is a broad term comprising various dermatologic conditions that predispose the external auditory canal to otitis externa. This list includes atopic dermatitis, seborrheic dermatitis, contact dermatitis, psoriasis, lupus erythematosus, neurodermatitis, and infantile eczema. The signs and symptoms of eczematous otitis externa are intense itching, scaly skin, crusting, oozing, erythema, and fissuring of the external auditory canal. Occasionally, vesicles and hives can be present. The diagnosis is by history and physical examination. The history should include a thorough dermatologic history. Upon physical examination of the external auditory canal one can appreciate the eczematous changes that yield the name eczematous otitis externa. The treatment of eczematous otitis externa is the management of the underlying dermatologic disease. This can entail removing a particular contact substance from the patient's environment or applying a corticosteroid preparation to relieve itching along with the use of oral antipruritics and antihistamines to treat the underlying dermatologic manifestation. The application of a drying agent may also be beneficial, since many of these dermatologic manifestations involve moist fissured skin.

OTOMYCOSIS

Otomycosis, also known as fungal otitis externa, accounts for approximately 10% of cases of otitis externa in the United States. The percentage is even higher in tropical climates. Fungal infections have three basic requirements to proliferate: moisture, warmth, and darkness. Fungal otitis externa is divided into two groups, primary disease, in which the fungus is the main and only pathogen, and secondary fungal otitis externa, in which a fungal infection is superimposed on a bacterial infection. Fungal otitis externa has also been associated with necrotizing otitis externa, called invasive mycosis.

The symptoms of primary and secondary fungal otitis externa differ. The major complaint in primary fungal otitis externa is intense itching, whereas secondary fungal otitis externa manifests as pain and complementary pruritus. Frequently, patients have been on weeks to months of topical antibacterial medication. Most cases of otomycosis are found in chronic states of resistant otitis externa.

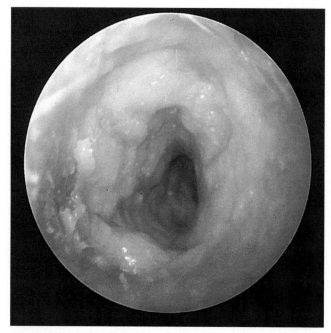

Figure 35–13. Chronic otitis externa. Accumulation of mucopurulent secretions and epithelial debris in the bony portion of the canal. Erythema and edema are noted along the canal walls.

The fungus most commonly associated with fungal otitis externa is the family of *Aspergillus* followed by candidal species.[27, 28] The three major species of *Aspergillus* are *Aspergillus niger* (black), *Aspergillus flavus* (yellow), and *Aspergillus fumigatus* (gray). Candidal species include *Candida albicans*, a white fungus, and *Candida parapsilosis*. Other fungi known to cause fungal otitis externa are *Phycomycetes, Rhizopus, Actinomyces,* and *Penicillium.*

Diagnosis of fungal otitis externa consists of history, physical examination, and cultures. Physical examination yields the diagnosis in the majority of the cases. The history may include a previous medical history of diabetes mellitus, an immunocompromised state, other known fungal infections, or a prior history of otitis externa with use of antibiotic and corticosteroid drops. Physical examination can reveal black, yellow, gray, or white fungal growth and debris in the external auditory canal, which is diagnostic for fungal otitis externa (Figs. 35–14 and 35–15). Cultures should be obtained to aid in differentiating primary from secondary infections.

Treatment of fungal infection includes removing the offending agent and altering the environment of the external auditory canal with acidifying agents and antifungal topical ear drops. Frequently, these infections are best managed with meticulous ear canal cleansing and painting of the ear canal with Merthiolate or gentian violet to promote acidification and drying. Gentian violet, in particular, not only has acidifying and drying properties but also possesses specific antibacterial and antifungal properties.

COMPLICATIONS OF OTITIS EXTERNA

Complications of otitis externa range from minor discomfort of the external auditory canal to severe life-threatening nec-

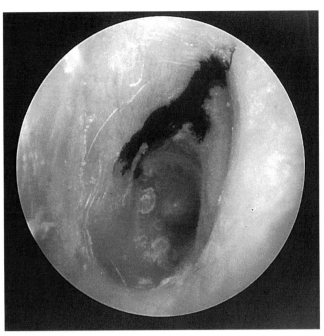

Figure 35–15. Fungal otitis externa. Figure 35–14 after application of gentian violet to aid in resolution of the fungal infection.

rotizing otitis externa. Otitis externa complications are due to (1) failure of patients to address the signs and symptoms of otitis externa and seek prompt medical attention, (2) rapid proliferation of pathogens as seen with diabetes mellitus and in immunocompromised patients, (3) attempts by patients to alleviate the itching and pain by applying over-the-counter medications, (4) patient manipulation of the external auditory canal with fingers and foreign objects, and (5) undertreatment by physicians by not seeing the patient on a frequent enough basis for proper follow-up care. Complications of otitis externa are ear canal stenosis, lateralization of the ear, tympanic membrane perforations, auricular cellulitis, chondritis, parotitis, and progression to necrotizing otitis externa.[2] Tympanic membrane perforations in otitis externa are of two etiologies: (1) chronic drainage has removed the protective pH barrier and provides a moist dark habitat promoting the growth of bacteria and fungi, and (2) mechanical manipulation of the ear by the patient, who places a foreign body or fingernail in the external auditory canal to alleviate itching, or by a physician, who places a wick too deeply into an obstructed external auditory canal. Auricular cellulitis and chondritis can be caused by edema. The edema inhibits the proper lymphatic drainage and venous flow, therefore promoting and complicating otitis externa. Parotitis from otitis externa is encountered when infection spreads through lymphatic channels at the anterior aspect of the auricle called the fissures of Santorini.[4]

OTOTOXICITY OF OTIC PREPARATIONS

The potential of ototoxicity from otic preparations, though extremely small, must be discussed. Ototoxicity from topical otic preparations has two routes of action, direct and indirect. The direct route implies a perforated tympanic membrane

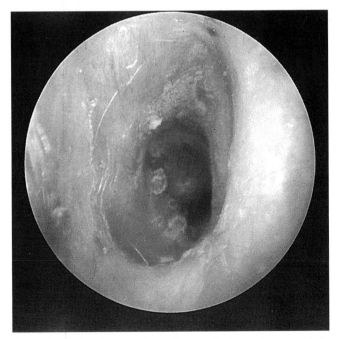

Figure 35–14. Fungal otitis externa. Saprophytic fungal infection of the inferior canal wall extending into the tympanic membrane. Thickening of the canal wall skin is appreciated.

that gives the preparation access to the middle ear. Within the middle ear space, the preparation comes in contact with the oval and round windows and is allowed to diffuse across the membranes to the cochlea. The indirect route is by systemic absorption of the topical otic preparation through the skin. This absorption is decreased in otitis externa owing to the inflammation of the skin. The ototoxic effects of medication include sensorineural hearing loss, tinnitus, and vertigo. The sensorineural hearing loss is noticed first in the higher frequencies and then progresses to the lower frequencies. This progression is due to the anatomic composition of the cochlea. The basal turn of the cochlea and the outer hair cells are affected first (i.e., higher-frequency sounds), progressing in an orderly fashion to the apical turn and the inner hair cells (i.e., the lower-frequency sounds). Ototoxic materials present in otic preparations include the vehicles, antibiotics, antifungals, acidic agents, and steroids. Materials proven to be ototoxic are propylene glycol, acetic acid, alcohol, benzalkonium chloride, iodochlorhydroxyquinolone, chlorhexidene acetate, povidone-iodine, *m*-cresyl acetate, chloramphenicol, colistin, gentamicin, neomycin, polymyxin B, and hydrocortisone.[29] Commonly used otologic and ophthalmic preparations that do not exhibit ototoxicity are nystatin, amphotericin B, clotrimazole, tolnaftate, sulfacetamide, ciprofloxacin, triamcinolone, and dexamethasone. Other agents currently used in otologic preparations have not been thoroughly tested.[30]

PREVENTION

Patient education is the key to the prevention of otitis externa. This education familiarizes the patient with the risk factors to aid in the prevention of otitis externa. Risk factors include a warm, humid climate; trauma from overzealous ear cleaning; scratching an itch with a foreign body or one's own fingernail; removal of excess cerumen; and retention of water from swimming, scuba diving, snorkeling, and bathing.[7] Patients who live in warm climates and have problems with water retention are prone to have frequent episodes of otitis externa and are instructed with precautionary measures. These measures are to instill 70% ethyl alcohol or acidic drops and to use a blow dryer on a low, warm setting to remove excess moisture on humid days and after water activities.[31] For water activities in ponds, lakes, and oceans, ear plugs are advised as long as they are placed and removed atraumatically. After removal of the plugs, excess water should be removed. Patients should be instructed not to place anything in the external auditory canal, including their own finger, because doing so can abrade and lacerate the canal. The patient should be cautioned about overzealous cleaning of the external auditory canal because of the removal of the protective pH barrier and the possibility of inducing trauma to the canal. This education and prevention are beneficial for the patient, who will not then have to endure the pain and discomfort of otitis externa. Prevention is also economically satisfying for the patient and the insurance carrier, because it involves fewer days lost from work, fewer physician appointments, and less money appropriated for medication. Prevention is truly the best treatment.

References

1. Friedman I, Arnold W: Pathology of the Ear. New York: Churchill-Livingstone, 1993.
2. Cassissi N, Cohn A, Davidson T, et al.: Diffuse otitis externa: Clinical and microbiologic findings in the course of a multicenter study on a new otic solution. Ann Otol Rhinol Laryngol 1977; 86(suppl 39): 1.
3. Johnson CM: Diagnosis and treatment of discharging ears. Br Med J 1966; 1: 1091–1093.
4. Lee KJ: Anatomy of the ear. In: Lee KJ (ed): Essential Otolaryngology, 5th ed. New York: Elsevier Science, 1991.
5. Main T, Lim D: The human external auditory canal secretory system—an ultrastructural study. Laryngoscope 1975; 86: 1164–1176.
6. Hyslop NE: Ear wax and host defense [editorial]. N Engl J Med 1971; 284: 1099–1100.
7. Petrakis NL, Doherty M, Lee RE, et al.: Demonstration and implications of lysozyme and immunoglobulins in human ear wax. Nature 1971; 229: 119–120.
8. Matsunaga E: The dimorphism in human normal cerumen. Hum Genet 1962; 25: 273–286.
9. American Medical Association: Drug Evaluations. Chicago: American Medical Association, 1993.
10. Youmans G, Paterson P, Sommers H: The Biologic and Clinical Basis of Infectious Diseases. Philadelphia: WB Saunders, 1975, pp 85–86.
11. Senturia BH: Etiology of external otitis. Laryngoscope 1945; 55: 227–293.
12. Singer DE, Freeman E, Hoffert ER, et al.: Otitis externa: Bacteriological and mycological studies. Ann Otol Rhinol Laryngol 1952; 61: 317–330.
13. Syverton JT, Hess WR, Krafchuk J, et al.: Otitis externa: Clinical observations and microbiological flora. Arch Otolaryngol 1946; 43: 213–225.
14. Saunders W: The microflora and the treatment of external otitis and otitis media. Postgrad Med 1959; 25: 176–179.
15. Reichard W: The microbiology of external otitis in Puerto Rico. Arch Otolaryngol 1962; 76: 19–29.
16. Chandler JR: Malignant external otitis: Further considerations. Ann Otol 1977; 86: 417–427.
17. Senturia BH: External otitis, acute diffuse: Evaluation of therapy. Ann Otol Rhinol Laryngol 1973; 82: 1–23.
18. Senturia BH, Marcus MD, Lucente FE: Disease of the External Ear, 2nd ed. New York: Grune & Stratton, 1980.
19. Hirsch BE: Infections of the external ear. Am J Otolaryngol 1992; 13: 145–155.
20. Hawke M, Wong J, Krajden S: Clinical and microbiological features of otitis externa. J Otolaryngol 1984; 13: 289–295.
21. Jahn A, Hawke M: Infections of the external ear. In: Cummings CW, Harker LA (eds): Otolaryngology–Head and Neck Surgery, 2nd ed. St Louis: CV Mosby, 1993.
22. Linstrom CJ, Lucente FE: External otitis. In: English GM (ed): Otolaryngology. Philadelphia: JB Lippincott, 1994.
23. Schuller DE, Schleuning AJ: DeWeese and Saunders' Otolaryngology—Head and Neck Surgery, 7th ed. St Louis: CV Mosby, 1988.
24. Ballenger JJ: Disease of the Nose, Throat, Ear, Head and Neck, 13th ed. Philadelphia: Lea & Febiger, 1985.
25. Martin-Hirsch DP, Smelt GJC: Conchal flap meatoplasty. J Laryngol Otol 1993; 107: 1029–1031.
26. Paparella MM: Surgical treatment of intractable external otitis. Laryngoscope 1966; 80: 1136–1147.
27. Lopez L, Evans R: Drug therapy of Aspergillus otitis externa. Otolaryngol Head Neck Surg 1980; 88: 649–651.
28. Fairbanks D: Otic topical agents. Otolaryngol Head Neck Surg 1980; 88: 327–331.
29. Rohn GN, Meyerhoff WL, Wright, CG: Ototoxicity of topical agents. Otolaryngol Clin North Am 1993; 26: 747–758.
30. Slattery W, Brownlee R: Otic preparations. In: Swarbrick J, Boylan J (eds): Encyclopedia of Pharmaceutical Technology, vol 11. New York: Marcel Dekker, 1995.
31. Lucente FE: External otitis. In: Gates GA (ed): Current Therapy in Otolaryngology–Head and Neck Surgery. Philadelphia: BC Decker, 1990.

32. Alfonso R. Gennaro (ed): Remington's Pharmaceutical Sciences, 18th ed. Easton, Pennsylvania: Mack Publishing, 1990.

33. Physician's Desk Reference, 49th ed. Montvale, New Jersey: Medical Economics Data Production, 1995.

34. McEvoy GK (ed): American Hospital Formulary Service Drug Information. Bethesda, Maryland: American Society of Health-System Pharmacists, 1995.

35. Pocket Guide to Antimicrobial Therapy in Otolaryngology–Head and Neck Surgery, 7th ed. Alexandria, VA: The American Academy of Otolaryngology–Head and Neck Surgery Foundation, 1993.

36. The United States Pharmacopeia, 22nd ed. Rockville, Maryland: USP Convention, 1990.

37. The Sanford Guide to Antimicrobial Therapy. Dallas: Antimicrobial Therapy, 1995.

38. Hoffman RA, Goldofsky E: Topical ophthalmologics in otology. Ear Nose Throat J 1970; 4: 201–220.

Jennifer Rubin Grandis
Victor L. Yu

CHAPTER THIRTY-SIX

Necrotizing (Malignant) External Otitis

▼

Necrotizing (malignant) external otitis can be a life-threatening infection of the external ear and base of skull that typically afflicts the elderly patient with diabetes mellitus. There are an increasing number of reports of necrotizing external otitis in patients with AIDS, suggesting that a generalized immune dysfunction may also predispose to this infection. *Pseudomonas aeruginosa* is almost universally the offending organism, although prior treatment with antipseudomonal antimicrobial agents may make its isolation difficult. Patients typically present with exquisite otalgia accompanied by otorrhea. Cranial neuropathies reflect disease that has progressed along the skull base. An elevated erythrocyte sedimentation rate (ESR) is the most characteristic laboratory abnormality. Diagnosis is made by isolation of the organism in the appropriate clinical setting. Computed tomography (CT) scanning and magnetic resonance imaging (MRI) may demonstrate bone erosion or subtemporal extension, thus aiding in diagnosis. Treatment consists of long-term administration (6–8 weeks) of systemic antipseudomonal antibiotics (e.g., ciprofloxacin 750 mg bid). Disease resolution may be confirmed by a repeat ESR in a patient who is symptom free. Repeat CT scan or MRI may be indicated in patients with persistent or worsening symptoms despite therapy. Moreover, it seems prudent to consider this diagnosis in any patient with AIDS who presents with painful otorrhea that is unresponsive to simple external otitis regimens.

ANATOMY

Necrotizing external otitis is an invasive infection of the external auditory canal and skull base. The external ear canal is a curved structure approximately 2.5 cm in length that extends from the external auditory meatus laterally to the tympanic membrane medially. The outer two thirds are composed of cartilage, whereas the inner one third is osseous. Necrotizing external otitis typically begins at the bony-cartilaginous junction of the external ear canal, which is pierced by small openings known as Santorini's fissures (Fig. 36–1). Spread of the infection typically follows a characteristic route from the external canal through these fissures into the mastoid bone and along the base of skull progressing from lateral to medial (Fig. 36–2).

The progressive skull base infection is often reflected by the pattern of cranial nerve palsies that characterize this disease. The facial nerve is typically the first (and often the only) cranial nerve involved as it exits the lateral skull base via the stylomastoid foramen. Children with necrotizing external otitis have a higher incidence of facial palsy, most

likely because of their relatively undeveloped mastoid process and to the more medial location of their bone-cartilage junction of the external auditory canal, both of which place the nerve in closer proximity to the canal.[1] Medially, the glossopharyngeal, vagal, and spinal accessory nerves are afflicted at the jugular foramen, and the hypoglossal nerve as it exits the hypoglossal canal. Less often, the trigeminal and abducens nerves may be affected at the petrous apex. There is a single case report of optic nerve involvement in a patient with necrotizing external otitis.[2] The olfactory, oculomotor, and trochlear nerves are not noted to be affected by this disease.

PATHOGENESIS

P. aeruginosa is the causative organism in more than 95% of cases. Although other organisms can be isolated concomitantly with *Pseudomonas*, they are generally inhabitants of normal skin, such as diphtheroids, *Staphylococcus aureus*, and *Staphylococcus epidermidis*. Isolated reports of other organisms causing necrotizing external otitis include cases of *Aspergillus fumigatus*,[3–7] *S. aureus*,[8] *Proteus mirabilis*,[9] and *Klebsiella oxytoca*.[10] Many of the hosts in these cases were immunocompromised.[3, 9] We have previously calculated that <1% of the reported cases in adults were *not* caused by *P. aeruginosa*.[11] Therefore, in cases in which organisms other than *Pseudomonas* are isolated, the diagnosis must be rigorously established by further objective criteria.

A gram-negative bacterium, *P. aeruginosa*, as a ubiquitous saprophyte, is widely distributed in soil, water, sewage, and plants.[12] It is also noted to be capable of proliferating in distilled water.[13] Despite its widespread presence in the environment, *P. aeruginosa* is not a component of normal skin flora in the external auditory canal.[14, 15] Moreover, when the canal flora of diabetics has been compared with the flora of nondiabetics, no difference is apparent.[16]

Pseudomonas contamination of water has been associated with the development of infections in the immunocompetent host. In one study, the *P. aeruginosa* isolated from the ear canals of patients with simple (noninvasive) external otitis was similar in phage type and serotype to the *Pseudomonas* isolated from the recreational water site in which the subjects had recently been swimming.[17] Other researchers have noted that the level of aural water exposure was directly correlated with the incidence of simple external otitis.[14]

EPIDEMIOLOGY

Necrotizing external otitis typically occurs in the elderly patient with diabetes mellitus. In fact, more than 90% of the

Figure 36-1. Necrotizing (malignant) external otitis occurs when infection crosses into the bony aspect of the external auditory canal and temporal bone. It enters the mastoid process and the base of the skull through Santorini's fissures. Facial nerve paresis is the most common cranial nerve abnormality seen.

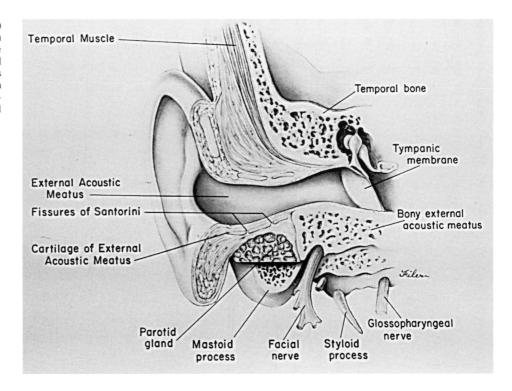

Temporal Muscle

Temporal bone

Tympanic membrane

External Acoustic Meatus

Fissures of Santorini

Bony external acoustic meatus

Cartilage of External Acoustic Meatus

Parotid gland

Mastoid process

Facial nerve

Styloid process

Glossopharyngeal nerve

adults with this disease are noted to display some form of glucose intolerance.[11] The mean age is generally more than 65 years; therefore, any viable pathogenetic theory must incorporate advanced age and diabetes with an increased predilection for *P. aeruginosa* infection. Aging and diabetes mellitus both contribute to abnormalities of small blood vessels.

Diabetic microangiopathy may explain the predilection of elderly diabetics to necrotizing external otitis.[11, 18] Histopathologic analysis of the capillaries of the skin and subcutaneous tissues overlying the temporal bone in diabetics has confirmed a thickening of periodic acid–Schiff–positive material in the subendothelial basement membrane. No direct relationship exists, however, between the level of glucose intolerance and susceptibility to or severity of infection. We and others have noted that patients with only glucose intolerance are as likely to develop this disease as individuals with insulin-dependent diabetes of long duration.[11]

Approximately two thirds of our patients with necrotizing external otitis had a history of aural irrigation with tap water (usually for a cerumen impaction) within a few days prior to the onset of symptoms. We undertook a case control study in diabetics with and without necrotizing external otitis who were matched for age, sex, and glucose intolerance. The only significant difference between the two populations was the higher incidence of aural irrigation in the diabetics with necrotizing external otitis.[19] Numerous reports worldwide have confirmed this association between aural irrigation and the onset of necrotizing external otitis.[18, 20–25]

Children with necrotizing external otitis most likely represent a different scenario. Fewer than 30 cases have been reported in the literature, making this a rare disease in the pediatric population. In contrast to affected adults, the majority of children with necrotizing otitis externa are not

diabetic, but they are immunocompromised on the basis of such conditions as leukemia, malnutrition, and solid tumors. Although they uniformly recover (no deaths have been reported), these children tend to be more toxic at onset than their adult counterparts, as manifested by fever, leukocytosis, and *P. aeruginosa* bacteremia.[11]

Patients infected with the human immunodeficiency virus (HIV) have a generalized immune dysfunction and are therefore prone to infections with common as well as uncommon microorganisms. Patients with AIDS appear to have some predilection for necrotizing external otitis. The handful of cases reported in the literature reveal a number of salient features in this population.[26–31] Five of the six cases have been in adults, with an isolated report in a child. The mean age of the adult patients was 35 years, and none was diabetic. The isolated microorganism was *P. aeruginosa* in three cases and *A. fumigatus* in two cases.

CLINICAL MANIFESTATIONS

The most common presenting complaints are otalgia and otorrhea. Although this disease may be difficult to distinguish from simple (noninvasive) external otitis, the pain in necrotizing external otitis is usually more severe and often disabling. The pain also tends to be nocturnal either awakening the patient from sleep or preventing the patient from sleeping. Headache and temporomandibular joint (TMJ) pain are often present and can also be extreme. Pain with chewing (TMJ-related) may be more severe than the reported otalgia and may lead to diminished oral intake and weight loss. Purulent aural drainage is usually present initially, although the amount of otorrhea is variable and tends to diminish as the disease becomes advanced.[11]

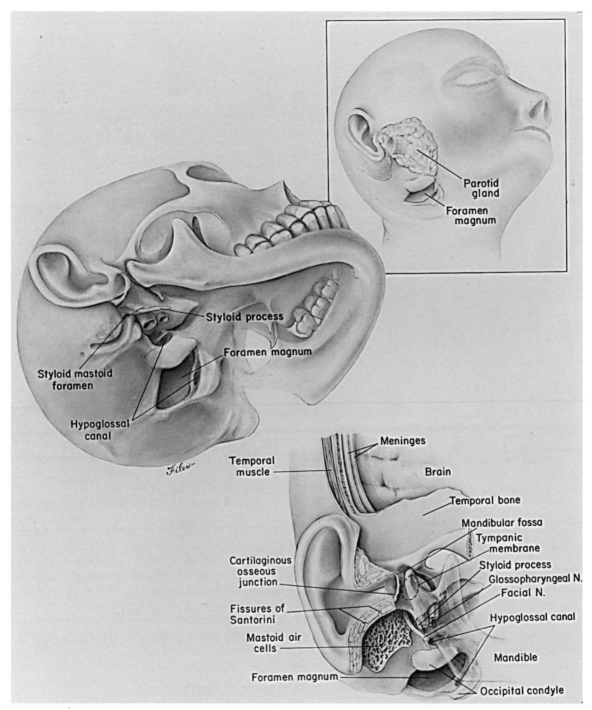

Figure 36–2. Anatomic sites of infection in malignant external otitis. The infection starts in the external ear canal, crosses the osseous-cartilaginous junction, and invades the temporal bone and adjoining structures. Cranial nerve involvement is directly related to its proximity to the path of infection. The cranial nerves affected, in order of frequency, are the facial nerve (VII) as it exits the stylomastoid foramen; the glossopharyngeal (IX), the vagus (X), and the spinal accessory nerves (XI) as they exit via the jugular foramen; and the hypoglossal nerve (XII) as it passes along the hypoglossal canal. Other sites of potential involvement include the temporomandibular joint, the meninges, sinuses, and parotid gland.

Granulation tissue at the bone-cartilage junction (Santorini's fissures) of the external auditory canal is the classic finding on physical examination. Often, patients present with an ulceration in this region or, more commonly, diffuse swelling of the soft tissues overlying the bony canal. If the patient has been previously treated (especially with antipseudomonal antibiotics) or a biopsy of the area has been performed, findings within the external auditory canal may be difficult to interpret. Cranial nerve palsies can characterize this disease but are more common in advanced cases. The pattern of cranial neuropathies is discussed previously (see "Anatomy"). The prognostic significance of cranial nerve defects has been debated.[32, 33] Because patients with multiple cranial nerve palsies have more advanced disease, the independent contribution of the neuronal dysfunction to morbidity and mortality is difficult to establish. Other central nervous system complications, including meningitis, brain abscess, and dural sinus thrombophlebitis, are rare but are fatal when they occur.[34]

DIFFERENTIAL DIAGNOSIS

The differential diagnosis includes other inflammatory conditions, such as simple external otitis and malignancy. Simple or noninvasive external otitis can usually be differentiated from necrotizing external otitis on the basis of clinical parameters (e.g., less severe otalgia in a nonclassic host). If one is still unable to rule out simple external otitis on the basis of symptoms and epidemiologic likelihood, an ESR determination may be helpful. The authors have found that the ESR, although nonspecific, is often extremely elevated (e.g., ESR >80 mm/hr) in necrotizing external otitis.[11] In contrast, patients with simple external otitis do not have an elevated ESR.

Squamous cell carcinoma of the temporal bone often manifests as a painful lesion of the external auditory canal. Because radiographic studies such as CT and MRI cannot differentiate between necrotizing external otitis and carcinoma, biopsy is the only definitive way to make this diagnosis. It should be noted that *P. aeruginosa* might rarely be a commensal within the external ear canal and that the ESR might be moderately elevated in a patient with malignancy. In these rare cases, the correct diagnosis requires the exclusion of a diagnosis of malignancy by negative results on histopathology and cytology and by an objective therapeutic response to antibacterial agents. Fortunately, the simultaneous occurrence of necrotizing external otitis and temporal bone cancer is extremely rare.[35, 36]

DIAGNOSIS

Laboratory

The majority of hematologic and laboratory parameters are unaffected in necrotizing external otitis with the exception of the ESR. For example, the white blood cell count and differential are usually normal. We have found the ESR to be valuable in both the diagnosis and follow-up of patients with this disease.[11] ESR also appears to reflect disease activity and may be the only objective piece of data to document recurrent or persistent disease.

Although there are a few reports of necrotizing external otitis in younger patients without diabetes mellitus[37, 38] we suggest that a glucose tolerance test be performed in all patients without previously documented diabetes who present with this infection.

Imaging

Most of the earlier radiographic studies have involved plain films and polytomography. However, the advent of newer imaging modalities such as CT has rendered obsolete the need for transmission radiography in the diagnosis of this disease.

Nuclear imaging studies such as bone and gallium scanning were applied to patients with this severe skull base infection in earlier studies. Bone scanning with technetium Tc 99m, in which the radionuclide tracer accumulates at sites of osteoblastic activity in response to bone destruction by the infection, is exquisitely sensitive in making the diagnosis of necrotizing external otitis.[39–44] The lack of specificity of bone scanning limits its utility, as noted in a study in which radiologists, blinded to the patient's diagnosis, were unable to differentiate simple (noninvasive) from necrotizing (invasive) external otitis.[45] It has been suggested that quantitative (rather than qualitative) bone scintigraphy may be a way of distinguishing necrotizing external otitis from its more benign counterpart.[46] Because increased osteoblastic activity can still be seen up to several years following successful recovery from necrotizing external otitis, bone scanning cannot be used to evaluate the efficacy of therapy or to assess possible recurrent disease.

Gallium (^{67}Ga) scanning citrate is more specific than bone scanning because the radioisotope is incorporated into granulocytes and bacteria, accumulating in areas of intense inflammation and infection. Again, earlier reports have noted that results of serial gallium scans in patients with necrotizing external otitis can demonstrate disease resolution.[39, 41, 44] Others, however, have reported patients with recurrent disease in whom gallium scans were normal.[47] As with bone scanning, gallium scanning is limited by the relatively imprecise anatomic localization of disease.

CT is currently the best imaging technique for defining the anatomic extent of disease in necrotizing external otitis.[48–51] It appears to be ideal for evaluating bone erosion and delineating fat and muscle planes in the subtemporal region. In a prospective study of serial CT scans in 11 patients, Rubin and colleagues[50] found that the presence of bone erosion (usually of the external auditory canal) and/or soft tissue disease in the area beneath the temporal bone was helpful in making the diagnosis of necrotizing external otitis. Although bone failed to remineralize with time (a limitation of this modality), soft tissue disease did coincide with clinical cure (Fig. 36–3). CT was particularly useful in documenting recurrent disease in that subset of patients who developed symptoms after receiving a full course of antipseudomonal therapy. We note that CT was unable to differentiate necrotizing external otitis from malignancy.

A single report suggested that MRI might be more sensitive than CT, because two of the four patients evaluated had evidence of contralateral skull base disease on MRI that was not apparent on CT.[47] In a long-term prospective study, we compared serial CT and MRI studies in seven patients with necrotizing external otitis.[51] Our study showed that MRI was slightly better at demonstrating medial skull base disease because of its ability to delineate changes in the fat content of marrow. Although it is possible that MRI was more sensitive in evaluating soft tissue changes, we found no case in which MRI was positive and CT negative. Thus, CT remains the initial radiographic imaging of choice, primarily because of the importance of evaluating the integrity of cortical bone in this disease. The role of MRI in the diagno-

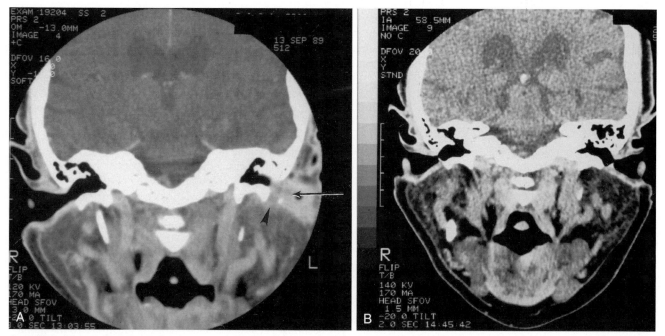

Figure 36–3. Necrotizing external otitis with early extension inferiorly. *A*, Coronal computed tomography (CT) scan shows an area of nonspecific attenuation *(arrow)* in the external auditory canal. Just at the bone-cartilaginous junction, there is a small area of soft-tissue attenuation *(arrowhead)* extending inferiorly below the limit of the canal (compare with the opposite side) that represents early extension through Santorini's fissures. *B*, CT scan obtained 1 year after initiation of therapy shows no evidence of abnormality in the soft tissues beneath the bone-cartilaginous junction.

sis and follow-up of patients with necrotizing external otitis remains to be clarified.

TREATMENT

It is often stated that meticulous control of serum glucose levels is beneficial in patients with necrotizing external otitis. Although this is a reasonable therapeutic approach in patients with diabetes and a serious infection, progression of the infection has never been correlated with the level of hyperglycemia.

Antimicrobial Agents

Systemic antipseudomonal antibiotics are the mainstay of therapy for patients with necrotizing external otitis. Prior to the availability of such agents, the mortality was approximately 50% and recurrences were frequent.[18] Since the advent of the semisynthetic penicillins, the mortality rate has dropped to approximately 20%.[37] Until the advent of the quinolone agents in 1990, the mainstay of therapy was prolonged (6–8 weeks) administration of intravenous antipseudomonal combination antibiotics (usually an antipseudomonal penicillin and an aminoglycoside). It should be noted that although this therapy was generally curative, the patient often required a prolonged hospitalization and not infrequently suffered serious side effects from the antimicrobials (e.g., hearing loss, vestibulopathy, and renal dysfunction from the aminoglycoside).

Third-generation cephalosporins have also been successfully used in patients with necrotizing external otitis, includ-

ing cefsulodin, moxalactam, and ceftazidime.[52–54] These agents appear to offer no higher success rate than traditional combination therapy, must still be administered intravenously, and may have other undesirable side effects (e.g., bleeding diathesis as a result of vitamin K deficiency with moxalactam).

The introduction of the quinolones has revolutionized the therapy of necrotizing external otitis. Not only has the cure rate increased from about 75% to more than 90%, but adverse effects are fewer. Ciprofloxacin (750 mg twice a day orally) is probably the antibiotic of choice,[55–60] although no comparative trials have been performed. Ciprofloxacin plus rifampin (600 mg twice a day) was used in one study, with the possible theoretical advantage of minimizing emergence of quinolone resistance.[61] Because this infection is essentially an osteomyelitis of the skull base, long-term therapy is required. We have elected to treat our patients with antimicrobial agents for a minimum of 6–8 weeks. Therapy for 8–12 weeks is appropriate if the disease has recurred.

The widespread availability of the fluoroquinolones, most likely combined with an increased awareness of this diagnosis on the part of the primary care physician and otolaryngologist, has changed the presentation of necrotizing external otitis. Patients now more commonly present relatively early in the course of the infection (e.g., prior to the development of cranial nerve palsies) and often after having been partially treated. It should be kept in mind when one is making the diagnosis under these circumstances that the ESR, radiographic findings, symptoms, physical findings, and the ability to recover the organism from the external canal may all be affected.

For patients with disease caused by *Aspergillus* species, amphotericin B is indicated. The encapsulated forms of amphotericin B are preferred, because nephrotoxicity is minimized, an advantage in these patients, who often have underlying nephropathy due to diabetes mellitus. We have used itraconazole as maintenance therapy for 4–8 weeks following 16 weeks of amphotericin B colloidal dispersion therapy.

Topical antibiotics probably have no role in the treatment of this deep-seated pseudomonal infection. Frequently, patients are given ear drops with antipseudomonal activity at the time of initial presentation, which only makes it more difficult to isolate the offending organism from external auditory canal cultures.

Surgery

Prior to the availability of antipseudomonal antibiotics in the late 1960s, necrotizing external otitis was a surgically treated disease with mortality rates approaching 50%.[18] Although there are still occasional reports of cases requiring extensive débridement for a skull base abscess,[62] the role of surgery in necrotizing external otitis should generally be limited to débridement and biopsy. There is currently no indication for routine mastoidectomy or facial nerve decompression, even in the presence of neuropathy.[11]

Hyperbaric Oxygen

There have been a few anecdotal reports on the use of the hyperbaric oxygen chamber in patients with necrotizing external otitis, with most series reporting mixed results.[63–66] The biologic rationale is unclear, although it has been suggested that aminoglycoside agents are more active in high-oxygen environments. We suggest that the role of this modality be restricted to those occasional cases in which standard therapy fails.

COMPLICATIONS

Complications of necrotizing external otitis are generally a result of the cranial nerve dysfunction that can characterize advanced disease. Exposure keratitis may result from facial nerve palsy if eye protection measures are not taken. Weakness of the cranial nerves around the jugular foramen (glossopharyngeal, vagus, and spinal accessory nerves) may lead to swallowing problems, aspiration, and vocal dysfunction). Other complications generally arise from the agents used for treatment but tend to be limited to mild gastrointestinal disturbances in the case of the oral quinolones. Recurrence rates as high as 27% have been reported, but it should be noted that this was prior to the availability of the quinolones.[11] Death, usually from a combination of unrelenting skull base infection and multiple cranial nerve palsies, is fortunately rare today; the exceptions are in HIV patients, who often have multifactorial causes of death.

PREVENTION

Epidemiologic data suggest that one possible way to prevent the development of necrotizing external otitis is to avoid aural irrigation with *Pseudomonas*-containing water in high-risk populations (e.g., the elderly patient with diabetes mellitus).[35] If the ears must be irrigated (e.g., for cerumen impaction) in these patients, one can use either sterile water or tap water that has been heated (and then cooled) to kill the organism.

References

1. Horn KL, Gherini S: Malignant external otitis of childhood. Am J Otol 1981; 2: 402–404.
2. Holder CD, Gurucharri M, Bartels LJ, Colman MF: Malignant external otitis with optic neuritis. Laryngoscope 1986; 96: 1021–1023.
3. Petrak RM, Pottage JC, Levin S: Invasive external otitis caused by *Aspergillus fumigatus* in an immunocompromised patient. J Infect Dis 1985; 151: 196.
4. Gordon G, Giddings NA: Invasive otitis externa due to *Aspergillus* species: case report and review. Clin Infect Dis 1994; 19: 866–870.
5. Cunningham MJ, Yu VL, Turner J, Curtin HD: Necrotizing otitis externa due to *Aspergillus* in an immunocompetent patient. Arch Otolaryngol Head Neck Surg 1988; 114: 554–556.
6. Phillips P, Bryce G, Shepherd J, Mintz D: Invasive external otitis caused by *Aspergillus*. Rev Infect Dis 1990; 12: 277–281.
7. Lyos AT, Malpica A, Estrada R, et al.: Invasive aspergillosis of the temporal bone: An unusual manifestation of acquired immunodeficiency syndrome. Am J Otolaryngol 1993; 14: 444–448.
8. Bayardelle P, Jolivet-Granger M, Larochelle D: Staphylococcal malignant external otitis. Can Med Assoc J 1982; 126: 155–156.
9. Coser PL, Stamm AEC, Lobo RC, Pinto JA: Malignant external otitis in infants. Laryngoscope 1980; 90: 312–315.
10. Garcia Rodriguez JA, Montes Martinez I, Gomez Gonzalez JL, et al.: A case of malignant external otitis involving *Klebsiella oxytoca*. Eur J Clin Microbiol Infect Dis 1992; 11: 75–77.
11. Rubin J, Yu VL: Malignant external otitis: Insights into pathogenesis, clinical manifestations, diagnosis, and therapy. Am J Med 1988; 85: 391–398.
12. Yoshpe Purer Y, Golderman S: Occurrence of *Staphylococcus aureus* and *Pseudomonas aeruginosa* in Israeli coastal waters. Appl Environ Microbiol 1987; 53: 1138–1141.
13. Favero MS, Carson LA, Bond WW, Petersen NJ: *Pseudomonas aeruginosa* growth in distilled water from hospitals. Science 1971; 173: 836–838.
14. Wright DN, Alexander JM: Effect of water on the bacterial flora of swimmers' ears. Arch Otolaryngol 1974; 99: 15–18.
15. Manni JJ, Kuylen K: Clinical and bacteriological studies in otitis externa in Dar es Salaam, Tanzania. Clin Otolaryngol 1984; 9: 351–354.
16. Salit IE, Miller B, Wigmore W, Smith JA: Bacterial flora of the external canal in diabetics and non-diabetics. Laryngoscope 1982; 92: 672–673.
17. Seyfried PL, Cook RJ: Otitis externa infections related to *Pseudomonas aeruginosa* levels in five Ontario lakes. Can J Public Health 1984; 75: 83–91.
18. Chandler JR: Malignant external otitis. Laryngoscope 1968; 78: 1257–1294.
19. Rubin J, Yu VL, Kamerer DB, Wagener M: Aural irrigation with water: A potential pathogenic mechanism for inducing malignant external otitis? Ann Otol Rhinol Laryngol 1990; 99: 117–119.
20. Dinapoli RP, Thomas JE: Neurologic aspects of malignant external otitis: Report of three cases. Mayo Clin Proc 1971; 46: 339–344.
21. Schwarz GA, Blumenkrantz MJ, Sundmaker WLH: Neurologic complications of malignant external otitis. Neurology 1971; 21: 1077–1084.
22. Wilson DF, Pulec JL, Linthicum PH: Malignant external otitis. Arch Otolaryngol 1971; 93: 419–422.
23. John AC, Hopkin NB: An unusual case of necrotizing otitis externa. J Laryngol Otol 1978; 92: 259–264.
24. Ford GR, Courtney-Harris RG: Another hazard of ears syringing: Malignant external otitis. J Laryngol Otol 1990; 104: 709–710.
25. Zikk D, Rapoport Y, Himelfarb MZ: Invasive external otitis after removal of impacted cerumen by irrigation [letter]. N Engl J Med 1991; 325: 969–970.
26. Scott GB, Buck BE, Letterman JG, et al.: Acquired immunodeficiency syndrome in infants. N Engl J Med 1984; 310: 76–81.

27. Reiss P, Hadderingh R, Schot LJ, Danner SA: Invasive external otitis caused by *Aspergillus fumigatus* in two patients with AIDS. AIDS 1991; 5: 605–606.

28. Rivas-Lacarte MP, Pumarola-Segura F: Malignant otitis externa and HIV antibodies: A case report. Ann Otorhinolaringol Ibero Am 1990; 17: 505–512.

29. McElroy EA, Marks GL: Fatal necrotizing externa in a patient with AIDS. Rev Infect Dis 1991; 13: 1246–1247.

30. Kielhofner M, Atmar RL, Hamill RJ, Musher DM: Life-threatening *Pseudomonas aeruginosa* infections in patients with human immunodeficiency virus infection. Clin Infect Dis 1992; 14: 403–411.

31. Weinroth SE, Schessel D, Tuazon CU: Malignant otitis externa in AIDS patients: Case report and review of the literature. Ear Nose Throat J 1994; 43: 772–778.

32. Chandler JR: Pathogenesis and treatment of facial paralysis due to malignant external otitis. Ann Otol 1972; 81: 648–658.

33. Chandler JR: Malignant external otitis: Further consideration. Ann Otol 1977; 86: 417–428.

34. Schwarz GA, Blumenkrantz MJ, Sundmaker WLH: Neurologic complications of malignant external otitis. Neurology 1971; 21: 1077–1084.

35. Grandis JR, Hirsch BE, Yu VL: Simultaneous presentation of malignant external otitis and temporal bone cancer. Arch Otolaryngol Head Neck Surg 1993; 119: 687–689.

36. Matucci KF, Setzen M, Galantich P: Necrotizing otitis externa occurring concurrently with epidermoid carcinoma. Laryngoscope 1986; 96: 264–266.

37. Soliman AE: A rare case of malignant external otitis externa in a non-diabetic patient. J Laryngol Otol 1978; 92: 811–812.

38. Shpitzer T, Levy R, Stern Y, et al.: Malignant external otitis in non-diabetic patients. Ann Otol Rhinol Laryngol 1993; 102: 870–872.

39. Ostfeld E, Aviel A, Pelet D: Malignant external otitis: The diagnostic value of bone scintigraphy. Laryngoscope 1981; 91: 960–964.

40. Reiter D, Bilaniuk LT, Zimmerman RA: Diagnostic imaging in malignant otitis externa. Otolaryngol Head Neck Surg 1982; 90: 606–609.

41. Parisier SC, Lucente FE, Hirschman SZ, et al.: Nuclear scanning in necrotizing progressive "malignant" external otitis. Laryngoscope 1982; 92: 1016–1020.

42. Mendelson DS, Som PM, Mendelson MH, Parisier SC: Malignant external otitis: The role of computed tomography and radionuclides in evaluation. Radiology 1983; 149: 745–749.

43. Strashun AM, Nejatheim M, Goldsmith SJ: Malignant external otitis early scintigraph detection. Radiology 1984; 150: 541–545.

44. Garty I, Rosen G, Holdstein Y: The radionuclide diagnosis, evaluation and follow-up of malignant otitis externa (MOE)—the value of immediate blood pool scanning. J Laryngol Otol 1985; 99: 109–115.

45. Levin WJ, Shary JH, Nichols LT, Lucente FE: Bone scanning in severe external otitis. Laryngoscope 1986; 96: 1193–1195.

46. Uri N, Gips S, Frant A, et al.: Quantitative bone and 67Ga scintigraphy in the differentiation of necrotizing external otitis from severe external otitis. Arch Otolaryngol Head Neck Surg 1991; 117: 623–626.

47. Cherini SG, Brackmann DE, Bradley WG: Magnetic resonance imaging and computerized tomography in malignant external otitis. Laryngoscope 1986; 96: 542–548.

48. Gold S, Som PM, Lawson W, et al.: Radiographic findings in progressive necrotizing "malignant" external otitis. Laryngoscope 1984; 94: 363–366.

49. Curtin HD, Wolf P, May M: Malignant external otitis: CT evaluation. Radiology 1982; 145: 383–388.

50. Rubin J, Curtin MD, Yu VL, Kamerer DB: Malignant external otitis: Utility of CT in diagnosis and follow-up. Radiology 1990; 174: 391–394.

51. Grandis JR, Curtin HD, Yu VL: Necrotizing (malignant) external otitis: A prospective comparison of CT and MRI in diagnosis and follow-up. Radiology 1995; 196: 499–504.

52. Haverkos HW, Caparosa R, Yu VL, Kamerer D: Moxolactam therapy—its use in chronic suppurative otitis media and malignant external otitis. Arch Otolaryngol 1982; 108: 329–333.

53. Mendelson MH, Meyers BR, Hirschman SZ, et al.: Treatment of invasive external otitis with cefsulodin. Rev Infect Dis 1984; 6: S698–S704.

54. Johnson MP, Ramphal R: Malignant external otitis: Report on therapy with ceftazidime and review of therapy and prognosis. Rev Infect Dis 1990; 12: 173–180.

55. Sade J, Lang R, Goshen S, Kitzes-Cohen R: Ciprofloxacin treatment of malignant external otitis. Am J Med 1989; 87(suppl 5A): 138S–141S.

56. Joachims HZ, Danino J, Raz R: Malignant external otitis: Treatment with fluoroquinolones. Am J Otolaryngol 1988; 9: 102–105.

57. Leggett JM, Predergast K: Malignant external otitis: The use of oral ciprofloxacin. J Laryngol Otol 1988; 102: 53–54.

58. Morrison GAJ, Bailey CM: Relapsing malignant otitis externa successfully treated with ciprofloxacin. J Laryngol Otol 1988; 102: 872–876.

59. Hickey SA, Ford GR, O'Connor AF, et al.: Treating malignant otitis with oral ciprofloxacin. Br J Med 1989; 299: 550–551.

60. Levenson MJ, Parisier SC, Dolitsky J, Bindra G: Ciprofloxacin: Drug of choice in the treatment of malignant external otitis (MEO). Laryngoscope 1991; 101: 821–824.

61. Rubin J, Stoehr G, Yu VL, et al.: Efficacy of oral ciprofloxacin plus rifampin for treatment of malignant external otitis. Arch Otolaryngol Head Neck Surg 1989; 115: 1063–1069.

62. Raines JM, Schindler RA: The surgical management of recalcitrant malignant external otitis. Laryngoscope 1980; 90: 606–609.

63. Mader JR, Love JT: Malignant external otitis—cure with adjunctive hyperbaric oxygen therapy. Arch Otolaryngol 1982; 108: 38–40.

64. Lucente FE, Parisier SC, Som PM, Arnold LM: Malignant external otitis: A dangerous misnomer? Otolaryngol Head Neck Surg 1982; 90: 266–269.

65. Lucente FE, Parisier SC, Som PM: Complications of the treatment of malignant external otitis. Laryngoscope 1983; 93: 279–281.

66. Davis JC, Gates GA, Lerner C, et al.: Adjuvant hyperbaric oxygen in malignant external otitis. Arch Otolaryngol Head Neck Surg 1992; 118: 89–93.

Jane L. Weissman

CHAPTER THIRTY-SEVEN

Imaging the Paranasal Sinuses

Computed tomography (CT) is the study of choice for most patients with paranasal sinus infections. Magnetic resonance imaging (MRI) is more useful than CT for evaluating neoplasms of the paranasal sinuses. Occasionally, MRI studies provide complementary information about infections. Considering price, radiation exposure, and diagnostic information provided, plain films and multidirectional tomograms are rarely indicated.[1]

PLAIN FILMS AND TOMOGRAMS

A Waters's radiographic view is a frontal projection with the petrous ridge at or below the floor of the maxillary sinuses (Fig. 37–1A). Waters's views provide a clear picture of the maxillary sinuses.[2] A Caldwell's view is a posteroanterior projection that places the petrous ridge at the level of the orbital floor. It shows the frontal and ethmoid sinuses well.[2] Lateral views are labeled "right" or "left" according to which side was closer to the film cassette. Structures closer to the film are magnified less and so are more sharply defined. The lateral view shows the nasopharynx as well as the paranasal sinuses.[2] The submentovertical (base) view shows the sphenoid and posterior ethmoid sinuses well.[2]

Ideally, plain films should be obtained with the patient upright,

so fluid levels are most conspicuous.[3] (Fig. 37–1B). With CT imaging readily available today, tomography is rarely indicated.

Partial or complete opacification of a paranasal sinus is readily apparent on plain films, though these films offer little information about the composition of material filling a sinus. Fluid can usually be differentiated from thickened mucosa or a soft tissue mass by the presence of a meniscus (Fig. 37–1B). However, a completely opacified sinus might contain obstructed secretions, edematous mucosa, one or more retention cysts, or a neoplasm.

Plain films delineate osseous detail well. Thickening (sclerosis) of a sinus wall and blurring or obliteration of the normal mucoperiosteal line suggests chronic inflammation. However, a neoplasm may also cause sclerosis.[2, 4] Frank bone destruction may be the result of a malignancy, an aggressive benign neoplasm, or an inflammatory process. Once osseous walls are breached, involvement of adjacent structures (orbit, anterior cranial fossa, infratemporal fossa) is not assessed well with plain films.

CT SCANNING TECHNIQUE

For axial CT images, the patient lies supine on a table that moves by increments through the scanner gantry (Fig. 37–

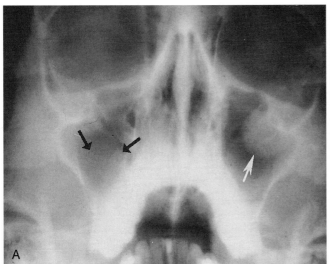
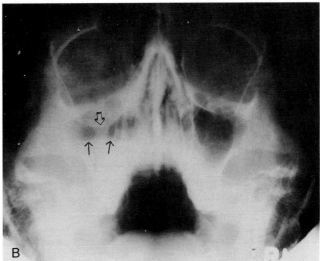

Figure 37–1. Plain films, Waters's views. *A*, The study shows a retention cyst *(white arrow)* in the left maxillary sinus and mucosal thickening *(black arrows)* in the right maxillary sinus. *B*, There is fluid *(solid arrows)* in the right maxillary sinus. In this case, the fluid is blood from an orbital floor blowout fracture *(open arrow)*.

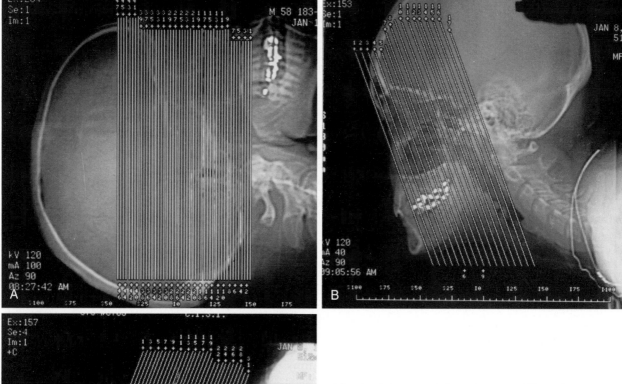

Figure 37–2. Scout views from computed tomography (CT) scans. *A,* On this supine scout view, the numbered lines correspond to locations of the axial images. *B,* For this scout view from a prone coronal CT study, the patient's chin rests on a cushion. The numbered lines are angled (compare to Fig. 37–2*A*) so the slices are as close to coronal as possible. *C,* For a supine coronal CT study, the patient's head is held in a specially designed cradle.

2*A*). For coronal images, the patient can lie prone (Fig. 37–2*B*) or supine (Fig. 37–2*C*) but must be able to hyperextend the neck. The scanner gantry is tilted to obtain coronal images.

Modern scanner software can obtain slices as thin as 1 mm. For paranasal sinuses, slices 3–5 mm thick are usually adequate. Slices can be contiguous (no interslice gap) or separated by 1–2 mm.

Modern scanners can obtain a single slice in 1 or 2 seconds. It may take 10 minutes or less to acquire the data for an entire coronal study. "Helical" scanners scan continuously as the table glides through the gantry; images can be reconstructed from this data in any plane.

An intravenous contrast agent is not necessary for CT scanning of most inflammatory diseases of the paranasal sinuses. However, contrast is useful to assess extension of infection beyond the sinuses into the orbits, infratemporal fossa, or brain and to delineate the relationship of an abscess to blood vessels. CT contrast agents are water-soluble iodinated media.

After a patient is scanned once, the data can be processed to generate images called algorithms. Algorithms are computer manipulations of the image data created through processes called convolution and backprojection that are beyond the province of this chapter. It is important to recognize that bone algorithms emphasize bone detail (Fig. 37–3*A*) and soft tissue algorithms delineate soft tissue detail (Fig. 37–3*B*). Similarly, there are lung algorithms, liver algo-

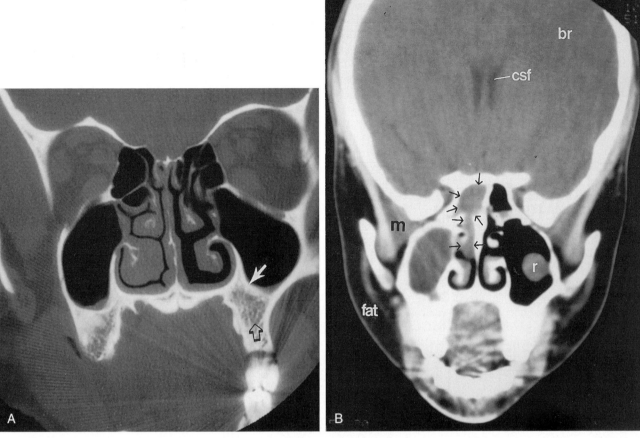

Figure 37–3. Algorithms. *A*, Coronal computed tomography (CT) scan (bone algorithm) of the paranasal sinuses shows detail of cortical *(white arrow)* and medullary *(open arrow)* bone. Soft tissues are indistinct shades of gray. *B*, Coronal CT scan (soft tissue algorithm) emphasizes differences between soft tissues: brain (br), cerebrospinal fluid (csf), fat (fat), muscle (m), and retention cyst (r). Bone is homogeneously dense; bone detail is minimal. There is a sphenochoanal polyp *(arrows)* on the right.

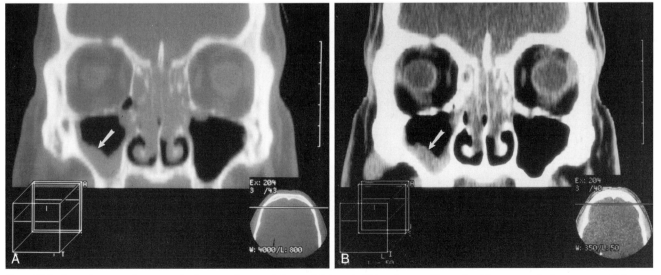

Figure 37–4. Coronal computed tomography images reformatted from axial data. *A*, This reformatted bone algorithm was made from many axial images like the one in the right lower corner. Close inspection reveals the jagged or step-like edges *(arrow)* characteristic of reformatted images. *B*, On this coronal reformatted soft tissue algorithm, the reformation artefact is less conspicuous *(arrow)*.

rithms, and so on. Bone algorithms demonstrate normal osseous anatomy (cortex, medullary cavity), bone destruction, and even subtle bone erosion. However, on bone algorithms, most soft tissues are a homogeneous dark gray color. Using the same data, the software can create soft tissue algorithms (Fig. 37–3*B*) that show subtle differences in densities of muscle, obstructed secretions, retention cysts, thickened mucosa, and neoplasm. Bone detail is minimal on soft tissue algorithms. All images from sinus CT studies should be viewed at bone and soft tissue algorithms.

If a patient is unable to hyperextend the neck for direct coronal images, the computer software can reformat axial images to generate coronal images (Fig. 37–4). These may not be as detailed and refined as direct coronal images, but often reformatted coronal images are quite adequate. Coronal reformatted images can also be viewed at bone and soft tissue settings (see Fig. 37–4).

Many radiology departments have developed a "mini-CT" scan of the sinuses (Fig. 37–5). This limited study is designed to look for sinus disease in patients who are not surgical candidates but who can be treated medically. For a "mini-CT" scan, limited thick axial or coronal images are obtained through the sinuses.[1] Slices can be 5–10 mm thick and up to 5 mm apart. The images are filmed at a level intermediate between bone and soft tissue.

A "mini-CT" scan provides greater anatomic information than plain films and irradiates the lens of the eye less than five or six plain films. An axial mini-CT scan is acquired more easily and quickly than coronal CT scans. In theory, a mini-CT scan should cost no more than the series of plain films of the sinuses it is designed to replace.

MRI TECHNIQUES

MRI studies are rarely indicated in the evaluation of infection confined to the paranasal sinuses. Occasionally, MRI studies add important information about orbital and intracranial involvement, although these features are seen well on CT scans. It is important to be aware of pitfalls in MRI of the sinuses.

Axial, coronal, and sagittal MR images can be acquired without repositioning the patient, who lies supine throughout the study, but the patient must lie quietly within the magnet for an hour or longer. The patient is not exposed to ionizing radiation. MRI studies are almost always more expensive than CT scans.

The MR images obtained depend on the clinical question to be answered. Axial T_1-weighted, T_2-weighted, and proton density sequences through the sinuses, orbits, and brain are often useful, as are coronal T_1-weighted images through the sinuses and orbits. Cortical bone is a signal void (black) on MRI studies, an important limitation in evaluating the paranasal sinuses.

After administration of intravenous contrast agent (various chelates of the element gadolinium), additional T_1-weighted sequences are obtained. If extension of infection into the orbits is a concern, fat-suppression techniques allow enhanc-

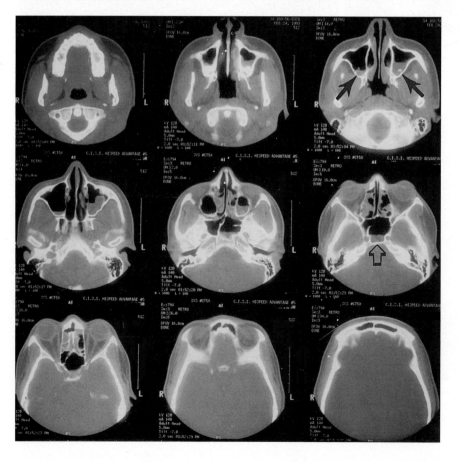

Figure 37–5. These nine axial images make up one complete mini–computed tomography scan. There is fluid in both maxillary antra (*solid arrows*) and the sphenoid (*open arrow*) sinus, and there is mucosal thickening of very viscous fluid in the ethmoid sinuses.

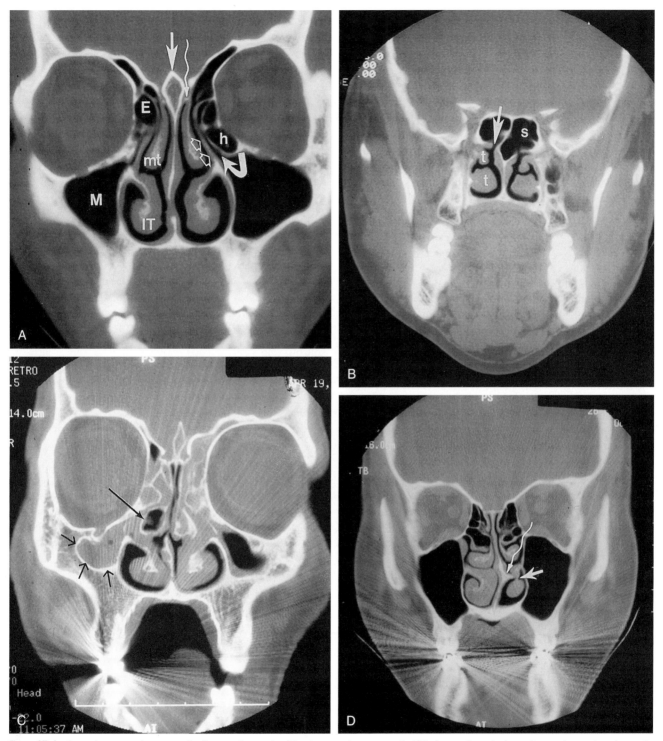

Figure 37–6. Coronal computed tomography images (bone algorithms): normal anatomy. *A,* This image through the ostiomeatal complex shows the maxillary sinus (M), infundibulum *(curved arrow),* uncinate process *(open arrows),* middle (mt) and inferior (IT) turbinates, ethmoid sinuses (E), crista galli *(straight arrow),* and cribriform plates *(wavy arrow).* A Haller's air cell (h) makes up the lateral wall of the left infundibulum. *B,* A more posterior image shows the sphenoid sinus (S), right sphenoid ostium *(arrow),* and turbinates (t). *C,* This image shows a hypoplastic right maxillary sinus *(small arrows).* There is a concha bullosa (aerated middle turbinate) on the right *(long arrow). D,* This image shows a large spur of the nasal septum *(wavy arrow).* The spur touches the left inferior turbinate *(straight arrow).* The turbinate mucosa on the right is more swollen than the mucosa on the left; this reflects the normal nasal cycle.

ing abscess (hyperintense or white) to be distinguished from normal orbital fat (which is also hyperintense).

NORMAL RADIOGRAPHIC ANATOMY

Coronal CT images of the paranasal sinuses are ideal for evaluating the osteomeatal complex (OMC).[5-7] The uncinate process, infundibulum, and middle meatus (Fig. 37–6A) are clearly delineated, often on the same slice. On a more anterior coronal slice, agger nasi air cells[7] are apparent. The posterior ethmoid air cells and sphenoid sinus are seen on more posterior slices (Fig. 37–6B). The fovea ethmoidalis and cribriform plates can be appreciated on axial images but are seen best on coronal images (see Fig. 37–6A and C). CT scans also detect normal variants such as a Haller air cell (an infraorbital ethmoid air cell)[5] (see Fig. 37–6A), concha bullosa (pneumatized middle turbinate) (Fig. 37–6C), and paradoxic turbinates. Accessory ostia of the maxillary sinus are small openings into the nasal cavity along the medial wall of the sinus.

The osseous and cartilaginous portions of the nasal septum can be evaluated on both axial and coronal images. Nasal septal deviation and nasal septal spurs (Fig. 37–6D) are seen well. A spur may contact an adjacent turbinate. The inferior and middle turbinates are usually seen well. Asymmetric swelling of turbinate mucosa on one side of the nose usually reflects the normal nasal cycle[8] (see Fig. 37–6D).

On MR images, the cortical bone is a signal void identical to air, and cartilage is nearly a signal void. Overlying mucosa enables turbinates, cartilaginous nasal septum, and sinus walls to be seen on MR images.

Axial MR images clearly delineate the anterior and posterior walls of the frontal sinuses and the anterior and posterolateral walls of the maxillary antra. The OMC is not optimally seen on axial MR images.

MUCOSA

Benign inflammatory disease of the paranasal sinuses is readily apparent on CT scans. Edematous mucosa has low to intermediate density on CT scans without intravenous contrast. Without contrast, viscous secretions adherent to the sinus wall may look identical to thickened mucosa.[9] After contrast administration, the thin mucosa enhances, but the underlying edematous submucosa (and viscous fluid) does not.

On MR images, edematous mucosa and submucosa are hyperintense (white) on T_2-weighted images (Fig. 37–7), and the mucosa enhances intensely after administration of gadolinium. Mucosal thickening is a common "incidental" observation on MRI studies of the brain obtained for reasons other than sinus disease (see Fig. 37–7).

Thickened mucosa may be linear or polypoid. Unless the underlying bone is sclerotic, it is not possible to determine whether the findings are acute or chronic.[6]

SECRETIONS

Thin fluid pools along the dependent wall of a sinus (Fig. 37–8A and B). In an acutely obstructed sinus, secretions are

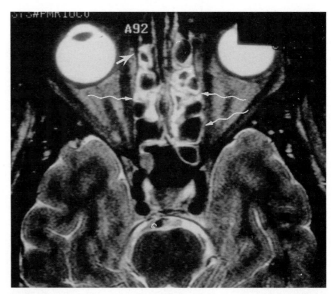

Figure 37–7. Axial T_2-weighted magnetic resonance image shows high-signal mucosal thickening *(wavy arrows)* throughout the ethmoid air cells. Bone is a thin, linear signal void *(straight arrow)*.

mostly water[6] and so are hypodense on CT scans. Bacterial sinusitis and viral sinusitis may have similar appearances on CT scans.[9]

Hyperdense sinus contents may be blood, calcified fungal hyphae, or desiccated secretions (Fig. 37–8C). It may not be possible to differentiate these possibilities.

On T_1-weighted MR images, watery obstructed secretions are hyperintense on T_2-weighted images (see Fig. 37–8B) and hypointense (dark) on T_1-weighted images (Fig. 37–8D). After administration of gadolinium, T_1-weighted images can distinguish normally enhancing mucosa from retained secretions (which do not enhance) (see Fig. 37–8D). However, in a chronically obstructed sinus, the mucosa resorbs water.[6] Goblet cells, which make mucous glycoproteins, proliferate.[6] The obstructed secretions become less watery, more proteinaceous, and increasingly hyperintense on T_1-weighted images.[10] High concentrations of glycoproteins seem to be responsible for the hyperintensity.[11] Methemoglobin (a metabolite of blood seen after hemorrhage) is also hyperintense on T_1-weighted images.

Very desiccated secretions become so proteinaceous that they lack enough mobile hydrogen protons to generate a signal. These inspissated secretions yield a signal void on all MRI sequences.[10] This signal void cannot be distinguished from the signal void of air in a sinus lumen on MRI[6] (Fig. 37–8D and E). It is important to be aware of this limitation on MRI. In this setting, CT scans may provide important complementary information.

FUNGUS AND GRANULOMATOUS DISEASE

Fungus colonization and infection usually occur in completely opacified sinuses.[3] An air-fluid level suggests bacterial infection.[3, 6] Fungal infections may cause both bone erosion and reactive thickening (sclerosis).[6]

Calcification in a sinus lumen is very suggestive of a

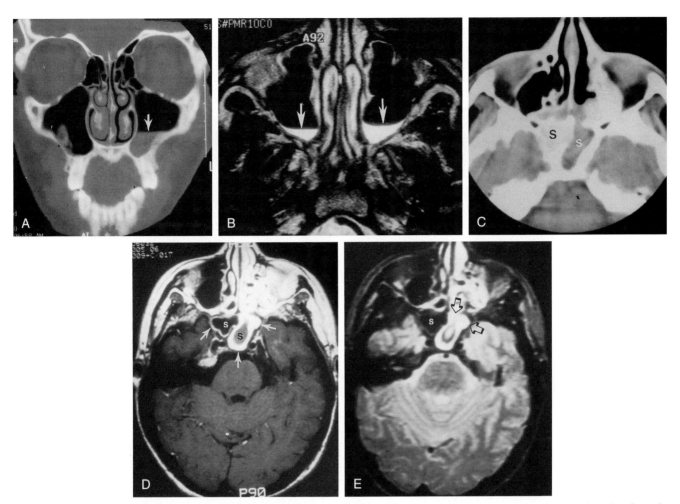

Figure 37–8. Secretions. *A,* Prone coronal computed tomography (CT) image (bone algorithm) shows fluid *(arrow)* pooling along the dependent floor of the left maxillary sinus. *B,* Supine axial T_2-weighted magnetic resonance image (MRI) shows high-signal fluid pooling along the dependent posterior walls of both maxillary sinuses *(arrows). C,* Axial CT image (tissue algorithm) shows low-density material filling the left sphenoid air cell (white S) and high-density material (black S) in right sphenoid air cell. *D,* Axial gadolinium-enhanced T_1-weighted MRI of the same patient as Figure 37–8C shows enhancing mucosa lining both sphenoid air cells *(arrows).* The left side also contains intermediate-signal material, presumably secretions more proteinaceous than cerebrospinal fluid (black S). The signal void in the right air cell lumen (white S) looks like air. However, this image was obtained immediately after the CT scan (Fig. 37–8C); this air cell is not clear. At surgery, the contents were very desiccated material. *E,* Axial T_2-weighted MRI at the same level as Figure 37–8D shows the misleading signal void in the right sphenoid lumen (S). The left sphenoid is lined by edematous mucosa *(arrows),* and its contents have a mixed signal on this pulse sequence.

mycetoma.[3] Both the fungus (mycetoma) and the desiccated secretions may be quite dense on CT images. Calcified fungus and fungal colonization can yield a signal void or near-void, which may be confused with an aerated sinus (see Fig. 37–8D and E). Iron, manganese, and magnesium in the fungi create the signal void.[10]

Granulomatous diseases such as tuberculosis, rhinoscleroma, actinomycosis, and nocardiosis have no diagnostic characteristics on CT or MRI studies.[3, 6] Thickening of the mucosa throughout the paranasal sinuses and soft tissue in the nasal cavity is frequently seen but is not specific.[6]

RETENTION CYSTS AND POLYPS

Retention cysts and polyps may vary in density from low (Fig. 37–9A) to high (Fig. 37–9B) on CT scans, and from hypointense to hyperintense on MRI studies (Fig. 37–9C

and *D).* A long-standing, desiccated retention cyst or polyp tends to be hypointense on T_2-weighted images. Overlying mucosa enhances (see Fig. 37–9A and D), but polyps and retention cysts enhance little if at all.

Polyposis of the nasal cavity and paranasal sinuses has a characteristic appearance on CT scans (see Fig. 37–9B). In addition to opacification of all or most of the sinuses, soft tissue fills the nasal cavity. The polyps may have a flowing or swirling appearance (see Fig. 37–9B). Often the bones are intact, though aggressive polyposis may remodel or erode bone and may extend intracranially (Fig. 37–9E). Intracranial extension can be appreciated on coronal CT scans with contrast (see Fig. 37–9E) but is evaluated in greatest detail with contrast-enhanced MRI studies that assess dura and brain.

Coronal CT scans clearly delineate the origin and extent of an antronasal or antrochoanal polyp (Fig. 37–9F and G). Because it is important to identify the sinus of origin of a polyp before surgical resection, CT studies are useful to

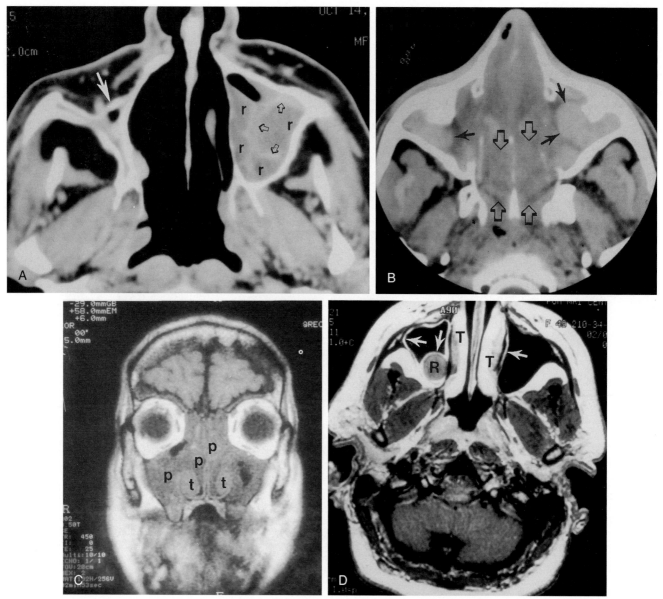

Figure 37–9. Retention cysts and polyps. *A*, Axial computed tomography (CT) image (tissue algorithm) with contrast agent shows several low-density retention cysts (r) in the left maxillary sinus. The overlying mucosa enhances *(open arrows)*. The contracted lumen and defect in the anterior wall of the right maxillary sinus *(white arrow)* reflect a prior Caldwell-Luc procedure. The right middle turbinate was also removed. *B*, Axial CT image (tissue algorithm) without contrast agent of a patient with polyposis. Both maxillary sinuses and both sides of the nasal cavity are completely filled with inhomogeneous soft tissue. The foci of high density *(solid arrows)* and flowing appearance *(open arrows)* are characteristic of polyposis. *C*, Coronal T$_1$-weighted magnetic resonance image (MRI) shows inhomogeneous soft tissue filling the nasal cavities and maxillary sinuses (p). Inferior turbinates (t). *D*, Axial T$_1$-weighted MRI with gadolinium shows an intermediate-signal retention cyst (R) in the right maxillary sinus. The smooth sinus mucosa enhances intensely *(arrows)* as does the turbinate mucosa (T).

identify the rare ethmochoanal or sphenochoanal[12] polyp (see Fig. 37–3*B*).

MUCOCELE AND PYOCELE

On CT scans, a mucocele is an expanded, opacified sinus or air cell (Fig. 37–10*A*). The contents may range from low density (approximately isodense to fluid such as cerebrospinal fluid) to the high density of inspissated contents. A mucocele may be quite hyperintense on an unenhanced T$_1$-weighted MRI study. CT images show displacement of adjacent normal structures by a mucocele (see Fig. 37–10*A*).

A pyomucocele is an infected mucocele (Fig. 37–10*B*). Intravenous contrast makes inflamed mucosa more conspicuous on a CT study. There is also infiltration (edema) of the surrounding soft tissues (muscles and fat) (see Fig. 37–10*B*). Small discontinuities in the osseous walls of a mucocele or pyomucocele are best seen on CT images.

ORBITAL CELLULITIS

Ethmoid infections may infiltrate through the lamina papyracea to involve the orbit.[13] Clinically, it may be difficult to

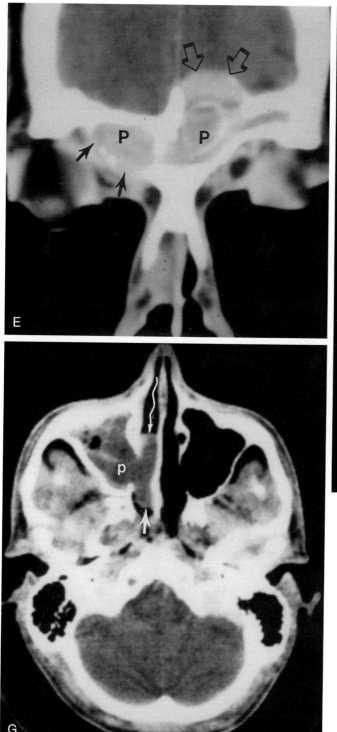

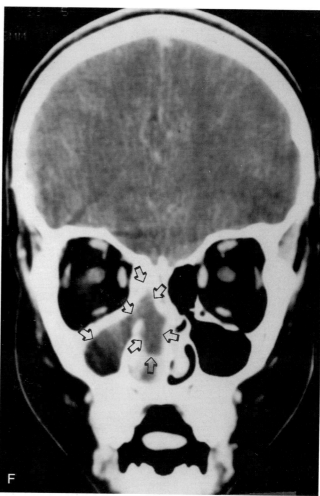

Figure 37–9 *Continued E*, Coronal CT image (tissue algorithm) shows aggressive polyposis (P) extending through the roof of the frontal sinus intracranially *(open arrows)* and through the sinus floor *(solid arrows). F*, Coronal CT image (tissue algorithm) of an antrochoanal polyp extending from the right maxillary sinus, through the infundibulum, into the right nasal cavity *(arrows). G*, Axial CT image of another patient shows an antrochoanal polyp extending from the right maxillary sinus (p) into the nasal cavity *(wavy arrow)* and back through the posterior choana into the nasopharynx *(straight arrow).*

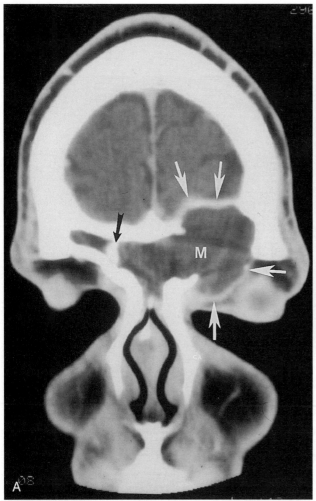

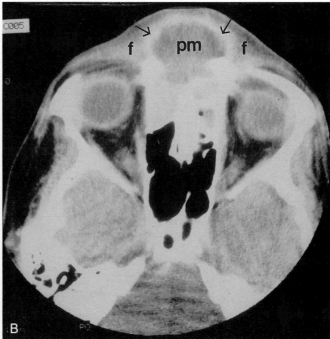

Figure 37–10. Mucoceles. *A*, Coronal computed tomography (CT) image with contrast agent (tissue algorithm) shows an expansile, low-density mucocele (M) enlarging the left frontal sinus. The intersinus septum is displaced to the right *(black arrow)*. The walls of the sinus are so thin in places that only the enhancing mucosa can be seen *(white arrows)*. *B*, Axial CT image with contrast agent (tissue algorithm) of a pyomucocele. The pyomucocele (pm) is more dense than the mucocele in Figure 37–10*A*, and the rim is thick and enhances *(arrows)*. The surrounding fat is edematous (f).

distinguish between orbital cellulitis and an orbital abscess. CT scans make this distinction easy (Fig. 37–11). This is one setting in which an intravenous contrast agent may be quite useful. The rim of the abscess usually enhances, whereas pus does not. Extension back through the orbital apex to cavernous sinus is also seen best after intravenous administration of contrast.

POSTOPERATIVE IMAGING

After functional endoscopic sinus surgery (FESS), patients may be referred for CT imaging to evaluate their persistent or recurrent complaints of sinusitis. The appearance of the paranasal sinuses after FESS is characteristic: uncinectomy, infundibulotomy, internal ethmoidectomy, and resection of

Figure 37–11. Axial computed tomography image with contrast agent (tissue algorithm) of a patient with left ethmoiditis (e) and a left orbital abscess *(arrows)*. The abscess has a thick rim and low-density contents. The appearance suggests pus in an abscess rather than orbital cellulitis.

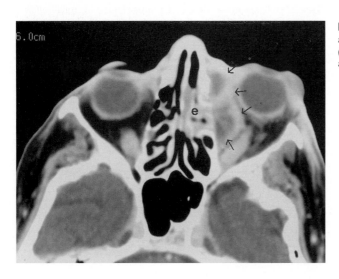

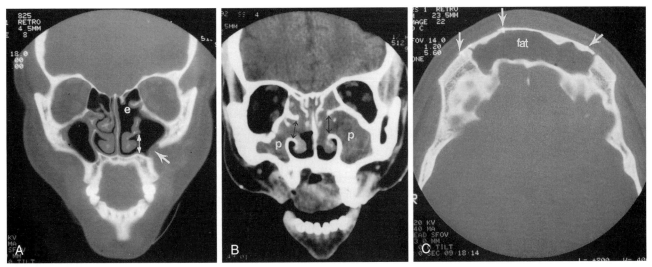

Figure 37–12. *A*, Coronal computed tomography (CT) image (bone algorithm) of a patient who had a left maxillary Caldwell-Luc procedure *(large arrow)*, nasoantral window *(double-headed arrow)*, ethmoidectomy (e), and resection of the left middle turbinate and uncinate process. *B*, Coronal CT image (tissue algorithm) of a patient with recurrent polyposis (p) despite prior bilateral endoscopic sinus surgery. The polyps occlude the surgical ostia *(double-headed arrows)*. *C*, Axial CT image (bone algorithm) of a patient who had an osteoplastic frontal sinus flap. The lumen was packed with fat (fat). The anterior wall of the sinus was removed, then replaced and plated with small screws *(arrows)*.

the middle turbinate are all readily apparent (Fig. 37–12*A*), as is a prior Caldwell-Luc procedure (Figs. 37–9*A* and 37–12*A*). Recurrent mucosal thickening, retention cysts, and obstructed secretions can also be seen (Fig. 37–12*B*). The surgical ostia may be obstructed or clear (see Fig. 37–12*B*).

Coronal CT scans show nasoantral windows well (see Fig. 37–12*A*). Other sinus procedures, such as external ethmoidectomy and frontal sinus osteoplastic flap (Fig. 37–12*C*)

may be incidental observations on patients studied for other reasons. It is useful to recognize these findings on CT scans.

INFLAMMATION VERSUS TUMOR

Delineation of the extent of tumor includes determining what is not tumor. On CT scans, it may be difficult to separate

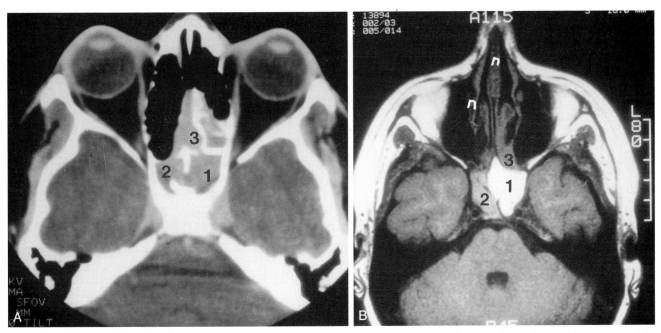

Figure 37–13. *A*, Axial computed tomography image with contrast agent (tissue algorithm) of a patient with an esthesioneuroblastoma. The contents of the left sphenoid sinus (1), right sphenoid sinus (2), and nasal cavity (3) have the same density. Tumor cannot be distinguished from obstructed secretions. *B*, Axial T_1-weighted magnetic resonance image of the same patient shows that the left sphenoid contents are hyperintense, indicating chronically obstructed secretions (1). The right sphenoid contents are not as hyperintense but are brighter than cerebrospinal fluid (2). The tissue in the nasal cavity (3) is hypointense to both of these. The tumor was confined to the nasal cavity but had obstructed both sides of the sphenoid sinus.

tumor in the paranasal sinuses or nasal cavity from obstructed secretions in a sinus lumen (Fig. 37–13*A*). MR images, with their greater inherent tissue contrast and multiple pulse sequences, can usually facilitate this distinction (Fig. 37–13*B*).

As described previously, the signal intensity of obstructed secretions depends on the composition of the secretions. Watery secretions are hypointense on T_1-weighted images and hyperintense on T_2-weighted images. Unlike tumors, secretions do not enhance after administration of gadolinium (see Fig. 37–13*B*). The contents of a chronically obstructed sinus may be more desiccated and proteinaceous. These secretions are hyperintense on T_1-weighted and T_2-weighted studies (see Fig. 37–13*B*).

References

1. Mafee MF: Modern imaging of paranasal sinuses and the role of limited sinus computerized tomography; considerations of time, cost, and radiation. Ear Nose Throat J 1994; 73: 532–546.
2. Dodd GD, Jing B-S: Radiology of the Nose, Paranasal Sinuses, and Nasopharynx. Baltimore: Williams & Wilkins, 1977.
3. Som PM: Sinonasal Cavity. In: Bergeron RT, Som PM (eds): Head and Neck Imaging, 2nd ed. St Louis: Mosby–Year Book, 1991, pp 51–276.
4. Silver AJ, Baredes S, Bello JA, et al.: The opacified maxillary sinus: CT findings in chronic sinusitis and malignant tumors. Radiology 1987; 163: 205–210.
5. Mafee MF, Chow JM, Meyers R: Functional endoscopic sinus surgery: Anatomy, CT screening, indications, and complications. AJR Am J Roentgenol 1993; 160: 735–744.
6. Som PM, Curtin HD: Chronic inflammatory sinonasal diseases including fungal infections: The role of imaging. Radiol Clin North Am 1993; 31: 33–44.
7. Mafee MF: Preoperative imaging anatomy of nasal-ethmoid complex for functional endoscopic sinus surgery. Radiol Clin North Am 1993; 1: 1–20.
8. Zinreich SJ, Kennedy DW, Kumar AJ, et al.: MR imaging of normal nasal cycle. Comparison with sinus pathology. J Comput Assist Tomogr 1988; 12: 1014–1019.
9. Gwaltney JM, Phillips CD, Miller RD, Riker DK: Computed tomographic study of the common cold. N Engl J Med 1994; 330: 25–30.
10. Som PM, Dillon WP, Curtin HD, et al.: Hypointense paranasal sinus foci: Differential diagnosis with MR imaging and relation to CT findings. Radiology 1990; 176: 777–781.
11. Som PM, Dillon WP, Sze G, et al.: Benign and malignant sinonasal lesions with intracranial extension: Differentiation with MR imaging. Radiology 1989; 172: 763–766.
12. Weissman JL, Tabor ET, Curtin HD: Sphenochoanal polyps. Radiology 1991; 178: 145–148.
13. Samad I, Riding K: Orbital complications of ethmoiditis: B.C. Children's Hospital experience, 1982–1989. J Otolaryngol 1991; 20: 400–403.

CHAPTER THIRTY-EIGHT

Management of Acute Bacterial Sinusitis in Children

▼

When considering a diagnosis of sinusitis in a child or an adult, the major problem is to distinguish between simple upper respiratory tract infection (URI) or allergic inflammation and secondary bacterial infection of the paranasal sinuses. The former categories of URI and allergy may prompt consideration of symptomatic treatment, whereas patients with sinusitis benefit from specific antimicrobial therapy. Both URI and allergic inflammation are recognized risk factors for acute sinusitis, with URI the most common.[1]

ANATOMY

A brief review of the anatomy and physiology of the paranasal sinuses will help clarify certain clinical features of sinus infection. Figure 38–1 shows a coronal and a sagittal view demonstrating the relationship between the nose and the paranasal sinuses. The nose is divided in the midline by the nasal septum. From the lateral wall of the nose are projected three shelflike structures designated according to their anatomic position as inferior, middle, and (seen best on the sagittal view) superior turbinate. Beneath both the middle and superior turbinates is a meatus that drains two or more of the paranasal sinuses. The maxillary, anterior ethmoids, and frontal sinuses drain to the middle meatus, and the posterior ethmoids and sphenoid sinuses drain to the superior meatus. Only the lacrimal duct drains to the inferior meatus.

The maxillary and ethmoid sinuses form during the third to fourth gestational month and, accordingly, although very small, are present at birth. Initially the maxillary sinus is a slitlike cavity running parallel to the middle turbinate. It gradually enlarges and forms a quadrilateral shape with a volume of approximately 15 mL. It is important to note the position of the outflow tract of the maxillary sinus, which sits high on the medial wall of the sinus cavity. This awkward positioning impedes gravitational drainage and probably predisposes to frequent infections of the maxillary sinus as a complication of viral upper respiratory infections.

The ethmoid sinus is composed of multiple air cells (3–15 on each side) separated by thin bony partitions. Each air cell drains by an independent ostium (measuring 1–2 mm) into the middle meatus. The small size of the air cells and the narrow caliber of these draining ostia predispose to retention of secretions if there is even modest inflammation of the mucosal lining as is the case in viral respiratory infection or allergy.

The frontal sinus develops from an anterior ethmoid cell and moves to a position above the orbital ridge by the 5th

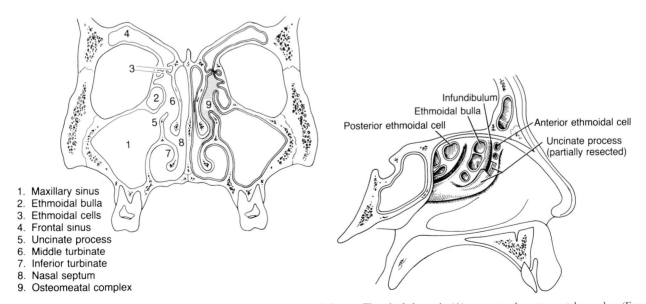

1. Maxillary sinus
2. Ethmoidal bulla
3. Ethmoidal cells
4. Frontal sinus
5. Uncinate process
6. Middle turbinate
7. Inferior turbinate
8. Nasal septum
9. Osteomeatal complex

Figure 38–1. Coronal *(A)* and sagittal *(B)* sections of the nose and paranasal sinuses. The stippled area in *(A)* represents the osteomeatal complex. (From Wald ER: Sinusitis in Children. N Engl J Med 1992; 326: 319–323.)

or 6th birthday. Development of the frontal sinuses is not complete until late adolescence. The frontal sinus is not a frequent site of bacterial infection but may be a focus for spread of infection to the orbit or central nervous system. The sphenoid sinuses are immediately anterior to the pituitary fossa and just behind the posterior ethmoids. Isolated bacterial infection of the sphenoid sinuses is unusual; they are usually infected as part of a pansinusitis.

Recently interest has focused on the so-called osteomeatal complex (Fig. 38–1). This is the area between the middle and inferior turbinates that represents the confluence of the drainage areas of the frontal, ethmoid, and maxillary sinuses. In the osteomeatal complex there are several areas in which two mucosal layers come into contact and thereby are predisposed to local impairment of mucociliary clearance. This may result in the retention of secretions at the site and the potential for infection even without actual ostial closure.[2]

PHYSIOLOGY

Three key elements are important to the normal physiology of the paranasal sinuses: the patency of the ostia, the function of the ciliary apparatus, and, integral to the latter, the quality of secretions.[3] Retention of secretions in the paranasal sinuses is usually due to one or more of the following: obstruction of the ostia, reduction in the number or impaired function of the cilia, or overproduction or change in the viscosity of secretions.

Sinus Drainage

The drainage of the paranasal sinuses is the key to abnormality in the sinus area. The drainage passages (infundibula) of the maxillary sinuses are small, tubular structures with a diameter of 2.5 mm (cross-sectional area approximately 5 mm) and a length of 6 mm.[4] The diameter of the ostium of each of the individual ethmoid air cells that drain independently into the middle meatus is even smaller, measuring 1–2 mm; the anterior ostia are smaller than the posterior ostia. The narrow caliber of these individual ostia sets the stage for obstruction to occur easily and often.

The factors predisposing to ostial obstruction can be divided into those that cause mucosal swelling and those due to mechanical obstruction.[5] The various factors that may cause mucosal swelling, consequent either to systemic illness or to local insults, are shown in Table 38–1. In addition, those conditions that predispose to mechanical obstruction of sinus ostia are listed. Although many conditions may lead to ostial closure, viral upper respiratory infection and allergic inflammation are by far the most frequent and most important.

When complete obstruction of the sinus drainage passages occurs, there is a transient increase in intrasinal pressure followed by the development of a negative intrasinal pressure.[6] When the drainage passage opens again, the negative pressure within the sinus relative to atmospheric pressure may allow the introduction of bacteria into the usually sterile sinus cavity. Alternatively, sneezing, sniffing, and nose blowing with altered intranasal pressure may facilitate the entry

Table 38–1. FACTORS PREDISPOSING TO OBSTRUCTION OF SINUS DRAINAGE

Mucosal Swelling	Mechanical Obstruction
Systemic disorder	Choanal atresia
Viral upper respiratory infection (URI)	Deviated septum
Allergic inflammation	Nasal polyps
Cystic fibrosis	Foreign body
Immune disorders	Tumor
Immotile cilia	Ethmoid bullae
Local insult	**Mucus Abnormalities**
Facial trauma	Viral URI
Swimming, diving	Allergic inflammation
Rhinitis medicamentosa	Cystic fibrosis

of bacteria from a heavily colonized posterior nasal chamber into the sinus cavity. The mucosa of the paranasal sinus continues to secrete actively even after obstruction occurs. Clearance of secretions is impossible when the ostium is totally obstructed. If the ostium is patent but reduced in size, the removal of secretions is delayed.

Mucociliary Apparatus

Disorders of the mucociliary apparatus in conjunction with reduced patency of the sinus ostia are major pathophysiologic events in acute sinusitis. In the posterior two thirds of the nasal cavity and within the sinuses, the epithelium is pseudostratified columnar in which most of the cells are ciliated.

The normal motility of the cilia and the adhesive properties of the mucous layer usually protect respiratory epithelium from bacterial invasion. However, certain respiratory viruses may have a direct cytotoxic effect on the cilia. The alteration of cilia number, morphology, and function may facilitate secondary bacterial invasion of the nose and the paranasal sinuses.

Sinus Secretions

Cilia can beat only in a fluid medium. There appears to be a double layer of mucus in the airways: the gel layer (superficial viscid fluid) and the sol layer (underlying serous fluid). The gel layer traps particulate matter such as bacteria and other debris. The tips of the cilia touch the gel layer during forward movement and thereby move the particulate matter along. The bodies of the cilia, however, move through the sol layer, a fluid thin enough to allow the cilia to beat.

Alterations in the volume or character of the mucus, as may occur in cystic fibrosis or asthma, appear to be an important factor impairing clearance of secretions during a common cold. The presence of purulent material in the acutely infected sinus may also impair ciliary movement and further compound the effects of ostial closure.

EPIDEMIOLOGY

Acute bacterial sinusitis is most commonly a complication of viral URIs. Accordingly, episodes of acute bacterial sinusitis occur most often during the viral respiratory season and in the age groups most susceptible to recurrent viral infections. It has recently been estimated that approximately 5%–10% of URIs are complicated by bacterial infection of the sinuses.[7] Attendance at daycare centers and the presence of older school-age siblings in the household are risk factors for sinusitis.

CLINICAL MANIFESTATIONS

Symptoms and Signs

During the course of an apparent viral URI, there are two common clinical presentations that suggest that the patient has acute bacterial sinusitis. These can be designated *persistent* and *severe*.[8] The most common presentation is with persistent respiratory symptoms. In the context of acute bacterial sinusitis, persistent symptoms are those that last more than 10 but fewer than 30 days and have not begun to improve. The 10-day mark separates a simple viral URI from bacterial sinusitis, and the 30-day mark separates acute from subacute or chronic sinusitis. Most uncomplicated viral URIs last 5–7 days. Although patients may not be asymptomatic by the 10th day, they are virtually always improved. The persistence of respiratory symptoms beyond the 10-day mark, without appreciable improvement, suggests a bacterial complication of the URI. The nasal discharge may be of any quality (thin or thick; clear, mucoid, or purulent) and the cough (which may be dry or wet) must be present in the daytime, although it is often noted to be worse at night. Malodorous breath is often reported by parents of preschoolers. Complaints of facial pain and headache are rare, although occasional painless morning eye swelling may have been noted by the parent. The child may not appear very ill, and usually if fever is present it is low-grade. In this case, it is not the severity of the clinical symptoms but their persistence that calls for attention.

The second less common presentation is a "cold" that seems more severe than usual. The severity is defined by a combination of high fever (at least 39.0° C) and purulent nasal discharge. The quality of nasal discharge undergoes frequent changes during the course of an uncomplicated viral URI. It begins as a watery discharge that becomes thicker, colored, and opaque after a few days. Most often the nasal discharge remains purulent for several days and then clears again to a mucoid or watery consistency before resolving. If fever is present at all during the course of a viral URI, it is at the outset in association with other constitutional symptoms such as headache and myalgias. Usually the fever disappears and the respiratory symptoms begin. Accordingly, the combination of high fever and purulent nasal discharge for at least 3–4 days signals a secondary bacterial infection of the paranasal sinuses. This group of patients may suffer from headaches behind or above the eye and occasionally experience periorbital swelling.

Physical Findings

On physical examination, the patient with bacterial sinusitis may be found to have mucopurulent discharge present in the nose or posterior pharynx. The nasal mucosa is usually erythematous but may on occasion be pale and boggy; the throat may show moderate injection. Examination of the tympanic membranes may show evidence of acute otitis media or otitis media with effusion. This occurs more often in chronic than in acute sinusitis. The cervical lymph nodes are usually not significantly enlarged or tender. Occasionally, there is either tenderness, as the examiner palpates over or percusses the paranasal sinuses, or appreciable periorbital edema—soft, nontender swelling of the upper and lower eyelid with discoloration of the overlying skin, or both. Unfortunately, facial tenderness is neither sensitive nor specific. Malodorous breath (in the absence of pharyngitis, poor dental hygiene, or a nasal foreign body) may suggest bacterial sinusitis. None of these characteristics differentiates viral rhinosinusitis from bacterial sinusitis.

In general, for most children younger than 10 years of age, the physical examination is not very helpful in making a specific diagnosis of acute bacterial sinusitis. However, if the mucopurulent material can be removed from the nose and the nasal mucosa is treated with topical vasoconstrictors, pus may be seen coming from the middle meatus. This observation and periorbital swelling are probably the most specific findings in acute bacterial sinusitis.

Key elements of the physical examination include

- Assessment of the nasal mucosa for erythema, edema, and discharge; the use of a local vasoconstrictor to optimize visualization of the middle meatus is helpful in some cases

- Assessment of the pharynx for mucopurulent discharge

- Transillumination of maxillary and frontal sinuses in patients older than 10 years of age

- Palpation and percussion of the face for tenderness

- Percussion of the teeth for tenderness

- Notation of malodorous breath

- Auscultation of lungs; chest compression for wheezing

Differential Diagnosis

The major symptoms that prompt the consideration of the diagnosis of acute bacterial sinusitis are persistent and/or purulent nasal discharge and persistent cough. Alternative diagnoses to consider in patients with purulent nasal discharge are uncomplicated viral URI, group A streptococcal infection, adenoiditis, and nasal foreign body. In uncomplicated URI, the purulent nasal discharge is usually accompanied by low-grade fever and other elements of upper respiratory inflammation such as pharyngitis and conjunctivitis. The symptoms usually begin to improve after a few days. Streptococcal infection in children younger than 3 years of age, so-called streptococcosis, may present with persistent respiratory symptoms such as nasal discharge, low-grade fever, lassitude, and poor appetite. The diagnosis can be excluded by culturing the nasopharynx or throat for group A streptococci. Adenoiditis is suggested when purulent nasal discharge is persistent beyond 10 days without improvement in a patient with normal sinus radiographs. A nasal foreign body is usually characterized by unilateral nasal discharge, which is purulent and often bloody. Most strikingly, the nasal discharge is very foul smelling—usually noticeable from the doorway of the examining room.

Patients who present with persistent cough as the most troublesome symptom prompt the consideration of several diagnoses including reactive airways disease, *Mycoplasma pneumoniae* bronchitis, cystic fibrosis, and gastroesophageal reflux (GER). URI-triggered reactive airways disease may cause dramatic cough without accompanying wheezing. This may occasionally occur in conjunction with acute bacterial sinusitis but more often is a residual symptom after URI that substantially prolongs the clinical course of the illness. *Mycoplasma* bronchitis, occurring most commonly in children between 5 and 15 years of age, begins with prominent sore throat and fever. As the upper respiratory symptoms subside, cough begins and becomes prominent and persistent. Cystic fibrosis needs to be considered in children with persistent cough, although it is unlikely to explain the symptom in a previously thriving child who presents with an intercurrent illness. GER may be responsible for pulmonary and neurologic symptoms as well as failure to thrive. It should be considered most seriously in children with night-time cough only or who have had poorly controlled asthma or previous episodes of pneumonia.

DIAGNOSIS

When the clinical history suggests a diagnosis of sinusitis the following procedures may help confirm the diagnosis.

Sinus Aspiration

Although maxillary sinus aspiration is not a routine procedure, it can be safely performed by a skilled otolaryngologist on carefully selected patients in the ambulatory setting using a transnasal approach. Sedation or general anesthesia may be required for adequate immobilization in the young child. Current indications for maxillary sinus aspiration include (1) failure to respond to multiple courses of antibiotics, (2) severe facial pain, (3) orbital or intracranial complications, and (4) evaluation of an immunoincompetent host. There must be careful decontamination and anesthesia of the area beneath the inferior turbinate through which the trocar is passed. Material aspirated from the maxillary sinus should be sent for quantitative aerobic and anaerobic cultures (if possible) and Gram's stain. The recovery of bacteria in a density of at least 10^4 colony-forming units per milliliter is considered to represent true infection.[9, 10] The finding of at least one organism per high-power field on Gram's stain of sinus secretions correlates with the recovery of bacteria in a density of 10^5 colony-forming units per milliliter.

Imaging

Radiography has traditionally been used to evaluate the presence of sinus disease. Standard radiographic projections include an anteroposterior, a lateral, and, for the maxillary sinuses, an occipitomental view. Radiographic findings in patients with acute sinusitis are diffuse opacification, mucosal thickening of at least 4 mm, or an air-fluid level. Although these radiographic findings are not specific for acute bacterial sinusitis, they are helpful in confirming the presence of acute sinusitis in patients with suggestive signs and symptoms.

Much has been written about the frequency of abnormal sinus radiographs in asymptomatic populations of children; however, most studies have been flawed by either inattention to the presence of symptoms and signs of respiratory inflammation or failure to classify abnormal radiographic findings as major or minor.[11, 12] When children older than 1 year of age have neither respiratory signs nor symptoms, their sinus radiographs are almost always normal.[13] On the other hand, when children with persistent or severe respiratory symptoms have radiographs demonstrating the presence of an air-fluid level, complete opacification of the sinus cavities or mucosal thickening of at least 4–5 mm, bacteria in high density are present in a maxillary sinus aspirate 75% of the time.[10]

Sinus radiographs are significantly abnormal in 88% of children younger than 6 years of age with persistent respiratory symptoms.[14] Accordingly, sinus radiographs need not be performed in this age group in children with uncomplicated sinus infection. Plain radiographs should be obtained to confirm the presence of sinus infection in children younger than 6 years of age who present with severe symptoms and in all children of at least 6 years of age with suspected bacterial sinusitis. The clinician can feel confident that plain radiographs provide sufficient information in patients with signs and symptoms of acute uncomplicated bacterial sinus infection.[15]

Several studies have examined the frequency of incidental paranasal sinus abnormalities on computerized tomographic (CT) scans of pediatric patients.[16, 17] Again there has been a failure to obtain information regarding recent signs or symptoms of respiratory infection[16] or to classify the degree and significance of radiographic abnormalities.[17] A recent study showed frequent abnormalities on CT scan in patients with a "fresh common cold."[18] McAlister and colleagues have highlighted the observation that CT scans are superior to plain radiographs in the delineation of sinus abnormalities particularly in patients with chronic or recurrent disease.[19] This is not surprising, as plain radiographs are a summation of overlapping structures, whereas CT scans provide many individual images. CT scans are not necessary for the management of children with uncomplicated acute bacterial sinusitis; they should be reserved for the evaluation of children with (1) complicated sinus disease (either orbital or central nervous system complications), (2) numerous recurrences, or (3) protracted or nonresponsive symptoms (i.e., circumstances in which sinus surgery is contemplated).

The osteomeatal complex is the area of abnormality in patients with recurrent acute bacterial sinusitis or chronic sinusitis. This area is best examined with the CT scan. Persistent or residual changes in the sinuses, especially the ethmoids, may be seen even after antimicrobial therapy in many patients despite the absence of clinical signs and symptoms of disease. These abnormalities indicate persistent inflammation or slow clearance of secretions but not necessarily bacterial infection.

MICROBIOLOGY

Data on the microbiology of sinusitis in pediatric patients is best organized according to the duration of clinical symptoms. However, literature review is complicated by varied definitions of acute, subacute, and chronic sinusitis. Several studies done on ambulatory patients with acute (10–30 days) and subacute (30–120 days)[20] illnesses have highlighted the important bacterial pathogens as *Streptococcus pneumoniae, Haemophilus influenzae,* and *Moraxella catarrhalis.* Other much less frequently recovered bacterial species include group A streptococci, group C streptococci, viridans streptococci, peptostreptococci, *Moraxella* species and *Eikenella corrodens.*[10] A similar distribution of bacterial pathogens is observed in asthmatic patients with sinusitis. *S. pneumoniae* is most common in all age groups and accounts for 30%–40% of isolates. *H. influenzae* and *M. catarrhalis* are similar in prevalence and account for approximately 20% of cases. Both *H. influenzae* and *M. catarrhalis* may be beta-lactamase-producing and thereby amoxicillin-resistant. Neither staphylococci nor anaerobic bacteria are commonly recovered from these patients. Respiratory viral isolates include adenovirus, parainfluenza, influenza virus, and rhinovirus in approximately 10% of patients. This number might be higher if diagnostic aspirates were performed earlier in the course of respiratory symptoms.

TREATMENT

Antibiotic

The prescription of antimicrobials is the backbone of the medical management of acute bacterial sinusitis. Table 38–2 shows a list of antimicrobials potentially useful in patients with acute sinusitis. Amoxicillin is acceptable and desirable for the treatment of most cases of uncomplicated sinusitis in children. It is effective most of the time, inexpensive, and safe. The latter characteristic is particularly important when treating a condition that has a high spontaneous cure rate.[14]

Although amoxicillin is preferred in most cases, there are several clinical situations in which a broader-spectrum regimen is appropriate. These include (1) failure to improve

Table 38–2. TREATMENT OF SINUSITIS IN CHILDREN

Antimicrobial	Dosage
Amoxicillin	40 mg/kg/day in 3 divided doses
Amoxicillin/potassium clavulanate	40/10 mg/kg/day in 3 divided doses
Erythromycin/sulfisoxazole	50/150 mg/kg/day in 4 divided doses
Sulfamethoxazole/trimethoprim	40/8 mg/kg/day in 2 divided doses
Cefaclor	40 mg/kg/day in 3 divided doses
Cefuroxime axetil	30 mg/kg/day in 2 divided doses
Cefprozil	30 mg/kg/day in 2 divided doses
Cefixime	8 mg/kg/day in 1 dose
Cefpodoxime proxetil	10 mg/kg/day in 2 divided doses
Loracarbef	30 mg/kg/day in 2 divided doses

while being treated with amoxicillin, (2) residence in a geographic area with a high prevalence of beta-lactamase-producing *H. influenzae,* (3) the occurrence of frontal or sphenoidal sinusitis, (4) the occurrence of complicated ethmoidal sinusitis, and (5) presentation with very protracted (more than 30 days) symptoms. Antimicrobials with the most comprehensive coverage for patients with acute bacterial sinusitis are amoxicillin–potassium clavulanate, erythromycin-sulfisoxazole, and cefuroxime axetil. Five new antimicrobial agents are available for the management of respiratory infections but have not been evaluated in published studies of sinusitis in children: cefixime, cefprozil, cefpodoxime, loracarbef, and clarithromycin; cefprozil and loracarbef have performed well when evaluated in adult patients with acute sinusitis.[21, 22]

Several antimicrobial agents have been compared in the treatment of children with acute bacterial sinusitis in published studies or abstracts. Theoretically, antimicrobials that are effective against beta-lactamase-producing bacterial species should offer a therapeutic advantage over amoxicillin in treating approximately 20% of patients with acute sinusitis. (In Pittsburgh 35% of *H. influenzae* and approximately 100% of *M. catarrhalis* are beta-lactamase-producing.) However, it is known that patients with acute sinusitis have a spontaneous clinical cure rate of 40%–50%.[14] Therefore, nearly half the patients harboring beta-lactamase-producing organisms in their maxillary sinuses will recover even when not receiving an optimal antimicrobial agent. Accordingly, we can expect to see at most about a 10% difference between regimens that are effective and those that are not effective against beta-lactamase-producing bacterial species. To demonstrate a 10% difference between any two treatments would require the study of hundreds of patients in each group of a controlled clinical trial. Most studies of antimicrobial efficacy have involved small numbers of patients—usually between 25 and 30 patients. Therefore, not surprisingly, most antimicrobials have appeared to perform similarly in studies evaluating the clinical outcome of patients with sinusitis.

The serious emerging problem in the antimicrobial management of acute or recurrent sinusitis is infection caused by penicillin-resistant pneumococci.[23] The frequency of penicillin-resistant pneumococci varies geographically, and many isolates of pneumococci are resistant to other commonly used antimicrobials such as sulfamethoxazole-trimethoprim and erythromycin. The optimal therapy for these infections is not known; selection should be guided by susceptibility results when available. The oral agents to which most penicillin-resistant pneumococci remain susceptible are clindamycin and rifampin.[24]

Patients with acute bacterial sinusitis may require hospitalization because of systemic toxicity or inability to take oral antimicrobials. These patients may be treated with cefuroxime at a dosage of 100–200 mg/kg/day, intravenously, in three divided doses or ampicillin-sulbactam at a dose of 150–200 mg/kg/day intravenously.

Clinical improvement is prompt in nearly all children treated with an appropriate antimicrobial agent. Patients febrile at the initial encounter become afebrile, and there is a remarkable reduction of nasal discharge and cough within 48 hours. If the patient does not improve, or worsens, in 48 hours, clinical reevaluation is appropriate. If the diagnosis is unchanged, sinus aspiration may be considered for precise bacteriologic information. Alternatively, an antimicrobial agent effective against beta-lactamase-producing bacterial species and penicillin-resistant pneumococci should be prescribed. If parenteral therapy is being used, vancomycin may need to be added.

The appropriate duration of antimicrobial therapy for patients with acute bacterial sinusitis has not been systematically investigated. Many patients have a brisk response to antimicrobial intervention and experience dramatic improvement in respiratory symptoms in 3–4 days. For these patients 10 days of treatment is adequate. For patients who respond more slowly, a reasonable recommendation is to treat until the patient is symptom-free and then for an additional 7 days.

Surgery

Patients with acute bacterial sinusitis hardly ever require surgical intervention unless they present with orbital or central nervous system complications. Rarely, sinus aspiration may be required to ventilate a sinus that has not responded to aggressive antimicrobial management.

When patients with acute sinusitis or complications of sinusitis fail to improve with maximal medical therapy, sinus surgery should be considered. Early surgical efforts focused on the creation of a nasoantral window within the maxillary sinus.[25] This additional dependent ostium was thought to facilitate gravitational drainage. However, these proved to be relatively ineffective, in part because cilia that line the maxillary sinus still transport secretions toward the natural meatus. In addition, patency of the window was usually brief.

At present the focus of surgical therapy is on the osteomeatal unit highlighted in Figure 38–1. Using an endoscope, most current surgical efforts attempt enlargement of the natural meatus of the maxillary outflow tract (by excising the uncinate process and the ethmoid bullae) and performance of an anterior ethmoidectomy.[26, 27] When central nervous system or orbital complications are present, an ophthalmologist and neurosurgeon join the multidisciplinary team.

Other Medications

Adjuvant therapies such as antihistamines, decongestants, and anti-inflammatory agents have not been systematically studied in children.[28] Limited evaluation of systemic decongestants has shown their effect to be an increase in the patency of the maxillary sinus ostium and a decrease in nasal airway resistance.[6] Their overall impact on the clinical course of episodes of viral rhinosinusitis or acute bacterial sinusitis has not been reported. Topical decongestants such as oxymetazoline may be used for 1 or 2 days for symptomatic relief of nasal congestion. Longer use is discouraged because of the concern about rhinitis medicamentosa. Antihistamines should be reserved for patients with recognized allergies. Intranasal steroids do not have a role in acute bacterial sinusitis.

Some children experience recurrent episodes of acute bacterial sinusitis. The most common cause of recurrent sinusitis is recurrent viral URI, often a consequence of daycare attendance or the presence of an older school-age sibling in the household. Other predisposing conditions include allergic and nonallergic rhinitis, cystic fibrosis, an immunodeficiency disorder (insufficient or dysfunctional immunoglobulins), ciliary dyskinesia, or an anatomic problem. Evaluation of children with recurrent acute bacterial sinusitis should include consideration of consultation with an allergist, a sweat test, quantitative measurement of immunoglobulin levels, and a mucosal biopsy to assess ciliary function and structure. If specific allergens are identified or an allergic diathesis documented, therapy might include desensitization, antihistamines, or topical intranasal steroids. If a treatable immunodeficiency is identified, specific immunoglobulin therapy should be initiated. Otherwise, a trial of antimicrobial prophylaxis may be appropriate in highly selected patients. Although antimicrobial prophylaxis has not been studied in patients with recurrent acute sinusitis, it has proved to be a useful strategy in reducing symptomatic episodes of acute otitis media in patients with recurrent ear disease. If patients do not respond to maximal medical therapy, surgical intervention may be appropriate.

CYSTIC FIBROSIS

Cystic fibrosis is the most common life-threatening genetic disorder in whites, with a gene frequency of 1 in 25.[29] Children with cystic fibrosis usually present in infancy with manifestations of pulmonary disease or intestinal malabsorption resulting from pancreatic insufficiency. Rarely, sinonasal symptoms lead to the diagnosis of cystic fibrosis in a child with minimal or no evidence of lower respiratory tract involvement.[30] Although many papers have been written about cystic fibrosis and sinusitis, there has only been a single prospective systematic and comprehensive otolaryngologic evaluation of a population of patients with cystic fibrosis.[31]

Clinical Presentation

The presence of bacterial sinusitis or nasal polyps in patients with cystic fibrosis is usually signaled by the onset and persistence of purulent nasal discharge, nasal obstruction (mouth breathing, halitosis, and morning sore throat), and postnasal drainage (manifest by increase in morning cough).[32] Prominent morning headaches may be another clinical problem. Impairment of taste and smell with a resulting decrease in appetite is frequent. It is difficult to attribute the complaint of increased cough to sinus infection in patients with cystic fibrosis as cough may be a result of lower airway abnormality rather than paranasal sinus disease. The usual time of onset of nasal polyposis is between 5 and 14 years of age. In adults, the prevalence of polyps actually decreases.[33]

Purulent nasal discharge and a swollen intranasal cavity (characterized by erythematous nasal mucosa with or without polyps) are confirmed on physical examination. When polyps are present they frequently cause displacement of the middle turbinate and deviation of the nasal septum.[34] The turbinates may be hyperplastic and show polypoid changes. There may be cobblestoning of the posterior pharynx. A widened nasal bridge may result from chronic sinusitis.

Diagnosis

A specific diagnosis of bacterial sinusitis may be difficult in patients with cystic fibrosis because of the universality of abnormalities of the paranasal sinuses found on imaging studies.[31, 35, 36] Complete opacification of maxillary and ethmoid sinuses is the rule, and these sinuses may be smaller than average. There is often failure of the frontal sinuses to develop and relatively small sphenoid sinuses.[37] When computerized axial tomographic images of the paranasal sinuses are performed in patients with cystic fibrosis, they are nearly always abnormal.[33]

Direct examination of the nose often demonstrates the presence of mucopus. Endoscopic examination may show retention of secretions in the paranasal sinuses and obstruction of the osteomeatal complex. There may be an enormous number of polyps with deviation of the nasal septum.[34]

Microbiology

The bacteriology of sinusitis in patients with cystic fibrosis has been systematically evaluated in only a single study of 20 patients.[38] *Pseudomonas aeruginosa, H. influenzae, Staphylococcus aureus,* and alpha streptococci were the usual isolates. In another investigation, 15 sinus irrigations were performed on 10 patients; bacterial isolates including *Pseudomonas* species, *H. influenzae, S. pneumoniae,* and *Escherichia coli* were recovered from 5.[39] Jaffe and colleagues also reported the isolation of *P. aeruginosa, E. coli, H. influenzae,* and *Streptococcus faecalis* from the sinus aspirates of selected children with cystic fibrosis.[34]

Therapy

Medical Therapy

Medical therapy of paranasal sinusitis consists of appropriate antibiotics.[32] Sinus aspiration is rarely performed before the initiation of therapy; accordingly, antibiotics are selected empirically. These antibiotics may be the same as those usually chosen to treat exacerbations of lower respiratory tract infection. The selection of parenteral antibiotics might include an expanded-spectrum penicillin plus a beta-lactamase inhibitor (e.g., ticarcillin and potassium clavulanate) with or without an aminoglycoside or an advanced-generation cephalosporin (e.g., ceftazidime) with clindamycin. If oral therapy is preferred, only the quinolones have the capability of covering both *Pseudomonas* and *Staphylococcal* species. Although, previously there has been concern about the use of quinolones in children, the accumulation of recent data is reassuring regarding safety.[40] The duration of therapy is a minimum of 3 weeks and frequently 4–6 weeks.[32]

Allergic rhinitis, as an inflammatory condition of the upper respiratory tract, has been documented to occur no more often in children with cystic fibrosis than in a population of children without cystic fibrosis.[41, 42] Ancillary therapy for the management of nasal symptoms includes intranasal steroids. Regression of nasal polyps has been observed after the use of intranasal steroids but may also occur spontaneously.

Surgical Therapy

Many patients with cystic fibrosis and bacterial paranasal sinusitis are not successfully treated medically and must be considered for surgical procedures. Persistent purulent nasal discharge, chronic nasal obstruction, and headaches that are unresponsive to antibiotic therapy and intranasal steroids are an indication for surgical intervention.[32]

The extent of surgical intervention for sinonasal problems in patients with cystic fibrosis has been debated. Initially, only polypectomy and limited sinus procedures were recommended because of concern for prolonged anesthesia; however, later reports showed that these limited operative interventions resulted in only short-term benefit. In contrast, comprehensive surgical efforts including Caldwell-Luc procedures with ethmoidectomy or functional endoscopic sinus surgery lead to prolonged periods of symptomatic improvement and the need for fewer subsequent operations.[43–45]

Although the role of surgical management in children with chronic sinusitis is in general controversial (and probably rarely indicated),[46] children with cystic fibrosis may benefit dramatically. This has been best illustrated in programs in which patients with cystic fibrosis are considered for lung transplantation. In 1989, investigators began performing sinus surgery and subsequent sinus lavage in cystic fibrosis patients expected to be undergoing lung transplantation.[47] Preliminary data suggested that the procedures were beneficial. A similar approach using endoscopic sinus surgery plus monthly tobramycin sinus irrigations was recently reported from Stanford University.[48] Although their study compared prospectively evaluated patients with historical controls, the results were encouraging. In another center, the performance of functional endoscopic sinus surgery before transplant followed by daily irrigation of the maxillary sinuses with a tobramycin solution has been effective in maintaining symptom-free patients for many months.[37] Tobramycin appears to reduce growth and colonization of *Pseudomonas* organisms in the paranasal sinuses. The long-term efficacy of the management of refractory chronic sinusitis in adult cystic fibrosis patients with endoscopic sinus surgery and antimicrobial lavage and its application to children awaits prospective evaluation in a multicentered clinical trial.

References

1. Wald ER: Sinusitis in children. N Engl J Med 1992; 326: 319–323.
2. Kennedy DW, Zinreich JS, Rosenbaum AE, Johns ME: Functional endoscopic sinus surgery. Arch Otolaryngol 1985; 111: 576–582.
3. Reimer A, von Mecklenburg C, Tormalm NG: The mucociliary activity of the upper respiratory tract: III. A functional and morphological study of human and animal material with special reference to maxillary sinus disease. Acta Otolaryngol 1978; 335(suppl): 3–20.
4. Drettner B: Pathophysiology of paranasal sinuses with clinical implications. Clin Otolaryngol 1980; 5: 272–284.
5. Rachelefsky GS, Katz RM, Siegel SC: Diseases of paranasal sinuses in children. Curr Prob Pediatr 1982; 12: 1–57.
6. Aust R, Drettner B, Falck B: Studies of the effect of peroral fenylpropa-

nolamin on the functional size of the human maxillary ostium. Acta Otolaryngol 1979; 88: 455–458.

7. Wald ER, Guerra N, Byers C: Upper respiratory tract infections in young children: Duration of and frequency of complications. Pediatrics 1991; 87: 129–133.

8. Wald ER, Reilly JS, Casselbrant M, et al.: Treatment of acute maxillary sinusitis in childhood: A comparative study of amoxicillin and cefaclor. J Pediatr 1984; 104: 297–302.

9. Evans FO, Sydnor B, Moore WEC, et al.: Sinusitis of the maxillary antrum. N Engl J Med 1975; 293: 735–739.

10. Wald ER, Milmoe GJ, Bowen AD, et al.: Acute maxillary sinusitis in children. N Engl J Med 1981; 304: 749–754.

11. Maresh M, Washburn AH: Paranasal sinuses from birth to late adolescence: II. Clinical and roentgenographic evidence of infection. Am J Dis Child 1940; 60: 841–861.

12. Shopfner CE, Rossi JO: Roentgen evaluation of the paranasal sinuses in children. AJR 1973; 118: 176–186.

13. Kovatch AL, Wald ER, Ledesma-Medina J, et al.: Maxillary sinus radiographs in children with nonrespiratory complaints. Pediatrics 1984; 73: 306–308.

14. Wald ER, Chiponis D, Ledesma-Medina J: Comparative effectiveness of amoxicillin and amoxicillin–clavulanate potassium in acute paranasal sinus infections in children: A double-blind, placebo-controlled trial. Pediatrics 1986; 77: 795–800.

15. Lusk RP, Lozar RH, Muntz HR: The diagnosis and treatment of recurrent and chronic sinusitis in children. Pediatr Clin North Am 1989; 36: 1411–1421.

16. Diament MJ, Senac MO, Gilsanz V, et al.: Prevalence of incidental paranasal sinuses opacification in pediatric patients: A CT study. J Comput Assist Tomogr 1987; 11: 426–431.

17. Glasier CM, Ascher DP, Williams KD: Incidental paranasal sinus abnormalities on CT of children: Clinical correlation. AJNR 1986; 7: 861–864.

18. Gwaltney JM, Philips CD, Miller RD, Riker DK: Computed tomographic study of the common cold. N Engl J Med 1994; 330: 25–30.

19. McAlister WH, Lusk R, Muntz HR: Comparison of plain radiographs and coronal CT scans in infants and children with recurrent sinusitis. AJR 1989; 153: 1259–1264.

20. Wald ER, Byers C, Guerra N, et al.: Subacute sinusitis in children. J Pediatr 1989; 115: 28–32.

21. Gwaltney JM Jr, Scheld MW, Sande MA, Sydnor A: The microbial etiology and antimicrobial therapy of adults with acute community-acquired sinusitis: A fifteen year experience at the University of Virginia and review of other selected studies. J Allergy Clin Immunol 1992; 90: 457–462.

22. Van den Wijngaart W, Verbrugh H, Theopold HM, et al.: A non-comparative study of cefprozil at two dose levels in the treatment of acute uncomplicated bacterial sinusitis. Clin Ther 1992; 14: 306–313.

23. Leggiadro RJ: Penicillin and cephalosporin-resistant *Streptococcus pneumoniae*: An emerging microbial threat. Pediatrics 1994; 93: 500–503.

24. Nelson CT, Mason EO Jr, Kaplan SL: Activity of oral antibiotics in middle ear and sinus infections caused by penicillin-resistant *Streptococcus pneumoniae*: Implications for treatment. Pediatr Infect Dis J 1994; 13: 585–589.

25. Muntz HR, Lusk RP: Nasal antral windows in children: A retrospective study. Laryngoscope 1990; 100: 643–646.

26. Lusk RP: Surgical management of chronic sinusitis. In: Lusk RP (ed): Pediatric Sinusitis. New York: Raven Press, 1992, pp 77–125.

27. Lusk RP, Muntz HR: Endoscopic sinus surgery in children with chronic sinusitis: A pilot study. Laryngoscope 1990; 100: 654–658.

28. Zieger RS: Prospects for ancillary treatment of sinusitis in the 1990s. J Allergy Clin Immunol 1992; 90: 478–495.

29. Wood RE, Boat TF, Doershuk CF: Cystic fibrosis (state-of-the-art). Am Rev Respir Dis 1976; 113: 833–878.

30. Wiatrak BJ, Myer CM III, Cotton RT: Cystic fibrosis presenting with sinus disease in children. Am J Dis Child 1993; 147: 258–259.

31. Neely JG, Harrison GM, Jerger J, et al.: The otolaryngologic aspects of cystic fibrosis. Trans Am Acad Ophthalmol Otolaryngol 1972; 76: 313–324.

32. Ramsey B, Richardson MA: Impact of sinusitis in cystic fibrosis. J Allergy Clin Immunol 1992; 90: 547–552.

33. Cuyler JP, Monghan AJ: Cystic fibrosis and sinusitis. Otolaryngol 1989; 18: 173–175.

34. Jaffe BF, Strome M, Khaiv KT, Schwackman H: Nasal polypectomy and sinus surgery for cystic fibrosis—A 10-year review. Otolaryngol Clin North Am 1977; 10: 81–90.

35. Gharib R, Allen RP, Joos HA, Bravo LR: Paranasal sinuses in cystic fibrosis. Am J Dis Child 1964; 108: 499–502.

36. Ledesma-Medina J, Osman MZ, Hirdany BR: Abnormal paranasal sinuses in patients with cystic fibrosis of the pancreas. Pediatr Radiol 1980; 9: 61–64.

37. Davidson TM, Murphy C, Mitchell M, et al.: Management of chronic sinusitis in cystic fibrosis. Laryngoscope 1995; 105: 354–358.

38. Shapiro ED, Milmoe GJ, Wald ER, et al.: Bacteriology of the maxillary sinuses in patients with cystic fibrosis. J Infect Dis 1982; 146: 589–593.

39. Drake-Lee AB, Morgan DW: Nasal polyps and sinusitis in children with cystic fibrosis. J Laryngol Otol 1989; 103: 753–755.

40. Kubin R: Safety and efficacy of ciprofloxacin in paediatric patients—Review. Infection 1993; 21: 413–421.

41. Warner JO, Taylor BW, Normal AP, et al.: Association of cystic fibrosis with allergy. Arch Dis Child 1976; 51: 507–511.

42. Wilmott RW: The relationship between atopy and cystic fibrosis. Clin Rev Allergy 1991; 9: 29–46.

43. Jones JW, Parsons DS, Cuyler JP: The results of functional endoscopic (FES) surgery on the symptoms of patients with cystic fibrosis. Intern Pediatr Otolaryngol 1993; 28: 25–32.

44. Crockett DM, McGill TJ, Friedman EM, et al.: Nasal and paranasal sinus surgery in children with cystic fibrosis. Ann Otol Rhinol Laryngol 1987; 96: 367–372.

45. Cepero R, Smith RJH, Catlin FI, et al.: Cystic fibrosis—An otolaryngologic perspective. Otolaryngol Head Neck Surg 1987; 97: 356.

46. Wald ER: Chronic sinusitis in children. J Pediatr 1995; 127: 339–347.

47. Lewiston NJ, King V, Umetsu D, et al.: Cystic fibrosis patients who have undergone heart-lung transplantation benefit from maxillary sinus antrostomy and repeated sinus lavage. Transplant Proc 1991; 23: 1207–1208.

48. Moss RB, King VV: Management of sinusitis in cystic fibrosis by endoscopic surgery and serial antimicrobial lavage. Arch Otolaryngol Head Neck Surg 1995; 121: 6566–6572.

Jack M. Gwaltney

Management of Acute Sinusitis in Adults

▼

Sinus involvement is an inherent part of the common cold syndrome itself,[1] making the viral rhinosinusitis of the common cold the most frequently occurring acute infectious illness of humans. Having this knowledge helps one better understand the pathogenesis of secondary acute bacterial sinusitis and also explains why symptoms of the common cold and of acute bacterial sinusitis are so similar. A classification of acute sinusitis comprises several distinct etiologic entities (Table 39–1). Understanding the distinctions made in such a classification is important in developing a rational plan for clinical management of patients with acute sinusitis. Available information supports the concept that an initial viral rhinosinusitis (common cold or influenza-like illness) predisposes, in a small percentage of cases, to secondary bacterial infection of the sinus cavity. The possibilities are then present for a mixed viral-bacterial infection or for a bacterial infection alone. Factors such as allergy and obstruction may also predispose to acute bacterial sinusitis. Other conditions, such as acute community-acquired fungal sinusitis and nosocomial sinusitis, complete the classification of acute sinusitis.

ANATOMY AND PHYSIOLOGY

The anatomy and physiology of the paranasal sinuses and the steps in their embryonic development are reviewed in Chapter 38. Of special interest in the pathogenesis of acute sinusitis is the mucociliary drainage systems of the various sinus cavities and the passageways through which drainage into the nasal cavity is effected.

Of particular interest is the maxillary sinus because of its size, location, and accessibility to study. The maxillary sinus cavity of an adult, on average, has a volume of approximately 30 mL.[2] Drainage from this structure is directed through the infundibulum, a small tubular passageway with an average diameter in the adult of approximately 3 mm. Under normal conditions, material is propelled at a rate of approximately 1 cm/min. Clearance is sufficient to prevent accumulation of fluid in the sinus cavity. This is because mucus secretion in the normal maxillary sinus is very scanty.[3] The density of seromucous glands in the maxillary and other sinus cavities is quite low compared with the nasal cavity (Table 39–2).[4–6] Most of the small amount of mucus secreted into the sinus cavity comes from goblet cells in the epithelium. Mucus secretion is changed in as yet poorly understood ways by the events associated with a cold.[7] The sinus drainage system cannot handle the increased amount of viscous fluid that is deposited in the cavity. This material is not effectively propelled to the infundibulum by the cilia, and the infundibulum itself becomes occluded. Thick, tenacious fluid accumulates in the sinus cavity, where on computed tomography (CT) examination it appears in irregular distributions on the floor and along the walls (Fig. 39–1).[1]

EPIDEMIOLOGY

The incidence of viral rhinosinusitis (the common cold and influenza-like illness) has been well studied, occurring on an annual basis of two to three episodes per year in adults and six to eight in children.[8] There is a well-defined seasonal pattern of occurrence in temperate areas, with a period of high prevalence extending from September through March.

Table 39–1. CLASSIFICATION OF ACUTE SINUSITIS

Community-acquired

Viral (as part of the rhinosinusitis of colds and influenzal illness)
Bacterial (secondary to viral, allergic, obstructive causes)
Viral/bacterial (simultaneous viral and bacterial infection)
Fungal (in normal or immunosuppressed host)

Nosocomial

Bacterial (associated with nasal tubes)
Fungal (in immunosuppressed host)

Table 39–2. DENSITY (mm²) of Mucus-Producing Structures in the Nose and Sinuses

Seromucous glands[4,5]	
Nose	8
Sinuses	
maxillary	0.2
ethmoid	0.5
frontal	0.08
sphenoid	0.05
Goblet cells[6]	
Nose	5700–11000
Sinuses	
maxillary	9700
ethmoid	6500
frontal	5900
sphenoid	6200

*Superscript numbers indicate chapter references.

341

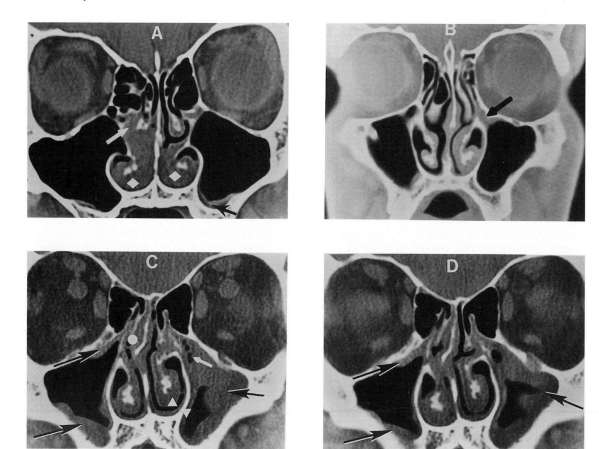

Figure 39–1. Computed tomography (CT) scans of adults with early (2–4 day) natural colds, showing abnormalities of the nasal passages and sinuses. *A,* Bilateral engorgement of inferior turbinates *(diamonds)*; obstruction of ostiomeatal complex *(white arrow)*; abnormality on floor of sinus cavity, probably thick secretion *(black arrow). B,* Occlusion of infundibulum *(black arrow). C,* Edema of nasal mucosa *(paired arrow heads)*; obstruction of ostiomeatal complex *(white dot)*; thick secretions *(black and white arrows)* with bubbles *(white arrow). D,* Same patient. CT scan repeated 2 hours later shows failure to move thick secretions effectively *(black and white arrows)* toward infundibulum.

Several different families of respiratory viruses contribute to the syndrome, and each viral family, more or less, has a period of heightened prevalence.

The incidence of acute bacterial sinusitis is less well defined, primarily because of the difficulty in accurately making the diagnosis. In a large longitudinal study of Cleveland families, 0.5% of persons with colds were thought to have a secondary bacterial sinusitis on the basis of a clinical diagnosis (Table 39–3).[9] In a more selected population of adult otolaryngology patients with common cold–like illness, 2.2% were found to have purulent secretions in the maxillary sinus by sinus puncture.[10] Culture results were not reported.

The seasonal trend in the incidence of sinusitis has been shown to correlate with that of the common cold and other acute respiratory infections, but not with that of allergic rhinitis, supporting the idea that viral rhinosinusitis is the major predisposing cause of the condition.[11] However, cases of acute bacterial sinusitis occur throughout the year and are associated with other activities and conditions, such as nasal allergy, swimming, and obstruction of the nasal and sinus passages by masses such as polyps, foreign bodies, and tumors. Other risk factors for bacterial sinusitis are cystic fibrosis and AIDS. Risk factors for nosocomial sinusitis include nasal intubation, nasal packing, cranial and facial fractures, and mechanical ventilation.

PATHOGENESIS

Three key factors play a role in the pathogenesis of the usual case of acute bacterial sinusitis: (1) the normal bacterial flora of the nasopharynx, which supplies a reservoir of the bacterial pathogens that cause acute bacterial sinusitis (Table 39–4),[12] (2) the ongoing occurrence of common colds and influenza-like illness, which create the conditions for bacterial invasion of the sinus, and (3) the inability of the sinus drainage apparatus to deal with the changes that take place during a cold, the event that facilitates bacterial growth in the sinus.

Table 39–3. ACUTE BACTERIAL SINUSITIS COMPLICATING THE COMMON COLD

Population	Method of Diagnosis	No. Patients With Colds	No. Cases of Sinusitis
Cleveland families[9]	clinical	11134	53 (0.5%)
Adult ENT patients[10]	sinus puncture†	89	2 (2.2%)

*Superscript numbers indicate chapter references.
†Diagnosis based on finding purulent secretions.

Table 39–4. INDIGENOUS BACTERIAL FLORA OF THE NOSE IN ADULTS[1]

	Frequency of Recovery (%)
Nasal vestibule	
Staphylococcus aureus	25–40
Posterior nasopharynx	
Streptococcus pneumoniae	15–25
Haemophilus influenzae	6–40
Streptococcus pyogenes	6
S. aureus	12

[1]From Gwaltney JM Jr, Hayden FG: The nose and infection. In: Proctor DF, Andersen I (eds): The Nose: Upper Airway Physiology and the Atmospheric Environment. Amsterdam: Elsevier Biomedical, 1982, pp 399–422.

The pathogenesis of the common cold syndrome is far from being understood in its entirety, nor is it an appropriate subject for the current discussion.[13] However, certain important features can be summarized, including viral deposition in the nose and viral transport to the posterior nasopharynx to the region of the adenoid, where, in the case of rhinovirus, it encounters the rhinovirus receptor (intercellular adhesion molecule I [ICAM-1]). Following initiation of infection, various inflammatory pathways and neurologic reflexes are triggered, resulting in dilation of blood vessels, intercellular leakage of plasma, discharge of seromucous glands and goblet cells, and stimulation of pain nerve fibers and of sneeze and cough reflexes. Sneezes and coughs may be an important mechanism for depositing nasopharyngeal bacteria into the sinus cavity against the outwardly directed flow of sinus mucociliary clearance.

That these events lead to entrapment of thick secretions in the sinus cavity during a cold or influenza is clearly demonstrated on computed tomography (CT) examination of the sinus. The primary importance of the disease in the sinuses versus the nasal passages is shown by the frequency of abnormality observed in the respective areas (Table 39–5). In a study of 31 adults with early (2–4 days) natural colds, some of which were due to rhinovirus, 77% of the patients had infundibular occlusion, and 87% and 64.5% had abnormalities in the maxillary and ethmoid sinus cavities, respectively.[1] Surprisingly, only 23% had engorged turbinates at the time of CT examination, and 42% had thickening of the nasal walls due to modest and nonoccluding mucosal swelling.

The sinus cavity abnormalities appeared to be due mainly

Table 39–5. FREQUENCY OF CT SCAN ABNORMALITIES IN THE NASAL PASSAGES AND SINUSES

	Percentage (%)
Nasal	
Engorged turbinates	23
Thickening of nasal walls	42
Sinus	
Occlusion of maxillary infundibulum	77
Abnormality of sinus cavity	
Maxillary	87
Ethmoid	64.5
Frontal	32
Sphenoid	39

to thick secretions because the material contained bubbles (see Fig. 39–1). Also, it had an irregular distribution, which would be unlikely with mucosal thickening. That mucosal thickening also played a role in the sinus cavity findings could not be excluded, because unenhanced CT does not distinguish between the two processes. However, there was no thickening in many parts of the sinus cavity walls, indicating that mucosal edema, if present, was not evenly distributed throughout the cavity.

The final event in the pathogenesis of acute bacterial sinusitis occurs when entrapped bacteria multiply and, in turn, produce the deleterious effects associated with the different species. Some, such as *Moraxella (Branhamella) catarrhalis* and unencapsulated *Haemophilus influenzae*, are of a low order of virulence and invasiveness, whereas others, such as *Staphylococcus aureus, Streptococcus pyogenes*, and *Streptococcus pneumoniae*, have multiple determinants of virulence and/or invasiveness. One event that may take place is that bacterial enzymes attack the thick fluid associated with viral rhinosinusitis, making it less viscous. This would result in thinner fluid, which is perceived as a classic air-fluid level on imaging. An air-fluid level is considered highly suggestive of bacterial sinusitis. In one series, 16 (89%) of 18 patients with acute community-acquired sinusitis who had an air-fluid level on sinus radiography had a positive bacterial culture on sinus aspiration.[14]

In a small percentage of cases, acute bacterial sinusitis may also be complicated by intracranial extension of the infection. This problem is discussed in Chapter 42. Also, acute bacterial sinusitis, especially when not treated or inadequately treated, may have a role in the development of chronic sinus disease, but the understanding of this event, if it does occur, is poor.

MICROBIAL ETIOLOGY

Viral Etiology

Viruses causing the rhinosinusitis of the common cold and influenza-like illness are found in the rhinovirus, coronavirus, adenovirus, parainfluenza virus, influenza virus, and respiratory syncytial virus groups.[8] Among these several groups of viruses are over 200 antigenically distinct immunotypes. Viruses from the rhinovirus, influenza, and parainfluenza groups have been recovered from sinus aspirates of patients with acute sinusitis, either alone or in association with bacteria such as *S. pneumoniae* and *H. influenzae*.[14, 15] In the limited amount of viral culturing that has been done of sinus aspirates from patients with acute sinusitis, viruses have been recovered alone or in combination with bacteria in 16% of cases. It is possible that viruses may not have to be present in the sinus cavity itself to cause the changes seen on CT.

Bacterial Etiology

The bacterial causes of acute community-acquired sinusitis were first established in the 1950s and 1960s by investigators in Scandinavia doing sinus puncture studies.[16–20] Since then,

Table 39–6. BACTERIAL ETIOLOGY

	Percentage of Cases (Range)
Streptococcus pneumoniae	20–41
Haemophilus influenzae	6–50
S. pneumoniae and *H. influenzae*	1–9
Anaerobic bacteria	0–10
Moraxella (Branhamella) catarrhalis	2–4
Streptococcus pyogenes	1–8
Other streptococcal species	2
Staphylococcus aureus	0–8

other investigations in the United States and elsewhere have confirmed this work and have shown that the bacterial etiology of acute community-acquired sinusitis has not changed.[14, 15, 21] *S. pneumoniae* and *H. influenzae* continue to cause up to three quarters of all cases (Table 39–6). Following these in importance are mixed anaerobic infection, *M. catarrhalis*, alpha-hemolytic streptococci, *S. pyogenes*, and *S. aureus*.

Anaerobic sinusitis is usually associated with dental infection. Such infections may contain complex mixtures of anaerobic and microaerophilic species, including *Bacteroides* and streptococci.[15] Sinus infections due to alpha-hemolytic streptococci, when identified, have shown pyogenic species such as *Streptococcus intermedius*. There is no evidence that *Mycoplasma* species cause acute sinusitis. *Mycoplasma* have not been recovered from sinus aspirates, and sinusitis is not a characteristic feature of illness associated with known *Mycoplasma pneumoniae* infection. The role of *Chlamydia*, if any, is still under investigation.

Although the relative importance of the different bacteria has not changed over the past 40 years, there have been, and are continuing to be, important changes in their antimicrobial sensitivities. These changes first involved strains of *S. aureus* that became resistant initially to penicillin and later to methicillin (Table 39–7). Because *S. aureus* is a relatively uncommon, although potentially serious, cause of acute community-acquired sinusitis, the emergence of high-level resistance did not present a common problem. Next, resistance to ampicillin-like drugs emerged in strains of *H. influenzae* and

emerged or was recognized in *M. catarrhalis*, causing a more common problem. Fortunately, most sinusitis strains of *H. influenzae* are nonencapsulated, and these bacteria and *M. catarrhalis* are usually noninvasive when in the sinus. Low-level and high-level penicillin resistance also has emerged in *S. pneumoniae*, a very serious problem.[22–25] The effect this development has in the future on the management of acute community-acquired sinusitis is currently unknown but will probably be considerable.

Fungal Etiology

Fungi can also cause sinusitis in the community setting, and acute fungal sinusitis has been recognized with growing frequency. The fungal groups involved are *Aspergillus*,[26–28] *Homobasidiomyces*,[29] *Hyalohyphomyces*,[15, 30] *Phaeohyphomyces*,[31–35] *Pseudallescheria*,[36] *Sporothrix*,[36] and the zygomycetes[26] (Table 39–8). Fungal infections are responsible for only a very small percentage of cases of acute community-acquired sinusitis, but when they are encountered, it is important to make the correct diagnosis, because effective treatment requires surgical débridement of the sinus cavity. Fungi also cause acute invasive infection of the sinus in immunocompromised patients in community and hospital settings. Fungal sinusitis is discussed in Chapter 43.

CLINICAL PRESENTATION

The clinical presentations of viral rhinosinusitis (the common cold and influenzal illness) and of acute bacterial sinusitis share many characteristics and are often very similar. The classically described features of acute bacterial sinusitis, which include fever and facial pain, tenderness, swelling, and erythema, are not common when measured against the gold standard of a positive sinus aspirate culture.[15] Both colds and acute bacterial sinusitis share the features of mucopurulent nasal discharge, nasal obstruction, facial "pressure" or "tightness," sore throat, and cough. In contrast, intermittent, low-grade fever is present in approximately half of adult patients with acute bacterial sinusitis, and fever is

Table 39–7. ANTIMICROBIAL SENSITIVITIES

		Sensitivities		
Bacteria	Resistance(s)	Trimethoprim/Sulfamethoxazole, Cefuroxime, Amoxicillin/clavulanate Loracarbef, Cefixime	Cefotaxime, Ceftriaxone	Vancomycin
Staphylococcus aureus	Penicillin	+	+	+
	Methicillin	− *	−	+
Haemophilus influenzae	Ampicillin	+	+	−
Moraxella (Branhamella) catarrhalis	Ampicillin	+	+	−
Streptococcus pneumoniae	Penicillin			
	Low level	±	+	+
	High level	− †	±	+

*+ = susceptible; − = resistant, ± = variably susceptible.
†Trimethoprim/sulfamethoxazole active against some strains.

Table 39–8. FUNGAL INFECTIONS

Aspergillosis*
   Aspergillus fumigatis
   Aspergillus flavus
   Aspergillus niger
   Aspergillus oryzae
   Aspergillus nidulans
Pseudallescheriasis
   Pseudallescheria boydii
Sporothrichosis
   Sporothin schenckii
Homobasidiomycosis
   Schizophyllum commune
Hyalohyphomycosis
   Penicillium melini
Phaeohyphomycosis*
   Bipolaris hawaiiensis
   B. spicifera
   Exserohilum rostratum
   E. mcginnisii
   Alternaria alternata
   Curvularia lunata
Zygomycosis
   Mucor species
   Rhizophus species
   Cunninghamella bertholletiae

*Associated with allergic syndrome.

unusual in adults with colds. However, fever also occurs in adults with uncomplicated influenza and adenovirus infection.

Physical examination may or may not show pharyngeal inflammation or exudate, depending on the etiology of the infection. Streptococcal pharyngitis and adenovirus infection (acute respiratory disease, pharyngoconjunctival fever) may cause pharyngeal erythema and exudate, but rhinovirus and coronavirus colds and influenza do not. Pharyngeal erythema and exudate are not characteristic features of acute bacterial sinusitis. Mucopurulent nasal secretions may be present in the nasal passages with either viral or bacterial sinusitis. Secretions may be seen draining down into the middle meatus on endoscopic examination, but the sensitivity and specificity of this finding for acute bacterial sinusitis have not been rigorously examined. The sensitivity and specificity of tenderness on sinus percussion have also not been formally compared with results of sinus aspirate culture, but clinical experience suggests that this sign is not very sensitive.

Most cases of viral colds or influenzal illnesses are over or have improved in a week.[37] The duration of untreated, aspirate-positive, acute bacterial sinusitis has not been studied for ethical reasons, but the illness usually extends for longer than a week.

DIAGNOSIS

The diagnosis of acute infectious sinusitis can be viewed as a two-step process. The first step is to determine the presence of disease in the sinus cavity and/or its drainage passage, and the second is to determine the microbial etiology. It is particularly important to distinguish a viral rhinosinusitis from an acute bacterial sinusitis, because the latter requires antimicrobial treatment for optimal management.

Establishment of Disease

Sinus CT examination is an exquisitely sensitive diagnostic test for detecting disease of the sinus. However, in the absence of an air-fluid level, CT does not reliably distinguish viral from bacterial etiology (see Chapter 37). On the basis of the findings of the previously mentioned study in adults with colds,[1] it can be assumed that most patients with colds (and influenza) have sinus CT abnormalities. Because in the absence of an air-fluid level, CT and other imaging techniques do not reliably distinguish viral from bacterial etiology, imaging examinations are not sufficiently specific or cost-effective for the routine diagnosis of acute community-acquired sinusitis. However, if a complication such as intracranial extension of the infection is suspected, imaging studies are essential for proper patient management, as discussed in Chapter 42.

The classic findings for the diagnosis of acute bacterial sinusitis are fever ($\geq$38° C), facial erythema and edema, and sinus pain and tenderness (Table 39–9). Also, maxillary toothache is a highly specific complaint when dental infection is the precipitating event. Patients with intracranial extension of the infection and resultant meningitis or brain abscess have the clinical features of those conditions.

Attempts to identify other sensitive and specific items for diagnosing acute bacterial sinusitis from the history and physical examination have not been particularly successful (Table 39–10). In one study of adult males with nasal discharge, histories of colored nasal discharge, cough, and sneezing were most sensitive but were not specific, whereas poor response to decongestants, maxillary toothache, and temperature >38° C were specific but not sensitive.[38] In another study of adult emergency ward patients with paranasal symptoms, purulent rhinorrhea with unilateral predominance, sinus tenderness on percussion, and pus in the nasal cavity were moderately sensitive findings.[39] In the first study, the criterion standard was a positive sinus radiograph, and in the second, purulence of a sinus aspirate; neither study used the gold standard of positive bacterial culture from a sinus aspiration specimen.

In the absence of the previously listed classic signs and symptoms, duration of illness appears to be as good as any one clinical item for distinguishing viral from acute bacterial sinusitis. Most uncomplicated colds or influenza infections are over or definitely improved by 10–14 days. An acute upper respiratory illness with the features of an acute rhinosinusitis *that has not improved or is worse* after 10–14 days should raise the suspicion of a bacterial etiology.

Sinus transillumination, although worth doing, gives no information about the ethmoid and sphenoid sinuses. Also, it cannot distinguish with certainty between viral and bacterial infection. It can roughly quantify the amount of disease in the frontal and maxillary sinuses. In one study of adult males, sinus transillumination had a sensitivity of 73% and specificity of 54% compared with a positive sinus radiograph.[38] In another study, when compared with positive sinus aspirate culture, transillumination performed surprisingly well.[15] The results of that study suggest that when findings of transillumination are completely normal, this test considerably reduces, but does not exclude, the possibility of acute bacterial sinusitis. When transillumination demonstrates

Table 39–9. CATEGORIES OF SEVERITY AND MANAGEMENT PLANS FOR SUSPECTED ACUTE COMMUNITY-ACQUIRED BACTERIAL SINUSITIS*

	Category		
	Emergent	*Urgent*	*Elective*
Features	Signs and symptoms suggesting intracranial extension (meningitis, brain abscess)	Fever ≥38° C, facial edema and erythema, maxillary toothache, air-fluid level	A cold or "flu"-like illness that has persisted for >10–14 days with no improvement or with worsening
Management plan	Emergency diagnostic measures: head CT, LP, surgical consultation	Cefuroxime axetil, 250 mg bid,† or amoxicillin/clavulanate, 500/125 mg three times daily plus	Antibiotic and supportive treatment as for urgent
	Intravenous antibiotics (a 3rd-generation cephalosporin and vancomycin) while awaiting culture and sensitivity results Surgical decompression as needed	An oral decongestant (pseudoephedrine) and a mucoevacuant (guaifenesin)	

*In the setting of an illness beginning as a common cold, "flu"-like illness, or allergic rhinitis or associated with swimming or other risk factors.
†Or other antibiotics with a favorable profile of activity against intermediately resistant *Streptococcus pneumoniae;* adult dose.

complete opacity in a previously normal sinus, it increases the probability of bacterial infection. Dullness without complete opacity was less useful in predicting a bacterial etiology.

Establishment of Microbial Etiology

The sinus cavities are inaccessible to sampling by noninvasive procedures. Sinus puncture is the gold standard for collecting sinus cavity specimens for bacterial culture, although in approximately one quarter to one half of patients with a clinical diagnosis of acute community-acquired sinusitis, culture from specimens collected by antral sinus puncture is negative.[21, 40] Most of the bacterial culture–negative cases are presumably viral. Also, some patients with negative cultures may have bacterial infection in other sinuses, such as the ethmoid. Sinus puncture is used in experimental studies and selected clinical cases but is not feasible for routine diagnosis. Physicians managing cases of acute community-acquired sinusitis should know its bacterial causes and their antibiotic susceptibility when selecting antimicrobial treatment (see Tables 39–6 and 39–7).

Endoscopic collection of samples for bacterial culture from the middle meatus is not known to be similar in diagnostic accuracy to sinus aspiration. A direct comparison of the two methods is currently being conducted. It is not possible to insert an endoscope into the maxillary sinus cavity without puncturing the wall, unless a large accessory ostium is present or the patient has undergone surgical antrostomy. Bacterial culture from a nasal swab specimen is not a sufficiently accurate predictor of conditions in the sinus cavity to be useful in antimicrobial selection. Nasal cultures yield a falsely high recovery of *S. aureus*,[15, 20, 41] are poor for recovery of *M. catarrhalis*, and are not accurate for *H. influenzae* and *S. pneumoniae*.[15, 41] Also, a small proportion of patients with acute community-acquired sinusitis have more than one bacterial pathogen recovered from the same sinus cavity or have bilateral sinus infection due to different bacterial species.[15, 41, 42]

Diagnostic sinus puncture is indicated in the infrequent case of acute community-acquired sinusitis with suspected intracranial extension, in selected treatment failures, and in cases of nosocomial sinusitis. In these situations, it is important to establish microbial etiology and antimicrobial sensitivities. Sinus puncture is very safe when performed by a physician experienced in the procedure (Table 39–11). Sinus puncture is not excessively painful but does cause the psy-

Table 39–10. SENSITIVITY AND SPECIFICITY OF CLINICAL FINDINGS IN ADULTS WITH ACUTE SINUSITIS

Population	Finding	Sensitivity (%)	Specificity (%)
Male with Nasal Discharge[38] (positive sinus radiograph)	History of colored nasal discharge	72	52
	Cough	70	44
	Sneezing	70	34
	Poor response to decongestants	41	80
	Maxillary toothache	18	93
	Purulent secretion	51	76
	Sinus tenderness	48	65
	Temperature >38° C	16	85
Emergency ward patients[39] with paranasal symptoms (purulent sinus aspirate)	Purulent rhinorrhea, unilateral predominance	48	—
	Unilateral pain	37	
	Purulent rhinorrhea, bilateral	35	
	Sinus tenderness on percussion	43	
	Pus in nasal cavity	41	

*Superscript numbers indicate chapter references.

Table 39–11. SINUS PUNCTURE TECHNIQUE

1. Anterior nares and area below the inferior turbinate cleansed with an antiseptic solution.
2. Puncture site below the inferior turbinate anesthetized.
3. Medial wall of antrum punctured with 12-guage needle.*
4. Sinus contents aspirated with a syringe or 1 mL normal saline instilled and aspirated if necessary to provide a specimen.†
5. Capped syringe transported promptly to the laboratory for processing.

*Insertion of a plastic catheter through the needle runs the risk of shearing off the end of the catheter in the sinus cavity when the catheter is removed.

†Positioning of the head by flexion of the neck in different directions improves the specimen yield. The normal saline should not contain antibacterial preservatives.

chological stress associated with needle puncture in the facial area.

Sinusitis developing in the hospital setting has been associated with methicillin-sensitive and methicillin-resistant strains of *S. aureus* and with a variety of gram-negative bacteria, including *Pseudomonas aeruginosa, Enterobacter* species, *Klebsiella pneumoniae, Proteus mirabilis,* and *Escherichia coli.*[43-47] Also, *Bacteroides* species, beta-hemolytic streptococci (group A and non–group A). *S. pneumoniae* and *Haemophilus* species have caused nosocomial sinusitis.

TREATMENT

Viral Rhinosinusitis

The treatment of viral rhinosinusitis, with the exception of influenza type A, is primarily based on decongestion and facilitation of mucus drainage. Influenza A should be prevented by vaccination and treated with amantadine or rimantadine. These antivirals are very effective when given within the first 48 hours of an influenza type A illness (see Chapter 14).

Shrinkage of the nasal turbinates with resultant decongestion of the nasal passages can be readily achieved with topically applied drugs such as phenylephrine, oxymetazoline, and xylometazoline. Although the effects of pseudoephedrine and other orally administered decongestants are not as dramatic, these drugs may give more sustained though less immediate decongestion in the nose.[48] Topical decongestant therapy should not be prolonged past 3 or 4 days to avoid rebound nasal congestion from rhinitis medicamentosa.

The effectiveness of decongestants for opening the infundibulum and other sinus drainage passages has not been well studied. How much decongestion by itself can open sinus ostia and facilitate removal of the highly viscous material in the sinus cavity is problematic. The diameter of the small tubular structure composing the infundibulum is limited by the dimensions of its bony walls, which are not subject to decongestant activity. It is not surprising that in one study in which a manometric method was used to study the functional size of the infundibulum in patients with "acute rhinosinusitis," 100 mg of phenylpropanolamine given orally had a minimal, nonsignificant decongestant effect.[49]

Mucoevacuants, including oral guaifenesin,[50] and iodinated glycerol[51, 52] and topical acetylcysteine,[53] are available

to reduce mucus viscosity. These drugs have been evaluated primarily for their effectiveness in clearing lower airway secretions. There is little information on what, if any, benefit they may provide for mobilizing viscous material in the sinus cavity. Because of their safety and theoretic value, it seems reasonable to try them in patients with acute sinusitis, although topical application of medication into the nose is unlikely to have much effect on secretions in the sinus cavity. Other supportive treatments should include hydration and analgesics as needed for headache, fever, and malaise.

Information on the value of topical steroids for treating viral rhinosinusitis (common cold and influenzal illness) is limited. In one controlled, blinded clinical trial, 168 μg of intranasal beclomethasone given twice a day had little if any effect on nasal symptoms and nasal mucus secretion weights in young adults with experimental rhinovirus colds.[54]

Bacterial Sinusitis

The therapeutic management of acute bacterial sinusitis is based primarily on giving an antimicrobial drug with an appropriate spectrum of antibacterial activity at an adequate dose and for a sufficient period (Table 39–9). The bacterial causes of acute sinusitis and their resistance patterns were discussed previously. No one antibiotic currently available covers the entire etiologic spectrum of acute community-acquired sinusitis, including methicillin-resistant *S. aureus* and highly resistant *S. pneumoniae.* However, several antibiotics have been proven effective against the important bacterial causes of acute community-acquired sinusitis in clinical studies using pretreatment and posttreatment sinus puncture for proof of bacteriologic cure.[40] These drugs and the doses used are shown in Table 39–12. It should be remembered that resistant pneumococci and staphylococci may not be covered by these drugs.

A duration of therapy of 10–14 days is recommended. Ten days of treatment was used in the sinus puncture studies with approximately 90% bacteriologic cure rates, but the sinus aspiration itself may have had some therapeutic value. Also, in some cases, low concentrations of viable bacteria were still present in the sinus cavity after 10 days of treatment. Therefore, a 2-week course of treatment may be advisable. There is little or no information from clinical trials employing pretreatment and posttreatment sinus aspirate cultures on which to base recommendations for longer or shorter courses of antimicrobial treatment. Other important considerations in the selection of antimicrobial agents are the patient's allergic history and the cost of the drug. In the small percentage of patients who do not show a satisfactory response to initial treatment, CT examination of the sinuses and diagnostic sinus aspiration for bacterial culture and sensitivities should be considered as the next steps in management.

Attempts to measure antibiotic concentrations in the sinus cavity have produced inconsistent results.[55, 56] Also, the concentrations measured have not correlated well with bacteriologic cure rates based on sinus aspirate culture.[57] The value of pretreatment and posttreatment sinus puncture cultures in evaluating the effectiveness of antibiotic treatment is supported by several examples. Clindamycin was not effective

Table 39–12. RESULTS OF ANTIMICROBIAL TREATMENT STUDIES[40]

Study	Agent	Dosage	No. of Bacteriologic Cures/No. of Evaluations (%)
Charlottesville, Virginia	Trimethroprim/sulfamethoxazole	Double strength twice daily	18/19 (95)
	Cefuroxime axetil	250 mg twice daily	36/38 (95)
	Amoxicillin/clavulanate	500/125 mg three times daily	11/12 (92)
	Loracarbef	400 mg twice daily	13/14 (93)
Nordic Multicenter Trial	Cefixime	200 mg bid	105/115 (91)

Pretreatment and posttreatment sinus aspirates were obtained from all patients.
*Superscript numbers indicate chapter references.

in eradicating *H. influenzae* infection in the sinus cavity in one study, and inadequate doses of cefaclor (1 g and 1.5 g) were ineffective in two other studies.[40, 58] Because of the self-limited nature of most cases of acute community-acquired sinusitis, clinical observation alone would have been unlikely to have detected these failures.

Other antibiotic regimens are not currently recommended. Azithromycin has not undergone testing with pretreatment and posttreatment sinus aspirate cultures in patients with acute community-acquired sinusitis, and thus, effective dosing regimens have not been established. Clarithromycin has been shown effective for sensitive strains of *S. pneumoniae* in acute community-acquired sinusitis, but pretreatment and posttreatment sinus aspirate cultures results for *H. influenzae* have not been made available to the author. Studies of quinolones employing pretreatment and posttreatment sinus aspirate cultures are in progress and will be published soon. Some of these antibiotics may prove useful because of their activity against intermediately resistant strains of *S. pneumoniae*.

A recent study of the effectiveness of a three-day course of trimethroprim-sulfamethoxazole in the treatment of radiographically diagnosed acute community-acquired sinusitis gave an unacceptably low rate ($\simeq$ 75%) of clinical cure and a 12% relapse rate.[59] The study did not employ sinus aspirate cultures before (or after) treatment. It would be expected from previous sinus puncture studies[40] that approximately half of the 39 cases receiving the 3-day course of treatment were nonbacterial (negative aspirate culture), leaving only 20 true bacterial cases. If the nine reported failures were in the latter group, then the real clinical cure rate would be no better than 55%, which is an even less acceptable therapeutic outcome. That the reported failures were in bacterial cases seems reasonable, because the nonbacterial (presumed viral) cases would have recovered promptly without antibiotic treatment, as observed in an earlier study.[1]

Effective treatment of acute nosocomial sinusitis requires selection of antimicrobials with a broad spectrum of activity against gram-negative bacteria and *S. aureus* and/or treatment based on results of bacterial culture and antimicrobial sensitivities from a sinus aspirate. Nasal tubes and packing should be removed when possible. In sinus infections in which there is suspected extension into surrounding structures, surgical intervention is usually required (see Chapter 42). Surgery is also indicated in cases of sinusitis of fungal etiology (see Chapter 43).

Supportive treatment of acute bacterial sinusitis is based on the same principles of decongestion and mucoevacuation

discussed for the treatment of viral rhinosinusitis. The approach to the treatment of acute bacterial sinusitis is summarized in Table 39–9. There is no convincing evidence that topical steroids are useful in the treatment of acute bacterial sinusitis, and they are not recommended as part of routine management.

References

1. Gwaltney JM Jr, Phillips CD, Miller RD, Riker DK: Computed tomographic study of the common cold. N Engl J Med 1994; 330: 25–30.
2. Graney DO, Rice DH: Anatomy (paranasal sinuses). In: Cummings CH (ed): Otolaryngology Head Neck Surgery. St Louis: Mosby–Year Book, 1993, pp 901–906.
3. Tos M, Mogensen C: Mucus production in chronic maxillary sinusitis: A quantitative histopathological study. Acta Otolaryngol (Stockh) 1984; 97: 151–159.
4. Morgensen C, Tos M: Quantitative histology of the maxillary sinus. Rhinology 1977; 55: 129.
5. Morgensen C, Tos M: Quantitative histology of the normal sphenoid sinus. Rhinology 1978; 56: 203.
6. Mogensen C, Tos M: Density of goblet cells in the normal adult human nasal septum. Anat Anz 1977; 141: 237.
7. Kim KC: Epithelial goblet cell secretion. In: Takishima T, Shimura S (eds): Airway Secretion: Physiological Bases for the Control of Mucous Hypersecretion. (Lung Biology in Health and Disease, vol 72.) New York: Marcel Dekker, 1994, pp 433–449.
8. Gwaltney JM Jr: The common cold. In: Mandell GL, Douglas RG Jr, Bennett JE (eds): Principles and Practice of Infectious Diseases, 3rd ed. New York: Churchill Livingstone, 1990, pp 489–493.
9. Dingle JH, Badger GF, Jordan WS Jr: Illness in the Home: A Study of 25,000 Illnesses in a Group of Cleveland Families. Cleveland: The Press of Western Reserve University, 1964.
10. Berg O, Carenfelt C, Rystedt G, Änggård A: Occurrence of asymptomatic sinusitis in common cold and other acute ENT infections. Rhinology 1986; 24: 223–225.
11. Gable CB, Jones JK, Lian JF, et al.: Chronic sinusitis: Temporal occurrence and relationship to medical claims for upper respiratory infections and allergic rhinitis. Pharmacoepidemiol Drug Safety 1994; 3: 337–349.
12. Gwaltney JM Jr, Hayden FG: The nose and infection. In: Proctor DF, Andersen I (eds): The Nose: Upper Airway Physiology and the Atmospheric Environment. Amsterdam: Elsevier Biomedical, 1982, pp 399–422.
13. Gwaltney JM Jr: Rhinovirus. In: Mandell GL, Bennett JE, Dolin R (eds): Principles and Practice of Infectious Diseases, 4th ed. New York: Churchill Livingstone, 1995, pp 1656–1663.
14. Hamory BH, Sande MA, Sydnor A Jr, et al.: Etiology and antimicrobial therapy of acute maxillary sinusitis. J Infect Dis 1979; 139: 197–202.
15. Evans FO Jr, Sydnor JB, Moore WEC, et al.: Sinusitis of the maxillary antrum. N Engl J Med 1975; 293: 735–739.
16. Urdal K, Berdal P: The microbial flora in 81 cases of maxillary sinusitis. Acta Otolaryngol (Stockh) 1949; 37: 20–25.
17. Björkwall T: Bacteriological examinations in maxillary sinusitis: Bacterial flora of the maxillary antrum. Acta Otolaryngol Suppl (Stockh) 1950; 83: 33–58.

18. Lystad A, Berdal P, Lund-Iverson L: The bacterial flora of sinusitis with an in vitro study of the bacterial resistance to antibiotics. Acta Otolaryngol Suppl (Stockh) 1964; 188: 390–399.

19. Rantanen T, Arvilommi H: Double-blind trial of doxicycline in acute maxillary sinusitis: A clinical and bacteriological study. Acta Otolaryngol (Stockh) 1973; 76: 58–62.

20. Axelsson A, Brorson JE: The correlation between bacteriological findings in the nose and maxillary sinus in acute maxillary sinusitis. Laryngoscope 1973; 83: 2003–2011.

21. Jousimies-Somer HR, Savolainen S, Ylikoski JS: Bacteriological findings of acute maxillary sinusitis in young adults. J Clin Microbiol 1988; 26: 1919–1925.

22. Jacobs MR: Treatment and diagnosis of infections caused by drug-resistant *Streptococcus pneumoniae*. Clin Infect Dis 1992; 15: 119–127.

23. Appelbaum PC: Antimicrobial resistance in *Streptococcus pneumoniae*: An overview. Clin Infect Dis 1992; 15: 77–83.

24. Friedland IR, McCracken GH Jr: Management of infections caused by antibiotic-resistant *Streptococcus pneumoniae*. N Engl J Med 1994; 331: 377–382.

25. Pankuch GA, Visalli MA, Jacobs MR, Appelbaum PC: Activities of oral and parenteral agents against penicillin-susceptible and -resistant pneumococci. Antimicrob Agents Chemother 1995; 39: 1499–1504.

26. Stevens MH: Primary fungal infections of the paranasal sinuses. Am J Otolaryngol 1981; 2: 348–357.

27. Romett J, Newman R: Aspergillosis of the nose and paranasal sinuses. Laryngoscope 1982; 92: 764–766.

28. Rinaldi MG: Invasive aspergillosis. Rev Infect Dis 1983; 5: 1061–1077.

29. Kern ME, Uecker FA: Maxillary sinus infection caused by the homobasidiomycetous fungus *Schizophyllum commune*. J Clin Microbiol 1986; 23: 1001–1005.

30. Morriss FH Jr, Spock A: Intracranial aneurysm secondary to mycotic orbital and sinus infection: Report of a case implicating penicillium as an opportunistic fungus. Am J Dis Child 1970; 119: 357–362.

31. Zieske LA, Kipke RD, Hamill R: Dematiaceous fungal sinusitis. Otolaryngol Head Neck Surg 1991; 105: 567–577.

32. Padhye AA, Ajello L, Wieden MA, Steinbronn KK: Phaeohyphomycosis of the nasal sinuses caused by a new species of *Exserohilum*. J Clin Microbiol 1986; 24: 245–249.

33. MacMillan RH III, Cooper PH, Body BA, Mills AS: Allergic fungal sinusitis due to *Curvularia lunata*. Hum Pathol 1987; 18: 960–964.

34. Killingsworth SM, Wetmore SJ: *Curvularia/Drechslera* sinusitis. Laryngoscope 1990; 100: 932–937.

35. Aviv J, Lawson W, Bottone E, et al.: Multiple intracranial mucoceles associated with *Phaeophyphomycosis* of the paranasal sinuses. Arch Otolaryngol Head Neck Surg 1990; 116: 1210–1213.

36. Morgan MA, Wilson WR, Neel B III, Roberts GD: Fungal sinusitis in healthy and immunocompromised individuals. Am J Clin Pathol 1984; 82: 597–601.

37. Gwaltney JM Jr, Hendley JO, Simon G, Jordan WS Jr: Rhinovirus infections in an industrial population. II: Characteristics of illness and antibody response. JAMA 1967; 202: 494–500.

38. Williams JW Jr, Simel DL, Roberts L, Samsa GP: Clinical evaluation for sinusitis: Making the diagnosis by history and physical examination. Ann Intern Med 1992; 117: 705–710.

39. Berg O, Carenfelt C: Analysis of symptoms and clinical signs in the maxillary sinus empyema. Acta Otolaryngol (Stockh) 1988; 105: 343–349.

40. Gwaltney JM Jr, Scheld WM, Sande MA, Sydnor A: The microbial etiology and antimicrobial therapy of adults with acute community-acquired sinusitis: A fifteen-year experience at the University of Virginia and review of other selected studies. J Allergy Clin Immunol 1992; 90: 457–462.

41. Jousimies-Somer HR, Savolainen S, Ylikoski JS: Comparison of the nasal bacterial floras in two groups of healthy subjects in patients with acute maxillary sinusitis. J Clin Microbiol 1989; 27: 2736–2743.

42. Wald ER, Milmoe GJ, Bowen A, et al.: Acute maxillary sinusitis in children. N Engl J Med 1981; 304: 749–754.

43. Pope TL, Stelling CB, Leitner YB: Maxillary sinusitis after nasotracheal intubation. South Med J 1981; 74: 610–612.

44. Via-Reque E, Rattenborg CC: Prolonged oro- or nasotracheal intubation. Crit Care Med 1981; 9: 637–639.

45. Caplan ES, Hoyt NJ: Nosocomial sinusitis. JAMA 1982; 247: 639–641.

46. Deutschman CS, Wilton PB, Sinow J, et al.: Paranasal sinusitis: A common complication of nasotracheal intubation in neurosurgical patients. Neurosurgery 1985; 17: 296–299.

47. Linden BE, Aguilar EA, Allen SJ: Sinusitis in the nasotracheally intubated patient. Arch Otolaryngol Head Neck Surg 1988; 114: 860–861.

48. Dressler WE, Myers T, London SJ, et al.: A system of rhinomanometry in the clinical evaluation of nasal decongestants. Ann Otol Rhinol Laryngol 1977; 86: 310.

49. Aust R, Drettner B, Falck B: Studies of the effect of peroral fenylpropanolamin on the functional size of the human maxillary ostium. Acta Otolaryngol 1979; 88: 455–458.

50. Kuhn JJ, Hendley JO, Adams KF, et al.: Antitussive effect of guaifenesin in young adults with natural colds: Objective and subjective assessment. Chest 1982; 82: 713–718.

51. Petty TL: The national mucolytic study: Results of a randomized double-blind placebo-controlled study of iodinated glycerol in chronic obstructive bronchitis. Chest 1990; 97: 75–83.

52. Pavia D, Agnew JE, Glassman JM, et al.: Effects of iodopropylidene glycerol on tracheobronchial clearance in stable, chronic bronchitic patients. Eur J Respir Dis 1985; 67: 177–184.

53. Ziment I: Acetylcysteine: A drug that is much more than a mucolytic. Biomed Pharmacother 1988; 42: 513–520.

54. Farr BM, Gwaltney JM Jr, Hendley JO, et al.: A randomized controlled trial of glucocorticoid prophylaxis against experimental rhinovirus infection. J Infect Dis 1990; 162: 1173–1177.

55. Gullers K: Penicillin in paranasal sinus secretions. Chemotherapy 1969; 14: 303–307.

56. Carenfelt C, Eneroth C-M, Lundberg C, et al.: Evaluation of the antibiotic effect of treatment of maxillary sinusitis. Scand J Infect Dis 1975; 7: 259–264.

57. Scheld WM, Sydnor A Jr, Farr B, et al.: Comparison of cyclacillin with amoxicillin in the therapy of acute maxillary sinusitis. Antimicrob Agents Chemother 1986; 30: 350–353.

58. Gwaltney JM Jr, Sydnor A, Sande MA: Etiology and antimicrobial treatment of acute sinusitis. Ann Otol Rhinol Laryngol 1981; 90: 68–71.

59. Williams JW Jr, Holleman DR Jr, Samsa GP, Simel DL: Randomized controlled trial of 3 vs 10 days of trimethoprim/sulfamethoxazole for acute maxillary sinusitis. JAMA 1995; 273: 1015–1021.

Chronic Sinusitis

▼

Most of the available literature on sinusitis has targeted acute sinusitis in evaluating microbiology and pharmacologic treatment. Information for these same parameters on chronic sinusitis is much scantier. In the past 10 years, diagnosis and surgical treatment of chronic sinusitis have received considerable attention, with little research being done into the epidemiology, natural history, etiology, histopathology, and medical treatment. In fact, no guidelines exist for the appropriate medical treatment of chronic sinusitis, just recommendations.[1] With changes in the medical practice environment in place and on the horizon, it will become increasingly important to develop appropriate guidelines for medical and surgical treatment of chronic sinusitis based on scientific data and experience. The problem of sinusitis is immense for our patients. Sinusitis brought almost 25 million patients to see physicians in 1993–1994.[2] Prescribed medications for upper respiratory infection (URI) amounted to an expense of 200 million dollars in 1992. Of the 25 million people who saw a physician in 1993–1994, 97% received a prescription. Up to 20% of these patients were offered a surgical solution. Gliklich and Metson[3] have shown that the amount of morbidity related to chronic sinusitis rivals that for heart disease and arthritis as the major causes of missed work, school, and social activities. This chapter attempts to inform the reader about the current state of chronic sinusitis from a medical and surgical therapy standpoint.

DEFINITIONS

No uniform definitions have been decided upon for chronic sinusitis, but recommendations are available from the American Academy of Otolaryngology–Head and Neck Surgery (Rhinology and Paranasal Sinus Committee) and the International Conference on Sinus Disease: Terminology, Staging, Therapy, held July 24–25, 1993, in Princeton, New Jersey. The two groups have agreed upon the following definitions.[2]

- **Acute sinusitis:** An acutely symptomatic bacterial sinus infection in which symptoms persist no longer than 6–8 weeks or fewer than four episodes occur per year consisting of acute symptoms of 10 days' duration that resolve with medical therapy.

- **Chronic sinusitis:** Persistent disease that cannot be alleviated by observation or previous medical therapy alone, with evidence of mucosal hyperplasia on radiographic evaluation.

- **Chronic sinusitis in the adult:** At least 8 weeks of persistent signs and symptoms or four episodes per year of

recurrent acute bacterial sinusitis, each lasting at least 10 days, in association with persistent changes on computerized tomography (CT). In the case of the use of medical therapy, CT changes should be present 4 weeks after medical therapy without intervening acute infection.

- **Chronic sinusitis in children:** 12 weeks of persisting signs and symptoms or six episodes per year of recurrent acute bacterial sinusitis, each lasting at least 10 days, in association with changes in a CT scan. When medical therapy is used, persistent change on CT 4 weeks after medical therapy without intervening infection should be noted.

- **Recurrent acute sinusitis:** Repeated acute episodes of bacterial sinusitis that resolve with medical therapy leaving no significant mucosal change (damage).

Without appropriate definitions, an understanding of chronic sinusitis and how it relates to acute and recurrent acute sinusitis is not possible. These definitions relate directly to the therapy used for treatment and are important for guideline development.

PATHOPHYSIOLOGY

A normal healthy sinus requires a balance of multiple factors. Mucus secretion amount and composition must be normal. The mucus secretions, enzymes, and immunoglobulins must be appropriate to deal with microorganisms, antigens, and pollutants that are trapped in the mucus blanket.[4] An intact mucociliary system is most important for the clearance of bacteria, debris, and other organic matter gaining entrance to the sinus. The infundibula and ostia have to be patent to achieve drainage. Disease occurs when mucus becomes static secondary to overproduction or anatomic obstruction causing stagnation, pH changes, poor gas exchange, and, eventually, mucociliary paralysis and disruption.[4] Bacterial growth takes place in a closed-off sinus cavity (obstructed environment). The retained secretions and developing bacterial infection produce inflammation, causing mucosal edema and swelling that further obstruct drainage. Changes of pressure (and gas) in the nasal passages and sinuses are believed to contribute to ingress of bacteria and development of infection.[4] Positive pressure results from nasal obstruction due to congestion of the turbinates. Infundibular and ostial occlusion contributes to negative pressure (suction) in the sinus cavities.[4] Bacteria enter the sinuses by a pushing, or positive pressure, on the nasal side and a suction, or negative pressure, on the sinus side. Once ostial occlusion occurs, there is no gaseous exchange in the sinus cavity, oxygen is absorbed, and an anaerobic environment is created.[4]

Patients who have abnormal mucociliary function or are immunocompromised have major problems with maintaining healthy sinus physiologic function and are much more susceptible to acute and chronic sinus infection.

Sinusitis that occurs after sinus surgery is still often related to inadequate drainage of the sinus cavity. Uncontrolled healing with scarring and obstruction, failure to remove the uncinate process, failure to locate the natural ostia and include it in the surgical antrostomy, middle turbinate lateralization with maxillary or frontal sinus obstruction, walled-off posterior ethmoids, and a blocked sphenoid sinus are causes of inadequate postsurgical drainage. Mucociliary transport is altered, secretions are blocked and become static, and patients develop acute or persistent infections.

It should be recognized that sinus surgery, although helpful in unblocking drainage areas of the sinus, may sometimes interfere with the anatomy and physiology necessary for normal functioning, such as interrupting normal drainage pathways with scarring. Once this has occurred, affected patients are still subject to occasional bouts of sinusitis. The second group of patients who continue to have postsurgical problems are those who are immunocompromised, have mucociliary dysfunction, or are metabolically compromised, e.g., by diabetes or thyroid disease. Persistent crusting and/or purulent drainage is a cause of postoperative pathophysiology. This may be associated with specific infections, such as cystic fibrosis strains of *Pseudomonas aeruginosa* or strains of *Staphylococcus aureus*. Many of these patients are additionally compromised owing to complete turbinate (inferior and middle) removal, which creates an atrophic dysfunctional mucosa. Sinusitis in this latter group of patients is often the most difficult to control medically and surgically.

HISTOPATHOLOGY

The mucosa of the sinus undergoes several levels of histopathologic change, as noted here. Beginning with localized acute edema and loss of cilia, progression of disease continues to bacterial infection with influx of inflammatory cells and mucosal hypertrophy if infection is not reversed.[4] Although most mucosal changes are reversible with adequate treatment, in some cases, bony hypertrophy with sinus contraction and eventual mucosal fibrosis leads to so-called irreversible or irretrievable chronic sinusitis.[4] Today, this entity is rarely seen, because diagnostic techniques and medical and/or surgical treatment allow for earlier diagnosis and treatment.

Two studies have been reported that looked at changes occurring in the nasal cavity and sinuses in chronic sinusitis. Milbrath and colleagues[5] examined the middle turbinate by biopsy in various stages of sinusitis and found that the histopathology changed in direct relationship to the extent of disease. Stage 1 sinusitis had minimal inflammation and edema of the turbinate, whereas stage 4 often showed marked inflammation, edema, and polypoid degeneration.[5] Goldwyn and colleagues[6] showed that the histologic appearance of sinuses differed between patients with and without

sinusitis and that the degree (severity) of inflammation was variable and unpredictable. For instance, a patient may have a localized area of intense inflammation with the remainder of the sinuses showing mild inflammation. Anterior ethmoid disease with osteomeatal complex involvement and all other sinuses being normal is an example. Diffuse disease with a low level of inflammation was also observed, such as is noted with minimal mucosal thickening in multiple sinuses.[6]

Studies are available that nicely show histologic change in the mucus blanket and cilia related to chronic sinusitis, cystic fibrosis, and previous surgery.[7] In cystic fibrosis, mucus consistency and ciliary dysfunction are responsible for chronic sinusitis.

MICROBIOLOGY

The microbiology of chronic sinusitis is not well understood, unlike that of acute sinusitis. Factors that complicate research into this area are the precise and accurate classification of study groups, the need to perform sinus aspiration to collect uncontaminated specimens for culture, and microbiologic testing in patients who have usually received multiple courses of antibiotics during the course of their illness.[8–11] These factors have led to confusion about which organisms are truly pathogenic in chronic sinusitis.

Chronic sinusitis has been associated with a mixed flora of anaerobic and aerobic organisms, depending on which study is quoted. Some studies have recovered anaerobic bacteria, but other studies have not confirmed these results.[12] Muntz and Lusk[13] cultured ethmoid mucosal specimens obtained at surgery from children and found mainly alpha-hemolytic *Streptococcus* (23%) and *S. aureus* (19%) as single organisms noted, respectively. Thirty percent of specimens grew multiple organisms. Another study of a small group of children with chronic sinusitis and allergies found *Moraxella (Branhamella) catarrhalis* most commonly, with 25% of patients having polymicrobial infection.[14] Orobello and colleagues,[15] in another study using surgical specimens from the ethmoid in children, found *Staphylococcus epidermidis* and viridans streptococci to predominate. In adults, a similarly confusing picture is noted. Frederick and Braude[16] recovered anaerobic bacteria in 52% and aerobic bacteria in 43% of their subjects. A Finnish study by Karma and colleagues,[17] in patients with chronic maxillary sinusitis, found a polymicrobial flora with only *Haemophilus influenzae* showing consistent heavy growth. Doyle and Woodham[18] noted in chronic maxillary sinusitis that anaerobes and viridans streptococci predominated. In chronic ethmoid sinusitis, coagulase-negative staphylococci (70%) and streptococci (33%) predominated, with no anaerobes cultured. In a subset of patients with chronic sinusitis, *P. aeruginosa* and *S. aureus* appear to have a definitely pathogenic role, whereas in most patients with chronic disease, the pathogenic role of ongoing bacterial infection is by no means clear.[8, 18]

Some experts consider antibiotic treatment a mainstay of therapy in chronic sinusitis, but there is abundant evidence from experience that antibiotic treatment alone does not cure the disease in most cases.[8, 10, 19, 20] This evidence indicates that the ongoing pathologic process in chronic sinusitis is not due solely to bacterial infection.

Patients with chronic sinusitis also have acute exacerbations. Evans and colleagues[19] in adults and Wald and colleagues[21] in children demonstrated a spectrum of bacteria that closely resembled that seen with acute sinusitis, with *Streptococcus pneumoniae* and *Haemophilus influenzae* predominating.[19, 21]

Additionally, the microbiology of postsurgical sinusitis has been investigated. The microbiologic flora includes gram-negative organisms such as *Enterobacter* and *Pseudomonas*.[22, 23] Although this flora may on occasion represent a true bacterial infection requiring intravenous antibiotics, it is this author's experience that often, these organisms represent contamination due to postsurgical nasal debris and/or exposed or devitalized bone. Patients who truly have infection with *Pseudomonas* species and *S. aureus* are often the most difficult to cure.

DIAGNOSIS

History

Patients with chronic sinusitis most commonly present with nasal obstruction, drainage, and postnasal drip usually of several months' duration. Nighttime cough, headache, bad breath, and loss of smell can also be present. In children, cough and bad breath are more prominent (Table 40–1). A history of previous sinus surgery, of extensive disease, and of being immunocompromised, asthmatic, or allergic are risk factors for severe and intractable chronic sinusitis.

Physical Signs

A complete head and neck examination should be performed with special focus on the nasal cavity. Anterior rhinoscopy is sufficient to identify only anterior disease and septal deviation. Examination of the nasal cavity using the otoscope may identify disease in the middle turbinate–anterior meatal areas and is very helpful in small children, in whom endoscopy cannot be performed. The examination of choice is flexible or rigid endoscopy of the nose and nasopharynx.[24] Although flexible endoscopy does not provide as good illumination and breadth of examination as rigid endoscopy, it nevertheless provides a more thorough, less painful examination, particularly in children, because more of the examination can be performed. The examiner should look for anatomic abnormalities, mucosal changes, purulence, septal deformities, masses, and other nasopharyngeal pathology.

Every patient suspected of having chronic sinusitis should undergo an endoscopic examination prior to any consideration for surgery in order to qualify and quantify anatomic abnormalities. This is especially important in the chronic sinusitis patient being considered for surgical revision. It is important to note that a normal-appearing nasal cavity on endoscopy does not rule out chronic sinusitis, and these patients should undergo CT scanning for definitive diagnosis. It is important that the clinical picture correlate with imaging findings.

Imaging

Numerous studies have indicated the need for appropriate imaging to establish the diagnosis of chronic sinusitis. Coronal CT scan represents the radiologic gold standard in the diagnosis of chronic sinusitis.[25–27] The CT scan is the most sensitive, economical, and noninvasive means of diagnosing disease in the sinus cavity and upper reaches of the nasal passages. With the availability of fast, low-cost CT screening using 5-mm cuts in the coronal view, much more information can be gained than from plain films and magnetic resonance imaging (MRI) without exposing the patient to needless radiation. Axial CT scans are often easier to obtain in children. Coronal CT scans can be reconstructed from axial views if necessary. Full 2- to 3-mm cut sinus CT scans are very helpful in difficult or complicated cases requiring surgical revision. Sagittal reconstruction can be helpful for the frontal recess. Fungal sinusitis often has a typical mottled appearance, especially in the maxillary sinus. Reducing the

Table 40–1. SIGNS AND SYMPTOMS OF UPPER RESPIRATORY INFECTION, ALLERGIES, AND SINUSITIS

	Cold	Allergies	Acute Sinusitis	Chronic Sinusitis
Symptoms				
Runny, watery nose	Yes	Yes	Uncommon	Uncommon
Stuffy nose and congestion	Yes	Yes	Yes	Yes
Facial pain	Possible	No	Yes	Possible
Pain or pressure over sinus	Often	Possible	Yes	Possible
Headache	Often	No	Yes	Possible
Bad breath[1]	No	No	Yes	Yes
Fever	No	No	Not common in adults	No
Cough[1]	Possible	Uncommon	Common in children	Often
Other Clues	Viral infection that lasts 5–7 days; generally not severe enough to send patient to bed with fever and pressure.	Itchy eyes; can be either chronic or brought on by exposure to allergens, such as certain foods, dust, pollen, or animal dander; postnasal drip.	Lasts up to 3 months; caused by bacteria; cough; thick yellow or green puslike nasal drainage; postnasal drip.	Lasts 3 months or longer; primary role of bacteria unclear; cough; postnasal drip; fatigue.

[1]Symptoms especially noted in children.

windows to 100–300 Hounsfield units is helpful to delineate the fungal infection. CT scans in patients requiring revision surgery can reveal surgically altered anatomy along with the severity of the sinusitis. Small mucoceles may be missed in these types of patients unless suspicions are raised by physician experience or examination. Sinus radiographic abnormalities may be seen in asymptomatic patients because of previous colds or other undetermined causes and do not require treatment.[28–31]

MRI is too costly to be used in the routine diagnosis of chronic sinusitis and does not show fine anatomic detail as well as CT.[32] Its main benefit is to distinguish sinusitis from tumor or to help in the diagnosis of fungal sinusitis.[33, 34] The T_2-weighted image is often the more decisive in diagnosing tumor. Fungal lesions that are dehydrated may appear as a normal image or with a rim of mucosal thickening surrounding a radiolucent area. Correlation with other T_1-weighted or T_2-weighted images and contrast-enhanced sections is helpful. MRI is also important for the evaluation of extranasal/extrasinus sinusitis or mucocele.

In summary, the diagnosis of chronic sinusitis depends upon the history, physical examination including endoscopic evaluation, and CT scanning. This is the appropriate database needed in order to take the next step for the patient, which is selection of appropriate therapy.

THERAPY

Medical Therapy: Antibiotics

Unlike acute sinusitis, for which antibiotic therapy aimed at specific groups of organisms is usually successful in uncomplicated cases, chronic sinusitis does not usually respond with permanent or sustained improvement to antibiotic therapy. In using antimicrobial treatment of chronic sinusitis, there is no consensus about length of treatment, which organisms need coverage, and which antibiotics are most effective.

Rachalefsky and colleagues,[35] in a double-blind study of 84 children with chronic sinusitis, found amoxicillin more effective than trimethoprim-sulfamethoxazole (TMP/SMX) and erythromycin. They also found all antibiotic groups superior to a decongestant/antihistamine alone. Of note, only 2 patients showed no response to two consecutive 3-week courses of antibiotics, and sinus puncture showed resistant organisms. Of interest, Dohlman and colleagues[20] did a similar comparison but used amoxicillin-clavulanate as one of the drugs. They, however, found antibiotics to have no advantage over decongestants in subacute sinusitis. These studies contradict each other. Huck and colleagues[36] described 15 adult patients with chronic sinusitis treated with either amoxicillin or cefaclor in whom there was no difference in clinical response but only 56% improvement after a 10-day course of antibiotics. Another study by Gehenno and Rohen[37] found ofloxacin effective in 94% of patients with chronic sinusitis. Both of these studies were not controlled, and organisms were not identified by puncture technique (Table 40–2).

No studies have been conducted to examine the question of optimum length of treatment. For instance, in the Huck study noted previously, antibiotics were given for only 10 days.[36] A study by Meltzer and colleagues[38] that looked at a 3-week course of antibiotics with or without topical nasal steroid showed that 33% of patients developed a recurrence of symptoms after antibiotics were stopped. The Rachalefsky study showed all but 2 patients to respond to two 3-week courses of antibiotics.[35]

In summary, it is not clear what are the best antibiotic choices for treating patients with chronic sinusitis nor what is the optimum duration of therapy. A course of treatment of 3–6 weeks seems reasonable but is not based on the results of adequate clinical testing.

Husfeldt and colleagues[39] compared ofloxacin with erythromycin for acute and chronic sinusitis and found a 95% cure rate with ofloxacin after 14 days. In contradiction, another study employing ampicillin-sulbactam for chronic sinusitis demonstrated only 45% improvement.[40]

Maisel and Kimberly[41] showed cefaclor effective for chronic maxillary sinusitis when combined with a Caldwell-Luc procedure. Cefotetan given intramuscularly has been reported to have excellent results in chronic sinusitis.[42] Cephalexin was reported to have an 83% cure rate in 69 patients with acute and chronic sinusitis, a finding that flies in the face of most antibiotic recommendations for chronic sinusitis.[43]

Ciprofloxacin alone and ciprofloxacin versus amoxicillin-clavulanate given for 10 days were evaluated for chronic sinusitis and found to have clinical success rates of 75% and 60% for ciprofloxacin and 50% for amoxicillin clavulanate.[44, 45] Ciprofloxacin was well tolerated compared with amoxicillin-clavulanate. Otten and colleagues,[46] in one of two interesting studies in children, showed that 24 of 26 children followed for 6 years with chronic sinusitis improved over time with medical therapy alone and by age 7 years stabilized their sinusitis. The second study comparing sinus irrigation with antibiotic treatment in children showed no difference between treatments for chronic sinusitis.[47]

Ghandi and colleagues[48] looked at 86 children with recurrent acute and chronic sinusitis to see whether antibiotic prophylaxis was worthwhile if used over 1 year; they found that 74% of patients experienced a 50% or greater reduction in sinus infections in comparison with the previous year, including children with immunodeficiency. Although this approach is a consideration for this particular type of patient, the idea of prophylaxis is at present being reconsidered because of the increase in resistant *S. pneumoniae*.

In summary, the bacteriology of chronic sinusitis has been shown to be variable, with polymicrobial anaerobic and aerobic organisms present. Also, the role of antibiotic therapy is confusing. Data as to which antibiotics if any are most effective in providing significant clinical benefit are not available for either children or adults, nor is optimal treatment duration established. The literature, however, does give some insights. It is apparent that in those studies in which antibiotics were given for only 10–14 days, the clinical "cure" rate was about 60%; the few studies in which antibiotics were given 4–6 weeks reported improvement in 80% or more of patients. Therefore, one can extrapolate from this information that antibiotic treatment should be given for a minimum of 3 weeks for chronic sinusitis. Antibiotic choice is another matter. Although one would think that antibiotics with good anaerobic coverage perform

Table 40–2. ANTIBIOTIC TRIALS IN PATIENTS WITH CHRONIC SINUSITIS

Study	Number	Inclusion	Antibiotics and Other Modalities	Dose and Duration	How Controlled	How Evaluated	Results
Adults							
Huck et al.[36]	108 (15 chronic sinusitis)	Acute/recurrent chronic sinusitis	Amoxicillin Cefaclor	500 mg tid 10 days 500 mg bid	Double-blind, randomized	(1) clinical symptoms; (2) radiologic clearance; (3) bacterial eradication	Amoxicillin = cefaclor 33% chronic, 50% recurrent acute "cure"
Gehanno and Rohen[37]	198	Chronic sinusitis	Ofloxacin	200 mg bid 10 days	Uncontrolled	Clinical symptoms, bacteriologic sampling	40% improved, 53% cured
Meltzer et al.[38]	116	Maxillary sinusitis, chronic	Amoxicillin-clavulanate with/without topical nasal steroids	3 weeks 500 mg tid	Multicenter double-blind, randomized, controlled	(1) clinical symptoms; (2) radiography	Amoxicillin/ clavulanate improved sinusitis in both groups (+ stat significant)
Husfeldt et al[39]	280 total; 136 ofloxacin, 144 erythromycin	Acute exacerbation chronic sinusitis	Ofloxacin vs Erythromycin	400 mg 14 days 500 mg bid	Double-blind, uncontrolled	Clinical symptoms	Ofloxacin: 58% cured, 37% improved Erythromycin: 62% cured, 33% improved
Nicolett et al.[40]	22	Acute/chronic sinusitis	Ampicillin-sulbactam	1.5 gm bid IV 5–10 days	Uncontrolled	Clinical symptoms, bacterial eradication	100% bacterial eradication 55% clinical recovery 45% improved findings
Maisel and Kimberly[41]	50	Chronic maxillary sinusitis	Cefaclor with antrostomy vs. Caldwell-Luc procedure and cefaclor	250 mg tid 7–10 days PO	Uncontrolled	Clinical symptoms	Antrostomy or Caldwell-Luc 85%–90% curative if covered by cefaclor Worth of cefaclor vs. placebo not evaluated

Study	No.	Condition	Drug	Dose	Study Design	Outcome Measures	Results
Bassetti et al.[42]	20	Chronic maxillary sinusitis	Cefotetan	1 gm bid 7 days	Uncontrolled	Clinical symptoms	19/20 subjective and objective symptoms gone
Schaefer and Ronis[43]	69	Acute/chronic maxillary sinusitis	Cephalexin	250 mg 10 days qid / 500 mg bid 9 days	Uncontrolled / Uncontrolled	Clinical symptoms, bacterial eradication	85% improved or cured, 75% "cure," 12% improved, 90% bacterial eradication
Frombeur et al.[44]	56	Chronic sinusitis	Ciprofloxacin	500 mg bid 9 days	Uncontrolled	Bacterial eradication, clinical symptoms	75% cure, 12% improved, 90% bacterial eradication
Legent et al.[45]	251	Chronic sinusitis	Ciprofloxacin vs. Amoxicillin-clavulanate	500 mg bid 9 days / 500 mg tid 9 days	Double-blind, placebo-controlled	Clinical symptoms, bacterial eradication	Ciprofloxacin: 60% "cure," 90% bacterial eradication; Amoxicillin/clavulanate: 50% "cure," 90% bacterial eradication
Children							
Dohlman et al.[20]	96	Subacute sinusitis	Decongestant/nasal spray; Amoxicillin vs. trimethoprim-sulfamethoxazole (TMP/SMX) vs. amoxicillin-clavulanate	3 weeks; Amoxicillin 30–40 mg/kg/day; TMP 8 mg/kg/day; SMX 40 mg/kg/day; Amox.-clav. 30–40 mg/kg/day	Random double-blind, controlled	Clinical symptoms, radiologic clearance	Amox = 72%; Amox/Clav = 73%; TMP/SMX = 69%; Non-antimicrob. = 63%; No statistical diff.
Rachalefsky et al.[35]	84	Chronic sinusitis	Amoxicillin, trimethoprim-sulfamethoxazole (TMS) erythromycin (ERY)	Up to three 2-week courses (crossover)	Double-blind controlled	Symptom improvement, medication reduction	Amoxicillin best drug of 3 evaluated, TMS second, ERY = placebo
Otten et al.[46]	79	Chronic sinusitis	Placebo vs. cefaclor	20 mg/kg/day for 1 week; Divided doses	Double-blind, randomized, controlled	Clinical symptoms, radiologic clearance	No difference between treatment; 64% cefaclor; Placebo 52%
Ghandi et al.[48]	26	Chronic sinusitis	Amoxicillin, amoxicillin/clavulanate, trimethoprim-sulfamethoxazole, cefaclor	1-year prophylaxis 1/3–1/2 full dose daily	Uncontrolled	Clinical symptoms	74% patients noted 50% or greater reduction in infection

the best, this does not appear to be the case. The recommendation, therefore, is to treat with a broad-spectrum antibiotic that may or may not have good anaerobic coverage. Prophylaxis can be utilized in high-risk groups with some success but should be considered with caution, especially in view of the very serious problem of the development of drug-resistant pneumococci. Table 40–3 contains recommendations for the medical treatment of chronic sinusitis.

Adjunctive Treatment

Adjunctive treatment for chronic sinusitis consists of decongestants, antihistamines, corticosteroids, irrigations, saline sprays, mucolytics, humidity, and allergy management. Although adjunctive treatments are widely recommended, few prospective studies have been directed toward evaluating their effectiveness.[49, 50] However, because most otolaryngologists and others treating chronic sinus disease believe in the value of adjunctive therapy, the characteristics of these drugs are reviewed here.

Corticosteroids

Topical steroids have been used successfully for the treatment of rhinitis, in particular allergic rhinitis, but the benefits of the treatment of either acute or chronic sinusitis have not been established. Meltzer and colleagues[38] reported a prospective double-blind study comparing flunisolide nasal spray to placebo in 116 adults with documented acute maxillary sinusitis. All patients received 3 weeks of amoxicillin-clavulanate in addition. Less turbinate congestion and greater symptom improvement were noted with the topical steroid spray, but no significant difference in the rate of recurrence of sinus symptoms was noted after completion of the study. Four other studies have shown weak support for topical corticosteroids in sinusitis.[51] Other studies show no benefit to topical nasal corticosteroids.[52]

Of interest is a study reported by Sykes and colleagues,[8]

who combined antibiotics and corticosteroids together in a topical spray and found that 70% of patients with chronic mucopurulent rhinosinusitis responded positively in a double-blind controlled study. Steroid spray alone resulted in a 60% response rate compared with placebo, which had a 20% response rate.

In summary, there appears to be evidence that topical steroid spray alone or in conjunction with topical antibiotic therapy may have some benefit for the treatment of chronic sinusitis, especially in those patients with allergic rhinosinusitis, but more prospective documentation is necessary to support its use.[53, 54]

There is *no* study in the literature reporting the benefits of oral corticosteroids for the treatment of chronic sinusitis. It is, however, this author's experience that oral corticosteroids are as important to the treatment of chronic sinusitis as antibiotics. High-dose corticosteroid therapy (60 mg/day prednisone) given in a 6- to 7-day burst has been used for years with excellent clinical results in chronic sinusitis. Excellent clinical results are defined as significant improvement or cure with avoidance of surgery. The underlying reason for success is marked reduction of mucosal edema and inflammation, which allows for better drainage and possibly better antibiotic performance. All patients in the author's practice with chronic sinusitis receive oral and topical corticosteroids as part of treatment for chronic sinusitis. Although prospective studies weighing the true benefit of oral corticosteroids for the treatment of chronic sinusitis are pending, experience indicates that oral corticosteroids are, indeed, a consideration for chronic sinusitis.

Decongestants

Topical and systemic decongestants are commonly prescribed for the treatment of chronic sinusitis. Minimal data are available in the literature to confirm their benefit. Concern about the occurrence of rhinitis medicamentosa from prolonged use of topical decongestants in patients with chronic sinusitis has been discussed.[52] This author, however,

Table 40–3. SUGGESTED MEDICAL THERAPY FOR CHRONIC SINUSITIS IN ADULTS AND CHILDREN

Therapy	Type and Route	Duration	Dosage
Antibiotic	Anti–beta-lactamase antibiotics Broad-spectrum Oral	3–6 wks	High full dosage
Corticosteroids			
Topical and	Topical nasal	3–6 wks	Medication and disease dependent (4 sprays qd–bid)
Oral	Oral prednisone[1]	5–7 days	40–80 mg qAM
Decongestants			
Topical (spray) or	Oxymetazoline	3–6 wks	8-day rotation: 5 days on, 3 days off 2 sprays bid
Oral	Pseudoephedrine or phenylpropanolamine	3–6 wks	Usual or high dose
Mucolytics[2]	Guaifenesin	3–6 wks	High dose
Allergy treatment	1. If history positive for consideration of allergy, begin allergy work-up and consider long-term treatment.		
	2. Topical and oral corticosteroids in most cases will nicely cover short-term allergy management.		
	3. Antihistamines cause drying and thickening of nasal/sinus secretions and ciliary dysmotility; they should be used only if necessary.		

[1]Prednisone much cheaper and more potent than Medrol Dosepak.
[2]Often, mucolytics are available combined with pseudoephedrine or phenylpropanolamine.

has found that topical decongestants such as oxymetazoline work well for chronic sinusitis, especially when combined with a topical steroid spray. Decongestant sprays are used in an 8-day rotation (5 days using spray, 3 days not) throughout the course of treatment without the occurrence of rhinitis medicamentosa.

Systemic decongestants (pseudoephedrine and phenylpropanolamine) appear to influence the maxillary sinus ostial patency in normal and diseased patients.[55] Aust and colleagues,[56] however, looked at 20 patients with acute sinusitis and found no benefit. Pseudoephedrine seems to be better tolerated than phenylpropanolamine.[57]

On the basis of clinical experience, decongestants appear to have a role in the treatment of chronic sinusitis.

Mucolytics and Humidity

Mucolytic agents, either in combination with decongestants or alone, have theoretical advantages in the treatment of sinusitis because of the thickened secretions found in the sinuses and nasal passages seen in this disease. Although the hypothesis is interesting, again, minimal objective data have been obtained to show the effectiveness of currently available compounds in reducing secretion viscosity and enhancing clearance. Everything from cysteine derivatives to chicken soup has been evaluated to improve nasal mucous flow.[58, 59]

A study in children showed a clinical and radiologic benefit of nebulized saline and bromhexine for sinusitis and asthma.[60] Panosetti[61] did not find any benefit to mucolytics for chronis sinusitis. Wawrose and colleagues[62] reported that patients with acquired immunodeficiency syndrome (AIDS) noted significant improvement with guaifenesin compared with placebo for chronic rhinosinusitis.

Nasal irrigations can help clear secretions. A study by Grossan[63] showed that using a Water Pik improved mucociliary clearance and decreased purulence. Proetz irrigations have been noted to be helpful in acute purulent sinusitis, but no data are available for chronic sinusitis.

Humidity has been noted to be beneficial for acute sinusitis since before the introduction of antibiotics.[64] No data are available regarding the benefit of humidity for chronic sinusitis.

In summary, there appears to be some evidence that mucolytics may be helpful for the treatment of chronic sinusitis. Humidity and nasal irrigations may also be helpful.

Allergy Management

Experienced sinus surgeons recognize that patients with chronic sinusitis who also have allergy and/or asthma are often the most difficult patients to treat medically. If allergic management is not incorporated into the therapeutic regimen of such patients, sinusitis cannot be controlled. Several studies have shown a definite association between allergy and sinusitis.[65, 66] Indeed, it is not uncommon in acute seasonal allergy to have an associated bout of acute sinusitis. Many allergic patients also have an underlying chronic sinusitis.[67, 68] Three treatment modalities have demonstrated efficacy in allergic rhinosinusitis: environmental control, phar-

macotherapy, and allergic desensitization.[69] Antihistamines should be considered for allergic patients with sinusitis, although one should keep in mind the drying effects and ciliary immobilization associated with these medications. Oftentimes, desensitization injections along with topical nasal medication like corticosteroids and/or cromolyn sodium will work even better. Asakura and colleagues[70] noted, in 37 children who were randomized to antibiotics and immunotherapy versus antibiotics alone, that the former group had a more rapid clinical and radiologic resolution of symptoms.

Desensitization as a long-term treatment can often take months to work and has to be supplemented with topical and/or oral medications. Waiting to decide on surgery according to desensitization results may be impractical, but desensitization certainly can be utilized postoperatively to keep sinusitis from recurring because of allergy. Environmental control and food allergy analysis may also be very important in the treatment of chronic sinusitis.

Attempts to try to control allergy to aid in the treatment of chronic sinusitis are important and deserve consideration. A limited literature suggests the use of desensitization for this purpose. Environmental control, food allergy management, and pharmacologic treatment have received little objective evaluation for chronic sinusitis and allergy but are the best short-term treatments available.

Sinus Surgery

Patients for whom appropriate medical therapy for chronic sinusitis fails become surgical candidates. In the past, it was often believed that chronic sinusitis was a surgical disease, but better medical therapy is now available, allowing for improvement of chronic sinusitis and avoidance of surgery. For the medical failure cases, endoscopic sinus surgery has become the main surgical technique for treatment with backup by external ethmoidectomy, transantral ethmoidectomy, or a Caldwell-Luc procedure as necessary. Several outcome studies have shown symptomatic improvement and/or cure in up to 80%–90% of adults and children.[71–77] However, complications of endoscopic sinus surgery may be substantial, warranting a full trial of medical therapy prior to surgery.[78, 79]

The American Academy of Otolaryngology–Head and Neck Surgery, the American Rhinological Society, and other related groups have determined that guidelines for surgical therapy of chronic sinusitis are necessary.[80] These guidelines are under analysis and are not final. However, an attempt is made here to outline special elements of these guidelines so that the reader can gain some understanding about what is forthcoming. Definitions of disease are similar to those summarized in the early part of the chapter. Twelve hundred clinical scenarios have been reviewed in an effort to identify patients who require sinus surgery. Scenarios were evaluated individually, graded, and incorporated into a computer data bank. Factors for each scenario looked at were history, history of asthma, duration and type of medical treatment, CT scan findings, physical examination findings, allergy history and treatment, and age. Patients with a low score are not candidates for surgery, whereas those who fulfill entry criteria are the best surgical candidates. The adult patients who have the following characteristics are the best surgical candidates: (Table 40–4):

1. Strong history for sinusitis.
2. Failure of 3–6 weeks of appropriate antibiotic therapy (anti–beta-lactamase antibiotic).
3. Failure of a course of immunotherapy and/or pharmacotherapy, if the patient is allergic.
4. Failure of topical and/or oral corticosteroid therapy.
5. Failure of treatment with adjunctive methods of therapy, i.e., decongestants, mucolytics.
6. Anatomic or radiologic abnormalities causing mechanical obstruction.
7. Evidence of pansinusitis or marked sinus involvement on CT scanning.

An intermediate group who could be classified as equivocal surgical candidates would be those patients with the following criteria:

1. Moderate or suggestive history for sinusitis.
2. Failure of appropriate antibiotic treatment given for up to 2–3 weeks.
3. Failure of adjunctive measures of therapy, i.e., decongestant, mucolytics.
4. CT scanning shows persistent evidence of sinusitis.
5. Evidence of anatomic variant or ostiomeatal complex obstruction.

Patients who are definitely not surgery candidates are the following:

1. Questionable or minimal history of sinusitis.
2. Less than 2-week treatment of an appropriate antibiotic or an inappropriate antibiotic.
3. No adjunctive therapy.
4. No corticosteroid therapy.
5. No allergy management, if allergic.
6. Normal or minimal disease CAT scans.
7. No evidence of anatomic variant.

Note: Sinusitis in patients with the features described in items 2 and 7 tends to clear up with medical treatment, since minimal disease is present. Persistent symptoms should be treated aggressively for longer times to help change the patient's scoring into an equivocal or definite surgery category.

CONCLUSIONS

The following points can be summarized from this chapter and the scientific literature:

- The patient's history, physical examination including endoscopy, and radiologic evaluation are all part of the database necessary to make a diagnosis of chronic sinusitis.

- The microbiologic flora of chronic sinusitis is variable and includes anaerobic and aerobic bacteria. Few scientific studies are in agreement about the exact microbiologic flora and what role these organisms play in chronic sinusitis. Postsurgical bacteriologic flora is different from that in chronic sinusitis and may reflect actual infection and/or contamination.

- Antibiotics may be helpful in the treatment of some cases of chronic sinusitis, but scientifically sound information on which antibiotics to use, dosage, and duration is not established. Current recommendations are that antibiotics should be broad-spectrum and given at high doses for a minimum duration of 3–4 weeks.

- Adjunctive treatments, particularly corticosteroids, are believed to be helpful in treating sinusitis, but their effectiveness is not scientifically proven.

- Surgery guidelines for medical treatment failures are in development. Severity of disease as well as intensity and duration of medical therapy are used to determine whether a patient is an appropriate surgical candidate.

References

1. Stankiewicz JA, Osguthorpe JD: Medical treatment of sinusitis [editorial]. Otolaryngol Head Neck Surg 1994; 110: 361–362.
2. Kennedy DW: Sinus Disease: Guide to First Line Management. Darien, Connecticut: Health Communication, Inc., 1994, p 10.
3. Gliklich RE, Metson R: Health impact of chronic sinusitis in patients seeking otolaryngologic care. Otolaryngol Head Neck Surg 1995; 113: 104–109.
4. Draf W: Endoscopy of the Paranasal Sinuses. New York: Springer-Verlag, 1983, p 32.
5. Milbrath MM, Madiedo G, Toohill RJ: Histopathological analysis of the middle turbinate after ethmoidectomy. Am J Rhinol 1994; 8: 37–42.
6. Goldwyn BG, Sakr W, Marks SC: Histopathologic analysis of chronic sinusitis. Am J Rhinol 1995; 9: 27–30.
7. Ramsey B, Richardson MA: Impact of sinusitis in cystic fibrosis. J Allergy Clin Immunol 1992; 90: 547–552.
8. Sykes DA, Wilson R, Chan KL, et al.: Relative importance of antibiotic and improved clearance in topical treatment of chronic mucopurulent rhinosinusitis. Lancet 1986; 16: 359–360.
9. Arruda LK, Mimica IM, Sole D, et al.: Abnormal maxillary sinus radiographs in children. Pediatrics 1990; 85: 553–558.
10. Gwaltney JM, Scheld WM, Sande MA, et al.: The microbial etiology and antimicrobial therapy of adults with acute community acquired sinusitis. J Allergy Clin Immunol 1992; 90: 457–462.
11. Wald ER, Reilly JS, Casselbrant M, et al.: Treatment of acute maxillary sinusitis in childhood. J Pediatrics 1984; 104: 297–302.

Table 40–4. GUIDELINES FOR SINUS SURGERY FOR CHRONIC SINUSITIS

In Children (younger than 13 years):

1. A strong history for sinusitis.
2. A positive CT scan after treatment for sinus disease.
3. Antibiotic treatment with broad-spectrum anti–beta-lactamase for 28 days.
4. Allergy should be ruled out. If allergic, patient should have allergy management. If immunotherapy has not been initiated, it can be initiated after surgery if patient is a surgical candidate.
5. Adenoidectomy prior to formal sinus surgery.
6. Topical steroids or oral steroids should be considered if potential benefits outweigh risks.

In Adults (13 years and older):

1. Antibiotic treatment with broad-spectrum anti–beta-lactamase for 28 days.
2. A strong history for sinusitis.
3. Positive CT scan for sinus disease after treatment.
4. If allergic, patient should receive appropriate medical therapy.
5. Trial of oral and topical steroids and decongestants as part of medical therapy.

12. Brook I: Bacteriologic features of chronic sinusitis in children. JAMA 1981; 246: 967–969.

13. Muntz HR, Lusk RP: Bacteriology of the ethmoid bulla in children with chronic sinusitis. Otol Head Neck Surg 1991; 117: 179–181.

14. Goldenhersh MJ, Rachelefsky GS, Dudley J, et al.: The microbiology of chronic sinus disease in children with respiratory allergy. J Allergy Clin Immunol 1990; 85: 1030–1039.

15. Orobello PW, Park RI, Belcher LJ, et al.: The microbiology of chronic sinusitis in children. Arch Otolaryngol Head Neck Surg 1991; 117: 980–992.

16. Frederick J, Braude AI: Anaerobic infection of the paranasal sinuses. N Engl J Med 1974; 290: 135–140.

17. Karma P, Jokipii L, Sipila P, et al.: Bacteria in chronic maxillary sinusitis. Arch Otolaryngol Head Neck Surg 1979; 105: 386–390.

18. Doyle PW, Woodham JD: Bacterial flora in acute and chronic sinusitis. J Clin Neurol 1991; 29: 2396–2399.

19. Evans FO, Sydnor JB, Moore WE, et al.: Sinusitis of the maxillary antrum. N Engl J Med 1975; 293: 735–739.

20. Dohlman AW, Hemstreet MP, Odrezin GT, et al.: Subacute sinusitis: Are antimicrobials necessary? J Allergy Clin Immunol 1993; 91: 1015–1023.

21. Wald ER, Byers C, Guerra N, et al.: Subacute sinusitis in children. J Pediatr 1989; 115: 28–32.

22. Bolger WE: Gram negative sinusitis: Emerging clinical entity? Am J Rhinol 1994; 8: 279–283.

23. Hsu J, Lanza DC, Kennedy DW: Antimicrobial resistance in bacterial chronic sinusitis [abstract]. Presented to American Rhinologic Society; April 30, 1995; Palm Desert, California.

24. Woodham JD, Doyle PW: Endoscopic diagnosis, medical treatment, and a working classification of chronic sinusitis. J Otolaryngol 1991; 20: 6–10.

25. Babbel R, Harnsberger HR, Nelson B, et al.: Optimization of techniques in screening CT of the sinuses. AJNR 1991; 12: 849–854.

26. Gross GW, McGeady SJ, Kerut T, et al.: Limited slice CT in the evaluation of paranasal sinus disease in children. Am J Roentgenol 1991; 156: 367–369.

27. Bingham B, Shankar L, Hawke M: Pitfalls in computed tomography of the paranasal sinuses. J Otolaryngol 1991; 20: 414–418.

28. Gwaltney JM, Phillips CD, Miller RD, et al.: Computed tomographic study of the common cold. N Engl J Med 1994; 330: 25–30.

29. McAlister WA, Lusk RP, Muntz HR: Comparison of plain radiographs and coronal CT scans in infants and children with recurrent sinusitis. Am J Roentgenol 1989; 153: 1259–1264.

30. Havas TE, Motbey JA, Guillane DJ: Prevalence of incidental abnormalities on computerized tomography of the paranasal sinuses. Arch Otolaryngol Head Neck Surg 1988; 114: 856–859.

31. Lloyd G: CT of the paranasal sinuses: Study of a control series in relation to endoscopic sinus surgery. J Laryngol Otol 1990; 104: 477–481.

32. Kennedy DW, Zinreich SJ: Physiologic mucosal changes within the nose and ethmoid sinus: Imaging of the nasal cycle by MRI. Laryngoscope 1988; 98: 928–933.

33. Som PM, Shapiro MD, Biller HF, et al.: Sinonasal tumors and inflammatory tissues: Differentiation with MRI imaging. Radiology 1991; 167: 803–808.

34. Weissman JL, Tabor EK, Curtin HD: Sphenochoanal polyps: Evaluation with CT and MR imaging. Radiology 1991; 173: 145–148.

35. Rachelefsky GS, Katz RM, Siegel SC: Chronic sinusitis in children with respiratory allergy. J Allergy Clin Immunol 1982; 69: 382–387.

36. Huck W, Reed BD, Nielsen RW, et al.: Cefaclor vs amoxicillin in the treatment of acute, recurrent, and chronic sinusitis. Arch Fam Med 1993; 2: 497–503.

37. Gehenno P, Rohen B: Effectiveness and safety of ofloxacin in chronic otitis media and chronic sinusitis in adult outpatients. Eur Arch Otorhinolaryngol 1993; 250: 573–574.

38. Meltzer EO, Orgel HA, Backhaus JW, et al.: Assessment of flunisolide nasal spray vs placebo as an adjunct to antibiotic treatment of sinusitis. J Allergy Clin Immunol 1992; 89: 301–304.

39. Husfeldt P, Egede F, Nielsen PB: Antibiotic treatment of sinusitis in general practice. Eur Arch Otorhinolaryngol 1993; 250: 523–525.

40. Nicolett G, Speciale A, Caccomo F, et al.: Sulbactam/ampicillin in the treatment of otitis and sinusitis. J Int Med Res 1991; 19(suppl): 29A–35A.

41. Maisel RH, Kimberly BP: Treatment of chronic sinusitis with open drainage and cefaclor. Am J Otolaryngol 1988; 9: 30–33.

42. Bassetti D, Concia E, Solbiati M, et al.: Multidisciplinary approach to chronic sinusitis. Drugs Exp Clin Res 1988; 14: 559–560.

43. Schaefer SD, Ronis ML: Cephalexin in the treatment of acute and chronic maxillary sinusitis. South Med J 1985; 78: 45–47.

44. Frombeur JP, Barrault S, Koubbi G, et al.: Study in the efficicy and safety of ciprofloxacin in the treatment of chronic sinusitis. Chemotherapy 1994; 40(suppl 1): 24–28.

45. Legent F, Bordure P, Beauxillain C, et al.: A double blind comparison of ciprofloxacin and amoxicillin clavulanate and in the treatment of chronic sinusitis. Chemotherapy 1994; 40(suppl): 8–15.

46. Otten HW, Antvelink JB, Ruyter de Wildt H, et al.: Is antibiotic treatment of chronic sinusitis effective in children? Clin Otolaryngol 1994; 19: 215–217.

47. Otten FW, Van Aarem A, Grotte JJ: Long-term follow-up chronic maxillary sinusitis in children. Int J Pediatr Otorhinolaryngol 1991; 22: 81–84.

48. Ghandi A, Brodsky C, Ballow M: Benefits of antibiotic prophylaxis in children with chronic sinusitis. Allergy Proc 1993; 14: 37–43.

49. Druce HM: Diagnosis of sinusitis in adults: History, physical examination, nasal cytology, echo, and rhinoscope. J Allergy Clin Immunol 1992; 90: 936–941.

50. Zeiger RS: Prospects for ancillary treatment of sinusitis in the 1990's. J Allergy Clin Immunol 1992; 90: 478–495.

51. Quarnberg Y, Kantola O, Solo J: Influence of topical steroid treatment on maxillary sinusitis. Rhinology (Eur) 1992; 30: 103–112.

52. Malm L: Pharmacological background to decongesting and anti-inflammatory treatment of rhinitis and sinusitis. Acta Otolaryngol 1994; 515(suppl): 53–55.

53. Krouse HA, Phung ND, Klaustermeyer WB: Intranasal beclomethasone in severe rhinosinusitis and nasal polyps. Ann Allergy 1983; 50: 385–388.

54. Rebhun J: Effectiveness of antibiotic nasal sprays on the treatment of severe chronic bacterial sinusitis. Immunol Allergy Pract 1993; 40: 164–169.

55. Melen I, Lindahl L, Andreasson L: Effects of phenylpropanolamine on ostial and nasal patency in patient treatment for chronic sinusitis. Acta Otolaryngol (Stockh) 1979; 88: 455–458.

56. Aust R, Drettner B, Falck B: Studies of the effect of peroral phenylpropanolamine in the functional size of the human maxillary ostia. Acta Otolaryngol (Stockh) 1979; 88: 455–458.

57. Porta M, Jick H, Habakangas JS: Follow-up study of pseudoephedrine users. Ann Allergy 1986; 57: 340–342.

58. Ziment I: Acetylcysteine: A drug that is much more than a mucokinetic. Biomed Pharmacother 1988; 42: 513–520.

59. Saketkoo K, Januszkiewicz A, Sackner MA, et al.: Effects of drinking hot water, cold water, and chicken soup on nasal mucosis velocity and nasal airflow resistance. Chest 1978; 74: 408–410.

60. Van Bever HPS, Bosmans J, Stevens NJ: Nebulization treatment with saline compared to bromhexine in treating chronic sinusitis in asthmatic children. Allergy 1987; 42: 33–36.

61. Panosetti E: Clinical trial of oral acetylcysteine in chronic sinusitis. Eur J Resp Dis 1980; 61: 159–161.

62. Wawrose SF, Tami TA, Amoils P: The role of guaifenesin in the treatment of sinonasal disease in patients with HIV. Laryngoscope 1992; 102: 1225–1228.

63. Grossan M: A device for nasal irrigation. Trans Am Acad Ophthalmol Otol 1974; 47: 279–281.

64. Macknin ML, Matthews S, Vanderburg S: Effects of inhaling heated vapor on symptoms of the common cold. JAMA 1990; 264: 989–991.

65. Spector SL: The role of allergy in sinusitis in adults. J Allergy Clin Immunol 1992; 90: 518–520.

66. Furukawa CT: The role of allergy in sinusitis in children. J Clin Allergy Immunol 1992; 90: 515–517.

67. Lawson W: The intranasal ethmoidectomy: An experience with 1077 procedures. Laryngoscope 1991; 101: 367–371.

68. Matthews BL, Smith LE, Jones R, et al.: Endoscopic sinus surgery: Outcome in 155 cases. Otolaryngol Head Neck Surg 1991; 104: 244–246.

69. Trevino RJ, Gordon BR: Allergic rhinosinusitis: The total rhinologic disease. Ear Nose Throat J 1993; 72: 116–125.

70. Asakura K, Kojima T, Shirasaki H, Kataura A: Evaluation of the effects

of antigen specific immunotherapy on chronic sinusitis in children with allergy. Auris Nasus Larynx 1990; 17: 33–38.

71. Gross CW, Gurucharri MJ, Lazar RH, Long TE.: Functional endoscopic sinus surgery (FESS) in the pediatric age group. Laryngoscope 1989; 99: 272–275.

72. Lusk RP, Muntz HR: Endoscopic sinus surgery in children with chronic sinusitis: A pilot study. Laryngoscope 1990; 100: 654–658.

73. Kennedy DW: Prognostic factors, outcomes and staging in ethmoid sinus surgery. Laryngoscope 1992; 102: 1–18.

74. Hoffman SR, Dersarkissian RM, Buck SH, et al.: Sinus disease and surgical treatment: A results-oriented quality assurance study. Otolaryngol Head Neck Surg 1989; 100: 573–577.

75. Toffel PH, Aroesty DJ, Weinmann RH: Secure endoscopic sinus surgery as an adjunct to functional surgery. Arch Otol Head Neck Surg 1989; 115: 822–825.

76. Rice DH: Endoscopic sinus surgery: Results at 2-year follow up. Otolaryngol Head Neck Surg 1989; 101: 476–479.

77. May M, Levine HL, Shaitkin B: Results of endoscopic sinus surgery. In: Levine HL, May M (eds): Endoscopic Sinus Surgery. New York: Thieme Medical Publishers, 1993, pp 178–192.

78. Stankiewicz JA: Complications of endoscopic intranasal ethmoidectomy. Laryngoscope 1987; 97: 1270–1273.

79. Maniglia AJ: Fatal and other major complications of endoscopic sinus surgery. Laryngoscope 1991; 101: 349–354.

80. Dana ST: VHS sinus panel report. Bull Am Acad Otolaryngol Head Neck Surg 1994; 13: 12–14.

CHAPTER FORTY-ONE

Special Problems in Sinusitis

Sinusitis is an important and potentially lethal source of sepsis in the hospitalized patient. This is especially true in patients admitted with major craniofacial trauma, in patients with severe immunosuppressive diseases, and in patients subjected to nasotracheal or nasogastric intubation. Features that seem to be associated with an increased incidence of sinusitis in the hospitalized patient are severe underlying disease, use of invasive monitoring devices, alterations in normal flora (perhaps due to antimicrobial use), and proximity to other critically ill, infected individuals.

Sinusitis in this patient population is commonly owing to resistant organisms; over half of these organisms may be aerobic gram-negative bacilli.

NOSOCOMIAL SINUSITIS

Sinusitis has long been recognized as a potential complication of nasal instrumentation and insertion of nasogastric and nasotracheal tubes.[1-11] Early reports suggest that 2%–5% of patients with nasal intubation may develop sinusitis.[1, 3] Later reports of patients studied with the use of modern imaging for diagnosis suggest the incidence of nasal intubation–associated sinusitis to be 27%–42%.[6, 11] Desmond and colleagues[10] prospectively evaluated 65 patients requiring insertion of the nasogastric (NG) tube. Seventy-four percent of patients demonstrated radiographic abnormality after 48 hours of NG intubation. The most common radiographic abnormalities were present on the side of the NG tube. Holzapfel and colleagues,[12] in a prospective randomized trial of orotracheal versus nasotracheal intubation, demonstrated a trend (p = .08) toward increased incidence of infectious maxillary sinusitis. Other authors present even more conclusive evidence for an etiologic relationship between nasal instrumentation and subsequent development of sinusitis.[1, 4–7, 13]

Pathogenesis

Nasal intubation with a nasotracheal or NG tube, nasal packing, and the presence of concurrent craniofacial fracture have been associated with a higher incidence of paranasal sinus infection. Trauma to the nasal mucosa with subsequent edema and mechanical obstruction of the paranasal sinuses predisposes to retention of secretions in the sinuses, providing an ideal medium for bacterial proliferation. Maxillofacial trauma results in sinus hemorrhage and occasional introduction of foreign material into the sinuses, which may further promote sinusitis.

The use of high-dose corticosteroids has been reported as a frequent association in patients who develop nosocomial sinusitis.[13] It is unclear whether this represents an independent risk factor or merely serves to promote development of infection in patients with nasal intubation.

The maxillary sinus is the site most commonly affected in clinical studies; however, computed tomography (CT) imaging suggests that the ethmoid, sphenoid, and frontal sinuses may all be affected, either independently or in a pansinusitis.[9-11]

Clinical Manifestations

The presence of fever, rhinorrhea, nasal congestion, and pain or tenderness over the sinuses was associated with bacteriologically documented sinusitis in 86% of patients with fever of unknown origin in a study reported by Lebeda and colleagues.[14] Many critically ill intubated patients are unable to voice complaints that localize the site of infection to the paranasal sinuses. The presence of fever, leukocytosis, and purulent rhinorrhea in a hospitalized patient may be indicative of sinusitis. CT is commonly used to evaluate the critically ill patient. Opacification or the presence of an air-fluid level is abnormal and further suggests the diagnosis in the presence of the clinical findings. However, an abnormal CT scan should not be considered out of the context of the clinical situation.

Duration of nasal intubation correlates with the likelihood of developing sinusitis. Linden and colleagues[1] report an average of 6 days of intubation in patients who develop sinusitis. Caplan and Hoyt[5] note that the average such patient has had either nasotracheal or nasogastric intubation for 13 days, with a range of 5–35 days.[5] Deutschman and colleagues,[7] in a prospective study of 27 nasally intubated patients, noted that patients who had elective nasotracheal intubation developed sinusitis an average of 15 days after intubation, whereas those who required emergency intubation after trauma or shock developed sinusitis after only 8 days.[7]

Microbiology

Bacteriology of nosocomial sinusitis in the patient with nasal intubation does not correspond to the bacteriology of community acquired sinusitis. In some series, *Staphylococcus aureus* is the most commonly encountered bacterium; however, *Enterobacter, Pseudomonas aeruginosa*, and *Klebsiella* are commonly isolated (Table 41–1). Polymicrobial infections are identified commonly in patients who undergo sinus

Table 41–1. REPRESENTATIVE ORGANISMS FOR NOSOCOMIAL SINUSITIS IN PATIENTS WITH NASAL INTUBATION

Series	Organisms in Order of Frequency
Holzapfel et al.[12]	*Escherichia coli* *Streptococcus* species *Staphylococcus aureus* *Haemophilus influenzae* *Proteus* species *Bacteroides* species
Lebeda et al.[14]	*S. aureus* *Moraxella (Branhamella) catarrhalis* *Pseudomonas aeruginosa* *Haemophilus* species *Bacteroides* species
Rouby et al.[15]	*S. aureus* *Candida* species *Streptococcus* species *Pseudomonas* species *E. coli*
Deutschman et al.[16]	*Staphylococcus epidermidis* *Streptococcus* species *P. aeruginosa* *Acinetobacter calcoaceticus*

aspiration for culture.[1, 5, 6, 11, 15, 16] *Bacteroides* species and fungi may occasionally be encountered.[15, 17]

Culture of the anterior nares does not correlate with cultures obtained by direct sinus aspiration.[18, 19] Samples obtained through selective sampling of secretions in the middle meatus adjacent to the maxillary and ethmoid ostia correlate closely with direct sinus aspiration, but these samples must be carefully obtained. Decontamination with antibacterial agents should be performed prior to endoscopic guidance through the nose. The optimal technique for obtaining material for culture is to aspirate the involved sinus directly.

Diagnosis

In the clinical setting of fever, rhinorrhea, and facial discomfort, sinusitis should be considered. Imaging with computed tomography is most appropriate in the critical care setting. Demonstration of sinus opacification or air-fluid levels is highly suggestive of sinusitis. Rouby and colleagues[15] report that direct sinus aspiration results in a diagnosis of infectious maxillary sinusitis in only 38% of patients with abnormal sinus radiographs, suggesting that radiography should not be used as an exclusive diagnostic measure. The presence of purulent rhinorrhea in the setting of fever and leukocytosis is highly suggestive. Aspiration of purulent material from the affected sinus remains the sine qua non of diagnosis.

Treatment

Removal of the offending instrument, nasal decongestion, and the administration of antibiotics are sufficient therapy for most patients. Sinusitis in the patient with nasogastric or nasotracheal intubation is an indication to establish an alternative form of either alimentation or respiration. This may require insertion of a gastrostomy tube (or percutaneous endoscopic gastrostomy) or a tracheotomy in some patients.

An essential component of the therapy of sinusitis is drainage of the involved sinus. Either topical or systemic decongestants promote relief of obstruction at the site of the natural ostia, which may serve as sufficient drainage in many patients.

Broad-spectrum empiric antibiotic therapy is appropriate in hospitalized patients with nosocomial sinusitis. This measure reflects the vast array of organisms that may be encountered. Sepsis in critically ill patients, especially in those already receiving antimicrobial therapy, should be considered an indication for direct aspiration of the affected sinus to confirm the diagnosis and establish the etiologic organism and its antimicrobial susceptibility.

At the time of sinus aspiration, irrigation with sterile saline serves to mechanically displace the infected secretions, which is therapeutic in and of itself. A more formal sinusotomy aimed at widely establishing the patency of the sinus ostium may be required occasionally in patients who are critically ill or have recalcitrant sinusitis.

SINUSITIS IN THE NON-AIDS IMMUNOSUPPRESSED PATIENT

It is generally acknowledged that patients with significant immunosuppression are at risk for increased incidence of septic complications. These complications may be due to unusual or opportunistic organisms. This is especially true in hospitalized patients subjected to invasive testing and monitoring, who may have altered flora owing to antibiotic use and are in close proximity to critically ill infected individuals.[20] Likewise, an increased risk of sinusitis has been recognized in patients with immunosuppression[21]: patients with severe debilitating diseases, such as disseminated malignancy and uncontrolled diabetes; patients who are therapeutically immunosuppressed, such as transplant patients; patients with acquired or inherited immunosuppression, such as hypogammaglobulinemia; and patients with severe trauma, such as head injury or shock.

The incidence of sinusitis in patients undergoing heart transplantation has been reported to be 26%[22] and 37%.[23] Shibuya and colleagues[24] report the observed incidence of sinus disease in patients following bone marrow transplantation to be 31% overall. In two thirds of these patients, pretreatment sinus radiographs had been normal.[24] In contrast, sinusitis in the kidney transplant population is reported to be only 4%.[25]

Microbiology

Community-acquired sinusitis is associated with *Streptococcus pneumoniae*, *Haemophilus influenzae*, and *Moraxella catarrhalis* in more than 75% of cases. This relatively consistent picture of bacteriology *is not* dependable in the population of immunosuppressed patients, in whom gram-negative aerobic bacilli and fungi may be encountered in more than 50%. Organisms reported include *P. aeruginosa*, *Escherichia coli*, *Klebsiella pneumoniae*, *Bacteroides melaninogenicus*, *Aspergillus*, and Phycomycetes.[20, 21]

Diagnosis

The correct diagnosis of sinusitis requires an adequate index of suspicion. Nasal congestion and rhinorrhea with pain or tenderness over the paranasal sinuses are highly suggestive. Under most circumstances, the diagnosis of sinusitis can be established on the basis of the clinical constellation of signs and symptoms as well as an intranasal examination. Infection in the paranasal sinuses results in edema, erythema of the mucosa of the turbinates and lateral nasal wall, and purulent rhinorrhea. Endoscopic evaluation of the intranasal structures commonly demonstrates purulent debris coming from the affected sinus. Radiographic confirmation of the diagnosis is especially important in critically ill patients and patients with severe immunosuppression and in situations in which the diagnosis may be in question. CT is the study of choice. Additionally, CT may serve to identify the specific sinus involved such that direct aspiration for culture and sensitivity can be efficiently targeted to the likely site of infection.

Treatment

Treatment of sinusitis consists of eradication of the offending organism and establishment of normal ventilation of the involved sinus. Community-acquired infection in the immunocompetent patient is undertaken through empiric administration of antibiotics appropriate to the "big three" bacteria. Concomitant administration of either a systemic or a topical decongestant is accepted as the standard of therapy. The broad spectrum of organisms that may be associated with sepsis in the immunocompromised patient suggests that specific therapy directed at the offending organism may be advantageous in most cases. Under these circumstances, material can be obtained through an endoscopically guided culture directed at the sinus ostium. An alternative is direct puncture of the involved sinus. This measure also enables irrigation of the sinus with saline, resulting in mechanical clearance of the infected material and promotion of resolution under most circumstances.

Shaw and colleagues[26] recommend that patients with sinus abnormalities have surgery prior to chemotherapy if the sinus disease is refractory to medical treatment.

Surgery for sinusitis is usually limited to endoscopically directed débridement of the natural ostium with improvement of the drainage of the involved sinus. More aggressive and extensive surgery may be necessary for invasive mycosis; this is discussed in Chapter 43.

The prognosis of immunocompromised patients with infectious sinusitis depends upon early and appropriate therapy and successful management of concurrent disease. This fact further supports the call for routine aspiration of the infected sinus in patients with severe immunosuppression. Administration of culture-directed antimicrobial therapy with concurrent management of associated disease will result in the best outcome.

References

1. Linden BE, Aguilar EA, Allen SJ: Sinusitis in the nasotracheally intubated patient. Arch Otolaryngol Head Neck Surg 1988; 114: 860–861.
2. Arens JF, LeJeune FE Jr, Webre DR: Maxillary sinusitis, a complication of nasotracheal intubation. Anesthesiology 1974; 40: 415–416.
3. Gallagher TJ, Civetta JM: Acute maxillary sinusitis complicating nasotracheal intubation: A case report. Anesth Analg 1976; 55: 885–886.
4. Kronberg FG, Goodwin WJ: Sinusitis in intensive care unit patients. Laryngoscope 1985; 95: 936–938.
5. Caplan ES, Hoyt NJ: Nosocomial sinusitis. JAMA 1982; 247: 639–641.
6. O'Reilly MJ, Reddick EJ, Black W, et al.: Sepsis from sinusitis in nasotracheally intubated patients: A diagnostic dilemma. Am J Surg 1984; 147: 601–604.
7. Deutschman CS, Wilton P, Sinow J, et al.: Paranasal sinusitis associated with nasotracheal intubation: A frequently unrecognized and treatable source of sepsis. Crit Care Med 1986; 14: 111–114.
8. Hansen M, Poulsen MR, Bendixen DK, Hartmann-Andersen F: Incidence of sinusitis in patients with nasotracheal intubation. Br J Anaesth 1988; 61: 231–232.
9. Fassoulaki A, Pamouktsoglou P: Prolonged nasotracheal intubation and its association with inflammation of paranasal sinuses. Anesth Analg 1989; 69: 50–52.
10. Desmond P, Raman R, Idikula J: Effect of nasogastric tubes on the nose and maxillary sinus. Crit Care Med 1991; 19: 509–511.
11. Bach A, Boehrer, Schmidt H, Geiss HK: Nosocomial sinusitis in ventilated patients. Anaesthesia 1992; 47: 335–339.
12. Holzapfel L, Chevret S, Madinier G, et al.: Influence of long-term oro- or nasotracheal intubation on nosocomial maxillary sinusitis and pneumonia: Results of a prospective, randomized, clinical trial. Crit Care Med 1993; 21: 1132–1138.
13. Bell RM, Page GV, Bynoe RP, et al.: Post-traumatic sinusitis. J Trauma 1988; 28: 923–930.
14. Lebeda MD, Haller JR, Graham SM, Hoffman HT: Evaluation of maxillary sinus aspiration in patients with fever of unknown origin. Laryngoscope 1995; 105: 683–685.
15. Rouby JJ, Laurent P, Gosnach M, et al.: Risk factors and clinical relevance of nosocomial maxillary sinusitis in the critically ill. Am J Respir Crit Care Med 1994; 150: 776–783.
16. Deutschman CS, Wilton PB, Sinow J, et al.: Paranasal sinusitis: A common complication of nasotracheal intubation in neurosurgical patients. Neurosurgery 1985; 17: 296–299.
17. Wolf M, Zillinsky I, Lieberman P: Acute mycotic sinusitis with bacterial sepsis in orotracheal intubation and nasogastric tubing: A case report and review of the literature. Otolaryngol Head Neck Surg 1988; 98: 615–617.
18. Gwaltney JM Jr, Syndor A Jr, Sande MA: Etiology and antimicrobial treatment of acute sinusitis. Ann Otol Rhinol Laryngol 1981; 90: 68–71.
19. Evans FO, Syndor JB, Moore WE, et al.: Sinusitis of the maxillary antrum. N Engl J Med 1975; 293: 735–739.
20. Humphrey MA, Simpson GT, Grindlinger GA: Clinical characteristics of nosocomial sinusitis. Ann Otol Rhinol Laryngol 1987; 96: 687–690.
21. Berlinger NT: Sinusitis in immunodeficient and immunosuppressed patients. Laryngoscope 1985; 95: 29–33.
22. Teixido M, Kron TK, Plainse M: Head and neck sequelae of cardiac transplantation. Laryngoscope 1989; 100: 231–236.
23. Ganzel TM, Brohm J, Nechtman CM, et al.: Otolaryngologic problems in cardiac transplant patients. Laryngoscope 1989; 99: 158–161.
24. Shibuya TY, Momin F, Abella E, et al.: Sinus disease in the bone marrow transplant population: Incidence, risk factors, and complications. Otolaryngol Head Neck Surg 1995; 113: 705–711.
25. Reyna J, Richardson JM, Mattox DE, et al.: Head and neck infection after renal transplantation. JAMA 1982; 247: 3337–3339.
26. Shaw GY, Panje WR, Corey JP, et al.: Risk factors in the development of acute sinusitis in immunocompromised patients. Am J Rhinol 1991; 5: 103–108.

Norris K. Lee
Richard L. Mabry

CHAPTER FORTY-TWO

Complications of Sinusitis

▼

The major complications associated with sinusitis are directly correlated with their anatomic location. The severity of a complication depends largely on the significance of the neighboring structure. Because of the central location of the paranasal sinuses, several important areas are at risk. The infectious agent affects neighboring anatomic areas by contiguous spread, either directly through bony dehiscences or via soft tissue channels within the surrounding bones.

The possible complications of acute sinusitis include cellulitis and abscess of the facial soft tissues, intraorbital contents, and intracranial contents. Chronic sinusitis, a complication of acute sinusitis discussed in Chapter 40, can cause any of the aforementioned complications, as well as nasal polyposis, osteomyelitis of facial bones, and mucocele or pyocele causing bony and soft tissue space-occupying deformities of the orbit, intracranial contents, or midface. The clinical recognition, management, and pathogenesis of these complications are addressed from an anatomic perspective.

ANATOMY

The anatomic relationships of the paranasal sinuses can be appreciated in Figures 42–1A and B; a computed tomography (CT) scan with appropriate soft tissue and bony windows demonstrates the same anatomy. Coronal and axial views of the sinuses reveal the close proximity of the sinuses to the following key regions: orbit, anterior cranial fossa, cavernous sinus, nasal cavity, and superficial midface.

Transmission of infection to adjacent structures can occur through both thin and thick bony areas. Each of the sinuses has bony margins; however, some of these bones not only are thin but also can be dehiscent in some areas. The thinnest bones are the most likely to have natural dehiscences. Thus, the lamina papyracea, fovea ethmoidalis, and lateral wall of the sphenoid sinus are particularly predisposed to transmission of infection (Fig. 42–1A). A CT scan that shows lack of calcified bone in these areas may indicate truly dehiscent bone, or there may be translucent, malleable bone that is intact. These areas are remarkably thin and susceptible to transgression by either infection or surgical instrumentation (purposeful or inadvertent). The posterior wall of the frontal sinus is usually relatively thick, but both tables of the frontal bone are pierced by diploic veins. These veins can be conduits for spread of infection anteriorly into the soft tissues of the forehead or posteriorly into the anterior cranial fossa.

Because spread of sinus infection is by contiguous invasion, the structures within the orbit and cranial cavity that are most often affected are those that are immediately adjacent to the infected sinus. For anterior ethmoiditis, this includes the medial orbital fat and medial rectus muscle. For posterior ethmoiditis, the contents of the orbit at its apex are particularly susceptible to inflammation or infection owing to the closed space and lack of room for edematous expansion (see Fig. 42–1B). Hence, the ophthalmic artery and vein, and optic, oculomotor, and abducens nerves are at risk; the trochlear nerve is located more lateral in the superior orbital fissure and thus is slightly less vulnerable. In the case of sphenoid sinusitis, the entire contents of the cavernous sinus are at risk, including the cavernous portion of the internal carotid artery, the ophthalmic artery and vein, the venous plexus that forms the cavernous sinus itself, and cranial nerves III, IV, V_1, V_2, and VI (Fig. 42–1C). For the frontal sinus, inferior intraorbital extension may affect the superior rectus, superior oblique, and levator palpebrae muscles as well as the supratrochlear and supraorbital sensory nerves.[1] Posterior extension of frontal sinusitis may affect the meninges of the anterior cranial fossa as well as the brain parenchyma itself. Maxillary sinusitis rarely causes intraorbital disease even though the antrum is subjacent to the orbit. However, in patients with a history of maxillofacial trauma, there can be soft tissue contiguity between the antrum and orbit, thereby predisposing the orbit to infectious complications. The most common complications of maxillary sinusitis involve the infraorbital nerves superiorly or the roots of the maxillary teeth, which may protrude into the floor of the antrum. Specific symptoms and signs are discussed with each complication.

COMPLICATIONS OF ACUTE SINUSITIS

Chronic Sinusitis

Chronic sinusitis can be considered the most common complication of untreated acute sinusitis. It is addressed fully in Chapter 40. Suffice it to say here that one of the classic presenting signs of chronic sinusitis is nasal polyposis. Chronic polyposis, especially in the lower or anterior nasal cavity where air currents are more direct, can engender chronic epithelial changes, causing masses that appear to be solid and fleshy and, therefore, can be mistaken for tumors. Polyps of very long duration can develop mineral salt precipitation, yielding bony densities on CT scan, which can be misinterpreted to be osteosarcoma-like malignancies (Fig. 42–2). By the time a polyp appears in the nose, it is unlikely that medical therapy alone will cause it to regress totally; however, we have witnessed some rare occasions of complete resolution of small polyps with purely medical therapy.

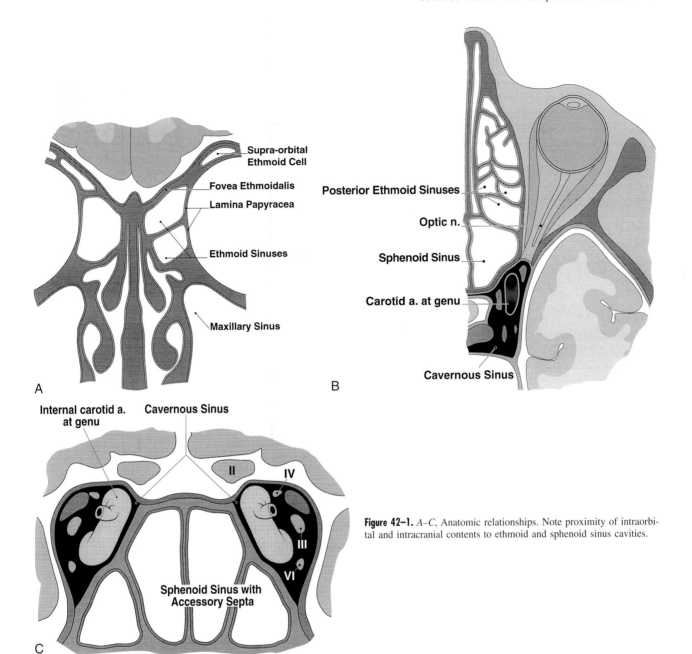

A

B

C

Internal carotid a. at genu

Cavernous Sinus

Sphenoid Sinus with Accessory Septa

Supra-orbital Ethmoid Cell

Fovea Ethmoidalis

Lamina Papyracea

Ethmoid Sinuses

Maxillary Sinus

Posterior Ethmoid Sinuses

Optic n.

Sphenoid Sinus

Carotid a. at genu

Cavernous Sinus

Figure 42–1. *A–C*, Anatomic relationships. Note proximity of intraorbital and intracranial contents to ethmoid and sphenoid sinus cavities.

Nasal polypectomy alone can be performed as a palliative procedure for relieving nasal obstruction, if mitigating circumstances suggest avoidance of sinus surgery; however, the complications of chronic sinusitis are still possible in such cases.

Cultures should be more routinely taken if a complication is apparent or suspected, especially with the rising incidence of multidrug resistance and the ease of endoscope-directed sampling of purulent material. Often, the otorhinolaryngologist is consulted by a patient who has already been treated with all available classes of antibiotic. The specialist should then confirm that the patient was compliant with all the antibiotics. Reasons for noncompliance include excessive cost or noncoverage by insurance plan formulary, side effects (most commonly gastrointestinal reactions), secondary gains,

and confusion with other medications that are often prescribed simultaneously (e.g., antihistamines, decongestants). If noncompliance has been ruled out, but the patient has had some improvement in symptoms at the beginning of a course of antibiotic, then consideration should be given to the possibility that antibiotic levels were inadequate, because of either dosing or duration of treatment. Extending treatment schedules out to 3 weeks or longer, instead of the usual 10 days, can be helpful. In patients with ciliary dysmotility, cystic fibrosis, or acquired immunodeficiency syndrome (AIDS) and in patients hospitalized for long periods, *Pseudomonas* species are also common; appropriate therapy would include oral ciprofloxacin or intravenous aminoglycosides, if warranted. Infections by other gram-negative organisms are rare but notable in the pediatric age group.[2]

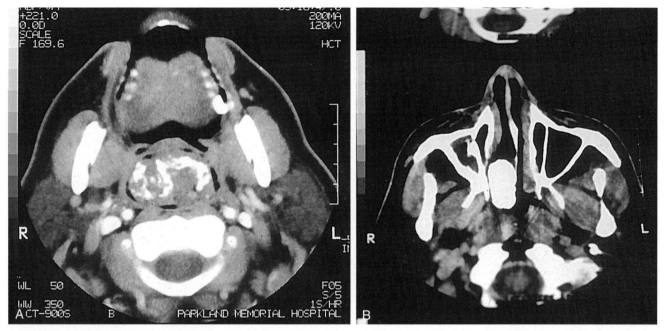

Figure 42–2. *A* and *B*, Chronic antrochoanal polyp, coronal and axial CT. Calcific deposits were so thick that this polyp could not be excised en bloc. Calcified polyp required bone-cutting scissors for removal.

Immunology

Defects in immunity should be sought in patients who have persistent chronic sinusitis despite maximal medical therapy. For those patients who eventually undergo surgical therapy yet still fail to show response to wide-open sinusotomies, other defects in immune status should be evaluated. Typically, work-up of immunoglobulin (Ig) subclass deficiency includes: total IgE, total IgG, and determination of IgG subclasses 1–4. Treatment of subclass deficiency may include intravenous immunoglobulin supplementation and/or long-term antibiotic prophylaxis. It is also necessary to determine the patient's ability to mount an adequate immunologic response to stimuli such as a polysaccharide vaccine.

Orbital Complications

Intraorbital Infections

Orbital extension of acute sinus infections occurs most commonly through bony dehiscences in the lamina papyracea or the frontal sinus floor. The orbit may be involved without any prior history of recurrent sinusitis. Orbital complications can sometimes be the only presenting sign of sinusitis, with little or no associated nasal symptoms. In a study of 129 pediatric patients presenting with an "acute orbit," only 16 (12.4%) were attributable to sinusitis, predominantly ethmoid in origin; this low prevalence of sinusitis may be due to the fact that the series was reported from an ophthalmologic service.[3] Other alternatives in the differential diagnosis were not listed but presumably included common causes such as facial infections, dacryocystitis, trauma with or without alloplastic implants, iatrogenic causes, and tumors.[4] In a combined study of 303 cases of orbital cellulitis admitted

to a general pediatric and a specialty otorhinolaryngology hospital, at least 75% of cases were radiologically documented to be of sinus origin;[5] this latter prevalence seems more realistic. In a retrospective review of 6770 pediatric sinusitis hospital admissions over a 25-year period, 2.3% of patients were found to have orbital or periorbital complications.[6] In younger children, orbital complications of acute ethmoiditis are more common than in adulthood, owing to developmental dehiscences in the lamina papyracea. In older children, intraorbital complications can also involve the superior aspect of the orbit from the later-developing frontal sinuses (Fig. 42–3). Sinusitis in a previously healthy child or young adult can be associated with a history of air or water forced into the sinus cavities or orbit under pressure, such as experienced in jumping into water feet first or riding a steep thrill slide in a water amusement park. Any prior history of nasal or maxillofacial trauma, either iatrogenic or accidental, may predispose the patient to orbital complications resulting from breaks in the integrity of the lamina papyracea or orbital floor.

The practitioner should be familiar with the standard classification system for intraorbital infection as described by Chandler and colleagues.[7] Signs of group 1 orbital involvement are upper eyelid edema with or without erythema (Fig. 42–4). At this stage, there is usually not serious infectious infiltration of orbital soft tissues, but venous outflow is hindered by inflammation in the orbit. Group 2 orbital involvement (cellulitis) demonstrates signs of chemosis, restricted ocular movement, and proptosis, with symptoms of diplopia and possible visual loss. Group 3 infection (subperiosteal abscess) can be limited by the tough periorbita but can also coexist with components of group 2 because of surrounding inflammation. Group 4 infection (intraorbital abscess) is characterized by progression of orbital cellulitis to an organized abscess in the orbital soft tissues, resulting

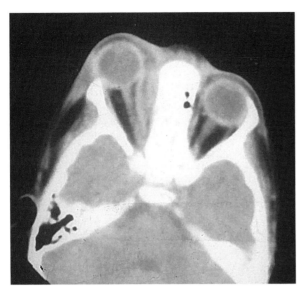

Figure 42–3. Medial orbital subperiosteal abscess, secondary to acute ethmoiditis. Note early intraorbital cellulitis, edema of medial rectus muscle, and impingement of abscess on medial rectus. Involvement of the muscle caused diplopia.

through thin or dehiscent bone, pushing the orbital periosteum laterally or inferiorly (Fig. 42–5). In such cases, the infectious process is technically intraorbital (within the confines of the bony orbit), but the patient's symptoms are not as marked as in the case of infection that has spread within the soft tissues of the orbit. A sizable subperiosteal abscess may cause signs of an intraorbital space-occupying mass, with displacement of the globe laterally if the abscess originated in the ethmoids or inferiorly in cases of frontal sinusitis (Fig. 42–6). If the displacement is severe enough, impairment of the nearest extraocular muscle may cause limitation of eye movement and diplopia. As long as the infection is limited to the subperiosteal plane, there should be no impairment of vision or ophthalmoplegia, nor will there be any conjunctival signs, such as chemosis and vascular injection. Bacteriology varies by age group: specimens from children younger than 9 years grow single aerobic flora *(Streptococcus, Staphylococcus)* or yield negative cultures. Children older than 15 years yield polymicrobial cultures, including anaerobes *(Bacteroides, Veillonella, Peptostreptococcus, Fusobacterium)* and routine aerobes *(Streptococcus, Staphylococcus, Eikenella)*. Children between ages 9 and 14 grow fewer anaerobes but more varied aerobic flora *(Streptococ-*

in proptosis, ophthalmoplegia, pain, and visual loss. Patients with group 5 infection (cavernous sinus thrombosis) are severely ill and have a poor prognosis. Patients in groups 4 and 5 may have long-term visual loss if they survive the initial infection.

Clinical examination can diagnose orbital infection but cannot reliably differentiate between abscess and cellulitis. The best method of evaluating the severity and extent of intraorbital infection is by CT scan of the sinuses and orbits. Coronal and axial views should be obtained, preferably at intervals less than 5 mm.[8] Soft tissue windows usually diagnose an abscess, and the convex pushing of the periorbita by a subperiosteal abscess can often be appreciated. However, in diagnosing abscesses, CT scanning can have a false-negative rate (CT suggests cellulitis but intraoperative findings are of intraorbital abscess) in up to 17% of cases.[9, 10] Therefore, a high level of suspicion must be maintained to rule out abscess. Inflammatory involvement of the intraorbital soft tissues is indicated by "muddy" opacification of the orbital fat signal, edema of the extraocular muscles, and generalized hyperemia of the soft tissues. If possible, bone windows should be obtained, with special attention paid to evaluation of the lamina papyracea, frontal sinus floor, and anterior cranial fossa floor. It is highly important to maintain ongoing vigilance, especially in cases in which the original clinical presentation does not improve rapidly, because the natural history of cellulitis-phlegmon can proceed to abscess. Additionally, in previously surgically drained abscesses, purulent pockets can reaccumulate. The consequences of a misdiagnosis or nondiagnosis of abscess based on a false-negative CT scan can be profound, so serial clinical examinations remain the most important indicator for surgical intervention.[9]

Subperiosteal Abscess. Subperiosteal abscess (Chandler group 3) refers to infection limited to the subperiosteal plane. This usually occurs by extension of an expanding infection

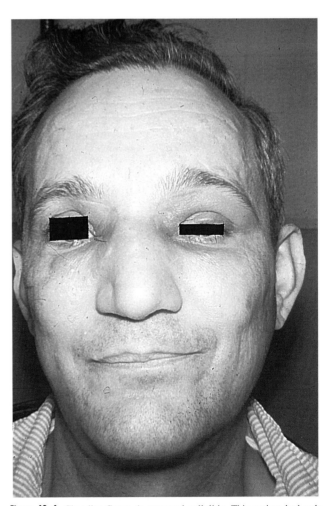

Figure 42–4. Chandler Group 1: preseptal cellulitis. This patient had only edema and cellulitis of the left upper eyelid with no signs or symptoms of intraorbital inflammation.

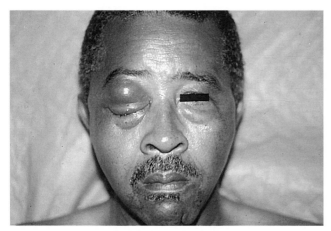

Figure 42–5. Chandler Group 3: right frontal subperiosteal abscess. This patient presented with ophthalmoplegia, diplopia, and proptosis. He had full recovery postoperatively.

cus, *Staphylococcus, Haemophilus influenzae, Moraxella, Eikenella, Klebsiella).*[11] A clinical scenario that can mimic subperiosteal abscess is subperiosteal hematoma in the presence of ethmoiditis; for this condition, the treatment is the same.[12]

Treatment for subperiosteal abscess comprises antibiotics, surgical resection of infected tissues, and surgical drainage of the abscess cavity. Because of the rapid course of untreated intraorbital infection, surgical drainage of subperiosteal abscesses should be performed in a timely, emergent manner. If an abscess is suspected or documented on CT scan, the role of antibiotic therapy is no longer primary but rather is adjunctive. Because the definitive treatment for any abscess is surgical, intravenous antibiotics are part of the preoperative routine only if a (logistical or unforeseen) delay is encountered. For a better chance of isolating the offending

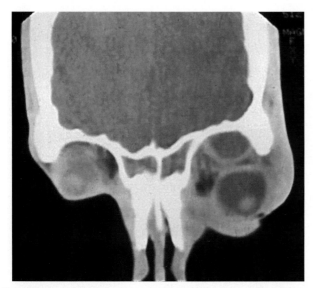

Figure 42–6. Subperiosteal abscess originating from lateral aspect of frontal sinus in 16-year-old male. This patient had severe proptosis, ophthalmoplegia, Chandler class 3 involvement, but no visual loss. He had full recovery postoperatively.

organism, antibiotics can be delayed until after the abscess is drained, if the operation is not unduly delayed.

The surgical approach should be carefully planned, with precise measurements taken to assist the surgeon in the exact localization of the abscess. Depending on the location of the abscess, and the expertise and experience of the surgeon, either an endoscopic and/or an external approach can be undertaken. The transcutaneous approach via a Lynch-type external frontoethmoidectomy is standard, particularly for abscesses located more laterally in the orbit.[13] Typically, endoscopic assistance can be helpful for abscesses at the far anterior and posterior regions of the ethmoid sinus, which are not easily approached externally. This added endoscopic precaution is wise, because the medial prolapse of the orbital soft tissues may obliterate the anterior ethmoidal and frontoethmoidal recess regions. Blocked drainage in that region can lead quickly to further infection, which can then progress rapidly to orbital cellulitis because of the surgical removal of bone between the sinus cavity and orbital contents. When possible, a transnasal endoscopic approach alone can be employed.[14, 15]

In the endoscopic approach, it is wise to leave the lamina papyracea intact during the ethmoidectomy, so that all landmarks remain firm and clear. Premature removal of the lamina papyracea may cause prolapse of the orbital soft tissues into the surgical field, thereby obscuring definitive identification of the abscess cavity. To ensure that the proper part of the lamina papyracea is endoscopically removed, one should remember that close examination of the lamina should reveal natural bony dehiscences through which purulent abscess contents can be noted to be oozing. If the source of pus is not easily seen, gentle pressure on the pliable lamina papyracea may identify areas of weakness that are the most likely sites of purulent extension.

Adequately drained abscesses should resolve quickly, with recovery and hospital discharge expected in a few days. Intravenous antibiotics may often be continued at home. Slower orbital recovery may be due to associated cellulitis or to inadequately drained or reaccumulated abscess. A low threshold for obtaining a repeat CT scan should be maintained in the presence of slow resolution of orbital findings. Full recovery with few or no sequelae can be expected in these cases if the diagnosis and surgical treatment are accomplished in timely fashion, particularly before infection spreads into the intraorbital soft tissues.

Orbital Cellulitis and Intraorbital Abscess. When sinusitis progresses to cause infection of the intraorbital soft tissues, either via direct invasion or via spread of infection from an acute subperiosteal abscess, it can cause induration and/or cellulitis of orbital soft tissues. The time course of orbital cellulitis can be very rapid, worsening quickly from chemosis to visual field loss to total blindness over the course of hours. The reason for this can be attributed to either the increased intercellular fluid pressure, which causes ophthalmic vein collapse, or ophthalmic or retinal artery insufficiency due to spasm or direct thrombosis. Involvement of orbital soft tissues at the orbital apex is termed orbital apex syndrome. Cranial nerves II, III, IV, V_1, and VI are involved, with a clinical picture dominated by visual loss and ophthalmoplegia with associated proptosis and/or ptosis.[16] However, associated proptosis, chemosis, or lid edema can be absent.[17, 18] Surgical decompression of the orbital apex should be combined with removal of infected sinus tissues if symptoms do not rapidly resolve with antibiotic therapy.

The role of the otolaryngologist is to differentiate between an abscess and cellulitis-phlegmon. The presence of an abscess is an indication for surgical intervention, whereas cellulitis without abscess should initially be treated medically. Evaluation of a suspected orbital soft tissue complication of acute sinusitis begins with a physical examination documenting the presence or absence of chemosis, diplopia, ophthalmoplegia, and gross visual acuity. If there is suspicion of early intraorbital cellulitis or abscess, time can be taken to obtain a formal ophthalmologic consultation with complete visual acuity testing. However, if rapidly advancing orbital cellulitis or abscess is suspected, time is of the essence, and visual acuity testing should not delay imaging studies or therapeutic measures.

Intraorbital cellulitis itself is not necessarily a surgical problem. Serial documentation of visual acuity performed on an hourly basis by an ophthalmologist is important. Intravenous antibiotics should be promptly started, with broad-spectrum coverage; typically, 2nd-generation cephalosporins are used. Progression of symptoms after 24 hours of antibiotics or lack of improvement after 72 hours should indicate surgical intervention, both for débridement of the involved sinuses and for orbital decompression and/or exploration. Postoperatively, close monitoring of the eye examination, with serial visual acuity documentation, is very important for the first several hours to days. In contradistinction to subperiosteal abscess, orbital cellulitis typically resolves slowly, with hospital stays sometimes extending beyond 1 week.

Because development of an intraorbital abscess is a possible complication of orbital cellulitis, a low threshold for repeating serial CT scans should be maintained, even after surgical intervention. If an abscess develops within the soft tissues of the orbit, a transorbital approach is usually required for drainage. Surgical consultation should be obtained from an experienced ophthalmologist who is accustomed to working within the soft tissues of the orbit, because this area is unfamiliar territory to many otorhinolaryngologists. Because of intraorbital manipulations and the possible change in intraorbital volume, diplopia is a complication that may not be avoidable, both immediately and in the long term. The patient should be forewarned of this eventuality; preoperative evaluation by an ophthalmologist should include counseling regarding the possible need for corrective strabismus surgery at a later time.

The prognosis for intraorbital cellulitis and abscess is worse than for subperiosteal abscess. Long-standing diplopia is theoretically possible because of fibrosis in the extraocular muscles. The retina has a low regenerative capacity; therefore, any visual loss sustained during the orbital infection may not return, even if the infection is cured before total blindness occurs. The incidence of permanent blindness is 2%, highly associated with undiagnosed abscess that remains undrained.[9]

Retro-orbital Complications

Cavernous Sinus Thrombosis. The cavernous sinus is prone to infection from several sources. Owing to its poste-rior and central location, the cavernous sinus is susceptible to direct spread of infection from the sphenoid sinus as well as indirect spread from the posterior ethmoid sinuses or orbital contents via the ophthalmic veins. The presenting symptoms of untreated or undertreated cavernous sinus infection include nausea/vomiting, fever with spiking chills ("picket fence fever"), decreased visual acuity, diplopia, and hypesthesia, dysesthesia, or parasthesia along cranial nerve V_1 or V_2. Also characteristic are severe headaches located in the middle of the head, behind the eyes, or in a location difficult for the patient to accurately localize. Infection in the slow-moving blood pools of the cavernous sinus can progress very rapidly to cause cavernous sinus thrombosis, which is a life-threatening condition. Signs of cavernous sinus thrombosis are proptosis, ophthalmoplegia, papilledema, chemosis, venous stasis in the orbital soft tissues, visual loss or blindness, and decreased mental acuity. The mortality for this complication is approximately 20% because of ensuing intracranial infection. The incidence of bilateral thrombosis of the cavernous sinuses is significant; therefore, total blindness is a possible complication if the patient does not succumb to the infection. Further complications include meningitis, intracerebral abscess(es), cerebritis, and carotid–cavernous sinus fistula.[19]

Any patient in whom cavernous sinus involvement is suspected should undergo an immediate CT scan with intravenous contrast material. Positive findings include contrast enhancement in the cavernous sinus, intraorbital soft tissue venous congestion, and sinusitis in any paranasal sinus (most commonly the sphenoid or ethmoid sinuses). Full angiography is also helpful in the definitive diagnosis.

After the CT scan defines the anatomy, endoscopic examination can be performed using local anesthesia to obtain cultures from the middle meatus or sphenoid ostium. Microbiology typically identifies *Staphylococcus aureus* (50%–70%), streptococci (20%), and gram-negative anaerobes (e.g., *Bacteroides, Fusobacterium*).[20, 21] Lumbar puncture may yield leukocytosis and increased protein, but cultures may eventually be negative. Blood cultures may be positive, especially if obtained during a fever spike. Multidrug, intravenous antibiotics should be started early. A synthetic penicillin such as nafcillin is needed to cover most *Staphylococcus* species, including *S. aureus*. In addition, a broader-spectrum coverage, including anaerobes, is provided by 3rd-generation cephalosporins, chloramphenicol, and metronidazole, all of which have good blood-brain barrier penetration.

If there is strong suspicion of progression to cavernous sinus thrombosis, neurosurgical and ophthalmologic consultations should be obtained. The role of anticoagulant therapy is still debated. Theoretically, such measures may help prevent progression of the clot. Constant vigil should be maintained on an hourly basis for evidence of extension of infection into other intracranial compartments (see later). Surgical intervention for drainage of the offending sinus and orbital decompression may be indicated for salvaging vision, but if the intracranial complications have progressed significantly, surgery may be futile. Timely diagnosis and treatment may yield survival in 70%–75% of cases.[20] However, survivors may have permanent sequelae, including blindness and other cranial nerve palsies.[22]

Intracranial Complications

Because a common site of intracranial infection is the frontal lobe region, which is clinically a relatively silent area, a high suspicion must be maintained for frontal sinus symptoms that do not resolve quickly. Thus, acute sinusitis in the frontal or sphenoid sinuses must be observed very closely, with vigilant monitoring of vital signs and mental faculties. There can be a relatively high degree of discordance between clinical findings and actual intracranial disease, until late stages of involvement are present. The best method of treating intracranial complications is to prevent them from occurring through timely use of antibiotics and surgical intervention while the acute sinusitis is still limited to the sinus cavity. This early recognition of potentially dangerous complications is of such importance that we will briefly review the symptoms and signs of advanced acute (frontal and sphenoid) sinusitis just prior to its progression to intracranial disease.

Symptoms of uncomplicated acute frontal sinusitis are frontal region headache/pain, local tenderness, mild fever, and nasal congestion in the ethmoid region. Patients with acute frontal sinus symptoms should undergo endoscopically guided culture of the frontonasal recess if possible, started on broad-spectrum oral antibiotics, and watched closely. Those patients whose symptoms do not resolve on oral antibiotics within 48 hours should be started on broad-spectrum intravenous antibiotics to cover *S. aureus* and resistant anaerobic streptococci; use of a semisynthetic penicillin plus chloramphenicol, metronidazole, or a 3rd-generation cephalosporin for good central nervous system penetration is recommended.[21, 23] If another 48 hours of observation with intravenous antibiotics do not obtain improvement, regardless whether cultures demonstrate pathogens that may be sensitive to the empirically chosen antibiotics in vitro, surgical drainage of the frontal sinus is indicated, either endoscopically or transcutaneously via a Lynch incision. Care must be taken to ensure adequate frontal sinus drainage in the postoperative period via the frontonasal duct. In pediatric patients, the majority of intracranial complications occur in males (78%), older than 9 years (89%), who have no prior sinusitis history (78%).[24] The younger pediatric population is not so prone to intracranial complications because of the late development of the frontal sinuses.

Symptoms of acute sphenoid sinusitis are much more protean, including intense headache at the cranial vertex or occiput, or pain that is difficult to describe or localize. Unfortunately, nonfocal pain may be treated lightly if the physician does not have a high degree of suspicion. Often, these patients do not give a history of recurrent episodes of sinusitis, but they generally do have a history of recent upper respiratory infection. Simple sinus radiographs identify an air-fluid level in the sphenoid sinus. Treatment should consist of broad-spectrum antibiotics, decongestant, and mucolytics for 24–48 hours. If there is no resolution, intravenous antibiotics should be started and close observation continued, to rule out cavernous sinus or other intracranial infection. Failure of symptoms to resolve in another 36 hours should suggest the need for surgical drainage via an endoscopic approach in the vicinity of the natural ostium or through the posterior ethmoid region (e.g., Wigand approach).

Intracranial spread of sinusitis can occur indirectly via a hematogenous route from the sphenoid or frontal sinuses, directly via the cavernous sinus, or, more commonly, from frontal sinusitis by direct posterior extension or through the diploic veins in the posterior table of the frontal bone. Frontal sinusitis has been reported to be the single most common cause (23%) of cerebral abscess in a series of 74 cases.[25]

Progressive frontal sinusitis can lead to meningitis, cerebritis, subdural or epidural empyema/abscess, or intraparenchymal brain abscess. Although we discuss them separately, any or all of the complications can occur together. Thus, although meningitis and cerebritis are treated medically, they can evolve into or be associated with localized purulent collections that require neurosurgical drainage. For all of these complications, the bacteria responsible include *Streptococcus* and *Staphylococcus* species, *H. influenzae, Neisseria,* and anaerobes.

Meningitis

Meningitis manifests as classic symptoms of fever, headache, photophobia, stiff neck, and behavioral changes or obtundation. Seizures can also occur, because of inflammation and irritation of the underlying parenchyma. The altered mental status may make diagnosis unclear, but a clear history of recent upper respiratory infection with frontal headache can usually be elicited. Cerebrospinal fluid shows leukocytosis, elevated opening pressure, elevated protein level, depressed glucose level, and bacteria identifiable on Gram's stain. Specimens for blood culture should also be drawn concomitantly.

Abscesses: Epidural, Subdural, Intraparenchymal

An abscess or empyema of the epidural potential space almost always is adjacent to the frontal sinus and is often due to direct suppuration around an osteomyelitic focus (Fig. 42–7). The tough dura may limit the purulent material to an extradural location, but symptoms arise from the mass effect as well as from the surrounding inflammation, causing localized symptoms such as dull frontal headache, drowsiness, fever, and other nonspecific complaints. Because these symptoms are similar to those associated with uncomplicated acute frontal sinusitis or osteomyelitis, a high level of suspicion should be maintained by the rhinologist. Additionally, the frontal regions of the brain are the most likely areas to be affected first, but the nonspecific nature of the associated symptoms contributes to difficulty in diagnosis.[26]

Subdural abscesses occur in the potential space between the dura and the arachnoid space. The route of infection can be either direct, from the diploic veins or an osteomyelitic focus, or indirect, from meningitis. Because they are located deep to the dura, such abscesses are more likely to cause localizable symptoms as well as changes in mental status. Inflammation of the underlying pia mater, thrombosis of the meningeal veins, and rapid spread within the subdural space to other areas of the brain cause symptoms of fever, seizures, hemiplegia, aphasia, and obtundation. Because of the space-occupying mass, lumbar puncture is debatable.

In contrast to a direct route of spread from the frontal

Figure 42–7. Epidural and subdural abscesses adjacent to posterior table of frontal sinus.

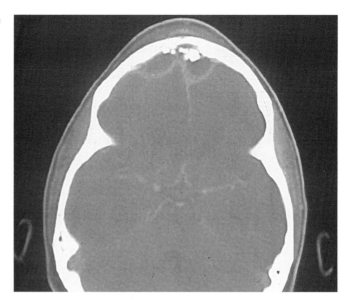

sinus, intraparenchymal brain abscess is seeded by the hematogenous route and thus may be located in any region of the brain, although the frontal lobes are still the most likely to be involved (Fig. 42–8). Brain abscesses are likely to cause marked shifts in the cerebrum, due to localized cerebritis and edema, leading to more severe symptoms. Additionally, brain abscesses can affect specific regions of the central nervous system, causing localizable dysfunctions. More than half of all intracranial abscesses of sinus origin have been reported in patients less than 30 years old without predisposing factors of systemic immunodeficiency.[27, 28] Brain ab-

scesses are usually single but are multiple in 13% of cases.[29] Seizure activity is relatively common (33%), especially in children.[24]

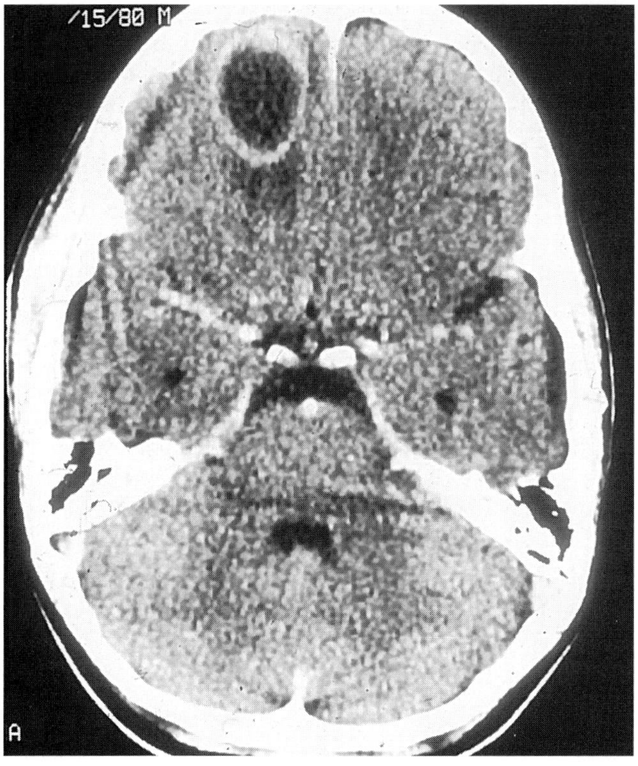

Diagnosis

Work-up for intracranial complications includes CT scan with intravenous contrast material, blood cultures, and routine blood work. The indication for lumbar puncture is debatable because of the high incidence of false-negative results in cases of abscesses as well as the danger of transtentorial herniation.[29, 30] CT scanning has lowered the incidence of mortality in these cases through earlier diagnosis.[31] Magnetic resonance imaging (MRI) may offer superior soft tissue details intracranially.[32] If sphenoid sinusitis is diagnosed, there is a danger of pituitary failure; thus, vigilance against thyroid dysfunction and adrenal insufficiency should be instituted by obtaining baseline studies.

Treatment

Meningitis and cerebritis are treated by broad-spectrum antibiotics that are capable of penetrating the blood-brain barrier. Third-generation cephalosporins, chloramphenicol, and metronidazole penetrate the blood-brain barrier and also provide broad coverage, but staphylococcal species are not covered well enough. Therefore, a semisynthetic penicillin must be added. There is less urgency than with intracranial abscesses to proceed to surgical drainage of the paranasal sinuses if meningitis is the only complication. However, vigilance for synchronous intracranial sites of disease must be maintained.

Abscesses are surgical disorders, so all therapy should be directed toward stabilizing the patient as quickly as possible, with the endpoint being drainage of the abscess. In a series of 13 pediatric patients with intracranial abscesses, 3 required emergent neurosurgical drainage, and 10 were observed and started on antibiotics. All 10 medically treated patients demonstrated enlarging abscesses, all of which eventually needed neurosurgical intervention.[33] During the same period of general anesthesia, endoscopic drainage of the

Figure 42–8. Intraparenchymal brain abscess, secondary to frontal sinusitis.

Table 42-1. INTRACRANIAL COMPLICATIONS OF SINUSITIS: OUTCOMES

	Empyema/ Abscess	Meningitis	Venous Thrombosis	Osteomyelitis	Total
Number of cases	12	8	3	3	24†
Number of cases with residual sequelae	5	2	3	0	10
Incidence	42%	25%	100%	0%	42%

Derived from Clayman GL, Adams GL, Paugh DR, Koopman CF Jr: Intracranial complications of paranasal sinusitis: A combined institutional review. Laryngoscope 1991; 101: 234–239.

†Some patients manifested more than one complication.

involved sinuses should be accomplished.[29] This combined approach has been shown to decrease hospital stay and incidence of neurosurgical reexploration.[34] The specific neurosurgical approaches for intracranial abscesses are beyond the scope of this chapter, but options include open drainage as well as radiologically guided or stereotactically controlled procedures.

In a retrospective review of 649 sinusitis patients hospitalized for acute or chronic sinusitis, Clayman and colleagues[28] documented a 3.7% incidence of intracranial complications. Table 42–1 presents a meta-analysis of their data, depicting the incidence of serious intracranial complications and their associated long-term sequelae. Almost half developed permanent sequelae of varying degrees. Venous sinus thrombosis is the most serious intracranial complication, with 100% of affected patients developing serious long-term sequelae, including mortality. Empyema/abscess in any location resulted in residual sequelae in 5 of 12 cases (42%). Meningitis carried a 25% incidence of residual defects. Other series reported higher incidences of mortality, up to 20%–25%.[35, 36]

COMPLICATIONS OF CHRONIC SINUSITIS

Mucocele

Intraorbital mucocele is a complication of chronic sinusitis. The most common source of the mucocele is the frontal sinus or a supraorbital ethmoid cell, with the intrasinus pressure eroding the floor or lateral aspect of the sinus

(Fig. 42–9). Typically, the patient has no ophthalmologic complaints until the mucocele is large enough to cause proptosis, diplopia, or vision loss; however, enlargement of a mucocele can be so gradual that the patient and family may not recognize any abnormality. Pain associated with a mucocele is rare, but signs and symptoms of chronic sinusitis may be long-standing: nasal obstruction, congestion, postnasal drip, midface headaches, recurrent infections requiring antibiotics, and nasal polyposis. CT scanning with bony and soft tissue windows delineates the relationship of the mucocele to the orbital tissues. Special attention should be paid to the integrity of the orbital roof and the relationship of the mass to intracranial contents. Mucoceles can extend posteriorly into the anterior cranial fossa.

Osteomyelitis

Chronic osteomyelitis of facial bones, secondary to chronic sinusitis, is rare with the widespread use of broad-spectrum antibiotics. The bone most commonly involved is the frontal bone, causing tenderness and frontal bossing, historically known as Pott's puffy tumor (Fig. 42–10). In our experience, the maxilla is the next most commonly involved bone. Diagnosis is made by physical examination that reveals local tenderness and dull pain; definitive diagnosis is made by CT scan and nuclear isotope scanning. A surgical procedure is usually needed, to obtain adequate cultures of the sinus mucosa and bone. Treatment consists of intravenous antibiotics for at least 6 weeks. Hyperbaric oxygen therapy, given either preoperatively or perioperatively, may be helpful; however, there are no controlled, prospective trials proving its merits.[37] If necessary, surgical débridement of nonviable bone is warranted. Postoperative antibiotics and hyperbaric oxygen are indicated in severe cases. Close monitoring for intracranial complications is prudent, because the recommended medical therapy is so lengthy that the aforementioned intracranial complications may have time to develop.

Allergic Fungal Sinusitis

The presence of persistent pale, edematous mucosa, and thick, inspissated, green-brown, greasy secretions should

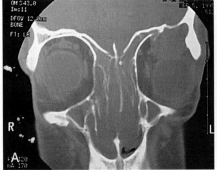
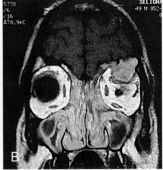
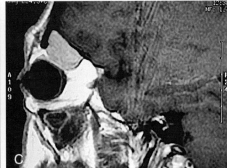

Figure 42–9. *A,* Computed tomography (CT): mucocele originating from lateral aspect of left supraorbital ethmoid cell, displacing globe inferiorly. This patient had 3 mm proptosis but no other complaints. Mucocele was approached transorbitally, but all other sinuses were addressed endoscopically. *B,* Coronal magnetic resonance imaging (MRI): bone of orbital roof was intact, demonstrated on CT and intraoperatively. *C,* Parasagittal MRI: cultures grew *S. faecalis.*

suggest allergic fungal sinusitis (AFS); affected patients typically have other atopic reactivity as well. Their underlying problem is allergic, not infectious. This fungal "infection" is not a truly invasive infection of soft or bony tissues; it is to be distinguished from the invasive fungal sinusitis associated with immunocompromise or diabetic ketoacidosis. Patients with AFS are not gravely ill but may present with proptosis and impressively enlarged or destroyed sinus cavities full of mucoid secretions. They can have coexisting chronic bacterial sinusitis and allergic fungal sinusitis, so the intranasal findings can vary from pale allergic mucosa to inflamed mucosa and polyps.

Geographically, the area of greatest prevalence of AFS lies in a belt of hot, humid weather along the southern United States. Pathophysiologically, affected patients are not immunocompromised but manifest severe allergic reactions to dematiaceous fungi such as *Aspergillus, Helminthosporium, Alternaria, Bipolaris, Curvularia,* and *Exserohilum* species, which do not invade soft tissues (in contradistinction to invasive fungal infections, e.g., mucormycosis in diabetics). They frequently have a characteristic CT scan with findings that are almost pathognomonic: hazy densities in the middle of extensive soft tissue thickening, often with deformed or absent bony margins (Fig. 42–11). In general, these infections are not more serious than slowly expanding masses. Rarely, they can produce intracranial and intraorbital complications, both alone and in concert with a coexisting bacterial sinusitis.[38, 39]

Because patients with AFS suffer from a complex combi-

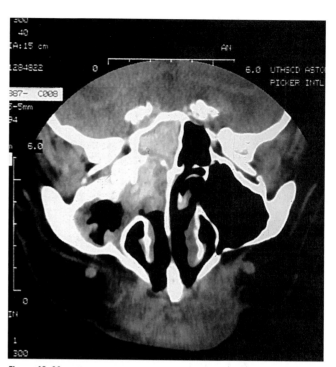

Figure 42–11. Allergic fungal sinusitis, computed tomography scan. Soft tissue opacification of any sinus can occur, with areas of hazy, high-density mucoid concretions (not calcifications) located in central regions.

nation of allergic and infectious sinusitis, they need maximal medical therapy in conjunction with surgical intervention. Therapy is directed at surgical extirpation of disease, in conjunction with controlling the allergies with appropriate medical means. Preoperative antibiotics, antihistamines, and local and systemic steroids are necessary to maximize the chances of improvement with surgery. Surgically, despite the impressive CT appearance, a thick rind of reactive mucosa envelops the mucoid secretions. Even with destruction of the lateral walls of the sphenoid sinus or posterior table of the frontal sinus, there is little fear of transgressing the dura mater, if the rhinologist is careful to remove only the diseased secretions and obstructing mucosa; there is usually no need for neurosurgical consultation.

Usually, all of the sinus surgery can be performed endoscopically by an experienced sinus surgeon, but the procedure may require resection of the lamina papyracea to provide adequate drainage of any intraorbital mucocele(s). Mucoceles located laterally in the orbit may need an additional external approach. Extensive postoperative care is necessary to ensure that the cavities remain open. Daily high-pressure and voluminous nasal/sinus irrigation is helpful to mechanically clear out allergens, while maximal medical therapy is continued, including systemic steroids for at least 3 weeks postoperatively. Immunotherapy with relevant fungal antigens shows promise in clinical trials that are ongoing.[40]

References

1. Garcia CE, Cunningham MJ, Clary RA, Joseph MP: The etiologic role of frontal sinusitis in pediatric orbital abscesses. Am J Otolaryngol 1993; 14: 449–452.

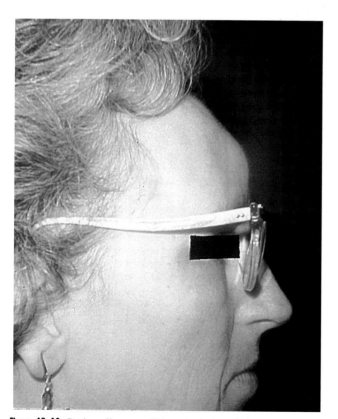

Figure 42–10. Pott's puffy tumor. This patient's frontal sinus extended relatively high. The usual location of Pott's puffy tumor is immediately superior to the glabella.

2. Hemady R, Zimmerman A, Katzen BW, Karesh JW: Orbital cellulitis caused by *Eikenella corrodens*. Am J Ophthalmol 1992; 114: 584–588.
3. Williams BJ, Harrison HC: Subperiosteal abscesses of the orbit due to sinusitis in childhood. Austr N Z J Ophthalmol 1991; 19: 29–36.
4. Moloney JR, Badham NJ, McRae A: The acute orbit. J Laryngol Otol 1987; 101(suppl 12): 1–18.
5. Schramm VL, Curtin HD, Kennerdell JS: Evaluation of orbital cellulitis and results of treatment. Laryngoscope 1982; 92: 732–738.
6. Fearon B, Edmonds B, Bird R: Orbital-facial complications of sinusitis in children. Laryngoscope 1979; 89: 947–952.
7. Chandler JR, Langenbrunner DJ, Stevens ER: The pathogenesis of orbital complications in acute sinusitis. Laryngoscope 1970; 80: 1414–1428.
8. Williams SR, Carruth JA: Orbital infection secondary to sinusitis in children: Diagnosis and management. Clin Otolaryngol 1992; 17: 550–557.
9. Patt BS, Manning SC: Blindness from orbital complications of sinusitis. Otolaryngol Head Neck Surg 1991; 104: 789–795.
10. Clary RA, Cunningham MJ, Eavey RD: Orbital complications of acute sinusitis: Comparison of computed tomography scan and surgical findings. Ann Otol Rhinol Laryngol 1992; 101: 598–600.
11. Harris GJ: Subperiosteal abscess of the orbit: Age as a factor in the bacteriology and response to treatment. Ophthalmology 1994; 101: 585–595.
12. Zalzal G: Periorbital hematoma secondary to sinusitis in a child. Arch Otolaryngol Head Neck Surg 1991; 117: 557–559.
13. Arjmand EM, Lusk RP, Muntz HR: Pediatric sinusitis and subperiosteal orbital abscess formation: Diagnosis and treatment. Otolaryngol Head Neck Surg 1993; 109: 886–894.
14. Elverland HH, Melheim I, Anke IM: Acute orbit from ethmoiditis drained by endoscopic sinus surgery. Acta Otolaryngol Suppl (Stockh) 1992; 492: 147–151.
15. Manning SC: Endoscopic management of medial subperiosteal orbital abscess. Arch Otolaryngol Head Neck Surg 1993; 119: 789–791.
16. Kronschnabel EF: Orbital apex syndrome due to sinusitis. Laryngoscope 1974; 84: 353–371.
17. Tarazi AE, Shikani AH: Irreversible unilateral visual loss due to acute sinusitis. Arch Otolaryngol Head Neck Surg 1991; 117: 1400–1401.
18. el-Sayed Y, al-Muhaimed H: Acute visual loss in association with sinusitis. J Laryngol Otol 1993; 107: 840–842.
19. Oktedalen O, Lilleas F: Septic complications to sphenoidal sinus infection. Scand J Infect Dis 1992; 24: 353–356.
20. Southwick F, Richardson EP Jr, Swartz MN: Septic thrombosis of the dural venous sinuses. Medicine 1986; 65: 82–106.
21. Baker AS: Role of anaerobic bacteria in sinusitis and its complications. Ann Otol Rhinol Laryngol Suppl 1991; 154: 17–22.
22. Yarington CT: The prognosis and treatment of cavernous sinus thrombosis. Ann Otol Rhinol Laryngol 1961; 70: 263–267.
23. Bluestone CD, Steiner R: Intracranial complications of acute frontal sinusitis. South Med J 1965; 58: 1–10.
24. Rosenfeld EA, Rowley AH: Infectious intracranial complications of sinusitis, other than meningitis, in children: 12-year review. Clin Infect Dis 1994; 18: 750–754.
25. Chalstrey S, Pfleiderer AG, Moffat DA: Persisting incidence and mortality of sinogenic cerebral abscess: A continuing reflection of late clinical diagnoses. J Royal Soc Med 1991; 84: 193–195.
26. Daya S, To SS: A 'silent' intracranial complication of frontal sinusitis. J Laryngol Otol 1990; 104: 645–647.
27. Nunez DA: Presentation of rhinosinugenic intracranial abscesses. Rhinology 1991; 29: 99–103.
28. Clayman GL, Adams GL, Paugh DR, Koopman CF Jr: Intracranial complications of paranasal sinusitis: A combined institutional review. Laryngoscope 1991; 101: 234–239.
29. Kratimenos F, Crockard HA: Multiple brain abscess: A review of fourteen cases. Br J Neurosurg 1991; 5: 153–161.
30. Singer JI: An aseptic meningitis picture from incipient brain abscess. Pediatr Emerg Care 1992; 8: 238–240.
31. Small M, Dale BA: Intracranial suppuration 1968–1982—a 15 year review. Clin Otolaryngol 1984; 9: 315–321.
32. Press GA, Weindling SM, Hesselink JR, et al: Rhinocerebral mucormycosis: MR manifestations. J Comput Asst Tomog 1988; 12: 744–749.
33. Johnson DL, Markle BM, Wiedermann BL, Hanahan L: Treatment of intracranial abscesses associated with sinusitis in children and adolescents. J Pediatr 1988; 113: 15–23.
34. Hoyt DJ, Fisher SR: Otolaryngologic management of patients with subdural empyema. Laryngoscope 1991; 101: 20–24.
35. Maniglia AJ, Goodwin WJ, Arnold JE, Ganz E: Intracranial abscess due to nasal sinus and orbital infections in adults and children. Arch Otolaryngol Head Neck Surg 1989; 115: 1424–1429.
36. Bradley PJ, Manning KP, Shaw MD: Brain abscess secondary to paranasal sinusitis. J Laryngol Otol 1984; 98: 719–725.
37. Strauss MB: Refractory osteomyelitis. J Hyperbar Med 1987; 2: 146–159.
38. Aviv JE, Lawson W, Bottone EJ, et al: Multiple intracranial mucoceles associated with phaeohyphomycosis of the paranasal sinuses. Arch Otolaryngol Head Neck Surg 1990; 116: 1210–1213.
39. Daghistani KJ, Jamal TS, Zaher S, Nassif OI: Allergic *Aspergillus* sinusitis with proptosis. J Laryngol Otol 1992; 106: 799–803.
40. Mabry RL, Manning SC, Mabry CS: Immunotherapy for allergic fungal sinusitis. Otolaryngol Head Neck Surg 1995 (in press).

Andrew Blitzer
William Lawson

CHAPTER FORTY-THREE

Fungal Sinusitis

▼

Fungal sinusitis produces significant disability and mortality. It is important for the clinician to understand this group of relatively uncommon forms of sinusitis, since the symptoms may easily be overlooked and the condition misdiagnosed. Early diagnosis and treatment may prevent permanent disability and possible death.

The evaluation and management of these infections require close communication between specialists, including otolaryngologist, infectious disease consultant, microbiologist, and pathologist.

OVERVIEW

The incidence and prevalence of fungal infections of the nose and paranasal sinuses are increasing, as is the diversity of pathogenic organisms. Table 43–1 gives an overview of the incidence of various fungal organisms in the etiology of sinusitis. *Aspergillus* is still the most common, but the incidence and number of pathogenic organisms are changing, likely owing to the increasing numbers of persons rendered immunocompromised by transplant surgery or infections such as acquired immunodeficiency syndrome (AIDS).

The published incidence of fungal sinusitis varies much and is very high as reported in the European literature. In a review of 600 cases of maxillary sinusitis, 81 were caused by a fungus, principally *Aspergillus fumigatus*.[1] In another study 22 fungal infections and 97 mixed fungal and bacterial infections were found among 414 children with maxillary sinusitis, for a prevalence of 28.7%.[2] Fungi from 24 genera were isolated, the most common being *Penicillium* organisms (49 cases), followed by *Aspergillus* (30 cases), *Candida* (20 cases), and *Dematium* (12 cases). Other fungal organisms

isolated were *Alternaria*, *Cephalosporium*, *Chaetomium*, *Chrysosporium*, *Cladosporium*, *Dendrostilbella*, *Epicoccum*, *Gliocladium*, *Graphium*, *Mortierella*, *Mucor*, *Mycelia*, *Paecilomyces*, *Rhodotorula*, *Scopulariopsis*, *Stemphylium*, *Stachyboris*, *Torulopsis*, *Trichoderma*, and *Trichosporon* organisms.

Stammberger describes having treated over 140 patients with massive fungal sinusitis in the period from 1976 to 1985.[3] Among 48 patients he studied, 10 had diabetes and 10 were receiving prolonged antibiotic therapy. *A. fumigatus* appeared to be the most common offending organism, being present in pure culture in 31 cases and in mixed cultures in 8 cases (in 3 with *Pencillium* organisms, 3 with *Cladosporium*, 1 with *Fusarium*; 1 with *Aspergillus niger*). In 6 other cases in which fungi were cultured, there were pure cultures of *Cladosporium* (4 cases), *Penicillium* (1 case), and a mixed culture of *Cladosporium* and *Fusarium* organisms (1 case).

In Northern India, over a 2-year period, Chakrabarti and colleagues isolated fungi in 50 of 119 clinically suspected cases.[4] The organism was *Aspergillus flavus* in 40 cases, *A. fumigatus* in 3 cases, other *Aspergillus* species in 2 cases, *Alternaria* species in 2 cases, *Rhizopus arrhizus* in 2 cases, and *Candida albicans* in 1 case. The authors characterized the infections as noninvasive in 31 cases, invasive in 17 cases, and allergic in 2 cases.

This chapter will review aspergillosis, mucormycosis, and the dematiaceous fungi. Blastomycosis, candidiasis, histoplasmosis, and paracoccidioidomycosis also occur in the paranasal sinuses, and information about these fungi may be found elsewhere in this book or in the articles by Blitzer and Lawson.[5, 6, 7] Information about fusariotoxicosis, sporotricosis, paecilomycosis, basidiomycosis, and cryptococcosis can be found in Table 43–2. Other less common invasive and noninvasive fungal infections can be found in Table 43–3.

Sinusitis caused by multiple organisms is very rare. There are five documented cases of sinonasal infections by multiple dematiaceous fungi (Table 43–4). These mixed infections showed a predilection for young males, and four of five patients had normal immune status.

There are too few reported cases of infections with multiple fungal organisms to allow investigators to draw definite conclusions. As in single-fungus sinus disease, however, multiple sinuses tend to be infected in immunocompetent hosts, and surgical débridement is usually adequate to cure noninvasive cases. The patient of Washburn and colleagues nevertheless experienced an aggressive infection with a protracted clinical course from a tissue-invasive organism that was controlled with difficulty by radical surgery and systemic antifungal therapy.[8] The case reported by Zieske and colleagues involved bone erosion and required multiple surgical procedures and intravenous amphotericin B for con-

Table 43–1. CAUSATIVE ORGANISMS IN FUNGAL SINUSITIS

Genus	Prevalence (%)
Aspergillus	Most common
Mucor	Numerous
Dematiaceous fungi	95
Bipolaris	47
Curvularia	22
Alternaria	10
Exserohilum	9
Cladosporium	7
Fusarium	5
Sporothrix	4
Paecilomyces	3
Basidiomyces	2
Cryptococcus	2

Table 43–2. OTHER FUNGAL INFECTIONS

Fungus	Patients (No.)	Site	Underlying Disease	Treatment	Comment
Fusarium (noninvasive) [45, 126–129]	3	Maxillary sinus	Status post bone marrow transplant, leukemia	Amphotericin B (failed to control disease; rapid death)	Infection occurs mostly in immunocompromised hosts; organism produces myocotoxin causing myelosuppression
	1	Nasal septum	Status post bone marrow transplant		
	1	Middle turbinate	Diabetes mellitus		
Sporotrichosis (invasive) [130–134]	1	Maxillary sinus	Systemic spread of mucocutaneous disease	Surgery plus systemic antifungal therapy	Uncommon infection of an invasive fungus; nasal lesions usually related to visceral dissemination
	1	Septum, lateral nasal wall	Systemic spread of mucocutaneous disease	Surgery plus systemic antifungal therapy	
	1	Ethmoid and orbit	Diabetes mellitus	Surgery plus systemic antifungal therapy	
	1	Ethmoid	Immunocompromised patient	Lateral rhinotomy, amphotericin B	
Paecilomyces (noninvasive) [33, 135–137]	1	Maxillary sinus	Status post endodontic therapy	Curettage	Generally follows ophthalmic, cardiac, or neurosurgery with placement of implant or prosthesis
	1	Maxillary sinus	None	Caldwell-Luc	
	1	Sphenoid sinus	None	Sphenoidotomy	
Basidiomyces (noninvasive) [33, 138–141]	1	Nasal septum	Chronic lung disease	Local surgery	Low-virulence infection; none in immunocompromised patients; all cases with chronic sinusitis
	1	Palatal ulcer	None	Local surgery	
	3	Maxillary sinus	Chronic sinusitis, diabetes mellitus	Caldwell-Luc (surgical débridement adequate therapy)	
Cryptococcus (invasive and noninvasive) [33, 143–146]	1	Nasal septum	None	None	Sinonasal form extremely rare
	1	Nasal vestibule	None	Went on to produce meningoencephalitis	
	2	Maxillary, ethmoid, sphenoid	AIDS (one case)	Surgery, amphotericin B, 5-flucytosine	

trol.[9] In the immunocompromised patient of Loveless and colleagues, the infection remained limited to the nasal cavity, the portal of entry; the infection responded to local surgical drainage and control of the underlying systemic disease by chemotherapy.[10]

ETIOLOGY

A number of environmental and host factors have been cited as causative to the development of fungal sinusitis. In both

Table 43–3. FUNGAL INFECTIONS NOT INCLUDED IN DISCUSSION

Allescheria (Pseudoallescheria, Petriellidium) (invasive)[8, 33, 130, 147–158]
Basidiobolus (invasive/noninvasive)[159, 160]
Cephalosporium (invasive/noninvasive)[161]
Cercospora (invasive/noninvasive)[162]
Chromoblastomycosis (noninvasive)[91, 163–169]
Chrysosporium (invasive/noninvasive)[170]
Coccidioides (noninvasive)[35, 171–174]
Conidiobolus (noninvasive)[159, 175]
Cunninghamella (invasive)[176]
Emericella (noninvasive)[177]
Entomophthoroa (noninvasive)[159]
Loboa (noninvasive)[178]
Malbranchea (noninvasive)[179]
Myospherulosis (noninvasive)[180, 181]
Myriodontium (invasive)[182]
Penicillium (invasive/noninvasive)[45, 127, 183, 184]
Rhinosporidium (invasive/noninvasive)[5, 12, 24, 73, 185–192]
Stemphylium (noninvasive)[7, 184]
Streptomyces (invasive/noninvasive)[193]

normal healthy persons and those who have impaired local or systemic defenses, the most common condition that allows conversion of usually ubiquitous, saprophytic organisms to pathogenic ones seems to be sinus obstruction with impaired ventilation. Climate also appears to be a factor, as there are geographic areas where fungal sinusitis is endemic, including the Sudan,[11] Northern India,[4] and Saudi Arabia.[12] All of these areas have a warm, dry climate. In the United States, many cases of dematiaceous fungal sinusitis occur in the Southwest[13–15] or Hawaii.[16] Allergic mucosal thickening seems to be a strong predisposing factor for the development of *Aspergillus* and dematiaceous fungal sinusitis. Other factors are prolonged antibiotic therapy, long-term steroid therapy (local and/or systemic), chronic bacterial sinusitis, and host factors such as diabetes mellitus, carcinoma, blood dyscrasias, immunosuppression, and immunodeficiency states.

Stammberger believes that, in addition to host resistance factors, local anatomic factors in the middle meatus of the lateral nasal wall produce regional obstruction and predispose the patient to bacterial infection.[3] The mucosal changes, ostial obstruction, and decreased mucociliary transport cause reduced sinus ventilation, which lowers sinus pH and favors fungal colonization and growth.

RADIOLOGY

Usually, the radiographs of patients with fungal sinusitis show total opacification of one or several sinuses. The dis-

Table 43–4. SINONASAL INFECTION WITH MULTIPLE FUNGI

Author	Sex/Age (yr)	Pathogen	Signs	Involved Sinus(es)	Therapy	Result
Loveless et al. (1981)[10]	M/47	*Curvularia, Alternaria* spp.	Nasal septal abscess	—	Surgery	Cure
Adam et al. (1986)[57]	M/10	*Exserohilum rostratum, Alternaria* spp.	Nasal polyp, nasal mass	Left maxillary, ethmoid, sphenoid	Surgery	Cure (17 mo)
Washburn et al. (1988)[8]	F/44	*Drechslera biseptata, Curvularia lunata*	Nasal polyps, headache, anosmia	Pansinusits	Surgery, systemic antifungal therapy	Recurrence; cure (2 yr)
Jay et al. (1988)[38]	M/17	*Bipolaris spicifera, Curvularia* spp.	Unilateral nasal mass, proptosis	Right ethmoid and sphenoid	Surgery	Cure (2 yr)
Zieske et al. (1991)[19]	M/16	*Exserohilum rostratum; Bipolaris spicifera*	Nasal polyps	Bilateral maxillary and ethmoid	Surgery, systemic antifungal therapy	Cure (18 mo)

ease tends to be unilateral except for the allergic form, in which bilateral involvement is common. In a comparative computed tomography (CT) and magnetic resonance imaging (MRI) study of patients with fungal sinusitis, Zinreich and coworkers reported that the more inspissated mucus characteristic of fungal sinusitis showed greater attenuation (mean of 122 Hounsfield units) than that associated with bacterial sinusitis.[17]

On MRI, watery secretions show a low T_1-weighted signal intensity, high T_2-weighted signal, and low to intermediate proton density signal intensity. In cases of chronic sinusitis the secretions become desiccated, and the T_2-weighted signal intensity is the first to change, eventually becoming a signal void. When this happens, the T_1-weighted signal intensity also becomes a signal void. The surrounding mucous membranes may be edematous, with a high T_2-weighted signal.[18] The decreased signal intensity noted, especially in the T_2-weighted image, has been shown to be the result of increased levels of magnesium, manganese, and iron in the fungal mucin.[17] The reported incidence of bone erosion varies much. Because of the chronicity of the infection, expansion of the sinus with remodeling of bone occasionally is seen.[17, 18]

NONINVASIVE FUNGAL SINUSITIS

Fungal infections of the paranasal sinuses may present as benign colonization of the sinuses marked by swelling of sinus linings, obstruction with fluid, mucoid secretions, and/or green-brown waxy material. *Aspergillus* is the most common fungal pathogen in the nose and paranasal sinuses.

The nose and paranasal sinuses have local processes that may promote fungal infection, including nasal polyps, recurrent bacterial infections, and chronic rhinitis with stagnation of nasal secretions. Some authors have felt that the occlusion of the natural ostia of the sinuses creates an anaerobic environment that may promote fungal pathogenicity.[19, 20] The infectious nature of *Aspergillus* in the nose and paranasal sinuses was described before 1900. The disease has been very well-studied in the Sudan, where the disorder is endemic.[21–23]

Most persons who develop aspergillosis have no underlying disease. Green and colleagues found only 1 of 20 patients with orbital aspergillosis to have diabetes.[24] Zinneman failed to discover any systemic disease in a review of 37 cases of sino-orbital disease, and Jahrsdoerfer's group could identify an underlying disease (alcoholic cirrhosis) in only 1 of 17 lethal cases.[25, 26] There have been only occasional reports of sinus aspergillosis in diabetes or leukemia patients.[27–29] Three of the eight patients in Jahrsdoerfer's series were receiving immunosuppressive therapy for leukemia. The disease runs a more fulminant course in patients who are immunocom-

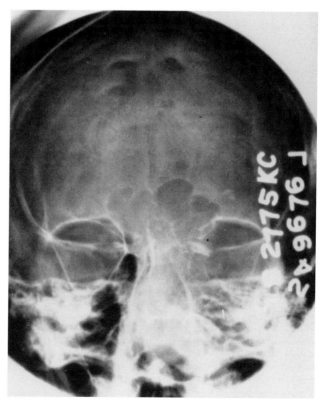

Figure 43–1. Caldwell's view of the sinuses showing opacification of frontal sinuses, ethmoid sinuses, and left maxillary sinus in a patient with allergic fungal sinusitis. Cultures grew *Alternaria*.

promised; reported mortality in bone marrow transplant patients is 100%.[19, 20, 26, 30] Recent reports of aspergillosis have included patients with aplastic anemia and cancer with neutropenia.[31] There is also a more recent association of *Aspergillus* sinusitis with nasal allergies. This material is described in detail in the section on allergic fungal sinusitis. Axelsson and colleagues found that a number of patients with fungal sinusitis had been taking prolonged antibiotic therapy for sinusitis.[32] Titche attributed the increasing incidence to the increased use of antibiotics and immunosuppressive agents.[5, 23]

Similarly, patients who have noninvasive sinus infections caused by the dematiaceous fungi *(Bipolaris, Curvularia, Alternaria, Exserohilum, Cladosporium)* are immunocompetent, often with a history of atopy. Most of the patients had a history of nasal polyps, nasal obstruction, or anosmia, and some allergic rhinitis, with or without serum eosinophilia (Figs. 43–1 to 43–3). Many of the patients complained of discolored mucoid rhinorrhea. Others presented with ocular complaints (proptosis, blurred vision, hypertelorism, diplopia, epiphora, papilledema, eyelid mass).[6, 8, 14, 33–47]

Generally, only one sinus is involved with *Aspergillus*, most often the maxillary sinus. The others, in decreasing order of frequency, are the ethmoid, sphenoid, and frontal. In a review of 103 cases, 67 patients were found to have solitary involvement (46 maxillary, 8 sphenoidal, 8 nasal, 3 ethmoidal, 2 frontal).[48, 49] Aspergillosis of the sphenoid sinus can be confusing (stone formation and cavernous sinus syndrome have been reported), or it can mimic a pituitary tumor.[50, 51]

Nasal, postnasal, sinus, and orbital symptoms are all found in sinus infections with *Aspergillus* organisms and dematiaceous fungi. The nasal symptoms are associated with a

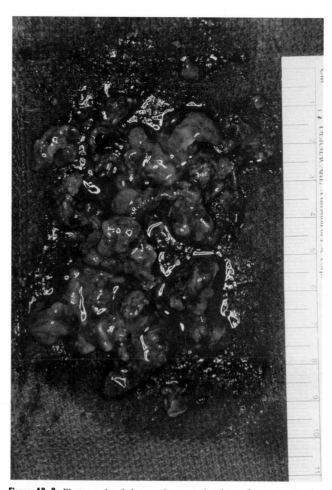

Figure 43–3. Photograph of the specimen at the time of surgery showing nasal polyps, hyperplastic sinus mucosa, and green-brown clay-like material found in the sinuses.

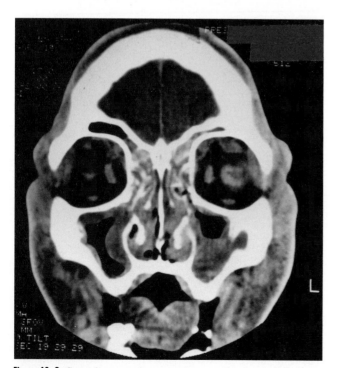

Figure 43–2. Coronal computed tomography scan of patient in Figure 43–1 showing pan-sinus involvement of *Alternaria*.

mucoid or mucopurulent discharge, swollen nasal mucosa and enlarged turbinates, and, occasionally polyps and/or facial pain. In some cases the secretions are gelatinous, containing necrotic tissue. In the noninvasive type, the patient complains of nasal obstruction, rhinorrhea, and a sensation of fullness of the face.[33]

Radiographically, there may be an air-fluid level with either the invasive or noninvasive form. CT has been very useful in defining the full extent of the disease. *Aspergillus* sinusitis often has a mixture of high- and low-density areas within the sinuses. Bone windows allow very accurate assessment of possible invasion. MRI can be used better to define the high and low signals produced by a mycetoma ("fungus ball").[5, 50, 52–56] With infection caused by the dematiaceous fungi, multiple sinuses were usually involved. Bilateral disease was present in 16 of the 29 cases with complete radiographic findings. Bone erosion was present in 23 cases: the skull base was involved in 12,[8, 34, 37–39, 57–61] the orbital wall in 8,[8, 37, 59, 62–67] and the frontal bone in 5.[9, 37, 41, 42, 61, 68, 69] Despite this high incidence of bone destruction, tissue invasion was uncommon. Nevertheless, the frequent occurrence of bone loss, combined with orbital and intracranial findings, invited the misdiagnosis of malignancy. In some cases, the slowly progressive growth of the fungal inflammatory mass resulted in bone remodeling.[8, 38, 70]

Treatment for the noninvasive fungal sinusitis usually consists of sinusotomy and curettage of all diseased and necrotic tissue. This alone is usually curative.[23, 71] Some authors have suggested instillation of nystatin.[23, 72, 73] In *Bipolaris* infections Manning and colleagues found surgical débridement to be curative in all instances.[33] One patient was given antifungal therapy, which, retrospectively, the author believed to be unnecessary. This study is at variance with the other cases in the literature, however, which show that this condition tends to be chronic and recurrent, even following wide-field débridement. Among the 13 patients cured primarily, 6 received antifungal therapy in addition to surgery. Fifteen other patients experienced one or several recurrences requiring multiple operative procedures as well as systemic fungicidal agents in all cases. Four patients underwent craniotomy in attempts to control the disease.[33, 59, 61, 65] It is important to note that surgical débridement must be complete because residual disease will result in recurrence. Similarly, in cases of *Curvularia* infection most authors' treatment consists solely of surgical débridement, which appears to be curative. A patient of Killingsworth and Wetmore required surgical revision.[64] Seven patients received antifungal therapy with amphotericin in addition to surgical débridement. Four of the five recurrences appeared within several months,[66, 67, 69, 74] In the case reported by Brummond and colleagues, recurrence developed after 4 years.[69]

MYCETOMA

Mycetoma, or fungus ball, is a benign colonization of the sinus. It occurs most often in a single sinus cavity, usually the maxillary. The mycetoma often provokes little or no inflammatory response unless it causes obstruction of the ostia and stasis of secretions with secondary bacterial sinusitis. The mycetoma does not invade; however, bone loss may occur owing to pressure resorption from the expanding mass. Most individuals who develop mycetomas have no underlying disease.[24]

CT is useful in defining the size and extent of a mycetoma (Fig. 43–4). Bone resorption can easily be identified with bone windows. MRI can be used to better define the high and low signals most often produced by mycetomas. This may be important when a large mycetoma could be confused with other lesions.[18]

Histopathologically, the sinus epithelium is ulcerated. There is usually an inflammatory infiltrate of variable size consisting of lymphocytes, plasma cells, and neutrophils. There may be some bone resorption. Mycelia of dichotomous branching and septate hyphae can be found in the mucopurulent exudate. The finding of a fungus ball consisting of mycelia and necrotic debris led to coining of the term "aspergilloma."[23, 28, 32, 75] A mycetoma caused by *Mucor* organisms has also been reported.[111] Granulomas may also be found within the sinus. These granulomas have been classified by Veress and colleagues[76] as (1) proliferative with pseudotubercles in a fibrous stroma, (2) a necrotizing type with large areas of edema and necrosis, or (3) a mixed type. The treatment for the mycetoma is generally sinusotomy,

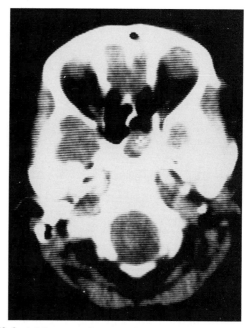

Figure 43–4. Axial computed tomography scan of patient with headache who was found to have an isolated "fungus ball" of *Aspergillus* in the sphenoid sinus.

irrigation, and curettage of all the material and any necrotic tissue. This alone is generally curative.[23, 71]

INVASIVE FUNGAL SINUSITIS

A number of fungi may become tissue invasive and destroy soft tissue and bone. These may present as an ulcerative lesion of the mucosa or a red or black area or can masquerade as tuberculosis or as carcinoma. Invasive fungal cases are more frequently observed in patients with an underlying condition such as diabetes, leukemia, chronic renal failure, or an immunosuppressive disease such as AIDS. Others are found in patients receiving immunosuppressants after transplant surgery.

When aspergillosis becomes invasive it usually spreads from the maxillary sinus to the ethmoid and extends to the orbit and nasal cavity. Most of the cases of orbital aspergillosis were found to have originated in the maxillary and ethmoidal sinuses. Green and colleagues found orbital involvement in 16 of 20 cases (6 from the Sudan) and Zinneman found 36 of 37 with orbital involvement (17 from the Sudan).[24, 25] *Aspergillus* invasion of the sphenoid sinus was found to be a lethal sign when it occurred. The invasive form has also been reported in pediatric patients.[51, 77]

Patients with invasive aspergillosis may have symptoms that vary from discolored nasal discharge and/or crusting to destruction of the inferior turbinates and sinuses. There may be bleeding or necrosis from angioinvasion. When the disease extends to the orbit and brain, it generally becomes terminal. Once angioinvasive, the fungus may produce thromboses or mycotic aneurysms. It may also disseminate to the lungs, liver, and spleen.[78, 79] Aspergillosis has been found to progress to the middle ear and spread to the mas-

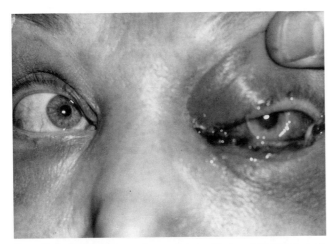

Figure 43–5. Diabetic woman who was in ketoacidosis and developed ptosis, proptosis, chemosis, and ophthalmoplegia of the left eye. The patient was found to have invasive mucormycosis.

toid, causing otomastoiditis. This is associated with severe ear pain. The temporal lobes may be involved secondarily. In Jahrsdoerfer's series were 17 deaths among 103 patients, all of which were caused by intracranial extension.[26] Interestingly, in almost all of these cases there was no known underlying disease. Invasive sinus aspergillosis may or may not occur together with facial nerve paralysis, optic neuritis, arteritis, and/or rupture of the carotid artery. Involvement of the skull base can simulate a malignancy.[80–84]

Many disorders predispose patients to invasive *Aspergillus* infections. Ketoacidosis of diabetes mellitus allows for high levels of glucose as well as an acid environment; both favor fungal growth. Diabetes also alters neutrophil function and causes small vessel disease, giving poor tissue oxygenation. In chronic renal failure, acidosis is also produced, which is favorable for fungal growth. Hematologic malignancies are associated with poor white blood cell function. AIDS patients have specific immunoglobulin G (IgG) abnormalities, complement consumption, and neutrophil dysfunction, all of which predispose the patient to fungal growth.[78, 85]

The largest group (70%) of patients who develop mucormycosis have diabetes mellitus. This affinity for diabetes patients is related to the fact that *Rhizopus* organisms thrive in an environment that is rich in glucose and has an acid pH, since they have an active ketone reductase system. This theory was tested in animals with experimentally induced diabetes with ketosis; that environment was found to promote invasion of *Mucor* organisms. Diabetes patients also have decreased phagocytic activity of their polymorphonuclear leukocytes. The organisms also grow in patients with chronic renal failure or diarrhea in which there is a metabolic acidosis.[5, 85–89]

Patients with adrenal suppression, hematologic dyscrasias, and other immunologically compromising conditions are at great risk for developing mucormycosis. If animals with chronic leukopenia are subjected to intranasal instillation of spores they develop mucormycosis. Intravenous drug abuse has also been reported in 17 patients with mucormycosis, 3 of whom had AIDS. A few perfectly healthy patients have developed mucormycosis.[87, 90–92]

Once the spores have entered the tissues, the organism becomes angioinvasive and has a predilection for the internal elastic lamina of the arteries. Later it invades veins and lymphatics. This invasion causes thrombosis with secondary ischemic infarction and hemorrhagic necrosis. The organism thrives in the necrotic tissue and spreads by direct extension along injured blood vessels. Histologically, there is abundant necrosis of tissue, neutrophil infiltration, and hyphae, which may or may not be prominent. The tissue-invasive nonseptate hyphae (cellophane tubules) are best demonstrated with a silver methenamine stain.[5, 85, 93]

The most common clinical signs of patients with mucormycosis in our review of 179 cases were cranial nerve deficit (especially blindness, ophthalmoplegia, and facial paralysis), proptosis, facial swelling, palatal ulcer, coma, and stupor. The presenting signs of prognostic value seemed to be hemiplegia, facial necrosis, and nasal deformity, which all seemed to carry a poor prognosis.[5, 85, 93–95] The physical examination is important, since early diagnosis and prompt treatment are correlated with a more favorable prognosis. Examination of the nose may show brick-red or black areas along the nasal turbinates. When this finding is encountered, a biopsy should be performed to look for nonseptate hyphae (representing fungal invasion) (Figs. 43–5 to 43–8).[85, 94]

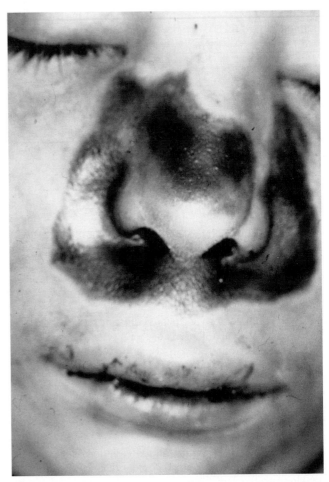

Figure 43–6. An adolescent male with leukemia who developed nasal erythema that progressed to necrosis within 1 day. Biopsy (Fig. 43–7) showed invasive mucormycosis. The patient died the next day.

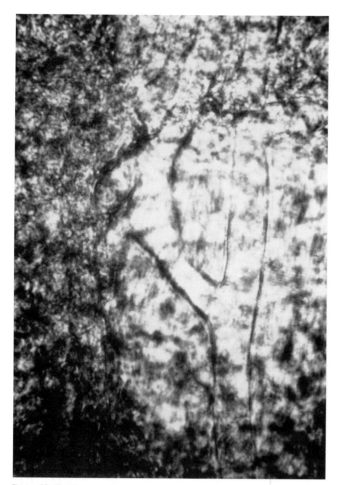

Figure 43–7. Silver methenamine stain of biopsy of patient in Figure 43–6 showing the "cellophane" tubules with non–septate hyphae characteristic of mucormycosis.

Radiographically, invasive aspergillosis shows bone destruction, usually involving the floor or medial orbital wall. The erosion may involve the basisphenoid and the pituitary fossa, the temporal bone and pterygopalatine fossa, the alveolus with loosening of teeth, and the frontal bone. An air-fluid level in the invasive form is rare. CT has been very useful in defining the full extent of the disease. *Aspergillus* sinusitis often has a mixture of high- and low-density areas within the sinuses. Bone windows allow very accurate assessment of possible invasion. MRI can be used better to define the high and low signals and central nervous system involvement.[18]

In patients with mucormycosis, radiographic analysis of the patients did not seem to correlate with prognosis but did allow evaluation of the extent of disease. The most common finding on routine sinus radiographs was clouding of multiple sinuses. Mucosal thickening and bone erosion may also be found. CT better defines soft tissue invasion and necrosis, early bone erosion, and cavernous sinus thrombosis.[96–98] MRI, with or without gadolinium, is the best way of evaluating early changes in major vessels, including carotid artery thrombosis and cavernous sinus thrombosis. MRI is also the best way of evaluating intracranial extension.[50, 99–102]

In general terms, the treatment of invasive fungal sinusitis includes management of the underlying disease to reverse predisposing factors, surgical removal of necrotic tissue, and systemic antifungal therapy.

In patients with mucormycosis the most important determinant of survival seems to be the underlying disease rather than age, sex, or laterality. Among patients with no underlying disease (8 cases) survival was 75%. In diabetes patients (126 cases) overall survival was 60%. Among patients with other systemic disorders (45 cases) overall survival was 20%. Leukemia, infant diarrhea, and renal disease carry an extremely poor prognosis. Medical management of the underlying condition appears to contribute significantly to survival. Correction of acidosis and hyperglycemia, which generally can be accomplished in diabetes patients, contributes to their high survival rate; however, the underlying disability cannot be easily reversed in persons with AIDS or other types of immune compromise, those receiving systemic steroids, those with hematopoietic malignancies or chronic renal failure, or those taking cyclosporine following organ transplant. When they develop mucormycosis, these patients have an extremely poor prognosis.[5, 81, 85, 103, 104]

The medical management of invasive *Aspergillus* sinusitis utilizes systemic amphotericin B as the predominant agent. It is unclear whether local irrigation with amphotericin has

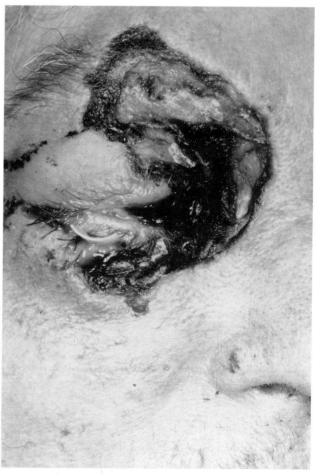

Figure 43–8. A diabetic man who developed sinusitis followed by necrosis of the medial portion of the eyelids and nasal skin. Biopsy revealed invasive mucormycosis.

any effect on the disease. Amphotericin B has been used in combination with rifampin and/or flucytosine effectively in vitro, but a significant increase in survival has not been demonstrated.[105] A report has demonstrated a favorable response with the use of liposomal amphotericin B. Five cases of seven with invasive *Aspergillus* rhinosinusitis whom conventional amphotericin B therapy failed were cured with a course of liposomal amphotericin B. The ketoconazoles have been found to play some role in the medical management of aspergillosis.[50, 106, 107] Itraconazole has been found in vitro and in vivo to have activity against *Aspergillus*, but its effectiveness in treating invasive *Aspergillus* sinusitis is unknown.[5, 50] Likewise unknown is the effect of combining amphotericin B and itraconazole in invasive aspergillosis of the sinuses.[78]

Perhaps the most important addition to the treatment of mucormycosis is the administration of amphotericin B, which raised the survival in diabetes patients from 37% to 79%. In the "nondiabetes" group, amphotericin B raised survival from 0% to 47%. Patients receiving combined treatment—surgery and amphotericin B—had an overall survival rate of 81%. For diabetes patients survival with combined therapy and management of the ketoacidosis was 89%. Other antifungal agents alone have no place in the management of *Mucor* infections.[5, 50, 85, 108]

The critical nature of mucormycosis warrants rapid infusion of effective doses of amphotericin B, *not* gradually incremental dosing as is generally used for less lethal fungal diseases. A test dose should be given first, with careful monitoring of the patient to avoid anaphylaxis. The usual dose is 0.3 mg/kg dissolved in 500 mL of 5% dextrose in water (D5W) over 1–3 hours daily; it is increased to 0.5 or 0.6 mg/kg/day or as toxicity permits. The creatinine clearance rate or serial creatinine determinations are monitored to detect the development of toxicity. Once the renal parameters have stabilized, a double dose (1 mg/kg) is given on alternate days to prevent toxicity. Since the agent is fungistatic rather than fungicial, long-term treatment (weeks to months) is necessary, to a cumulative dose of 2500–4000 mg. The clinical signs and symptoms, including reduction of fever, wound healing, negative cultures, and decreasing white blood count, may be the best guide for cessation of treatment.[5, 85, 108]

Combined drug therapy continues to be evaluated. There are some interesting data utilizing interferon-α_2 and amphotericin B in patients with mucormycosis and hairy cell leukemias. Combination therapy may be of particular value in patients who have an underlying disease associated with a high mortality rate from mucormycosis.[109]

The toxicity of amphotericin B is an important consideration in the treatment of mucormycosis, particularly in patients with metabolic disorders. Whereas renal toxicity is directly related to serum concentrations and total dose of the drug, some decrease in glomerular filtration is expected in all cases. To prevent irreparable nephrotoxicity the dose should be adjusted to keep the blood urea nitrogen (BUN) value less than 50 mg/100 mL and the creatinine value less than 3.5 mg/mL.[85, 109]

Rigor and fever, with occasional hypotension and delirium, may be seen in the patient who is already febrile. The appearance of these signs may be confused with intracranial extension of the disease. Fever, chills, headache, nausea, and vomiting have been described in as many as 80% of the patients. Hypokalemia has been reported in approximately 20% of patients. Amphotericin B may also produce a normochromic, normocytic anemia from bone marrow suppression, although this condition is usually reversible.[85, 108] Some patients who appear to have a dramatic response to the agents may still succumb from damage to the carotid artery. Early and late cavernous-carotid fistulas and mycotic aneurysms of the carotid have been reported. Patients should, therefore, be followed for some time after the initial response to therapy is observed.[85, 110]

Surgery has an important role in the management of the patient with invasive fungal sinusitis. Since the fungus thrives in devitalized and necrotic tissue, rigorous débridement is indicated. Areas of tissue that are ischemic should also be removed, since vascular thrombosis prevents chemotherapeutic agents from reaching the diseased tissues. In early cases in which there is no necrosis, simple nasal, transantral, or ethmoidal biopsy and curettage should be performed to establish a diagnosis early and allow adequate drainage of the sinuses. Simple débridement appears to be adequate treatment for the noninvasive or benign form.[111] Once necrosis has occurred, more radical débridement is necessary. The extent of the resection depends on the extent of the disease and the condition of the patient. Orbital exenteration in cases of mucormycosis may be required if there are signs of retinal artery thrombosis, orbital apex necrosis, or ocular invasion. The eye should not be routinely sacrificed to achieve a better survival rate, since there are no data to show that survival is increased by orbital exenteration. Some authors have advocated routine removal of a blind eye, since it is useless, and provides a portal for intracranial extension. In our review and that of Ochi, surgical débridement or resection seemed to enhance survival.[5, 85, 112] Our review demonstrated a 78% survival rate for patients who had radical débridement, as compared with 57.5% for patients who had no surgery or only biopsy. In diabetes patients, surgery enhanced survival to a rate of 82%, as compared with surgery in patients without diabetes, who had a survival rate of only 62.5%. Although surgery seems to enhance survival, the interval between diagnosis and the surgical procedure did not appear to be a factor. At least 35% of the survivors had surgery later than 1 week after the diagnosis was established.[85]

ALLERGIC FUNGAL SINUSITIS

Allergic fungal sinusitis is a relatively new entity, having been elucidated within the last decade. Our knowledge of the true prevalence and the actual pathogens has also expanded only recently. The existence of this class of fungal disease underscores the necessity for serologic testing and isolation of the fungus in culture to establish the correct diagnosis (see Figs. 43–9 to 43–12).

Millar and colleagues in 1981 were the first to report a relationship between allergic bronchopulmonary aspergillosis and allergic aspergillosis of the paranasal sinuses.[113] They noted a histologic similarity between the material found in five cases of maxillary sinus aspergillosis and the expelled

Figure 43–9. Young immunocompetent female with *Petriellidium boydii* sinonasal infection having intracranial extension. Axial computed tomography scan: Note ethmoid, antral, and sphenoid disease with erosion of skull base and involvement of the cavernous sinus. Débridement through a lateral rhinotomy and miconazole therapy were curative.

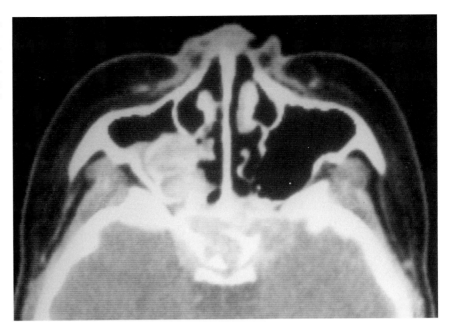

plugs from pulmonary cases they studied. Two years later, Katzenstein and colleagues amplified on this observation and described the entity of allergic aspergillosis sinusitis on the basis of a retrospective study of 113 patients, 7 of whom had green, viscous secretions in the sinuses that contained eosinophils, Charcot-Leyden crystals, and fungal hyphae.[114, 115] Of these 7 patients, all had nasal polyps and radiographic evidence of multiple sinus involvement, 6 had asthma, 3 were atopic, and 1 had serum eosinophilia. Four of 5 had precipitins to *A. fumigatus*. In 1987, Waxman and colleagues[116]

reported 8 more cases of this condition. Collective review of these 15 cases revealed equal sex distribution and a mean age of 29 years (range 13–56 years) for the group. Among the 15 patients, 14 had polyps, 11 had asthma, and 1 had aspirin sensitivity. Radiographically, there was generally multisinus involvement, and bone erosion was noted in 2 cases. Skin reactivity to *Aspergillus* species was present in 6 of 10 patients tested, and 5 of 7 patients tested had precipitins to *A. fumigatus*.

It should be noted that, although allergic bronchopulmonary aspergillosis and allergic *Aspergillus* sinusitis are not uncommon entities, the occurrence of both in a single person is rare. Such cases were reported by Safirstein and Sher and Schwartz.[117, 118] The designation of *Aspergillus* as the pathogen was based on fungal morphology (nonseptate hyphae) and serologic findings rather than on isolation of the fungus and culture. In the period 1981–1992, both allergic pulmo-

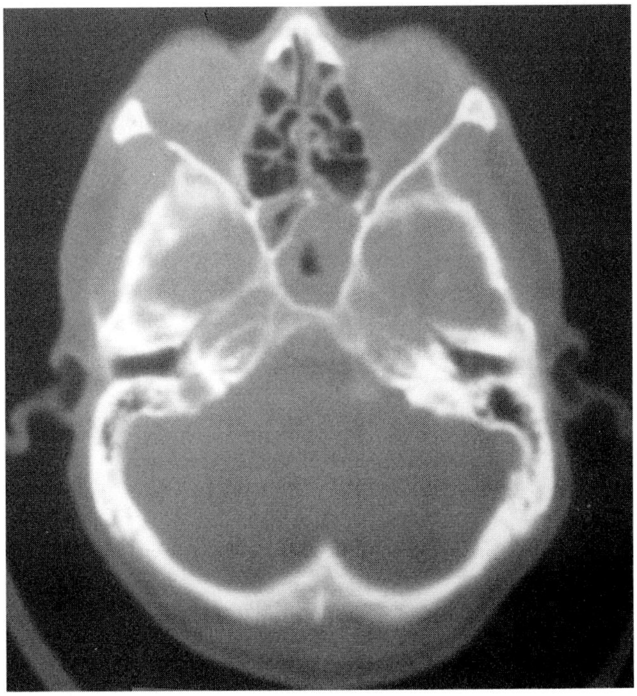

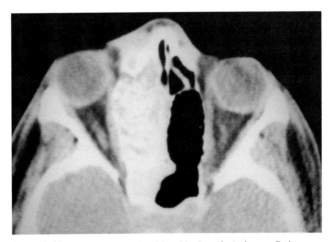

Figure 43–10. AIDS patient with a history of recurrent cryptococcal meningitis. Axial computed tomography scan: Note extensive sphenoid sinus disease. Biopsy revealed *Cryptococcus neoformans*.

Figure 43–11. Allergic fungal sinusitis with *Curvularia lunata*. Patient presented with unilateral proptosis, nasal polyps, and a history of atopy and asthma. Axial computed tomography scan: Note expansion of ethmoid labyrinth.

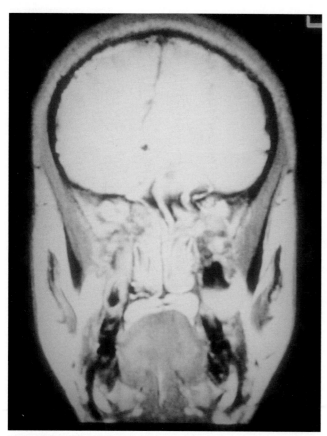

Figure 43–12. Young immunocompetent male presenting with bilateral nasal polyps and proptosis. Coronal computed tomography scan: Note bilateral pansinusitis with multiple intracranial mucoceles. Patient underwent craniotomy and external sphenoethmoidectomies. Culture of biopsy material revealed *Exserohilum rostratum.*

nary and paranasal sinus infections have been reported with other mycotic agents.[13, 119–122]

Ence and colleagues reported 14 cases of allergic fungal sinusitis produced by five different organisms.[14] Cultures were positive in 11 patients; *Bipolaris spicifera* was present in 5 patients, *Alternaria alternaria* in 2, *Curvularia lunata* in 2, and *Bipolaris australiensis* in 1; 1 patient had a mixed infection with *B. spicifera* and *A. fumigatus.* In this series, the average age was 31 years (range 11–58 years) with an equal sex distribution. All 14 patients had nasal polyps, 6 had asthma, and 11 were atopic. Ence's group found elevated serum precipitins and fungus-specific IgE and IgG antibodies in patients infected with *B. spicifera.*[14] A review of 44 cases of allergic fungal sinusitis by Friedman and colleagues[123] revealed 24 female and 19 male patients, whose age range was 8–56 (mean 26) years. A history of allergy, chronic rhinitis, and asthma was present in 50% of patients. Friedman's group calculated that this organism was demonstrated by culture in only 4 of 30 reported cases of allergic *Aspergillus* sinusitis.[123]

Microscopically, the thick mucoid matrix contains masses of eosinophils, necrotic debris, and Charcot-Leyden crystals. The last are composed of lysophospholipase derived from the membranes of released granules of eosinophils.[7, 14, 33] Ence and colleagues recommended the use of the Brown and Brenn stain to facilitate their identification.[14] Gram's

stain is also useful, as it stains the Charcot-Leyden crystals purple. Hartwick and Batsakis[124] believed that lamination of cells and debris in the mucus should suggest a fungal pathogen. Hyphae are generally inconspicuous and must be sought. Their identification is facilitated by special stains, such as Gomori's methenamine silver stain and the Fontana-Masson stain. Friedman and colleagues stressed the importance of the Fontana-Masson stain for melanin because it stains the dematiaceous fungi, which in tissue are morphologically indistinguishable from *Aspergillus.*[123] The exception is *A. niger,* which is a pigment producer. Mucosal and bone invasion by fungal elements is absent. The sinus mucosal lining is edematous and infiltrated by eosinophils, lymphocytes, and plasma cells.

Radiographically, multiple sinuses are generally involved and bone destruction is present in 30%–50% of the cases. Handley and colleagues reported multifocal bone erosion in 7 of their 11 cases, secondary to resection and remodeling rather than tissue invasion.[125] Common sites of destruction are the medial antral wall, the ethmoid septae, and the lamina papyracea. Manning and colleagues reported the occurrence of facial deformity in all 6 of their pediatric cases secondary to expansile sinus changes.[33] CT reveals increased attenuation within the sinus, often with serpiginous opacities of metallic density.

Allergic fungal sinusitis is generally managed with conservative surgery because of its noninvasive nature. Surgery consists of curettage and ventilation of the involved sinuses by intranasal ethmoidectomy, sphenoid sinusotomy, sublabial antrotomy (Caldwell-Luc procedure), or frontal sinusotomy, depending on the site of involvement. External approaches are reserved for more aggressive lesions with bone erosion and patients whom conservative management has failed.[7, 33] Antibiotics are often employed because of intercurrent bacterial infection; however, systemic antifungal therapy is usually reserved for the few cases that show clinical evidence of orbital or intracranial invasion. The use of systemic steroids has been advocated, because this condition represents a hypersensitivity reaction to the fungal allergen. The efficacy of steroid therapy has not been completely established, however. Allphin and colleagues reported that all three of their patients whom surgery and topical corticosteroid therapy had failed nevertheless improved with systemic use of steroids.[66]

In summary, patients with allergic fungal sinusitis typically have a history of atopy, with positive skin tests, serum eosinophilia, elevated total serum IgG, elevated fungus-specific IgE and IgG, multisinus involvement, allergic mucin, and common bone erosion without tissue invasion.

References

1. Grigoriu D, Brambule J, Delaacretaz J, et al.: La sinusite maxillaire fungique. Dermatologica 1979; 159:180–186.
2. Laskownick AA, Kurdzielewisc J, Macura A, et al.: Mycotic sinusitis in children. Mykosen 1978; 21:407–411.
3. Stammberger H: Endoscopic surgery for mycotic and chronic recurring sinusitis. Ann Otol Rhinol Laryngol 1985; 94(Suppl 119): 1–11.
4. Chakrabarti A, Sharma SC, Chandler J: Epidemiology and pathogenesis of paranasal sinus mycoses. Otolaryngol Head Neck Surg 1992; 107:745–750.

5. Blitzer A, Lawson W: Mycotic infections of the nose and paranasal sinuses. In: English G (ed): Otolaryngology. Philadelphia: JB Lippincott, 1992, pp 1–23.

6. Lawson W, Blitzer A: Fungal infections of the nose and paranasal sinuses: Part II. Otol Clin North Am 1993; 26:1037–1069.

7. Blitzer A, Lawson W: Fungal infections of the nose and paranasal sinuses: Part I. Otol Clin North Am 1993; 26:1007–1037.

8. Washburn RG, Kennedy DW, Begley MG, et al.: Chronic fungal sinusitis in apparently normal hosts. Medicine (Baltimore) 1988; 67:231–247.

9. Zieske LA, Kopke RD, Hamill R: Dematiaceous fungal sinusitis. Otolaryngol Head Neck Surg 1991; 105:567–577.

10. Loveless MO, Winn RE, Campbell M, et al.: Mixed invasive infection with *Alternaria* species and *Curvularia* species. Am J Clin Pathol 1981; 76:491–494.

11. Milosev B, Margoob ES, Abdel A, et al.: Primary aspergilloma of the paranasal sinus in the Sudan—a review of seventeen cases. Br J Surg 1969; 56:132–137.

12. Moses JS: Ocular rhinosporidiosis in Tamil Nadu, India. Mycopathologia 1990; 111:5–8.

13. Gourley DS, Whisman BA, Jorgansen N, et al.: Allergic *Bipolaris* sinusitis: Clinical and immunopathologic characteristics. J Allergy Clin Immunol 1990; 85:583–591.

14. Ence BK, Gourley DS, Jorgensen NL, et al.: Allergic fungal sinusitis. Am J Rhinol 1990; 4:169–178.

15. Manning SC, Vuitch F, Weinberg AG, et al.: Allergic aspergillosis: A newly recognized form of sinusitis in the pediatric population. Laryngoscope 1989; 99:681–685.

16. Zieske LA, Kopke RD, Hamill A: Dematiaceous fungal sinusitis. Otolaryngol Head Neck Surg. 1991; 105:567–577.

17. Zinreich SJ, Kennedy DW, Malat J, et al.: Fungal sinusitis: Diagnosis with CT and MRI imaging. Radiology 1988; 169:439–444.

18. Som PM: Imaging of paranasal sinus disease. Otol Clin North Am 1993; 26:983–995.

19. Armstrong D: Life threatening opportunistic fungal infection in patients with AIDS. Ann NY Acad Sci 1988; 544:443–450.

20. Martino P, Raccah R, Gentile G, et al.: *Aspergillus* colonization of the nose and pulmonary aspergillosis in neutropenic patients: A retrospective study. Haematologica 1989; 74:263–265.

21. Mahgoob ES: Mycosis of the Sudan. Trans R Soc Trop Med Hyg 1977; 71:184.

22. Milroy CM, Blanshard JD, Lucas S, et al.: Aspergillosis of the nose and paranasal sinuses. J Clin Pathol 1989; 42:123.

23. Titche LL: Aspergillosis of the maxillary sinus. Ear Nose Throat J 1978; 57:398.

24. Green WR, Font RL, Zimmerman LE: Aspergillosis of the orbit. Arch Ophthalmol 1969; 82:302.

25. Zinneman HH: Sino-orbital aspergillosis. Minn Med 1972; 55:661.

26. Jahrsdoerfer RA, Ejercito VS, Johns MM, et al.: Aspergillosis of the nose and paranasal sinsuses. Am J Otolaryngol 1979; 1:6.

27. McGill TJ, Simpson G, Healy GB: Fulminant aspergillosis of the nose and paranasal sinuses: A new clinical entity. Laryngoscope 1980; 90:748.

28. Nash CS: Fulminating infection of the nose due to *Monilia* or *Aspergillus*. Arch Otolaryngol 1938; 28:234.

29. Smolansky SJ: Aspergillosis of the paranasal sinuses. Ear Nose Throat J 1978; 57:320.

30. Meyers JD: Fungal infections in bone marrow transplant patients. Semin Oncol 1990; 17:10–13.

31. Brown AE: Overview of fungal infections in cancer patients. Semin Oncol 1990; 17:2–5.

32. Axelsson H, Carlsoo B, Weibring J, et al.: Aspergillosis of the maxillary sinus: Clinical and histopathological features of 4 cases and a review of the literature. Acta Otolaryngol 1978; 86:303.

33. Manning SC, Schaefer SD, Close LG, et al.: Culture-positive allergic fungal sinusitis. Arch Otolaryngol 1991; 117:174–178.

34. Gourley DS, Whisman BA, Jorgensen NL, et al.: Allergic *Bipolaris* sinusitis: Clinical and immunopathologic characteristics. J Allergy Clin Immunol 1990; 85:583–591.

35. Koshi G, Anandi V, Kurien M, et al.: Nasal phaeohyphomycosis caused by *Bipolaris hawaiiensis*. J Med Vet Mycol 1987; 25:397–402.

36. Pingree TF, Holt GR, Otto RA, et al.: *Bipolaris*-caused fungal sinusitis. Otolaryngol Head Neck Surg 1992; 106:302–305.

37. Gourley DS, Whisman BA, Martin ME, et al.: Clinical and immuno-

38. logical characteristics of allergic fungal sinusitis caused by *Bipolaris spicifera*. J Allergy Clin Immunol 1988; 81:285–292.

38. Jay WM, Bradsher RW, LeMay B, et al.: Ocular involvement in mycotic sinusitis caused by *Bipolaris*. Am J Ophthalmol 1988; 105:366–370.

39. Robson JMB, Benn RAV, Hogan PG, et al.: Allergic fungal sinusitis presenting a paranasal tumor. Aust NZ J Med 1989; 19:351–353.

40. Sobol SM, Love RG, Stutman HR, et al.: Phaeohyphomycosis of the maxilloethmoidal sinus caused by *Drechslera spicifera*: A new fungal pathogen. Laryngoscope 1984; 94:620–627.

41. Young CN, Swart JG, Ackermann D, et al.: Nasal obstruction and bone erosion caused by *Drechslera hawaiiensis*. J Laryngol Otol 1978; 92:137–143.

42. Rinaldi MG, Phillips P, Schwartz JG, et al.: Human *Curvularia* infections: Report of 5 cases and review of the literature. Diagn Microbiol Infect Dis 1987; 6:27–29.

43. Nishioka G, Schwartz JG, Rinaldi MG, et al.: Fungal maxillary sinusitis caused by *Curvularia lunata*. Arch Otolaryngol Head Neck Surg 1987; 113:665–666.

44. Phillips P, Rinaldi MG, Holt GR, et al.: Phaeohyphomycotic sinusitis caused by *Curvularia lunata*. Presented at the Annual Meeting of the American Society for Microbiology, Washington, DC, March 23–28, 1986.

45. Stammberger H: Endoscopic surgery for mycotic and chronic recurring sinusitis. Ann Otol 1985; 94(Suppl 199):1–11.

46. Brown JW, Nadell J, Sanders CV, et al.: Brain abscess caused by *Cladosporium irichoides* (bantianum). A case with paranasal sinus involvement. South Med J 1976; 69:1519–1521.

47. Ismail Y, Johnson RH, Wells MV, et al.: Invasive sinusitis with intracranial extension caused by *Curvularia lunata*. Arch Intern Med 1993; 153:1604–1606.

48. Elagina MI, Skorodumova IV, Shatskaia NK: A case of fungal lesions in the paranasal sinuses with formation of an aspergilloma in the nasal cavity. Vestn Otolaryngol 1985; 4:70.

49. Gil-Carcedo LM, Benito JL, Santos P, et al.: Aspergiloma de ethmoides. Acta Otorhinolaryngol Esp 1990; 41:99.

50. Kwon-Chung KJ, Bennett JE: Aspergillosis. In: Kwon-Chung KJ, Bennett JE (eds): Medical Mycology. Philadelphia: Lea & Febiger, 1992, pp 201–247.

51. Roser SM, Canalis RF, Hanna CJ: Aspergillosis of the maxillary antrum. J Oral Med 1976; 31:91.

52. Carrazana EJ, Rossitch E, Morris J: Isolated central nervous system aspergillosis in the acquired immunodeficiency syndrome. Clin Neurol Neurosurg 1991; 93:227–230.

53. Gershon SL: Prolonged granulocytopenia: The major risk factor for invasive pulmonary aspergillosis in patients with acute leukemia. Ann Intern Med 1984; 100:345–351.

54. Hora JF: Primary aspergillosis of the paranasal sinuses and associated areas. Laryngoscope 1965; 75:768.

55. Loidolt D, Mangge H, Wilders-Truschnig M, et al.: In vivo and in vitro suppression of lymphocyte function in paranasal sinus mycoses. Laryngol Rhinol Otologie 1989; 68:407–410.

56. Peterson DE, Schimpff SC: *Aspergillus* sinusitis in neutropenic patients with cancer: A review. Biomed Pharmacother 1989; 43:307–312.

57. Adam RD, Paquin ML, Peterson EA, et al.: Phaeohyphomycosis caused by the fungal genera *Bipolaris* and *Exserohilum*: A report of 9 cases and review of the literature. Medicine 1986; 65:203–217.

58. Friedman GC, Hartwick RW, Ro JY, et al.: Allergic fungal sinusitis: Report of three cases associated with dematiaceous fungi. Am J Clin Pathol 1991; 96:368–372.

59. Pratt MF, Burnett JR: Fulminant *Dreschslera* sinusitis in an immunocompetent host. Laryngoscope 1988; 98:1343–1347.

60. Rolston KVI, Hopfer RL, Larson DL: Infections caused by *Dreschslera* species: Case report and review of the literature. Rev Infect Dis 1985; 7:525–529.

61. Ruben SJ, Scott TE, Seltzer HM: Intracranial and paranasal sinus infection due to *Dreschslera*. South Med J 1987; 80:1057–1058.

62. Frenkel L, Kuhls TL, Nitta K, et al.: Recurrent *Bipolaris* sinusitis following surgical and antifungal therapy. Pediatr Infect Dis 1987; 6:1130–1132.

63. Harpster WH, Gonzales C, Opal SM: Pansinusitis caused by the fungus *Dreschslera*. Otolaryngol Head Neck Surg 1985; 93:683–685.

64. Killingsworth SM, Wetmore SJ: *Curvularia/Dreschslera* sinusitus. Laryngoscope 1990; 100:932–937.

65. Markin SL, Fetchick RJ, Leone CR, et al.: *Bipolaris hawaiiensis*–caused phaeohyphomycotic orbitopathy: A devastating fungal sinusitis in an apparently immunocompetent host. Ophthalmology 1989; 96:175–179.

66. Allphin AL, Strauss M, Abdul-Karim FW: Allergic fungal sinusitis: Problems in diagnosis and treatment. Laryngoscope 1991; 101:815–820.

67. Bartynski JM, McCaffrey TV, Frigas E: Allergic fungal sinusitis secondary to dematiaceous fungi—*Curvularia lunata* and *Alternaria*. Otolaryngol Head Neck Surg 1990; 103:32–39.

68. Antoine GA, Raterink MH: *Bipolaris:* A serious new fungal pathogen of the paranasal sinus. Otolaryngol Head Neck Surg 1989; 100:158–162.

69. Brummond W, Kurup VP, Harris GJ, et al.: Brief reports: Allergic sino-orbital mycosis: A clinical and immunologic study. JAMA 1986; 256:3249–3253.

70. Scully RE: Case records of the Massachusetts General Hospital: Case 20–1991. N Engl J Med 1991; 324:1423–1429.

71. Larranaga J, Fandino J, Gomez-Bueno J, et al.: Aspergillosis of the sphenoid sinus simulating a pituitary tumor. Neuroradiology 1989; 31:362.

72. Harris GJ, Will BR: Orbital aspergillosis. Conservative débridement and local amphotericin irrigation. Ophthal Plast Reconstr Surg 1989; 5:207–211.

73. Weller WA, Joseph DJ, Hora JF: Deep mycotic involvement of the right maxillary and ethmoid sinuses, the orbit, and adjacent structures. Laryngoscope 1960; 70:999–1002.

74. McMillan RH III, Cooper PH, Body BA, et al.: Allergic fungal sinusitis due to *Curvularia lunata*. Hum Pathol 1987; 18:960–964.

75. Warder FR, Chikes PG, Hudson WR: Aspergillosis of the paranasal sinuses. Arch Otolaryngol 1975; 101:683.

76. Veress B, Malik OA, Tayeb AA, et al.: Further observations on the primary paranasal *Aspergillus* granuloma in the Sudan: A morphological study of 46 cases. Am J Trop Med 1973; 22:765.

77. Lavelle WG: Aspergillosis of the sphenoid sinus. Ear Nose Throat J 1988; 67:266.

78. Teh W, Matti BS, Marisiddaiah H, et al.: *Aspergillus* sinusitis in patients with AIDS: Report of three cases and review. Clin Infect Dis 1995; 21:529–535.

79. Sarti EJ, Lucente FE: Aspergillosis of the paranasal sinuses. Ear Nose Throat J 1988; 67:824–831.

80. Caroli A, Joosen E, Van Huynehhem L, et al.: A case of sinus aspergillosis associated with peripheral facial paralysis. Acta Stomatol Belg 1985; 82:167.

81. Corvisier N, Gray F, Gherardi R, et al.: Aspergillosis of the ethmoid sinus and optic nerve, with arteritis and rupture of the internal carotid artery. Surg Neurol 1987; 28:311.

82. Sarti EJ, Blaugrund SM, Lin PT, et al.: Paranasal sinus disease with intracranial extension: Aspergillosis versus malignancy. Laryngoscope 1988; 98:632.

83. Strauss M, Fine E: *Aspergillus* otomastoiditis in AIDS. Am J Otol 1991; 12:49–53.

84. Hall PJ, Farrior JB: *Aspergillus* mastoiditis. Otolaryngol Head Neck Surg 1993; 108:167–170.

85. Blitzer A, Lawson W, Myers BR, et al.: Patient survival factors in paranasal sinus mucormycosis. Laryngoscope 1980; 90:635.

86. Abramson E, Wilson D, Arky RA: Rhinocerebral phycomycosis in association with diabetic ketoacidosis. Ann Intern Med 1967; 66:735.

87. Bauer H, Sheldon WH: Leukopenia and experimental mucormycosis. Am J Pathol 1957; 33:617.

88. Karam F, Chmel H: Rhino-orbital cerebral mucormycosis. Ear Nose Throat J 1990; 89:187.

89. Sheldon WH, Bauer H: Tissue mast cells and acute inflammation in experimental cutaneous mucormycosis of normal 45/80 treated and diabetic rats. J Exp Med 1960; 112:1069.

90. Fong KM, Seneviratne EME, McCormack JG: *Mucor* cerebral abscess associated with intravenous drug abuse. Aust N Z J Med 1990; 20:74–77.

91. Kwon-Chung KJ, Bennett JE: Mucormycosis. In: Kwon-Chung KJ, Bennett JE (eds): Medical Mycology. Philadelphia: Lea & Febiger, 1992, pp 524–559.

92. Quatrocolo G, et al.: Rhinocerebral mucormycosis and internal carotid artery thrombosis in a previously healthy patient. Acta Neurol Belg 1990; 90:20–26.

93. Baker RD: Mucormycosis. In: Baker RD (ed): Human Infection with Fungi, Actinomycetes and Algae. Berlin: Springer-Verlag, 1971, pp 832–919.

94. Baker RD: Mucormycosis. In: Baker RD (ed): Human Infection with Fungi, Actinomycetes and Algae. Berlin: Springer-Verlag, 1971, pp 832–919.

95. Baker RD: Mucormycosis. In: Baker RD (ed): Human Infection with Fungi, Actinomycetes and Algae. Berlin: Springer-Verlag, 1971, pp 832–919.

96. Estrem SA, Tully R, Davis WE: Rhinocerebral mucormycosis: Computed tomographic imaging of cavernous sinus thrombosis. Ann Otol Rhinol Laryngol 1990; 99:160.

97. Gamba JL, Woodruff WW, Djang WT, et al.: Craniofacial mucormycosis: Assessment with CT. Radiology 1986; 160:207.

98. Ishida M, Noiri T, Taya N: Mucormycosis in paranasal sinuses. J Otolaryngol Soc Jpn 1989; 92:21.

99. Galetta SL, Wulc AE, Goldberg HI, et al.: Rhinocerebral mucormycosis: Management and survival after carotid occlusion. Ann Neurol 1990; 28:103.

100. Kaufman L, et al.: Detection of two *Blastomyces dermatitidis* serotypes by exoantigen analysis. J Clin Microbiol 1983; 18:110–114.

101. McDevitt GR, Brantley MJ, Cawthon MA: Rhinocerebral mucormycosis: A case report with magnetic resonance imaging findings. Clin Imaging 1989; 13:317.

102. Yousem DM, Galetta SL, Gusnard DA, et al.: MR findings in rhinocerebral mucormycosis. J Comput Assist Tomogr 1989; 13:878.

103. Kaplan AH, Poza-Juncal E, Shapiro R, et al.: Cure of mucormycosis in a renal transplant patient receiving cyclosporine with maintenance of immunosuppression. Am J Nephrol 1988; 8:139.

104. Maniglia AJ, Goodwin WJ, Arnold JE, et al.: Intracranial abscesses secondary to nasal, sinus, or orbital infections in adults and children. Arch Otolaryngol Head Neck Surg 1989; 115:1424.

105. Denning DW, Stevens DA: Antifungal and surgical treatment of invasive aspergillosis: A review of 2121 published cases. Rev Infect Dis 1990; 12:1147–1201.

106. Denning DW, Tucker RM, Hanson LH, et al.: Treatment of invasive aspergillosis with itraconazole. Am J Med 1989; 86:791.

107. Sugar AM, Alsip SG, Galgiani JN, et al.: Pharmacology and toxicity of high-dose ketoconazole. Antimicrob Agents Chemother 1987; 31:1874.

108. Battock DJ, Grausz H, Bobrowsky JS: Alternate day amphotericin B therapy in the treatment of rhinocerebral phycomycosis. Ann Intern Med 1968; 68:122.

109. Bennett CL, Westbrook CA, Gruber B, et al.: Hairy cell leukemia and mucormycosis: Treatment with alpha-2 interferon. Ann J Med 1986; 81:1065.

110. Saff G, Frau M, Murtagh FR, et al.: Mucormycosis associated with carotid cavernous fistula and cavernous mycotic aneurysm. J Fla Med Assoc 1989; 76:863.

111. Henderson LT, Robbins KT, Weitzner S, et al.: Benign *Mucor* colonization (fungus ball) associated with chronic sinusitis. South Med J 1988; 81:846.

112. Ochi JW, Harris JP, Feldman JL, et al.: Rhinocerebral mucormycosis: Results of aggressive surgical débridement and amphotericin B. Laryngoscope 1988; 98:1339.

113. Millar JW, Johnston A, Lamb D: Allergic aspergillosis of the maxillary sinuses [abstr]. Thorax 1981; 36:710.

114. Katzenstein AL, Sale SR, Greenberger PA: Allergic *Aspergillus* sinusitus: A newly recognized form of sinusitis. J Allergy Clin Immunol 1983; 72:89–93.

115. Katzenstein AL, Sale SR, Greenberger PA: Pathologic findings in allergic *Aspergillus* sinusitis: A newly recognized form of sinusitis. Am J Surg Pathol 1983; 7:439.

116. Waxman JE, Spector JG, Sale SR, et al.: Allergic *Aspergillus* sinusitis: Concepts in diagnosis and treatment of a new clinical entity. Laryngoscope 1987; 97:261–266.

117. Sher TH, Schwartz HJ: Allergic *Aspergillus* sinusitis with concurrent allergic bronchopulmonary *Aspergillus*: Report of a case. J Allergy Clin Immunol 1988; 81:844–846.

118. Safirstein B: Allergic bronchopulmonary aspergillosis with obstruction of the upper respiratory tract. Chest 1976; 70:788–790.

119. Halwig JM, Brueske DA, Greenberger PA, et al.: Allergic bronchopulmonary curvulariosis. Am Rev Respir Dis 1985; 132:186–188.

120. Hendrick DJ, Ellithorpe DB, Lyon F, et al.: Allergic bronchopulmonary helminthosporiosis. Am Rev Respir Dis 1982; 126:935–938.

121. Brummund W, Kurup VP, Harris GJ, et al.: Allergic sinoorbital mycosis. JAMA 1986; 256:3249–3253.

122. Macmillan RH, Cooper PH, Body BA, et al.: Allergic fungal sinusitis due to *Curvularia lunata*. Hum Pathol 1987; 18:960–964.

123. Friedman GC, Hartwick RW, Ro JY, et al.: Allergic fungal sinusitis. Report of three cases associated with dematiaceous fungi. Am J Clin Pathol 1991; 96:368–372.

124. Hartwick RW, Batsakis JG: Sinus aspergillosis and allergic fungal sinusitis. Ann Otol 1991; 100:427–430.

125. Handley GH, Visscher DW, Katzenstein AL, et al.: Bone erosion in allergic fungal sinusitis. Am J Rhinol 1990; 4:149–153.

126. Anaissie E, Kantarjian H, Ro J, et al.: The emerging role of *Fusarium* infections in patients with cancer. Medicine 1988; 67:77–83.

127. Laskownicka Z, Kurdzielewicz J, Macura A, et al.: Mycotic sinusitis in children. Mykosen 1978; 21:407–411.

128. Blazer BR, Hurd DD: *Fusarium* infections in bone marrow transplant recipients. Am J Med 1984; 77:645–651.

129. Valenstein P, Schell WA: Primary intranasal *Fusarium* infection: Potential for confusion with rhinocerebral zygomycosis. Arch Pathol Lab Med 1986; 110:751–754.

130. Morgan MA, Wilson WR, Neel HB, et al.: Fungal sinusitis in healthy and immunocompromised individual. Am J Clin Pathol 1984; 82:597–601.

131. Winn RE: Systemic fungal infections: Diagnosis and treatment. I. Sporotrichosis. Infect Dis Clin North Am 1988; 2(4):899–911.

132. Agger WA, Caplan RH, Maki DG: Ocular sporotrichosis mimicking mucormycosis in a diabetic. Ann Ophthalmol 1978; 10:767–771.

133. Castro RM, DeSabogal MD, Cuce LC: Disseminated sporotrichosis: Report of a clinical case with myocutaneous, osteoarticular and ocular lesions. Mykosen 1981; 24:92–94.

134. Ogura S: Sporotrichosis of the maxillary antrum that stimulated symptoms of a maxillary tumor. Otolaryngology 1955; 27:541–543.

135. Otcenasek M, Jirousek Z, Nozicka A, et al.: Paecilomycosis of the maxillary sinus. Mykosen 1984; 27:242–251.

136. Rockhill RC, Klein MD: *Paecilomyces lilicinus* as the cause of chronic maxillary sinusitis. J Clin Microbiol 1980; 11:737–739.

137. Rowley SD, Strom CG: *Paecilomyces* fungus infection of the maxillary sinus. Laryngoscope 1982; 92:332–334.

138. Catalano P, Lawson W, Bottone E, et al.: Basidiomycetous (mushroom infection) of the maxillary sinus. Otolaryngol Head Neck Surg 1990; 102:183.

139. Batista AD, Maia JA, Singer R: Basidioneuromycosis in man. Am Soc Biol Pernambuco 1955; 13:52–60.

140. Ciferri R, Batista AC, Campos S: Isolation of *Schizophyllum commune* from a sputum. Atti Ist Bot Lab Crittogam Univ Pavia 1956; 14:3–5.

141. Kern ME, Uecker FA: Maxillary sinus infection caused by the homobasidiomycetous fungus *Schizophyllum commune*. J Clin Microbiol 1986; 6:1001–1005.

142. Restrepo AD, Greer AD, Robledo M, et al.: Ulceration of the palate caused by a basidiomycete *Schizophyllum commune*. Sabouraudia 1973; 11:201–204.

143. Litman ML, Zimmerman LE: Cryptococcosis. New York, Grune & Stratton, 1956, pp 8–37.

144. Briggs DR, Barney PL, Bahu RM: Nasal cryptococcosis. Arch Otolaryngol 1974; 100:390–392.

145. Kohlemeier W: Torulose der Nasenebenhoehlen nasal. Zentralblt Allg Pathol Pathol Anat 1995; 93:92–93.

146. Choi SS, Lawson W, Bottone EJ, et al.: Cryptococcal sinusitis: A case report and review of literature. Otolaryngol Head Neck Surg 1988; 99:414–418.

147. Lutwick LI, Galgani JN, Johnson RH, et al.: Visceral fungal infections due to *Petriellidium boydii (Allescheria boydii)*: In vitro drug sensitivity studies. Am J Med 1976; 61:632–640.

148. Mader JT, Ream RS, Heath PW: *Petriellidium boydii (Allescheria boydii)* sphenoidal sinusitis. JAMA 1978; 239:2368–2369.

149. Winston DJ, Jordan MC, Rhodes J: *Allescheria boydii* infections in the immunosuppressed host. Am J Med 1977; 63:830–835.

150. Arnett JC, Hatch HB: Pulmonary allescheriasis: Report of a case and review of the literature. Arch Intern Med 1975; 135:1250–1253.

151. May LK, Knight RA, Harris HW: *Allescheria boydii* and *Aspergillus fumigatus* skin test antigens. J Bacteriol 1966; 91:2155–2159.

152. Bark CJ, Zaino LJ, Rossmiller K, et al.: *Petriellidium* sinusitis. JAMA 1978; 240:2339–1340.

153. Gluckman SJ, Ries K, Abrutyn E: *Allescheria (Petriellidium) boydii* sinusitis in a compromised host. J Clin Microbiol 1977; 5:481–484.

154. Hecht R, Montgomerie JZ: Maxillary sinus infection with *Allescheria boydii (Petriellidium boydii)*. Johns Hopkins Med J 1978; 142:107–109.

155. Bloom SM, Warner RR, Weitzman I: Maxillary sinusitis: Isolation of *Scedosporium (Monosporium) apiospermum*. Mt. Sinai J Med 1982; 49:492–494.

156. Bryan CS, DiSalvo AF, Kaufman L, et al.: *Petriellidium boydii* infection of the sphenoid sinus. Am J Clin Pathol 1980; 74:846–851.

157. Travis LB, Roberts GD, Wilson WR: Clinical significance of *Pseudallescheria boydii*: A review of 10 years' experience. Mayo Clin Proc 1985; 60:531–537.

158. Winn RE, Ramsey PD, McDonald JC, et al.: Maxillary sinusitis from *Pseudallescheria boydii*—efficacy of surgical therapy. Arch Otolaryngol Head Neck Surg 1983; 109:123–125.

159. Kwon-Chung KJ, Bennett JE: Entomophtoromycosis. In: Kwon-Chung KJ, Bennett JE (eds): Medical Mycology. Philadelphia: Lea & Febiger, 1992, pp 447–463.

160. Dworzack DL, Pollock AS, Hodges GR, et al.: Zygomycosis of the maxillary sinus and palate caused by *Basidiobolus haptosporus*. Arch Intern Med 1978; 128:1274–1276.

161. Cowen DE, Dine DE, Chessen J, et al.: *Cephalosporium* midline granuloma. Ann Intern Med 1965; 62:791–795.

162. Lie-Lian-Joe, Eng NT, Keropati S: A new verrucous mycosis caused by *Cercospora apii*. Arch Dermatol 1957; 75:864–870.

163. Kwon-Chung KJ, Bennett JE: Chromoblastomycosis. In: Kwon-Chung KJ, Bennett JE (eds): Medical Mycology. Philadelphia, Lea & Febiger, 1992, pp 337–354.

164. Yamamoto H, Caselitz J: Chromoblastomycosis of the maxillary sinus. Arch Otolaryngol 1985; 242:129–133.

165. Gardner JT, et al.: Chromoblastomycosis in Texas: Report of four cases. Tex State J Med 1964; 60:913.

166. Nakamura T: Primary chromoblastomycosis of the nasal septum. Am J Clin Pathol 1972; 58:365–370.

167. Zazor L: A case of primary nasal chromoblastomycosis. Mykosen 1987; 30:468–471.

168. Pavlidakey GP, Snow SN, Mohs FE: Chromoblastomycosis treated by Mohs' micrographic surgery. Dermatol Surg Oncol 1986; 12:1073–1075.

169. Silber JG, Gombert ME: Treatment of chromomycosis with ketoconazole and 5-flurocytosine. J Am Acad Dermatol 1983; 8:236–238.

170. Levy FE, Larson JT, George E, et al.: Invasive *Chrysosporium* infection of the nose and paranasal sinuses in an immunocompromised host. Otolaryngol Head Neck Surg 1991; 104:384–388.

171. Drutz DJ: Amphotericin B in the treatment of coccidioidomycosis. Drugs 1983; 26:337–346.

172. Galgiani JN, et al.: Ketoconazole therapy of progressive coccidioidomycosis. Am J Med 1988; 84:603–610.

173. Graybill JR, et al.: Itraconazole treatment of coccidioidomycosis. Am J Med 1990; 89:282–290.

174. Kwon-Chung KJ, Bennett JE: Coccidioidomycosis. In: Kwon-Chung KJ, Bennett JE (eds): Medical Mycology. Philadelphia: Lea & Febiger, 1992, pp 356–396.

175. Clark BM, Edington GM: Subcutaneous phycomycosis and rhinoentomophthoromycosis. In: Baker RD (ed): Human Infection with Fungi, Actinomycetes and Algae. New York: Springer-Verlag, 1971, pp 684–690.

176. Berman RO, Crain BJ, Proctor AM, et al.: Cunninghamella: A newly recognized cause of rhinocerebral mucormycosis. Am J Clin Pathol 1983; 80:98–102.

177. Mitchell RG, Chaplin AJ, Mackenzie DW: *Emericella nidulan* in a maxillary sinus fungal mass. J Med Vet Mycol 1987; 23:339–341.

178. Kwon-Chung KJ, Bennett JE: Lobomycosis. In: Kwon-Chung KJ, Bennett JE (eds): Medical Mycology. Philadelphia: Lea & Febiger, 1992, pp 514–523.

179. Benda TJ, Corey JP: *Malbranchea pulchella* fungal sinusitis. Otolaryngol Head Neck Surg 1994; 110:501–504.

180. Kyriakos M: Myospherulosis of the paranasal sinuses, nose and middle ear: A possible iatrogenic disease. Am J Clin Pathol 1977; 67:118–130.

181. Rosai J: The nature of myospherulosis of the upper respiratory tract. Am J Clin Pathol 1978; 69:475–481.

182. Maran AG, Kwong K, Milne LJ, et al.: Frontal sinusitis caused by *Myriodontium keratinophilum*. Br Med J 1987; 290:207–209.

183. Morriss FH, Spock A: Intracranial aneurysm secondary to mycotic orbital and sinus infection. Am J Dis Child 1970; 119:357–362.

184. Bassiouny A, Maher A, Bucci TJ, et al.: Noninvasive antromycosis. J Laryngol Otol 1982; 96:215–228.

185. Ahluwalia KB, Bahadur S: Rhinosporidiosis associated with squamous cell carcinoma of the tongue. J Laryngol Otol 1990; 104:648–650.

186. Aravindan KP, Viswanathan MK, Leelamma J: Rhinosporidioma of bone: A case report. Indian J Pathol Microbiol 1989; 32:312–313.

187. Chatterjee PK, Katua CR, Chatterjee SN, et al.: Recurrent multiple rhinosporidiosis with osteolytic lesions of the hands and feet. J Laryngol Otol 1977; 91:729.

188. Karunaratne WAE: Rhinosporidiosis in Man. London: Athlone Press, 1964.

189. Kwon-Chung KJ, Bennett JE: Rhinosporidiosis. In: Kwon-Chung KJ, Bennett JE (eds): Medical Mycology. Philadelphia: Lea & Febiger, 1992, pp 695–706.

190. Mohaptia LN: Rhinosporidiosis. In: Baker RD (ed): Human Infection with Fungi, Actinomyces, and Algae. Berlin: Springer-Verlag, 1971, pp 676–682.

191. Rajam RV, Viswanathan GC, Rao AR, et al.: Rhinosporidiosis, a study with a report of a fatal case of systemic dissemination. Indian J Surg 1955; 17:269.

192. Satyanarayana C: Rhinosporidiosis (with a record of 255 cases). Acta Otolaryngol 1960; 51:318.

193. Clarke PR, Warnock GB, Blowers R, et al.: Brain abscess due to *Streptomyces greseus*. J Neurol Neurosurg Psychiatr 1964; 227:553–555.

Margaret A. Kenna

C H A P T E R   F O R T Y - F O U R

Laryngotracheobronchitis

▼

Laryngotracheobronchitis (LTB), or croup, is a common viral illness in the pediatric population. The term "croup" was introduced in 1765 by Francis Home in a paper entitled "An Inquiry Into the Nature, Causes and Cure of the Croup" in which he described 12 cases of croup. The word is probably derived from the Scottish term "roup," meaning "to cry out in a shrill voice" or from the Anglo-Saxon word "kropan," "to cry aloud."[1, 2] Since the initial description of croup by Home in 1765, many other disease entities have been confused with viral LTB, including spasmodic croup, bacterial tracheitis, membranous laryngotracheobronchitis, epiglottitis, diphtheria, and angioneurotic edema (Table 44–1). Distinguishing between these entities is important because the causes and management vary significantly and if incorrect treatment is chosen it could have an adverse or even fatal outcome. Fortunately, significant strides have been made in the management of LTB; so, if the correct diagnosis is made a positive outcome can almost always be ensured.

EPIDEMIOLOGY

Viral LTB is a common illness in young children, accounting for 10%–15% of lower respiratory tract disease in children. Many studies over multiple years have been used to estimate that at least 580,000 cases of croup occur every year in the United States in children younger than 5 years of age. The disease is most prevalent from age 3 months to 3 years and peaks during the second year of life.[1, 2] The reported incidence in children younger than 6 years has varied from 3

Table 44–1. DIFFERENTIAL DIAGNOSIS OF ACUTE AIRWAY OBSTRUCTION IN CHILDREN

Infectious
  Viral laryngotracheobronchitis
  Supraglottitis
  Bacterial tracheitis
  Retropharyngeal abscess
  Diphtheria
  Peritonsillar abscess
Noninfectious
  Angioneurotic edema
  Foreign body
  Neoplasm
  Neurologic (vocal cord paresis/paralysis)
  Trauma (blunt, burns, thermal injury)

cases per 100 children per year in North Carolina to 7 cases per 1000 children per year in Seattle.[3–5] Croup has also been reported, though rarely, in adults, usually following an upper respiratory tract viral infection prodrome.[6] Most authors report a higher incidence of croup in boys than in girls (up to 2:1) for both emergency room visits and hospitalizations.[2–4, 7]

Most cases of viral LTB occur in the late fall and early winter, are often epidemic, and reflect the epidemiologic patterns of the various etiologic agents. Human parainfluenza virus types 1 and 2 (HPIV 1 and HPIV 2) account for most of the cases of LTB in young children. HPIV 1, the most common cause of LTB, accounts for up to 50% of croup cases worldwide, is most prevalent during the fall, and most recently has tended to cause outbreaks of infection every other year.[1, 8] HPIV 2 tends to cause smaller outbreaks of infection at less predictable intervals, but most often during the fall and early winter and uncommonly in outbreak form.[1, 8] Viral croup is the most common lower respiratory tract disease caused by HPIV 2. Sporadic, and sometimes severe, cases of LTB are commonly associated with HPIV 3.[1, 2] HPIV 3 has recently been noted to be most prevalent in the spring and summer, although in the even-numbered years when HPIV 1 and 2 were absent, HPIV 3 appeared in the fall.[8] A very small percentage of cases of croup have been attributed to HPIV 4A and 4B.

All HPIVs are RNA viruses that are members of the genus paramyxovirus and belong to the Paramyxoviridae family. Included in this family are other important human pathogens, including mumps, measles, and respiratory syncytial virus (RSV), and many important animal pathogens, including Newcastle disease virus, canine distemper, Sendai virus, and simian virus 5. All HPIVs share similarities in their structural, physiochemical, and biologic characteristics, although molecular analysis of all four types reveals more antigenic and genetic heterogeneity than had been appreciated in the past. There are five basic serotypes within the paramyxovirus genus that can be grouped into two divisions: (1) HPIV 1 and 3; (2) HPIV 2 and 4 and mumps. Although they all share common antigens, they can also be identified separately by monoclonal antibodies and specific hyperimmune animal serum. All four strains have shown antigenic change over the past several years, which raises concern about the possible utility of vaccines, especially ones based on older strains of the viruses.[1, 2, 8, 9]

Influenza virus types A and B have also been associated with outbreaks of croup.[10] Since this virus may result in very significant systemic illness as well, croup caused by influenza virus may be accompanied by involvement of many other organ systems.

RSV, which belongs to the pneumovirus genus of the paramyxoviridae family, may also cause viral LTB. While RSV is the major cause of lower respiratory tract infection in young children, croup is the least common clinical manifestation, accounting for 5%–15% of croup cases; however, since as many as 89% of young children admitted to the hospital with acute lower respiratory tract disease may have RSV isolated, this pathogen cannot be discounted as a cause of croup. As severe RSV infection is mainly a disease of very young, children with RSV croup tend to be slightly younger than children with other viral LTBs. RSV is an enveloped, single-strand RNA virus of 120–300 mm. There are two major strains of RSV, A and B, and subtypes within each group. The major antigenic differences between the two groups are due to the largest surface glycoprotein, the G protein. Both strains may be present simultaneously during outbreaks, although in varying proportions.[1, 2, 11]

The measles virus may also cause croup and has been associated with outbreaks leading to bacterial tracheitis.[12] Measles virus belongs to the genus Morbillivirus of the family Paramyxoviridae. It is closely related to the viruses causing canine distemper, rinderpest of cattle, and pest des petits ruminants of goats and sheep. Wild measles virus is pathogenic only for primate, and only one strain has been identified.[13] Other viruses that have been implicated in viral LTB include several strains of adenovirus, rhinovirus, coxsackievirus, herpes simplex virus, and reoviruses. Croup due to enteroviruses, while less common, may occur in the summer and early fall.

Moraxella catarrhalis has recently been implicated in the pathogenesis of croup.[14] Although this pathogen is more commonly associated with otitis media, sinusitis, and possibly pharyngitis, its role in the production of croup cannot be discounted. Other bacteria that have been implicated as a cause of bacterial croup include *Staphylococcus aureus*, *Streptococcus pneumoniae*, *Haemophilus influenzae*, *Streptococcus pyogenes*, *Mycoplasma pneumoniae*, and, very rarely, *Cryptosporidium* species. It is unclear whether these bacteria represent the primary pathogen or the agent of superinfection over a primary viral illness.[1, 2]

PATHOPHYSIOLOGY

Viral upper respiratory tract infections usually affect the mucosa of the nose and the nasopharynx first, then spread down to involve the larynx and tracheobronchial tree. The mucosa of the subglottis in the young child is loosely attached and therefore permits submucosal edema formation, with narrowing of the airway. The barking cough and stridor characteristic of croup generally result from edema of the subglottic airway. Because the cricoid cartilage is normally a complete ring, the airway is narrowest there and cannot swell outward. Therefore, even minimal (especially circumferential) edema can cause significant airway obstruction because resistance to air flow is inversely related to the fourth power of the radius of the airway. In the child 1–2 years old with an airway diameter of 6.5 mm, 1 mm of

circumferential edema decreases the cross-sectional area of the subglottis by 50%. In croup, stridor is most common on inspiration because the negative inspiratory pressure tends to narrow the already partially narrowed extrathoracic structures. Biphasic stridor can occur if the subglottis is extremely narrow, especially if there is significant glottic and/or supraglottic involvement as well. Copious secretions produced secondary to acute inflammation may also clog both small and large airways, producing secondary obstruction in an already narrowed area. Histologically, inflammatory changes are noted in the epithelium, mucosa, and submucosa of the glottis, subglottis, and throughout the tracheobronchial tree, even including the alveoli. Atelectasis may also be present.

During the first few years of life children may be especially susceptible to viral LTB, for several reasons. First, they have anatomically small, and somewhat collapsible, airways. Second, crying and concomitant nasal obstruction may aggravate the symptoms in a child with an already narrowed airway. Third, a primary viral infection may be more likely to spread throughout the entire respiratory tract, causing more extensive disease.

DIFFERENTIAL DIAGNOSIS

Spasmodic croup is an ill-defined entity that can be difficult to differentiate from viral LTB. The dry, barking cough of spasmodic croup also usually starts at night; stridor is inspiratory but rarely severe. A viral upper respiratory tract infection (URI) prodrome is not always present. Fever is low-grade or absent. Many patients with spasmodic croup have a history of atopy, although a precipitating cause is frequently obscure. The symptoms very often resolve spontaneously or with cold mist, over a period of hours rather than days (the latter is more usual in viral LTB). Spasmodic croup is often recurrent, especially in very young children. Some authors feel that spasmodic croup represents the very mild end of the clinical spectrum of viral LTB; others regard it as a separate disease process that may be allergic in nature.[15, 16]

The most common bacterial diseases of the airway to be confused with viral LTB are epiglottis (supraglottitis) and bacterial tracheitis. *H. influenzae* type B (HIB) used to be the most common bacterial pathogen of epiglottitis, but since the introduction of the HIB vaccine epiglottitis has declined precipitously in incidence.[17] Other organisms, however, including group A beta-hemolytic streptococci (GABHS) and *M. catarrhalis*, may still cause this disease. Atypical presentations of epiglottitis may occur in children immunized against HIB who do not develop immunity and in immunocompromised children whose epiglottitis may be due to unusual organisms. Children with supraglottitis tend to be slightly older and more "toxic" in appearance with high (>38.5° C) fever; they sit leaning forward and drool, and suffer very significant respiratory distress. These patients are less likely to have a clear history of an antecedent viral URI.

Bacterial tracheitis or membranous laryngotracheobronchitis may involve the entire tracheobronchial tree; the organisms most commonly reported are *S. aureus*, *H. influenzae*, and GABHS. Bacterial tracheitis may have as a prodrome mild URI, with gradual or sudden worsening of the clinical picture. Most authors feel that it is a bacterial superinfection of a viral URI; influenza virus, parainfluenza virus, measles virus, RSV, and enteroviruses all have been reported as antecedents of bacterial tracheitis. Both epiglottitis and bacterial tracheitis often present with high fever and a generally more toxic appearance than that associated with viral croup. On endoscopy, often needed for diagnosis and airway management, children with bacterial tracheitis are found to have involvement of the larynx, trachea, and bronchi, and a distinct purulent membrane lining the airway in many cases. At the time of bronchoscopy, removal of the membrane may be necessary for clinical improvement.[18–20]

Another bacterial disease process that can be mistaken for croup is retropharyngeal abscess. Affected children are also often very ill, with high fever, forward-sitting posture, and drooling, not unlike the signs of supraglottitis. They may develop laryngeal edema as well as significant enlargement of the retropharyngeal lymph nodes, and occasionally of the parapharyngeal space. These children are also very young, usually younger than 4 years, so they still have a significant amount of retropharyngeal lymphoid tissue. Physical examination may reveal a bulging retropharyngeal space, usually unilateral owing to the median raphe, and may also show significant cervical lymphadenopathy. Lateral soft tissue radiographs of the neck demonstrate widening of the prevertebral soft tissue space and, in rare cases, an air-fluid level. On endoscopy, findings include enlargement of the retropharyngeal space, and occasionally laryngeal edema. The subglottic space is normal.

Foreign bodies in the aerodigestive tract may also be confused with viral LTB, especially if the child with the foreign body also has a viral URI. The patient's history and response to medial management for croup usually help to differentiate the two entities, but occasionally endoscopy is needed for definitive diagnosis. Although foreign bodies of the tracheobronchial tree are more likely to be confused with croup, esophageal foreign bodies impinging on the tracheoesophageal party wall occasionally present with a barking cough and stridor.

Hereditary angioedema, caused by C1-esterase deficiency, may mimic recurrent croup. The airway obstruction can be severe, and often will not respond to the usual croup measures. This is one case of "croup" in which diligent laboratory investigation may yield a diagnosis.

Gastroesophageal reflux (GER), especially in small children, may cause airway symptoms and recurrent croup. The lack of correlating URI, fever, and time of year, along with other symptoms of GER, should suggest the diagnosis. In obscure cases of recurrent croup, GER should be considered.[21]

DIAGNOSIS AND CLINICAL PRESENTATION
(Table 44–2)

The diagnosis of viral LTB can usually be made on the basis of clinical characteristics and the epidemiologic setting. A

Table 44–2. CLINICAL DIAGNOSIS OF SUPRAGLOTTITIS, LARYNGOTRACHEOBRONCHITIS, BACTERIAL TRACHEITIS, AND FOREIGN BODY ASPIRATION

	Supraglottitis	Laryngotracheobronchitis	Bacterial Tracheitis	Foreign Body Aspiration
History				
Relative incidence in children presenting with stridor	8%	88%	2%	2%
Onset	Rapid, 4–12 h	Prodrome, 1–7 d	Prodrome, 3 d, then 10 h	Acute or chronic
Age	1–6 yr	3 mo–3 yr	3 mo–12 yr	Any
Male: female	1:1	2:1	1:1	2:1
Season	None	October-May	None	None
Etiology	*H. influenzae*	Parainfluenza viruses	*Staphylococcus* spp.	Many
Pathology	Acute inflammatory edema of epiglottis and supraglotittis	Subglottic edema with variable inflammation of trachea and bronchial tree	Tracheal bronchial edema, necrotic debris	Site dependent
Signs and Symptoms				
Dysphagia	Yes	No	No	Rare
Difficulty swallowing	Yes	No	Rare	No
Drooling	Yes	No	Rare	No
Stridor	Inspiratory	Inspiratory and expiratory	Inspiratory	Variable
Voice	Muffled	Hoarse	Normal	Variable
Cough	No	Barking	Variable	Yes
Temperature	Markedly elevated	Minimally elevated	Moderate	Rare
Respiratory rate	Increased early	Increased late	Normal	Increased if bronchial obstruction present
Heart rate	Increased early	Increased late	Proportional to fever	Normal
Position	Erect, anxious, "air hungry"; supine position exacerbates obstruction	No effect on airway obstruction	No effect	No effect
Retractions	Supraclavicular, substernal, and intercostal retractions	Most cases mild; can be severe	Present, variable severity	Variable

From Custer JR: Croup and related disorders. Pediatr Rev 1993; 14: 19–29.

1–3 day viral URI prodrome of low-grade fever and rhinorrhea followed by barking cough, hoarseness, stridor, and retractions is usually enough to suggest the diagnosis. The characteristic barking cough usually appears during the night, and in more severe cases is accompanied by inspiratory stridor. Extremely severe cases may be accompanied by expiratory stridor as well. If there is marked airway obstruction the child may also be pale, apprehensive, and wanting to sit forward. Often, however, children with croup who "sound terrible" may be playing happily in little apparent distress, in contrast to those with epiglottitis or bacterial tracheitis, who usually both sound and look extremely ill. The symptoms of croup may wax and wane, marked airway obstruction and more severe stridor being present at one time and minimal stridor in the next hours. Children are often worse at night and better in the morning. This fluctuating course may go on for several days, especially in those with milder disease.

In the child with croup, anteroposterior soft tissue radiographs of the neck often demonstrate a "steeple sign" in the subglottic area: the normally convex lateral "shoulders" become convex medially (Fig. 44–1). Soft tissue lateral neck films may also show narrowing of the subglottis with a wider air column noted on expiration in comparison with inspiration, hypopharyngeal overdistention, and thickening of the vocal cords. In contrast, thickening of the aryepiglottic folds or epiglottis suggests a diagnosis of supraglottitis (Fig. 44–2). Films, however, are not a substitute for detailed clinical assessment, as they can be misinterpreted.[22] Taking the child to the x-ray suite from the emergency room for

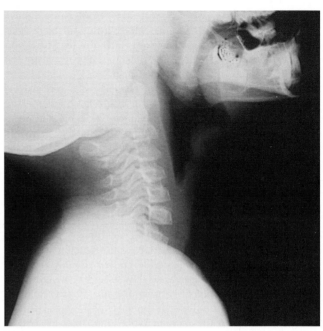

Figure 44–1. Lateral soft tissue radiograph of the neck illustrating thickening of the aryepiglottic folds and epiglottis (or "thumb sign") classically seen with supraglottitis (epiglottitis).

airway films is not advised, because if the child has acute airway compromise this is not the best place to handle it. If the treating physician feels that radiographic evaluation is indicated, the technologist should come to the patient in the emergency room to obtain films.

If needed, confirmation can be made by viral isolation or by use of one of the new rapid diagnostic tests. For RSV, nasal wash specimens produce the highest rate of virus recovery, although swabs of the throat and nasopharynx together can also be used. In addition to culture, direct and indirect fluorescent antibody techniques and enzyme immunoassay may be used. The disadvantage of the cultures, as compared with the more rapid methods, is reporting time; the advantage is possible isolation of other pathogens. Newest detection methods include the polymerase chain reaction and in situ hybridization.

If the patient with signs and symptoms of croup does not exhibit a significant clinical response to medical management, endoscopy may be needed for further diagnostic evaluation, and sometimes stabilization of the airway. Tan and Manoukian reported on 500 children admitted to Montreal Children's Hospital from 1984 to 1988 with a diagnosis of croup. Eighteen of these children underwent diagnostic rigid endoscopy for recurrent croup or worsening respiratory condition (or both). Seven of the eighteen had lesions in addition to their croup, including two with subglottic hemangioma, two with subglottic stenosis, one with vocal cord paralysis, and one with epiglottitis.[23] In the 1991 paper by Gallagher and Myer, the diagnosis of bacterial membranous laryngotracheobronchitis was definitively distinguished from severe viral croup by either flexible or rigid endoscopy rather than solely on the basis of clinical characteristics or radiography.[20] Flexible laryngoscopy and bronchoscopy have the advantages of not requiring general anesthesia and of providing

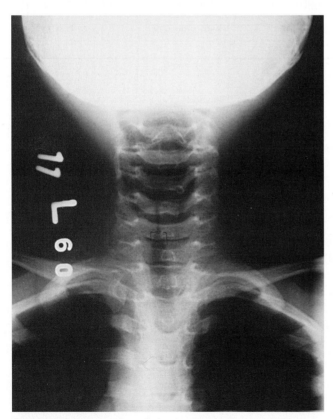

Figure 44–1. Anteroposterior soft tissue radiograph of the neck illustrating the "steeple sign" seen with LTB.

an immediate diagnosis; the disadvantages include requiring a cooperative patient, not always being able to suction out thick secretions or remove membranes, and inability to stent open a tenuous airway. Rigid endoscopy, though it requires general anesthesia, affords the ability to suction easily, remove membranes, perform cultures, and secure the airway.

MANAGEMENT

Supportive treatment with cool mist remains the cornerstone of the treatment of croup. At home, mist can be administered by cool mist vaporizer, by placing the child in a bathroom filled with steam from the shower, or by taking the child outdoors in the cool night air. In the hospital, mist can be administered by a parent or other caregiver. Occasionally croup tents are used, but they have the disadvantage of obscuring the view of the child.

In the hospital, initial management may consist of hydration, cool mist with or without supplemental oxygen, and racemic epinephrine. Some authors have recommended use of helium-oxygen mixtures, which, theoretically, should improve gas flow because helium is less dense than air; however, helium should not be used if the patient has a significant oxygen requirement, as it may lead to or exacerbate hypoxia.[24]

Many physicians, especially in the emergency room setting, use a "croup score," both for initial triage and to evaluate response to medical therapy.[25] Most croup scores use some weighted combination of color, respirations, pulse rate, presence of stridor, severity of retractions, and level of consciousness to evaluate the child. Whatever method is used, sound medical judgment is needed to predict the onset of respiratory failure, hypoxia, and hypercarbia. Questions that should be asked include these: Is the child's color normal or cyanotic? On auscultation, is air entry normal or decreased? If stridor is present, is it mild or severe? If stridor is present, are retractions also present and are they mild or severe? Is the child alert, agitated, or hard to arouse? Increasing respiratory rate, increasing pulse rate, cyanosis, and lethargy are ominous signs, although cyanosis as the sole measure of hypoxemia is not always reliable (i.e., cyanosis in children with darker skin or anemia may be especially difficult to appreciate). All children with significant symptoms need to be reevaluated frequently, even during the course of 1 or 2 hours, as significant worsening may occur with little warning. Pulse oximetry, a noninvasive method for assessing oxygenation, may help monitor for hypoxia, although technical problems with the machines themselves mean that constant clinical reassessment is needed, in addition to pulse oximetry.[26] Transcutaneous carbon dioxide measurements may also be useful, especially in the assessment of response to medical therapy.[27] Invasive measures, such as blood gas determinations, should usually be avoided, as they may provoke crying and increased respiratory effort, all of which can exacerbate the existing obstructive symptoms.

Aerosolized racemic epinephrine has become a mainstay of croup management, and if the patient does not have a prompt clinical response to cool mist, racemic epinephrine is indicated. It is thought to act by stimulating alpha-adrenergic receptors in the subglottic mucosa, producing vasoconstric-

tion and decreasing edema. The main drawback of racemic epinephrine is the rebound phenomenon: symptoms return after a significant clinical response (this may represent only return of edema after the medication's effects wear off). Therefore, patients should not be discharged from the emergency room immediately after a racemic epinephrine treatment, as further treatment with epinephrine or steroids may be indicated. The usefulness of L-epinephrine, which is less expensive and more readily available worldwide, in the treatment of croup has also been demonstrated.[28, 29]

The most recent important advance in the medical management of viral LTB is the use of systemic steroids. A meta-analysis in 1989 by Kairys and colleagues examined 10 randomized controlled trials of steroids in the treatment of croup published since 1960. Their analysis indicated that the use of steroids was associated with a significantly increased percentage of patients who showed clinical improvement at both 12 and 24 hours after steroid administration. Additionally, the number of endotracheal intubations in the steroid-treated group was significantly decreased.[30] A 1989 editorial in the Lancet critiqued this article and pointed out several areas of concern, including various doses and types of steroids, nonstandard criteria for croup severity, stratification for LTB versus spasmodic croup, and standard outcome measure.[31]

Since 1989 several other prospective randomized studies have definitively demonstrated the efficacy of steroids in the treatment of croup.[32–34] Two other studies from the Royal Melbourne Hospital in Australia showed that the administration of systemic prednisolone prior to extubation increased the chances of successful extubation in children who had been intubated for croup but had failed a previous extubation, reduced the duration of intubation for croup, and also decreased the need for reintubation of children who had been intubated for croup.[33, 35]

Two recent studies addressed the use of nebulized budesonide in the treatment of children with mild to moderate or moderate to severe croup.[36, 37] Both studies found a significant improvement in the steroid group as compared with the saline group, although some patients in both groups (fewer in the budesonide group) required systemic dexamethasone for progressive or recurrent symptoms.

The studies cited above showed definitively that steroids given to children with croup are beneficial; dexamethasone is the preparation used most frequently. Usual doses of dexamethasone range from 0.3–1.0 mg/kg. Steroids now are commonly administered in the emergency room and in doctors' offices to children with significant symptoms of croup, to try to avoid intubation and, at times, even to try to avoid admission to the hospital. Questions that still remain about the use of steroids include route of administration (oral, nebulized, or intravenous), criteria for administration, and the relative effectiveness of different doses.

As already noted, in patients with impending airway obstruction rigid endoscopy can be used for both diagnosis and airway stabilization. Before intubation became routine tracheotomy was a life-saving intervention in patients with croup and it continues to be utilized for either extubation failures or as a primary modality. Drawbacks to tracheotomy included the need for a surgical procedure and care and complications of the tracheotomy tube itself (including granulation tissue, suprastomal collapse, bleeding, accidental decannulation, and plugging of the tube). A review of 208 children who required airway intervention for LTB at The Children's Hospital in Camperdown, New South Wales from 1979 to 1988 showed that 181 (87%) were intubated and later extubated; 13% underwent tracheotomy. Tracheotomy was performed if there was difficulty with the initial intubation or if the patient "failed" extubation. Five children developed acquired subglottic stenosis. Factors thought to be related to endotracheal tube trauma leading to subglottic stenosis included absence of a leak at the time of extubation, intubation for longer than 5 days, pre-existing subglottic stenosis, previous intubation for LTB, previous neonatal intubation and ventilation, too large endotracheal tube, and difficult initial intubation. The presence of inflammation has also been suggested as a factor in the development of subglottic stenosis after endotracheal intubation.[35, 38–40]

Guidelines for management of croup are these:

1. Cool mist. If stridor worsens or develops, medical intervention should be obtained.

2. Nebulized racemic epinephrine should be utilized if mist alone fails. If the child has a prompt response with decreased stridor, increased air exchange, and improved score, discharge from the emergency room can be considered.

3. If the child requires frequent doses of racemic epinephrine systemic steroids should be administered. In addition, children considered for discharge after one or two racemic epinephrine treatments may receive "prophylactic" steroids before discharge.

4. If the child is clearly tiring, has a significant oxygen requirement, and is not responding to the medical measures cited above, intubation should be seriously considered.

SUMMARY

Viral LTB continues to be a very common problem in childhood. Successful diagnosis and management still depend primarily on careful history taking and physical examination. Treatment includes cool air, cool mist, racemic epinephrine, and steroids. Bronchoscopy, intubation, and (uncommonly) tracheotomy, may be needed for airway management. Most children with correctly diagnosed and managed croup have a satisfactory outcome and no long-term sequelae.

References

1. Hall CB: Acute laryngotracheobronchitis (croup). In: Mandell GL, Bennett JE, Dolin R (eds): Principles and Practice of Infectious Disease, 4th ed. New York: Churchill Livingstone, 1995, pp 573–779.
2. Cherry JD: Croup. In: Feigin RD, Cherry JD (eds): Textbook of Pediatric Infectious Diseases, 3rd ed, vol 1. Philadelphia: WB Saunders, 1992, pp 209–220.
3. Denny FW, Murphy TF, Clyde WA, et al.: Croup: An 11-year study in a pediatric practice. Pediatrics 1983; 71: 871–876.
4. Foy HM, Cooney MK, Maletzky AJ, et al.: Incidence and etiology of pneumonia, croup and bronchiolitis in pre-school children belonging to a pre-paid medical care group over a four year period. Am J Epidemiol 1973; 97: 80–84.
5. Hoekelman RA: Infectious illness during the first year of life. Pediatrics 1977; 59: 119–121.
6. Deeb ZE, Einhorn KH. Infectious adult croup. Laryngoscope 1990; 100: 455–457.
7. Henrickson KJ, Suhn SM, Savatski LL: Epidemiology and cost of infection with human parainfluenza virus types 1 and 2 in young children. Clin Infect Dis 1994; 18: 770–779.
8. Knott AM, Long CE, Hall CB: Parainfluenza viral infections in pediatric outpatients: Seasonal patterns and clinical characteristics. Pediatr Infect Dis J 1994; 13: 269–273.
9. Henrickson K, Ray R, Belshe R: Parainfluenza viruses. In: Mandell GL, Bennett JE, Dolin R (eds): Principles and Practice of Infectious Diseases, 4th ed. New York: Churchill Livingstone, 1995, pp 1489–1496.
10. Sugaya N, Nerome K, Ishida M, et al.: Impact of influenza virus infection as a cause of pediatric hospitalization. J Infect Dis 1992; 165: 373–375.
11. Hall CB, McCarthy CA: Respiratory syncytial virus. In: Mandell GL, Bennett JE, Dolin R (eds): Principles and Practice of Infectious Diseases, 4th ed. New York: Churchill Livingstone, 1995.
12. Ross LA, Mason WH, Lanson J, et al.: Laryngotracheobronchitis as a complication of measles during an urban epidemic. J Pediatr 1992; 121: 511–515.
13. Gershon AA: Measles virus (rubeola). In: Principles and Practice of Infectious Diseases, 4th ed. New York: Churchill Livingstone, 1995, pp 1519–1526.
14. Dudley JP: *Branhamella catarrhalis* and croup: Toxicity in the upper respiratory tract. Am J Otolaryngol 1991; 12: 113–116.
15. Hide DW, Guyer BM: Recurrent croup. Arch Dis Child 1985; 60: 585–586.
16. Zach M, Erben A, Olinsky A: Croup, recurrent croup, allergy, and airways hypersensitivity. Arch Dis Child 1981; 56: 336–341.
17. Senior BA, Radkowski D, MacArthur C, et al.: Changing patterns in pediatric supraglottitis: A multi-institutional review, 1980–1992. Laryngoscope 1994; 104: 1314–1322.
18. Korppi M, Leinonen M, Makela PH, et al.: Bacterial involvement in parainfluenza virus infection in children. Scand J Infect Dis 1990; 22: 307–312.
19. Sendi K, Crysdale WS, Yoo J: Tracheitis: Outcome of 1,700 cases presenting to the emergency department during two years. J Otolaryngol 1991; 21: 20–24.
20. Gallagher PG, Myer CM: An approach to the diagnosis and treatment of membranous laryngotracheobronchitis in infants and children. Pediatr Emerg Care 1991; 7: 337–342.
21. Putnam P: Gastroesophageal Reflux. In: Bluestone CD, Stool SE, Kenna MA (eds): Pediatric Otolaryngology, 3rd ed. Philadelphia: WB Saunders Co, 1995, 1144–1156.
22. Stankiewicz JA, Bowes AK: Croup and epiglottitis: A radiologic study. Laryngoscope 1985; 95: 1159–1160.
23. Tan AKW, Manoukian JJ: Hospitalized croup (bacterial and viral): The role of rigid endoscopy. J Otolaryngol 1991; 21: 48–53.
24. Custer JR: Croup and related disorders. Pediatr Rev 1993; 14: 19–29.
25. Westley CR, Cotton EK, Brooks JG: Nebulized racemic epinephrine by IPPB for the treatment of croup: A double-blind study. Am J Dis Child 1978; 132: 484–487.
26. Stoney PJ, Chakrabarti MK: Experience of pulse oximetry in children with croup. J Laryngol Otol 1991; 105: 295–298.
27. Fanconi S, Burger R, Maurer H, et al.: Transcutaneous carbon dioxide pressure for monitoring patients with severe croup. J Pediatr 1990; 117: 701–705.
28. Kelly PB, Simon JE: Racemic epinephrine use in croup and disposition. Am J Emerg Med 1992; 10: 181–183.
29. Waisman Y, Klein BL, Boenning DA, et al.: Prospective randomized double-blind study comparing L-epinephrine and racemic epinephrine aerosols in the treatment of laryngotracheitis (croup). Pediatrics 1992; 89: 302–306.
30. Kairys SW, Olmstead EM, O'Connor GT: Steroid treatment of laryngotracheitis: A meta-analysis of the evidence from randomized trials. Pediatrics 1989; 83: 683–693.
31. Steroids and croup. Lancet, 1989; 2: 1134–1136.
32. Super DM, Cartelli NA, Brooks LJ, et al.: A prospective randomized double-blind study to evaluate the effect of dexamethasone in acute laryngotracheitis. J Pediatr 1989; 115: 323–329.
33. Tibballs J, Shann FA, Landau LI: Placebo-controlled trial of prednisolone in children intubated for croup. Lancet 1992; 340: 745–748.
34. Kuusela AL, Vesikari TA. A randomized double-blind, placebo-con-

trolled trial of dexamethasone and racemic epinephrine in the treatment of croup. Acta Paediatr Scand: 1988; 77: 99–104.

35. Freezer N, Butt W, Phelan P. Steroids in croup: Do they increase the incidence of successful extubation? Anaesth Intensive Care 1990; 18: 224–228.

36. Klassen TP, Feldman ME, Watters LK, et al.: Nebulized budesonide for children with mild-to-moderate croup. N Engl J Med 1994; 331: 285–289.

37. Husby S, Agertoft L, Mortensen S, et al.: Treatment of croup with nebulised steroid (budesonide): A double blind, placebo controlled study. Arch Dis Child 1993; 68: 352–355.

38. Prescott CAJ, Vanlierde MJRR: Tracheostomy in the management of laryngotracheobronchitis. South African Med J 1990; 77: 63–66.

39. McEniery J, Gillis J, Kilham H, et al.: Review of intubation in severe laryngotracheobronchitis. Pediatrics 1991; 87: 847–853.

40. Sofer S, Dagan R, Tal A: The need for intubation in serious upper respiratory tract infection in pediatric patients (a retrospective study). Infection 1991; 19: 131–133.

J. Mark Reed
Robin T. Cotton

CHAPTER FORTY-FIVE

Supraglottitis

▼

Few conditions arouse the sense of urgency in a clinician more than that produced by a child or adult in respiratory distress. The very nature of an airway emergency demands a rapid response as well as an established protocol to deal effectively with the circumstances. Supraglottitis (epiglottitis) is one such condition that elicits extreme concern, if not fear, not only for the patient and family but possibly for the health care provider. Since Sinclair's description of the disorder in 1941, little has changed[1]:

A review . . . reveals a constant clinical picture of severe prostration in addition to the obstructive symptoms of acute laryngitis. The features of this picture were the abrupt appearance of respiratory distress in a previously well child without a history of croup, often accompanied by a complaint of severe sore throat probably due to the greatly swollen epiglottis. High fever, leukocytosis and the appearance of "shock" out of proportion to the duration of symptoms completed the picture.

Supraglottitis results from an infectious process, but in this condition time and cooperation are of the essence, as they are not in most infectious processes. Because the airway is in jeopardy a careful assessment is necessary to establish the diagnosis, and an institutional protocol involving multiple disciplines should be initiated. The planned, coordinated intervention of otolaryngologist, pediatrician, emergency medicine physician, anesthesiologist, and other support personnel helps to ensure a successful outcome. Surgery plays a lesser role, except in the most extreme circumstances.

Theisen was the first to identify supraglottitis ("angina epiglottidea anterior") as an acute infectious process (in the *Albany Medical Annals* in 1900).[2] It was he who credited Marsh with the first case report on record in 1838, stating, "In his cases the attacks came on very suddenly. The pharynx in all cases was entirely normal, while the epiglottis was greatly reddened and oedematous. The epiglottis could be easily seen in the one case when the tongue was depressed. The patients were feverish. His accurate description and recognition of the condition are all the more remarkable when we consider that it was long before laryngology become an exact science." Theisen added three of his own patients to the medical literature and advocated the use of "early scarifications" as well as "iced ichthyol spray, one-half per cent solution . . . every twenty minutes, with an ice pack around the neck." In his small series, *Staphylococcus, Streptococcus,* and *Pneumococcus* organisms were identified as pathogens and there were no deaths.

In the July 8, 1916, edition of the *Journal of the American Medical Association,* Key identified *Bacillus influenzae* as the primary pathogen of supraglottitis in a stricken physician.[3] This organism, now known as *Haemophilus influenzae*

type B, is recognized as the leading cause of the disease worldwide.

ANATOMY AND PATHOPHYSIOLOGY

Laryngeal anatomy is classified according to established landmarks and includes the following well-known regions: supraglottis, glottis, and subglottis. This discussion is limited to the first. The supraglottic larynx is defined by the structures found superior to a horizontal line drawn through the laryngeal ventricle and is composed of the epiglottis, aryepiglottic folds, arytenoids, and false vocal cords. These structures form the aditus laryngis, or laryngeal inlet. The mucous membrane that covers the supraglottis is loosely attached to the lingual surface of the epiglottis and tightly bound to the laryngeal surfaces of the epiglottic and arytenoid cartilages.[4] It is this loose mucosal arrangement, as well as abundant areolar tissue that fills the aryepiglottic folds, that foster edema when inflammatory conditions arise (Fig. 45–1). Therefore, because of the circumferential nature of the laryngeal inlet, a dramatic decrease in the effective respiratory area is produced. Work of breathing is substantially increased, and this eventually results in fatigue. The principle is based on a mathematical formula that relates resistance inversely to the 4th power of the radius. The thick secretions which tend to spill into the airway, only serve to narrow the inlet, compounding the obstruction. The vibratory nature of the edematous tissues produces low-pitched stridor as well as a muffled voice ("hot potato"). The effect is confined mainly to the supraglottis, owing to the tightly bound mucosal covering and scant areolar tissue within the glottic tissues; however, histologic evidence supports inflammatory involvement of the paraglottic space in some cases.[5]

PATHOGENS

The bacteriology of childhood supraglottitis differs from that of the adult form and involves a relatively narrow spectrum of organisms. The pathogen most commonly encountered among all ages is *H. influenzae* type B. This organism, an encapsulated gram-negative, pleomorphic coccobacillus with the type B capsular polysaccharide, has been responsible for as many as 20,000 cases of systemic infections per year. In general, risk factors associated with *H. influenzae* type B include household contacts younger than 4 years of age, immune deficiencies, attendance in daycare, and the Alaskan Eskimo race.[6] In addition to its role in supraglottitis, *H.*

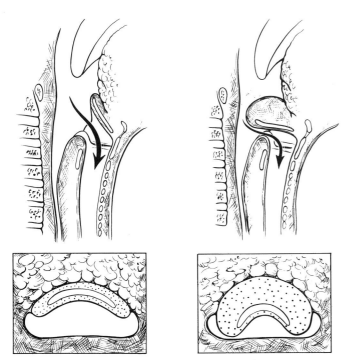

Figure 45–1. *A,* Sagittal and transverse views of the normal supraglottic airway. *B,* Sagittal view of the larynx demonstrating marked epiglottic edema and reduction of the functional airway in supraglottitis. The transverse view demonstrates massive edema of the submucosal tissues of the lingual surface of the epiglottis. The mucosa is tightly adherent to the vocal surface.

influenzae type B is also responsible for other severe invasive infections, including septicemia, pneumonia, and meningitis. Before the development of *H. influenzae* type B vaccine in 1985 (a conjugated vaccine was approved in 1990) the vast majority of pediatric cases of supraglottitis were caused by this organism.[1, 7–15] In recent years the causative role of *H. influenzae* type B has been diminished in the pediatric age group. Nevertheless, beta-lactamase production has been found in over a third of cases associated with childhood supraglottitis.[7]

Gram-positive organisms and anaerobes play a much greater role in adult supraglottitis. Commonly cultured pathogens include mixed oral flora that comprise a wide range of organisms: alpha-hemolytic streptococci, group A beta-hemolytic streptococci, *Staphylococcus aureus, Streptococcus pneumoniae, Neisseria, Bacteroides,* and *Peptostreptococcus species, Escherichia coli,* and *Candida albicans.*[10, 16–18] Different series in the literature report widely differing incidence figures for *H. influenzae* type B in the adult age group. In a review of 48 patients by Shih and colleagues, throat cultures in 27 yielded only one case of *H. influenzae* type B. No evidence of *H. influenzae* type B was found in 30 patients studied by Wolf and colleagues, and only one culture was positive among 17 patients reported by Kass and colleagues.[16, 18, 19] Other studies find a majority of cases attributable to *H. influenzae* type B in adults.[10, 20–22] In a comprehensive review by Khilanani and Khatib, *H. influenzae* was found in 37.6% of isolates, and in a study by MayoSmith and colleagues, all isolates were consistent with *H. influenzae* bacteremia.[21, 22]

Viral infections have been implicated as the cause of supraglottitis in immunocompromised persons. Scattered case reports recognize herpes simplex virus 1, infectious mononucleosis and parainfluenza and influenza viruses in the development of airway obstruction from supraglottic edema.[23–25]

EPIDEMIOLOGY

Supraglottitis primarily affects younger children. The vast majority of cases are found among those 2–4 years of age, males being more commonly affected than females (1.5:1).[8, 14, 20, 26] Some studies support a recent shift toward younger patients, whereas others show a trend toward older children.[7, 8, 14, 15] Gorelick and colleagues found a median age of 35.5 months for the period 1979–1990, as compared with a median of 80.5 months for the period of 1990–1992.[8] They attribute the difference to the administration of the conjugate *H. influenzae* type B vaccine to younger children.

The annual incidence of supraglottitis in the adult population has remained relatively stable. Estimates range from approximately 0.22 cases per 100,000 per year to 1.8 cases per 100,000 per year.[22, 27, 28] Until rather recently, the pediatric-adult ratio was approximately 2.5:1.[20, 27]; however, reports now suggest a shift toward a higher rate in the adult population.[27] This may be explained by greater awareness of the disease in that age group rather than a true increase.

The most remarkable finding to date is the reported decrease in the incidence of pediatric supraglottitis since the introduction in 1985 of the *H. influenzae* type B vaccine (see the final section, Prevention). In 1992 Frantz and Rasgon reported their findings of a study examining the pediatric members of a large health maintenance organization.[27] Before 1990, the annual incidence of supraglottitis was estimated to be 3.47 cases per 100,000 members. Subsequently, the incidence was found to decline to 0.63 cases per 100,000 members. Another study found an annual incidence of 10.9 cases per 10,000 admissions before 1990, as compared with 1.8 cases per 10,000 after that time.[8] Other studies, although they did not cite population figures, noted a substantial decrease in the number of supraglottitis admissions.[15] These reductions were not felt to be secondary to a change in referral patterns or hospital admissions. Seasonal preponderance has been described in the literature; however, reports favoring an increased incidence of supraglottitis in the spring and summer, fall, and winter fail to support a preponderance in any one season.[7, 11–14, 20, 26]

CLINICAL MANIFESTATIONS

Signs and Symptoms

The "typical" presentation of supraglottitis in a child differs from that in adults. The most impressive feature may not be one particular symptom or sign; rather, the overall presentation promotes a sense of urgency, immediately suggesting the diagnosis. One of the most distinguishing features of the illness in the pediatric age group is its rapid progression. Typically, it takes 12 hours or less for a previously healthy child to present in respiratory extremis. Throughout this brief period, the child usually complains of sore throat and odynophagia as the initial complaints. In the majority of cases fever is present. As the inflammatory process continues, edema develops within the loose connective tissues of the epiglottis and aryepiglottic folds, limiting the functional area of the laryngeal inlet. This results in turbulence of the tissues and audible vibrations. The resulting stridor is primarily inspiratory and low pitched.

In contrast to young children, adolescents and adults usually exhibit a more indolent disease course. The illness is commonly preceded by an upper respiratory tract infection, and over the course of several days symptoms develop. Therefore, one must have a high index of suspicion in dealing with adult patients, to avoid a delay in diagnosis. Features that are shared by both groups include persistent sore throat and odynophagia. Stridor may or may not develop during the course of the illness. Exceptions may be seen, however: some persons present with a more fulminant course typical of the pediatric age group's disease.

Physical Findings

The physical examination, combined with the history, provide most of the information needed to make an accurate diagnosis in the majority of cases. At the time of presentation, the general appearance is suggestive of marked toxemia (Fig. 45–2). The child typically assumes the position most favorable to sustaining an adequate airway: seated with the back angled forward and the chin extended in the sniffing position. The arms are pushed back to support the upper body. There is a strong tendency to avoid the supine position. No effort should be made by the treating physician or nurse to alter this natural "tripod position." The combination of a sore throat and difficulty swallowing with thick oropharyngeal secretions make drooling a common finding. Gagging associated with emesis may be present. The voice is described as normal or muffled, and hoarseness usually is not consistent with the diagnosis because of the lack of involvement of the true vocal cords. The act of breathing tends to be slow, in order to allow greater entry of air with less resistance and stridor. Unlike croup, cough is an infrequent symptom.

On examination of the oropharynx erythema may or may not be present, but if it is not the examiner should not discount the diagnosis of supraglottitis nor the possibility of eventual airway obstruction. The most important feature is a large, "cherry red" epiglottis, which on direct examination may be seen rising above the level of the base of the tongue. If the epiglottis is especially large, consideration should also be given to an epiglottic abscess. If the findings described are observed in children, examination of the oral cavity may precipitate laryngeal spasm and should be avoided; however, adult patients usually tolerate a full oral cavity examination and indirect or direct fiberoptic laryngoscopy. The use of either technique in adults has not been found to cause laryngospasm or airway obstruction. In expert hands the use of a small-caliber fiberoptic laryngoscope may be tolerated in selected pediatric cases. Therefore, endoscopic examination

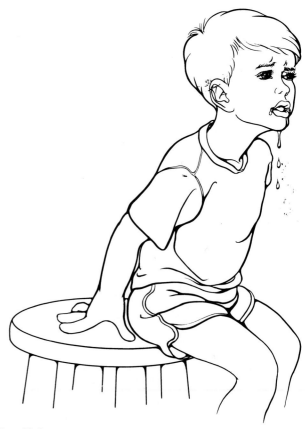

Figure 45–2. The typical "tripod" position associated with supraglottitis. All efforts by the child are directed toward maintaining an adequate airway. To alter this favorable position places the child in danger of airway obstruction and should be avoided.

of the oropharynx and larynx should be encouraged in most adults and some children, to promote an early diagnosis.

Other features of airway compromise may also be seen—suprasternal and intercostal retractions, restlessness, mental status changes, or frank cyanosis. An ominous finding is the often sudden decrease in stridor that precedes total airway obstruction. This should not be mistaken for improvement in the airway.

If time allows, a complete physical examination should be performed. Care should be directed especially to observation and palpation of the neck musculature because of the reported association with meningitis. Lumbar puncture should not be performed until the airway has been stabilized. Auscultation of the lungs may reveal findings such as rales, rhonchi, or evidence of consolidation that may suggest intercurrent pneumonia. Fever (temperature >38° C) is a relatively common finding; nevertheless, as many as 40% of patients remain afebrile.[26]

Imaging

When the diagnosis of supraglottitis is in doubt, the question of a soft tissue lateral neck film may be posed. Other questions include, What is the sensitivity of a soft tissue lateral film, and does it change the approach to management? Controversies regarding these issues are found in the literature

CHAPTER FORTY-FIVE / Supraglottitis | **399**

and vary among institutions. Whetmore and Handler reported a positive radiographic finding suggestive of supraglottitis in 77% of pediatric cases.[12] Others reported rates greater than 90%.[14, 16] In a review of adult patients by MayoSmith and colleagues 79% of films were predictive of supraglottitis[22]; however, they concluded that this was not a reliable substitute for direct examination. The main issue of concern lies in the fact that a patient in respiratory distress usually does not find the radiology suite a suitable place to obstruct the airway. Personnel may be inexperienced in dealing with airway emergencies, and appropriate equipment may not be available. In many institutions, the radiology department is located some distance from the emergency department or operating room; this makes the situation even riskier if transport is required. A useful guideline is that, in *most* situations, routine use of lateral soft tissue films is not indicated if the clinical situation supports the diagnosis of supraglottitis. The delay while obtaining the film could be too costly. However, if the patient has minimal symptoms and the diagnosis is unclear, a radiograph may prove helpful. In this situation, the patient must be accompanied to the radiology suite by one who is experienced in airway management and adequate supplies must be available in case resuscitative measures are required. The bottom line is that good common sense should prevail.

In the event that a lateral soft tissue film is obtained in the face of supraglottitis, the findings reveal an air–soft tissue interface bordering a large epiglottis—the so-called thumbprint sign (Fig. 45–3). Enlargement of the aryepiglottic folds may also be apparent. Other conditions that mimic supraglottitis, such as viral laryngotracheobronchitis, retropharyngeal abscess, or membranous laryngotracheobronchitis can also be detected.

Radiology plays a much more vital role once the airway is established. A routine chest radiograph not only confirms proper placement of the endotracheal or tracheotomy tube but is also useful for detecting the presence of pulmonary infiltrates. The sudden reversal of high inspiratory pressures may lead to the radiographic finding of bilateral interstitial infiltrates. This, in conjunction with the physical findings of pulmonary rales, is suggestive of "postobstructive" pulmonary edema, which is discussed later. Consolidation of a lung field suggests intercurrent pneumonia and is not uncommonly seen in conjunction with *H. influenzae*. Both findings warrant immediate medical management.

Differential Diagnosis

Several conditions that affect the upper respiratory tract may be confused with supraglottitis. Both infectious and noninfectious causes pose life-threatening risks of their own and must be considered in the initial assessment. Noninfectious causes are numerous and include congenital or acquired subglottic stenosis and intrinsic or extrinsic masses such as hemangiomas, lymphangiomas, papillomas, and various cysts. Ingestion of a foreign body should always be considered. Included in the differential diagnosis for infectious agents are viral laryngotracheobronchitis or "croup," retropharyngeal abscess, and membranous laryngotracheobron-

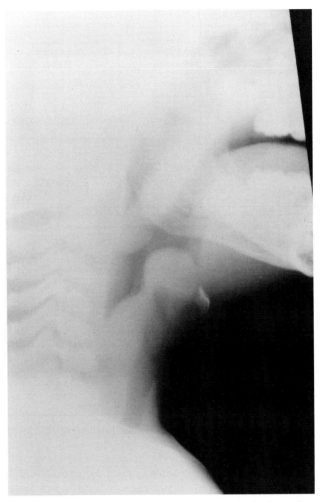

Figure 45–3. Soft tissue lateral radiograph of the neck showing a large rounded epiglottis typical of supraglottitis. This finding is known as the "thumb print" sign.

chitis (Table 45–1). These are more likely to be confused with supraglottitis and are discussed in greater detail later.

Viral Laryngotracheobronchitis

Viral laryngotracheobronchitis, or "croup," accounts for the majority of cases of infectious upper airway obstruction and affects 3%–5% of the pediatric age group. Five to ten percent of persons so affected eventually require hospitalization.[29] Although children of any age can be affected, the peak incidence appears to be in the second year of life.[30]

The illness commonly begins as an upper respiratory tract infection and progresses to various degrees of respiratory difficulty and stridor. The process develops over the period of 1–2 days and may last as long as 1–2 weeks before resolving.[29] Laryngeal involvement is heralded by the development of a barking cough and hoarseness. Stridor occurs in the majority of cases and is usually inspiratory and high pitched. The child certainly looks less "toxic" than one who has supraglottitis.

The agent primarily responsible for the disorder is parainfluenza virus type 1. Others included, in order of frequency,

Table 45–1. DIFFERENTIAL DIAGNOSIS OF SUPRAGLOTTITIS

	Supraglottitis (Epiglottitis)	Viral Laryngotracheobronchitis (Croup)	Retropharyngeal Abscess	Membranous Laryngotracheobronchitis
Etiology	*Hemophilus influenzae* type b	Parainfluenzae virus types	gram $+/-$, anaerobes	*Staphylococcus aureus*
Age range	1–6 years	½–4 years	1–6 years	Few weeks–early teens
Onset of illness	Generally <12 hours	24–48 hours	1–2 days	Several days (rapid progression)
Level of obstruction	Epiglottis, aryepiglottic folds, false vocal cords	Subglottic space	Oropharynx, hypopharynx	Subglottic space, trachea
Stridor	Inspiratory	Inspiratory, high pitched	Late finding	Biphasic
Dysphagia	Present	Absent	Present	Absent
Drooling	Present	Absent	Present	Absent
Treatment	Airway intervention, antibiotics	Cool mist, racemic epinephrine, steroids	Surgical drainage	Therapeutic bronchoscopy, antibiotics, intubation

are parainfluenza virus types 3 and 2, respiratory syncytial virus, and influenza virus A.

Radiographic studies are not indicated routinely unless the diagnosis is suspected. Lateral soft tissue films show narrowing of the subglottic space secondary to subglottic edema. Associated findings include dilatation of the hypopharynx and a normal-looking retropharynx and epiglottis. An anteroposterior chest radiograph reveals symmetric narrowing of the subglottis, the so-called steeple sign (Fig. 45–4).

Treatment of viral laryngotracheobronchitis depends on the clinical findings of the child. In mild cases—those limited to a barky cough and minimal or no stridor—management consisting of cool mist may be given at home by reliable parents. Symptoms such as audible stridor, retractions, or anxiety warrant admission to the hospital.

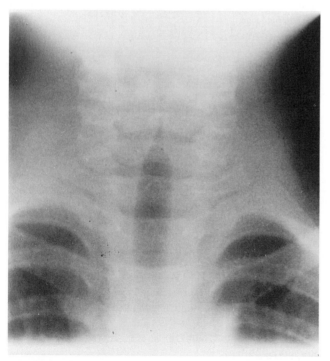

Figure 45–4. The "steeple" sign as seen on an anteroposterior radiograph of the neck.

In room air children with croup are prone to hypoxemia through a ventilation and perfusion mismatch. Although oxygen is not used routinely, in conjunction with water vapor mist it is helpful for documented hypoxemia or respiratory distress. The use of corticosteroids, formerly considered controversial, is now a routine part of the management of croup. Critical reviews have established that corticosteroids, primarily dexamethasone, are safe and effective when given early in the course of disease.[31–34] In a meta-analysis review of 1286 patients by Kairys and colleagues patients in the steroid-treated group had an 80% reduction in the need for endotracheal intubation and had noted improvement at both 12 and 24 hours after treatment.[33] The effect of steroids appears to be dose related (i.e., larger doses are more beneficial). Dexamethasone, 0.6–1.0 mg/kg, has been recommended as the initial starting dose.[34]

Other medical treatment rests in the use of nebulized racemic epinephrine, which contains equivalent amounts of the D- and L-isomers of epinephrine, the L-form being 15–20 times more potent.[30] It has a strong vasoconstrictive effect on the subglottic mucosa, owing to an alpha-adrenergic effect, but often treatment must be repeated, owing to its transient effect. This is known as the "rebound phenomenon," and children who receive a course of racemic epinephrine must be admitted to the hospital for observation. In severe cases of croup, the airway must be maintained by artificial means—either endotracheal intubation or tracheotomy.

Retropharyngeal Abscess

A retropharyngeal abscess consists of a collection of pus extending from the skull base to the region of the sixth cervical vertebra posterior to the pharynx. This usually results from suppuration of the retropharyngeal lymph node chain. The condition affects children in the earlier years; 71% are younger than 6 years.[35] The majority have no history of previous illness, although a previous upper respiratory tract infection is not uncommon. Presenting symptoms include neck swelling and stiffness, fever, dysphagia, odynophagia, drooling, and occasionally torticollis. Stridor associated with respiratory difficulty is a late finding.

Physical examination is significant for cervical adenopathy and unilateral bulging of the posterior pharyngeal wall. Care must be taken in the examination of the oropharynx, to avoid premature rupture of the abscess cavity. Palpation or probing of the posterior pharynx should be avoided. Tonsillitis is a common associated finding.[35]

Adjunctive laboratory and radiographic studies may prove beneficial. Alpha-hemolytic streptococci were found to be the predominant organism in one series of 65 patients.[35] Soft-tissue lateral radiographs demonstrate swelling, and, occasionally, air in the retropharyngeal space. Edema greater than the width of one vertebral body, in the absence of neck flexion and expiration, is suggestive of a retropharyngeal process. Computed tomography can be helpful in differentiating cellulitis from abscess.

Most retropharyngeal abscesses require surgical drainage, although up to 25% of patients may be treated medically.[35] Protection of the airway is of utmost importance during intubation, to prevent rupture of the abscess and potential aspiration. Broad-spectrum antibiotic coverage should precede surgical drainage and continue throughout the recovery period.

Membranous Laryngotracheobronchitis

Membranous laryngotracheobronchitis has features of both viral laryngotracheobronchitis and supraglottitis. The age range of affected children extends from a few weeks to the early teenage years, and the mortality rate is approximately 4%. The cause is unclear, but the disease is thought to be a complication of viral laryngotracheobronchitis.[36]

Membranous laryngotracheobronchitis is often preceded by several days by an upper respiratory tract infection. Without warning, symptoms may progresses rapidly over several hours to respiratory distress. Stridor is usually biphasic and is associated with a harsh cough. Like supraglottitis, the patient appears toxic, and high fever is commonly present. Contrasting features include the absence of drooling and the ability to lie flat.[37] Soft-tissue lateral radiographs are useful if irregularities of the airway suggesting membrane-like debris are present after an effective cough. Therefore, radiography may or may not be useful in establishing the diagnosis.

The diagnosis of membranous laryngotracheobronchitis is usually entertained only after an unsuccessful trial of racemic epinephrine. This finding should alert the clinician to the fact that endoscopy is required and must not be delayed. After removal of purulent secretions, aggressive pulmonary toilet is maintained by endotracheal intubation.

Antibiotic therapy is directed toward the most common organism, *S. aureus;* however, modifications should be made according to culture and sensitivity results. *H. influenzae, Streptococcus pyogenes,* and *S. pneumoniae* have also been reported with the disorder.[36]

Extubation can usually be successfully accomplished in 2–six days; however, some advocate tracheotomy as the only technique for airway support, to avoid the complication of subglottic stenosis.[36]

DIAGNOSIS

The diagnosis of supraglottitis is based on clinical findings; definitive judgment is reserved for endoscopy. Other investigations that are commonly used in the diagnosis of infectious processes, including laboratory studies and radiography, play a secondary role. In fact, obtaining additional studies before endoscopy may jeopardize the airway and result in sudden obstruction. Children are especially at risk, owing to the increased anxiety associated with phlebotomy or parental separation for transfer to the radiography suite. Thus, ancillary testing should be done only after stabilization of the airway or in mild cases when the diagnosis is in doubt.

Laboratory Findings

The function of the laboratory in the diagnosis and management of supraglottitis is twofold: measurement of the white blood cell count (WBC) and culture and sensitivity of pathogens. The majority of all patients exhibit some degree of leukocytosis. Most commonly, the leukocyte count ranges between 15 and 20 $\times$ 10^9/L to more than 50 $\times$ 10^9/L.[8, 11, 14, 17, 22] The WBC has little practical use in diagnosis or management, and attempts to correlate it with the severity of disease have been unsuccessful.[11]

One of the most helpful laboratory procedures involves culture of the infecting organism and determination of its antibiotic sensitivity. Specimen collection—blood and supraglottis swab—may proceed once the airway is secured. Blood cultures yield positive results in the majority of pediatric patients. In a study by Kessler and colleagues 72.7% of blood cultures were positive, results that compare favorably with studies by Wetmore and Handler, who found 64% positive results, and Gorelick and Baker, who had 67%.[7, 8, 12] Higher percentages were found by Briggs and Altenau and Trollfors and Strangert, who both reported yields of 92%.[10, 13] Therefore, in the pediatric age group, blood cultures are a reliable and valuable technique and should be part of the standard protocol. In contrast, direct culture of the epiglottis may not be as diagnostic. *H. influenzae,* the primary pathogen of pediatric supraglottitis, was recovered from only 16%–21% of cases, to a high of 67%.[7, 8, 13, 14] Other organisms, such as normal oral cavity flora, are common contaminants with direct swab techniques and add little to the diagnosis.

Blood cultures taken from adult populations generally have a lower yield than those from the pediatric age group. Wolf and colleagues had no positive blood cultures in a review of 30 adults with supraglottitis, and other large series report less than 25% success.[16–19, 22, 38] In a review of 185 patients whose blood was cultured Trollfors and Strangert reported 66% positive results, 94% of those produced by *H. influenzae.*[10]

TREATMENT

Treatment of supraglottitis cannot be passive. From observation in the intensive care unit to tracheotomy, some form of intervention is almost always required. Support of the airway and appropriate antibiotic coverage produce a baseline of safety and yield good results in most circumstances. Conversely, any management protocol that fails to include these basic principles may place the patient at risk and jeopardize a successful outcome. Treatment of supraglottitis is not done on an outpatient or clinic basis. Inpatient treatment is the standard of care for all patients with this disorder, and the appropriate management protocol is addressed in the following sections.

Indications

Once a timely initial evaluation has been completed, definitive intervention is usually required. Few would argue that the airway should always be secured in the pediatric age group, although the topic stirs more debate in adults. A mortality rate of 6.1% has been associated with the practice of observation in children, as compared with less than 1% when a secure airway exists.[39] A general underlying principle regarding the management of anyone with supraglottitis is that it is a *clinical diagnosis* and, so, measures that waste time or pose risk of airway obstruction must be avoided. Children tend to become anxious when separated from their parents. Every effort should be made to keep the child close to at least one parent or, if necessary, in the parent's arms. No effort should be made to change the position of the child, whether sitting or lying face down. Venipuncture, arterial blood gases, and blood cultures can wait. These serve only to increase anxiety and respiratory effort, which can potentiate airway obstruction. The child, however, usually tolerates oxygen given by nasal cannula and an oxygen saturation probe placed on a finger.

From the moment the diagnosis has been entertained, certain steps must be taken. First, the team responsible for dealing with airway emergencies must be called. In most institutions this group includes the otolaryngologist, pediatrician, emergency medicine physician, and anesthesiologist, as well as other support personnel such as nurses and respiratory therapists. Second, the operating room is notified that the patient is awaiting transport. In the event that the operating room is unable to take the patient at that time, arrangements are made to secure a space in the intensive care unit or recovery room. All required supplies are prepared for transport, including a crash cart with intubation tools and various sized endotracheal tubes, oxygen tank with Ambu-bag and mask, and a tracheotomy tray. The physician most skilled in airway management leads the team—in most circumstances the otolaryngologist or anesthesiologist. In the event of sudden complete airway obstruction, an important point to remember is that in most circumstances masked ventilation can overcome the obstruction and allow time for intubation.

Anesthesia is induced by having the patient spontaneously breathe a mixture of halothane and oxygen. This usually takes longer than normal because of the extent of airway compromise. Again, depending on experience, the otolaryngologist or anesthesiologist is responsible for the initial intubation, which is first by the oral route. Once the airway is secured, direct laryngoscopy can be performed prior to nasotracheal intubation or tracheotomy (Fig. 45–5). Other measures, such as placement of intravenous lines, blood cultures, and antibiotic therapy, should be initiated at this time.

Before the adoption of endotracheal intubation as a com-

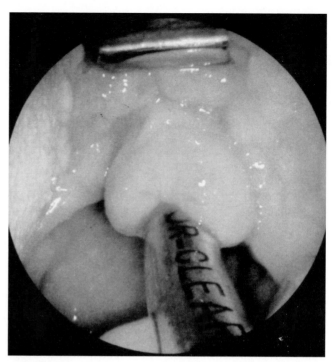

Figure 45–5. Endoscopic view of supraglottitis. An endotracheal tube is seen passing through an inflamed and erythematous supraglottis. In the event of premature extubation, distraction of the tissues by the tube usually allows time for reintubation.

mon procedure in the 1960s, most patients underwent tracheotomy for airway control.[39] Ease of suctioning, security of the airway, and avoidance of subglottic stenosis were considered advantages of this technique. Now largely replaced by nasotracheal intubation in elective situations, tracheotomy is still the procedure of choice for the difficult airway that cannot be secured by intubation. Other factors that contribute to the choice of tracheotomy include unavailability of an experienced endoscopist (in the event the endotracheal tube becomes dislodged) and inexperienced nursing staff. Complications of tracheotomy are well-known; however, mortality is not statistically higher as compared with endotracheal intubation in the treatment of supraglottitis.[39] Removal of the tracheotomy tube can usually be accomplished in 4–10 days.[11, 14, 26]

Endotracheal intubation is the preferred way to secure the airway in most cases.[7, 8, 12–15, 26, 40] With the advent of the modern intensive care unit, most physicians and nurses are comfortable in caring for these tubes. This technique avoids a surgical procedure and may be protective by maintaining a transient supraglottic lumen in the event extubation occurs prematurely. Accidental extubation occurs in approximately 5%–13% of cases, but untoward complications have not been reported.[7, 12, 13, 15, 40] By utilizing leakage of air around the tube as an indicator of edema resolution, successful extubation can be predicted.[40] The average time of intubation is approximately 2 days; therefore, long-term complications such as subglottic stenosis have not been found to be a problem.[12, 13, 15, 40] This finding is probably related to the fact that supraglottitis spares the subglottic space, thus transmitting little pressure from the endotracheal tube.

Duration of hospitalization varies, according primarily to the method of airway protection. Endotracheal intubation generally affords a shorter course (average 5–7 days).[7, 8, 14, 40] Patients who have required tracheotomy are generally discharged from the hospital after 9 days.[12, 13]

Alternatives

Much debate has focused on the appropriate mode of airway intervention for adults. Various reports support a conservative approach; others, an interventionist approach.[16–19, 21, 22, 41] A conservative approach is generally defined as close observation of a patient in conjunction with appropriate antibiotic and supportive therapy, without invasive airway support. Interventionists favor the addition of endotracheal intubation or tracheotomy in concert with medical management. In a report by Frantz and colleagues, 110 of 129 patients were managed successfully without endotracheal intubation or tracheotomy.[17] They also found that an upright posture and the presence of stridor were indicators that airway intervention would be required (15%). Others have described conservative approaches to those who present with a less fulminant course, defined as symptoms present over a period of several days.[18, 19] Those presenting with dyspnea or stridor of sudden onset were more likely to require intervention in this group. Fever is not statistically associated with the need for airway support[16, 17]; however, positive blood cultures are positively correlated.[22]

Mortality rates for adult patients who are managed without airway intervention range from 7%–13%.[21, 22, 41] This represents on average, a 10-fold increase over the mortality for the pediatric age group. Close observation, as advocated in the conservative approach, may not always be successful. In a study by MayoSmith and colleagues,[22] two patients were initially observed in the emergency department and were subsequently transferred to a hospital bed. Both developed sudden respiratory arrest and died in spite of resuscitative efforts. Another report shows that, despite close observation in the intensive care unit, two patients died of sudden respiratory arrest.[42] Reports such as these serve to fuel the controversy over appropriate airway management in the adult population. One should understand the important fact that as the airway becomes more severely compromised the difficulty of intubation increases substantially. A guiding principle is that if one entertains the possibility of needing airway intervention, the task should be completed in a timely fashion.

Antibiotics

Because supraglottitis is primarily an infectious disease, therapy directed against the offending organism must be initiated after stabilization of the airway. In children, antibiotics are directed toward *H. influenzae* type B. Ampicillin has long been regarded as a safe and effective treatment for *H. influenzae* type B infections; however, during the past two decades concern has been raised about the emergence of resistant strains. Production of the beta-lactamase enzyme is the primary mode of resistance, followed by a smaller group

of organisms that show alterations in penicillin-binding proteins. In recent series of pediatric supraglottitis patients, more than one third of *H. influenzae* type B cultures exhibit resistance to ampicillin.[7, 14] Chloramphenicol has been used as an adjunct to ampicillin therapy, yet concerns about bone marrow depression and resistance by some strains of *H. influenzae* type B have limited its use.

Single-drug therapy utilizing second- or third-generation cephalosporins has become an accepted mode of treatment. Cefuroxime is a second-generation cephalosporin that has proven efficacy against *H. influenzae* type B, including ampicillin-resistant strains and most gram-positive and gram-negative organisms. Central nervous system penetration, which is important in the selection of antibiotics against *H. influenzae* type B, is adequate. Many now consider cefuroxime the initial drug of choice in the treatment of supraglottitis,[17, 26] especially for the adult age group, who may require a broader range of coverage owing to the variety of infecting organisms. Cefotaxime and ceftriaxone are third-generation cephalosporins that achieve greater penetration of the central nervous system but have reduced efficacy against gram-positive organisms. These drugs are especially useful for *H. influenzae* type B–related supraglottitis and meningitis; however, their use as first-line drugs in the adult age group may not be warranted. Ampicillin-resistant strains of *H. influenzae* type B currently remain sensitive to cefuroxime, cefotaxime, and ceftriaxone. Of course, the use of cephalosporins, as well as any antibiotic should be modified according to the culture and sensitivity results. Patients should complete a 10-day course of therapy.

Because of the risk of secondary spread of *H. influenzae* type B, use of rifampin has been advocated for selected contacts of invasive *H. influenzae* type B disease. Households with children younger than 4 years and all contacts should receive the appropriate prophylactic dose. Children are administered 20 mg/kg, and parents are given 600 mg/day for 4 consecutive days. The index case receives rifampin at the completion of antibiotic therapy, to eradicate colonization of the nasopharynx.[43]

COMPLICATIONS

Although a relatively localized process anatomically, supraglottitis not uncommonly results in complications that have systemic effects. These are primarily related to the airway and lungs but also involve hematologic dissemination of the infecting organism with involvement of distant sites. This is not an unexpected finding in light of the high rate of positive blood cultures. Great care must be taken in the initial patient evaluation to avoid overlooking a developing complication. In the same manner, diligent observation and anticipation are required in the hospitalization period once initial management is completed.

After death, airway obstruction, with or without anoxic brain injury, is the most serious complication of supraglottitis. Emergency measures such as tracheotomy increase the rate of complications when performed outside the controlled atmosphere of the operating room; therefore, in this instance, an ounce of prevention *is* worth a pound of cure.

One of the most rapid complications to occur after stabilization of the airway is pulmonary edema. In children with supraglottitis, pulmonary edema develops as many as 7%–12% of patients and mortality may approach 40%.[43] Several mechanisms have been proposed. One concerns the formation of interstitial edema as a consequence of the sudden reversal of upper airway obstruction. The process is thought to be mediated by improvement in pulmonary vascular return resulting in higher pressures within the vascular bed. Another possibility suggests that a hypoxic state results in increased sympathetic tone, leading to systemic vasoconstriction and higher perfusion pressures within the lung. This, then, results in edema formation. Last, direct hypoxic injury of the pulmonary microcirculation may lead to loss of capillary integrity and subsequent pulmonary edema.[43] The adult respiratory distress syndrome (ARDS) has been described as a similar pulmonary complication in the adult age group, although the mechanism is currently unclear.[43]

H. influenzae type B is the leading cause of bacterial meningitis in children in the United States and is an ominous complication of supraglottitis. Friedman and colleagues reviewed 15 cases of meningitis associated with supraglottitis and found a 40% mortality rate.[43] The combination of nuchal rigidity and symptoms of upper airway obstruction certainly warrant further investigation once the airway has been stabilized. Lumbar puncture may be performed in the operating room before transfer to the intensive care unit. The mechanism of a synchronous infection is most likely related to the magnitude of bacteremia within the host. A much higher blood level of organisms has been associated with meningitis.[43]

Epiglottic abscess is a relatively common occurrence in adults with supraglottitis: as many as one-fourth of patients are affected.[19] The complication may be detected at the time of initial laryngoscopy or may develop later in the course. Failure to extubate in a timely fashion leads one to suspect residual infection, and in this instance, direct laryngoscopy should be performed in the operating room, as both a diagnostic and a therapeutic measure. A simple incision of the epiglottis relieves the purulence and speeds resolution of edema. Spontaneous rupture is also common.

Pneumonia has been associated with supraglottitis in as many as 25% of cases.[43] Other thoracic complications include empyema, pneumothorax, pleural effusion, pericardial effusion, and congestive heart failure.[17, 40, 43] Additional complications are related to the mode of therapy, most dealing with endotracheal intubation or tracheotomy. The most obvious complication involves dislodgement or blockage of the respiratory tube. Fortunately, in most circumstances replacement is accomplished readily and without untoward effects. Complications associated with tracheotomy are well-known and include bleeding, pneumothorax, and mucus plugging. One of the most serious late complications of endotracheal intubation is subglottic stenosis. Fortunately, today, this is a rare finding with short-term intubation.

PREVENTION

Recent studies indicate that the incidence of supraglottitis has dramatically decreased in the pediatric age group since the introduction of the conjugate vaccine.[8, 15, 27] This trend likely will continue and should affect the incidence in the adult age group as the population ages. Because not all children receive appropriate vaccinations, however, eradication of *H. influenzae* type B supraglottitis is unlikely, and in the future other invasive organisms will probably play a greater role. Clinicians must remain diligent in their suspicion and at all times remain ready to deal with this potentially fatal disease.

References

1. Sinclair SE: *Haemophilus influenzae* type b in acute laryngitis with bacteremia. JAMA 1941; 117: 170–173.
2. Theisen CF: Angina epiglottidea anterior. Report of three cases. Albany Med Ann 1900; 21: 395–405.
3. Key SN: Angina epiglottidea, report of a case caused by the bacillus influenzae. JAMA 1916; 67: 116.
4. Splanchnology. In: Johnson TB, Davies DV, Davies F (eds): Gray's Anatomy, Descriptive and Applied. London: Longmans, Green and Co, 1958, pp 1305–1319.
5. Healy GB, Hyams VJ, Tucker GF: Paraglottic laryngitis in association with epiglottitis. Ann Otol Rhinol Laryngol 1985; 94: 618–621.
6. Kaplan SL: *Haemophilus influenzae*. In: Oski FA, DeAngelis CD, Feigin RD, McMillan JA, Warshaw JB (eds): Principles and Practice of Pediatrics, 2nd ed. Philadelphia: JB Lippincott, 1994, pp 1187–1191.
7. Kessler A, Wetmore RF, Marsh RR: Childhood epiglottitis in recent years. Int J Pediatr Otorhinolaryngol 1993; 25: 155–162.
8. Gorelick MH, Baker MD: Epiglottis in children, 1979 through 1992, effects of *Haemophilus influenzae* type b immunization. Arch Pediatr Adolesc Med 1994; 148: 47–50.
9. Walker P, Crysdale WS: Croup, epiglottitis, retropharyngeal abscess, and bacterial tracheitis: Evolving patterns of occurrence and care. Int Anesthesiol Clin 1992; 30: 57–70.
10. Trollfors B, Nylen O, Strangert K: Acute epiglottitis in children and adults in Sweden. 1981–83. Arch Dis Child 1990; 65: 491–494.
11. Vetto RR: Epiglottitis, report of thirty-seven cases. JAMA 1960; 173: 88–92.
12. Wetmore RF, Handler SD: Epiglottitis: Evolution in management during the last decade. Ann Otol Rhinol Laryngol 1979; 88: 822–826.
13. Briggs WH, Altenau MM: Acute epiglottitis in children. Otolaryngol Head Neck Surg 1980; 88: 665–669.
14. Emerson SG, Richman B, Spahn T: Changing patterns of epiglottitis in children. Otolaryngol Head Neck Surg 1991; 104: 287–292.
15. Ryan M, Hunt M, Snowberger T: A changing pattern of epiglottitis. Clin Pediatr 1992; 31: 532–535.
16. Kass EG, McFadden EA, Jacobson S, et al: Acute epiglottitis in the adult: Experience with a seasonal presentation. Laryngoscope 1993; 103: 841–844.
17. Frantz TD, Rasgon BM, Quesenberry CP: Acute epiglottitis in adults, analysis of 129 cases. JAMA 1994; 272: 1358–1360.
18. Shih L, Hawkins DB, Stanley RB Jr: Acute epiglottitis in adults, a review of 48 cases. Ann Otol Rhinol Laryngol 1988; 97: 527–529.
19. Wolf M, Strauss B, Kronenberg J, et al.: Conservative management of adult epiglottitis. Laryngoscope 1990; 100: 183–185.
20. Wuertele P: Acute epiglottitis in children and adults: A large-scale incidence study. Otolaryngol Head Neck Surg 1990; 103: 902–908.
21. Khilanani U, Khatib R: Acute epiglottitis in adults. Am J Med Sci 1984; 287: 65–70.
22. MayoSmith MF, Hirsch PJ, Wodzinski SF, et al: Acute epiglottitis in adults, an eight year experience in the state of Rhode Island. N Engl J Med 1986; 314: 1133–1139.
23. Bogger-Goren S: Acute epiglottitis caused by herpes simplex virus. Pediatr Infect Dis J 1987; 6: 1133–1134.
24. Biem J, Roy L, Halik J, et al.: Infectious mononucleosis complicated by necrotizing epiglottitis, dysphagia, and pneumonia. Chest 1989; 96: 204–205.
25. Grattan-Smith T, Forer M, Kilham H, et al.: Viral supraglottitis. J Pediatr 1987; 110: 434–435.
26. Crysdale WS, Sendi K: Evolution in the management of acute epiglottitis: A 10-year experience with 242 children. Int Anesthesiol Clin 1988; 26: 32–37.

27. Frantz TD, Rasgon BM: Acute epiglottitis: Changing epidemiologic patterns. Otolaryngol Head Neck Surg 1993; 109: 457–460.

28. Takala AK, Eskola J, VanAlphen L: Spectrum of invasive *Haemophilus influenzae* type b disease in adults. Arch Intern Med 1990; 150: 2573–2576.

29. Battaglia JD: Severe croup: The child with fever and upper airway obstruction. Pediatr Rev 1986; 7: 227–233.

30. Levison H, Tabachnik E, Newth CJL: Wheezing in infancy, croup, and epiglottitis. Curr Probl Pediatr 1982; 12: 38–65.

31. Baugh R, Gilmore BB Jr: Infectious croup: A critical review. Otolaryngol Head Neck Surg 1986; 95: 40–46.

32. Hawkins DB: Corticosteroids in the management of laryngotracheobronchitis. Otolaryngol Head Neck Surg 1980; 88: 207–210.

33. Kairys SW, Olmstead EM, O'Connor GT: Steroid treatment of laryngotracheitis: A meta-analysis of the evidence from randomized trials. Pediatrics 1989; 83: 683–693.

34. Hawkins DB, Crockett DM, Shum TK: Corticosteroids in airway management. Otolaryngol Head Neck Surg 1983; 91: 593–596.

35. Thompson JW, Cohen SR, Reddix P: Retropharyngeal abscess in children: A retrospective and historical analysis. Laryngoscope 1988; 98: 589–592.

36. Donaldson JD, Maltby CC: Bacterial tracheitis in children. J Otolaryngol 1989; 18: 101–104.

37. Rabie I, McShane D, Warde D: Bacterial tracheitis. J Laryngol Otol 1989; 103: 1059–1062.

38. Shapiro J, Eavey RD, Baker AS: Adult supraglottitis. JAMA 1988; 259: 563–567.

39. Cantrell RW, Bell RA, Morioka WT: Acute epiglottitis: Intubation versus tracheostomy. Laryngoscope 1978; 88: 994–1005.

40. Crockett DM, Healy GB, McGill TJ, et al.: Airway management of acute supraglottitis at the Children's Hospital, Boston: 1980–1985. Ann Otol Rhinol Laryngol 1988; 97: 114–119.

41. Friedman M, Toriumi DM, Grybauskas V, et al.: A plea for uniformity in the staging and management of adult epiglottitis. Ear, Nose Throat J 1988; 67: 873–880.

42. American Academy of Pediatrics: *Haemophilus influenzae* infections. In: Peter G (ed): 1991 Red Book: Report of The Committee on Infectious Diseases, 22nd ed. Elk Grove Village, IL: American Academy of Pediatrics; 1991, pp 225–229.

43. Gonzalez C, Gartner JC, Casselbrant ML, et al: Complication of acute epiglottitis. Int J Pediatr Otorhinolaryngol 1986; 11: 67–71.

44. Bonadio WA, Losek JD: The characteristics of children with epiglottitis who develop the complication of pulmonary edema. Arch Otolaryngol Head Neck Surg 1991; 117: 205–207.

45. Sternbach GL, Goldschmid D: Adult respiratory distress syndrome associated with adult epiglottitis. J Emerg Med 1993; 11: 23–26.

46. Friedman EM, Damion J, Healy GB, et al.: Supraglottitis and concurrent hemophilus meningitis. Ann Otol Rhinol Laryngol 1985; 94: 470–472.

47. LaScolea LJ Jr, Rosales SV, Welliver RC, et al.: Mechanisms underlying the development of meningitis or epiglottitis in children after *Haemophilus influenzae* type B bacteremia. J Infect Dis 1985; 151: 1162–1165.

48. Molteni RA: Epiglottitis: Incidence of extraepiglottic infection: Report of 72 cases and review of the literature. Pediatrics 1976; 58: 526–531.

49. Hussan WU, Keaney NP: Bilateral thoracic empyema complicating adult epiglottitis. J Laryngolo Otol 1991; 105: 858–859.

CHAPTER FORTY-SIX

Group A Beta-hemolytic Streptococcal Tonsillopharyngitis

▼

Despite numerous clinical studies and microbiologic advances, group A beta-hemolytic streptococcal (GABHS) tonsillopharyngitis continues to be a major problem with controversial aspects regarding diagnosis and treatment.

ANATOMY

The pathologic changes of acute streptococcal throat infection are usually confined to the tonsils, posterior pharynx, uvula, posterior soft palate, and the draining anterior cervical lymph nodes of Waldeyer's ring. Changes in the infected tissues reflect an inflammatory process that includes erythema, edema, and the presence of exudate from leukocyte migration to the mucosa. Vesicles and ulcerations are uncommon. In infants, the nasopharynx more typically manifests the infectious process.

Infection may be transferred from the posterior tonsillopharynx or the nasopharynx to the skin, causing facial erysipelas or pyoderma. GABHS infection may extend locally to adjacent sites, including the paranasal sinuses, eustachian tube and middle ear, peritonsillar and retropharyngeal tissues, epiglottis, and regional lymph nodes. Further direct extension may lead to mastoiditis, cavernous sinus thrombosis, osteomyelitis, or meningitis.

PATHOPHYSIOLOGY

GABHS infection produces a self-limited, localized inflammation of the tonsillopharynx generally lasting 3–5 days. The microbiology and virulence of this organism are discussed in Chapter 15. Antibiotic treatment, if prompt and appropriate, reduces the duration of symptoms, shortens the period of contagion, and reduces the occurrence of localized spread and suppurative complications. A major objective of administering antibiotics is to prevent rheumatic fever and, possibly, to reduce the incidence of poststreptococcal glomerulonephritis.

EPIDEMIOLOGY

GABHS infections are spread person to person; humans are the natural reservoir for this bacterium. The nasopharynx and oropharynx are the main colonization foci of this organism; the skin and feces are potential sites. Aerosolized upper respiratory tract secretions serve as the primary source of GABHS spread. Direct contact with infected nasopharyngeal and oropharyngeal mucosa is less important as is contact with contaminated objects such as toothbrushes. Rarely, food is a vehicle for dissemination of GABHS.

Spread of GABHS requires the presence of a susceptible host and is facilitated by close contact. Acquisition of infection is rare in infancy, probably owing to maternal immunity conferred transplacentally. Infection is uncommon before the age of 2 years, possibly owing to decreased attachment of GABHS to nasopharyngeal and oropharyngeal epithelial cells. When infection occurs during the toddler years it most often involves the nasopharynx. Close contact with an increased number of persons potentially infected with GABHS, as in day care and grade school, is associated with more frequent spread of illness. Adolescents and adults usually have had contacts with the organism over time to provide immunity, thus rendering GABHS tonsillopharyngitis uncommon in these populations. The frequency of isolation of GABHS and other tonsillopharyngeal pathogens in children and adults is shown in Table 46–1.[1]

CLINICAL MANIFESTATIONS

In most patients GABHS tonsillopharyngitis cannot be accurately diagnosed on clinical grounds.[2–7] The patient with a classic GABHS throat infection has fever, tonsillopharyngeal erythema and exudate, swollen and tender anterior cervical adenopathy, absence of rhinorrhea and cough, and an elevated white blood cell (WBC) count during midwinter to

Table 46–1. CAUSES OF PHARYNGITIS

Cause	Peak Prevalence (%)	
	Children	Adults
Bacterial	30–40	5–10
GABHS	28–40	5–9
Group C, G, or F streptococci	0–3	0–18
N. gonorrhoeae	0–0.01	0–0.01
A. haemolyticum	0–0.05	0–10
M. pneumoniae	0–3	0–10
C. pneumoniae	0–3	0–9
Viral	15–40	30–60
Idiopathic	22–55	30–65

From Pichichero ME: Group A streptococcal tonsillopharyngitis: Cost-effective diagnosis and treatment. Ann Emerg Med 1995; 25: 390–403.

early spring. When this constellation of clinical symptoms is present, the likelihood of GABHS infection approaches 60%–70% in children and 20%–30% in adults.

A nine-factor probability estimator for diagnosing GABHS tonsillopharyngitis was derived by Breese (Table 46–2) after screening more than 20,000 acute respiratory illnesses in children associated with sore throat.[8] Children with fewer than 25 points in the Breese scoring system had a 6% probability of having GABHS tonsillopharyngitis; this represented 20% of the children from whom throat cultures were obtained. Children with 26–31 points (36% of the study population) had a probability of approximately 40%. Children with 32–38 points (44% of the study population) had a probability of 84%. It should be noted that the Breese scoring system requires a WBC count for every patient; epidemiologic factors (patient age and season of the year) are also important. Eliminating any factor, such as the WBC count, invalidates the applicability of the scoring.[5]

For young adults, the accuracy of experienced physicians' probability estimates for diagnosing GABHS tonsillopharyngitis has been assessed in a university health service setting.[6] When two general internists, three pediatricians, and five family physicians predicted the culture outcome on clinical grounds for 308 patients with sore throat, the likelihood of GABHS infection was overestimated for 81% of their patients. Typical of young adults, only 15 cultures (4.9%) were positive for GABHS. Overdiagnosis almost always led to the decision to treat.

In adults, culture-positive GABHS tonsillopharyngitis usually occurs in a patient with a history of GABHS exposure and physical findings of fever, pharyngotonsillar inflammation, pharyngotonsillar exudates, and swollen cervical lymph nodes. A discriminate scoring system has been developed by Walsh and colleagues.[9] In this model, the patient was assigned points for each of five characteristics of GABHS tonsillopharyngitis: +3 points for each degree of temperature above 36.1° C, +17 points for recent exposure to GABHS infection, −7 points for recent cough, +6 points for pharyngeal exudate, and +11 for enlarged or tender cervical lymph nodes. The predictive probability of GABHS tonsillopharyngitis was then calculated by summing the points assigned to each patient. Scores of 30 points or fewer produced a probability of less than 20% of GABHS tonsillopharyngitis (which occurred in about two-thirds of the adults with sore throats), whereas a score in excess of 30 points provided a probability of more than 40% of GABHS tonsillopharyngitis. A score in excess of 40 points (seen in about 10% of adults cultured) was associated with nearly 100% predictability of a positive GABHS culture.

From these and other carefully conducted studies, we can conclude that, for most patients, the clinical diagnosis of GABHS throat infections is unreliable; however, a subset of children (approximately 20%) and adults (approximately 67%) present with sore throat but few other symptoms of GABHS tonsillopharyngitis. They need neither a diagnostic test (culture or rapid antigen detection) nor treatment; they have sore throat as part of a viral upper respiratory tract infection. They can be clinically distinguished from the other patients because they have accompanying rhinorrhea, cough, hoarseness, and, often, absence of fever, tonsillopharyngeal erythema or exudate, and cervical lymphadenitis.

Differential Diagnosis

The largest proportion of children (15%–40%) and adults (30%–60%) with tonsillopharyngitis have a viral infection (see Table 46–1).[1, 10–12] About 8%–40% of children and 5%–9% of adults with sore throat, fever, and tonsillopharyngeal inflammation have GABHS infection. Other bacteria infrequently cause throat infection. Particularly among adolescents and young adults, the differential diagnosis of GABHS tonsillopharyngitis should include infection caused by group C and G *Streptococcus* species and *Neisseria gonorrhoeae*.[13–18] Anaerobes may be involved in deep-seated infections such as peritonsillar or retropharyngeal abscesses; however, there is no evidence that surface colonization with these organisms causes symptomatic tonsillopharyngitis.[19–22]

Table 46–2. BREESE STREPTOCOCCAL SCORE SYSTEM FOR CHILDREN*

I. Season	Score	II. Age (years)	Score	III. WBC Count (cells/μL)	Score	IV. Symptoms and Signs	Score (points) Yes	No	Unknown
Feburary March April	4	5–10	4	8–8.4	1	Fever 100.5° F	4	2	2
January May December	3	4, 11–14	3	8.5–10.4	2	Sore throat	4	2	2
June October November	2	3, or >15	2	10.5–13.4	3	Cough	2	4	4
July August September	1	≤2	1	13.5–20.4	5	Headache	4	2	2
				≥20.5	6	Abnormal pharynx	4	1	3
				Not done	3	Abnormal cervical glands	4	2	3

From Breese BB: A simple scorecard for the tentative diagnosis of streptococcal pharyngitis. Am J Dis Child 1977; 131: 514–517.
*Under the Score headings are the number of points included in the clinical score for the pediatric patient with sore throat. If the score is ≤25 points the chance of GABHS tonsillopharyngitis is 6%; if the score is 26–31 points the chance is 50%; and if the score is 32–38 points the chance is 84%.

Mycoplasma pneumoniae, Chlamydia pneumoniae (TWAR agent), and *Arcanobacterium hemolyticum* are occasional agents of symptomatic tonsillopharyngitis. In developing countries *Corynebacterium diphtheriae* remains a cause of tonsillopharyngitis. Sore throats are often "idiopathic." It is not clear whether these latter cases of tonsillopharyngitis are, in fact, caused by viruses that, at present, cannot be identified or whether they are due to other factors such as postnasal drip, allergy, active or passive smoking, and so on.

LABORATORY DIAGNOSIS

Throat Culture

In 1954, Breese and Disney first reported the use of throat cultures plated on sheep blood agar in an office setting.[23] Since then, the use of a throat culture to confirm the presence of GABHS has become common practice and has grown steadily, so that by the early 1980s the Centers for Disease Control estimated that between 28 and 36 million throat cultures were performed annually in the United States. The value of this simple laboratory test in avoiding unnecessary antibiotic therapy and in identifying patients who require treatment should not be underestimated.

False-Positive Throat Cultures

False-positive GABHS throat cultures in most cases represent misidentified beta-hemolytic streptococci belonging to Lancefield groups B, C, F, or G, or beta-hemolytic *Staphylococcus aureus*. The most widely used test for the differentiation of GABHS from non-GABHS strains is the bacitracin sensitivity test; it provides a presumptive identification of GABHS based on the observation that 95%–100% of GABHS organisms demonstrate a zone of inhibition around a disk containing 0.04 units of bacitracin, whereas 83%–97% of non-GABHS do not.[24] If there are sufficient numbers of GABHS in the area of the disk, the test can be interpreted adequately on a primary blood agar plate.

False-Negative Throat Cultures

Some 3.6%–17% of children with symptomatic sore throat develop an antibody rise in response to GABHS antigens, despite negative throat cultures.[25, 26] Discordance between duplicate throat cultures obtained at the time of an office visit has been offered as evidence that the throat culture is unreliable as a diagnostic test; however, discordance is actually quite uncommon. Discordance rates of 1%–10% typically are seen. In a study where three simultaneous throat cultures were obtained in consecutive patients between ages 2 and 20 years, concordance of positive or negative culture on all three swabs was seen in 102 (99%) of 103 patients.[27]

Other explanations for false-negative throat cultures include faulty culture technique, occult antibiotic therapy, and faulty bacteriologic methods. The optimal site for throat culture is the surface of the tonsil. The tongue, hard palate, teeth, and buccal mucosa are not satisfactory. In one study,

two culture methods were compared: vigorous swabbing of both tonsillar surfaces plus the posterior pharyngeal wall versus placement of the throat culture swab to the posterior pharyngeal wall with rotation of the swab 90 degrees (author's unpublished data). The isolation rates were identical with both techniques. Others have found that both tonsils must be sampled, since cultures taken from one tonsil are negative in as many as 20% of patients whose other tonsil is "positive."[28]

Patients frequently do not take the full amount of prescribed antibiotic and save leftover drug for the next episode of similar symptoms. In a hospital emergency room study, 10% of patients who forthrightly denied antibiotic use on direct questioning by a physician had antibacterial activity detected in their urine.[29] Because isolation of GABHS is difficult after one or two doses of antibiotic, the role of occult antibiotic use as a cause of false-negative throat cultures may be significant.

Quality assurance methods should be incorporated into laboratory routines. (This is now mandated by the Clinical Laboratories Improvement Amendment.) A known isolate of GABHS should be inoculated daily onto a plate and incubated as a positive control concurrently with other throat swab cultures from patients suspected of having GABHS infection. Duplicate throat swabs should be processed periodically in a reference laboratory (hospital) to corroborate office laboratory results.

Rapid GABHS Antigen Detection Tests

GABHS antigen detection tests can be performed quickly at a cost that is comparable to that of a 10-day supply of even the least expensive antibiotic. These tests all rely on extraction of carbohydrate antigen of GABHS followed by detection with an antibody-tagged reagent that produces a clumping effect or color change after interaction. Performed properly, the sensitivity (average, 76%–87%) and specificity (average, 90%–96%) of rapid antigen detection testing can approach those achievable with throat culture (Table 46–3). When the rapid GABHS antigen test is positive, this result can be deemed reliable and the patient can be treated appropriately. When rapid antigen detection testing reveals a negative result, use of a second swab for confirmatory culture is usually recommended to avoid missing an infection that might require therapy. To be used most effectively, the test

Table 46–3. STUDIES COMPARING ACCURACY OF LATEX AGGLUTINATION AND ENZYME IMMUNOASSAY GABHS ANTIGEN-DETECTION TESTS WITH THROAT CULTURE

Parameters	Hospital Based	Office Based
No. of patients/no. of publications*	7767/15	2798/11
Sensitivity (%)†	87 (75–95)	79 (45–93)
Specificity (%)†	96 (86–100)	90 (75–98)
Overall accuracy (%)†	92 (75–99)	86 (60–77)

From Pichichero ME: Group A streptococcal tonsillopharyngitis: Cost-effective diagnosis and treament. Ann Emerg Med 1995; 25: 390–403.

*Specific studies are cited in references 11, 12, 46, and 47.

†Value represents weighted mean based on number of subjects included in the published reports; the range of results is shown in parentheses.

should be performed near the area where patients are seen. Such availability allows integration of results of rapid GABHS antigen detection testing into clinical decision making, despite the heavy flow of patients in all types of care settings.[1] Performance of rapid GABHS antigen testing does not require a trained or certified microbiologist or laboratory technician. These tests can be performed by any properly trained physician, nurse, or allied health professional. It is essential that those performing the tests carefully review the package insert so as to comply fully with their instructions. Shortcuts and lack of attention to detail reduce the sensitivity and specificity of the test results.

Cost Effectiveness Analyses of Laboratory Confirmation of GABHS

When properly used throat cultures and rapid GABHS antigen detection testing can be cost effective. For the primary prevention of acute rheumatic fever, three treatment strategies might be considered: (1) treating only patients with GABHS-positive throat cultures, (2) treating all patients, and (3) treating none. When the prevalence of positive GABHS cultures in the patient population under treatment is 20% or more (rare in adults and uncommon in children), empiric treatment of all patients is most cost effective. In an epidemic situation treating all patients is most effective and least costly; however, treating only GABHS culture–positive patients is the optimal strategy when the prevalence of GABHS is within the typical range (between 5% and 20%).[30] Applying the clinical decision rules of Walsh and colleagues to the management of tonsillopharyngitis in adults is an alternative management strategy that is cost effective for diagnosis and treatment (see Clinical Diagnosis).[9] If cultures are not obtained for patients with fewer than 10 points, the culture rate is reduced by 25% and treatment by 94%, yet this approach leaves no culture-positive patient untreated.[31] Including rapid GABHS antigen detection testing in the clinical approach leaves four alternative strategies to be considered: (1) treating all patients, (2) treating on the basis of rapid GABHS antigen test results alone, (3) treating on the basis of culture alone, or (4) treating on the basis of antigen test results plus confirmatory culture of antigen test-negative patients. In this paradigm, the treat-all strategy is the least cost effective when the costs of treating antibiotic complications are included. Antigen test plus confirmatory culture may actually cost less than either one-test strategy because the confirmatory culture has the potential to detect a small but measurable number of patients with GABHS infection who are at risk for sequelae.[32]

For physicians who practice in a setting where longitudinal care is provided, a throat culture is a very useful alternative. After a throat culture is obtained, empirical treatment for 1 or 2 days can be undertaken pending culture results, or the patient can be advised to call the next day for a culture result, thus permitting laboratory confirmation of the presence or absence of GABHS. The latter approach is particularly useful when the physician doubts that GABHS is present but is not certain or when the patient remains concerned after being told that antibiotics appear to be unnecessary.

If follow-up contact is unlikely to occur or is impossible and compliance with an oral antibiotic regimen is questionable (e.g., with indigent care), the rapid test, if it is reliably performed, can become the definitive determination for treatment, and intramuscular benzathine penicillin is the preferred antibiotic. In the absence of rapid GABHS antigen detection capability, clinical scoring of disease likelihood might be considered to determine which patients are least likely and which most likely to benefit from empiric treatment. Although no physician wants to miss an opportunity to treat a GABHS throat infection, the costs of unnecessary antibiotic therapy (in terms of side effects, particularly with injectable penicillin) can be substantial.[30–32] Thus, the presence of GABHS tonsillopharyngitis in the population served at a particular point in time is relevant. In a low-prevalence epidemiologic time frame, no treatment is a reasonable strategy.[30]

TREATMENT

Treatment should relieve the symptoms of the acute illness, eliminate transmissibility, and prevent both suppurative and nonsuppurative sequelae. Ideally, the chosen antibiotic should be easy to administer, free of adverse side effects, and affordable for patients. No antibiotic currently used in the treatment of GABHS tonsillopharyngitis achieves all of these goals in all infected patients, not even the gold standard of therapy, penicillin. The physician considering treatment of GABHS tonsillopharyngitis is faced with a large number of generic and proprietary antibiotics whose efficacies, adverse effects, and costs vary. Treatment following the recommendations of the American Heart Association (Table 46–4) results in bacteriologic and clinical success in the majority of cases[32a]; however, there are a number of failures and exceptions to the rules.

Antibiotic Treatment

Antibiotic Susceptibility

GABHS are highly susceptible to penicillins and cephalosporins.[33, 34] In vivo activity of these drugs is significantly influenced by the level of antibiotic achieved at the site of infection. Antibiotics may exhibit varying degrees of absorption, absorption affected by food, or action mitigated by enzymatic breakdown through microbial resistance mechanisms. GABHS are usually susceptible to erythromycin, clarithromycin, azithromycin, lincomycin, and clindamycin.[35] GABHS resistance to the macrolides has occurred and may develop in a community or country as a consequence of antibiotic pressure from their extensive use.[36–39] Cross-resistance among macrolides is observed. Concurrent resistance to penicillin does not occur.

The minimal inhibitory concentration (MIC) of the aminoglycosides, sulfonamides, chloramphenicol, and tetracycline against most GABHS strains is consistent with the clinical observation that these agents are of limited value in the treatment of GABHS tonsillopharyngitis. Sulfadiazine is acceptable for secondary prophylaxis in rheumatic fever. This

Table 46–4. THERAPEUTIC RECOMMENDATIONS OF THE AMERICAN HEART ASSOCIATION

Agent*	Dose	Route	Duration of Treatment
Benzathine penicillin G			
Patients <27.3 kg	600,000 U	IM	Once
Patients ≥27.3 kg	1,200,000 U	IM	Once
Penicillin V (phenoxymethyl penicillin)	250 mg thrice daily	PO	10 days
Erythromycin†			
Estolate	20–40 mg/kg/day in 2–4 doses (maximum 1 g/day)	PO	10 days
or			
Ethylsuccinate	40 mg/kg/day in 2–4 doses (maximum 1 g/day)	PO	10 days

Reproduced with permission from Dajani AS, et al.: Prevention of rheumatic fever. Circulation 1988; 78: 1082–1086. Copyright 1988 American Heart Association.

*The following agents are acceptable but not usually recommended: amoxicillin, dicloxacillin, oral cephalosporins, and clindamycin. The following agents are not acceptable: sulfonamides, trimethoprim, tetracycline, and chloramphenicol.

†For penicillin-allergic individuals.

reflects the difference between antibiotic efficacy when bacterial colonization first begins (when prophylactic drugs might be effective) and when active infection is established (when agents effective in treatment are required).

Antibiotic Tolerance

The phenomenon of antibiotic tolerance has received extensive study in the laboratory and clinically over the past decade. A ratio of the MIC to the minimum bactericidal concentration (MBC) of ≥32 defines tolerance in bacterial strains[40]; other criteria have been employed.[41–45] Studies of the occurrence of penicillin tolerance by GABHS have produced conflicting results. Surveys of GABHS-tolerant strains have given a range of 0%–30%.[46–48] In large part these differences can be attributed to laboratory technique variables. A high prevalence of penicillin-tolerant GABHS may occur in epidemics among closed or semiclosed populations.[49–52] No relationship has been found between M or T serotype and tolerance among GABHS strains. A clear correlation between penicillin tolerance and treatment failure in animal studies and clinical cases has been demonstrated for *Streptococcus viridans* and *S. aureus;* such a correlation is lacking for GABHS. Clinical observations of tolerant GABHS strains have involved outbreaks where all strains were penicillin tolerant and all patients were penicillin treatment failures and where penicillin treatment failures occurred no more frequently in patients infected with tolerant as in those with susceptible strains.[49, 51, 52] Macrolides have been useful in halting epidemics caused by GABHS-tolerant strains.

Tissue and Blood Levels

For penicillin and the cephalosporins the duration of effective drug levels is much more important than the peak serum concentration. Increasing blood penicillin levels by concurrent administration of probenecid or addition of procaine penicillin to benzathine penicillin does not enhance bacteriologic or clinical efficacy. Once a concentration of penicillin is reached that ensures activity at the bacterial cell wall, increased concentrations of the drug do not eradicate GABHS more effectively. Beta-lactam antibiotics work against actively growing bacteria. After initial bactericidal activity, there is an interval before active bacterial growth

resumes during which the antibiotic is not essential. This makes intermittent oral therapy feasible as an alternative to the continuous levels of antibiotics achieved with injectable benzathine penicillin G.

Duration of Therapy

Injections of benzathine penicillin provide bactericidal levels against GABHS for 21 to 28 days.[53, 54] The addition of procaine alleviates some of the discomfort associated with benzathine injections and may favorably influence the initial clinical response. Eradication of GABHS is produced by the sustained levels of penicillin achieved with the benzathine formulation. As we discuss later in this chapter, the necessity for 10 days of oral penicillin and erythromycin therapy to achieve a maximum bacteriologic cure rate has been documented. Therapy for 5–7 days with injectable penicillin or oral penicillin does not adequately eradicate GABHS.

Since compliance with 10 days of therapy is often problematic, a shorter course of therapy is an attractive option. A shortened course—4–5 days of therapy—with one of several cephalosporins (cefadroxil, cefuroxime axetil, cefpodoxime proxetil, cefdinir) has been shown to produce a bacteriologic eradication rate similar or superior to that achievable with 10 days' administration of oral penicillin V (Table 46–5).[55–59] Azithromycin may be administered for 5 days because this antibiotic persists in tonsillopharyngeal tissues; thus, bacteriostatic levels are maintained for approximately 10 days after discontinuation of the drug (total, 15 days' therapy).[60] If bacteriologic eradication is the primary measure of effective GABHS treatment, as it is the only corollary for the prevention of acute rheumatic fever, then superior bacteriologic eradication with a compliance-enhancing short course of cephalosporin or azithromycin therapy may prove a significant advance.

Symptomatic Response to Antibiotic Therapy

In the patient's mind the major reason for antibiotic therapy for sore throat is to quell symptoms and shorten the clinical course of illness. For many years the clinical effect of ameliorating symptoms of GABHS tonsillopharyngitis through antibiotic use was deemed minimal. This assumption was refuted by several double-blind evaluations that showed greater clinical improvement in patients receiving penicillin

Table 46–5. SHORT-COURSE CEPHALOSPORIN TREATMENT

Agent	Reference	Duration of Treatment (days)	Bacteriologic Cure Rate	
			Cephalosporin	Penicillin (10 days)
Cefuroxime axetil	55	7	17/20 (84%)	Not available
Cefuroxime axetil	56	4	82/90 (96%)	77/80 (96%)
Cefadroxil	57	5	87/104 (84%)	93/105 (89%)
Cefpodoxime proxetil	58	5	59/61 (97%)	49/52 (94%)
Cefpodoxime proxetil	59	5	113/126 (90%)	101/130 (78%)*
Cefdinir	Unpublished	5	201/224 (92%)	155/216 (72%)†

*Significant difference (p = .017); 5 days' cefpodoxime superior to 10 days' penicillin.
†Significant difference (p<.001); 5 days' cefdinir superior to 10 days' penicillin.

than in those receiving a placebo. Subsequent study by our group showed that penicillin can relieve symptoms of GABHS tonsillopharyngitis better than acetaminophen alone.[61]

Although antibiotics alleviate symptoms of GABHS tonsillopharyngitis, all patients improve spontaneously, even without treatment. The natural course of GABHS tonsillopharyngitis is rapid onset of symptoms and signs of infection with spontaneous resolution in 2–5 days in most patients. Thus, patients who seek care after they have had a sore throat for more than a week usually do not have GABHS tonsillopharyngitis. It is spontaneous resolution of symptoms but persistence of the organism in the tonsillopharynx that sets the stage for ongoing contagion and risk of acute rheumatic fever (ARF). Even though the patient feels better, persistence of the organism elicits an ongoing immune response. If the strain is rheumatogenic and the host genetically predisposed, ARF may follow.

Failure to observe a prompt clinical response to antibiotic therapy in a patient thought to have GABHS tonsillopharyngitis should lead the physician to question the diagnosis. Prompt clinical improvement is to be expected, and when such a response is not observed it usually means that GABHS is not the cause of the tonsillopharyngeal infection: either GABHS is not present or the patient is only a carrier. The symptom-relieving effects of therapy are most marked if treatment is instituted early in the course of illness. If therapy is started after the first 24–48 hours, the symptoms and signs of GABHS tonsillopharyngitis may not disappear significantly more rapidly than if no treatment were given. The incidence of suppurative complications may not be affected appreciably by the time of initiation of therapy.

Prompt treatment is not vital to the prevention of rheumatic fever. Catanzaro and colleagues demonstrated in their study of military recruits with exudative GABHS tonsillopharyngitis that, even if treatment is delayed 9 days after onset of symptoms, ARF can be prevented.[62] Thus, after 9 days' GABHS infection, when nearly maximal antigenic stimulation has already occurred and after the acute symptoms of GABHS tonsillopharyngitis have subsided, prevention of ARF is achievable. This observation is in contrast with sulfadiazine treatment, which, given early in the course of illness, favorably influences the acute symptoms but does not eradicate GABHS from the respiratory tract and does not prevent ARF.

Contagion

The transmission rate of GABHS is approximately 35% in a family or school setting if the patient is not treated.[63] Appropriate, effective antibiotic treatment prevents transmission of GABHS to other susceptible persons. Penicillin renders an infected person minimally contagious to others in approximately 24 hours.[64] The duration of contagion when alternative antibiotics are used has not been studied systematically. If penicillin is discontinued after 3 days' therapy, there is a 50% likelihood that the patient will suffer relapse (i.e., a positive GABHS infection, which may be asymptomatic).[63] If the penicillin is discontinued after 6–7 days' treatment, the likelihood that GABHS will recur is approximately 34%.[63]

Prevention of Rheumatic Fever

The efficacy of penicillin for the primary prevention of ARF was established in the early 1950s.[65, 66] These studies occurred in military recruits with GABHS tonsillopharyngitis who were given injectable penicillin G mixed in peanut oil or sesame oil and 2% aluminum monostearate. The doses and intervals between injections are shown in Table 46–6. The 300,000-U dose of the penicillin in oil preparation provided sufficient antibacterial activity for GABHS eradication for 2–3 days, whereas the 600,000-U dose provided adequate penicillin levels for 4–5 days. Thus, the three-dose schedule in Group 1 with a 600,000-U dose on day 4 likely provided at least 10 days' anti-GABHS therapy. In Group 1 the bacteriologic cure rate was 87%; in Group 2 it was 82%; and in Group 3 (1 injection), 69%. Control patients showed a spontaneous cure rate of 43%–56%. The penicillin-treated groups showed a significant (sevenfold) reduction in ARF; men in group 1 did best.

Benzathine Penicillin G

Injections of penicillin G in oil with aluminum was abandoned between 1952 and 1960 in favor of benzathine penicillin G injections (reviewed in reference 67). To reduce the discomfort from injection, a preparation of injectable penicillin was developed that combined the long-acting effect of benzathine with procaine penicillin in varied mixtures. Procaine penicillin provides diminished injection site pain and rapidly produces a high level of penicillin in the blood

Table 46–6. GABHS TONSILLOPHARYNGITIS—TREATMENT AT WARREN AFB 1949–1950

Group	Immediate	Subsequent Dose at Interval (hours)			Posttreatment GABHS Bacteriologic Failure (%)	
		48	72	96	Treated	Control
I	3×10^5 U	3×10^5 U	——	6×10^5 U	13	52
II	3×10^5 U	——	3×10^5 U	——	18	44
III	6×10^5 U	——	——	——	31	57

Data from Denny FW, et al.: Prevention of rheumatic fever: Treatment of the preceding streptococcic infection. JAMA 1950; 143: 151. Wannamaker LW, et al.: Prophylaxis of acute rheumatic fever by treatment of the preceding streptococcal infection with various amounts of depot penicillin. Am J Med 1951; 10: 673.

stream and tonsillopharynx. A combination of 900,000 U of benzathine penicillin G plus 300,000 U of procaine penicillin is superior to a variety of other regimens (Table 46–7).

Oral Penicillin G and Penicillin V

Comparisons of penicillin in oil, benzathine penicillin G, and oral penicillin G were undertaken between 1953 and 1960, when oral therapy became available (reviewed in reference 67). Eradication rates were demonstrated to be similar with 10 days of oral penicillin G and with intramuscular penicillin (Table 46–8).

Studies of military recruits published in 1951–1952 demonstrated that eradication of GABHS by penicillin prevented ARF. Thereafter, acceptable treatment of GABHS tonsillopharyngitis was evaluated on the basis of bacteriologic eradication. It is an often forgotten fact that oral penicillin was never shown in a prospective controlled trial to prevent ARF. The logical assumption, successfully applied to GABHS tonsillopharyngitis treatment since 1951–1952, was to equate bacteriologic elimination of GABHS from the tonsillopharynx with likely prevention of ARF. The low incidence of ARF in patients given oral penicillin appears to validate this therapeutic routine.

Oral penicillin V was introduced in the early 1960s as an improvement over penicillin G; it is better absorbed and therefore produces higher blood and tonsil tissue levels. Various dosing regimens with oral penicillin G and V have been assessed (reviewed in reference 67) (Table 46–9). A daily dose of 500–1000 mg of penicillin V is preferable. Smaller doses have lower eradication rates, and larger doses are not beneficial (see Table 46–9). Twice-daily dosing with oral penicillin V may be adequate therapy for GABHS tonsillopharyngitis; once-daily treatment is not.

Nafcillin, Cloxacillin, and Dicloxacillin

The efficacy of oral penicillin G has been compared with that of oral nafcillin, and the latter is less effective. Cloxacillin and dicloxacillin are adequate therapy for GABHS eradication (reviewed in reference 67).

Ampicillin and Amoxicillin

Orally administered ampicillin and amoxicillin are equivalent but not superior to penicillin in bacteriologic eradication of GABHS from the tonsillopharynx (Table 46–10). Amoxicillin is more effective than penicillin against the common pathogens that cause otitis media. Middle ear infections are seen concurrently with GABHS tonsillopharyngitis in as many as 15% of pediatric patients. In patients younger than 4 years of age the prevalence of concurrent GABHS tonsillopharyngitis and otitis media may reach 40%. There is a second issue with regard to oral amoxicillin: in suspension formulation it tastes better than oral penicillin, which is compliance-enhancing for children.

Table 46–7. STUDIES ESTABLISHING ERADICATION OF GABHS BY BENZATHINE PENICILLIN G

Investigators	Population Studied (No.)	Therapeutic Regimens*	Cure Rate† (%)
Chamovitz and colleagues, 1954	Airmen (257)	IM benzathine penicillin G, single dose:	
		0.6 MU	94
		1.2 MU	99
Breese and Disney, 1955	Children (1021)	IM benzathine penicillin G (0.6 MU)	94
Breese and colleagues, 1960	Children (604)	IM benzathine penicillin G (0.6 MU)	92
		IM benzathine penicillin G (0.6 MU) + procaine penicillin G (0.6 MU)	86
Bass and colleagues, 1976	Children (400)	IM benzathine penicillin G (0.6 MU)	79
		IM benzathine penicillin G (1.2 MU)	89
		IM benzathine penicillin G (0.6 MU) + procaine penicillin G (0.6 MU)	85
		IM benzathine penicillin G (0.9 MU) + procaine penicillin G (0.3 MU)	94

From Pichichero ME: Antimicrobials for the treatment of group A β-hemolytic streptococcal pharyngitis. In: Tandy R, Reddy KS, Narula J (eds): Rheumatic Fever. Oxford: Oxford University Press, 1996.
*MU = million units; 0.2 MU = 125 mg for penicillin G or V.
†Measured as percentage of patients with eradication of GABHS from tonsillopharynx ≤ 5–6 weeks after therapy.

Table 46–8. SELECTED STUDIES SHOWING ERADICATION OF GABHS BY INTRAMUSCULAR AND ORAL DOSAGES OF PENICILLIN

Investigators	Therapeutic Regimens*	Cure Rate† (%)
Breese, 1953	IM procaine penicillin G	
	once, 0.3 MU	59
	twice at 3 day intervals, 0.3 MU	75
	thrice at 3 day intervals, 0.3 MU	83
	IM benzathine penicillin G, 0.6 MU, once	93
	Oral penicillin G, 1.2–3.6 MU/day, for 10 days	75
Wannamaker, 1953	IM procaine penicillin G in oil, 0.6 MU, once	33
	IM procaine penicillin G in oil, 0.6 MU, four doses every other day	100
	IM benzathine penicillin G, 0.6 MU, once	70
	IM benzathine penicillin G, 1.0 MU/day, for 5 days	82
Mohler and colleagues, 1956	IM benzathine penicillin G, 0.6–0.9 MU, once	94
	Oral penicillin G for 7 days, 0.6 MU/day	82
Breese and Disney, 1957	IM benzathine penicillin G, 0.6 MU, once	93
	Oral penicillin G, 0.6–0.8 MU/day, for 10 days	86
Markowitz and colleagues, 1957	IM benzathine penicillin G, 1.2 MU monthly, once	100
	Oral penicillin G daily, 0.2 MU/day	94
Breese and Disney, 1958	IM benzathine penicillin G, 0.6 MU, once	93
	Oral benzathine penicillin G, 0.6 MU/day	90
	Oral penicillin V, 0.6 MU/day, for 10 days	89
	Oral penicillin G, 0.6 MU/day, for 10 days	87
	Oral penicillin G + probenecid, 0.75 MU/day, for 10 days	82
Miller and colleagues, 1958	IM benzathine penicillin G, 0.6 MU, once	87
	Oral penicillin G, 0.4 MU/day, for 10 days	80
	Oral penicillin G, 1.2 MU/day, for 10 days	95
Stillerman and colleagues, 1960	IM benzathine penicillin G, 0.6 MU, once	84
	IM benzathine penicillin G, 1.2 MU, once	87
	Oral penicillin V, 0.6 MU/day, for 10 days	80
	Oral penicillin V, 1.2 MU/day, for 10 days	87
Stillerman, 1969	IM benzathine penicillin G, 0.8 MU, once	91
	Oral penicillin V, 0.8 MU/day, for 10 days	83
	Oral penicillin V, 1.6 MU/day, for 7 days	72
Howie and Ploussard, 1971	IM benzathine penicillin G, 0.6–1.2 MU, once	100
	Oral penicillin G, 0.75 MU/day, for 10 days	70
Colcher and Bass, 1972	IM procaine + benzathine penicillin G mixture (1.2 MU)	86
	Oral penicillin V, 250 mg thrice daily, for 10 days:	
	Normally informed patients	75
	Optimally informed patients	90
Shapera and colleagues, 1973	IM benzathine penicillin G, 0.3–1.2 MU, once	97
	Oral penicillin V, 0.8–1.6 MU/day, for 10 days	94
Lester and colleagues, 1974	IM benzathine penicillin G, 0.6–1.2 MU, once	94
	Oral penicillin V, 0.8–1.6 MU/day, for 10 days	95
Matsen and colleagues, 1974	IM benzathine penicillin G, 0.6–1.2 MU, once	96
	Oral penicillin V, 0.6–1.6 MU/day, for 10 days	97
Ginsberg, 1982	IM benzathine penicillin G, 0.9 MU, once	88
	Oral penicillin V, 24 mg/kg/day, for 10 days	88

From Pichichero ME: Antimicrobials for the treatment of group A β-hemolytic streptococcal pharyngitis. In: Tandy R, Reddy KS, Narula J (eds): Rheumatic Fever. Oxford: Oxford University Press, 1996.
*MU = million units; 0.2 MU = 125 mg of penicillin G or V.
†Measured as percentage of patients with eradication of GABHS from tonsillopharynx ≤ 4 weeks after therapy (carriers excluded if possible).

Amoxicillin plus Clavulanate

Amoxicillin plus clavulanate has been shown to improve outcomes in the treatment of GABHS tonsillopharyngitis, as compared with penicillin in three comparative studies but not in a fourth.[68–71] Amoxicillin is bactericidal against GABHS, and clavulanate is a potent inhibitor of beta-lactamase. Thus, amoxicillin plus clavulanate would be effective if copathogens were co-colonizing the tonsillopharynx in a GABHS-infected patient (discussed in the section, Copathogens).

Erythromycin

For penicillin-allergic patients, erythromycin emerged as the suggested agent for GABHS tonsillopharyngitis. Erythromycin estolate and ethylsuccinate have been consistently shown to compare more favorably with oral penicillin in bacteriologic eradication than erythromycin base or stearate (Table 46–11) (reviewed in reference 67). Dosing frequency studies with various erythromycin preparations have shown twice, three times, or four times daily administration to produce equivalent bacteriologic eradication rates.

Clindamycin and Lincomycin

Clindamycin and lincomycin have been evaluated as primary treatment for GABHS tonsillopharyngitis (reviewed in reference 67) (Table 46–12). Clindamycin and lincomycin have a spectrum of activity that includes GABHS and potential copathogens *S. aureus* and anaerobic bacteria. Clindamycin

Table 46–9. STUDIES OF ORAL DOSAGES OF PENICILLIN G AND V IN ERADICATING GABHS

Investigators	Penicillin Agent	Daily Dose (mg)	Schedule (×/day)	Cure Rate* (%)
Breese, Disney, 1956	V	375	3	89
Shalet and colleagues, 1958	G	500	3	86
	V	375	3	89
Breese and colleagues, 1964	G	500	3	75
	V	500	3	88
Stillerman, Bernstein, 1964	V	375	3	77
	V	750	3	89
Breese and colleagues, 1965	G	500	4	58
		500	2	85
		1000	2	84
		500	4	86
		1000	4	85
Rosenstein and colleagues, 1968	V	500	2	90
Vann and Harris, 1972	G	1000	2	89
Stillerman and colleagues, 1973	V	500	2	86
	V	375	3	79
Spitzer and Harris, 1977	V	1000	2	87
	V	750	3	86
Gerber and colleagues, 1985	V	500	2	72
	V	750	3	82
Gerber and colleagues, 1989	V	750	1	78
	V	750	3	92
Krober and colleagues, 1990	V	1000	4	89
		1000	2	94
		1000	1	69

From Pichichero ME: Antimicrobials for the treatment of group A β-hemolytic streptococcal pharyngitis. In: Tandy R, Reddy KS, Narula J (eds): Rheumatic Fever. Oxford: Oxford University Press, 1996.
*Cure rate defined as bacteriologic eradication at end of treatment.

is effective in eradicating the GABHS carrier state.[72–74] Routine use of these agents for GABHS tonsillopharyngitis is not recommended because of concern for infrequent but significant side effects (i.e., pseudomembranous colitis).

Azithromycin, Clarithromycin, and Roxithromycin

Clarithromycin has been assessed for treatment of GABHS tonsillopharyngitis and it has shown a bacteriologic eradication rate similar or superior to that of penicillin.[75–79] The efficacy of roxithromycin is unclear.[79a] Azithromycin has been evaluated for treatment of GABHS tonsillopharyngitis as a 5-day regimen.[60] This shorter course of treatment is effective because azithromycin persists in tissues and cells so that an effective antibiotic level is maintained for an additional 10 days beyond the completion of therapy (total 15 days' bacteriostatic levels in the oropharynx). All of the

newer macrolides produce fewer gastrointestinal side effects than erythromycin.

Rifampin

Rifampin with oral penicillin has been studied as a possible combination for eradication of GABHS in carriers. Successful results have been observed.[80, 81]

Cephalosporins

Oral cephalosporins have been studied since 1969 as alternative antibiotics for the treatment of GABHS tonsillopharyngitis. A consistently superior bacteriologic eradication rate, and in many cases clinical cure, has been observed with the cephalosporins, as compared with penicillin.[82–84] In 1991, a meta-analysis was published that compared the bacteriologic

Table 46–10. AMPICILLIN OR AMOXICILLIN TREATMENT

Authors	Agent	Daily Dose	Schedule (×/day)	Cure Rate* (%)	
				Ampicillin/Amoxicillin	Penicillin
Breese and colleagues, 1966	Ampicillin	10–20 mg/kg	3	78	83
Ström and colleagues, 1968	Ampicillin	375–750 mg	3	85	91
Stillerman and colleagues, 1972	Ampicillin	500 mg	3	73	74
Stillerman and colleagues, 1974	Amoxicillin	375 mg	3	87	80
Breese and colleagues, 1974	Amoxicillin	375 mg	3	85	89
Breese and colleagues, 1977	Amoxicillin	15–20 mg/kg	3	91	88

From Pichichero ME: Antimicrobials for the treatment of group A β-hemolytic streptococcal pharyngitis. In: Tandy R, Reddy KS, Narula J (eds): Rheumatic Fever. Oxford: Oxford University Press, 1996.
*Cure rate defined as bacteriologic eradication at end of treatment.

Table 46–11. ERYTHROMYCIN TREATMENT OF GABHS TONSILLOPHARYNGITIS IN CHILDREN

Investigators	Daily Dose (mg/kg)	Formulation	Schedule (×/day)	Cure Rate* (%) Erythromycin	Penicillin
Stillerman and colleagues, 1960	30–40	Propionate	4	48	82
Breese, 1961	30–40	Propionate	4	64	73
Stillerman and colleagues, 1963	30–40	Propionate	4	78	72
Moffett, 1963	15–30	Estolate	4	78	77
Breese and colleagues, 1966	20	Estolate	4	85	80
Hughes and colleagues, 1969	40	Ethylsuccinate	4	85	NA
Howie and Ploussard, 1972	40–50	Ethylsuccinate	3	92	88
	20–40	Estolate	3	92	
Levine and Berman, 1972	30	Estolate	3	85	NA
Shapera and colleagues, 1973	40	Estolate	4	91	97
Ryan and colleagues, 1973	30–50	Estolate	4	92	NA
		Stearate	4	90	
Lester and colleagues, 1974	15–30	Stearate	4	91	87
Breese and colleagues, 1974	30	Estolate	3	92	88
	50	Ethylsuccinate	3	94	
Janicki and colleagues, 1975	23–38	Estolate	3	95	NA
	23	Stearate	3	100	
Derrick and Dillon, 1976	20	Estolate	2	86	NA
Breese and colleagues, 1977	30	Estolate	3	98	95
Derrick and Dillon, 1979	20	Estolate	2	87	NA
	40	Ethylsuccinate	2	86	
Ginsburg and colleagues, 1982	30	Estolate	2	92	80
Ginsburg and colleagues, 1982	30	Ethylsuccinate	2	75	NA
	30	Estolate	2	95	
Ginsburg and colleagues, 1984	15	Estolate	2	94	NA
	25	Ethylsuccinate	2	65	
Disney and colleagues, 1990	30	Ethylsuccinate	4	76	NA
Milatovic, 1991	20	Ethylsuccinate	2	80	NA

From Pichichero ME: Antimicrobials for the treatment of group A β-hemolytic streptococcal pharyngitis. In: Tandy R, Reddy KS, Narula J (eds): Rheumatic Fever. Oxford: Oxford University Press, 1996.

*Percent cure defined as bacteriologic eradication at end of treatment.

NA = not available.

and clinical cure rates achieved with various cephalosporins and with various penicillin preparations.[82] The meta-analysis identified 19 studies that fulfilled stringent criteria for adequate study design and implementation and included approximately 1000 patients assigned prospectively and randomly to receive one of several cephalosporin antibiotics. Results were compared to those for approximately 1000 patients treated with one of several penicillin formulations. The mean bacteriologic failure rate was significantly higher among those treated with penicillin (16%) than for those treated with cephalosporins (8%, p<.001) (Table 46–13). Overall, in 17 of the 19 studies analyzed, the cephalosporins produced a higher bacteriologic cure rate than the penicillins. The mean clinical failure rate was also evaluated by meta-analysis; it was 11% with various penicillin formulations, as compared with 5% for the cephalosporins (p<.001) (see Table 46–13). Numerous subsequent prospective, double-blind, randomized trials comparing first-, second-, and third-generation cephalosporin antibiotics continue to confirm the meta-analysis' results (reviewed in reference 67) (Table 46–14).

Changes in the Success of Penicillin Treatment

A range of penicillin treatment failure of 5%–35% has been reported in various studies over the past 30 years.[85–87] In the past decade an increase in penicillin treatment failures among patients with GABHS tonsillopharyngitis has been noted but challenged.[85–87] A rise in penicillin failures could be reflected in a rise in ARF, which has not been observed consistently; however, declining efficacy with penicillin (and other antibiotics) may not necessarily manifest as an increased incidence of ARF because treatment failure must occur in the presence of a rheumatogenic GABHS strain and specific host susceptibility factors as yet undetermined.

Recent descriptions of GABHS toxic shock syndrome, and more recently GABHS-mediated necrotizing fasciitis, have increased concern that a resurgence of virulent GABHS infections may be occurring. Penicillin treatment failure has been noted in patients experiencing severe GABHS infections. While the site of infection for these severe infections is usually cutaneous, the tonsillopharynx has been the source in some cases. These penicillin failures may be due to the Eagle effect[88]; that is, virulent, toxin-producing strains of GABHS may divide rapidly, reach a stationary phase of growth (perhaps as a consequence of diminished nutrients in the immediate environment of the infection), and during the stationary phase may resist the bactericidal activity of penicillin and other beta-lactams. Antibiotics that produce their action by inhibiting bacterial protein synthesis (e.g., clindamycin) have proven useful in eradicating such GABHS strains.[89]

Table 46–12. CLINDAMYCIN OR LINCOMYCIN TREATMENT

Investigators	Daily Dose (mg/kg)	Agent	Schedule (×/day)	Cure Rate* (%) Clindamycin or Lincomycin	Penicillin
Schaffer and colleagues, 1963	30	Lincomycin	4	88	89
Jackson and colleagues, 1965	22–33	Lincomycin	4	93	89
Breese and colleagues, 1966	20–40	Lincomycin	3	88	75
Breese and colleagues, 1969	20–40	Lincomycin	3	84†	59†
Randolph and DeHaan, 1969	20–40	Lincomycin	4	92	86
Randolph and colleagues, 1970	NA	Clindamycin	3 or 4	93	79
Howie and Ploussard, 1971	27–33	Lincomycin	3	88	79
Stillerman and colleagues, 1973	10–20	Clindamycin	3	90	82
			2	90	
Breese and colleagues, 1974	10–15	Clindamycin	3	92	88
Lester and colleagues, 1974	12–18	Clindamycin	2, 3, 4	95	89
Randolph and colleagues, 1975	10–30	Clindamycin	4	88	76
Brook and Leyva, 1981	20	Clindamycin	4	95†	NA
Brook and Hirokama, 1985	10	Clindamycin	4	93†	13†
Raz and colleagues, 1990	20	Clindamycin	2	98	NA
Tanz and colleagues, 1991	20	Clindamycin	2	92†	55†

From Pichichero ME: Antimicrobials for the treatment of group A β-hemolytic streptococcal pharyngitis. In: Tandy R, Reddy KS, Narula J (eds): Rheumatic Fever. Oxford: Oxford University Press, 1996.
*Cure rate defined as bacteriologic eradication at end of treatment.
†GABHS carriers included in study group.
NA = not available

Explanations for Antibiotic Failure

Antibiotic Formulation Deficiencies

The quality of benzathine penicillin G produced by various manufacturers in various countries may not be uniform. Benzathine penicillin G preparations that produce lower or variable drug levels and shorter duration have been described.[90] The same could be true for oral antibiotics utilized in therapy of GABHS.

Compliance

Oral penicillin V is recommended for three times daily administration by the American Heart Association. For optimal absorption, oral penicillin V should be administered 1 hour before or 2 hours after meals. Minimizing the number of times a day a patient must take any medication and the ability to take doses at mealtime improve patient compliance. Thrice-daily dosing not at mealtime (recommended for penicillin) represents a significant compliance barrier. Three times daily dosing typically is associated with 30%–50%

Table 46–13. META-ANALYSIS OF PENICILLINS VERSUS CEPHALOSPORINS

Treatment Regimen	Patients (No.)	Bacteriologic Failure Rate* (%)	Patients (No.)	Clinical Failure Rate† (%)
Cephalosporins	1290	8.0	926	5.0
Penicillins	1169	16.0	865	11.0

From Pichichero ME, Margolis PA: A comparison of cephalosporins and penicillins in the treatment of group A beta-hemolytic streptococcal pharyngitis. Pediatr Infect Dis J 1991; 10(4): 275–281.
*p = .0001
†p < .001

compliance, whereas dosing 1–2 times daily produces 70%–90% compliance. Intramuscular benzathine penicillin injections obviate compliance issues.

A good-tasting suspension formulation for oral antibiotics can be compliance-enhancing for children. A child may refuse, spit out, or vomit an odd or outright bad-tasting drug. Penicillin V suspension does not have a pleasant flavor, whereas most children find the taste of amoxicillin quite pleasant. Perhaps this is why U.S. physicians prescribe amoxicillin more frequently than penicillin for tonsillopharyngitis. Taste comparisons of antibiotic suspensions have found cephalosporins to taste best.[91, 92]

Patients' perceptions of antimicrobial side effects strongly influence compliance. All of the antibiotics commonly employed to treat GABHS tonsillopharyngitis are notable for their low incidence of adverse side effects. Rash and gastrointestinal upset occur in 1%–2% of patients who take penicillins and cephalosporins. Macrolides, particularly erythromycin, more frequently produce gastrointestinal upset. Amoxicillin plus clavulanate is associated with a higher incidence of diarrhea than other agents commonly considered for GABHS treatment.

Repeated Exposure

The symptoms of GABHS tonsillopharyngitis resolve spontaneously within 2–5 days of onset, even when the patient is not treated. Infected persons remain contagious for weeks, and possibly months, thereafter. Crowded living conditions encourage transmission of GABHS within the family, at work, at school, or in day care settings. After treatment, if there is a recurrence of GABHS tonsillopharyngitis and the infection involves the same serotype, patients may exhibit milder symptoms.[93] These persons are contagious to others in their environment and are themselves susceptible to rheumatic fever.

Table 46-14. CEPHALOSPORINS FOR TREATMENT

Investigators	Agent	Daily Dose	Schedule (×/day)	Cure Rate* (%) 10 Days' Cephalosporin	10 Days' Penicillin
Stillerman, 1969	Cephaloglycin	1500 mg	3	91	83
Stillerman and Isenberg, 1970	Cephalexin	1500 mg	3	91	80
Disney and colleagues, 1971	Cephalexin	30–40 mg/kg	3	81	76
Stillerman and colleagues, 1972	Cephalexin	1500 mg	3	89	74
Gau and colleagues, 1972	Cephalexin	20–24 mg/kg	3	96	92
Rabinovitch and colleagues, 1973	Cephalexin	2000 mg	4	100	97
Matsen and colleagues, 1974	Cephalexin	2000 mg	4	97	97
Derrick and Dillon, 1974	Cephalexin	1125–2250 mg	3	99	92
Stillerman, 1978	Cefatrazine	1125 mg	3	96	84
Disney and colleagues, 1979	Cefaclor	20 mg/kg	3	93	87
Ginsburg and colleagues, 1980	Cefadroxil	30 mg/kg	3	93	71
Ginsburg and colleagues, 1982	Cefadroxil	30 mg/kg	2	86	80
Henness, 1982	Cefadroxil	30 mg/kg	2	96	81
Stillerman, 1986	Cefaclor	10–31 mg/kg	3	86	70
Gerber and colleagues, 1986	Cefadroxil	30 mg/kg	4	98	94
Pichichero and colleagues, 1987	Cefuroxime	2–17 mg/kg	2	85	88
Pichichero and colleagues, 1987	Cefadroxil	30 mg/kg	4	90	76
Gooch and colleagues, 1987	Cefuroxime	250–500 mg	2	92	77
Stromberg and colleagues, 1988	Cefadroxil	1000–2000 mg	2	97	94
Milatovic and colleagues, 1989	Cefadroxil	25 mg/kg	2	93	81
Milatovic, 1991	Cefadroxil	25 mg/kg	2	92	84
Holm and colleagues, 1991	Cefadroxil	5–25 mg/kg	2	96	77
Reed and colleagues, 1991	Cefaclor	20 mg/kg	3	85	76
Disney and colleagues, 1992	Cephalexin	27 mg/kg	4	93	89
Brown and colleagues, 1991	Cefpodoxime	200 mg	2	97	91
Disney and colleagues, 1992	Loracarbef	30 mg/kg	2	87	82
Block and colleagues, 1992	Cefixime	8 mg/kg	1	94	77
Ramet and colleagues, 1992	Cefetamat	20 mg/kg	2	94	85
Gooch and colleagues, 1993	Cefuroxime	20 mg/kg	2	94	84
Milatovic and colleagues, 1993	Cefproxil	30 mg/kg	2	91	87
Pichichero and colleagues, 1994	Ceftibuten	9 mg/kg	1	91	80
Dajani and colleagues, 1993	Cefpodoxime	10 mg/kg	2	93	81
Pichichero and colleagues, 1994	Cefpodoxime	10 mg/kg	1	95	78

From Pichichero ME: Antimicrobials for the treatment of group A β-hemolytic streptococcal pharyngitis. In: Tandy R, Reddy KS, Narula J (eds): Rheumatic Fever. Oxford: Oxford University Press, 1996.

*Cure rate based on bacteriologic eradication at end of therapy.

Early Treatment Suppresses Immunity

Prompt institution of antibiotic treatment with the onset of acute symptoms may suppress the anti-streptolysin (ASO) and anti-DNAse B antibody rises typically observed to follow GABHS infections. Antibody suppression has been associated with GABHS tonsillopharyngitis relapse and recurrence (Table 46–15).[94, 95] These observations have been challenged[96]; however, no study of similar design with placebo control has produced contrary results. Although delaying treatment probably is not necessary in most cases of GABHS tonsillopharyngitis, it may be a useful strategy for patients who have frequent, recurrent, mild to moderate infections. By delaying treatment for 2 or 3 days (maximum 9 days from onset of symptoms), the patient's natural immunity may be allowed to develop without risk of rheumatic

Table 46-15. ADVERSE EFFECTS OF IMMEDIATE TREATMENT OF GABHS TONSILLOPHARYNGITIS WITH PENICILLIN

Repeat Acute GABHS Tonsillopharyngitis	Treatment Group Immediate Penicillin (N=170) (No.)	(%)	Delayed (48–56 hours) Penicillin (N=173) (No.)	(%)	p Value
Early recurrence	32	19	14	8	.006*
Late recurrence	22	13	5	3	.001*
Total recurrence	54	32	19	11	<.001*

Data from Pichichero ME, et al.: Adverse and beneficial effects of immediate treatment of Group A beta-hemolytic streptococcal pharyngitis with penicillin. Pediatr Infect Dis 1987; 6: 635–643 and El-Dahar NT, et al.: Immediate vs. delayed treatment of group A β-hemolytic streptococcal pharyngitis with penicillin V. Pediatr Infect Dis 1991; 10: 126–130.

*Treatment groups compared by Chi-square or Fisher's exact test, as appropriate, one-tailed probability.

fever. Such a strategy should not be considered if the patient is toxic or severely ill or if highly virulent or rheumatogenic strains are actively circulating in a community.

Copathogens

The presence of co-colonizing bacteria, termed "copathogens," that elaborate beta-lactamase in the tonsillopharynx has been proposed as a possible mechanism by which penicillin is inactivated before its bactericidal action affects GABHS (Fig. 46–1).[82, 83, 97] *S. aureus, H. influenzae, Moraxella catarrhalis* and beta-lactamase–producing anaerobic sp. are common flora in the tonsillopharynx. The prevalence of these beta-lactamase–producing bacteria may be increased as a consequence of penicillin treatment of patients with GABHS tonsillopharyngitis, thus leading to an increased incidence of penicillin treatment failures.

Indirect evidence suggests that when copathogens are present in the tonsillopharynx, use of antibiotics that are effective despite the presence of beta-lactamase may enhance bacteriologic and clinical success, but this is not a universal finding.[71, 82–84] It is not necessary to eradicate the copathogens that produce beta-lactamase; rather, it is necessary for the antibiotic employed to remain active despite the presence of beta-lactamase in vivo. Patients who have recurrent bouts of GABHS tonsillopharyngitis and/or whose GABHS is not eradicated by penicillin may be colonized with copathogens. Selecting an alternative antibiotic that is beta-lactamase stable and can be bactericidal to GABHS despite the presence of beta-lactamase in some cases proves an important therapeutic strategy in copathogen-colonized patients who experience GABHS tonsillopharyngitis.

Alteration of Microbial Ecology

Eradication of the normal oropharyngeal flora, especially alpha-hemolytic streptococci, may enhance the susceptibility

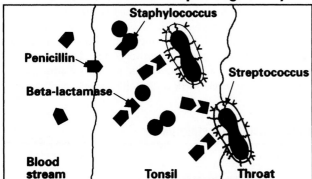

The mechanism of copathogenicity

Figure 46–1. Beta-lactamase copathogen or permissive pathogen hypothesis. Pathogenic group A beta-hemolytic streptococcus (GABHS) *(Streptococcus)* and copathogen, e.g., *Staphylococcus aureus (Staphylococcus)*, co-colonize the tonsils and throat. Parenterally or orally administered penicillin leaves the blood stream, enters the tonsillopharyngeal tissue, and is inactivated by the beta-lactamase elaborated by the *S. aureus* before the penicillin can produce its bactericidal action on the GABHS. It is proposed that the beta-lactamase stability of the cephalosporins and amoxicillin/clavulanate compared with that of penicillin provides a clinical advantage in the treatment of GABHS tonsillopharyngitis. (Pichichero M: Pediatr Inf Dis J 1993; 12: 268–274)

of patients to subsequent infection with GABHS; their presence has been shown to be associated with resistance to GABHS infection.[98] Antibiotics may eradicate or suppress the host's indigenous bacterial flora. Such alterations may result in clinical superinfections or may be subclinical, resulting in quantitative and qualitative changes in the oropharyngeal ecosystem. Penicillin treatment causes a significant quantitative decrease in alpha-hemolytic streptococci in the throat, and, thus, the ecologic balance in the throat is disturbed. These effects can persist weeks after therapy. Elimination of alpha-hemolytic streptococci from the throat eliminates their ability to produce bacteriocins that are part of the natural host resistance to GABHS colonization. Throat gargles of live alpha-hemolytic streptococci prepared from a patient's own throat bacteria have been suggested as a possible therapeutic strategy for prevention of GABHS infection, particularly for prevention of relapse or recurrent disease.[99, 100]

The Streptococcal Carrier State

A patient who has a positive GABHS throat culture but shows neither symptoms nor a demonstrable rise in streptococcal antibody titers, is likely a GABHS carrier. This operational definition is complicated by the fact that early institution of antibiotic therapy prevents an antibody response following GABHS infection. Thus, the absence of an antibody response does not rule out a bona fide GABHS infection if treatment has been rendered. Furthermore, patients experiencing a relapse with the same strain of GABHS (a homologous serotype) soon after a primary infection often have milder symptoms of GABHS infection that they do not remember, even though such patients have been shown to demonstrate an antibody rise that identifies them as being susceptible to ARF.

Treated or untreated, symptoms of acute infection with GABHS resolve but the patient may continue to carry the organism. In the early stages of this carrier state, patients are contagious to others. After some 1–2 months the carrier state is associated with diminished numbers of GABHS organisms in the tonsillopharynx, reduced bacterial virulence, and diminished transmissibility to others. A high prevalence of GABHS carriers may account for increased penicillin failures in a semiclosed community. The presence of GABHS on throat culture or as detected through rapid diagnostic testing does not distinguish between the patient with bona fide GABHS tonsillopharyngitis who is at risk for ARF and the patient with an acute viral sore throat who happens to be a GABHS carrier. The asymptomatic GABHS carrier state may persist despite intensive antibiotic treatment. Eradication of the GABHS carrier state is infrequently achievable with penicillin.

GABHS Strain Differences

A significantly higher incidence of GABHS relapse has been described following penicillin therapy in patients harboring certain M-typable strains (especially serotypes 3 and 12) as compared with patients harboring nontypable strains.[100a]

Disadvantages and Advantages of Penicillin Alternatives

The alternatives to penicillin for the treatment of GABHS tonsillopharyngitis typically are more expensive and have a broader antibiotic activity spectrum than that traditionally considered necessary for effective eradication of GABHS. Increased empiric use of broad-spectrum antibiotic therapy for treatment of sore throat with macrolides, cephalosporins, or amoxicillin plus clavulanate has the potential to contribute further to the escalating problem of antibiotic resistance among respiratory tract pathogens. Considerations of the cost of antibiotic therapy must be viewed in the light of differing bacteriologic cure rates. If enhanced bacteriologic eradication can be achieved with a more expensive agent and the enhanced eradication results in a reduction in illness burden, recurrence rates, morbidity, and/or mortality then the differential cost of the antibiotic may be small in comparison to the overall cost of failed therapy.

Criteria for Evaluation of New Agents

Guidelines have been developed for future studies of new agents for treatment of GABHS tonsillopharyngitis.[101] It has been recommended that the clinical and bacteriologic assessment of patients included in GABHS tonsillopharyngitis trials should provide for (1) bacteriologic identification of GABHS before institution of therapy, (2) repeat GABHS throat cultures performed within 4–7 days after conclusion of therapy and whenever clinical symptoms recur (additional cultures of throat specimens are indicated for subjects receiving antibiotics with prolonged serum or tissue concentrations), (3) documentation of a clinical response at 3–5 days after initiation of therapy, (4) subsequent evaluation at weekly intervals until the patient is asymptomatic and for monitoring of relapse of disease and/or poststreptococcal nonsuppurative sequelae, (5) retention of all isolates for serotyping, if possible, and (6) adequate evaluation of medication compliance. A serologic evaluation for antibody response to the GABHS infection is not viewed as essential.

Surgical Treatment

The frequency of tonsillectomy as specific therapy for children who suffer repeated episodes of GABHS infection has continued to decline over the past decade. Prospective study has demonstrated the benefit of tonsillectomy for children who have repeated episodes of culture-documented GABHS tonsillopharyngitis. Six or seven GABHS infections in a single year or three to four episodes in each of 2 years should prompt consideration of surgery.[102]

COMPLICATIONS

Suppurative Complications

Antibiotic therapy can prevent suppurative complications of GABHS, which include peritonsillar abscess, cervical adenitis, supraglottitis, cellulitis, fasciitis, peritonitis, arthritis, os-teomyelitis, thyroiditis, pneumonia, bacteremia, and meningitis.

Nonsuppurative Complications

That penicillin prevents primary and recurrent rheumatic fever is well-established. Whether antibiotic therapy prevents acute poststreptococcal glomerulonephritis is open to debate. Antibiotic therapy that successfully eradicates GABHS from the skin and/or tonsillopharynx prevents the spread of nephritogenic strains of GABHS within the community.

PREVENTION

The use of prophylactic antibiotic therapy and of tonsillectomy to prevent recurrent GABHS tonsillopharyngitis is discussed above and in Chapter 47. During the past decade research to develop a vaccine to enhance anti-GABHS immunity has been ongoing; such efforts show promise for the future.

References

1. Pichichero ME: Group A streptococcal tonsillopharyngitis: Cost-effective diagnosis and treatment. Ann Emerg Med 1995; 25: 390–403.
2. Breese BB, Disney FA: The accuracy of diagnosis of beta streptococcal infections on clinical grounds. J Pediatr 1954; 44: 670–673.
3. Stillerman M, Bernstein S: Streptococcal pharyngitis: Evaluation of clinical syndromes in diagnosis. Am J Dis Child 1961; 101: 476–489.
4. Honikman LH, Massell BF: Guidelines for the selective use of throat cultures in the diagnosis of streptococcal respiratory infection. Pediatrics 1971; 48: 573–581.
5. Funamuta JL, Berkowitz CD: Applicability of a scoring system in the diagnosis of streptococcal pharyngitis. Clin Pediatr 1983; 22: 622–626.
6. Poses RM, Cebul CD, Collins M, et al.: The accuracy of experienced physicians' probability estimates for patients with sore throats: Implications for decision making. JAMA 1985; 254: 925–929.
7. Pichichero ME, Disney FA, Green JL, et al.: Comparative reliability of clinical, culture, and antigen detection methods for the diagnosis of group A beta-hemolytic streptococcal tonsillopharyngitis. Pediatr Ann 1992; 21: 798–805.
8. Breese BB: A simple scorecard for the tentative diagnosis of streptococcal pharyngitis. Am J Dis Child 1977; 131: 514–517.
9. Walsh BT, Brookheim WW, Johnson RC, et al.: Recognition of streptococcal pharyngitis in adults. Arch Intern Med 1975; 135: 1493–1497.
10. McMillan JA, Sandstrom C, Weiner LB, et al.: Viral and bacterial organisms associated with acute pharyngitis in a school-aged population. J Pediatr 1986; 109: 747–752.
11. Putto A: Febrile exudative tonsillitis: Viral or streptococcal? Pediatrics 1987; 80: 6–11.
12. Huovinen P, Lahtonen R, Zeigler T, et al.: Pharyngitis in adults: The presence and coexistence of viruses and bacterial organisms. Ann Intern Med 1989; 110: 612–616.
13. Turner JC, Hayden GF, Kiselica D, et al.: Association of group C β-hemolytic streptococci with endemic pharyngitis among college students. JAMA 1990; 264: 2644–2647.
14. Cimolai N: β-hemolytic non–group A streptococci and pharyngitis. Am J Dis Child 1990; 144: 452–453.
15. Gerber MA, Randolph MF, Martin NJ, et al.: Community-wide outbreak of group G streptococcal pharyngitis. Pediatrics 1991; 87: 598–603.
16. Cimolai N, Elford RW, Anand BC, et al.: Do the β-hemolytic non–group A streptococci cause pharyngitis? Rev Infect Dis 1988; 10: 587–601.

17. Hayden GF, Murphy TF, Hendley JO: Non–group A streptococci in the pharynx: Pathogens or innocent bystanders? Am J Dis Child 1989; 143: 794–797.

18. Weisner PJ, Tronca E, Bonin P, et al.: Clinical spectrum of pharyngeal gonococcal infection. N Engl J Med 1973; 288: 181–185.

19. Thom DH, Grayston JT, Wang S-P, et al.: *Chlamydia pneumoniae* strain TWAR, *Mycoplasma pneumoniae,* and viral infections in acute respiratory disease in a university student health clinic population. Am J Epidemiol 1990; 132: 248–256.

20. Gerber MA, Ryan RW, Tilton RC, et al.: Role of *Chlamydia trachomatis* in acute pharyngitis in young adults. J Clin Microbiol 1984; 20: 993–994.

21. Waagner DC: *Arcanobacterium haemolyticum:* Biology of the organism and diseases in man. Pediatr Infect Dis J 1991; 10: 933–939.

22. Karpathios T, Drakonaki S, Zervoudaki A, et al.: *Arcanobacterium haemolyticum* in children with presumed streptococcal pharyngotonsillitis or scarlet fever. J Pediatr 1992; 121: 735–737.

23. Breese BB, Disney FA: The accuracy of diagnosis of beta streptococcal infections on clinical grounds. J Pediatr 1954; 44: 670–673.

24. Murray PR, Wold AD, Hall MM, et al.: Bacitracin differentiation for presumptive identification of group A beta-hemolytic streptococci: Comparison of primary and purified plate testing. J Pediatr 1976; 89: 576–579.

25. Moffett HL, Cramblett GH, Black JP: Group A streptococcal infections in a children's home. Pediatrics 1964; 33: 5–10.

26. Krober MS, Bass JW, Michaels GN: Streptococcal pharyngitis: Placebo-controlled, double-blind evaluation of clinical response to penicillin therapy. JAMA 1985; 253: 1271–1274.

27. Macknin M, Hall G, Rutherford I, et al.: Three simultaneously obtained throat cultures for beta-hemolytic group A streptococcus. Pediatr Infect Dis J 1987; 6: 575–576.

28. Brook I: Recovery of group A beta-hemolytic streptococci from both tonsillar surfaces. Pediatr Infect Dis J 1988; 7: 438.

29. Barnett ED, Pelton SI, Vinci R, et al.: Use of unprescribed antibiotics in an urban pediatric population. Interscience Conference on Antimicrobial Agents Chemotherapy 1990; 30: 178.

30. Tompkins RK, Burnes DC, Cable WE: An analysis of the cost-effectiveness of pharyngitis management and acute rheumatic fever prevention. Ann Intern Med 1977; 86: 481–492.

31. Cebul RD, Poses RM: The comparative cost-effectiveness of statistical decision rules and experienced physicians in pharyngitis management. JAMA 1986; 256: 3353–3357.

32. Lieu TA, Fleisher GR, Schwartz JS: Cost-effectiveness of rapid latex agglutination testing and throat culture for streptococcal pharyngitis. Pediatrics 1990; 85: 246–256.

32a. Dajani AS, Bisno AL, Chung KJ, et al: Prevention of rheumatic fever. A statement for health professionals by the Committee on Rheumatic Fever, Endocarditis, and Kawasaki Disease of the Council on Cardiovascular Disease in the Young, the American Heart Association. Circulation 1988; 78: 1082–1086.

33. Betriu C, Sanchez A, Gomez M, et al: Antibiotic susceptibility of group A streptococci: A 6-year follow-up study. Antimicrob Agents Chemother 1993; 37: 1717–1719.

34. Coonan KM, Kaplan EL: In vitro susceptibility of recent North American Group A streptococcal isolates to eleven oral antibiotics. Pediatr Infect Dis J 1994; 13: 630–635.

35. Wittler RR, Yamada SM, Bass JW, et al.: Penicillin tolerance and erythromycin resistance of group A β-hemolytic streptococci in Hawaii and the Philippines. Am J Dis Child 1990; 144: 587–589.

36. Stingemore RC, Francis GRJ, Toohey M, et al.: The emergence of erythromycin resistance in *Streptococcus pyogenes* in Fremantle, Western Australia. Med J Aust 1989; 150: 626–631.

37. Holmström L, Nyman B, Rosengren M, et al.: Outbreaks of infections with erythromycin-resistant group A streptococci in child day care centers. Scand J Infect Dis 1990; 22: 179–185.

38. Phillips G: Erythromycin-resistant *Streptococcus pyogenes.* J Antimicrob Chemother 1990; 25: 723–724.

39. Seppälä H, Nissinen A, Järvinen H, et al.: Resistance to erythromycin in group A streptococci. N Engl J Med 1992; 326: 292–297.

40. Van Asselt GJ, Mouton RP: Detection of penicillin tolerance in *Streptococcus pyogenes.* J Med Microbiol 1993; 38: 197–202.

41. Handwerger S, Tomasz A: Antibiotic tolerance among clinical isolates of bacteria. Rev Infect Dis 1985; 7: 368–386.

42. Sherris JC: Problems in in vitro determination of antibiotic tolerance in clinical isolates. Antimicrob Agents Chemother 1986; 30: 633–637.

43. Stratton CW, Cooksey RC: Susceptibility test: Special tests. In: Balows A, Hausler WJ Jr, Herrmann KL, et al. (eds): Manual of Clinical Microbiology, 5th ed. Washington, DC: Amer Soc Microbiology, 1991, pp 1153–1165.

44. Kim KS, Anthony BF: Use of penicillin-gradient and replicate plates for the demonstration of tolerance to penicillin in streptococci. J Infect Dis 1983; 148: 488–491.

45. Kim KS, Kaplan EL: Association of penicillin tolerance with failure to eradicate group A streptococci from patients with pharyngitis. J Pediatr 1985; 107: 681–684.

46. Michel MF, Van Leeuwen WB: Degree and stability to penicillin in *Streptococcus pyogenes.* Eur J Clin Microbiol Infect Dis 1989; 8: 225–232.

47. Betriu C, Campos E, Cabronero C, et al.: Penicillin tolerance of group A streptococci. Eur J Clin Microbiol Infect Dis 1989; 9: 799–800.

48. Krasinski K, Hanna B, LaRussa P, et al.: Penicillin tolerant group A streptococci. Diagn Microbiol Infect Dis 1986; 4: 291–297.

49. Stjernquist-Desatnik A, Orrling A, Schalén C, Kamme C: Penicillin tolerance in group A streptococci and treatment failure in streptococcal tonsillitis. Acta Otolaryngol (Stockh) 1992; (suppl)492: 68–71.

50. Grahn E, Holm SE, Roos K: Penicillin tolerance in beta-streptococci isolated from patients with tonsillitis. Scand J Infect Dis 1987; 19: 421–426.

51. Dagan R, Ferne M, Scheinis M, et al.: An epidemic of penicillin-tolerant group A streptococcal pharyngitis in children living in a closed community: Mass treatment with erythromycin. J Infect Dis 1987; 156: 514–516.

52. Dagan R, Ferne M: Association of penicillin-tolerant streptococci with epidemics of streptococcal pharyngitis in closed communities. Eur J Clin Microbiol Infect Dis 1989; 8: 629–631.

53. Kaplan EL, Berrios X, Speth J, et al.: Pharmacokinetics of benzathine penicillin G: Serum levels during the 28 days after intramuscular injection of 1,200,000 units. J Pediatr 1989; 115: 146–150.

54. Currie BJ, Burt T, Kaplan EL: Penicillin concentrations after increased doses of benzathine penicillin G for prevention of secondary rheumatic fever. Antimicrob Agents Chemother 1994; 38: 1203–1204.

55. Hebbelthwaite EM, Brown GW, Cox DM: A comparison of the efficacy and safety of cefuroxime axetil and Augmentin in the treatment of upper respiratory tract infections. Drugs Exp Clin Res 1987; 13: 91–94.

56. Gehanno P, Pangon P, Moisy N, et al.: Les angines: Enquête épidémiologique. Med Mal Infect 1987; 2: 75–79.

57. Milatovic D: Evaluation of cefadroxil penicillin and erythromycin in the treatment of streptococcal tonsillopharyngitis. Pediatr Infect Dis J 1991; 10: S61–S63.

58. Portier H, Chavanet P, Gouyon JB, et al.: Five-day treatment of pharyngotonsillitis with cefpodoxime proxetil. J Antimicrob Chemother 1990; 26: 79–85.

59. Pichichero ME, Gooch WM, Rodriguez W, et al.: Effective short-course treatment of acute group A beta hemolytic streptococcal tonsillopharyngitis: A comparison of five days vs ten days cefpodoxime proxetil vs ten days penicillin VK in children. Arch Pediatr Adolesc Med 1994; 148: 1053–1060.

60. Still JG: Management of pediatric patients with group A beta-hemolytic *Streptococcus* pharyngitis: Treatment options. Pediatr Infect Dis J 1995; 14: S57–S61.

61. Pichichero ME, Disney FA, Talpey WB, et al.: Adverse and beneficial effects of immediate treatment of Group A beta-hemolytic streptococcal pharyngitis with penicillin. Pediatr Infect Dis J 1987; 6: 635–643.

62. Catanzaro FJ, Stetson CA, Morris AJ, et al.: The role of streptococcus in the pathogenesis of rheumatic fever. Am J Med 1954; 17: 749–756.

63. Breese BB, Disney FA: Factors influencing the spread of beta hemolytic streptococcal infections within the family group. Pediatrics 1956; 17: 834–838.

64. Snellman LW, Stang HJ, Stang JM, et al.: Duration of positive throat cultures for Group A streptococci after initiation of antibiotic therapy. Pediatrics 1993; 91: 1166–1170.

65. Denny FW, Wannamaker LW, Brink WR, et al.: Prevention of rheumatic fever: Treatment of the preceding streptococcic infection. JAMA 1950; 142: 151–153.

66. Wannamaker LW, Rammelkemp CR Jr, Denny FW, et al.: Prophylaxis of acute rheumatic fever by treatment of the preceding streptococcal infection with various amounts of depot penicillin. Am J Med 1951; 10: 673–695.

67. Pichichero ME: Antimicrobials for the treatment of group A β-hemolytic streptococcal pharyngitis. In: Tandy R, Reddy KS, Narula J (eds): Rheumatic Fever. Oxford: Oxford University Press, 1996 (in press).

68. Smith TD, Huskins WC, Kim KS, et al.: Efficacy of β-lactamase–resistant penicillin and influence of penicillin tolerance in eradicating streptococci from the pharynx after failure of penicillin therapy for group A streptococcal pharyngitis. J Pediatr 1987; 110: 777–782.

69. Kaplan EL, Johnson DR: Eradication of group A streptococci from the upper respiratory tract by amoxicillin with clavulanate after oral penicillin V treatment failure. J Pediatr 1988; 113: 400–403.

70. Brook I: Treatment of patients with acute recurrent tonsillitis due to group A β-haemolytic streptococci: A prospective randomized study comparing penicillin and amoxycillin/clavulanate potassium. J Antimicrob Chemother 1989; 24: 227–233.

71. Tanz RR, Shulman ST, Sroka PA, et al.: Lack of influence of beta-lactamase–producing flora on recovery of group A streptococci after treatment of acute pharyngitis. J Pediatr 1990; 117: 859–863.

72. Brook I, Leyva F: The treatment of the carrier state of group A beta-hemolytic streptococci with clindamycin. Chemotherapy 1981; 27: 360–367.

73. Brook I, Hirokawa R: Treatment of patients with a history of recurrent tonsillitis due to Group A beta-hemolytic streptococci. A prospective randomized study comparing penicillin, erythromycin, and clindamycin. Clin Pediatr 1985; 24: 331–336.

74. Tanz RR, Poncher JR, Corydon KE, et al.: Clindamycin treatment of chronic pharyngeal carriage of group A streptococci. J Pediatr 1991; 119: 123–128.

75. Scaglione F: Comparison of the clinical and bacteriological efficacy of clarithromycin and erythromycin in the treatment of streptococcal pharyngitis. Curr Med Res Opin 1990; 12: 25–33.

76. Levenstein JH: Clarithromycin versus penicillin in the treatment of streptococcal pharyngitis. J Antimicrob Chemother 1991; 27: 67–74.

77. Bachand RT Jr: A comparative study of clarithromycin and penicillin VK in the treatment of outpatients with streptococcal pharyngitis. J Antimicrob Chemother 1991; 27: 75–82.

78. Schrock CG: Clarithromycin vs penicillin in the treatment of streptococcal pharyngitis. J Fam Pract 1992; 35: 622–626.

79. Still JG, Hubbard WC, Poole JM, et al.: Comparison of clarithromycin and penicillin VK suspensions in the treatment of children with streptococcal pharyngitis and review of currently available alternative antibiotic therapies. Pediatr Infect Dis J 1993; 12: S134–S141.

79a. Melcher GP, Hadfield TL, Gaines JK, et al.: Comparative efficacy and toxicity of roxithromycin and erythromycin in ethyl succinate in the treatment of streptococcal pharyngitis in adults. J Antimicrob Chemother 1988; 22: 549–556.

80. Chaudhary S, Bilinsky SA, Hennessy JL, et al.: Penicillin V and rifampin for the treatment of group A streptococcal pharyngitis: A randomized trial of 10 days penicillin vs 10 days penicillin with rifampin during the final 4 days of therapy. J Pediatr 1985; 106: 481–486.

81. Tanz RR, Shulman ST, Barthel MJ, et al.: Penicillin plus rifampin eradicates pharyngeal carriage of group A streptococci. J Pediatr 1985; 106: 876–880.

82. Pichichero ME, Margolis PA: A comparison of cephalosporins and penicillins in the treatment of group A beta-hemolytic streptococcal pharyngitis: A meta-analysis supporting the concept of microbial co-pathogenicity. Pediatr Infect Dis J 1991; 10: 275–281.

83. Pichichero ME: Cephalosporins are superior to penicillin for treatment of streptococcal tonsillopharyngitis: Is the difference worth it? Pediatr Infect Dis J 1993; 12: 268–274.

84. Deeter RG, Kalman DL, Rogan MP, et al: Therapy for pharyngitis and tonsillitis caused by group A beta-hemolytic streptococci: A meta-analysis comparing the efficacy and safety of cefadroxil monohydrate versus oral penicillin V. Clin Ther 1992; 14: 740–754.

85. Kaplan EL: Benzathine penicillin G for treatment of Group A streptococcal pharyngitis: A reappraisal in 1985. Pediatr Infect Dis 1985; 4: 592–596.

86. Pichichero ME: The rising incidence of penicillin treatment failures in Group A streptococcal tonsillopharyngitis: An emerging role for the cephalosporins? Pediatr Infect Dis J 1991; 10: S50–S55.

87. Markowitz M, Gerber MA, Kaplan EL: Treatment of streptococcal pharyngotonsillitis: Reports of penicillin's demise are premature. J Pediatr 1993; 123: 679–685.

88. Eagle H, Fleischman R, Masselman AD: Effective schedule of administration of the therapeutic efficiency of penicillin—importance of the aggregate time penicillin remains at effectively bactericidal levels. Am J Med 1950; 9: 280–299.

89. Stevens DL, Gibbons AE, Bergstrom R, et al.: The Eagle effect revisited: Efficacy of clindamycin, erythromycin, and penicillin in the treatment of streptococcal myositis. J Infect Dis 1988; 158: 23–28.

90. Zaher SR, Kassem AS, Abou-Shleib H, et al.: Differences in serum penicillin concentrations following intramuscular injection of benzathine penicillin G (BPG) from different manufacturers. J Pharmacol Med 1992; 2: 17–23.

91. Ruff ME, Schotik DA, Bass JW, et al.: Antimicrobial drug suspensions: A blind comparison of taste of fourteen common pediatric drugs. Pediatr Infect Dis J 1991; 10: 30–33.

92. Demers DM, Schotik D, Bass JW: Antimicrobial drug suspensions: A blinded comparison of taste of twelve common pediatric drugs including cefixime, cefpodoxime, cefprozil and loracarbef. Pediatr Infect Dis J 1994; 13: 87–89.

93. Woodin KA, Lee LH, Pichichero ME: Milder symptoms occur in recurrent episodes of streptococcal infection. Am J Dis Child 1991; 145: 389–390.

94. Pichichero ME, Disney FA, Talpey WB, et al.: Adverse and beneficial effects of immediate treatment of group A beta-hemolytic streptococcal pharyngitis in an emergency department. Pediatr Infect Dis J 1986; 5: 655.

95. El-Dahar NT, Hijazi SS, Rawashdeh NM, et al.: Immediate vs delayed treatment of group A beta-hemolytic streptococcal pharyngitis with penicillin V. Pediatr Infect Dis J 1991; 10: 126–130.

96. Gerber MA, Randolph MF, DeMeo KK, et al.: Lack of impact of early antibiotic therapy for streptococcal pharyngitis on early recurrence rates. J Pediatr 1990; 117: 853–858.

97. Brook I: Penicillin failure and copathogenicity in streptococcal pharyngotonsillitis. J Fam Pract 1994; 38: 175–179.

98. Roos K, Grahn E, Holm SE, et al.: Interfering α-streptococci as a protection against recurrent streptococcal tonsillitis in children. Intern J Pediatr Otorhinolaryngol 1993; 25: 141–148.

99. Lilja H, Grahn H, Holm SE, et al.: Alpha-streptococci–inhibiting beta-streptococci group A in treatment of recurrent streptococcal tonsillitis. Adv Otorhinolaryngol 1992; 47: 168–171.

100. Roos K, Holm SE, Grahn E, et al.: Alpha-streptococci as supplementary treatment of recurrent streptococcal tonsillitis: A randomized placebo-controlled study. Scand J Infect Dis 1993; 25: 31–35.

100a. Stillerman M, Bernstein SH: Streptococcal pharyngitis therapy. Am J Dis Child 1964; 107: 73–84.

101. Peter G: Streptococcal pharyngitis: Current therapy and criteria for evaluation of new agents. Clin Infect Dis 1992; 14 (suppl 2): S218–223.

102. Paradise JL, Bluestone CD, Bachman RZ, et al.: Efficacy of tonsillectomy for recurrent throat infection in severely affected children. N Engl J Med 1984; 310: 674–683.

Ayal Willner
Kenneth M. Grundfast

CHAPTER FORTY-SEVEN

Tonsillitis

▼

Tonsillitis is one of the most common problems treated by pediatricians. Both tonsillitis and tonsillectomy were described centuries ago[1, 2]; however, the pathophysiology of chronic tonsillitis and indications for tonsillectomy remain controversial. During the preantibiotic era, tonsillectomy was often the definitive cure for frequently recurring and chronic tonsillitis, but in recent years there has been an increasing trend toward antibiotic therapy. Surgical intervention for infectious tonsillar disease has been reserved for patients who experience complications of tonsillitis or more severe recurrent or chronic disease. The appropriate indications for tonsillectomy are being reviewed carefully, although few firm guidelines have been published. As an alternative to tonsillectomy, some clinicians advocate prophylactic antibiotics. The exact roles of these different therapeutic modalities have yet to be determined.

Recent publications have given us a better understanding of the underlying problems that lead to chronic tonsillar disease. Today we have a much better understanding of the organisms involved in acute episodes of tonsillitis, as well as the mechanisms of failure of antimicrobial therapies. In addition, more is known about the associated immunologic changes that accompany chronic tonsillitis and their impact on the chances of recurrent infection. With this information an improved understanding of the pathophysiology of chronic tonsillitis can be developed, and more rational treatment plans created.

EPIDEMIOLOGY

Group A streptococci are normal inhabitants of the nasopharynx and 15%–20% of children are colonized by this organism.[3] The incidence of streptococcal infection is lowest in infants, possibly owing to maternal immunoglobulins. Streptococcal pharyngotonsillitis is most common between age 5 and 15 years. Spread is via airborne droplets and, occasionally, via direct contact or in food, milk, or water.

In a study of 429 office-based pediatricians in the United States, tonsillitis was found to be the third most commonly treated problem, after upper respiratory tract infections and ear problems. Tonsillitis accounted for as many as 17% of the visits, depending on the child's age.[4] Similarly, in a study by the Department of Health and Human Services, recurrent tonsillitis was the second most common disease treated by pediatricians.[5] Chronic adenotonsillar disease accounts for a significant portion of the office visits in other parts of the world as well.[6, 7]

In accordance with the significance of the problem of tonsillitis, tonsillectomy is one of the most common surgical procedures performed. While the number of these procedures has dropped from almost 1 million in 1972 to fewer than half that in 1983,[8] operations on the tonsils and adenoids continue to be the most common major procedure performed on children,[9] and in 1987 more than 250,000 tonsillectomies and adenoidectomies were performed in the United States.[10]

ANATOMY AND EMBRYOLOGY

The palatine tonsils are a collection of lymphoid follicles and, along with the adenoids and lingual tonsils, are the first sampling site for inhaled and ingested antigens. The surface epithelium of these almond-shaped structures is invaginated to form 10–20 crypts. These burrow down to differing depths, where a variety of cells involved in the early stages of immune response first come in contact with antigen. The tonsil is invested by a condensation of connective tissue that forms a dense "hemicapsule."[11] It lies in the tonsillar fossa bound anteriorly by the palatoglossus muscle (the anterior tonsillar pillar), posteriorly by the palatopharyngeus muscle (the posterior tonsillar pillar), and laterally by the superior constrictor muscle. The tonsil receives its blood supply from the ascending and descending palatine arteries as well as the lingual, tonsillar, and descending pharyngeal arteries. Blood drains via the peritonsillar plexus to the lingual and pharyngeal veins and then to the internal jugular vein. There are no afferent lymphatics, and the efferent system drains to the upper deep cervical lymph nodes. Innervation comes through the glossopharyngeal nerve, which, via its tympanic branch, accounts for the referred ear pain that accompanies acute infection.[12]

The tonsils begin development in the fourteenth week of gestation, when the mesenchyme underlying the tonsillar cavity becomes invaded by mononuclear stem cells (pre-B cells). In the fifteenth week, the epithelial crypts grow down from the surface into the connective tissue, and typical lymphoid structure develops as the pre-B cells are immobilized by the mesenchymal tissue. B cell–rich primary follicles are present by the sixteenth week, but parafollicular T-cell regions develop postnatally.[13] By 2 weeks after birth, activation of the tonsils has commenced.

ETIOLOGY

A variety of organisms can cause inflammation of the tonsils, including aerobic and anaerobic bacteria, viruses, and *Mycoplasma, Toxoplasma,* and *Candida* species (Table 47–1).

Table 47-1. INFECTIOUS AGENTS AFFECTING WALDEYER'S RING

I. Bacteria
  Aerobic
    Groups A, B, C, and G
      streptococci
    Streptococcus pneumoniae
    Staphylococcus aureus
    Branhamella catarrhalis
    Neisseria gonorrhoeae
    Neisseria meningitidis
    Corynebacterium
      diphtheriae
    Corynebacterium
      hemolyticum
    Bordetella pertussis
    Haemophilus influenzae
    Haemophilus
      parainfluenzae
    Salmonella typhi
    Francisella tularensis
    Yersinia
      pseudotuberculosis
    Treponema pallidum
    Mycobacterium species
  Anaerobic
    Peptococcus species
    Peptostreptococcus
      species
    Actinomyces species
    Bacteroides
      melaninogenicus group
    Bacteroides oralis
    Bacteroides ruminicola
    Bacteroides fragilis group

II. Mycoplasmas
  Mycoplasma pneumoniae
  Mycoplasma hominis
III. Viruses and Chlamydia
  Adenovirus
  Enteroviruses (polio-,
    ECHO, coxsackie-)
  Parainfluenza virus, types
    1–4
  Epstein-Barr virus
  Herpes simplex virus
  Respiratory syncytial virus
  Influenzae A and B viruses
  Cytomegalovirus
  Reovirus
  Measles virus
  Rubella virus
  Rhinovirus
  Chlamydia trachomatis
IV. Fungi
  Candida species
V. Parasites
  Toxoplasma gondii
VI. Rickettsia
  Coxiella burnetii

From Brook I: The clinical microbiology of Waldeyer's ring. Otolaryngol Clin North Am 1987; 20: 261.

Viruses

Most cases of viral pharyngitis and tonsillitis are mild, do not require treatment with antibiotics, and are self-limiting. An exception is coxsackievirus A, which is characterized by vesicles (which then become ulcers) over the tonsils, anterior pillars, palate, and posterior pharynx. Children with this type of viral pharyngitis generally appear more ill than those infected with other viruses. Another important virus is the Epstein-Barr virus, the agent of infectious mononucleosis. Infections with this agent can range from mild ones with symptoms only in the upper respiratory tract to multisystemic disease.

Bacteria

Many studies have been done in efforts to determine the microbiology of chronic tonsillitis. Fewer have determined the microbial ecology of the tonsils in healthy subjects. The establishment of the upper respiratory tract flora is initiated at birth. Within a few days there are large numbers of lactobacilli and anaerobic streptococci. *Actinomyces, Fusobacterium,* and *Nocardia* organisms are present by age 6 months, and *Bacteroides, Propionibacterium,* and *Candida* species become established shortly thereafter. Fusobacteria reach high numbers after the eruption of teeth and are most

numerous by age 1 year. In the steady state, the aerobic-anaerobic ratio is approximately 1:10.[14]

In addition to normal flora, tonsils of healthy children can harbor known pathogenic bacteria. *Haemophilus influenzae,* group A beta-hemolytic streptococci, *Streptococcus pneumoniae, Moraxella catarrhalis,* and *Staphylococcus aureus* have all been cultured in significant numbers from children who had no complaints referable to the tonsils.[15, 16] Brook and Foote compared the tonsillar microbiology of four patients undergoing tonsillectomy who had no tonsillar hypertrophy or history of recurrent infection with that of four children undergoing tonsillectomy for chronic tonsillitis. Examining the core bacteria, they found qualitatively similar bacteria in both groups (Table 47–2). The tonsils from patients with chronic tonsillitis, however, exhibited significantly higher numbers of beta-hemolytic streptococci and *Bacteroides* and *Peptostreptococcus* species. Of note, beta-lactamase production was detectable in three out of four "normal" tonsils and in all of the tonsils removed for chronic tonsillitis.

Acute tonsillitis traditionally has been considered a streptococcal disease.[17–20] This may be due to the ease of detection of the serum antibody response that follows streptococcal infection. This increase in antibody titer may not be seen after other infections that are resolved at the tonsillar level.[9] Much of the recent literature, however, has focused on the polymicrobial aspects of recurrent tonsillitis.[14, 18–29] Brook and Hirokawa examined the tonsillar microflora of 45 patients with a history of chronic tonsillitis.[21] They isolated 243 aerobic and 245 anaerobic bacteria (average, 5.4 aerobes and 5.4 anaerobes per specimen; Table 47–3). In addition, they cultured mixed aerobic and anaerobic bacteria from all specimens. The aerobes most frequently isolated in their study were alpha- and gamma-hemolytic streptococci, beta-hemolytic streptococci, *M. catarrhalis, S. aureus,* and *Haemophilus* species. The predominant anaerobic organisms were *Bacteroides* and *Fusobacterium* species, anaerobic gram-positive cocci, and *Veillonella parvula.* Bieluch and colleagues determined the tonsillar microflora of 10 patients aged 5–32 years who suffered recurrent tonsillitis.[18] They recovered 6.3 aerobic and 3.3 anaerobic bacteria per patient. The aerobic organisms most commonly isolated were alpha-hemolytic streptococci, but the most common potential aerobic pathogen was *H. influenzae.* Group A beta-hemolytic

Table 47-2. COMPARISON OF CORE BACTERIA IN PATIENTS WHO HAVE AND DO NOT HAVE A HISTORY OF CHRONIC TONSILLITIS

Bacterium	Isolates (No.)	
	Normal	Chronic
Aerobic		
α-Hemolytic streptococci	4	4
γ-Hemolytic streptococci	2	3
Group A β-hemolytic streptococci	1	3
Staphylococcus aureus	2	2
Anaerobic		
Peptostreptococcus species	4	4
Fusobacterium species	4	6
Bacteroides intermedius	3	2
Bacteroides melaninogenicus	2	2

Table 47–3. ANAEROBIC AND AEROBIC BACTERIA ISOLATED FROM 45 PATIENTS WITH A HISTORY OF CHRONIC TONSILLITIS

Organism	Isolates (No.)
Gram-positive cocci	
Streptococcus pneumoniae	7
Alpha-hemolytic streptococci	41
Gamma-hemolytic streptococci	40
Group A, beta-hemolytic streptococci	45
Group F, beta-hemolytic streptococci	5
Staphylococcus aureus	17
Staphylococcus epidermidis	6
Gram-negative cocci	
Branhamella catarrhalis	35
Gram-positive cocci	
Lactobacillus species	11
Diphtheroid species	19
Gram-negative bacilli	
Haemophilus influenzae type B	8
Haemophilus parahemolyticus	3
Haemophilus parainfluenzae	2
Eikenella corrodens	4
Gram-positive cocci	
Peptococcus species	37
Peptostreptococcus species	20
Gram-negative cocci	
Veillonella parvulla	11
Gram-positive bacilli	
Bifidobacterium adolescentis	5
Eubacterium species	15
Lactobacillus acidophilus	13
Propionibacterium acnes	9
Actinomyces species	3
Gram-negative bacilli	
Fusobacterium species	12
Fusobacterium nucleatum	27
Bacteroides species	13
B. melaningenicus	27
B. asaccharolyticus	12
B. intermedius	10
B. oralis	10
B. ruminicola ssp, *brevis*	6
B. fragilis	7
Total	488

streptococci were isolated in only one patient. This group also noted a high prevalence of anaerobic bacteria, and anaerobic gram-positive cocci were isolated from all 10 patients. Seven of the patients had *Bacteroides* organisms cultured from their tonsils. Kielmovitch and colleagues performed a qualitative and quantitative study on 51 patients with recurrent streptococcal tonsillitis (25 patients) and obstructive tonsillar hypertophy (26 patients).[23] They found that the microbial composition and density in these two groups were similar. From the tonsillar surfaces, 5.5 aerobic and 3.5 anaerobic isolates per patient were cultured. *Streptococcus viridans* organisms were cultured from 100% of the tonsillar surfaces in both groups and *H. influenzae* and *S. aureus* organisms were isolated in 73% and 36% of patients, respectively.

In addition to delineating the pathogens of tonsillitis, the work by Kielmovitch, Brook, and others has served to highlight the disparity between the surface and core microbial ecology. This is particularly important since most prior information concerning both the causative organisms and the

appropriate treatments for tonsillitis are based on surface cultures. Brodsky and colleagues characterized types and numbers of bacteria in 55 tonsils excised for chronic tonsillar disease.[30] Specimens were cultured at the surface and in the core. They found that only 62% of bacteria found in the core could be cultured from the surface. All surface bacteria, on the other hand, were isolated from core specimens. The species most frequently isolated were *H. influenzae, Streptococcus pyogenes, S. pneumoniae, S. aureus, Staphylococcus epidermidis, S. viridans,* and *Neisseria* species. Importantly, only 59% of the core bacteria that were capable of producing beta-lactamase were cultured from the tonsillar surface. Brodsky and colleagues compared the core and surface cultures of 97 children undergoing tonsillectomy for chronic tonsillar disease.[24] *S. aureus* was the most common core and surface organism isolated. For 43% of all patients, surface culture yielded only normal flora while core culture contained pathogenic organisms. Similarly, Uppal and Bais noted a discrepancy between the surface and core bacteria in 64% of the tonsillar specimens they examined.[27]

IMMUNOLOGY

Cellular Components

The surface of the tonsil is normally covered with stratified squamous epithelium that dips into the tonsil to form the tonsillar crypt. There are usually some 10–20 crypts per tonsil. Within the crypt, the epithelium is loosely arranged and has macrophages, dendritic cells, and lymphocytes interspersed with the epithelial cells. In addition, the crypt wall contains micropore (M) cells, which are tubovesicular in nature and aid in the internalization of antigen. Beneath the epithelium lies the interfollicular zone, which is rich in T cells. In addition, this is an area of antigen presentation by the interdigitating cells, macrophages, and follicular dendritic cells. The germinal centers in the lymphoid follicles are the site of B-cell differentiation and proliferation.

Normal Immune Function

Intact immune function begins with the effective internalization of antigens from the pharynx into the lymphatic tissue of the tonsil. After antigen has passed to the tonsil's interior it is processed and presented to T and B lymphocytes. The resultant interaction leads to terminal differentiation of B cells to antibody-producing cells and to the creation of memory T and B cells. Appropriate sensitization is necessary for effective immune function, and there are multiple systems and many molecules that can induce T- and B-cell functions to varying extents. These systems work in concert, but, importantly, inappropriate signaling may lead to downregulation of the immune responsiveness of T and B cells. It is therefore necessary to delineate the different factors that can lead to modulation of the immune response.

Antigen Internalization

Antigen is internalized into the extrafollicular areas of the tonsil by passing through the M cell located at the base of the tonsillar crypt. These tubovesicular cells transport antigen into the tonsil.[31] Dendritic cells and macrophages are also found in the crypt wall epithelium. Like the M cells, they internalize antigen; however, they are also involved in presentation of antigen to T cells in the extrafollicular area and to the B-cell follicles.[32]

Antigen Presentation

Antigen presentation is a complex interaction between the antigen-presenting cells and the T and B lymphocytes. Antigen-presenting cells process antigen and present it bound to antibody in such a way as to interact with specific molecules on the lymphocyte cell surface. The main antigen-presenting cells are macrophages, interdigitating cells, and follicular dendritic cells. Macrophages are present in both the crypt epithelium and the germinal centers, as measured by monoclonal antibodies (mAb) MAC 387 and CD68. MAC 387–positive cells are seen in the crypt epithelium, whereas CD68 cells are seen in the extrafollicular areas and the germinal centers. These two types of macrophages represent one pathway of signaling T and B cells.[33]

The exact nature of the macrophage-lymphocyte signal is not fully known; however, it does appear to involve direct cell-to-cell contact in which the macrophage extends a cytoplasmic process that surrounds the lymphocyte. This interaction is dependent on the expression by the macrophage of MHC class II antigens, which are expressed after activation by interferon-γ. In addition to the interaction with T and B cells, macrophages also interact with the follicular dendritic cell via direct contact.[34] While the above discussion indicates that the macrophage plays an important role in antigen presentation, its role in lymphocyte activation has not been completely determined.

Another antigen-presenting cell, the interdigitating cell, which contains the S-100 protein, is found mostly in the extrafollicular areas but has been found in the crypt epithelium. Unlike the macrophage, it expresses the MHC II antigens without priming by interferon-γ. Like the macrophage, it is found in close contact with helper T cells and is believed to present antigen to maturing T cells.[35]

Follicular dendritic cells, which contain C3b found on active immune complexes, are present in the germinal centers and mantle zones. In these areas, follicular dendritic cells deliver antigens to B cells, which, in turn, in the germinal centers, present immunogen to T cells. The interaction of the follicular dendritic cell with the B cell may lead to the B cell's developing into either a memory B cell or an immunoglobulin-secreting cell.[33]

Along with these antigen-presenting cells, other cells may play supporting roles in the activation of lymphocytes. Fibroblastic reticulum cells, for example, are found in the T-cell areas and form a dendritic network.[36] The function of these cells is not known; however, fibroblasts treated with interferon-γ have been shown to express major histocompatibility complex antigens on their surface.[37] With other signals, fibroblasts may play a role in augmenting the T-cell response to antigenic stimulation.

Lymphocyte Activation

Successful activation of the T and B lymphocytes is the result of complex interactions between (1) the antigen-presenting cells and the lymphocytes, (2) accessory cells and lymphocytes, and (3) T and B lymphocytes. These interactions occur via direct contact or via cytokines. Direct interactions between presentation cells and T cells involve multiple connections.[37] A partial list of T-cell determinants and their corresponding antigen-presenting cell ligands is given in Table 47–4. A principal lymphocyte surface molecule is the CD3 determinant. It is structurally related to the T-cell receptor (TCR) and undergoes tyrosine phosphorylation of one of its chains upon interaction of the TCR/CD3 complex with antigen. T-cell activation results in an increase in intracellular calcium. Association of other ligands on the antigen-presenting cell with the T-cell surface determinants leads to an increase in the concentration of intracellular calcium and acts synergistically with CD3-mediated events to augment T-cell activation. One of these determinants, CD2, is thought to play a role in both cell-to-cell adhesion and activation of the T cell. On the other hand, CD4 and CD8, when bound to their antigen-presenting cell ligands, cause an increase in intracellular calcium but not in T-cell activation as measured by the production of interleukin-2 (IL-2) or the induction of cell proliferation. Interestingly, if interaction with antigen leads to the association of CD4 and CD8 with CD3, then binding to determinants on the antigen-presenting cell does induce T-cell activation. Another surface molecule, CD54 (decay-accelerating factor [DAF]), does not by itself increase intracellular calcium, but cross-linking of these molecules can induce T-cell proliferation. Furthermore, cross-linking CD54 with CD3 leads to augmentation of the CD3-induced calcium concentration rise as well as to increased T-cell proliferation.

Table 47–4. T-CELL SURFACE MOLECULES AND THEIR ANTIGEN-PRESENTING CELL LIGANDS

T-Cell Surface Determinant	Early Activation Events	Additional Requirements	APC Ligand	CD3 Expression Required
TCR/CD3	Ca^{2+} increase	AC	Antigen-polymorphic MHC	Yes
CD2	Ca^{2+} increase	AC independent	LFA-3	Yes
CD4/CD8	Ca^{2+} increase	CD3	Class II/I MHC	Unknown
CD54(DAF)	Augment Ca^{2+} increase	AC + PMA or CD3	Complement components	Unknown

From Geppert TD, Davis LS, Gur H, et al.: Accessory cell signals involved in T-cell activation. Immunol Rev 1990; 117: 5–6. Copyright 1990, Munksgaard International Publishers Ltd., Copenhagen, Denmark.

Along with T-cell activation, B-cell activation within the tonsil is a necessary component of proper immune function. In the germinal centers, follicular dendritic cells are probably the most important antigen-presenting cells for B cells. The follicular dendritic cells retain large amounts of antigen in complement-containing immune complexes. Antigen-antibody complexes are bound to the follicular dendritic cells via complement and Fc receptors. This complex of macromolecules is incorporated into icosomes, which are membrane-bound bodies coated with immune complexes. They are released into the intercellular area, where they bind to B cells. The icosome-bound antigen interaction with the B cell is enhanced because the B-cell surface proteins interact with both the antigenic determinants and the complement factors. Such cross-linking of B-cell surface receptors leads to B-cell activation.

The involvement of complement factors may lead to the formation of terminal complement complexes, but these apparently do not cause any harm. The terminal complement complexes may result in release of inflammatory mediators and may lead to mild edema. Such edema within the tonsil may facilitate icosome dispersion and increase the likelihood of B-cell contact and activation. B cells are further activated by tonsillar helper T cells via cell-to-cell contact after the antigen presented to the B cell is further processed by that cell and is then presented to the T cell in the context of human leukocyte antigen (HLA) class II molecules.

Along with cell-to-cell interactions, the activation of the immune system is mediated by cytokines. At least 19 different cytokines are detectable in tonsils of patients with either infectious mononucleosis or recurrent tonsillitis (Table 47–5).[38] As can be seen in the table, cytokines are readily found in all areas from the surface epithelium to the germinal center. IL-2 is well-known for its ability to augment lymphocyte activation. Follicular dendritic cells induce IL-6 production and T-cell clonal proliferation.[39] Cytokines are also involved in the regulation of IL-1 production, the immunoglobulin switch to all IgG subclasses, IgA production, and the induction of the Bcl-2 gene, which prevents apoptosis of immune-activated B lymphocytes.

The formation of an appropriate immune response, therefore, depends on myriad complex interactions among crypt epithelium cells, macrophages, interdigitating cells, follicular dentritic cells, T cells, B cells, and cytokines. Successful interactions lead to the production of activated B cells, which either enter the circulation and become associated with glandular tissue and the lamina propria of the upper respiratory tract epithelium[31, 32, 40] or differentiate locally to immunoglobulin cells. IgA is the predominant immunoglobulin produced in the mucosa-associated lymphoid tissue (MALT), and in the areas of the upper respiratory tract IgA1 production is favored.[32] In the tonsils and adenoids, unlike in the rest of the MALT, IgG immunocytes predominate and IgA-producing cells account for 30%–35%. IgA exists as a dimer, the two molecules being joined by a J chain. In the tonsils, unlike the adenoids, the dimeric IgA does not pick up a secretory piece as it passes through the epithelium. Instead, both IgG and IgA pass directly into the pharyngeal secretions by leaking between epithelial cells. This is enhanced by inflammation.[31]

IMMUNOPATHOPHYSIOLOGY

Anatomic Changes

Recurrent and chronic infection leads to tonsillar hyperplasia and/or nodularity. Microscopically, there is expansion of the

Table 47–5. CYTOKINES PRODUCED IN VIVO IN PATIENTS WITH RECURRENT TONSILLITIS OR INFECTIOUS MONONUCLEOSIS

Cytokine	Antibody	Isotype	Producer
IL-1α	1277-89-7, 1277-82-29	Mouse IgG1	H. Towbin (Ciba-Geigy, Basel, Switzerland)
	1279-143-4	Mouse IgG1	
IL-1β	2-D-8	Mouse IgG1	H. Towbin (Ciba-Geigy)
IL-1ra	1384-92-17-19	Mouse IgG1	H. Towbin (Ciba-Geigy)
IL-2	MQ1-17H12	Rat IgG2a	J. Abrams (DNAX, Palo Alto, CA)
IL-3	BVD8-6G8	Rat IgG	J. Abrams (DNAX)
	BVD3-IF9	Rat IgG1	
IL-4	MP4-25D2	Rat IgG1	J. Abrams (DNAX)
IL-5	JES-39D10	Rat IgG2a	J. Abrams (DNAX)
IL-6	MQ2-6A3	Rat IgG	J. Abrams (DNAX)
IL-8	NAP-1	Mouse IgG1	M. Ceska (Sandoz, Vienna, Austria)
IL-10	JES3-19F1	Rat IgG2a	J. Abrams (DNAX)
	JES3-12G8	Rat IgG2a	J. Abrams (DNAX)
IL-13	JES8-5A2	Rat IgG2a	J. Abrams (DNAX)
	JES8-30F11	Rat IgG2a	J. Abrams (DNAX)
GM-CSF	BVD2-21C11	Rat IgG2a	J. Abrams (DNAX)
	BVD2-5A2	Rat IgG2a	J. Abrams (DNAX)
G-CSF	BVD13-3A5	Rat IgG	J. Abrams (DNAX)
	BVD11-37G10	Rat IgG	J. Abrams (DNAX)
TNF-α	MP9-20A4	Rat IgG	J. Abrams (DNAX)
TNF-β	LTX 21	Mouse IgG2b	G. Adolf (Boehringer-Ingelheim, Vienna, Austria)
	LTX 22	Mouse IgG1	
IFN-γ	DIK1	Mouse IgG1	G. Andersson (KABI, Stockholm, Sweden)
TGF-β1	96	Polyclonal rabbit IgG	K. Miyazono (Ludwig Inst., Uppsala, Sweden)
TGF-β2	94	Polyclonal rabbit IgG	K. Miyazono (Ludwig Inst.)
TGF-β3	95	Polyclonal rabbit IgG	K. Miyazono (Ludwig Inst.)

From Andersson J, Abrams J, Bjork J, et al.: Concomitant in vivo production of 19 different cytokines in human tonsils. Immunology 1994; 83: 16–24. Blackwell Science Ltd.

lymphoid follicles with prominent germinal center formation. Polymorphonuclear cells may be seen in the epithelium, and aggregates of inflammatory cells and bacteria may be present within the crypts. If there is a viral component to the infection multinucleated giant cells may also be seen (Fig. 47–1).

Cellular Changes

Chronic inflammation results initially in an increase in reticulated epithelium. Later, however, the crypts become lined with squamous epithelium, which lacks the M cells that facilitate antigen entry.[41] This may lead to a decrease in the amount of antigen processed for presentation to T cells. In addition, patients with focal tonsillar infection have fewer tonsillar follicular dendritic cells in the lymphoepithelial symbiosis area.[42] Since multiple interactions are necessary for correct T-cell response, decreased antigen presentation may lead to suppression of the immune response. It has been shown that suboptimal signaling of T cells leads to partial activation and that the partially activated T cells may produce cell surface receptors for cytokines but do not proliferate. This partial activation may actually lead to tolerance, inhibition of ongoing responsiveness, and defective IL-2 production.[37]

Berstein and colleagues illustrated decreased production of IL-2 in 34 patients who underwent adenoidectomy or adenotonsillectomy. In these patients, adenoidal T cells were found to support B-cell production of the major immunoglobulin isotypes poorly. This was attributed to decreased IL-2 production, in response to stimulation by both mitogens and specific antigens, by adenoidal and tonsillar lymphocytes, as compared with peripheral blood lymphocytes. Interestingly, this decreased IL-2 production was observed in the context of much spontaneous lymphoproliferative activity.

The authors suggested that continuous background stimulation of tonsillar and adenoidal lymphocytes may lead to an increase in unstimulated proliferative activity while it blunts the response to specific antigenic challenges.[43]

Koch and Brodsky also examined lymphocyte activation in patients with chronic tonsillar disease. They noted a decreased proliferative response to *H. influenzae* type B and *S. pyogenes* stimulation in diseased tonsils as compared with controls. In addition, after stimulation, the death rate of diseased tonsillar lymphocytes was accelerated. Their evidence suggests that lymphocytes from diseased tonsils become refractory or tolerant to immune activation by certain pathogens associated with chronic tonsillar disease.[44] This finding was further supported and expanded by other workers who examined the response of tonsillar and peripheral blood lymphocytes to mitogenic and antigenic stimulation. They found that, while baseline mitogenic activity was high, the response to stimulation in these two lymphocyte populations was blunted. This decreased response was attributed to continued release of immunosuppressive factors, and the proliferative response recovered after tonsillectomy.[45] Thus, in certain situations hyperplastic tonsils may be viewed as immunocompromised organs that may decrease the overall effectiveness of the local immune system.

Patients with recurrent tonsillitis also exhibit B-cell deficiencies. Underlying them may be the decrease of IL-2 discussed previously or other additional changes in the lymphokine profiles produced by the antigen-presenting cells and T-cell subsets. Such changes may lead to reduced maintenance of the memory B-cell clones and decreased production of secretory IgA.[32] This has been evidenced by the reduced generation of J chain–expressing B cells in children with recurrent tonsillitis.[46]

Another cell important to the immune response is the neutrophil, which phagocytoses and destroys opsonized microorganisms. Chronic infections negatively affect neutrophil

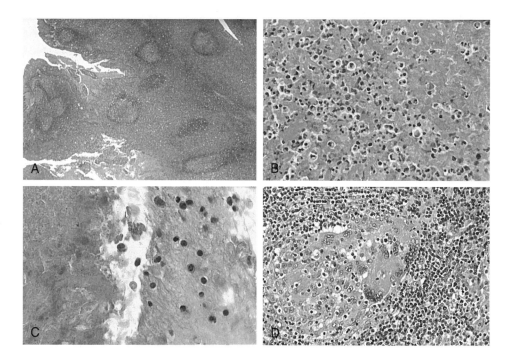

Figure 47–1. *A,* This low-power photomicrograph shows the typical lymphoid hyperplasia seen in chronic tonsillitis. Eccentric mantle zones around the germinal centers are typical for benign reactive hyperplasia. *B,* Polymorphonuclear (PMN) cells are seen in the crypt epithelium in this patient with chronic tonsillitis. *C,* Colonies of cocci are seen embedded in fibrinous material within the crypt. The crypt epithelium shows many PMN cells. *D,* This large multinucleated cell can be seen in fungal and in viral infection. Subsequent Gomori's methenamine silver staining of this sample failed to reveal fungal elements. Examination of the peripheral blood of this patient showed a large percentage of atypical lymphocytes, a finding consistent with a concomitant viral infection.

chemotactic functions.[47] Neutrophil function was studied in 17 patients aged 4–11 years who had chronic tonsillitis and adenoidal hypertrophy. In these patients, chemotaxis was significantly lower as compared with controls. Repeat evaluation 10 days after surgery showed no statistical difference between the two groups, but the increase in the chemotactic response in postoperative neutrophil function was significant as compared with preoperative values.[48]

Immunoglobulin Changes

The effect of chronic adenotonsillitis on immunoglobulins has been studied at the tonsillar and the peripheral blood level. Several changes are induced by chronic inflammation, and some can be correlated with the presence of bacteria typically seen in adenotonsillar infections. As has been stated previously, IgG and IgA are the principal antibodies produced in response to antigenic challenge; however, it is notable that IgD-producing cells are more prevalent in the MALT than in the gut-associated lymphoid tissue.[31] This may result from stimulation of resting B cells, which express IgD, by *H. influenzae* and *M. catarrhalis*. These bacteria, which frequently colonize the upper aerodigestive tract, produce an IgD-binding factor that cross-links IgD and human leukocyte antigen (HLA) class I molecules. This stimulates B-cell proliferation in a polyclonal manner and results in increased production of IgD and preferential production of secretory IgA1 (SIgA1) over production of secretory IgA2.

The production of IgD and the preferential production of SIgA1 have important implications for the local immune response. First, IgD cannot act as a secretory immunoglobulin. Thus, the cells that are directed to differentiate to produce this immunoglobulin are effectively removed from the immunoglobulin-producing cell pool. Second, *H. influenzae* produces a protease that cleaves IgA1. *S. pneumoniae* and *Neisseria meningitidis* also produce this protease. Thus, these bacteria, which are often found in patients with chronic adenotonsillitis, have developed both a mechanism to drive antibody production toward IgA1 and a mechanism to cleave this product with specific proteases.[32]

These immunoglobulin changes must be related to the common finding of increased immunoglobulin levels in the peripheral blood of patients with chronic tonsillitis. Significant elevations in IgG, IgA, IgM, and IgE have been found in patients with chronic tonsillitis. After tonsillectomy, these values returned to normal.[49–51] This seeming paradox of increased immunoglobulin levels in patients with chronic infection can be explained by the previously discussed T- and B-cell studies. Given the constant stimulation of the immune system in patients with chronic adenotonsillitis, there is background elevation of mitotic activity and antibody production. However, in response to stimulation by specific bacteria, production above this baseline is limited, as is shown by the decreased mitogenic activity of both tonsillar and peripheral blood lymphocytes. There may also be concomitant inability to increase the production of specific antibodies in response to specific infectious agents.

Kurono and colleagues illustrated this last point by examining SIgA levels and adherence of *S. pyogenes* to nasal mucosal cells. Secretory IgA inhibits bacterial adherence

to mucosal cells by attaching to the bacterial surface and interfering directly with the bacterial surface antigen component's adherence to the epithelium. In their study of 29 patients with chronic sinusitis they found elevated levels of SIgA as compared with 25 controls. Despite this, bacterial adherence to nasal mucosa was increased in patients with chronic sinusitis. It is apparent from these results that, though the immune system may produce large quantities of immunoglobulin, there may still be diminished activity in response to specific antigens.[52] A similar situation may exist in patients with chronic tonsillitis, but specific data are lacking.

The preceding discussion highlights the multiple immune defects that may be present in patients with chronic tonsillitis (Table 47–6). It can be seen that a cycle of infection leading to epithelial changes leading to decreased antigen presentation and immune function, which then leads to further infection, may be occurring in these patients. Other influences may further decrease the immune response. Which factors are the causative agents and which are responses or merely associated factors has not been fully delineated.

CLINICAL MANIFESTATIONS

Signs and Symptoms

The symptoms of acute tonsillar disease have been documented since the second and third centuries B.C.[2] The extreme throat discomfort, odynophagia, and tender cervical lymph nodes are familiar to every pediatrician and almost every parent. Symptoms, however, vary in different children. Toddlers may have a slight sore throat, low-grade fever, decreased appetite, lethargy, and anterior cervical lymphadenopathy. Older children, on the other hand, are more ill and have more severe pain and fever to 39° C or higher.[53] Dry throat, malaise, and otalgia may be accompanying symptoms.[12]

On physical examination the tonsils appear erythematous and swollen. Exudate may be seen on the entire surface of the tonsils or may be punctate and emanating from the tonsillar crypts. Petechiae may be seen on the soft palate, and a scarletiniform rash may be present. Dry mucous membranes with thickened secretions result from the decreased oral intake that characteristically accompanies an acute bout of tonsillitis. Usually there is no deviation of the uvula from the midline or associated trismus. The folds of the anterior tonsillar pillars are not effaced; that finding is more common in peritonsillar abscess. If the patient is quite ill from acute tonsillitis and requires hospital admission a complete blood

Table 47–6. IMMUNE DEFECTS IN PATIENTS WITH CHRONIC TONSIL DISEASE

M-cell loss	Impaired neutrophil chemotaxis
Decreased dendritic cells	Increased IgD production
Decreased activation of T cells	Preferential IgA1 production
Decreased IL-2 production	Reduced mucociliary clearance
Release of immunosuppressive factors	Beta-lactamase production
Reduced maintenance of B-cell clones	Loss of protective bacteria
Reduced J-chain–positive B cells	

count may be performed. This may show an elevated white cell count in the high teens or low twenty-thousand range, with a leftward shift. Recurrent infection leads to hyperplasia and tonsillar enlargement. Usually, adenoiditis that accompanies tonsillitis leads to adenoidal hypertrophy, and patients often complain of nasal congestion, rhinorrhea, chronic mild sore throat, halitosis, or disturbed breathing due to the obstructive hyperplasia. Their tonsils may be large and cryptic (Fig. 47–2), with thickening and nodularity of the epithelium or collections of debris emanating from the opening of a crypt. With fibrotic involution, however, the tonsils may appear small and the crypts accentuated. Examination of the neck reveals multiple small, nontender, lymph nodes.

Diagnostic Tests

In addition to a detailed history and thorough physical examination, throat culture has been used both to determine the causative organism of an episode of tonsillitis and to evaluate the success of medical therapy. Traditionally, culture of a throat swab is performed before institution of antibiotic therapy. More than 30 million throat swabs are processed annually for group A streptococci (GAS) in the United States[54]; however, culture has little effect on the treatment of a suspected group A streptococcal infection. In the majority of cases, antibiotic therapy is instituted before culture results are obtained, and, in half of these cases, therapy is continued regardless of culture results.[55] Over the last several years, a variety of in vitro immunologic diagnostic tests have been developed to detect GAS. These tests provide rapid results when performed as a point-of-care test and can eliminate the 48-hour turnaround time required to obtain results from culture methods.[56] All of these in vitro methods require the binding of GAS antigen to a specific antibody.[55] Reported sensitivity for these rapid test methods ranges from 54% to 100%, and specificities range from 45% to 99%.[57] The appropriate application for these immunoassays is not clear. Some authors suggest that the optical immunoassays are both sensitive and specific enough to obviate culture; others still recommend confirmatory cultures as part of the work-up for patients suspected to have bacterial tonsillitis.[55, 58]

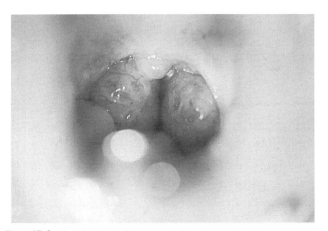

Figure 47–2. These large tonsils show prominent crypts with some thickening of the covering epithelium.

Differential Diagnosis

Diphtheria can present with throat pain and high fevers; however, the pseudomembranes associated with this disease can cover the tonsils, soft palate, and tonsillar pillars and may extend to the nose or larynx. They are gray, with distinct borders, and their removal leads to bleeding of the underlying mucosal surfaces. Swelling of the neck tissues may form a distinct collar, running from ear to ear, and may fill out the space beneath the jaw (bull neck).[59]

Infectious mononucleosis is a viral infection of the entire lymphoreticular system. Caused by the Epstein-Barr virus, it can lead to extreme swelling of the tonsils, which are often covered with a malodorous gray exudate. Infectious mononucleosis can be distinguished from acute bacterial tonsillitis with a determination of the white blood cell count and differential, which shows at least 50% lymphocytes with 10% atypical lymphocytes. Heterophile antibody testing, as well as determination of antibody titers against core and envelope antigens, can help determine if an acute immune response to this virus is being mounted.

TREATMENT

Antibiotic Therapy

Penicillin is considered the antibiotic of choice for acute tonsillitis, due to the belief that the majority of these cases are caused by group A beta-hemolytic streptococci (GABHS).[60] The mean inhibitory and bactericidal concentration of penicillin G to isolates of this organism is approximately 0.005 μg/mL. A single injection of benzathine penicillin G has been considered to be the "gold standard" in the treatment of acute tonsillitis. Oral penicillin, however, has been shown to be as effective as intramuscular penicillin and is now preferred by most primary care physicians.[61] A 10-day course of 250 mg for children younger than 12 and 500 mg for older children and adults, twice or thrice daily, has been shown to be equally effective therapy for acute tonsillitis.[62–64] Thus, the commonly practiced four times daily treatment with high-dose penicillin has not been proven necessary.[65]

In patients with chronic and recurrent tonsillitis, however, several theories have been put forward to explain the failure of treatment with penicillin. These include the appearance of penicillin-resistant alpha-hemolytic streptococci, increased incidence of infection with *H. influenzae* and *S. aureus,* and poor patient compliance.[66] When the bacterial pathogen may be resistant, therapy with erythromycin, clindamycin, or a cephalosporin has been suggested.[21, 67] Other reasons for treatment failure include bacterial co-pathogenicity, loss of protective bacteria, bacterial influences, and decreased immune function in the tonsillar tissues.

Several studies and meta-analysis of data have shown that cephalosporins are twice as effective as penicillins for treatment of GABHS pharyngitis. Clinical failure rates for cephalosporins and penicillins were 5% and 11%[68]; however, there are also concerns about the use of cephalosporins as first-line therapy for tonsillopharyngitis. These include their antimicrobial spectrum, which is broader than necessary, potential side effects, and price. Consideration of the local prevalence of resistant bacteria, the size of tonsil with respect to the likelihood that co-pathogenic bacteria are present in significant numbers, duration of the present infection, and number of previous tonsillitis episodes in a particular patient may allow the clinician to decide which antibiotic is best to use in a particular case.

Bacterial co-pathogenicity involves the protection of a pathogenic bacterial strain from antimicrobial therapies by nonpathogenic or mildly pathogenic bacteria that produce beta-lactamase. In these cases, the beta-lactamase produced by the nonpathogenic bacteria breaks down the penicillin (or amoxicillin) usually used to treat the acute tonsillar infection. Beta-lactamase–producing organisms have been cultured in a large percentage of patients with recurrent tonsillitis, and, as stated previously, more than 40% of patients with chronic tonsillar disease may have beta-lactamase–producing organisms in their tonsillar core that are not detected by surface culture.

In addition to co-pathogenicity, patients with chronic tonsillitis, by virtue of treatment of antecedent acute episodes, are likely to have lost some of the protective bacteria that are constituents of the normal oral flora. This change in the normal flora has been shown to contribute to increased sensitivity to invading microorganisms in the mucous membranes.[69] It has been found that frequent penicillin treatment of patients with recurrent tonsillitis leads to significant loss of alpha-hemolytic streptococci, specifically the alpha-hemolytic streptococci that have the capability to block injection with their own pathogenic group A streptococci.[70] This phenomenon is apparently reversible, and inoculation of interfering bacteria has been shown to decrease the risk of recurrence of tonsillar infection.[71]

Along with these changes, chronic adenotonsillar disease is associated with immunoglobulin changes that may increase the likelihood of recurrent tonsillitis. Pathogenic organisms can cause a shift in the antibody makeup of the local immunity by increasing the production of IgD and SIgA1. IgD is not effective in clearing or neutralizing pathogens, whereas SIgA1 is more easily destroyed by bacteria known to cause sinusitis in children. Thus, the pathogens have developed methods to protect themselves from the body's defenses.

Finally, antibiotic failure may be related to decreased tonsillar immune function and diminished local immune response. Chronic inflammation leads to a decrease in the amount of antigen processed for presentation to T cells and incomplete antigen-presenting cell–lymphocyte interaction. Suboptimal signaling of T cells may lead to partial activation of the T cells, which then produce cell surface receptors for cytokines but do not proliferate. Rather than effecting an immune response, this partial activation may actually lead to tolerance, inhibition of ongoing responsiveness, and defective proliferation and IL-2 production.[37]

Antibiotic Prophylaxis

Prophylactic antibiotic therapy has been used as an alternative to tonsillectomy in patients with recurrent and chronic tonsillitis. Prophylactic therapy with sulfadimidine has, dec-

ades ago, been shown to decrease the recurrences of GABHS tonsillitis.[72] A recent study of 179 patients treated with long-acting penicillin as prophylactic therapy against recurrent tonsillitis showed a significant reduction in the number of attacks of tonsillitis. However, because this study was performed in Sri Lanka the results may not be applicable to patients in the United States, where the prevalence of beta-lactamase–producing organisms may render this type of therapy less effective.

Tonsillectomy

Tonsillectomy has been performed for more than 3000 years, yet there is no consensus about the indications for the procedure.[73] This option should be considered when episodes of pharyngotonsillitis recur with disturbing frequency, whether or not they are caused by GABHS.[55] Paradise and colleagues examined 187 children who had seven episodes of throat infection in 1 year, five in each of 2 years, or three in 3 years. They found that 92% of tonsillectomy subjects had had no moderate or severe episodes of tonsillitis, as compared with 34% of controls. They concluded that the use of tonsillectomy was warranted in the patients that met their strict criteria.[74] Kavanagh and Beckford noted that patients with four or more episodes in a year would miss more than 2½ weeks of school, would require multiple visits to the doctor, and would be given numerous courses of antibiotics. They recommended tonsillectomy for these patients.[8]

Since tonsillectomy is such a common procedure, much attention has been focused on the indications for this procedure. Panels of physicians have participated in developing guidelines for tonsillectomy in patients with recurrent tonsillitis. Many agree that patients who have had four episodes of tonsillitis in the past year may be considered candidates for tonsillectomy. Fewer episodes may be considered an indication if one or more has been complicated by a peritonsillar abscess or airway obstruction, has led to hospitalization, or has caused the patient to miss 5 days or more of school or work (Table 47–7).[75]

Tonsillectomy is not without complication, and the risks of surgery must always be weighed when making the decision to operate. Complications are generally considered to be between 1% and 5%.[9, 76] In a study of 3340 cases, a major complication rate of 1.4% was found.[77] The most common complication is postoperative bleeding, which may be a minor amount of bleeding from the tonsillar fossa or a major life-threatening hemorrhage. Persistent hypernasality has been reported to occur in 1 in 1500 procedures, and results from a latent abnormality of the palate that is revealed during surgery. Surgical intervention is necessary in as many as 50% of these cases.[78] Other rare but important complications include mandibular fracture, nasopharyngeal stenosis, and torticollis (Table 47–8).

COMPLICATIONS OF TONSILLITIS

The many complications of tonsillitis include those that are obstructive, immune-mediated, toxin-mediated, and infectious. Patients with hyperplastic tonsils may develop respira-

Table 47-7. GUIDELINES FOR PRECERTIFICATION OF TONSILLECTOMY (REVISED JUNE 1995)

Tonsillectomy (With or Without Adenoidectomy) for Patients With Recurrent Acute Tonsillitis:	Number of Episodes of Tonsillitis (or Tonsillopharyngitis) Year Before Last		
	0–2	*3*	*≥4*
A. Age <16 years			
1. 1 or 2 episodes of tonsillitis (or tonsillopharyngitis) in the past year:			
a. None severe	Fail (1)		
b. 1 severe	Fail (2)		Pass (3)
c. 2 or more severe	Pass (4)		
2. 3 episodes of tonsillitis (or tonsillopharyngitis) in the past year:			
a. None severe	*Fail (5)		
b. 1 severe	*Fail (6)	Pass (7)	
c. 2 or more severe	Pass (8)		
3. 4 episodes of tonsillitis (or tonsillopharyngitis) in the past year:			
a. None severe	*Fail (9)	Pass (10)	
b. 1 or more severe	Pass (11)		
4. 5 or more episodes of tonsillitis (or tonsillopharyngitis) in the past year	Pass (12)		

*Pass if proposed in conjunction with an adenoidectomy appropriate for ear disease or chronic nasal obstruction.
From Pass-Fail Version of the Precertification Criteria for Tonsillectomy and Adenoidectomy. Santa Monica, California: Value Health Sciences, 1995.

tory distress when acute tonsillar inflammation leads to edema. In certain infections, for example, infection with the Epstein-Barr virus, the degree of swelling may be so severe that normally nonobstructive tonsils interfere with breathing. These patients may require a short course of steroids to decrease the swelling and resolve the airway problem. In some of these patients tonsillectomy may be required to alleviate the acute airway distress.

In certain patients, streptococcal tonsillitis can result in glomerulonephritis. Acute nephritic syndrome may develop 1–2 weeks after an acute streptococcal infection. Early administration of antibiotics does not prevent this sequela. This may vary from mild microhematuria with normal renal function to acute renal failure. Microscopically, all glomeruli appear enlarged and relatively bloodless, with diffuse mesangial cell proliferation and an increase in mesangial matrix. Antibodies to streptolysin O, DNase B, hyaluronidase, streptokinase, and NADase (streptozyme test) may confirm the diagnosis. The most frequent type of glomerulonephritis, however, is IgA nephropathy (IgAN), originally described by Berger and Hinglais in 1968.[79] This disease is slowly progressive and often leads to end-stage renal disease. In IgAN, infection of the upper respiratory tract leads to macroscopic hematuria. High levels of polymeric IgA circulating immune complexes may be detected in the blood of these patients. IgAN has been associated with chronic tonsillitis, and tonsillectomy has been effective in ameliorating this condition in many patients.[80]

Prior to the advent of antibiotics for the treatment of acute tonsillitis, acute rheumatic fever (ARF) was the most serious infectious complication of acute streptococcal infection. This entity is a syndrome encompassing three separate but related clinical entities: arthritis, carditis, and chorea (Table 47–9).[81] In addition, it can lead to continued valvular heart disease and valvular dysfunction.[82] With the introduction of sulfonamides, and later penicillin, the incidence as well as the severity of disease decreased from the 1950s through the 1980s. In fact, reports of the disappearance of ARF from Chicago and Baltimore appeared in the 1970s[74, 83]; however, beginning in the mid- to late 1980s, reports of increasing numbers of cases of ARF began to emerge from a variety of areas in the United States.[84–86] While nationally the number of cases has declined somewhat in the last several years, it is still above that of the mid-1970s to early 1980s.[87, 88] It is thought that the focal areas of increased incidence can be attributed to certain highly rheumatogenic strains of GABHS.[75] These strains may be highly mucoid and heavily encapsulated, making them intrinsically more capable of triggering the immune mechanisms that lead to ARF.[89] This

Table 47-8. COMPLICATIONS OF TONSILLECTOMY

Hemorrhage	Cardiac arrest
Major	Malignant hyperthermia
Minor	Aspiration pneumonitis
Hypernasality	Horner's syndrome
Airway obstruction	Mandibular fracture
Nasopharyngeal stenosis	Torticollis
Broken tooth	

Table 47-9. GUIDELINES FOR THE DIAGNOSIS OF AN INITIAL ATTACK OF RHEUMATIC FEVER (JONES CRITERIA, UPDATED 1992)

Major Manifestations	Minor Manifestations	Supporting Evidence of Antecedent Group A Streptococcal Infection
Carditis	Clinical findings	Positive result of a
Polyarthritis	Arthralgia	culture or a rapid
Chorea	Fever	streptococcal antigen
Erythema marginatum	Laboratory findings	test
Subcutaneous nodules	Elevated acute-phase	Elevated or rising titer
	reactants	of streptococcal
	Erythrocyte	antibody
	sedimentation	
	rate	
	C-reactive protein	
	Prolonged P-R	
	interval	

From Denny FW Jr: A 45-year perspective on the *Streptococcus* and rheumatic fever: the Edward H. Kass Lecture in Infectious Disease History. Clin Infect Dis 1994; 19: 1110–1122.

resurgence of cases of ARF underscores the importance of early and accurate diagnosis as well as effective antibiotic treatment of streptococcal respiratory tract infections to prevent the initial attack of ARF.

Scarlet fever is the classic toxin-mediated form of GABHS infection and was a major killer in past centuries and earlier this century.[90] This disease is characterized by fever, vomiting, toxicity, and chills, followed by the appearance in 12–24 hours of a red, punctate or finely papular exanthem. In addition to pharyngitis, the tongue may develop a thick white coat with red papillae, followed by a red tongue after desquamation of the white debris. Desquamation of the skin begins toward the end of the first week and may continue as long as 6 weeks, depending on the severity of the rash.[91] Fortunately, the incidence and severity of this entity have decreased dramatically, and by the early 1980s severe scarlet fever had become virtually extinct in the United States.

While scarlet fever has become rare, another toxin-mediated illness associated with GABHS has gained attention in recent literature.[92] These infections can lead to hypotension, renal impairment, coagulopathy, and death (Table 47–10).[93] This type of infection has been referred to as "toxic shock–like syndrome" because of its similarity to the *Staphylococcus*-induced toxic shock syndrome.

Today, the most common infectious complication is peritonsillar abscess, which may result from extension of an acute exudative tonsillitis or from abscess formation within Weber's salivary glands in the supratonsillar fossa.[2] Different treatments for peritonsillar abscess, in addition to antibiotic therapy, include needle aspiration, incision and drainage, and tonsillectomy (tonsillectomy à chaud, quinsy tonsillectomy). Another sequela of acute tonsillitis is parapharyngeal or retropharyngeal abscess (Fig. 47–3). This results from abscess formation within one of the nodes of these areas, which drain the tonsils and pharynx. Treatment requires antibiotics and, usually, incision and drainage of the abscess via an intraoral, external, or combined approach. If not successfully treated, the infection may spread to the surrounding neck spaces and into the chest. In all cases of infectious complications, therapy should include antibiotics that are beta-lactamase stable and effective against anaerobes.

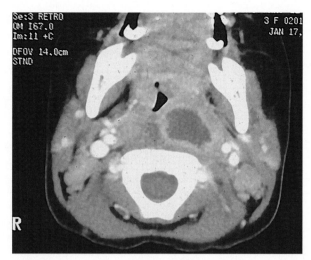

Figure 47–3. This axial computed tomography scan done with intravenous contrast enhancement shows a large hyperdense area surrounded by an enhancing rim in the left retropharynx. Spread of infection to lymph nodes can lead to abscess formation in either the retropharyngeal or parapharyngeal spores.

CONCLUSION

Tonsillitis continues to be a commonly treated entity. The microbiology, and the bacterial resistance against commonly used antimicrobials, have changed over the last several decades. Initial treatment regimens must be reevaluated, taking into consideration this changing microflora. Treatment of chronic tonsillitis involves correcting the deficiencies that have led to the cycle of repeated infections, including loss of protective bacteria, presence of co-pathogens, and changes in the immune function and immunoglobulin makeup. Therapies directed at reconstituting the normal microflora, such as inoculation of alpha-hemolytic streptococci into the oropharynges of patients with recurrent tonsillitis and restoring normal immune function, may lead to improved medical therapy and decreased need for operative treatment of this common disorder.

Table 47–10. CASE DEFINITION OF TOXIC SHOCK–LIKE SYNDROME (TSLS)

I. Isolation of group A streptococci
   A. From a normally sterile site
   B. From a normally nonsterile site
II. Clinical signs
   A. Hypotension (systolic blood pressure ≤90 mm Hg in adults or <5th percentile for age in children)
   B. At least two of the following:
     1. Renal impairment
     2. Coagulopathy
     3. Liver involvement
     4. Adult respiratory distress syndrome
     5. Generalized erythematous macular rash that may desquamate
     6. Soft tissue necrosis
A definite case fulfills I A and II (A and B).
A probable case fulfills I B and II (A and B).

From Working Group on Severe Streptococcal Infections: Defining the group A streptococcal toxic shock syndrome. JAMA 1993; 269: 390–391.

References

1. Bicknell P: Role of adenotonsillectomy in the management of pediatric ear nose and throat infections. Pediatr Infect Dis J 1994; 13:S75–S78.
2. Passy V: Pathogenesis of peritonsillar abscess. Laryngoscope 1994; 104:185–190.
3. Nelson W, Behrman R, Kliegman R, et al.: Infectious diseases: Bacterial infections. In: Behrman RE (ed): Nelson Textbook of Pediatrics, 14th ed. Philadelphia: WB Saunders, 1992, p 698.
4. Hoekelman RA, Starfield B, McCormick M, et al.: A profile of pediatric practice in the United States. Am J Dis Child 1983; 137:1057–1060.
5. Hardy AM: Department of Health and Human Services. Incidence and impact of selected infectious disease in children. Vital and Health Statistics, Series 10, No. 180. DHHS Publ. No. (PHS) 91-1508. Hyattsville, Maryland: Centers for Disease Control, 1991.
6. Stentstrom C, Ingvarsson L: General illness and need of medical care in otitis prone children. Int J Pediatr Otorhinolaryngol 1994; 19:23–32.
7. de Melker RA, Kuyvenhoven MM: Management of upper respiratory infections in Dutch family practice. J Fam Pract 1994; 38:353–357.
8. Kavanagh KT, Beckford NS: Adenotonsillectomy in children: Indications and contraindications. S Med J 1988; 81:507–511.
9. Brodsky L: Modern assessment of tonsils and adenoids. Pediatr Clin North Am 1989; 36:1551–1569.

10. Bluestone CD: Current indications for tonsillectomy and adenoidectomy. Ann Otol Rhinol Laryngol 1992; 101:58–64.

11. Wheater PR, Burkitt HG, Daniels VG: Functional Histology. New York; Churchill Livingstone, 1979.

12. Zalzal GH, Cotton RT: Adenotonsillar disease. In: Cummings CW (ed): Otolaryngology Head and Neck Surgery. St. Louis: CV Mosby, 1986.

13. Gaudecker B, Muller-Hermelink HK: The development of the human tonsilla palatina. Cell Tissue Res 1982; 224:579–600.

14. Brook I: The clinical microbiology of Waldeyer's ring. Otolaryngol Clin North Am 1987; 20:259–272.

15. Ingvarsson L, Lundgren K, Irving J: The bacterial flora in the nasopharynx in healthy children. Acta Otolaryngol (Suppl) 1982; 386:94–96.

16. Willard CY, Hansen AE: Bacterial flora of the nasopharynx in children. Am J Dis Child 1981; 97:318–325.

17. Ylikoski J, Karjalainen J: Acute tonsillitis in young men: Etiological agents and their differentiation. Scand J Infect Dis 1989; 21:169–174.

18. Bieluch VM, Martin ET, Chasin WD, et al.: Recurrent tonsillitis: Histologic and bacteriologic evaluation. Ann Otol Rhinol Laryngol 1989; 98:332–335.

19. Klein JO: Microbiology of diseases of the tonsils and adenoids. Ann Otol Rhinol Laryngol 1975; 84(Suppl 19):30.

20. Moffet HL, Siegel AC, Doyle HK: Nonstreptococcal pharyngitis. J Pediatr 1968; 73:51.

21. Brook I, Hirokawa R: Treatment of patients with a history of recurrent tonsillitis due to group A β-hemolytic streptococci. Clin Pediatr 1985; 24:331–336.

22. Brook I, Foote PA: Microbiology of "normal" tonsils. Ann Otol Rhinol Laryngol 1990; 99:980–982.

23. Kielmovitch IH, Keleti G, Bluestone CD, et al.: Microbiology of obstructive tonsillar hypertrophy and recurrent tonsillitis. Arch Otolaryngol Head Neck Surg 1989; 115:721–724.

24. Surow JB, Handler SD, Telian SA, et al.: Bacteriology of tonsil surface and core in children. Laryngoscope 1989; 99:261–266.

25. Manolis E, Tsakris A, Kandiloros D, et al.: Alterations to the oropharyngeal and nasopharyngeal microbial flora of children after tonsillectomy and adenoidectomy. J Laryngol Otol 1994; 108:763–767.

26. Nord CE, Heimdahl A, Tuner K: Beta-lactamase producing anaerobic bacteria in the oropharynx and their clinical relevance. Scand J Infect Dis 1988; 57(Suppl):50–54.

27. Uppal K, Bais AS: Tonsillar microflora—superficial vs deep. J Laryngol Otol 1989; 103:175–177.

28. Finegold S: Role of anaerobic bacteria in infection of the tonsils and adenoids. Ann Otol Rhinol Laryngol Suppl 1991; 154:30–33.

29. Ozawa A, Sawamura S: Microbial ecology of tonsillar infection. Acta Otolaryngol Suppl 1988; 454:178–184.

30. Brodsky L, Nagy M, Volk M, et al.: The relationship of tonsil bacterial concentration to surface and core cultures in chronic tonsillar disease in children. Int J Pediatr Otorhinolaryngol 1991; 21:33–39.

31. Scadding GK: Immunology of the tonsil: A review. J Roy Soc Med 1990; 83:104–107.

32. Brandtzaeg P, Halstensen TS: Immunology and immunopathology of tonsils. Adv Otorhinolaryngol 1992; 47:64–75.

33. Bernstein JM, Sendor S, Wactawski-Wende J: Antigen-presenting cells in the nasopharyngeal tonsil. Adv Otorhinolaryngol 1992; 47:80–90.

34. Yamamoto Y, Okato S, Nishiyama M, et al.: Function and morphology of macrophages in palatine tonsils. Adv Otorhinolaryngol 1992; 47:107–113.

35. von Gaudecker B: Development and functional anatomy of the human tonsilla palatina. Acta Otolaryngol 1988; (Suppl 454):28–32.

36. Hsu SM: Phenotypic expression of cells of stationary elements in human lymphoid tissue. A histochemical and immunohistochemical study. Hematol Pathol 1987; 1:45–56.

37. Geppert TD, Davis LS, Gur H, et al.: Accessory cell signals involved in T-cell activation. Immunol Rev 1990; 117:5–66.

38. Andersson J, Abrams J, Bjork L, et al.: Concomitant in vivo production of 19 different cytokines in human tonsils. Immunology 1994; 83:16–24.

39. Cortesina G, Carlevato MT, Bussi M, et al.: T-lymphocyte role in the immunological reactivity of palatine tonsil. Adv Otorhinolaryngol 1992; 47:101–106.

40. Wong DT, Ogra PL: Immunology of tonsils and adenoids—an update. Int J Pediatr Otorhinolaryngol 1980; 2:181–191.

41. Surgan L Jr: Tonsils and lymphoepithelial structures in the pharynx as immunobarriers. Acta Otolaryngol 1987; 103:369–372.

42. Yamamoto Y, Okato H, Takahashi H, et al.: The distribution and morphology of macrophages in the palatine tonsils. Acta Otolaryngol 1988; (Suppl 454):83–95.

43. Bernstein JM, Rich GA, Odziemiec C, et al.: Are thymus-derived lymphocytes (T cells) defective in the nasopharyngeal and palatine tonsils of children? Otolaryngol Head Neck Surg 1993; 109(4):693–700.

44. Koch RJ, Brodsky L: Effect of specific bacteria on lymphocyte proliferation in diseased and nondiseased tonsils. Laryngoscope 1993; 103:1020–1026.

45. Drucker MM, Agatsuma Y, Drucker I, et al.: Cell mediated immune response to bacterial products in human tonsils and peripheral blood lymphocytes. Infect Immunol 1979; 23:347–352.

46. Korsrud FR, Brandtzaeg P: Influence of tonsillar disease on the expression of J-chain by immunoglobulin-producing cells in human palatine and nasopharyngeal tonsils. Scand J Immunol 1981; 13:281–287.

47. Cazzola G, Valleta EA, Ciafonni S, et al.: Neutrophil function and humoral immunity in children with recurrent infections of the lower respiratory tract and chronic bronchial suppuration. Ann Allergy 1989; 63:213–218.

48. Sennaroglu L, Onerci M, Hascelik G: The effect of tonsillectomy and adenoidectomy on neutrophil chemotaxis. Laryngoscope 1993; 103:1349–1351.

49. Harbans L, Sachdeva OP, Mehta HR: Serum immunoglobulins in patients with chronic tonsillitis. J Laryngol Otol 1984; 98:1213–1216.

50. El-Ashmawy S, Taha A, Fatt-hi A, Basyouni A, et al.: Serum immunoglobulins in patients with chronic tonsillitis. J Laryngol Otol 1980; 94:1037–1045.

51. Yadav RS, Yadav SPS, Harbans L: Serum immunoglobulin E levels in children with chronic tonsillitis. Int J Pediatr Otorhinolaryngol 1992; 24:131–134.

52. Kurono Y, Fujiyoshi T, Mogi G: Secretory IgA and bacterial adherence to nasal mucosal cells. Ann Otol Rhinol Laryngol 1989; 98:273–277.

53. Shelov SP (ed): Caring for Your Baby and Young Child: Birth to Age 5. New York: Bantam, 1993, p 547.

54. Nadler H: Rapid detection of group A streptococci. Diagn Clin Testing 1989; 27:39–41.

55. Harbeck RJ, Teague J, Crossen GR, et al.: Novel, rapid optical immunoassay technique for detection of group A streptococci from pharyngeal specimens: Comparison with standard culture methods. J Clin Microbiol 1993; 31:839–844.

56. Heiter BJ, Bourbeau PP: Comparison of the Gen-Probe group A *Streptococcus* direct test with culture and a rapid streptococcal antigen detection assay for diagnosis of streptococcal pharyngitis. J Clin Microbiol 1993; 31:2070–2073.

57. Laubscher B, van Melle G, Dreyfuss N, et al.: Evaluation of a new immunologic test kit for rapid detection of group A streptococci, the Abbot Testpack Strep A Plus. J Clin Microbiol 1995; 33:260–261.

58. Dale JC, Vetter EA, Contezac JM, et al: Evaluation of two rapid antigen assays, Biostar Strep A OIA and Pacific Biotech CARDS O.S., and culture for detection of group A *Streptococcus* in throat swabs. J Clin Microbiol 1994; 32:2698–2701.

59. Remington J: Diphtheria. In: Behrman RE (ed): Nelson Textbook of Pediatrics, 14th ed. Philadelphia: WB Saunders, 1992, 720–724.

60. Paradise J: Etiology and management of pharyngitis and pharyngotonsillitis in children: A current review. Ann Otol Rhinol Laryngol 1992; 101:51–57.

61. Colcher IS, Bass JW: Penicillin treatment of streptococcal pharyngitis: A comparison of schedules and the role of specific counseling. JAMA 1972; 222:657–659.

62. Krober MS, Weir MR, Themelis NJ, et al.: Optimal dosing interval for penicillin treatment of streptococcal pharyngitis. Clin Pediatr 1990; 29:646–648.

63. Gerber MA, Randolph MF, DeMeo K, et al.: Failure of once daily penicillin V therapy for streptococcal pharyngitis. Am J Dis Child 1989; 143:153–155.

64. Gerber MA, Spadaccini LJ, Wright LL, et al.: Twice daily penicillin in the treatment of streptococcal pharyngitis. Am J Dis Child 1985; 139:1145–1148.

65. Bass JW: Antibiotic management of group A streptococcal pharyngotonsillitis. Pediatr Infect Dis J 1991; 10:S43–S49.

66. Brook I, Yocum P, Friedman E: Aerobic and anaerobic bacteria in tonsils of children with recurrent tonsillitis. Ann Otol 1981; 90:261–263.

67. Pichichero ME: The rising incidence of penicillin treatment failures in group A streptococcal tonsillopharyngitis: An emerging role for the cephalosporins? Pediatr Infect Dis J 1991; 10:S50–S55.

68. Pichichero ME: Cephalosporins are superior to penicillin for treatment of streptococcal pharyngitis: Is the difference worth it? Pediatr Infect Dis J 1993; 12:268–274.

69. Sanders CC, Sandres E: Enocin: An antibiotic produced by *Streptococcus salivarius* that may contribute to protection against infections due to group A streptococci. J Infect Dis 1982; 146:683–690.

70. Roos K, Grahn E, Holm SE: Evaluation of β-lactamase activity and microbial interference in treatment failures of acute streptococcal tonsillitis. Scand J Infect Dis 1986; 18:313–319.

71. Roos K, Grahn E, Holm SE, et al.: Interfering α-streptococci as a protection against recurrent streptococcal tonsillitis in children. Int J Pediatr Otorhinolaryngol 1993; 25:141–148.

72. Burke JB: Prophylactic sulphadimidine in children subject to recurrent infections of upper respiratory tract. Br Med J 1952; 1:538–541.

73. Bicknell P: Role of adenotonsillectomy in the management of pediatric ear, nose and throat infections. Pediatr Infect Dis J 1994; 13:S75–S78.

74. Paradise JL, Bluestone CE, Bachman RZ, et al.: Efficacy of tonsillectomy for recurrent throat infection in severely affected children: Results of parallel randomized and nonrandomized clinical trials. N Engl J Med 1984; 310:674–683.

75. Pass/Fail Version of the Precertification Criteria for Tonsillectomy and Adenoidectomy. Santa Monica, California: Value Health Sciences, 1995.

76. Richmond KH, Wetmore RF, Baranak CC: Postoperative complications following tonsillectomy and adenoidectomy—Who is at risk? Int J Pediatr Otorhinolaryngol 1987; 13:117.

77. Colclasure JB, Graham SS: Complications of outpatient tonsillectomy and adenoidectomy: A review of 3,340 cases. Ear Nose Throat J 1990; 69:155–160.

78. Donelly MJ: Hypernasality following adenoid removal. Ir J Med Sci 1994; 163:225–227.

79. Berger J, Hinglais N: Les depos intercapillaries d'IgA-IgG. J Urol Nephrol 1968; 74:694–695.

80. Sugiyama N, Shimizu J, Nakamura M, et al.: Clinicopathological study of the effectiveness of tonsillectomy in IgA nephropathy accompanied by chronic tonsillitis. Acta Otolaryngol 1993; 508(Suppl):43–48.

81. Denny FW Jr: A 45-year perspective on the *Streptococcus* and rheumatic fever: The Edward H Kass Lecture in infectious disease history. Clin Infect Dis 1994; 19:1110–1122.

82. Shulman ST: Complications of streptococcal pharyngitis. Pediatr Infect Dis 1994; 13:S70–S74.

83. Gordis L: The virtual disappearance of rheumatic fever in the United States: Lessons in the rise and fall of disease. T Duckett Jones Memorial Lecture. Circulation 1985; 72:1155–1162.

84. Veasy L, Weidmeier SE, Orsmond GS, et al.: Resurgence of acute rheumatic fever in the intermountain area of the United States. N Engl J Med 1987; 316:421–427.

85. Wald ER, Dashefsky B, Feidt C, et al.: Acute rheumatic fever in western Pennsylvania and the tristate area. Pediatrics 1987; 80:371–374.

86. Congeni B, Rizzo C, Congeni J, et al.: Outbreak of acute rheumatic fever in northeast Ohio. J Pediatr 1987; 111:176–179.

87. Veasy LG, Tani LY, Hill HR: Persistence of acute rheumatic fever in the intermountain area of the United States. J Pediatr 1994; 124:9–16.

88. Taubert KA, Rowley AH, Shulman ST: Nationwide survey of Kawasaki disease and acute rheumatic fever. J Pediatr 1991; 119:279–282.

89. Stollerman GH: The relative rheumatogenicity of strains of group A streptococci. Mod Concepts Cardiovasc Dis 1975; 44:35–40.

90. Weech AA: Scarlet fever in China. N Engl J Med 1931; 203:968–974.

91. Behrman RE (ed): Nelson Textbook of Pediatrics. Philadelphia: WB Saunders, 1992.

92. Stevens DL, Tanner MH, Winship J, et al.: Severe group A streptococcal infections associated with a toxic-shock–like syndrome and scarlet fever toxin. N Engl J Med 1989; 321:1–7.

93. Working Group on Severe Streptococcal Infections: Defining the group A streptococcal toxic shock syndrome. JAMA 1993; 269:390–391.

Scott P. Stringer

Peritonsillar Abscess

Peritonsillar abscess (PTA)—a collection of pus located between the fibrous capsule of the tonsil and the superior pharyngeal constrictor muscle—is the most common deep infection of the neck. Herzon determined, on the basis of a nationwide survey, that the incidence of PTA in the United States is 30.1 per 100,000 person-years or about 45,000 cases per year.[1] The first description of a PTA is most likely from the second and third century B.C. by Celsus, who recommended drainage of the abscess. Peritonsillar abscess has frequently been referred to in the past as "quinsy," a medieval English word for any throat affliction, and especially tonsillitis.[2] Before the advent of antibiotics and without proper management PTA represented a significant cause of mortality. George Washington may have died as a result of airway obstruction secondary to a peritonsillar abscess.[3]

ANATOMY

Bounded by the tonsil medially and the tonsillar fossa laterally, the peritonsillar space is a potential space. The tonsil is covered laterally by a fibrous capsule, which is a specialized portion of the pharyngobasilar fascia. The tonsillar fossa is defined by the palatoglossal fold anteriorly, the palatopharyngeal fold posteriorly, and the superior pharyngeal constrictor muscle laterally. Immediately deep to the superior pharyngeal constrictor muscle is the parapharyngeal space containing, in close proximity, the internal carotid artery and internal jugular vein.

PATHOPHYSIOLOGY

The most commonly held theory is that peritonsillar abscess occurs secondary to the penetration of bacteria from the tonsillar crypts through the tonsillar capsule and into the peritonsillar space. This is analogous to the formation of deep neck infections: it involves the seeding of a potential space or lymph node with bacteria and subsequent abscess formation, as do Ludwig's angina and retropharyngeal abscess. An alternative theory proposed by Passy involves a group of salivary glands in the supratonsillar space first described by Weber in 1927.[4] These glands send a ductal system to the surface of the tonsils and are thought to assist in the digestion of food particles in the tonsillar crypts. Passy noted that most peritonsillar abscesses occur in the supratonsillar region and, further, that peritonsillar abscess may occur without exudative tonsillitis. This theory seems unlikely, since (1) a number of authors have noted that a significant number of peritonsillar abscesses are located in the middle or inferior portion of the peritonsillar space[5–7]; (2) the obstruction and resultant infection of other salivary glands rarely form an abscess, especially when antibiotics are administered; and (3) an exudate on the tonsils is not required to make a diagnosis of tonsillitis. Fried and Forrest reported an association between dental caries and peritonsillar abscess in 27% of their patients, but this association could not be confirmed by others.[8, 9]

Pathogens

The results of cultures of peritonsillar abscess vary, particularly with respect to recovery of anaerobes, depending on the technique utilized. Anaerobes are particularly likely to be involved, as the peritonsillar space is a closed space and large numbers of anaerobes are present in the oral cavity and oropharynx. Brook and colleagues reported 18% of cultures grew anaerobes alone, 6% were exclusively aerobic, and 76% of cultures were mixed (aerobic and anaerobic).[10] Similar findings were noted by Savolainen and colleagues.[11] Specific bacterial species recovered and frequency of isolation vary by series, but the most common aerobic bacteria isolated include *Streptococcus pyogenes,* non–group A beta-hemolytic streptococci, *Streptococcus pneumoniae, Haemophilus influenzae, Streptococcus viridans,* and *Staphylococcus aureus.* Anaerobic species commonly cultured include *Peptostreptococcus, Fusobacterium* and *Actinomyces* species, *Bacteroides fragilis,* and *Bacteroides melaninogenicus.*[10–14] Brook's group noted an interesting pattern of culture results: in that *Bacteroides* species and *Peptostreptococcus* species as well *Bacteroides* species and *S. pyogenes* were almost exclusively isolated together.[10] Previous antibiotic therapy had no effect on the frequency or type of organisms cultured.[10, 14]

Jousimies-Somer and colleagues attempted to correlate culture results with clinical outcome. They noted that patients with pure aerobic cultures had had the fewest prior infections and were unlikely to need tonsillectomy or to experience a recurrence, whereas patients with the organism *Fusobacterium necrophorum* had a significant history of tonsillitis and their outcome was worse.[14]

Sugita and colleagues noted in 1982 that all of the organisms recovered were sensitive to penicillins or cephalosporins[12]; however, Brook and colleagues more recently noted the rising frequency of beta-lactamase–producing organisms, which they recovered in 15 of 52 isolates tested.[10] They further hypothesize that, given the large number of mixed cultures from peritonsillar abscesses, a single beta-lactamase–producing bacteria species may protect other species present in the abscess. Jousimies-Somer and colleagues noted that 38% of *Bacteroides* species tested produced beta-lactamases, and these organisms were present in 56% of patients.[14] Herzon reviewed the literature and found the reported incidence of penicillin-resistant organisms isolated from PTA to range from 0% to 68%.[1]

EPIDEMIOLOGY

PTA principally affects young people between the ages of 10 and 40 years (average age, mid-20s).[7, 13, 15–17] No consistent predilection for one side or sex has been demonstrated. Multiple authors have noted a bimodal seasonal pattern for PTA—in the late fall to early winter and again in the spring to early summer.[3, 15, 16, 18]

Bacterial tonsillitis may be confused with (and, rarely, occurs concurrently with) infectious mononucleosis. In a report of four cases of PTA in conjunction with infectious mononucleosis, Johnsen stated that fewer than 1% of PTA cases were associated with infectious mononucleosis.[19]

A number of series have demonstrated that the administration of antibiotics for tonsillitis does not necessarily prevent progression to PTA because 53%–89% of the patients seen with PTA were taking antibiotics at the time of diagnosis[11, 13, 15]; however, the sensitivities of the organisms to the initial antibiotics were not reported.

Patients presenting with PTA have been noted to have 21%–40% prevalence of a significant history of tonsillitis and a 0%–12% prevalence of prior PTA.[11, 13, 15, 17] Richardson and Birck noted a threefold increase in the incidence of PTA in children from 1969 to 1978, owing to the reduction in the number of tonsillectomies as a result of stricter operative indications.[20] The results from analyses of the incidence of PTA and recurrent tonsillitis following treatment of a PTA with methods other than tonsillectomy are discussed later in the chapter.

CLINICAL MANIFESTATIONS

Signs and Symptoms

The most common signs and symptoms associated with PTA are odynophagia, drooling, trismus, a "hot potato" voice, and fever. The symptoms typically have been present for 3–5 days before diagnosis.[13, 15, 17]

Physical Findings

Spires and colleagues detailed the prevalence of physical findings in 62 patients with PTA as follows: asymmetric peritonsillar swelling, 98%; deviation of uvula, 76%; trismus, 65%; hot potato voice, 61%; drooling, 57%; and tonsillar exudate, 51%.[16] The most common site of swelling is at the upper pole of the tonsil (Fig. 48–1), but Yung and Cantrell reported a 24% prevalence of abscesses in the middle to lower portion of the peritonsillar space.[7] Reports of a bilateral abscess range from 0% to 10%.[5, 7, 18, 20–22] The patients' temperatures varied between 36.4° and 39.5° C but

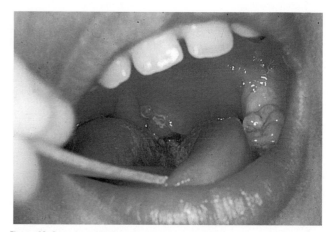

Figure 48–1. Intraoral photograph of a typical peritonsillar abscess demonstrating supratonsillar swelling pushing the tonsil inferomedially. Note also the deviation of the uvula and, in this case, exudative tonsillitis.

typically are around 38° C.[13, 17] Other series have confirmed the prevalence of trismus to be in the range of 55%–65%.[13, 23] Each patient should also be examined for signs of volume depletion, which is common with PTA.

DIFFERENTIAL DIAGNOSIS

Differentiating a peritonsillar abscess from most other disease processes is relatively straightforward. Infectious diseases that may mimic a peritonsillar abscess include buccal or masticator space abscess, parapharyngeal or retropharyngeal space abscess, and infectious mononucleosis. Examination of the oral cavity allows differentiation of buccal space or masticator space abscesses, which occur farther anterior in the oral cavity and are associated with a normal peritonsillar area. Confusion may result, owing to the common findings of trismus, odynophagia, fever, and perhaps drooling. If examination alone does not confirm the diagnosis, imaging studies will define the involved fascial compartment. Parapharyngeal and retropharyngeal abscesses independent of a peritonsillar abscess are usually the result of lymphadenitis that suppurates in the region. Signs and symptoms may be similar to those of PTA. Examination should reveal subtle differences in location and depth of the bulge in the pharynx. A combination of needle aspiration and imaging effectively distinguishes these entities. One of the more difficult infections to differentiate from PTA is infectious mononucleosis. The tonsils may be extremely enlarged as well as exudative and asymmetric, owing to infectious mononucleosis. Trismus, however, should not be present. Multiple enlarged and tender cervical lymph nodes should warrant consideration of a Monospot test. As previously mentioned, PTA may occur in association with infectious mononucleosis. If the patient with a positive Monospot does not respond to appropriate management, needle aspiration of the peritonsillar space may be indicated as a diagnostic maneuver.

The most difficult differential diagnostic decision is between PTA and peritonsillar cellulitis (PTC), an inflammation in the peritonsillar space without purulence. PTC and PTA may represent points on a continuum of peritonsillar infectious disease. PTC usually resolves with antibiotics alone, whereas, barring spontaneous rupture, PTA does not. Several attempts have been made to separate the two entities on the basis of signs and symptoms. Shoemaker and colleagues found that dysphagia, drooling, and greater age were suggestive of abscess, and trismus was associated with cellulitis.[9] They noted, however, that the differences were small and the symptoms were all quite common in both groups. Brodsky and colleagues were unable to differentiate PTA from PTC on the basis of age, duration of symptoms, temperature, white blood cell count, or the presence of trismus.[24] They did find that drooling was more commonly associated with PTA and that symptoms improved faster with PTC. Ophir and colleagues found that a "positive aspirate" did not correlate with temperature, trismus, or duration of symptoms.[13] Analysis of these and other series suggests that there is no reliable method for differentiating PTC from PTA on the basis of signs and symptoms alone.[2, 8, 25] In the absence of clear data to differentiate PTC from PTA, the use of diagnostic needle aspiration and the response of the patient to appropriate management remain the best methods for separation of these entities.

Neoplastic causes of a tonsillar swelling or deviation include lymphoma, tonsillar squamous cell carcinoma, parotid neoplasms, paragangliomas, neural neoplasms, and connective tissue neoplasms. Neoplasms occurring in the tonsil itself lack a peritonsillar bulge. Also, the history is typically protracted and other associated symptoms of infection are notably absent. Parapharyngeal space masses, if large enough, may cause the tonsil to deviate mediad. The absence of any symptoms or signs of infection speaks against peritonsillar abscess. Imaging studies easily differentiate these neoplasms from a peritonsillar abscess.

An internal carotid artery aneurysm or simply excessive tortuosity of the artery may cause tonsillar deviation. The lack of a history of acute illness, as well as of trismus, fever, and drooling, should allow differentiation of these anomalies. Confusion may result if tonsillitis occurred in the setting of an existing arterial malformation, but, again, trismus and drooling should rarely be present in this situation. Observation or palpation for a pulse may provide the answer, but if doubt remains, a computed tomographic (CT) scan allows differentiation. If on aspiration of a presumed peritonsillar abscess significant bright red blood is obtained, pressure should be applied and the patient observed for neurologic sequelae. Imaging studies are appropriate in this situation, to elucidate the vascular anatomy in the region.

DIAGNOSIS

Laboratory

An uncomplicated peritonsillar abscess does not require any routine laboratory evaluation. Specific situations may require ordering of an individual test. In the case of severe dehydration, electrolyte imbalances may exist and require analysis to guide replacement therapy. A history of significant bleeding suggests the need for coagulation and platelet studies. White blood cell count, as previously mentioned, is not diagnostic of PTA and is not therefore routinely indicated. If consider-

ation is given to immediate tonsillectomy for treatment of an abscess, the minimum preoperative laboratory depending on the patient's age and medical condition is appropriate.

Purulent material obtained from PTAs is routinely sent for culture and sensitivity, to exclude unusual organisms and to direct therapy, but several authors have noted that the culture and sensitivity results did not influence patient outcome in their series.[1, 13, 26] The increase in beta-lactamase–producing organisms might suggest that cultures are indicated to direct therapy; however, Tuner and Nord reported no difference in outcome between patients with and without beta-lactamase–producing bacteria. All patients were treated with penicillin alone or penicillin with metronidazole, and they concluded that surgical drainage was the most important factor in outcome.[27] The emergence of penicillin-resistant *S. pneumoniae* may provide another reason to continue to utilize culture-directed antimicrobial therapy. The cost effectiveness of culturing all PTAs remains to be examined.

Imaging

PTA may be diagnosed by history and physical examination in the overwhelming majority of cases and may be differentiated from PTC with needle aspiration in most cases; yet imaging may be of assistance in specified circumstances. Patel and colleagues demonstrated that CT with contrast was equal in accuracy to needle aspiration for diagnosing PTA, but the major drawback is cost.[2] CT may be useful for patients with severe trismus who cannot be examined or in the case of a negative needle aspirate when the index of suspicion for abscess remains high (Fig. 48–2). CT may also be useful in delineating atypical causes for medial displacement of the tonsil, as discussed previously. Both external and intraoral sonography have been demonstrated to have excellent accuracy in the diagnosis and differentia-

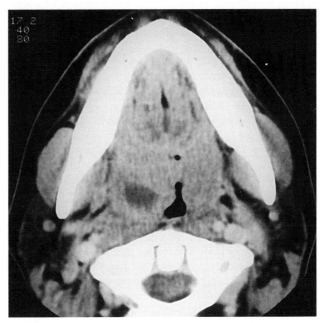

Figure 48–2. Computed tomographic scan demonstrating a peritonsillar abscess.

tion of PTA.[28, 29] The cost is less than that of CT. The use of either external or intraoral sonography requires local radiologic expertise (which may not be available in all areas) to properly interpret the sonogram. When a high index of suspicion exists in the face of a negative result from needle aspiration, sonography could be used for selected cases. Sonography does not provide as much information when atypical causes of tonsillar displacement are sought.

TREATMENT

Antibiotic

Evacuation of the purulence from a PTA is probably the key to its resolution, yet antibiotics are a necessary adjuvant, for a variety of reasons. Before the availability of antibiotics, sepsis, endocarditis, and brain abscess were dreaded complications considered to be associated with immediate tonsillectomy for a PTA. This led to the use of incision and drainage followed by serial dilatations as the primary treatment for PTA before the introduction of penicillin. It is not clear whether more septic complications occurred with tonsillectomy than with incision and drainage, but the use of antibiotics for preoperative systemic prophylaxis clearly played a role in reviving the use of immediate tonsillectomy for treatment of PTA. Antibiotics are also of benefit in curing the tonsillitis in the ipsilateral and contralateral tonsil when incision and drainage or needle aspiration has been used to evacuate the PTA. Antibiotic therapy alone may be expected to eradicate PTC. Finally, antibiotics may play a critical role in curing the PTA that is managed with needle aspiration alone. In this situation, complete and continued drainage is not assured, so antibiotics would of course play a more important role than in cases in which incision and drainage or immediate tonsillectomy is employed. No matter what the indication, antibiotic therapy typically is continued for 7–10 days after treatment, to ensure adequate treatment of associated tonsillitis.

The choice of antibiotic should be based on the expected microflora, which in this case most often are hemolytic streptococci, anaerobes, and *S. aureus*.[10] This would suggest the use of such antimicrobials as clindamycin, cefoxitin, imipenem, metronidazole plus a macrolide, or penicillin with a beta-lactamase inhibitor. Herzon surveyed 1362 otolaryngologists who treat PTA to determine their current management practices and found that the antibiotic utilized most often was penicillin, followed by cephalosporins, clindamycin, amoxicillin, and amoxicillin plus clavulanate potassium.[1] Most major needle aspiration series in the literature have simply used penicillin, a cephalosporin, or erythromycin and achieved nearly 100% resolution of the PTA, which again demonstrates the importance of evacuation of the pus, since, obviously, not all organisms were covered adequately by these antibiotics.[1, 13, 15–17, 26] Also, Maisel found that penicillin levels were detectable in the purulent material from only one-third of patients dosed prior to immediate tonsillectomy and cephalosporins were detectable in just over one-half of patients after injection.[30] The apparent lack of effect of beta-lactamase–producing organisms on outcome in patients treated with penicillin alone was mentioned previously.[27] It appears that penicillin (with or without a beta-lactamase inhibitor), clindamycin, or penicillin with metronidazole all remain effective, in a practical sense, as adjuvants to drainage in the management of PTA. Complete coverage of all potential organisms should be considered for any complicated or unusual cases, particularly if any septic complications are encountered. Finally, as local and global antimicrobial resistance patterns change, antibiotic selection may need to be reviewed.

Surgery

Indications

Every PTA is an indication for some sort of surgical procedure to drain the abscess, since, to date, no data support the efficacy of management of PTA with antibiotics alone. The decision as to whether a PTA exists is made on the basis of history, physical examination, perhaps needle aspiration, and, rarely, imaging. Patients deemed to have PTC are treated with antibiotics alone and are observed for signs of progression to abscess.

Alternatives

A nationwide survey of current PTA management practices by Herzon determined that the mean number of PTAs treated per practice per year was 7.01.[1] Prevalence figures for the treatment alternatives were, for needle aspiration, 32%; immediate tonsillectomy, 14%; and incision and drainage, 54%. The selection of a treatment is based on a variety of factors, including personal experience, cost, loss of productivity, pain, and prevention of future complications. The likelihood of a physician's using needle aspiration was inversely related to interval since board certification.[1]

Incision and drainage of a PTA was first described in the fourteenth century by the French surgeon Guy de Chauliac. This continued to be the treatment of choice for many centuries and remains one of the most commonly used treatments today. Another French surgeon, Chassaignac, reported the use of immediate tonsillectomy (also known as "tonsillectomy à chaud," "quinsy tonsillectomy," and "abscess tonsillectomy") for PTA in 1859[31]; however, the method did not gain favor immediately but was revitalized by a report from Winkler, of Germany, in 1911.[32] Reports of successful use of immediate tonsillectomy in the United States were published by Holinger, and then Baum, in the 1920s.[33, 34] While immediate tonsillectomy continued to gain popularity in most of Europe, acceptance in the United States was slow owing to the theoretic possibility of septic complications.[5, 6, 18] During the 1960s, however, immediate tonsillectomy began to be utilized more commonly in the United States, owing to the use of preoperative penicillin and because of the shorter hospital stay associated with immediate tonsillectomy as compared with incision and drainage followed by interval tonsillectomy.[7, 35, 36] These were the two treatment options used most frequently until the 1980s, when needle aspiration was evaluated in a number of clinical series.[13, 15–17, 26, 37]

Incision and Drainage. Incision and drainage is performed after the application of topical anesthetic spray and infiltration of local anesthetic into the area of the intended incision. Local anesthesia may not be maximally effective in the acid environment near the abscess, nor does it relieve the trismus, but it does provide some level of comfort and reassurance to most patients. An incision is made over the point of maximal fluctuance, which is then spread farther with a tonsil clamp to ensure that all areas of loculated pus are drained. This is generally quite painful for the patient, who is rarely willing to cooperate after the first attempt. Some physicians prefer to continue to dilate the abscess cavity daily, to make sure no more purulent matter collects.[38] Several trials that evaluated the effectiveness of needle aspiration used incision and drainage as a control. In four such series, incision and drainage was performed for 153 PTAs without complication and only five patients (3%) required repeat incision and drainage for a persistent abscess.[16, 17, 23, 38] Proponents of incision and drainage argue that it provides rapid relief of symptoms under local anesthesia in an outpatient setting; however, the procedure may be quite painful, and it expels purulence into a partially compromised airway.

Immediate Tonsillectomy. Immediate tonsillectomy removes the affected tonsil—and usually the contralateral tonsil—typically under general anesthesia for relief of PTA. Its major benefits are that all pus is drained and future PTA or recurrent tonsillitis is prevented. Opposition to the technique is based on considerations of increased intraoperative bleeding, the need for general anesthesia, and the unnecessary removal of a certain number of tonsils. Another consideration is that treatment may be delayed owing to logistical considerations for 8–72 hours, sometimes necessitating a preemptive incision and drainage or needle aspiration.[7, 18, 39]

Brandow reported a series of 156 immediate tonsillectomies in which he found the abscess to be located in the middle portion of the peritonsillar space in 22% of the patients and in the lower pole in 8% of the patients.[35] Similarly, Yung and Cantrell noted that at the time of quinsy tonsillectomy 24% of the abscesses were at the middle or inferior portion of the tonsil and that an unexpected abscess was noted in 8% of the contralateral tonsils.[7] They used these findings to contend that anything less than immediate tonsillectomy carried a high risk of residual abscess and treatment failure. In their series of 50 patients, average blood loss was 50 mL and there were two postoperative bleeds (4%). A number of series have confirmed the safety of—and specifically the lack of increased bleeding with—immediate tonsillectomy as compared with interval or delayed tonsillectomy.[6, 39–42] A number of authors have also demonstrated decreased total hospital time with immediate tonsillectomy as compared with incision and drainage followed by interval tonsillectomy.[40, 41] Of course, these data come from an era when hospitalization was not highly restricted and the conclusions were based on the assumption that all patients with a PTA should have their tonsils removed.

Most proponents of immediate tonsillectomy perform bilateral tonsillectomy, but some authors suggest removing only the affected tonsil, based on Bonding's finding of a higher incidence of pharyngitis in patients who had undergone bilateral tonsillectomy, particularly in patients over age 40.[22, 43, 44] Sorenson and colleagues reported their series of unilateral immediate tonsillectomies and found a 6% prevalence of recurrent PTA in the remaining tonsil, most frequently in the 10–19 year age group.[44]

Needle Aspiration. Needle aspiration has emerged as an alternative specifically to incision and drainage. Needle aspiration of PTA is not an entirely new concept, as it was frequently used to temporarily alleviate pain and before immediate tonsillectomy to decrease the risk of aspiration. Proponents of needle aspiration contend that it is easier to perform than incision and drainage and is less painful. The collection of the aspirate allows for culture if desired. Immediate relief of symptoms is provided, and the diagnosis is confirmed by the therapeutic maneuver itself. Finally, the risks of surgery and general anesthesia are avoided as they are not with immediate tonsillectomy.

Local anesthesia is attempted as previously described for incision and drainage. An 18- or 20-gauge needle is used, or, if extra length is needed for access, a spinal needle is selected. In either case, placing tape or cutting the plastic needle guard to leave only 1–1.5 cm of needle exposed provides a depth guard to prevent inadvertent vascular injury in an uncooperative patient. The use of a syringe pistol like that used for fine needle aspiration for cytologic examination allows the remaining hand to be free for depressing the tongue.[45] Aspiration is carried out at the point of maximal fluctuance. If no purulent material is obtained, a second and a third aspiration are performed in the middle and inferior portions of the peritonsillar space, which is generally tolerated well as compared with incision and drainage (Fig. 48–3). If no purulence is obtained, the patient is treated with antibiotics and is reexamined the next day. Repeat aspiration

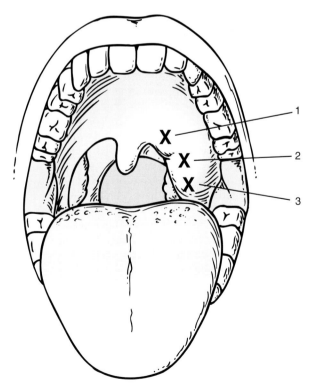

Figure 48–3. Recommended points for needle aspiration of peritonsillar abscess.

is performed if the patient is not improving and there is evidence of progression of the peritonsillar swelling.

Needle aspiration had traditionally been used only for diagnostic purposes. The observation that PTAs resolved with minimal drainage and antibiotics led to the use of needle aspiration for therapeutic purposes as well.[39] After some sporadic early reports on the effectiveness of needle aspiration, a large number of confirmatory series followed. The first description of needle aspiration as the sole surgical treatment for PTA was from a series of 39 patients reported by King in 1961.[46] There was only one failure in the series. Strome reported in 1973 a series of 20 patients managed with outpatient needle aspiration followed by interval tonsillectomy.[47] Four patients required repeat aspiration (initial failure rate, 20%), but all of the abscesses resolved after the second aspiration. The amount of purulent material collected ranged from 2–14 mL. In 1982 Schechter and colleagues published a retrospective analysis of 74 inpatients whose suspected PTA was managed with three-point needle aspiration.[15] The aspirate was positive in 52 cases, and the initial failure rate was 10%. Two of the initial twenty-two aspirate-negative patients subsequently developed an abscess, which was managed successfully with needle aspiration. In 1984 Herzon reported a similar experience but in an outpatient environment; only 2 of 41 patients required hospitalization.[26] Herzon also had an initial failure rate of 10%. The average amount of purulence obtained was 4.5 mL, and the mean time to complete resolution of symptoms was 2.6 days.

Spires and Stringer and their respective colleagues separately confirmed the efficacy of outpatient management of PTA with needle aspiration as compared with incision and drainage and obtained results similar to those from previous series using needle aspiration.[16, 17] Spires and colleagues noted a 95% success rate using three-point aspiration and found the following frequencies of positive aspirates by site: superior, 67%; midtonsil, 64%; and inferior, 25%. They calculated that if only the superior point were aspirated 33% of abscesses would be missed, but if two points were aspirated only 6% would be missed. In comparison, Snow and colleagues using a one-point aspiration technique had an initial failure rate of only 12%.[25] Stringer and colleagues utilized the technique of working inferiorly until purulence was obtained and had only an 8% initial treatment failure rate and a complete resolution rate with repeat aspiration of initial failures.[17] Most series have utilized either two- or three-point aspiration, and all have yielded initial treatment failure rates of 9%–15%.[11, 13, 23] Hospital admission rates have varied from 0% to 12%, mostly for reasons of volume depletion, and it may be possible in the emergency room or office setting to provide sufficient intravenous fluids to avoid hospitalization.

In 1993 Weinberg and colleagues confirmed the efficacy of needle aspiration, specifically in the pediatric population (aged 7–18 years).[48] Only 2 of 43 patients were unable to cooperate with the technique, which is much better tolerated than incision and drainage. At their institution needle aspiration for PTA reduced the immediate tonsillectomy rate from 72% in 1984–1985 to 12%. The need for subsequent tonsillectomy raised the incidence of tonsillectomy in the 1984–1985 group to 88% with follow-up of 6 years, as compared with 26% for the present series with follow-up ranging from 1 to 4 years.

Wolf and colleagues managed a group of 86 patients with single aspiration but repeated it daily until no pus was obtained.[38] The majority of patients continued to have pus, at least on the second day, and some had pus aspirated through 4 days. The initial failure rate cannot be compared with those of other series, but they noted a 20% PTA recurrence rate within the first month after treatment. This has never been documented in any other incision and drainage or needle aspiration series, which suggests that a single aspiration procedure may not remove all purulence or prevent some purulence from reaccumulating. Nevertheless, the large number of series reporting success with needle aspiration for PTA suggests that complete and permanent aspiration is not essential for initial cure.

In 1995 Herzon updated his series of patients with PTA managed by needle aspiration.[1] There were 130 abscesses in 123 patients who ranged in age from 6 to 55 years. The amount of purulence aspirated ranged from 1 to 20 mL on the first aspiration and 1 to 9 mL when a second aspiration was required for initial treatment failure. Outpatient management was possible for 86% of the patients. The abscess resolution rate was 96%, and incision and drainage was used to resolve the persistent lesions. The failure rate was higher for patients who required more than one aspiration: 28%, as compared with 3% for those who needed only one. A history of recurrent tonsillitis was documented in 22% of the patients and a previous PTA in 6%.

Advocates of quinsy tonsillectomy argue against needle aspiration and incision and drainage because without bilateral tonsillectomy as many as 20% of abscesses would be missed, based on the findings at the time of immediate tonsillectomy.[7] Meta-analysis by Herzon, however, of 10 series of PTAs numbering 464 patients revealed that needle aspiration as the single surgical modality was 94% effective in resolving PTA, which suggests that this theoretic concern is not of practical significance.[1] Approximately 10%–15% of patients will require a second aspiration the next day, which, once again, is performed on an outpatient basis, with minimal additional cost, and results in final resolution of the abscess. Purely from the standpoint of initial treatment, outpatient needle aspiration is less expensive than immediate tonsillectomy, even as outpatient surgery. Herzon determined the following costs for management of PTA: needle aspiration, $200; incision and drainage, $300; needle aspiration plus interval tonsillectomy, $3200; immediate tonsillectomy, $3600, and 2 days' inpatient intravenous antibiotics, $1400.[1] Annual nationwide costs for each procedure were estimated to be these: needle aspiration, $2.9 million; immediate tonsillectomy, $23.4 million; and incision and drainage, $7 million. The estimated 14% of patients who have to be admitted for an average of 2 days' intravenous antibiotics adds another $9 million to the cost.

COMPLICATIONS

Complications as a result of a PTA are, fortunately, quite rare in the antibiotic era. Historically common, the following septic complications may occur secondary to PTA: sepsis, endocarditis, polyarthritis, nephritis, and brain abscess. A second group of complications relates to progression of the abscess through the superior pharyngeal constrictor muscle via lymphatics or septic thrombophlebitis of the tonsillar vessels to the parapharyngeal space. An abscess in the parapharyngeal space may result in Horner's syndrome, lower cranial nerve palsies, or internal jugular thrombophlebitis. Further progression may lead to mediastinitis and necrotizing fasciitis. The most life-threatening complication in the parapharyngeal space is septic necrosis of the internal carotid artery. Initially, vasculitis of the vasa vasorum leads to weakening of the vessel wall, which may result in an internal carotid artery aneurysm. Further damage may result in spontaneous (and frequently fatal) hemorrhage. Salinger and Pearlman performed a literature review in 1933 of carotid hemorrhages secondary to PTA, in which 23 of 28 patients who had vessel ligation survived; without ligation the survival rate was 50%.[49] Autopsies in these patients demonstrated that instead of the internal carotid artery, external carotid branches may sometimes be the source of the bleeding. While the incidence of septic necrosis of the internal carotid artery has decreased in the antibiotic era, Blum and McCaffrey found reports of 23 cases of false aneurysm of the internal carotid artery secondary to PTA in the literature since 1933.[50]

More common complications include dehydration, spontaneous rupture of the abscess with aspiration, and impending airway obstruction. Intravenous fluids should be considered for all patients with PTA, even those managed as outpatients. Spontaneous rupture of an abscess may be prevented by prompt management or by decompression with needle aspiration, even if further therapy is planned. A suction device should be at the ready during any attempt at intubation of these patients. Moderate airway obstruction may also be alleviated by needle aspiration, but emergent loss of the airway may require tracheotomy.

PREVENTION

Although PTA has been reported to develop in "tonsillectomized" patients—usually when some tonsillar remnant is present—PTA after tonsillectomy is very rare.[51, 52] PTA is assumed to be secondary to tonsillitis, so the only way to prevent all PTAs is to remove everyone's tonsils, which is unreasonable. Instead, we can determine the likelihood of recurrent PTA or tonsillitis and selectively perform prophylactic tonsillectomy. The percentages of patients reported to develop a second PTA or recurrent tonsillitis have varied much. Herbild and Bonding followed 161 patients treated for a PTA for a median period of 5 years (range, 3.5–8 years) and found that 22% developed a second PTA, 20% had recurrent tonsillitis, 7% had recurrent pharyngitis, and 51% had no symptoms.[53] Patients older than 40 years had no symptoms in 70% of the cases, as compared with only 40% of patients younger than 40. On the basis of these data, they recommended immediate tonsillectomy for patients younger than 40 who had a history of tonsillitis. It is not clear from the study why the 7% with recurrent pharyngitis, apparently without tonsillitis, are considered candidates for tonsillectomy.

Nielson and Greisen noted an overall PTA recurrence rate of 22% at 4 years and similarly noted that the recurrence risk was greater for those younger than 30 years (33%) than for older persons (6%), especially those with a history of PTA or recurrent tonsillitis. The risk of combined recurrent tonsillitis and PTA in the younger group was 63%. The investigators recommended immediate tonsillectomy for all patients younger than 30, on the basis of these findings.[54]

Curley and Bates reported a series of similar findings in a series of patients managed with incision and drainage, noting that patients younger than 25 with a history of tonsillitis were most likely to develop a second PTA.[55] A number of other authors found the long-term recurrence rate for PTA to range from 6% to 25% and noted that increased risk was associated with a history of tonsillitis and younger age.[3, 8, 22, 56–58]

The prevalence of late recurrences after needle aspiration (≤17%) has been reported to be similar to that for incision and drainage.[11, 13, 15, 38] Savolainen and colleagues provided uniquely close follow-up of a series 98 patients with PTA at a military hospital in Helsinki, Finland, treated with needle aspiration.[11] At a minimum follow-up period of 8 months and a mean of 3 years, 83% of the patients had no further problems, whereas the other 17% underwent tonsillectomy for either recurrent PTA or tonsillitis. A history of tonsillitis was much more common in the group who required tonsillectomy. Interestingly, all cases of recurrent PTA occurred within 7 months, and most within 2 months. Based on these data they recommended immediate or interval tonsillectomy for all patients with multiple prior episodes of tonsillitis or a PTA.

Herzon completed meta-analysis of 19 studies of a total of 2083 patients with PTA treated by incision and drainage or needle aspiration and determined that the recurrence rate of PTA in the United States was 10% and in the rest of the world was 15%.[1]

Several approaches based on these data have been developed. Advocates of immediate tonsillectomy argue that it eradicates all risk of developing another PTA or further episodes of recurrent tonsillitis; however, this approach would result in the removal of tonsils from 85% to 90% of patients who never would have had recurrent PTA. The morbidity and cost associated with this unneeded surgery must be weighed against the morbidity and cost of taking care of 10%–15% of patients who would go on to develop a recurrent PTA. Consideration of recurrent tonsillitis in addition to recurrent PTA would make these figures differ as much as 20%–30%, but a majority of patients would still have their tonsils removed without significant likelihood of future morbidity. The finding that older patients who have had bilateral tonsillectomy are more likely to have pharyngitis should also be considered when entertaining a policy of immediate tonsillectomy for all PTA.[22]

A second approach is to treat the initial abscess with incision and drainage or needle aspiration and then to perform an interval tonsillectomy approximately 6 weeks later on all patients. This approach is based on the concern that bleeding and the risk of aspiration are greater with immediate tonsillectomy and that immediate tonsillectomy is inconvenient. The indiscriminate recommendation of tonsillectomy to all patients involves the same drawbacks as a policy of immediate tonsillectomy for all PTAs.

A policy of simply waiting to see who develops recurrent tonsillitis or PTA could be considered as well, but this approach would result in morbidity for at least 30%–35% of patients. Fortunately, we have data that will allow us reasonably to predict which patient is at greatest risk for having another PTA or recurrent tonsillitis. Patients younger than 40 years or perhaps those younger than 25 to 30 years who have a history of recurrent tonsillitis or of PTA are most likely to develop future morbidity. Some time after initial outpatient needle aspiration, outpatient tonsillectomy should be considered for this group. When convenient, immediate tonsillectomy is an alternative as initial treatment for selected patients at risk. Immediate tonsillectomy may also be appropriate, for example, in the military setting when waiting until later to perform tonsillectomy is not feasible. When the rare patient not deemed at risk develops another PTA or recurrent tonsillitis, it may be managed with tonsillectomy at that time.

Awareness of the cost of providing care to entire populations is increasingly important. If all patients with PTA had an abscess tonsillectomy or interval tonsillectomy, the annual cost in the United States would be an estimated $111 million.[1] Adding the cost of other initial treatment previously presented, the annual cost of managing PTA in the United States would be an estimated $150 million. Needle aspiration as initial treatment (reserving tonsillectomy for young patients with recurrent PTA or a history of tonsillitis) should reduce this annual cost to approximately $62 million.[1] It also eliminates the nuisance of urgent tonsillectomy and avoids a significant number of unnecessary tonsillectomies.

SUGGESTED MANAGEMENT STRATEGY

Based on the data and considerations discussed in this chapter, the following successful and cost-effective management strategy is proposed:

1. Suspected PTA should be managed with either outpatient needle aspiration or incision and drainage, depending on the physician's skill and preference.

2. Fluids are replaced if needed.

3. Antimicrobial therapy is instituted with penicillin or its derivatives, with or without a beta-lactamase inhibitor, cephalosporins, or clindamycin.

4. Initial treatment failures are re-treated in similar fashion.

5. Persistent treatment failures, immunocompromised patients, children who are unable to cooperate with treatment, and selected military personnel should be managed with immediate tonsillectomy.

6. Patients younger than 30 years who have a significant history of tonsillitis or PTA should be treated with interval tonsillectomy. Alternatively, patients in this category may be managed with immediate tonsillectomy in the unusual circumstance when this can be performed without delay solely on an outpatient basis.

References

1. Herzon FS: Peritonsillar abscess: Incidence, current management practices, and a proposal for treatment guidelines. Laryngoscope 1995; 105(suppl 74): 1–17.

2. Patel KS, Ahmad S, O'Leary G, et al.: Role of computed tomography in the management of peritonsillar abscess. Otolaryngol Head Neck Surg 1992; 107: 727–732.

3. Holt GR, Tinsley PP Jr: Peritonsillar abscesses in children. Laryngoscope 1981; 91: 1226–1230.

4. Passy V: Pathogenesis of peritonsillar abscess. Laryngoscope 1994; 104: 185–190.

5. Bateman GH, Kodicek J: Primary quinsy tonsillectomy. Ann Otol Rhinol Laryngol 1959; 68: 315–321.

6. Beeden AG, Evans JN: Quinsy tonsillectomy: A further report. J Laryngol Otol 1970; 84: 443–448.

7. Yung AK, Cantrell RW: Quinsy tonsillectomy. Laryngoscope 1976; 86: 1714–1717.

8. Fried MP, Forrest JL: Peritonsillitis: Evaluation of current therapy. Arch Otolaryngol Head Neck Surg 1981; 107: 283–286.

9. Shoemaker M, Lampe RM, Weir MR: Peritonsillitis: Abscess or cellulitis? Pediatr Infect Dis 1986; 5: 435–439.

10. Brook I, Frazier EH, Thompson DH: Aerobic and anaerobic microbiology of peritonsillar abscess. Laryngoscope 1991; 101: 289–292.

11. Savolainen S, Jousimies-Somer HR, Makitie AA, et al.: Peritonsillar abscess: Clinical and microbiologic aspects and treatment regimens. Arch Otolaryngol Head Neck Surg 1993; 119: 521–524.

12. Sugita R, Kawamura S, Icikawa G, et al.: Microorganisms isolated from peritonsillar abscess and indicated chemotherapy. Arch Otolaryngol 1982; 108: 655–658.

13. Ophir D, Bawnik J, Poria Y, et al.: Peritonsillar abscess: A prospective evaluation of outpatient management by needle aspiration. Arch Otolaryngol Head Neck Surg 1988; 114: 661–663.

14. Jousimies-Somer H, Savolainen S, Makitie A, et al.: Bacteriologic findings in peritonsillar abscesses in young adults. Clin Infect Dis 1993; (suppl 4): S292–S298.

15. Schechter GL, Sly DE, Roper AL, et al.: Changing face of treatment of peritonsillar abscess. Laryngoscope 1982; 92: 657–659.

16. Spires JR, Owens JJ, Woodson GE, et al.: Treatment of peritonsillar abscess: A prospective study of aspiration vs incision and drainage. Arch Otolaryngol Head Neck Surg 1987; 113: 984–986.

17. Stringer SP, Schaefer SD, Close LG: A randomized trial for outpatient management of peritonsillar abscess. Arch Otolaryngol Head Neck Surg 1988; 114: 296–298.

18. Bonding P: Tonsillectomy à chaud. J Laryngol Otol 1973; 87: 1711–1182.

19. Johnsen T: Infectious mononucleosis and peritonsillar abscess. J Laryngol Otol 1981; 95: 873–876.

20. Richardson KA, Birck H: Peritonsillar abscess in the pediatric population. Otolaryngol Head Neck Surg 1981; 89: 907–909.

21. Kristensen S, Juul A, Nielsen F: Quinsy: A bilateral presentation. J Laryngol Otol 1985; 99: 401–402.

22. Bonding P: Routine abscess tonsillectomy: Late results. Laryngoscope 1976; 86: 286–290.

23. Maharaj D, Rajah V, Hemsley S: Management of peritonsillar abscess. J Laryngol Otol 1991; 105: 743–745.

24. Brodsky L, Sobie SR, Korwin D, et al.: A clinical prospective study of peritonsillar abscess in children. Laryngoscope 1988; 98: 780–783.

25. Snow DG, Campbell JB, Morgan DW: The management of peritonsillar sepsis by needle aspiration. Clin Otolaryngol 1991; 16: 245–247.

26. Herzon FS: Permucosal needle drainage of peritonsillar abscesses: A five-year experience. Arch Otolaryngol 1984; 110: 104–105.

27. Tuner K, Nord CE: Impact of peritonsillar infections and microflora of phenoxymethylpenicillin alone versus phenoxymethylpenicillin with metronidazole. Infection 1986; 14: 129–133.

28. Ahmed K, Jones AS, Shah K, et al.: The role of ultrasound in the management of peritonsillar abscess. J Laryngol Otol 1994; 108: 610–612.

29. Buckley AR, Moss EH, Blokmanis A: Diagnosis of peritonsillar abscess: Value of intraoral sonography. Am J Roentgenol 1994; 162: 961–964.

30. Maisel RH: Peritonsillar abscess: Tonsil antibiotic levels in patients treated by acute abscess surgery. Laryngoscope 1982; 1: 80–87.

31. Chassaignac E: Traite Peratique de la Suppuration et du Drainage Chirurgical, vol 2. Paris: Masson, 1859.

32. Winkler E: Uber Therapie de phlegmonosen Entzundungen des Waldeyerschen Ringes. Dtsch Med Wochenschr 1911; 37: 21–39.

33. Holinger J: The removal of the tonsils in the presence of a peritonsillar abscess. Ann Otol Rhinol Laryngol 1921; 30: 195–198.

34. Baum HL: The radical cure of peritonsillar abscess. Ann Otol Rhinol Laryngol 1926; 35: 429–433.

35. Brandow EC Jr: Immediate tonsillectomy for peritonsillar abscess. Trans Am Acad Ophthalmol Otolaryngol 1973; 77: 412–416.

36. McCurdy JA Jr, Hays LL: Immediate tonsillectomy for peritonsillar abscess. Milit Med 1975; 140: 787–788.

37. Herzon FS, Aldridge JH: Peritonsillar abscess: Needle aspiration. Otolaryngol Head Neck Surg 1981; 89: 910–911.

38. Wolf M, Even-Chen I, Kronenberg J: Peritonsillar abscess: Repeated needle aspiration versus incision and drainage. Ann Otol Rhinol Laryngol 1994; 103: 554–557.

39. Templer JW, Holinger LD, Wood RP 2d, et al.: Immediate tonsillectomy for the treatment of peritonsillar abscess. Am J Surg 1977; 134: 596–598.

40. Lockhart R, Parker GS, Tami TA: Role of quinsy tonsillectomy in the management of peritonsillar abscess. Ann Otol Rhinol Laryngol 1991; 100: 569–571.

41. McCurdy JA Jr: Peritonsillar abscess: A comparison of treatment by immediate tonsillectomy and interval tonsillectomy. Arch Otolaryngol 1977; 103: 414–415.

42. Nielsen VM, Greisen O: Peritonsillar abscess. II. Cases treated with tonsillectomy à chaud. J Laryngol Otol 1981; 95: 805–807.

43. Christensen PH, Schonsted-Madsen U: Unilateral immediate tonsillectomy as the treatment of peritonsillar abscess: Results, with special attention to pharyngitis. J Laryngol Otol 1983; 97: 1105–1109.

44. Sorensen JA, Godballe C, Andersen NH, et al.: Peritonsillar abscess: Risk of disease in the remaining tonsil after unilateral tonsillectomy à chaud. J Laryngol Otol 1991; 105: 442–444.

45. Cannon CR: Syringe pistol aspiration of peritonsillar abscesses. Otolaryngol Head Neck Surg 1987; 96: 106–107.

46. King JT: Aspiration treatment of peritonsillar abscess. J Med Assoc Ga 1961; 50: 18–19.

47. Strome M: Peritonsillar abscess: A different approach. J Med Assoc Ga 1973; 62: 4–6.

48. Weinberg E, Brodsky L, Stanievich J, et al.: Needle aspiration of peritonsillar abscess in children. Arch Otolaryngol Head Neck Surg 1993; 119: 169–172.

49. Salinger S, Pearlman SJ: Hemorrhage from pharyngeal and peritonsillar abscesses: Report of cases, resume of the literature and discussion of ligation of the carotid artery. Arch Otolaryngol Head Neck Surg 1933; 18: 464–509.

50. Blum DJ, McCaffrey TV: Septic necrosis of the internal carotid artery: A complication of peritonsillar abscess. Otolaryngol Head Neck Surg 1983; 91: 114–118.

51. Randall CJ, Jefferis AF: Quinsy following tonsillectomy (five case reports). J Laryngol Otol 1984; 98: 367–369.

52. Roos K, Lind L: Peritonsillar abscess in spite of adequately performed tonsillectomy. Arch Otolaryngol Head Neck Surg 1990; 116: 205.

53. Herbild O, Bonding P: Peritonsillar abscess. Arch Otolaryngol 1981; 107: 540–542.

54. Nielsen VM, Greisen O: Peritonsillar abscess. I. Cases treated by incision and drainage: A follow-up investigation. J Laryngol Otol 1981; 95: 801–805.

55. Curley JW, Bates GJ: Rationalization of peritonsillar abscess as an indication for tonsillectomy. J Laryngol Otol 1988; 102: 37–38.

56. Litman RS, Hausman SA, Sher WH: A retrospective study of peritonsillar abscess. Ear Nose Throat J 1987; 66: 53–55.

57. Holt GR: Management of peritonsillar abscess in military medicine. Milit Med 1982; 147: 851–855.

58. Kronenberg J, Wolf M, Leventon G: Peritonsillar abscess: Recurrence rate and the indication for tonsillectomy. Am J Otolaryngol 1987; 8: 82–84.

James D. Cherry
Ulrich Heininger

CHAPTER FORTY-NINE

Whooping Cough (Pertussis)

▼

Pertussis (whooping cough) is an acute infection of the respiratory tract caused by *Bordetella pertussis* or, less frequently, by *Bordetella parapertussis*.[1–3] The illness occurs worldwide and affects all age groups, but primarily children; it is most serious in young, unprotected infants.

Effective whole-cell pertussis vaccines became available in the 1940s, and the rate of pertussis was reduced dramatically in countries where universal immunization of infants and children was implemented. Even with vaccine use, however, occasional local epidemics still occur and there is growing evidence of widespread, frequently atypical (and therefore unrecognized) illness in children, adolescents, and adults.[4–11] *B. pertussis* is one of the major causes of cough illness.

HISTORY

The clinical picture of pertussis was first reported in 1640 by Guillaume de Baillou, who described cases in a 1578 epidemic in Paris.[12] The isolation of *B. pertussis,* the main pathogen of pertussis was reported by Bordet and Gengou in 1906, and 30 years later *B. parapertussis* was recognized by Eldering and Kendrick as a different species that caused a similar illness.[13, 14]

Vaccines consisting of killed whole *B. pertussis* organisms were developed shortly after the bacterium was isolated, and first results of protection were reported by Madsen in 1925.[15] The mouse protection test, developed and reported by Kendrick and collaborators in 1947, allowed standardization of vaccine production.[16] Comprehensive studies conducted by the British Medical Council in the 1940s and 1950s demonstrated a good correlation between the potency of pertussis vaccines as determined in the mouse protection test and their clinical efficacy in children.[17] In consequence, immunization against pertussis, most commonly in combination with diphtheria and tetanus toxoids (DTP), became part of routine vaccination programs in many countries throughout the world.

Concerns about a relationship between pertussis vaccination and temporally associated serious adverse events (including sudden infant death syndrome [SIDS] and a variety of neurologic illnesses) led to a sharp decline in vaccination rates in Japan and several European countries during the 1970s.[1] These concerns, combined with well-documented high rates of unpleasant local and systemic reactions, led to development of new acellular vaccines. These vaccines cause fewer reactions and have been used in Japan since 1981[18]; however, clinical efficacy has only recently been demonstrated for some acellular vaccines used in infancy (see the section, Prevention).

MICROBIOLOGY

Organisms

B. pertussis and *B. parapertussis* are the etiologic agents of pertussis, and both bacteria are restricted to humans; 95% of illnesses are due to *B. pertussis.* In rare instances *Bordetella bronchiseptica,* which normally is enzootic in animals, has also been isolated from humans with pertussis-like cough illnesses.[19]

B. pertussis and *B. parapertussis* are closely related organisms with 98.5% genetic homology.[20] They are listed as distinct species because of important differences, the most important one being the failure of *B. parapertussis* to produce pertussis toxin. There are other antigenic differences, culture requirements, and metabolic characteristics.

Antigenic and Biologically Active Components of *Bordetella Pertussis*

B. pertussis contains a variety of components that are antigenic or biologically active (Table 49–1). The majority of these factors are part of the cell wall or surface of the organism. Depending on the presence or absence of specific agglutinogens, several serotypes of *B. pertussis* have been recognized; however, there is no evidence for differences in symptoms caused by the different serotypes.[1]

Culture and Serology

A laboratory diagnosis of pertussis can be made by culturing the organism, identifying its presence by direct fluorescent antibody (DFA) testing, or demonstrating the production of specific antibodies. *Bordetella* species can be recovered from nasopharyngeal specimens (Fig. 49–1); the rate of isolation is highest within the first 3 weeks of cough.[21] Specific swabs (calcium alginate) and media (Regan-Lowe or Bordet-Gengou agar and modified Stainer-Scholte broth) are required, and the laboratory should be experienced in isolating the organisms.[1, 3, 22, 23]

Recently the polymerase chain reaction (PCR) technique has been used to identify *B. pertussis* or *B. parapertussis* in nasopharyngeal specimens. This diagnostic tool has the

Table 49–1. BIOLOGICALLY ACTIVE AND ANTIGENIC COMPONENTS OF *Bordetella pertussis*

Component	Characteristics
Fimbriae	Two serologic types (types 2 and 3). Antibody to specific types cause agglutination of the organism. Organisms may contain type 2 fimbriae, type 3 fimbriae, types 2 and 3 fimbriae, or neither type 2 or 3 fimbriae. Fimbriae may play a role as adhesins.
Filamentous hemagglutinin	A cell-surface protein; functions as an adhesin
Pertussis toxin; also called "lymphocytosis-promoting factor"	A classic bacterial toxin with an enzymatically active A subunit and a B oligomer–binding protein. Toxic activity in animal model systems includes histamine sensitization, lymphocytosis promotion, stimulation of insulin secretion, and adjuvant and mitogenic activity. An envelope protein, it is an important adhesin; it adversely effects host immune cell functions.
Adenylate cyclase toxin	An extracytoplasmic enzyme which impairs host immune cell functions and may contribute to local tissue damage in the respiratory tract
Heat-labile toxin; also called "dermonecrotic toxin"	Cytoplasmic protein which causes skin necrosis in laboratory animals; may contribute to local tissue damage in the respiratory tract
Lipo-oligosaccharide; endotoxin	An envelope toxin with activities similar to those of endotoxins of other gram-negative bacteria. A significant cause of reactions to whole-cell pertussis vaccines. Antibody to lipo-oligosaccharide causes agglutination of the organism (agglutinogen type 1).
Tracheal cytotoxin	A disaccharide-tetrapeptide derived from peptidoglycan; causes local tissue damage in the respiratory tract
Pertactin	A 69-kD outer membrane protein that is an important adhesin; antibody to pertactin causes agglutination of the organism.

advantage of much greater sensitivity as compared with conventional culture[24]; however, since it is more expensive than culture and subject to easy contamination it has not yet been widely used as a routine procedure.

Serologic testing for *B. pertussis* infections in the clinical setting is neither standardized nor widely available.[1, 25] In the research setting the use of enzyme-linked immunosorbent assay (ELISA) has significantly contributed to the diagnosis of *B. pertussis* infections.[4–6, 8–11, 26] Most useful has been the determination of IgG and IgA antibodies to pertussis toxin (PT) and filamentous hemagglutinin (FHA). The most reliable proof of acute infection is the demonstration of a significant increase in antibody value between acute-phase and convalescent-phase serum specimens. Frequently acute-phase specimen collection is delayed, and therefore the acute-phase values are already elevated so that significant increases between first and second serum specimens cannot be demonstrated. Diagnosis *can* frequently be made on the basis of a high value or values from a single serum specimen.[5, 6, 8, 27]

B. parapertussis infection induces cross-reacting antibodies to *B. pertussis* filamentous hemagglutinin, so that use of this antigen alone cannot differentiate *B. pertussis* from *B. parapertussis* infections.[28] The measurement of agglutinating antibodies is also useful for the diagnosis of *B. pertussis* infections, and since the test is simple, cheap, and accurate it can be used in the clinical setting.[5, 6, 25, 27]

EPIDEMIOLOGY

Incidence

The incidence of pertussis and its mortality are markedly effected by pertussis vaccine use. In the prevaccine era in the United States the average reported attack rate of pertussis was 157 per 100,000 population (Fig. 49–2).[2] With the introduction and widespread use of pertussis vaccines, the attack rate fell about 150-fold between 1943 and 1976.

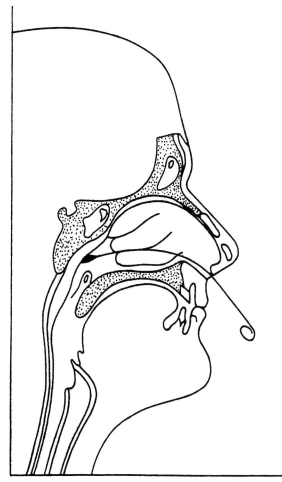

Figure 49–1. Method for obtaining a nasopharyngeal specimen: the swab is inserted into one of the nostrils and gently pushed forward into the nasopharynx. (Fig. 1 in Heininger U: Gemeinsamkeiten und Differenzen von Pertussis und Parapertussis. Published with permission from Pädiatr Präx 1995; 48: 437–445.)

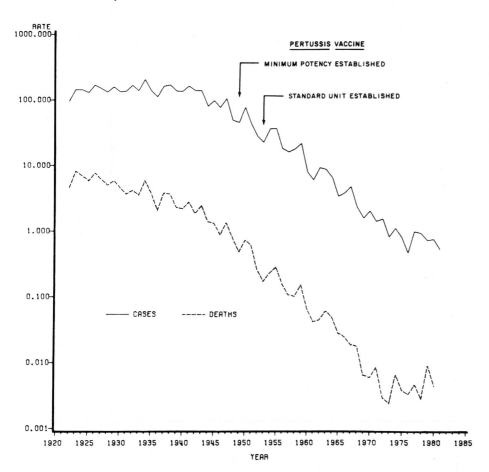

Figure 49–2. Pertussis: reported cases and deaths per 100,000 population, by year, United States, 1922–1981 (Centers for Disease Control and Prevention:, Annual summary 1981: Reported morbidity and mortality in the United States. MMWR 1982; 30: 65). With the introduction and widespread use of pertussis vaccines, the attack rate fell about 150-fold from 1943 to 1976.

For the 7-year period 1976–1982, the attack rate remained between 0.5 and 1.0 per 100,000 population (Fig. 49–3). From 1982–1993 the attack rate curve was modestly upward, reaching a rate of 2.3 per 100.000. The reason for this upward trend is unknown but most likely is due to heightened awareness of the disease.

In the prevaccine era about 85% of all cases in the United States were noted in children aged 1–9 years.[2] In contrast, today 41% of cases are reported in infants and 28% in children aged 10 years or older. In the prevaccine era there were, on average, 7000 pertussis deaths per year in the United States; presently about 10 are reported per year.[2, 29]

Pertussis epidemics in the prevaccine era occurred at 2–5 year intervals (average 3.2 years), and these cycles have continued in the vaccine era. As noted by Fine and Clarkson, the persistence today of the cycles that characterized the prevaccine era indicates that, although immunization has controlled disease, it has not reduced the transmission of the organism in the population.[30]

We found that 26% of university students with cough illnesses of at least 6 days' duration had *B. pertussis* infections and none was correctly diagnosed clinically.[5] The findings in this study led to the suggestion that *B. pertussis* infections are endemic in adults and are responsible for cyclic outbreaks in susceptible children. More recent studies in the United States and Germany support this hypothesis.[4, 6, 8, 11, 27]

Season, Geography, and Sex

Pertussis occurs throughout the world.[1, 2] Historically, there was no seasonal pattern to epidemic pertussis[2]; however, in the present vaccine era, in North America pertussis is most common in summer and fall.[31–33] In the past the incidence of pertussis was greater in females than in males.[2] More recently, between 1980 and 1989, this female predominance was observed again, but only in persons aged 15 years or older.[31]

Transmission

Transmission is believed to occur by droplets from a coughing patient to the upper respiratory tract of a susceptible person. It is also possible that indirect spread occurs. A symptomatic patient could contaminate the environment with respiratory tract secretions; then a new host-to-be comes in contact with the secretions and inoculates his or her own respiratory tract via the hands.[1] Attack rates in susceptible household contacts range from 70%–100%.[1–3] Antibody studies indicate that asymptomatic infections also occur in contacts.[27] These asymptomatic infections are likely to be short-lived and are probably not important in regard to contagion. Transmissibility is greatest early in the illness, during the catarrhal and early paroxysmal phases.

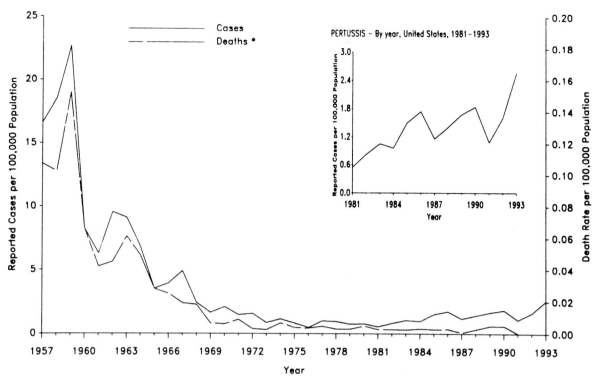

NOTE: DTP vaccine licensed 1948.
*Data on mortality are not yet available for 1992 and 1993.

Figure 49-3. Pertussis incidence rate per 100,000 population and death rate per 100,000 population, United States, 1957–1993 (Centers for Disease Control and Prevention: Summary of notifiable diseases, United States, 1993. MMWR 1993; 42(53): 43). For the 7-year period 1976–1982, the attack rate remained between 0.5 and 1.0 per 100,000 population. From 1982 to 1993, the attack rate curve was modestly upward, reaching a rate of 2.3 per 100,000. The reason for this upward trend is unknown, but it is most likely due to a heightened awareness of the disease.

PATHOGENESIS AND IMMUNITY

After exposure to *B. pertussis,* the pathogenesis of infection depends on four important steps: attachment, evasion of host defenses, local damage, and systemic disease.[1, 3, 34] Infection is initiated in the respiratory tract by the attachment of *B. pertussis* organisms to the cilia of the ciliated epithelial cells.[34] The adhesins (filamentous hemagglutinin, pertussis toxin, and pertactin) facilitate this attachment (see Table 49-1).[34–37]

Because fimbriae of some gram-negative bacteria are important for attachment, it has been assumed that *B. pertussis* fimbriae are important in attachment; however, in one tissue culture study, fimbriae did not mediate attachment of organisms to cells,[38] though in a more recent study, fimbriae did play a role in attachment in persistent infection.[39] Both adenylate cyclase and pertussis toxin affect immune cell functions adversely and therefore allow infection, once established, to continue.[1, 35, 40] Tracheal cytotoxin, heat-labile toxin, and adenylate cyclase have all been implicated as contributors to local tissue damage in the respiratory tract.[1, 41, 42] Of these toxins, tracheal cytotoxin is likely to be the most important.

Pertussis is a unique illness as there is only one manifestation of systemic disease in uncomplicated infection: leukocytosis with lymphocytosis due to pertussis toxin.[1, 43] The most important systemic complication of pertussis is encephalopa-

thy, and its cause is not known. The most likely explanation is anoxia associated with coughing paroxysms.

The prevailing opinion throughout this century is that immunity following *B. pertussis* infections is lifelong whereas vaccine-induced immunity is relatively short lived. The latter assumption is clearly true,[44] but studies by members of our research group suggest that the former opinion regarding infection-induced immunity is wrong.[6, 45] Using the fact that IgA antibodies to pertussis antigens (pertussis toxin, filamentous hemagglutinin, pertactin) result from infection and not vaccination, our group studied the prevalence of these antibodies in the sera of young male German and American age peers.[45] In Germany routine childhood immunization was not carried out during the 1970s and 1980s, and pertussis was epidemic. To our surprise, the rate and mean values of IgA antibodies in the two populations were similar, suggesting that adult infection rates were similar. In another study in Germany we found that *B. pertussis* infections were common in adults (incidence, 133 per 100,000 population), and they often occurred in persons with a known history of childhood pertussis.[6]

Today the nature of immunity in pertussis is not known. It has generally been assumed that serum antibody concentrations above some unknown value are responsible for protection.[27] At the present time no serologic correlates of immunity have been established. Recent animal studies suggest that cellular immunity may be important in bacterial clearance and that this immunity may augment protective antibody effects.[46]

Immunity following *B. pertussis* infection or pertussis vaccination does not protect against illness due to *B. parapertussis,* and, similarly, infection with *B. parapertussis* does not induce protection against disease caused by *B. pertussis.*[47–49]

CLINICAL MANIFESTATIONS

The clinical manifestations of *B. pertussis* infection are quite variable, depending on age, history of immunization or infection, passive acquisition of antibody, and perhaps other factors such as degree of exposure, host genetic and acquired factors, and genotype of the organism. The incubation period for pertussis varies between 6 and 20 days; for the majority of cases onset occurs 7–10 days after exposure.

Classic Illness

Classic illness occurs as a primary infection in unimmunized children who are between 1 and 10 years of age. The illness usually lasts 6–8 weeks and has three stages: catarrhal, paroxysmal and convalescent. Initial illness is characterized by rhinorrhea, lacrimation, and mild cough—signs that suggest a common cold. Body temperature is usually normal. The severity of the cough gradually increases over 1–2 weeks, but usually pertussis is not suspected until the cough becomes paroxysmal.

Following the catarrhal period the coughs increase in severity and number. Repetitive series of 5–10 or more forceful coughs during a single expiration occur. These paroxysms are followed by a sudden massive inspiratory effort, and a characteristic whoop may occur as air is inhaled forcefully through a narrowed glottis. Cyanosis, bulging eyes, protrusion of the tongue, salivation, lacrimation, and distention of neck veins occur during paroxysms. Several paroxysmal coughing episodes, with their associated massive inspiratory efforts, may occur sequentially, until the child succeeds in dislodging the obstructing mucus. Posttussive vomiting is common. Paroxysms may occur several times per hour during both day and nighttime.

The paroxysmal episodes are exhausting, and it is not unusual for the patient to appear dazed and apathetic. Weight loss may occur secondary to vomiting and because eating and drinking may be resisted because they trigger attacks. Attacks may also be triggered by yawning, sneezing, or physical exertion. Between attacks, the patient may appear normal and is usually in no distress.

Common and important complications of classic pertussis include pneumonia, otitis media, seizures, and encephalopathy. Pneumonia may be due to *B. pertussis* or to secondary bacterial invaders. Other complications include ulcer of the frenulum of the tongue, epistaxis, subconjunctival hemorrhages, and rectal prolapse.

The convalescent stage, which usually lasts 1–2 weeks, is characterized by decreasing frequency and severity of coughing episodes, whooping, and vomiting. Nearly all patients who have classic pertussis due to primary infection

have leukocytosis due to lymphocytosis. Fever and pharyngitis are not usual manifestations of pertussis; when they occur, a secondary cause should be sought. Except for the observation of typical paroxysms, physical examination of pertussis patients is usually unrewarding; on auscultation diffuse rhonchi may be noted. Infection with *B. parapertussis* causes an illness similar to that caused by *B. pertussis,* but it is generally less severe and shorter lived.[43]

Mild Illness

Mild nonclassical illness due to *B. pertussis* infection is common.[21, 24] This occurs in previously vaccinated children and as a primary infection in nonvaccinated children. We conducted a study in which we encouraged physicians to send to our laboratory nasopharyngeal specimens from children with any cough illness, whether or not the illnesses were typical of pertussis.[21] We found that, of 247 culture-positive cases, 47% had a total duration of cough illness of 28 days or less. In 26% the duration of cough was less than 3 weeks. The vast majority of these cases occurred in unvaccinated children.

In a study in which both culture and PCR were used for diagnosis of *B. pertussis* infection we found that many mild cases were PCR positive and culture negative.[24] Of cases that were PCR positive and culture negative only 68% had a cough illness of $\geq$ 4 weeks, and only 57% and 32%, respectively, had paroxysmal cough or whooping.

Infants

Pertussis in infancy is unique. Its spectrum of clinical manifestations varies by age, immunization, and the presence or absence of transplacentally acquired antibody.[1, 2, 7, 29, 31, 32, 50–52] In the United States the rates of hospitalizations, complications, and death for infants are hospitalization 69%, pneumonia 22%, seizures 3%, encephalopathy 0.9%, and death 0.6%.[31]

B. pertussis infection is particularly severe in neonates (death rate, 1.3%).[7, 31, 49–51] A common presenting finding is apnea, and typical coughing is not observed. Seizures in association with apnea are not infrequent. Severe disease in young infants is frequently associated with marked leukocytosis; total white blood cell counts in the range of 30,000–60,000 cells per microliter are seen, with lymphocytosis.

Whooping is a rare manifestation of illness in infants, and other respiratory tract manifestations are frequently confused with those due to respiratory tract viruses.[2] *B. pertussis* infection may be a cause of SIDS.[52]

Adults

In recent years awareness of adult pertussis has increased.[4–6, 8, 27, 29, 31, 32] Unrecognized pertussis cases in adults are often the primary cases from which infants and children become infected.[7, 32, 49–51] All adults have at some time been exposed to *B. pertussis* antigens, by either immunization or infection, or both, and this fact tends to modify the illness.[11, 27, 45] The illness appears to be different in those who were immunized as children. Of 31 university students with laboratory-confirmed *B. pertussis* infection in a United States study, the clinical diagnoses (and prevalence) by the primary case providers were as follows: upper respiratory tract infection (39%), bronchitis (48%), pertussis (0%), and other diagnoses (16%).[5] Although specific records were not available, it is likely that most of these students were vaccinated as children and that most had also had an unrecognized infection.[27, 45]

In contrast with these findings in the United States, we found that adults in Germany were more likely to have typical pertussis, even though our epidemiologic data suggested that all had had a previous infection.[6, 45] The rate of clinical manifestations in 64 laboratory-confirmed cases were as follows: paroxysms, 70%; whoop, 38%; posttussive phlegm, 66%; and posttussive vomiting, 17%. The clinical diagnosis was definite or probable pertussis in 39%; 14% were thought not to have pertussis.

DIAGNOSIS AND DIFFERENTIAL DIAGNOSIS

The clinical diagnosis of classic cases of pertussis should be made without difficulty; however the cause of the illness could be due to *B. pertussis* or *B. parapertussis*. The history of contact with a known case (i.e., a laboratory-confirmed one) also helps make the diagnosis when illness is mild or atypical. The presence of leukocytosis with lymphocyte predominance in a child with a cough illness or an infant with apnea is a strong indication that the illness is due to *B. pertussis*. There are few other diseases in which the level of lymphocytosis is 10,000 cells per microliter or more.

The definitive diagnosis is made by culture or specific antibody studies, as discussed previously in the Microbiology section. In classic disease the culture or a direct fluorescent antibody (DFA) study yields a positive result in about 80% of cases if the specimen was obtained within 2 weeks of onset of cough and if antibiotics were not previously administered.[21, 25] Routine laboratory diagnosis of *B. pertussis* infections in adults or in other atypical cases is hampered by the fact that care usually is not sought until the third or fourth week of the illness, and, frequently, antibiotics have been administered before the possibility of pertussis was considered.[5, 6]

Other infectious agents that cause illnesses with cough that can be confused with pertussis are *Mycoplasma pneumoniae; Chlamydia trachomatis, Chlamydia pneumoniae,* adenoviruses, and other respiratory viruses.[1–3] In addition, the cough associated with sinusitis can be confused with that due to *B. pertussis* infection. Airway foreign bodies can on occasion confound the diagnosis. One of us has seen a child with typical pertussis whose head and neck surgeon performed bronchoscopy because of concern that a foreign body was causing the problem.

TREATMENT

Several antibiotics have efficacy in vitro against *B. pertussis*.[53, 54] The first choice for treatment is oral erythromycin, which ameliorates the symptoms if given early during the course of the illness and eliminates the organism from the nasopharynx within a few days, thus shortening the period of contagion.[55] The dose for children is 50 mg/kg/day given every 6 hours for 14 days. For adults the dose is 2 g/day given every 6 hours for 14 days. Trimethoprim-sulfamethoxazole can be used as an alternative agent for patients who cannot tolerate erythromycin.[56]

Supportive care includes avoidance of factors that provoke attacks of coughing and maintenance of hydration and nutrition. In the hospital, gentle suction for removal of secretions and well-humidified oxygen may be required, particularly in infants with pneumonia and significant respiratory distress. For severe infections in neonates and young infants assisted ventilation may be necessary. Salbutamol and corticosteroids may be of some value, but definitive studies have not established these modes of treatment.[57, 58]

PROGNOSIS

The prognosis in pertussis is directly related to the patients' age. For older children and adults the prognosis is good. Infants are at significant risk for death (0.3%–1.3%) and encephalopathy (0.5%–1.4%).[31] In addition, long-term follow-up suggests that apnea or seizures at the time of disease may be associated with subsequent intellectual impairment.[59] The availability of pediatric intensive care units and assisted ventilation has reduced mortality for infants who get medical care. Unfortunately, many deaths occur outside the hospital.

PREVENTION

Present Vaccines

Whole-cell pertussis vaccines are used worldwide, and they effectively control pertussis in many countries.[1, 3] They consist of killed *B. pertussis* organisms that are adsorbed onto an adjuvant such as aluminum phosphate and contain a preservative such as thimerosal. In most countries the pertussis component is combined with diphtheria and tetanus toxoids (DTP) and is administered in three to five doses. The current recommendation in the United States is three doses at age 2, 4, and 6 months, a 4th dose at 12–18 months, and a 5th at 4–6 years of age.[60] Although three- and four-dose schedules that are completed at 10–18 months of age are somewhat effective in preventing severe disease in infants, they are inferior to the five-dose schedule used in the United States because they allow disease to occur in young school-aged children, who may spread the infection to unimmunized infants.[61, 62]

Several unpleasant, transient side effects can be attributed to the pertussis component in DTP vaccines.[1–3, 63] These include local reactions such as pain, erythema, and induration as well as systemic reactions, including fever, irritability, anorexia, persistent crying, hypotonic-hyporesponsive episodes, and seizures in seizure-prone children. All whole-cell vaccines contain endotoxin, and it is a major cause of fever and pain at the injection site and of other common reactions.[64] Persistent crying is initiated by painful local reactions.[65]

Since their early use in the 1940s whole-cell pertussis vaccines were thought to cause severe neurologic reactions and death.[1, 2] In the 1970s spectacular media reports in several countries and several scientifically flawed publications engendered general mistrust of pertussis vaccines; since then, however, several large epidemiologic studies have been published that establish without doubt that SIDS is not caused by pertussis vaccine and that the entity called "pertussis vaccine encephalopathy" does not exist.[3, 66, 67] Several societies and expert groups have concluded that there is no evidence to implicate pertussis vaccine as a cause of brain damage.[67]

New Acellular Vaccines

Research in the 1970s showed that three *B. pertussis* antigens (pertussis toxin, filamentous hemagglutinin, lipo-oligosaccharide) were liberated into the medium during culture and that these antigens could be concentrated and separated by density gradient centrifugation.[1, 68] This allowed for the development and production of vaccines by six different manufacturers in Japan. All six vaccines had minimal amounts of endotoxin but different amounts of "toxoided" pertussis toxin and filamentous hemagglutinin. In addition, it was found that five of the six vaccines also contained fimbriae-2 and pertactin.

Despite limited proof of efficacy, the six vaccines were put into routine use in Japan in 1981 and they have controlled epidemic pertussis during the ensuing 14 years. Since adequate data were not available on any single vaccine or on vaccine use in early infancy many extensive trials were subsequently carried out in Europe, Africa, and Japan. The results of early trials in Sweden and Japan resulted in licensure in the United States of two acellular vaccines for 4th and 5th doses.[69, 70]

During the last 5 years definitive trials in infants in four countries with eight different vaccines have been carried out.[67, 71] The results of some of these trials are presently becoming available. The present vaccines all contain different numbers and concentrations of antigens. A summary of the data available at present indicates that multicomponent vaccines that contain pertactin in addition to toxoided pertussis toxin and filamentous hemagglutinin have greater efficacy than the two-component (toxoided pertussis toxin, filamentous hemagglutinin) and single-component (toxoided pertussis toxin) products.

All acellular vaccines being evaluated today have been shown to be less "reactogenic" than whole-cell vaccines. It is our opinion that several multicomponent vaccines that contain toxoided pertussis toxin, filamentous hemagglutinin, and pertactin or toxoided pertussis toxin, filamentous hemagglutinin, pertactin, and fimbriae will be licensed in the United States in 1996. A three-component vaccine containing toxoided pertussis toxin, filamentous hemagglutinin, and pertactin was approved in Germany for use in infants in March 1995.

Because acellular vaccines are significantly less reactogenic than whole-cell vaccines they offer the possibility of booster immunizations for adolescents and adults.[76] It is our opinion that future programs with multicomponent acellular vaccines that include booster doses for adolescents and adults as well as universal childhood immunization will control disease—and perhaps the circulation of *B. pertussis.*

Isolation and Prophylactic Measures

In the index case erythromycin shortens communicability of the organisms and thus limits spread of the disease. During the first few days of treatment contact with susceptible persons should be avoided. In general, close (household, day care, playmate) contacts of the index patient should be protected from infection. This can be managed with prophylactic erythromycin[77] for 14 days and active immunization of children younger than 7 years who have not completed their immunization series for pertussis.[60]

Prophylactic use of erythromycin for exposed adults is frequently recommended. In the hospital setting this frequently involves many people and considerable expense. In our experience, the side effects of erythromycin are such that adult compliance is poor. Thus, it is our opinion that erythromycin should not be used prophylactically but should be used only at the first sign of respiratory illness for treatment of those exposed.

References

1. Cherry JD, Brunell PA, Golden GS, et al.: Report of the task force on pertussis and pertussis immunization—1988. Pediatrics 1988; 81: 939–984.
2. Cherry JD: The epidemiology of pertussis and pertussis immunization in the United Kingdom and the United States: A comparative study. Curr Probl Pediatr 1984; 14: 1–78.
3. Feigin RD, Cherry JD: Pertussis. In: Feigin RD, Cherry JD (eds): Textbook of Pediatric Infectious Diseases, 3rd ed. Philadelphia: WB Saunders Co, 1992, pp 1208–1218.
4. Mink C, Sirota NM, Nugent S: Outbreak of pertussis in a fully immunized adolescent and adult population. Arch Pediatr Adolesc Med 1994; 148: 153–157.
5. Mink C, Cherry JD, Christenson PD, et al.: A search for *Bordetella pertussis* infection in university students. Clin Infect Dis 1992; 14: 464–471.
6. Schmitt-Grohé S, Cherry JD, Heininger U, et al.: Pertussis in German adults. Clin Infect Dis 1995; 21: 860–866.
7. Heininger U, Stehr K, Cherry JD: Serious pertussis overlooked in infants. Eur J Pediatr 1992; 151: 342–343.
8. Wright SW, Edwards KM, Decker MD, et al.: Pertussis infection in adults with persistent cough. JAMA 1995; 273: 1044–1046.
9. Long S, Lischner H, Deforest A, et al.: Serologic evidence of subclinical pertussis in immunized children. Pediatr Infect Dis J 1990; 9: 700–705.
10. Long S, Welkon C, Clark J: Widespread silent transmission of pertussis in families: Antibody correlates of infection and symptomatology. J Infect Dis 1990; 161: 480–486.
11. Deville JG, Cherry JD, Christenson PD, et al.: Frequency of unrecognized *Bordetella pertussis* infections in adults. Clin Infect Dis 1995; 21: 639–642.
12. Cone TE: Whooping cough is first described as a disease sui generis by Baillou in 1640. Pediatrics 1970; 46: 522.
13. Bordet J, Gengou U: Le microbe de la coqueluche. Ann Inst Pasteur 1906; 20: 48–68.
14. Eldering G, Kendrick P: A group of cultures resembling both *Bacillus pertussis* and *Bacillus bronchisepticus* but identical with neither (abstract). J Bacteriol 1937; 33: 71.
15. Madsen T: Whooping cough: Its bacteriology, diagnosis, prevention and treatment. Boston Med Surg J 1925; 192: 50–60.

16. Kendrick PL, Eldering G, Dixon MK, et al.: Mouse protection tests in the study of pertussis vaccines. Am J Public Health 1947; 37: 803–810.

17. Medical Research Council: Vaccination against whooping cough. Br Med J 1959; 1: 994–1000.

18. Kimura M, Kuno-Sakai H: Pertussis vaccines in Japan. Acta Paediatr Jpn 1988; 30: 143–153.

19. Switzer WP, Mare CJ, Hubbari ED: Incidence of *Bordetella bronchisepticum* in wild life and man in Iowa. Am J Vet Res 1966; 27: 1134–1136.

20. Arico B, Rappuoli R: *Bordetella parapertussis* and *Bordetella bronchiseptica* contain transcriptionally silent pertussis toxin genes. J Bacteriol 1987; 169: 2847–2853.

21. Heininger U, Cherry JD, Eckhardt T, et al.: Clinical and laboratory diagnosis of pertussis in the regions of a large vaccine efficacy trial in Germany. Pediatr Infect Dis J 1993; 12: 504–509.

22. Regan J, Lowe F: Enrichment medium for the isolation of *Bordetella*. J Clin Microbiol 1977; 6: 303–309.

23. Wirsing von König CH, Tacken A, Finger H: Use of supplemented Stainer-Scholte broth for the isolation of *Bordetella pertussis* from clinical material. J Clin Microbiol 1988; 26: 2558–2560.

24. Schläpfer G, Cherry JD, Heininger U, et al.: Polymerase chain reaction identification of *Bordetella pertussis* infections in vaccinees and family members in a pertussis vaccine efficacy trial in Germany. Pediatr Infect Dis J 1995; 14: 209–214.

25. Onorato IM, Wassilak SG: Laboratory diagnosis of pertussis: The state of the art. Pediatr Infect Dis J 1987; 6: 145–151.

26. Hallander HO, Storsaeter J, Möllby R: Evaluation of serology and nasopharyngeal cultures for diagnosis of pertussis in a vaccine efficacy trial. J Infect Dis 1991; 163: 1046–1054.

27. Deen JL, Mink CM, Cherry JD, et al.: A household contact study of *Bordetella pertussis* infections. Clin Infect Dis 1995; 21: 1211–1219.

28. Granström M, Lindberg A, Askelöf P, et al.: Detection of antibodies in human serum against fimbrial haemagglutinin of *Bordetella pertussis* by enzyme-linked immunosorbent assay. J Med Microbiol 1982; 15: 85–96.

29. CDC: Pertussis—United States, January 1992–June 1995. MMWR 1995; 44: 525–529.

30. Fine PED, Clarkson JA: The recurrence of whooping cough: Possible implications for assessment of vaccine efficacy. Lancet 1982; 1: 666–669.

31. Farizo KM, Cochi SL, Zell ER, et al.: Epidemiological features of pertussis in the United States, 1980–1989. Clin Infect Dis 1992; 14: 708–719.

32. Nelson JD: The changing epidemiology of pertussis in young infants: The role of adults as reservoirs of infection. Am J Dis Child 1978; 132: 371–373.

33. Gordon M, Davies HD, Gold R: Clinical and microbiologic features of children presenting with pertussis to a Canadian pediatric hospital during an eleven-year period. Pediatr Infect Dis J 1994; 13: 617–622.

34. Weiss AA, Hewlett EL: Virulence factors of *Bordetella pertussis*. Ann Rev Microbiol 1986; 40: 661–686.

35. Munoz JJ: Action of pertussigen (pertussis toxin) on the host immune system. In: Wardlaw AC, Parton R (eds): Pathogenesis and Immunity in Pertussis London: John Wiley & Sons, 1988, pp 173–192.

36. Preston NW: Pertussis today. In: Wardlaw AC, Parton R (eds): Pathogenesis and Immunity in Pertussis. New York: John Wiley & Sons, 1988, pp 1–18.

37. Tuomanen E: *Bordetella pertussis* adhesins. In: Wardlaw AC, Parton R (eds): Pathogenesis and Immunity in Pertussis. New York: John Wiley & Sons, 1988, pp 75–94.

38. Urisu A, Cowell JL, Manclark CR: Filamentous hemagglutinin has a major role in mediating adherence of *Bordetella pertussis* to human WiDr cells. Infect Immun 1986; 52: 695–701.

39. Mooi FA, van der Heide HGJ, Willems R, et al.: *Bordetella pertussis* fimbriae: Role in pathogenesis and mechanism of phase variation. In: Manclark CR (ed): 1990 Sixth International Symposium on Pertussis Abstracts. Department of Health and Human Services. Bethesda, MD: United States Public Health Service, DHHS Publication No. (FDA) 90-1162-1163.

40. Hewlett EL, Gordon VM: Adenylate cyclase toxin of *Bordetella pertussis*. In: Wardlaw AC, Parton R (eds): Pathogenesis and Immunity in Pertussis. New York: John Wiley & Sons, 1988, pp 193–209.

41. Goldman WE: Tracheal cytotoxin of *Bordetella pertussis*. In: Wardlaw AC, Parton R (eds): Pathogenesis and Immunity in Pertussis. New York: John Wiley & Sons, 1988, pp 237–246.

42. Nakasa Y, Endoh M: Heat-labile toxin of *Bordetella pertussis*. In: Wardlaw AC, Parton R (eds): Pathogenesis and Immunity in Pertussis. New York: John Wiley & Sons, 1988, pp 217–229.

43. Heininger U, Stehr K, Schmitt-Grohé S, et al.: Clinical characteristics of illness caused by *Bordetella parapertussis* compared with illness caused by *Bordetella pertussis*. Pediatr Infect Dis J 1994; 13: 306–309.

44. Lambert HJ: Epidemiology of a small pertussis outbreak in Kent County, Michigan. Public Health Rep 1965; 80: 365–369.

45. Cherry JD, Beer T, Chartrand SA, et al.: Comparison of antibody values to *Bordetella pertussis* antigens in young German and American men. *Clin Infect Dis* 1995; 20: 1271–1274.

46. Mills KHG, Redhead K: Cellular immunity in pertussis. J Med Microbiol 1993; 39: 163–164.

47. Lautrop H: Observation on parapertussis in Denmark 1950–1957. Acta Pathol Microbiol Scand 1958; 43: 255–266.

48. Taranger J, Trollfors B, Lagergård T, et al: Parapertussis infection followed by pertussis infection. Lancet 1994; 344: 1703.

49. Beiter A, Lewis K, Pineda EF, et al.: Unrecognized maternal peripartum pertussis with subsequent fatal neonatal pertussis. Obstet Gynecol 1993; 82: 691–693.

50. Christie CDC, Baltimore RD: Pertussis in neonates. Am J Dis Child 1989; 143: 1199–1202.

51. McGregor J, Ogle JW, Curry-Kane J: Perinatal pertussis. Obstet Gynecol 1984; 68: 582–585.

52. Nicoll A, Gardner A: Whooping cough and unrecognized postperinatal mortality. Arch Dis Child 1988; 63: 41–47.

53. Hoppe J, Haug A: Antimicrobial susceptibility of *Bordetella pertussis* (Part I). Infection 1988; 16: 126–130.

54. Hoppe J, Eichhorn A: Activity of new macrolides against *Bordetella pertussis* and *Bordetella parapertussis*. Eur J Clin Microbiol Infect Dis 1989; 8: 653–654.

55. Bergquist S, Bernander S, Dahnsjö H, et al.: Erythromycin in the treatment of pertussis: A study of bacteriologic and clinical effects. Pediatr Infect Dis J 1987; 6: 458–461.

56. Hoppe J, Halm U, Hagedorn H, et al.: Comparison of erythromycin ethylsuccinate and co-trimoxazole for treatment of pertussis. Infection 1989; 17: 227–231.

57. Broomhall J, Herxheimer A: Treatment of whooping cough: The facts. Arch Dis Child 1984; 59: 185–187.

58. Zoumboulakis D, Anagnostakin D, Albanie V, et al.: Steroids in treatment of pertussis—a controlled clinical trial. Arch Dis Child 1973; 48: 51–54.

59. Swansea Research Unit of the Royal College of General Practitioners: Study of intellectual performance of children in ordinary schools after certain serious complications of whooping cough. Br Med J 1987; 295: 1044–1047.

60. American Academy of Pediatrics: Pertussis. In: Peter G (ed): 1994 Redbook: Report of the Committee on Infectious Diseases, 23rd ed. Elk Grove Village, IL: American Academy of Pediatrics, 1994, 355–362.

61. Cherry JD: Strategies for Diphtheria, Tetanus, and Pertussis (DTP) Immunization. Report of the 104th Ross Conference on Pediatric Research. Columbus, OH: Ross Products Division, Abbott Laboratories, 1994, 218–225.

62. Nielsen A, Larsen SO: Epidemiology of pertussis in Denmark: The impact of herd immunity. Int J Epidemiol 1993; 23: 1300–1308.

63. Cody CL, Baraff LJ, Cherry JD, et al.: Nature and rates of adverse reactions associated with DTP and DT immunizations in infants and children. Pediatrics 1981; 68: 650–660.

64. Baraff LJ, Manclark CR, Cherry JD, et al.: Analysis of adverse reactions to diphtheria and tetanus toxoids and pertussis vaccine by vaccine lot, endotoxin content, pertussis vaccine potency and percentage of mouse weight gain. Pediatr Infect Dis J 1989; 8: 502–507.

65. Blumberg DA, Lewis K, Mink CM, et al.: Severe reactions associated with diphtheria-tetanus-pertussis vaccine: Detailed study of children with seizures, hypotonic-hyporesponsive episodes, high fevers, and persistent crying. Pediatrics 1993; 91: 1158–1165.

66. Cherry JD: 'Pertussis vaccine encephalopathy': It is time to recognize it as the myth that it is. JAMA 1990; 263: 1679–1680.

67. Cherry JD: Pertussis: The trials and tribulations of old and new pertussis vaccines. Vaccine 1992; 10: 1033–1038.

68. Hewlett EL, Cherry JD: New and improved vaccines against pertussis. In: Woodrow GC, Levine MM (eds): New Generation Vaccines. New York: Marcel Dekker, 1990, pp 231–250.

69. Mortimer EA, Limura M, Cherry JD, et al.: Protective efficacy of the Takeda acellular pertussis vaccine combined with diphtheria and tetanus

toxoids following household exposure of Japanese children. Am J Dis Child 1990; 144: 899–904.

70. Ad Hoc Group for the Study of Pertussis Vaccines: Placebo-controlled trial of two acellular pertussis vaccines in Sweden: Protective efficacy and adverse events. Lancet 1988; 1: 955–960.

71. Schmitt HJ, Wagner S: Pertussis vaccines—1993. Eur J Pediatr 1993; 152: 462–466.

72. Schmitt HJ, Wirsing von König CH, Neiss A, et al.: Efficacy of acellular pertussis vaccine in early childhood after household exposure. JAMA 1996; 275: 37–41.

73. Trollfors B, Taranger J, Lagergård T, et al.: A placebo-controlled trial of a pertussis-toxoid vaccine. N Engl J Med 1995; 333: 1045–1050.

74. Greco D, Salmaso S, Mastrantonio P, et al.: A controlled trial of two acellular vaccines and one whole-cell vaccine against pertussis. N Engl J Med 1996; 334: 341–348.

75. Gustafsson L, Hallander HO, Olin P, et al.: A controlled trial of a two-component acellular, a five-component acellular and a whole-cell pertussis vaccine. N Engl J Med 1996; 334: 349–355.

76. Cherry JD: Acellular vaccines—a solution to the pertussis problem. J Infect Dis 1993; 168: 21–24.

77. Steketee R, Wassilak S, Adkins WN Jr, et al.: Evidence for a high attack rate and efficacy of erythromycin prophylaxis in a pertussis outbreak in a facility for the developmentally disabled. J Infect Dis 1988; 157: 434–440.

Chen-Chia Chiou

Diphtheria

▼

Diphtheria is an example of an infectious disease that has been conquered based on principles of microbiology and public health.[1] Diphtheria is characterized by the characteristic leathery membrane caused by *Corynebacterium diphtheriae*. Pierre Brettoneau in 1821 recognized diphtheria as a clinical entity. In 1883, Klebs described the diphtheria bacillus in the membrane of a patient with diphtheria. In 1884, Friedrich Loeffler isolated the micro-organism in pure culture. In 1888, Roux and Yersin showed that the cause of the disease was an extracellular protein (toxin) rather than the bacteria itself.[2] Diphtheria has gone from a major health problem to a rare, unfamiliar disease. Diphtheria shares many "firsts" in the history of medicine: the first bacterium to be established as a specific pathogen for a disease, the first bacterial disease for which a toxin was discovered, and the first to be treated with antitoxin and prevented by a toxoid vaccine in a public health setting. Research findings emanating from this disease led to major insights into pathology, bacteriology, and immunology in general.

THE PATHOGEN

C. diphtheriae is an irregularly staining, gram-positive, non-motile, nonsporulating, unencapsulated pleomorphic bacillus. Its name is derived from the Greek "korynee," or club, referring to its club shape, and "diphtheria," meaning leather hide, for the characteristic leathery pharyngeal membrane that it provokes. When this bacillus is grown in Loeffler's medium, which consists of coagulated serum with a high concentration of phosphate, granules of polymerized phosphate are produced that stain metachromatically with methylene blue (metachromatic granules). The club shape of the bacillus is not a universal morphologic feature but occurs when it is grown in nutritionally inadequate media, including Loeffler's media. *C. diphtheriae* organisms divide in such a way that in smears they form sharp angles with each other, demonstrating a palisading morphology ("Chinese characters") which differentiates it from other corynebacteria; this is more prominent on smears taken from colonies on Loeffler's medium than on direct smears taken from clinical specimens. The bacillus is recovered most readily on media containing tellurite, which retards the growth of other micro-organisms.

Colonies of *C. diphtheriae* appear grayish white on Loeffler's media. Three biotypes based on colonial morphology and biochemical characteristics can be distinguished: *gravis, intermedius,* and *mitis.* The *mitis* biotype causes less severe disease because it produces less toxin.[3]

The *C. diphtheriae* strains may be either toxigenic or nontoxigenic. The ability to produce toxin is mediated by a lysogenic β-phage carrying the gene for toxin production.[4] Strains of *C. diphtheriae* lacking lysogenic phage do not produce toxin, but they can be converted to toxigenicity in the laboratory and in nature by infecting them with the lysogenic toxin phage.[5] Toxin production can be increased by exposure to ultraviolet light and growth in iron-deficient media.[6] Toxigenicity of individual *C. diphtheriae* can be demonstrated by two tests: necrosis of tissue in guinea pigs or gel diffusion in agar. The latter test (Elek's test) demonstrates a precipitin band between toxin and antitoxin.

PATHOGENESIS

Diphtheria is initiated by entry of *C. diphtheriae* into the mouth or nose, and the bacilli remain localized on the mucosal surfaces of the upper respiratory tract. Occasionally, preexisting skin lesions as well as ocular or genital mucous membranes can serve as the portal of entry. The bacilli are unable to penetrate intact skin.

C. diphtheriae is not an invasive organism. The primary virulence factor is an exotoxin that inhibits protein synthesis in mammalian cells but not in bacteria. Following a 1–8 day period of incubation, lysogenized strains (strains infected with bacteriophage) may elaborate toxin. The toxin, a 62-kd-polypeptide, consists of two subunits. The larger B subunit

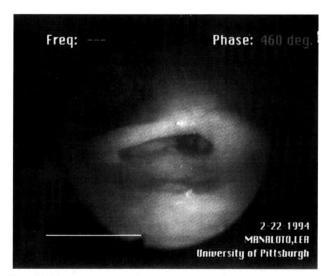

Figure 50–1. Long-standing laryngeal stenosis secondary to diphtheria at age 2 years. The posterior larynx is involved by a web of scar tissue that goes from arytenoid to arytenoid.

is involved in receptor binding, whereas the A subunit is enzymatically active. Following proteolytic separation, subunit A enters the mammalian cell and inactivates transfer RNA translocase (the elongation factor 2), thus preventing the addition of amino acids to the growing native polypeptide chain.[7] Diphtheria toxin is extremely potent: a single molecule can stop protein synthesis in a cell within several hours.[8] It is lethal for humans in an amount of about 130 μg/kg body weight.[9]

The toxin affects all cells in the body, but the most prominent effects are on the heart (myocarditis), nerves (demyelination), and kidneys (tubular necrosis). Although diphtheria antitoxin can neutralize circulating toxin or that adsorbed to cells, it is ineffective when cell penetration has occurred. There is a variable latent period. Myocarditis generally occurs 10–14 days after onset of illness. Peripheral neuritis usually does not occur until 3–7 weeks.[10]

Toxin-mediated tissue necrosis is severe in the vicinity of colonization. The local inflammatory response, coupled with the necrotic tissue, produces a fibrinous patchy exudate. As toxin production increases, a tough adherent pseudomembrane is formed that varies in color from gray to black, depending on the amount of blood it contains. The membrane contains fibrin, leukocytes, erythrocytes, organisms, and superficial epithelial cells. Since the epithelial cells are an integral part of the membrane, attempts to remove it provoke bleeding. The pseudomembrane sloughs spontaneously during the recovery period.

The membrane can be local (nasal, tonsillar, pharyngeal) or can extend far, forming a cast of the pharynx and the tracheobronchial tree. Edema of the soft tissue beneath the membrane may be extensive and contribute to the "bull neck" appearance. Occasionally secondary bacterial infection (usually streptococcal) develops. In both adults and children, a common cause of death is suffocation following aspiration of the membrane.

EPIDEMIOLOGY

Humans are the only known reservoir of *C. diphtheriae*. Sources of infection include secretions from the nose, throat, eyes, and skin lesions of infected persons. Transmission results after contact with a patient or carrier. The respiratory tract disease peaks in the colder months of autumn and winter. Skin infection is considered a problem principally in tropical areas. Skin carriers of *C. diphtheriae* may be more infectious than either nose or throat carriers.[11, 12] In areas where skin infections are endemic, levels of natural immunity may be high.[12, 13]

Diphtheria occurs worldwide. It is still endemic in developing countries (Brazil, Nigeria, eastern Mediterranean region, India, Indonesia, Thailand, and the Philippines).[14] The incidence of diphtheria has declined markedly following extensive use of diphtheria toxoid after World War II.[15, 16] Since 1980, five cases or fewer have been reported each year in the United States, and since 1988, all culture-confirmed cases in the United States have been imported[17]; however, the lower frequency of natural exposure to the disease is apparently leading to a decline in adult immunity. During periods of high incidence, diphtheria traditionally affected undervaccinated children. This profile is changing as lower levels of protective antitoxin are leaving adults susceptible to infection. Outbreaks have been reported among highly immunized populations.[18] Recent reports have cited pharyngeal carriage of nontoxigenic strains in homosexual men and invasive disease in intravenous drug abusers and children.[19–21] Epidemics have occurred among alcoholics and other disadvantaged groups.[22]

Prior immunization decreases the severity of disease.[23, 24] Disease was considered severe in 25% of nonimmunized patients as compared with 6.3% of fully immunized ones. Case fatality rate was also higher in unimmunized groups (19% versus 1.3%).[3]

Serum antitoxin levels can be measured by neutralization test in rabbit skin, in Vero cell culture, or by hemagglutination. Concentrations of 0.1–0.01 IU generally are thought to confer immunity against diphtheria.[22, 25] Seroprevalence studies in the United States, the Russian Federation, and other developed countries indicate that large numbers of adults remain susceptible to diphtheria, having serum antitoxin levels below the protective levels.[24–30] Epidemic diphtheria has reemerged in 14 of 15 New Independent States (NIS, the former Soviet Union). During 1994, almost 50,000 cases and 1,800 deaths occurred from diphtheria throughout the NIS.[31] High levels of susceptibility to diphtheria—particularly among adults—have played an important role in sustaining transmission in NIS.

CLINICAL MANIFESTATIONS

The clinical manifestations of diphtheria occur locally in the respiratory tract and skin at the port of entry and at distant sites secondary to the dissemination of the toxin. Diphtheria is classified clinically by the location of the membrane: nasal, tonsillar, pharyngeal, laryngeal, laryngotracheal, conjunctival, genital, or skin. More than one anatomic site may be involved. The incubation period ranges from 1–8 days.

Respiratory Tract Diphtheria

Nasal diphtheria may occur alone or as part of pharyngeal diphtheria; it may be unilateral or bilateral. Mild rhinorrhea resembling a common cold occurs first. Gradually, the nasal discharge becomes serosanguineous and mucopurulent. Erosions can develop on the anterior nares and upper lip. A foul odor may be notable. Careful inspection may reveal a white membrane on the nasal septum. Constitutional symptoms are usually very mild or absent because absorption of toxin from nasal mucosa is poor. This form occurs most often in infants.

The tonsils and the pharynx are the most common sites of diphtheria infection. Sore throat, pharyngeal injection, and low-grade fever (rarely higher than 103° F) can occur abruptly. Within 1–2 days the membrane develops on one or both tonsils with extension to the tonsillar pillars, uvula, soft palate, oropharynx, or nasopharynx. This characteristic extension distinguishes diphtheria from other forms of membranous tonsillitis. The membrane initially appears shiny white but soon evolves to a grayish color with patches of green or black necrosis. The borders of the membrane are sharply defined, and the membrane is adherent to the underlying tissue; attempts to remove it produce bleeding. There is marked swelling of the cervical lymph nodes and frequently extensive infiltration of the soft tissue of the neck, so the head is thrown back to relieve pressure on the airway. The swelling sometimes forms a distinct collar, reaching from ear to ear and filling out the whole space beneath the jaw, creating stridor and a bull neck appearance.

The extent of the membrane correlates with the severity of symptoms. In severe cases, respiratory failure may ensue. Relative bradycardia (the pulse rate is disproportionately increased in relation to body temperature) and hypotension may be seen. Palatal paralysis may occur. If there is bilateral paralysis, nasal regurgitation and difficulty in swallowing may occur. Stupor, coma, and death may follow within 7–10 days. In less severe cases, recovery may be slow or complicated by myocarditis or neuritis. In mild cases, the membrane sloughs off in 7–10 days and recovery is uneventful.

Laryngeal diphtheria can represent downward extension of the membrane from the pharynx or can be the original site of the disease (Fig. 50–1). Symptoms include hoarseness, dyspnea, respiratory stridor, and a brassy cough. These signs are indistinguishable from those of other types of infectious croup. A patient with laryngeal diphtheria may appear anxious and cyanotic, using accessory muscles of respiration. Suprasternal, subcostal, and supraclavicular retractions reflect severe laryngeal obstruction, which may be fatal if not alleviated. Edema and membrane involvement of the trachea may cause respiratory distress. Acute and fatal obstruction may occur if the airway becomes occluded by the membrane.

Cutaneous Diphtheria

Cutaneous diphtheria is characterized by chronic nonhealing ulcers that have a dirty grayish membrane and sharply demarcated edges. The lesions may last weeks or months and involve several parts of the body, including the umbilicus, genitocrural flexures, toe cleft, and the area behind the ears.[32] They are often associated with streptococcal or staphylococcal infections. Although cutaneous diphtheria is more common in tropical areas, outbreaks have occurred in the United States among alcoholic, homeless, and impoverished populations, such as native Americans. It should also be included in the differential diagnosis of skin lesions of travelers returning from tropical areas.[33] Skin carriers have very persistent diseases, and in endemic areas it probably contributes toward natural immunity.[11, 12, 34] Cutaneous diphtheria is an important source of person-to-person transmission, including respiratory forms.

Conjunctival Diphtheria

Conjunctival lesions usually are limited to the palpebral conjunctiva, which appears red, edematous, and membranous. Corneal lesions may also occur.[35]

Otic Diphtheria

Diphtheric infections of the ear have been reported in native American children in northern Canada.[15] The primary disease of these children was otitis media caused by streptococci; the *Corynebacterium* infection appeared to be secondary. Otic diphtheria can also present as otitis externa with a persistently purulent and foul-smelling discharge.

COMPLICATIONS

Airway obstruction and death may occur suddenly in patients with diphtheria. This is caused by aspiration of the dislodged pharyngeal membrane, by its extension to the larynx, or by external compression by enlarged nodes and edema. Systemic complications are due to toxin elaboration. Although almost any system may be affected, involvement of the heart and nervous system is most common. Myocarditis may follow both mild and severe forms of diphtheria. The risk of developing myocarditis is directly correlated with the extent and severity of local diseases. Generally, it is associated with delayed administration of antitoxin. Myocarditis most commonly occurs in the 2nd week of disease, when the local disease is improving. Tachycardia, muffled heart sounds, murmurs, and arrhythmia are indicative of myocardial involvement.[36] The most common arrhythmias are supraventricular and ventricular ectopy.[37]

Neurologic complications are also proportional to the severity of primary infection. It appears after a variable latent period, is predominantly bilateral, and usually is motor rather than sensory. Paralysis of the soft palate and pharyngeal muscles is common. Paralysis of ocular muscles or the diaphragm as well as peripheral neuropathy may also occur. Total resolution of diphtheric nerve damage usually follows therapy.

DIAGNOSIS

Knowledge of the patient's immune status is helpful: a recent immunization or booster injection with diphtheria toxoid makes the diagnosis of diphtheria unlikely. Definitive diagnosis depends on isolation of the organism. Rapid diagnosis can be made with immunofluorescent staining of a 4-hour culture, but the sensitivity and specificity of this test are not known for certain.[38, 39] The membrane should be cultured. The laboratory must be notified about the suspicion of diphtheria so that appropriate Loeffler's, tellurite, and blood agar media are inoculated. The recovery of beta-hemolytic streptococci from a culture dose not rule out the diagnosis of diphtheria since these bacteria have been found in 30% of diphtheria cases.[40]

Other laboratory studies have little diagnostic value. The white blood cell count may be normal or elevated. Anemia occasionally occurs, as a result of rapid hemolysis. Liver toxicity may present as hypoglycemia or glycosuria. In patients with diphtheric neuritis, slight elevation of protein and mild pleocytosis in cerebrospinal fluid can be documented. An elevated blood urea nitrogen value may develop in patients with acute tubular necrosis. An electrocardiogram may reveal ST-segment and T-wave changes, as well as supraventricular or ventricular ectopic beats.

Diphtheria bacilli that are recovered should be tested for toxigenicity. Toxin production can be demonstrated either by guinea pig neutralization test or Elek's test. In the former, two guinea pigs are inoculated with a broth suspension of the micro-organism. One of the animals is given diphtheria antitoxin before the intracutaneous challenge. At the site of inoculation, an inflammatory lesion will appear within 24 hours and will become necrotic in 72 hours in the control animal. No skin reaction occurs in the animal given antitoxin. In Elek's test, commercially available antiserum is placed on a filter paper strip that is laid across streaks of different colonies. After incubation, a precipitin reaction in the agar indicates toxin production.

The Schick test has been used to determine the immune status of the patient. In the Schick test, 0.1 mL of purified diphtheria toxin is injected intracutaneously. In the absence of circulating antitoxin, the injected toxin causes a local inflammatory response with erythema, swelling, and tenderness that peak at 5 days, as well as central pigmentation that persists. A positive Schick test consists of more than 10 mm induration and indicates susceptibility to diphtheria. The Schick test is not helpful in early diagnosis because it cannot be interpreted for several days.

DIFFERENTIAL DIAGNOSIS

Nasal diphtheria must be distinguished from a foreign body in the nose, adenoiditis, sinusitis, and the snuffles of congenital syphilis. Careful examination of the nose with a nasal speculum, sinus radiographs, and serologic tests for syphilis are helpful in excluding these conditions.

Tonsillar and pharyngeal diphtheria must be differentiated from streptococcal pharyngitis and infectious mononucleosis. Streptococcal pharyngitis is usually associated with higher temperature, more severe pain on swallowing, and a relatively nonadherent membrane limited to the tonsils. In about 30% of patients, pharyngeal diphtheria and streptococcal infection coexists. Infectious mononucleosis is characterized by lymphadenopathy, splenomegaly, skin rash, atypical lymphocytes, heterophil antibodies, and a membrane that does not extend beyond the tonsils or bleed when removed. Tonsillar and pharyngeal diphtheria should also be differentiated from other types of nonbacterial membranous tonsillitis (e.g., those caused by herpesvirus, adenovirus, coxsackievirus), from blood dyscrasia such as agranulocytosis and leukemia, from posttonsillectomy faucial membranes, and from oropharyngeal involvement by *Toxoplasma,* cytomegalovirus, and *Candida* organisms. Vincent's angina often affects gingival tissue; Gram's stain from ulcerative lesions within the pharynx shows mixed oropharyngeal flora.

Laryngeal diphtheria must be differentiated from viral croup, acute epiglottitis, aspirated foreign bodies, laryngotracheobronchitis, peripharyngeal and retropharyngeal abscesses, and laryngeal papillomas, hemangiomas, and lymphangiomas. A careful history and direct visualization of the larynx in the hospital should be diagnostic.

TREATMENT

Both antitoxin and antibiotics are mandatory in the treatment of diphtheria. The outcome of diphtheria depends on the location and extent of the membrane, the immunization status of the host, and the promptness with which antitoxin is administered. Antitoxin, a hyperimmune antiserum of equine origin, must be administered empirically on the basis of clinical suspicion. The antitoxin can neutralize the toxin only before it enters the cells, so it must be administered as early as possible. The Committee on Infectious Diseases of the American Academy of Pediatrics recommends 20,000–40,000 U of toxin for pharyngeal or laryngeal diphtheria of 48 hours' duration, 40,000–80,000 U for nasopharyngeal lesions, 80,000–100,000 U for extensive disease of 3 days' duration or more or for diffuse swelling of the neck.[41] Intravenous infusion over 1 hour is recommended for rapid inactivation of toxin. A single sufficient dose is used to avoid the risk of sensitization from repeated doses of horse serum. Tests for sensitivity to horse serum must be performed before administration of antitoxin.

Antimicrobial therapy is required to stop toxin production, to eradicate the organism, and to prevent its spread. Penicillin and erythromycin are the antibiotics of choice, although tetracycline, clindamycin, and rifampin are also effective. Erythromycin is given orally or parenterally (40–50 mg/kg/day for 14 days). Penicillin can be given as aqueous penicillin (100,000–150,000 U/kg/day intravenously in four divided doses) or procaine penicillin (12,500 to 50,000 U/kg/day intramuscularly in two divided doses for 14 days). Both of these antibiotics are also effective against group A beta-hemolytic streptococci. Eradication of the organism should be documented by two consecutive negative cultures after completion of treatment.[41]

Because clinical diphtheria may not induce protective immunity and patients are susceptible to reinfection, booster vaccination with an age-appropriate diphtheria toxoid is recommended during convalescence.[42] For cutaneous diphtheria, thorough cleansing of the lesion with soap and water and antimicrobial administration for 10 days are recommended.

Supportive care is also important. Serial ECGs should be obtained to detect possible myocardial complications. Hydration and adequate calorie intake should be maintained with either intravenous fluid or a liquid diet, since patients with diphtheria usually are unable to swallow. To prevent airway obstruction, intubation or tracheostomy should be performed for laryngeal diphtheria.

PREVENTION

The incidence of diphtheria has plummeted in response to active immunization on a mass scale. Recommendations from the Immunization Practices Advisory Committee are as follows[43]:

For children younger than 6 years, three 0.5-ml intramuscular injections of diphtheria-pertussis-tetanus (DPT) vaccine should be given at 2, 4, and 6 months of age, with booster doses at 15 or 18 months and again between 4 and 6 years of age. Most of the local and systemic reactions are to the pertussis component.

To persons older than 7 years, 0.5 mL of adult-type toxoid (Td) is given twice at a 4–8 week interval with a booster dose 1 year later. Td contains no more than 2 Lf (flocculation units) of diphtheria toxoid per dose, as compared with the 7–25 Lf in the pediatric DPT vaccine. If the recommended sequence of primary immunization is interrupted, normal levels of immunity can be achieved simply by administering the remaining doses instead of the whole series. Td boosters should be administered every 10 years.

Diphtheria immunization should be updated regularly for travellers to endemic or epidemic area.[17, 31, 44] Travellers should have completed a primary series of at least three doses of diphtheria toxoid and should have received the most recent dose of vaccine (either primary series or booster) within the previous 10 years. To improve specific immunity to diphtheria within the population, active vaccination against tetanus, given as a part of wound management, should involve a vaccine that contains both tetanus and diphtheria toxoid.[28]

The immediate prevention of diphtheria depends on the isolation of the patient and management of the contacts. Close contacts should have throat cultures and be observed for 7 days. Treatment should be instituted immediately if the cultures reveal the organism. The contact should also receive booster immunization. Travellers to affected countries should contact a health care provider promptly if they develop a sore throat or any skin lesion while traveling or during the 2 weeks after their return.[17]

The major manifestations of diphtheria can be prevented by immunization of the individual, but immunization is directed against the toxin, not against infection. Thus, both unimmunized and fully immunized persons may be carriers.[7, 18] If unimmunized, carriers should receive active immunization. If a carrier was immunized previously but did not receive a booster within 1 year, a booster dose of diphtheria toxoid should be given. A 7-day course of antibiotics (penicillin or erythromycin) or a single intramuscular dose of benzathine penicillin should also be given.

References

1. Kleinman LC: To end an epidemic: Lessons from the history of diphtheria. N Engl J Med 1992; 326: 773–777.
2. English PC: Diphtheria and theories of infectious disease: Centennial appreciation of the critical role of diphtheria in the history of medicine. Pediatrics 1985; 76: 1–9.
3. Brooks GF, Bennett JV, Feldman RA: Diphtheria in the United States, 1959–1970. J Infect Dis 1974; 129: 172–178.
4. Freeman VJ: Studies on the virulence of bacteriophage-infected strains of *Corynebacterium diphtheriae*. J Bacteriol 1951; 61: 675–688.
5. Pappenheimer AM, Murphy JR: Studies on the molecular epidemiology of diphtheria. Lancet 1983; 2: 923–926.
6. Collier RJ, Kandel J: Structure and activity of diphtheria toxin. I. Thiol-dependent dissociation of a fraction of toxin into enzymatically active and inactive fragments. J Biol Chem 1971; 246: 1496–1503.
7. Pappenheimer AM: Diphtheria studies on the biology of an infectious disease. Harvey Lect 1982; 76: 45–73.
8. Battistini A, Curatola AM, Gallinare P, et al.: Inhibition of protein synthesis by diphtheria toxin induces a peculiar pattern of synthesized protein species. Exp Cell Res 1988; 176: 174–179.
9. Feigin RD, Stechenberg BW, Strandgaard BH: Diphtheria. In: Feigin RD, Cherry JD (eds): Textbook of Pediatric Infectious Diseases, vol I, 3rd ed. Philadelphia WB Saunders, 1992, pp 1110–1116.
10. Dobie RA, Tobey DN: Clinical features of diphtheria in the respiratory tract. JAMA 1979; 242: 2197–2201.
11. Koopman JS, Campbell J: The role of cutaneous diphtheria infections in a diphtheria epidemic. J Infect Dis 1975; 131: 239–244.
12. Bowler ICJ, Mandell BK, Schlecht B, et al.: Diphtheria—the continuing hazard. Arch Dis Child 1988; 63: 194–195.
13. Bray JP, Burt EG, Potter EJ, et al.: Epidemic diphtheria and skin infections in Trinidad. J Infect Dis 1972; 126: 34–40.
14. World Health Organization: Expanded Programme on Immunization (EPI) Information System. Geneva: World Health Organization, 1993.
15. Dixon JMS: Diphtheria in North America. J Hyg (Camb) 1984; 93: 419–432.
16. Kwantes W: Diphtheria in Europe. J Hyg (Camb) 1984; 93: 433–437.
17. Centers for Disease Control and Prevention: Diphtheria acquired by U.S. citizens in the Russian Federation and Ukraine—1994. MMWR 1994; 12: 237–244.
18. Karzon DT, Edwards KM: Diphtheria outbreaks in immunized populations. N Engl J Med 1988; 318: 41–43.
19. Wilson APR, Efstratiou A, Weaver E, et al.: Unusual non-toxigenic *Corynebacterium diphtheriae* in homosexual men. Lancet 1992; 339: 998.
20. Millar OS, Cooper ON, Kakkar VV, et al.: Invasive infection with *Corynebacterium diphtheriae* among drug users. Lancet 1992; 339: 1359.
21. Tiley SM, Kociuba KR, Heron LG, et al.: Infective endocarditis due to nontoxigenic *Corynebacterium diphtheriae:* Report of seven cases and reviews. Clin Infect Dis 1993; 16: 271–275.
22. Harnisch JP, Tronca E, Nolan CM, et al.: Diphtheria among alcoholic urban adults. A decade of experience in Seattle. Ann Intern Med 1989; 111: 71–82.
23. Bjorkholm B, Bottiger M, Christenson B, et al.: Antitoxin antibody levels and the outcome of illness during an outbreak of diphtheria among alcoholics. Scand J Infect Dis 1986; 18: 235–239.
24. Chen RT, Broome CV, Weinstein RA, et al.: Diphtheria in the United States, 1971–1981. Am J Public Health 1985; 129: 172–178.
25. Christenson B, Bottiger M: Serological immunity to diphtheria in Sweden in 1978 and 1984. Scand J Infect Dis 1986; 18: 235–239.
26. Rappuoli R, Podda A, Giovannoni F, et al.: Absence of protective immunity against diphtheria in a large proportion of young adults. Vaccine 1993; 11: 576–577.
27. Bottiger M, Pettersson G: Vaccine immunity to diphtheria: A 20-year follow-up study. Scand J Infect Dis 1992; 24: 753–758.
28. Kjeldsen K, Simonsen O, Heron I: Immunity against diphtheria 25–30 years after primary vaccination in childhood. Lancet 1985; 1: 900–902.
29. Maple PA, Efstratiou A, George RC, et al.: Diphtheria immunity in UK blood donors. Lancet 1995; 345: 963–965.
30. Rix BA, Zhobakas A, Wachmann CH, et al.: Immunity from diphtheria, tetanus, poliomyelitis, measles, mumps, and rubella among adults in Lithuania. Scand J Infect Dis 1994; 26: 459–467.
31. Centers for Disease Control and Prevention: Diphtheria epidemic—New Independent States of the former Soviet Union, 1990–1994. MMWR 1995; 44: 180.
32. Highet AS, Hay RJ, Roberts SOB: Bacterial infections. In: Champion RH, Burton JL, Ebling FJH (eds): Textbook of Dermatology, vol II, 5th ed. Oxford: Blackwell Scientific Publications, 1992, pp 995–996.
33. Antos H, Mollison LC, Richards MJ, et al.: Diphtheria: Another risk of travel. J Infect 1992; 25: 307–310.
34. Belsey MA, LeBlanc DR: Skin infections and the epidemiology of diphtheria: Acquisition and persistence of C. diphtheriae infections. Am J Epidemiol 1975; 102: 179–184.
35. Rysselaere M, Vanneste L: Diphtheria of the eye. Bull Soc Belg Ophthalmol 1982; 201: 89–92.
36. Morgan BC: Cardiac complications of diphtheria. Pediatrics 1963; 32: 549–557.
37. Bethell DB, Dung NM, Loan HT, et al.: Prognostic value of electrocardiographic monitoring of patients with severe diphtheria. Clin Infect Dis 1995; 20: 1259–1265.
38. Brooks R, Joynson DHM: Bacteriological diagnosis of diphtheria. J Clin Pathol 1990; 43: 576–580.
39. Coyle MB, Hollis DG, Groman NB: *Corynebacterium* spp. and other coryneform organisms. In: Lennette EH, Balows A, Hausler WJ Jr, et al. (eds): Manual of Clinical Microbiology, 4th ed. Washington, D.C.: American Society for Microbiology, 1985, pp 193–204.

40. Hodes H: Diphtheria. Pediatr Clin North Am 1979; 26: 445–459.
41. Diphtheria. In: Report of the Committee on Infectious Diseases, 23rd ed. Elk Grove Village, IL: American Academy of Pediatrics, 1994, pp 177–181.
42. Farizo KM, Strebel PM, Chen RT, et al.: Fatal respiratory disease due to *Corynebacterium diphtheriae:* Case report and review of guidelines for management, investigation and control. Clin Infect Dis 1993; 16: 59–68.
43. Centers for Disease Control and Prevention: Diphtheria, tetanus, and pertussis: Recommendations for vaccine use and other preventive measures. MMWR 1991; 40: RR 10.
44. Centers for Diseases Control and Prevention: Diphtheria outbreak—Russian Federation, 1990–1993. MMWR; 1993; 42: 840–847.

Ronald B. Turner

CHAPTER FIFTY-ONE

The Common Cold

▼

Viral upper respiratory tract infections are the most common illnesses of humans. They account for approximately 50% of illnesses in the entire population and approximately 75% of illnesses in young infants.[1, 2] Although these illnesses are generally mild and self-limited, they are associated with an enormous economic burden, both in lost productivity and in costs of treatment. The common cold results in approximately 26 million days of school absence and 23 million days of work absence in the United States annually.[3] Each year consumers make approximately 27 million physician visits and purchase almost $2 billion worth of over-the-counter cough and cold medications for treatment of common cold symptoms.[4] A recent survey of a nationally representative sample of children aged 27–48 months found that 35% of them had received a cold remedy in the preceding 30 days.[5]

ANATOMY

The site of infection of common colds is generally limited to the mucosa of the upper respiratory tract. Some of the pathogens associated with common cold syndromes (e.g., parainfluenza viruses, respiratory syncytial virus [RSV]) may produce different clinical syndromes by infecting the lower respiratory tract. Rhinovirus, the pathogen most commonly associated with common cold symptoms, appears to be limited to infection of the nasal cavity. Rhinovirus has been isolated from the trachea of infected volunteers by bronchoscopy; however, it is difficult to exclude the possibility of contamination from the upper respiratory tract.[6] Following inoculation into the nasal cavity, virus is first detected by cultures of the posterior nasopharynx.[7] As the cold progresses, virus is detected at sites farther anterior in one or both nares.[7, 8] Abnormalities of the paranasal sinuses may frequently be detected by computed tomography (CT) or magnetic resonance imaging (MRI) during both natural colds and experimentally induced rhinovirus colds. Studies to isolate virus from the sinuses during uncomplicated colds have not been done.[9, 10]

PATHOPHYSIOLOGY

Pathogens

The rhinoviruses are the single most important cause of common cold symptoms, although RSV, adenovirus, and the parainfluenza and influenza viruses may all cause this clinical syndrome.[11] The coronaviruses are also thought to be frequent causes of the common cold; however, little definitive information is available about these agents because they cannot be isolated with routine virologic methods.

Pathogenesis

Much of the information relevant to the pathogenesis of the common cold is derived from studies in subjects infected experimentally with rhinovirus. The prominent symptoms of the common cold are rhinorrhea and nasal obstruction. It is clear that increased vascular permeability with leakage of serum into the nasal mucosa and nasal secretions is a major contributor to these symptoms.[12, 13] The contribution to the rhinorrhea of glandular secretions from the nose becomes more important later in the course of the illness.[13]

The mechanisms by which rhinovirus infection of the nasal epithelium results in increased vascular permeability and glandular secretions is not clear. Rhinovirus infection of the nasal epithelium is not associated with demonstrable histopathologic damage. Specimens of nasal secretions from human volunteers infected with rhinovirus contain small numbers of rhinovirus-infected and uninfected ciliated epithelial cells; however, examination of specimens of the nasal epithelium by light or electron microscopy reveals no consistent lesions.[14–16] Similarly, no morphologic changes were seen in monolayers of human nasal epithelium infected with rhinovirus.[17] The absence of detectable histopathology during rhinovirus infection led to the suggestion that the host response to the virus may play a primary role in the production of common cold symptoms.

Early studies of the host response to rhinovirus infection concentrated on the humoral immune response. Viral neutralizing activity, apparently associated with immunoglobulin A (IgA), first appears in nasal secretions 2–3 weeks after infection, at about the same time that neutralizing activity is detected in serum.[18–21] This neutralizing antibody in serum or nasal secretions is associated with serotype-specific protection from rhinovirus infection.[19, 20, 22] A recent study reported nonneutralizing rhinovirus-specific IgG and IgA in nasal secretions by the 3rd day of rhinovirus illness.[23]

There is evidence that the cellular immune response may

459

play a role in rhinovirus pathogenesis. The peripheral white blood cell (WBC) count increases in infected, ill subjects during the first 2–3 days after virus challenge.[24] This increase in the WBC count is the result of an increase in the concentration of neutrophils. Infected "non-ill" subjects have no change in the WBC count. A polymorphonuclear leukocyte response to rhinovirus infection is also seen in the nasal mucosa and nasal secretions.[14, 25] As with the change in peripheral neutrophil count, the increase in PMNs is seen in infected symptomatic subjects but not in asymptomatically infected ones.[25]

The correlation between lymphocytic response to rhinovirus infection and symptomatic illness is less clearly characterized. There are conflicting data about the effect of rhinovirus infection on the peripheral lymphocyte count.[24, 26, 27] Modest increases in T-lymphocyte concentrations have been reported in both the nasal mucosa and nasal secretions during rhinovirus infection.[28, 29] Few B lymphocytes are found in the nasal mucosa.

The role of inflammatory mediators has been the focus of several recent studies of rhinovirus pathogenesis. The similarity between the symptoms of allergic rhinitis and those of the common cold has prompted repeated attempts to establish the role of histamine in the common cold. Several studies have reported no detectable increase in histamine in nasal secretions during rhinovirus infection.[25, 30, 31] A recent study reported increases in histamine levels in 4 of 15 normal subjects and 13 of 17 subjects with a history of allergic rhinitis following rhinovirus inoculation.[13] Attempts to detect prostaglandin D_2, another mast cell–derived mediator, in rhinovirus-infected subjects have also been unsuccessful.[13, 25] The kinins bradykinin and lysylbrady-kinin have been found in the nasal secretions of volunteers with rhinovirus colds, both experimentally induced and naturally acquired.[25, 32] The concentration and time course of kinin production were roughly correlated with the severity and time course of symptoms in these subjects. The concentration of kinins in the nasal secretions did not increase in subjects who were infected with rhinovirus but did not develop symptoms. Intranasal challenge of uninfected volunteers with increasing concentrations of bradykinin resulted in symptoms of nasal obstruction, rhinorrhea, and sore throat.[33] The interleukins IL-1β and IL-8 have also recently been identified in the nasal secretions of symptomatic subjects with experimental rhinovirus colds.[10, 34] As with the kinins, the concentration of these proteins increases and then decreases, as symptom severity is increasing and then decreasing. Administration of intranasal IL-8 to normal, uninfected volunteers results in nasal obstruction.[35]

The neurologic response of the host may also play a role in the pathogenesis of rhinovirus colds. Neurologic pathways appear to be involved in the reactive airway disease associated with rhinovirus infection.[36, 37] Recent studies of nasal secretions have shown that glandular secretions in the nose, also under the control of cholinergic neurologic pathways, contribute to rhinorrhea, especially in the later stages of the illness.[13] Substance P, an inflammatory neuropeptide, appears to play a role in some forms of noninfectious rhinitis, and there has been speculation that this or other similar substances could contribute to the pathogenesis of the common cold. This hypothesis remains to be examined.

EPIDEMIOLOGY

Colds occur year-round, but their incidence is decreased during the summer months.[2, 11] The "respiratory virus season" usually begins with an increase in incidence of rhinovirus infections in the fall, usually August or September, and ends following the spring peak of rhinovirus infections in April or May. This period of increased incidence of disease is caused by sequential and relatively discrete outbreaks of different viral pathogens.[11] An increased incidence of common cold symptoms is associated with each of these outbreaks; however, other clinical syndromes are usually also present in the community during epidemics caused by pathogens other than rhinovirus.

The average incidence of the common cold in preschool children is 5–7 per child per year, but 10%–15% of children have at least 12 infections per year.[1, 38, 39] The incidence of illness decreases with age and averages 2–3 per person per year by adulthood. The incidence of common colds in young children is affected by conditions that increase exposure, such as other children in the home or extensive contact with children outside the home (e.g., daycare centers).[40–42] The difference in the incidences of illness between these groups of children decreases as the length of time spent in daycare increases; however, the incidence of illness remains higher in the daycare group through at least the first three years of life.[41]

The frequency of common colds might suggest that person-to-person spread must be fairly efficient. In fact, natural transmission of rhinovirus appears to be relatively inefficient. A transmission rate of 38% was reported in a study in which one partner of a married couple was infected with rhinovirus and, then, the spouse, documented to be susceptible to the virus, was observed for acquisition of infection.[43] Exposure of susceptible recipients to experimentally infected donors resulted in an infection rate of 44% in the recipients after 150 donor-hours of exposure.[44] Several studies of relatively brief exposure (3–36 hours) to virus-infected subjects found virus transmission rates of less than 10%.[45]

There are three general mechanisms by which common cold viruses might be spread: (1) small-particle aerosols, (2) large-particle aerosols, and (3) direct contact. Although the various common cold viruses presumably may be spread by any of these mechanisms, some routes of transmission may be more efficient than others for particular viruses. Studies of experimental rhinovirus colds in human volunteers suggest that direct contact is the most efficient mechanism of transmission of the virus, although transmission by large-particle aerosols has also been documented.[46, 47] A study of natural colds found that treatment of the hands with a virucidal compound significantly reduced transmission of colds.[48] There were no rhinovirus infections in the subjects who used the virucidal hand treatment in this study, a finding that supports the hypothesis that hand-to-hand transmission may be important in a natural setting.

Regardless of the route of transmission, contact between rhinovirus and the nasal mucosa appears to be important for establishment of infection. Very small inocula of virus applied to the nasal cavity consistently result in infection. In contrast, inoculation of virus into the oral cavity is an inefficient route for production of rhinovirus infection. The inoculum required for a 50% infection rate was calculated to be 0.3 tissue culture infectious dose 50 ($TCID_{50}$) by the nasal route and 2260 $TCID_{50}$ by the oral route.[20, 45, 49] Conjunctival inoculation of virus is also an efficient mechanism for initiation of rhinovirus infection, presumably because virus reaches the nasal cavity via the nasolacrimal duct.[7, 49]

CLINICAL MANIFESTATIONS

Signs and Symptoms

The onset of common cold symptoms typically occurs 1–3 days after viral infection. Nasal obstruction, rhinorrhea, and sneezing are frequently reported early in the course of the cold; however, sore or "scratchy" throat is most frequently reported as the most bothersome symptom on the first day of illness.[50, 51] The sore throat resolves quickly, and by the 2nd and 3rd day of illness nasal symptoms predominate. Cough is associated with approximately 30% of colds and typically does not become the most bothersome symptom until the 4th or 5th day of illness, when the nasal symptoms decrease in severity.[50, 51] The usual cold lasts about a week, although 25% last 2 weeks.[50]

Physical Findings

Physical findings of the common cold are limited to the upper respiratory tract. The increased nasal secretions may be obvious to the examiner. A change in the color or consistency of the secretions is common during the course of the illness and is not an indication of sinusitis or bacterial superinfection. The nasal obstruction reported by the patient usually is not obvious on physical examination.

DIFFERENTIAL DIAGNOSIS

The most important task of the physician caring for a patient with a cold is to exclude other conditions that are potentially more serious and/or are treatable. The most difficult illnesses to distinguish from the common cold are allergic rhinitis and sinusitis. The nasal symptoms of allergic rhinitis are very similar to those of the common cold. Recognition of a seasonal occurrence of symptoms by the patient or the presence of itching of the eyes and nose suggests the diagnosis of allergic rhinitis. Sneezing, which may be present in both illnesses, is usually more prominent in allergic rhinitis than in colds. The presence of eosinophilia (>20% of all cells) in a smear of nasal secretions is a relatively insensitive but specific finding in allergic rhinitis.[52]

There are two recognized syndromes of bacterial sinusitis—persistent and severe.[53] The severe syndrome is characterized by fever, purulent rhinorrhea, and headache or facial pain. This syndrome is unlikely to be misdiagnosed as a common cold. The persistent syndrome, on the other hand, is characterized by prolonged rhinorrhea with associated cough. This syndrome is differentiated from the common cold only by the duration of symptoms. The character of the

nasal secretions is not useful for distinguishing the common cold from sinusitis.

Other conditions that need to be considered in the differential diagnosis of the common cold, particularly in children, are nasal foreign bodies, streptococcal nasopharyngitis, pertussis, and congenital syphilis. Nasal foreign bodies usually produce a unilateral discharge that may be foul smelling and bloody. Streptococcal nasopharyngitis is a syndrome of Group A streptococcal infection that has been associated with nasal symptoms in infants younger than 3 years of age. These patients may have a clinical syndrome indistinguishable from that of the common cold. The illness is characterized by a mucopurulent or purulent discharge that may cause excoriation of the nares. Fever is an inconstant finding. The diagnosis of streptococcal nasopharyngitis is established by the isolation of group A streptococci from the nasal secretions in the appropriate clinical setting. The catarrhal phase of pertussis may also be indistinguishable from a cold. The diagnosis usually becomes evident with the onset of paroxysmal cough. A history of a chronic or severe cough in an adolescent or young adult contact or awareness of other pertussis infections in the community may suggest this diagnosis before onset of cough in an infant. The "snuffles" of congenital syphilis present as clear rhinorrhea beginning in the first 3 months (usually the first month) of life. A persistent or excoriating rhinorrhea in this age group should prompt evaluation of the patient and the mother for the possibility of syphilis. Although rhinorrhea may be a part of the clinical presentation of other infections (e.g., measles) the severity of the illness and the associated systemic manifestations generally readily differentiate these infections from the common cold.

DIAGNOSIS

Laboratory Evaluation

Routine laboratory studies generally are not helpful for the diagnosis and management of the common cold. A nasal smear for eosinophils, as described above, may be useful when allergic rhinitis is suspected. A predominance of polymorphonuclear leukocytes in the nasal secretions is characteristic of uncomplicated colds and does not support a diagnosis of bacterial superinfection or sinusitis.

The viral pathogens associated with the common cold may be detected by culture, antigen detection, or serologic methods. These studies are not indicated for patients with colds, since a specific etiologic diagnosis has no value in the management of these patients. Bacterial cultures and antigen detection are useful only when group A streptococcal or *Bordetella pertussis* infection or nasal diphtheria is suspected. The isolation of other bacterial pathogens from the nose is not an indication of bacterial nasal infection and is not a specific predictor of the etiologic agent in sinusitis.[54, 55]

TREATMENT

No effective antiviral agents are available for the treatment of the common cold, and symptomatic therapy remains the mainstay of treatment. The use of symptomatic therapies available over the counter and directed at specific symptoms of rhinovirus colds has been the subject of some controversy.[56] Although some of these medications have been found to be effective in adults, studies in children have been limited by the logistic and design problems presented by the inability to measure common cold symptoms objectively in noncompliant subjects. It is reasonable to conclude that the effects of these various preparations should be similar in adults and children. The use of these medications in children, however, must be balanced against the potential side effects of each drug.

The symptoms of the common cold that are perceived as most bothersome vary over the course of the cold. Ideally, the treatment regimen should be targeted to relieve the different symptoms as they occur. Many over-the-counter common cold remedies are formulations of multiple drugs. The use of products that contain combinations of drugs interferes with adjustment of the dosage to effectively treat the target symptom and increases the risk of side effects. The specific agents that have been found to be effective for treatment of the different symptoms of the common cold (Table 51–1) are as follows:

Nasal Congestion

Both topical and oral adrenergic agents are effective nasal decongestants.[57–59] Comparative studies of the common cold have not been done, however, it is generally accepted that the topical agents are more potent than the oral drugs.[60] Prolonged use of the topical adrenergic agents should be avoided, to prevent the development of rhinitis medicamentosa, an apparent rebound effect that causes the sensation of nasal obstruction when the drug is discontinued. Systemic absorption of the imidazolines (e.g., oxymetazoline and xylometazoline) has rarely been associated with bradycardia, hypotension, and coma. The systemic side effects of the oral adrenergic agents are central nervous system stimulation, hypertension, and palpitations. Although the oral adrenergic agents are frequently marketed in combination with antihistamines, the antihistamines have no effect on nasal congestion.

Table 51–1. EFFECTIVE TREATMENTS FOR COMMON COLD SYMPTOMS

Symptom	Treatment
Nasal obstruction	Topical adrenergic agents
	Oral adrenergic agents
Rhinorrhea	Antihistamines
	Ipratropium
Sneezing	Antihistamines
Sore throat/ myalgia	Acetaminophen
	Nonsteroidal anti-inflammatory drugs
Cough	Topical adrenergic agents*
	Bronchodilators*
	Dextromethorphan
	Codeine

*See text for specific indications for these agents.

Rhinorrhea

Rhinorrhea is treated primarily by blockade of cholinergic stimulation of glandular secretion. Atropine or ipratropium bromide treatment of experimental rhinovirus colds produced a small decrease in rhinorrhea or nasal mucus weight that was not statistically significant.[61, 62] In a larger study of natural colds, ipratropium produced approximately a 22% decrease in rhinorrhea, as compared with placebo.[63] Ipratropium has recently been approved for use in the treatment of rhinorrhea of common colds. The most common side effects of intranasal ipratropium are nasal irritation and bleeding.

A modest but statistically significant effect of first-generation antihistamines on rhinorrhea has been found in several small studies in adults, although other studies failed to detect any therapeutic effect.[64–67] Meta-analysis of some of these studies concluded that the antihistamines were significantly more likely than placebo to reduce rhinorrhea by at least 50% (findings presented at the Joint Meeting of the Nonprescription Drugs Advisory Committee and the Pulmonary-Allergy Drugs Advisory Committee of the FDA, November 15, 1994). Recently a large study of experimental colds found that antihistamines reduce rhinorrhea by approximately 27% as compared with placebo.[68] The second-generation (or nonsedating) antihistamines have had no effect on common cold symptoms in a limited number of studies; this suggests that the effect of the antihistamines on rhinorrhea is related to the anticholinergic—rather than the antihistaminic—properties of these drugs.[69, 70] The major side effect associated with the use of the antihistamines is sedation.

Sneezing

Sneezing is frequently reported as a symptom during the common cold; however, it is rarely considered bothersome by the patient. The antihistamines are effective for treatment of sneezing.[67, 68]

Sore Throat

The sore throat associated with colds generally is not severe, but treatment with mild analgesics is occasionally indicated, particularly if there is associated myalgia or headache. Aspirin and acetaminophen treatment for rhinovirus colds has been reported to be associated with a less rigorous serum antibody response and prolonged viral shedding.[71, 72] The clinical significance of these findings is not known.

Cough

Cough in some patients appears to be due to nasal obstruction or postnasal drip. Cough in these patients is most prominent during the time of greatest nasal symptoms and may be relieved by effective nasal decongestion.[73] In other patients, cough may be a result of virus-induced reactive airway disease.[36] These patients may have cough that persists for days to weeks after the acute illness and may benefit from bronchodilator therapy. For patients who do not respond to these interventions, cough suppression, with either codeine or dextro-methorphan hydrobromide, may be useful. Expectorants such as guaifenesin are not effective antitussive agents.[74]

A new approach to the treatment of colds that examined the effect of combining anti-inflammatory and antiviral compounds was recently reported. Gwaltney reported effective treatment of established rhinovirus infections with a combination of naproxen, ipratropium bromide, and interferon-α_{2b}.[75] The effect of this combination appeared to be greater than the effects usually seen with available common cold therapies.

COMPLICATIONS

The most common complication of the common cold, otitis media, develops in approximately 5% of affected children. The frequency of otitis media complicating colds may be greater in children who are in day care.[76] The use of oral decongestants during the cold does not alter the incidence of otitis media.[77] Antibiotic prophylaxis during the cold may be useful for prevention of otitis media in children who have frequent ear infections.[78, 79] This approach is less effective than continuous antibiotic prophylaxis.[80]

Sinusitis also appears to be a relatively frequent complication of the common cold. Mild sinusitis may present simply as prolonged rhinorrhea, and it is reasonable to treat empirically for sinusitis when, after 10–14 days, rhinorrhea is not improving and other illnesses in the differential diagnosis have been excluded.[53]

Exacerbation of asthma is a relatively uncommon ($<1\%$) but serious complication of the common cold. The pathogenesis of this complication may be related to sensitization of neurologic receptors in the upper respiratory tract that stimulate reflex bronchoconstriction.[37]

PREVENTION

The recognition that direct contact was an important mechanism of transmission of rhinovirus led to efforts to prevent contamination of the hands of infected or susceptible persons. A variety of chemical compounds have been evaluated for efficacy in inactivation of rhinovirus on environmental surfaces or on skin.[81–83] Although some of these agents were found to have activity, a practical and effective hand treatment has not been developed. Facial tissues treated with a combination of citric acid, malic acid, and sodium lauryl sulfate were found to inactivate a number of different viruses readily, and there was some evidence that these tissues would reduce or prevent transmission of colds.[84–86] In spite of the potential utility of this product, it was never made commercially available.

The large number of rhinovirus serotypes has long been recognized as an obstacle to the development of vaccines for protection against rhinovirus infections. In 1984, Abraham and Colonno reported that different rhinovirus serotypes shared the same cellular receptor.[87] Subsequent studies have shown that all rhinoviruses but one attach to cells via only two different receptors.[87, 88] The majority of serotypes bind by a single receptor that has been identified as intercellular adhesion molecule 1 (ICAM-1).[89, 90] Blockade either of the receptor site on the cells with antibody to ICAM-1 or of the receptor-binding site on the virus with soluble ICAM-1 has been shown to inhibit viral infection in vitro and suggests possible interventions for the common cold.[88, 91–94] The logistics of maintaining an appropriate concentration of either of these proteins in the nasal cavity over prolonged periods presents formidable obstacles to effective use of these agents, however. Prophylaxis of experimental rhinovirus colds with monoclonal antibody to ICAM-1, the major cellular receptor, delayed but did not prevent infection.[95]

Prevention of rhinovirus infections has also been attempted with a variety of antiviral agents. Both pirodavir, a virus capsid–binding agent, and interferon-alfa (IFN-α) are effective for prevention of rhinovirus infection.[96–103] The cost and the side effects of IFN-α preclude its use as an agent for the prevention of rhinovirus colds.[103–107] The ultimate role for pirodavir or receptor blockade for prevention of colds remains to be determined. Until these newer prophylactic treatments are available, handwashing remains the most effective measure for prevention of colds.

References

1. Dingle JH, Badger GF, Jordan WS Jr: Illness in the home: A study of 25,000 illnesses in a group of Cleveland families. Cleveland: Case Western Reserve University, 1964, p 398.
2. Gwaltney JM Jr, Hendley JO, Simon G, et al.: Rhinovirus infections in an industrial population: I. The occurrence of illness. N Engl J Med 1966; 275: 1261–1268.
3. Health and Human Services Vital Health Statistics 10. Washington, DC: 1986.
4. Rosenthal I: Expense of physician care spurs OTC, self-care market. Drug Topics 1988; 132: 62–63.
5. Kogan MD, Pappas G, Yu SM, et al.: Over-the-counter medication use among US preschool-age children. JAMA 1994; 272: 1025–1030.
6. Halperin SA, Eggleston PA, Hendley JO, et al.: Pathogenesis of lower respiratory tract symptoms in experimental rhinovirus infection. Am Rev Respir Dis 1983; 128: 806–810.
7. Winther B, Gwaltney JM Jr, Mygind N, et al.: Sites of rhinovirus recovery after point inoculation of the upper airway. JAMA 1986; 256: 1763–1767.
8. Turner RB, Winther B, Hendley JO, et al.: Sites of virus recovery and antigen detection in epithelial cells during experimental rhinovirus infection. Acta Otolaryngol Suppl 1984; 413: 9–14.
9. Gwaltney JM Jr, Phillips CD, Miller RD, et al.: Computed tomographic study of the common cold. N Engl J Med 1994; 330: 25–30.
10. Turner RB: Elaboration of interleukin 8 from fibroblast cells and human nasal epithelium in response to rhinovirus challenge. 34th Interscience Conference on Antimicrobial Agents and Chemotherapy. Orlando, Florida: American Society for Microbiology, 1994: 65.
11. Monto AS, Cavallaro JJ: The Tecumseh study of respiratory illness. II. Patterns of occurrence of infection with respiratory pathogens, 1965–1969. Am J Epidemiol 1971; 94: 280–289.
12. Douglas RG Jr: Pathogenesis of rhinovirus common colds in human volunteers. Ann Otol Rhinol Laryngol 1970; 79: 563–571.
13. Igarashi Y, Skoner DP, Doyle WJ, et al.: Analysis of nasal secretions during experimental rhinovirus upper respiratory infections. J Allergy Clin Immunol 1993; 92: 722–731.
14. Winther B, Farr B, Turner RB, et al.: Histopathologic examination and enumeration of polymorphonuclear leukocytes in the nasal mucosa during experimental rhinovirus colds. Acta Otolaryngol Suppl (Stockh) 1984; 413: 19–24.
15. Winther B, Brofeldt S, Christensen B, et al.: Light and scanning electron microscopy of nasal biopsy material from patients with natu-

rally acquired common colds. Acta Otolaryngol (Stockh) 1984; 97: 309–318.

16. Turner RB, Hendley JO, Gwaltney JM Jr: Shedding of infected ciliated epithelial cells in rhinovirus colds. J Infect Dis 1982; 145: 849–853.

17. Winther B, Gwaltney JM Jr, Hendley JO: Respiratory virus infection of monolayer cultures of human nasal epithelial cells. Am Rev Respir Dis 1990; 141: 839–845.

18. Cate TR, Couch RB, Johnson KM: Studies with rhinovirus in volunteers: Production of illness, effect of naturally acquired antibody, and demonstration of a protective effect not associated with serum antibody. J Clin Invest 1964; 43: 56–67.

19. Cate TR, Rossen RD, Douglas R Jr, et al.: The role of nasal secretion and serum antibody in the rhinovirus common cold. Am J Epidemiol 1966; 84: 352–363.

20. Hendley JO, Edmonson WP Jr, Gwaltney JM Jr: Relation between naturally acquired immunity and infectivity of two rhinoviruses in volunteers. J Infect Dis 1972; 125: 243–248.

21. Rossen RD, Kasel JA, Couch RB: The secretory immune system: Its relation to respiratory viral infection. Prog Med Virol 1971; 13: 194–238.

22. Perkins JC, Tucker DN, Knopf HL, et al.: Comparison of protective effect of neutralizing antibody in serum and nasal secretions in experimental rhinovirus type 13 illness. Am J Epidemiol 1969; 90: 519–526.

23. Barclay WS, Al-Nakib W: An ELISA for the detection of rhinovirus specific antibody in serum and nasal secretions. J Virol Methods 1987; 15: 53–64.

24. Douglas RG Jr, Alford RH, Cate TR, et al.: The leukocyte response during viral respiratory illness in man. Ann Intern Med 1966; 64: 521–530.

25. Naclerio RM, Proud D, Lichtenstein LM, et al.: Kinins are generated during experimental rhinovirus colds. J Infect Dis 1988; 157: 133–142.

26. Levandowski RA, Ou DW, Jackson GG: Acute-phase decrease of T lymphocyte subsets in rhinovirus infection. J Infect Dis 1986; 153: 743–748.

27. Skoner DP, Whiteside TL, Wilson JW, et al.: Effect of rhinovirus 39 infection on cellular immune parameters in allergic and nonallergic subjects. J Allergy Clin Immunol 1993; 92: 732–743.

28. Winther B: Effects on the nasal mucosa of upper respiratory viruses (common cold). Dan Med Bull 1994; 41: 193–204.

29. Levandowski RA, Weaver CW, Jackson GG: Nasal-secretion leukocyte populations determined by flow cytometry during acute rhinovirus infection. J Med Virol 1988; 25: 423–432.

30. Eggleston PA, Hendley JO, Gwaltney JM Jr, et al.: Histamine in nasal secretions. Int Arch Allergy Appl Immunol 1978; 57: 193–200.

31. Eggleston PA, Hendley JO, Gwaltney JM Jr: Mediators of immediate hypersensitivity in nasal secretions during natural colds and rhinovirus infection. Acta Otolaryngol Suppl 1984; 413: 25–35.

32. Proud D, Naclerio RM, Gwaltney JM Jr, et al.: Kinins are generated in nasal secretions during natural rhinovirus colds. J Infect Dis 1990; 161: 120–123.

33. Proud D, Reynolds CJ, LaCapra S, et al.: Nasal provocation with bradykinin induces symptoms of rhinitis and a sore throat. Am Rev Respir Dis 1988; 137: 613–616.

34. Proud D, Gwaltney JM Jr, Hendley JO, et al.: Increased levels of interleukin-1 are detected in nasal secretions of volunteers during experimental rhinovirus colds. J Infect Dis 1994; 169: 1007–1013.

35. Douglass JA, Dhami D, Gurr CE, et al.: Influence of interleukin-8 challenge in the nasal mucosa in atopic and nonatopic subjects. Am J Respir Crit Care Med 1994; 150: 1108–1113.

36. Aquilina AT, Hall WJ, Douglas RG Jr, et al.: Airway reactivity in subjects with viral upper respiratory tract infections: The effects of exercise and cold air. Am Rev Respir Dis 1980; 122: 3–10.

37. Empey DW, Laitinen LA, Jacobs L, et al.: Mechanisms of bronchial hyperreactivity in normal subjects after upper respiratory infection. Am Rev Respir Dis 1976; 113: 131–139.

38. Monto AS, Ullman BM: Acute respiratory illness in an American community: The Tecumseh study. JAMA 1974; 227: 164–169.

39. Monto AS, Sullivan KM: Acute respiratory illness in the community. Frequency of illness and the agents involved. Epidemiol Infect 1993; 110: 145–160.

40. Wald ER, Dashefshy B, Byers C, et al.: Frequency and severity of infections in day care. J Pediatr 1988; 112: 540–546.

41. Hurwitz ES, Gunn WJ, Pinsky PF, et al.: Risk of respiratory illness associated with day-care attendance: A nationwide study. Pediatrics 1991; 87: 62–69.

42. Fleming DW, Cochi SL, Hightower AW, et al.: Childhood upper respiratory tract infections: To what degree is incidence affected by day-care attendance. Pediatrics 1987; 79: 55–60.

43. D'Alessio DJ, Peterson JA, Dick CR, et al.: Transmission of experimental rhinovirus colds in volunteer married couples. J Infect Dis 1976; 133: 28–36.

44. Meschievitz CK, Schultz SB, Dick EC: A model for obtaining predictable natural transmission of rhinoviruses in human volunteers. J Infect Dis 1984; 150: 195–201.

45. D'Alessio DJ, Meschievitz CK, Peterson JA, et al.: Short-duration exposure and the transmission of rhinoviral colds. J Infect Dis 1984; 150: 189–194.

46. Dick EC, Jennings LC, Mink KA, et al.: Aerosol transmission of rhinovirus colds. J Infect Dis 1987; 156: 442–448.

47. Gwaltney JM Jr, Moskalski PB, Hendley JO: Hand-to-hand transmission of rhinovirus colds. Ann Intern Med 1978; 88: 463–467.

48. Hendley JO, Gwaltney JM Jr: Mechanisms of transmission of rhinovirus infections. Epidemiol Rev 1988; 10: 243–258.

49. Hendley JO, Wenzel RP, Gwaltney JM Jr: Transmission of rhinovirus colds by self-inoculation. N Engl J Med 1973; 288: 1361–1364.

50. Gwaltney JM Jr, Hendley JO, Simon G, et al.: Rhinovirus infections in an industrial population. II. Characteristics of illness and antibody response. JAMA 1967; 202: 494–500.

51. Tyrrell DA, Cohen S, Schlarb JE: Signs and symptoms in common colds. Epidemiol Infect 1993; 111: 143–156.

52. Lans DM, Alfano N, Rocklin R: Nasal eosinophilia in allergic and non-allergic rhinitis: Usefulness of the nasal smear in the diagnosis of allergic rhinitis. Allergy Proc 1989; 10: 275–280.

53. Wald ER, Reilly JS, Casselbrant M, et al.: Treatment of acute maxillary sinusitis in childhood: A comparative study of amoxicillin and cefaclor. J Pediatr 1984; 104: 297–302.

54. Todd JK, Todd N, Damato J, et al.: Bacteriology and treatment of purulent nasopharyngitis: A double-blind, placebo-controlled evaluation. Pediatr Infect Dis J 1984; 3: 226–232.

55. Evans FO Jr, Sydnor JB, Moore WEC, et al.: Sinusitis of the maxillary antrum. N Engl J Med 1975; 293: 735–739.

56. Smith MBH, Feldman W. Over-the-counter cold medications. A critical review of clinical trials between 1950 and 1991. JAMA 1993; 269: 2258–2263.

57. Akerlund A, Klint T, Olen L, et al.: Nasal decongestant effect of oxymetazoline in the common cold: An objective dose-response study in 106 patients. J Laryngol Otol 1989; 103: 743–746.

58. Doyle WJ, Riker DK, McBride TP, et al.: Therapeutic effects of an anticholinergic-sympathomimetic combination in induced rhinovirus colds. Ann Otol Rhinol Laryngol 1993; 102: 521–527.

59. Sperber SJ, Sorrentino JV, Riker DK, et al.: Evaluation of an alpha agonist alone and in combination with a nonsteroidal antiinflammatory agent in the treatment of experimental rhinovirus colds. Bull NY Acad Med 1989; 65: 145–160.

60. Connell JT, Linzmayer MI: Comparison of nasal airway patency changes after treatment with oxymetazoline and pseudoephedrine. Am J Rhinol 1987; 1: 87–94.

61. Gaffey MJ, Gwaltney JM Jr, Dressler WE, et al.: Intranasally administered atropine methonitrate treatment of experimental rhinovirus colds. Am Rev Respir Dis 1987; 135: 241–244.

62. Gaffey MJ, Hayden FG, Boyd JC, et al.: Ipratropium bromide treatment of experimental rhinovirus infection. Antimicrob Agents Chemother 1988; 32: 1644–1647.

63. Duckhorn R, Grossman J, Posner M, et al.: A double-blind, placebo-controlled study of the safety and efficacy of ipratropium bromide nasal spray versus placebo in patients with the common cold. J Allergy Clin Immunol 1992; 90: 1076–1082.

64. Sakchainanont B, Chantarojanasiri T, Ruangkanchanasetr S, et al.: Effectiveness of antihistamines in common cold. J Med Assoc Thai 1990; 73: 96–101.

65. Howard JC Jr, Kantner TR, Lilienfield LS, et al.: Effectiveness of antihistamines in the symptomatic management of the common cold. JAMA 1979; 242: 2414–2417.

66. Gaffey MJ, Gwaltney JM Jr, Sastre A, et al.: Intranasally and orally administered antihistamine treatment of experimental rhinovirus colds. Am Rev Respir Dis 1987; 136: 556–560.

67. Doyle WJ, McBride TP, Skoner DP, et al.: A double-blind, placebo-controlled clinical trial of the effect of chlorpheniramine on the response of the nasal airway, middle ear and eustachian tube to provocative rhinovirus challenge. Pediatr Infect Dis J 1988; 7: 229–238.

68. Gwaltney JM Jr, Park J, Paul RA, et al.: A randomized controlled trial of clemastine fumarate in experimental rhinovirus colds. 34th Interscience Conference on Antimicrobial Agents and Chemotherapy. Orlando, Florida, American Society for Microbiology, 1994.

69. Gaffey MJ, Kaiser DL, Hayden FG: Ineffectiveness of oral terfenadine in natural colds: Evidence against histamine as a mediator of common cold symptoms. Pediatr Infect Dis J 1988; 7: 223–228.

70. Berkowitz RB, Tinkelman DG: Evaluation of oral terfenadine for treatment of the common cold. Ann Allergy 1991; 67: 593–597.

71. Stanley ED, Jackson GG, Panusarn C, et al.: Increased virus shedding with aspirin treatment of rhinovirus infection. JAMA 1975; 231: 1248–1251.

72. Graham NM, Burrell CJ, Douglas RM, et al.: Adverse effects of aspirin, acetaminophen, and ibuprofen on immune function, viral shedding, and clinical status in rhinovirus-infected volunteers. J Infect Dis 1990; 162: 1277–1282.

73. Curley FJ, Irwin RS, Pratter MR, et al. Cough and the common cold. Am Rev Respir Dis 1988; 138: 305–311.

74. Kuhn JJ, Hendley JO, Adams KF, et al.: Antitussive effect of guaifenesin in young adults with natural colds. Objective and subjective assessment. Chest 1982; 82: 713–718.

75. Gwaltney JM Jr: Combined antiviral and antimediator treatment of rhinovirus colds. J Infect Dis 1992; 166: 776–782.

76. Wald ER, Guerra N, Byers C: Upper respiratory tract infections in young children: Duration of and frequency of complications. Pediatrics 1991; 87: 128–133.

77. Randall JE, Hendley JO: A decongestant-antihistamine mixture in the prevention of otitis media in children with colds. Pediatrics 1979; 63: 483–485.

78. Biedel CW: Modification of recurrent otitis media by short-term sulfonamide therapy. Am J Dis Child 1978; 132: 681–683.

79. Prellner K, Fogle-Hansson M, Jorgensen F, et al.: Prevention of recurrent otitis media in otitis-prone children by intermittent prophylaxis with penicillin. Acta Otolaryngol (Stockh) 1994; 114: 182–187.

80. Berman S, Nuss R, Roark R, et al.: Effectiveness of continuous vs. intermittent amoxicillin to prevent episodes of otitis media. Pediatr Infect Dis J 1992; 11: 63–67.

81. Sattar SA, Jacobsen H, Springthorpe VS, et al.: Chemical disinfection to interrupt transfer of rhinovirus type 14 from environmental surfaces to hands. Appl Environ Microbiol 1993; 59: 1579–1585.

82. Hendley JO, Mika LA, Gwaltney JM Jr: Evaluation of virucidal compounds for inactivation of rhinovirus on hands. Antimicrob Agents Chemother 1978; 14: 690–694.

83. Hayden GF, DeForest D, Hendley JO, et al.: Inactivation of rhinovirus on human fingers by virucidal activity of glutaric acid. Antimicrob Agents Chemother 1984; 26: 928–929.

84. Dick EC, Hossain SU, Mink KA, et al.: Interruption of transmission of rhinovirus colds among human volunteers using virucidal paper handkerchiefs. J Infect Dis 1986; 153: 352–356.

85. Hayden GF, Hendley JO, Gwaltney JM Jr.: The effect of placebo and virucidal paper handkerchiefs on viral contamination of the hand and transmission of experimental rhinoviral infection. J Infect Dis 1985; 152: 403–407.

86. Hayden GF, Gwaltney JM Jr, Thacker DF, et al.: Rhinovirus inactivation by nasal tissues treated with virucide. Antiviral Res 1985; 5: 103–109.

87. Abraham G, Colonno RJ: Many rhinovirus serotypes share the same cellular receptor. J Virol 1984; 51: 340–345.

88. Colonno RJ, Callahan PL, Long WJ: Isolation of a monoclonal antibody that blocks attachment of the major group of human rhinoviruses. J Virol 1986; 57: 7–12.

89. Greve JM, Davis G, Meyer AM, et al.: The major human rhinovirus receptor is ICAM-1. Cell 1989; 56: 839–847.

90. Staunton DE, Merluzzi VJ, Rothlein R, et al.: A cell adhesion molecule, ICAM-1 is the major surface receptor for rhinoviruses. Cell 1989; 56: 849–853.

91. Marlin SD, Staunton DE, Springer TA, et al.: A soluble form of intercellular adhesion molecule-1 inhibits rhinovirus infection. Nature 1990; 344: 70–72.

92. Crump CE, Arruda E, Hayden FG: In vitro inhibitory activity of soluble ICAM-1 for the numbered serotypes of human rhinovirus. Antiviral Chem Chemother 1993; 4: 323–327.

93. Condra JH, Sardana VV, Tomassini JE, et al.: Bacterial expression of antibody fragments that block human rhinovirus infection of cultured cells. J Biol Chem 1990; 265: 2292–2295.

94. de Arruda E, Crump CE, Marlin SD, et al.: In vitro studies of the antirhinovirus activity of soluble intercellular adhesion molecule-1. Antimicrob Agents Chemother 1992; 36: 1186–1191.

95. Hayden FG, Gwaltney JM Jr, Colonno RJ: Modification of experimental rhinovirus colds by receptor blockade. Antiviral Res 1988; 9: 233–247.

96. Barrow GI, Higgins PG, Tyrrell DAJ, et al.: An appraisal of the efficacy of the antiviral R 61837 in rhinovirus infections in human volunteers. Antiviral Chem Chemother 1990; 1: 279–283.

97. Hayden FG, Andries K, Janssen PA: Safety and efficacy of intranasal pirodavir (R77975) in experimental rhinovirus infection. Antimicrob Agents Chemother 1992; 36: 727–732.

98. Douglas RM, Moore BW, Miles HB, et al.: Prophylactic efficacy of intranasal alpha$_2$-interferon against rhinovirus infections in the family setting. N Engl J Med 1986; 314: 65–70.

99. Hayden FG, Gwaltney JM Jr: Intranasal interferon alpha$_2$ for prevention of rhinovirus infection and illness. J Infect Dis 1983; 148: 543–550.

100. Hayden FG, Gwaltney JM Jr: Intranasal interferon-alpha$_2$ treatment of experimental rhinovirus colds. J Infect Dis 1984; 150: 174–180.

101. Hayden FG, Albrecht JK, Kaiser DL, et al.: Prevention of natural colds by contact prophylaxis with intranasal alpha$_2$-interferon. N Engl J Med 1986; 314: 71–75.

102. Higgins PG, Al-Nakib W, Willman J, et al.: Interferon-beta ser as prophylaxis against experimental rhinovirus infection in volunteers. J Interferon Res 1986; 6: 153–159.

103. Monto AS, Shope TC, Schwartz SA, et al.: Intranasal interferon-α$_{2b}$ for seasonal prophylaxis of respiratory infection. J Infect Dis 1986; 154: 128–133.

104. Hayden FG, Mills SE, Johns ME: Human tolerance and histopathologic effects of long-term administration of intranasal interferon-α$_2$. J Infect Dis 1983; 148: 914–921.

105. Samo TC, Greenberg SB, Couch RB, et al.: Efficacy and tolerance of intranasally applied recombinant leukocyte A interferon in normal volunteers. J Infect Dis 1983; 148: 535–542.

106. Samo TC, Greenberg SB, Palmer JM, et al.: Intranasally applied recombinant leukocyte A interferon in normal volunteers. II. Determination of minimal effective and tolerable dose. J Infect Dis 1984; 150: 181–188.

107. Scott GM, Onwubalili JK, Robinson JA, et al.: Tolerance of one-month intranasal interferon. J Med Virol 1985; 17: 99–106.

CHAPTER FIFTY-TWO

Heidi D. Remulla
Peter A. D. Rubin

Dacryocystitis

▼

ANATOMY OF THE LACRIMAL EXCRETORY SYSTEM

The lacrimal excretory system is generally made up of three parts: the canaliculi, the lacrimal sac, and the nasolacrimal duct (Fig. 52–1). Tears enter the drainage system through the openings of the canaliculi called the puncta (~0.3 mm in diameter), which are located at the posterior margins of the medial aspect of the upper and lower lids. The first 2 mm of the canaliculi are oriented vertically, followed by an 8-mm horizontal portion. The upper and lower canaliculi usually meet and form a common canaliculus before entering the lacrimal sac through the common internal punctum. The valve of Rosenmüller, which is a mucosal fold found between the common canaliculus and the lacrimal sac, prevents backflow of tears from the sac. The lacrimal sac is located in a bony depression of the medial orbit called the lacrimal sac fossa and is bound medially by portions of the maxilla and lacrimal bones. It extends 12–14 mm vertically. Only a small portion (3–5 mm) of the lacrimal sac, termed the fundus, extends superior to the medial canthal tendon. Thus, infectious processes of the lacrimal sac characteristically point below the medial canthal tendon. Lacrimal sac masses that extend predominantly above the medial canthal tendon should increase the suspicion of a neoplastic process.

The lacrimal sac is separated from other orbital contents by the periosteum medially, the orbital septum posteriorly and the tripartite heads of the medial canthal tendon and its

fascial covering laterally. The location of the lacrimal sac anterior to the orbital septum is an important concept in understanding why cases of dacryocystitis do not typically result in orbital cellulitis. Inferiorly, the lacrimal sac extends into the 12-mm-long intraosseous nasolacrimal duct oriented posterolaterally within the frontal process of the maxilla and opens into the nasal cavity through the inferior meatus. The valve of Hasner, another important mucosal fold, is situated around this opening. Obstruction at this distal terminus of the membranous portion of the nasolacrimal duct is the most common cause of neonatal epiphora and dacryocystitis.

DACRYOCYSTITIS

Dacryocystitis, or infection of the lacrimal sac, occurs as a consequence of tear stagnation in the lacrimal sac secondary to obstruction to normal drainage of the tears through the nasolacrimal duct. Acute dacryocystitis presents as a painful swelling of the lacrimal sac with surrounding erythema, hyperthermia, and soft tissue edema, associated with tearing. In contrast, chronic dacryocystitis is characterized by a prolonged infection of the lacrimal sac with minimal or no signs of inflammation except for tearing and chronic ipsilateral conjunctivitis. These patients with chronic dacryocystitis, however, may develop intermittent recurrent bouts of the acute process. Dacryocystitis is most commonly seen in infants and elderly women. The predominance in females is thought to be due to their narrower and more tortuous nasolacrimal duct as well as to hormonal changes that may affect the vascular plexus surrounding the duct, resulting in edema and cicatricial changes.[1]

The obstruction may be present from birth, and this has been attributed to the presence of a membrane (the valve of Hasner) covering the distal portion of the nasolacrimal duct. Congenital nasolacrimal duct obstruction is a fairly common condition, affecting up to 20% of infants less than 1 year old.[2] Acute dacryocystitis is observed in less than 3% of infants with congenital nasolacrimal duct obstruction.[3] Most of these children (up to 96% of these affected infants[2]) have spontaneous improvement within the first year of life.

Acquired obstruction of the nasolacrimal duct may be primary or may occur as a result of trauma, infection/inflammation, or tumor infiltration. The primary acquired nasolacrimal duct obstruction (PANDO) in adults described by Linberg and McCormick[4] occurs with no known underlying cause. The changes in the nasolacrimal duct vary from dense chronic inflammatory infiltrates to fibrotic connective tissue changes obliterating the duct lumen with no evidence of stenosis of the osseous canal.[4, 5] A study by Blicker and

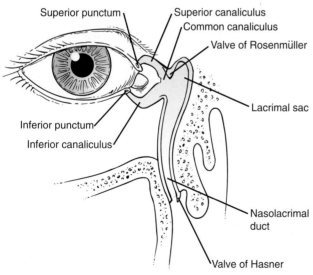

Superior punctum
Superior canaliculus
Common canaliculus
Valve of Rosenmüller
Lacrimal sac
Inferior punctum
Inferior canaliculus
Nasolacrimal duct
Valve of Hasner

Figure 52–1. The lacrimal excretory system.

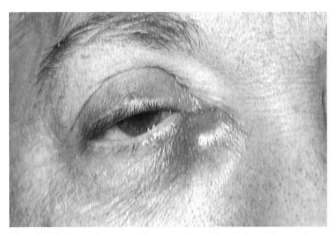

Figure 52–2. Acute dacryocystitis presenting with pain, swelling, and erythema in the region of the lacrimal sac.

Buffam[6] tried to explain the cause of PANDO as secondary to an unrecognized low-grade infection.

Facial trauma causing fracture of the bony nasolacrimal canal can result in ductal damage. Nasal or sinus surgery performed near the area of the tear-draining system may alter the normal anatomy. Even improper probing of the nasolacrimal duct can cause scarring and strictures of the duct. Infectious and inflammatory changes in the nasolacrimal duct and nasal mucosa secondary to a local or systemic disease can cause duct obstruction. Acute dacryocystitis has been reported in the setting of exudative rhinitis,[7] and infectious mononucleosis,[8] as well as following Kawasaki's disease[9] (Fig. 52–2). Tumor infiltration within the lacrimal system and its surrounding structures is also a known cause of obstruction. Malignant lymphoma of the lacrimal sac is unusual but commonly manifests as signs and symptoms of dacryocystitis.[10] Extrinsic neoplastic infiltration of the lacrimal drainage system can occur in the setting of primary maxillary sinus neoplasms. In some of these cases, the presenting sign may be epiphora or dacryocystitis. All these secondary causes of nasolacrimal duct obstruction result in stagnation of tears and secretions in the lacrimal sac, which can then be secondarily infected.

Bacteriology

The more common organisms isolated in infants with dacryocystitis include *Streptococcus pneumoniae*[11] and *Haemophilus influenzae*[12]. In adults, gram-positive organisms— *Staphylococcus epidermidis* and *Staphylococcus aureus*—are most common.[1, 12, 13] Among the gram-negative organisms, *Pseudomonas aeruginosa, H. influenzae,* and *Escherichia coli* have been reported to be most frequent.[1, 13] Anaerobic organisms such as *Propionibacterium acnes, Bacteroides* species and *Proteus* species should be suspected in resistant cases.[1, 14] *Candida albicans* is the most common fungal organism isolated.[1, 13, 15, 16] Other unusual reported cases of dacryocystitis have been caused by *Pasteurella multocida*[17] and *Mycobacterium fortuitum.*[18, 19] In separate studies, Coden and colleagues[1] and by Huber-Spitzy and colleagues[13] noted the decrease in prevalence of *S. pneumoniae*. This list of

common organisms may guide the clinician in planning for treatment; however, it should be borne in mind that the spectrum of organisms causing disease can change with time and may vary depending on geographic location.

Diagnosis

The diagnosis of dacryocystitis is usually straightforward in a tearing patient with a swelling in the medial canthal region. The differential diagnoses include lacrimal sac tumors, mucopyocele arising from infected ethmoid air cells (Fig. 52–3), ruptured dermoid cyst, and other medially located anterior orbit cysts. In dacryocystitis, mucus and pus may or may not be expressed from the puncta when pressure is applied over the lacrimal sac swelling. Palpation of an irreducible swelling without inflammation in a patient with a history of a malignant condition should alert the clinician as to the possibility of a neoplasm. Obstruction to the drainage of tears can be documented by the dye disappearance test (instilling 2% sodium fluorescein in the lower conjunctival cul-de-sac and grading the amount of the remaining dye staining the eye after 5 minutes) and/or irrigation of the lacrimal excretory system. In cases of acute dacryocystitis, canalicular probing and irrigation should be deferred until the inflammation has subsided. Adjunctive diagnostic tests such as dacryocystography, computerized tomography (CT), and magnetic resonance imaging (MRI)[20] can be helpful in evaluating abnormalities of the lacrimal system and its surrounding structures. However, adjunctive imaging increases the patient's expense and therefore should be requested only in selected cases.

Treatment

Medical Management

Management of dacryocystitis depends on the stage of the disease—acute or chronic—and on the age of the patient—

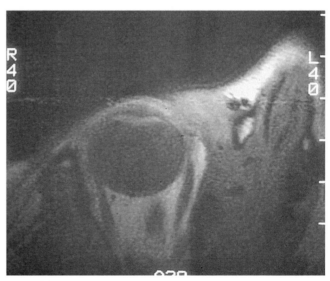

Figure 52–3. Dacryocystitis misdiagnosis. Magnetic resonance imaging demonstrating increased soft tissue density in the region of the lacrimal sac with direct communication from the opacified ethmoid air cells. This patient had a mucopyocele secondary to ethmoiditis.

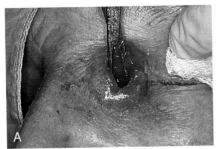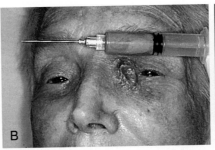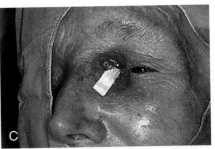

Figure 52–4. *A,* A fine hemostat placed into the lacrimal sac abscess to break up deep loculations and facilitate drainage of pus. *B,* Purulent material obtained from the lacrimal sac abscess. *C,* A drain placed into the abscess cavity to prevent closure of the wound and allow continuous drainage of pus.

infant or adult. Ultimately, the goal of treatment is to reestablish drainage of tears collected in the lacrimal sac into the nose. But prior to the definitive surgical management, treatment of the acute infection is recommended. Performing surgery on inflamed tissues carries the increased risk of spreading the infection to adjacent tissues and may be associated with problems such as increased bleeding and poor wound healing.

Treatment of an infection largely depends on the proper identification of the offending organism and administration of the appropriate antibiotic therapy. Pus expressed from the puncta or aspirated or drained directly from the lacrimal sac must be sent for Gram-stained smears, culture, and sensitivity studies. During the wait for the results of these studies, empiric treatment may be started and modified later. For adults, Cahill and Burns[21] have suggested the use of ciprofloxacin and trimethoprim-sulfamethoxazole for empiric treatment of acute dacryocystitis. Majahan[11] and Hurwitz and Rodgers[12] believe that cloxacillin is the best for these predominantly staphyloccocal infections. Again, it is emphasized that these are not the only or best antibiotics needed for treatment; the patient can be changed to the appropriate antimicrobial medication according to the culture and sensitivity results. If there is no response to the initial therapy, culture studies should be repeated.

Surgical Intervention

Patients with limited lacrimal sac infection may be initially treated with oral antibiotics with or without sac drainage. Those patients with an obvious pointing lacrimal sac abscess should undergo surgical drainage promptly. In equivocal cases, hot compresses will help localize the sac abscess prior to drainage. After adequate anesthesia, a transcutaneous stab incision is performed using a No. 11 blade through the area of pointing to release the pus. A fine hemostat is placed into the depths of the lacrimal sac and spread to break up any deeper loculations of purulent material and to facilitate drainage (Fig. 52–4*A*). In some cases, up to 5 mL of purulent material can be drained (Fig. 52–4*B*). The lacrimal sac contents should be sent for Gram's stain, culture, and sensitivity studies. In occasional cases, a dacryolith, which may have served as a nidus for the infection, may be recovered. A drain is placed to prevent immediate closure of the wound and to allow continuous egress of the purulent sac contents (Fig. 52–4*C*). Cahill and Burns[21] advocate lavage of the lacrimal sac with antibiotic solution (using neomycin-poly-

mixin-bacitracin, polymixin-trimethoprim, or ciprofloxacin) after the stab incision, then filling the sac with antibiotic ointment (neomycin-polymixin-bacitracin, gentamicin, or tobramycin) prior to placement of a drain.

For adults, upon resolution of the infection, the definitive dacryocystorhinostomy (DCR) procedure can be performed. For patients who have undergone incision and drainage of the sac abscess, the DCR is performed about 2 weeks following the drainage. DCR is a procedure that creates an opening from the lacrimal sac directly into the nasal cavity and thereby bypasses the obstruction in the nasolacrimal duct (Fig. 52–5). This procedure is typically performed through an external incision with suturing of the lacrimal sac flap to the nasal mucosal flap with a very high success rate (~95%). There is growing interest among ophthalmologists and otolaryngologists to perform this surgery using an endoscopic approach. Although the technique obviates a skin incision, the lacrimal and nasal flaps are not directly anastomosed, and the success rate of using this approach, to date, is less than that of conventional external surgery. In patients suspected of having a malignant process, it is wise to do a lacrimal sac biopsy during the DCR.[10]

Dacryocystectomy, or the removal of the lacrimal sac, is another surgical option in patients without tearing due to a secondary dry-eye condition. The goal of this procedure is removal of the sac, which is a potential space for the infec-

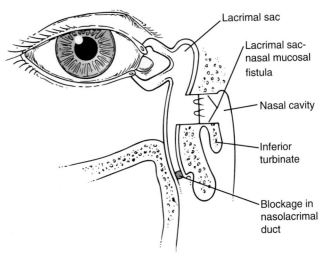

Figure 52–5. The lacrimal sac. Nasal mucosal fistula created after a dacryocystorhinostomy procedure.

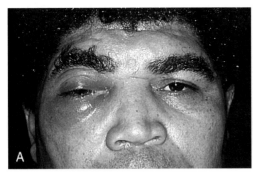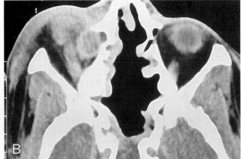

Figure 52-6. *A,* A 41-year-old male with chronic conjunctivitis and tearing who developed pain, swelling, decreased motility, and deterioration of vision in the right eye within a few days. *B,* Computerized tomography revealed a right lacrimal sac abscess extending posteriorly into the orbit. A dacryocystorhinostomy with intubation was necessary to drain the abscess and create a permanent drainage for tears.

tion to recur. Dacryocystectomy requires a shorter operating time and no bone removal and therefore may be preferred for patients unable to withstand the stress of prolonged surgery. The patient, however, should be clearly informed that tearing may occur as a result of the surgery.

Uncomplicated congenital nasolacrimal duct obstruction in infants is managed conservatively with massage and topical antibiotics when needed until the patient is 1 year of age, because most of these obstructions open spontaneously. In infants who develop dacryocystitis, probing of the lacrimal excretory system may be enough to open the very localized membranous obstruction. Unlike in adults, probing is usually unsuccessful, because most of the nasolacrimal duct lumen is obliterated with inflammation or fibrosis. Pollard[3] believes that probing can be performed safely in newborns with acute dacryocystitis. Through probing, the lacrimal sac is decompressed through an internal drainage. However, most experts believe that probing should be avoided during the acute inflammatory stage because of the increased risk of spreading the infection through false passages. For children older than 1 year, silicone intubation of the lacrimal system is highly suggested to decrease failure rate due to secondary closure. If probing and intubation are unsuccessful, a dacryocystorhinostomy should then be considered.

Complications

Patients with tear duct obstruction can develop complications such as chronic ipsilateral conjunctivitis and corneal ulcers. Because of the anatomic location of the lacrimal sac, untreated acute dacryocystitis usually spreads along the preseptal space. Uncommonly, the infection can break through the lateral side of the lacrimal sac wall and spread posteriorly into the orbit, forming an orbital abscess[22, 23] (Fig. 52-6). These cases should then be aggressively treated with immediate drainage of the orbital abscess and definitive DCR/intubation as well as appropriate intravenous antibiotic coverage such as ampicillin-sulbactam or nafcillin. Failure to control the infection and relieve the pressure in the orbit may lead to visual compromise and potentially life-threatening complications. Another possible complication related to dacryocystitis is seen in patients undergoing intraocular surgery. It is very important to assess the status of the lacrimal

excretory system prior to surgery. The presence of dacryocystitis is a contraindication to intraocular surgery. With nasolacrimal duct obstruction, the eye can be seeded with organisms originating from the lacrimal sac, even if not acutely infected clinically, resulting in an increased risk for endophthalmitis.[15]

Prevention

It is difficult to determine which patients with nasolacrimal duct obstruction will develop dacryocystitis. Topical antibiotics have only a minor role in prevention of the lacrimal sac infection. Establishing a proper drainage for tears by performing a DCR (in adults) or probing and intubation (in infants) to prevent stagnation of secretions in the lacrimal sac is still the best recommendation for prevention of dacryocystitis in patients with blocked tear ducts. Because spontaneous opening of the duct occurs in a high percentage of infants less than a year old, conservative management by massaging over the medial canthal region overlying the lacrimal sac to keep the sac empty and possibly to help rupture the obstructing membrane is an option for prevention of dacryocystitis in this age group.

References

1. Coden DJ, Hornblass A, Haas BD: Clinical bacteriology of dacryocystitis in adults. Ophthal Plast Reconstr Surg 1993; 9: 125–131.
2. MacEwan CJ, Young JDH: Epiphora in the first year of life. Eye 1991; 5: 596–600.
3. Pollard ZF: Treatment of acute dacryocystitis in neonates. J Pediatr Ophthalmol Strabismus 1991; 28: 431–343.
4. Linberg JV, McCormick SA: Primary acquired nasolacrimal duct obstruction. A clinicopathologic report and biopsy technique. Ophthalmology 1986; 93: 1055–1063.
5. Mauriello JA, Palydowycz S, DeLuca J: Clinicopathologic study of lacrimal sac and nasal mucosa in 44 patients with complete acquired nasolacrimal duct obstruction. Ophthal Plast Reconstr Surg 1992; 8: 13–21.
6. Blicker JA, Buffam FV: Lacrimal sac, conjunctival, and nasal culture results in dacryocystorhinostomy patients. Ophthal Plast Reconstr Surg 1993; 9: 43–46.
7. Goldberg SH, Fedok FG, Botek AA: Acute dacryocystitis secondary to exudative rhinitis. Ophthal Plast Reconstr Surg 1993; 9: 51–52.
8. Atkinson PL, Ansons AM, Patterson A: Infectious mononucleosis presenting as acute dacryocystitis. Br J Ophthalmol 1990; 74: 750.

9. Mauriello JA, Stabile C, Wagner RS: Dacryocystitis following Kawasaki's disease. Ophthal Plast Reconstr Surg 1986; 2: 209–211.

10. Karesh JW, Perman KI, Rodrigues MM: Dacryocystitis associated with malignant lymphoma of the lacrimal sac. Ophthalmology 1993; 100: 669–673.

11. Mahajan VM: Acute bacterial infections of the eye: Their aetiology and treatment. Br J Ophthalmol 1983; 67: 191–194.

12. Hurwitz JJ, Rodgers KJA: Management of acquired dacryocystitis. Can J Ophthalmol 1983; 18: 213–216.

13. Huber-Spitzy V, Steinkogler FJ, Huber E, et al.: Acquired dacryocystitis: Microbiology and conservative therapy. Acta Ophthalmol (Copenh) 1992; 70: 745–749.

14. Evans AR, Strong JD, Buck AC: Combined anaerobic and coliform infection in acute dacryocystitis. J Pediatr Ophthalmol Strabismus 1991; 28: 292.

15. Purgason PA, Hornblass A, Loeffler M: Atypical presentation of fungal dacryocystitis. Ophthalmology 1992; 99: 1430–1432.

16. Codere F, Anderson RL: Bilateral *Candida albicans* dacryocystitis with facial cellulitis. Can J Ophthalmol 1982; 17: 176–177.

17. Meyer DR, Wobig JL: Acute dacryocystitis caused by *Pasteurella multocida.* Am J Ophthalmol 1990; 110: 444–445.

18. Artenstein AW, Eiseman AS, Campbell GC: Chronic dacryocystitis caused by *Mycobacterium fortuitum.* Ophthalmology 1993; 100: 666–668.

19. Katowitz JA, Kropp TM: *Mycobacterium fortuitum* as a cause for nasolacrimal obstruction and granulomatous eyelid disease. Ophthalmic Surg 1987; 18: 97–99.

20. Rubin PAD, Bilyk JR, Shore JW, et al.: Magnetic resonance imaging of the lacrimal drainage system. Ophthalmology 1994; 101: 235–243.

21. Cahill KV, Burns JA: Management of acute dacryocystitis in adults. Ophthal Plast Reconstr Surg 1993; 9: 38–42.

22. Weiss GH, Leib ML: Congenital dacryocystitis and retrobulbar abscess. J Pediatr Ophthalmol Strabismus 1993; 30: 271–272.

23. Molgat YM, Hurwitz JJ: Orbital abscess due to acute dacryocystitis. Can J Ophthalmol 1993; 28: 181–183.

Andrew Blitzer
William Lawson
Anthony Reino

CHAPTER FIFTY-THREE

Sialadenitis

▼

ANATOMY

The salivary glands consist of three pairs of major glands and numerous minor salivary glands. The minor salivary glands are responsible for resting levels of moisture and lubrication of the oral cavity and pharynx. The major salivary glands are responsible for stimulated salivary production necessary for deglutition, digestion, and swallowing.

The saliva is composed of mucins, proteins, and lipids responsible for lubrication and protection of the hard and soft tissues of the oral cavity and pharynx. The liquid portion of the saliva serves a cleansing function for food remnants. There are also buffers and other elements that help to control the pH of acids or bases that enter the mouth. The saliva also contains a set of special phosphor-proteins that regulate the calcium and phosphate concentration of the teeth and maintain mineral salts at a saturated level. The saliva, through immunologic (immunoglobulins [Igs] IgA, IgG, and IgM) and nonimmunologic antibacterial proteins, minimizes bacterial growth and/or metabolism.[1]

The saliva also serves a digestive function. Its major component is alpha-amylase (ptylin), which is a starch-splitting enzyme. It also contains ribonuclease and oxyribonuclease, which split nucleic acids.[2] Saliva also contains peptide-splitting kallikreins, nonspecific esterases, and acid and alkaline phosphatases.[3]

The parotid gland is a pyramidal structure standing on its apex in the parapharyngeal space. The ductal system, a confluence of tributaries of the gland, leaves the gland at its anterior border. Stenson's duct crosses the masseter muscle to pierce the buccinator muscle and then enters the oral cavity at a papilla, which usually lies opposite the second molar tooth. There occasionally is a separate piece of salivary tissue attached to the distal duct called the accessory lobe. The entire gland is covered by a thick investing fascia that restricts its expansion and causes pain with swelling or abscess formation within the gland. An important regional structure is the facial nerve, which runs through the gland, causing arbitrary division into deep and superficial lobes.[4]

The submandibular gland is configured like a horseshoe around the posterior border of the mylohyoid muscle. The smaller portion of the gland is above the mylohyoid and follows the duct (Wharton's duct) into the floor of the mouth. This portion may merge with the sublingual portion in some persons. Wharton's duct runs upward from the gland hilum and then courses anteriorly over the edge of the mylohyoid muscle. This dependent position of the gland favors salivary stasis and is conducive to sialolith formation.[4]

The sublingual gland lies above the mylohyoid, along the course of the submandibular duct in the floor of the mouth.

The sublingual gland is drained by multiple ducts that open into the submandibular duct or empty directly into the oral cavity. There is also a very small cluster of apical or anterior lingual glands (Nuhn's glands), which lie on the undersurface of the apex of the tongue near the midline.[4]

The salivary glands are composed of acinar units that produce the saliva. Among the acini are serous elements that produce amylase and mucous elements that produce sialomucin. Other substances, such as lysozyme and lactoferrin, are also produced in the parotid acini. The acini are surrounded by myoepithelial cells, which act as contractile elements to increase the pressure within the ductal system. The ductal system is made up of intercollated ducts, which are short and surrounded by the myoepithelial cells, and the striated ducts. The striated ducts serve to secrete the saliva rapidly. There is also a mesenchymal system of interstitial connective tissue that holds the acini together in a lobular formation, allows for transport of electrolytes via the arterioles and venules, and carries the neural parasympathetic supply to the glandular tissue.[5]

Hypersecretion of saliva is associated with a wide variety of conditions, including rabies infection, mercury poisoning, acrodynia, tetanus, teething, and mucosal inflammation, and with such medications as anticholinesterases. Hyposecretion may be caused by numerous medications, such as antihistamines, parasympatholytic drugs, antiemetics, antidepressants, chemotherapeutic drugs, muscle relaxants, and diuretics. Radiation therapy and a number of disease states that destroy glandular tissue (e.g., Sjögren's syndrome and AIDS) will lead to hyposalivation. Patients suffering from bulimia and anorexia nervosa may have dehydration, electrolyte imbalances, bradycardia, and enlarged salivary glands with diminished salivary flow.[1]

Several host defense mechanisms operate through saliva. The gland makes sialomucins, which form a viscous, elastic layer to prevent penetration of the duct by antigenic substances. The gland also makes lysozyme in the acini and intercollated ducts, which hydrolyzes mucopolysaccharides or mucopolypeptides of the cell walls of gram-positive bacteria. The saliva contains peroxidase and thiocyanide ion, which has a bacteriostatic action. Additionally, the oxidative products iodine, bromine, and chlorine may be virucidal. The saliva also contains secretory IgA as well as some IgG and IgM. The secretory IgA of saliva is stimulated by bacteria and viruses and may be 100 times greater than that of serum.[1, 5]

EPIDEMIOLOGY

The most common salivary gland infection is the viral disease mumps. The peak incidence is in children 4 to 6 years of age. The infection rate is very high, with approximately 90% of people having antibody by age 14. About 50% of all mumps infections are clinically silent. Less common are the viral infections from cytomegalovirus and coxsackievirus.[6, 7]

Less common than viral infection are acute bacterial infections of the salivary gland. The parotid gland is most frequently involved, with an incidence estimated at 0.9%–0.8%.[7] About 20% of the acute cases are bilateral. It has been calculated that 0.03% of hospital infections are related to salivary gland infections. About 30%–40% of these cases of acute sialadenitis occur in postoperative patients, especially following gastrointestinal surgery. The onset of infection is generally 3–5 days after the procedure. Other acute infections are related to trauma, Stenson's or Wharton's duct trauma, oral infections, presence of calculi, or acquired ductal strictures.[6, 7]

PATHOPHYSIOLOGY

The bacterial pathogen most commonly found in sialadenitis is coagulase-positive *Staphylococcus aureus.* Less common bacterial pathogens include *Streptococcus pneumoniae, Escherichia coli, Haemophilus influenzae,* and the anaerobic pathogens *Bacteroides melaninogenicus* and *Peptostreptococcus micros.* Other agents include acid-fast bacteria, *Spirochaeta,* gonococci, and *Actinomyces.*[6, 7]

The most common viral pathogen, as already mentioned, is mumps; however, cytomegalovirus also may cause primary salivary infection. Other viruses that may affect the salivary glands as part of a systemic infection are those producing measles, coxsackievirus, echovirus, infectious mononucleosis, whooping cough, lymphochoriomeningitis, and encephalomyocarditis virus infection. A latent salivary infection may be caused by the cytomegalovirus and Epstein-Barr virus.[6, 7]

The pathophysiology of acute bacterial sialadenitis is most often related to dehydration leading to hyposalivation and stasis. The bacteria travel from the oral cavity in a retrograde fashion and multiply within the gland. The leak of toxic fluids containing proteolytic enzymes spills into the gland parenchyma, which are activated by tissue kinases, causing autodigestion of parenchymal tissue and the formation of multiple microabscesses.[6, 7]

Cases of sialadenitis arising in patients on antibiotic therapy suggest that other etiologic factors are operative. A similarity between parotitis and pancreatitis has been noted, and it has been suggested that autonomic nervous system dysfunction leads to increased vascular permeability, causing changes in the gland parenchyma with further extravasation of fluids from the vessels. Trypsinogen is then converted to trypsin, which causes autodigestion of the glandular tissue with secondary infection. The submandibular gland is rarely involved (unless obstructed by stone, tumor, or stricture), perhaps because of a high mucin content, which helps to aggregate bacteria and act as a protective agent.[6, 7]

Acute sialadenitis may progress to abscess formation. Although the parotid gland is the site most frequently involved by abscesses, submandibular gland abscess has been reported. When the abscess forms, there is progressive edema and induration of the overlying tissues. If no improvement is noted with antimicrobial therapy within a few days, if the swelling is rapidly increasing, or if a cavity is identified on radiographic studies, surgical incision and drainage should be performed. The dense glandular capsule often makes palpation of the abscess difficult, if not impossible. Rarely, a parotid abscess may also rupture into the external auditory canal or into the parapharyngeal space.[7]

Patients who have received radiation therapy for management of tumors of the head and neck are susceptible to sialadenitis, especially of the parotid gland. Radiation damage seems to affect the protein of the saliva rather than the protein synthesis itself. There occurs a 90% reduction of salivary flow and a permanent loss of secretory gland parenchyma. Histopathologically, there is swelling, vacuolization, and degranulation of the acinar cells, leading to acinar necrosis, parenchymal atrophy, interstitial fibrosis, ductal ectasia, ductal epithelial degeneration, and goblet cell metaplasia. This is followed by a loss of enzyme and electrolyte disturbances in the saliva, leading in turn to ductal obstruction and infection.[7–9]

Another cause of sialadenitis is related to the administration of iodinated glycerol, a mucolytic and expectorant used in the management of bronchitis and sinusitis. The resulting increase in the iodine concentration within the ducts causes mucosal edema and obstruction. This condition has an acute onset and may last from hours to days. The swelling can be unilateral or bilateral and is often tender. There is rapid resolution of the condition with the cessation of the iodinated glycerol.[10]

Obstruction of the salivary ducts by strictures, stones, or tumors will also lead to ductal ectasia, fibrosis, parenchymal atrophy, and salivary stasis with secondary infection. The majority of salivary stones occur in the submandibular gland (Figs. 53–1 and 53–2). This may be because the submandibular secretions are more viscous from their high mucous content; additionally, the deflection of the duct around the mylohyoid favors stasis. The majority of the stones are formed by secondary calcification around a nidus of mucus in the duct. Increasing pH and increased mucus (binds calcium better) tend to favor calcification and stone formation (Fig. 53–3). The calculi form at the ostium (30%), in the middle third (20%), at the mylohyoid (35%), and beyond the mylohyoid (15%). Obstruction leads to ductal destruction from secondary infection and stenosis. Parotid calculi are much less common. They can be palpated if they occur near the ostia, but most often, radiography or sialography is necessary to confirm their presence.[6, 7, 11–13]

Patients with cystic fibrosis experience recurrent parotid infections. The extremely viscous mucus causes ductal ectasia secondary to mucus inspissation with obstruction. With continued obstruction, further ductal dilation and parenchymal cyst formation occurs. The mucus particles laminate in an onion ring–like formation, with mucoprotein-calcium complexes producing lumpy microlith.[7]

Some patients suffer from electrolyte sialadenitis or dyschylia. This syndrome affects the submandibular gland in 90% of cases. In this condition, the increase in the salivary viscosity leads to retention of mucus in the terminal ducts, which in turn causes sialolithiasis. There is initially thick mucus and ductal ectasia. With time, spheroliths are precipi-

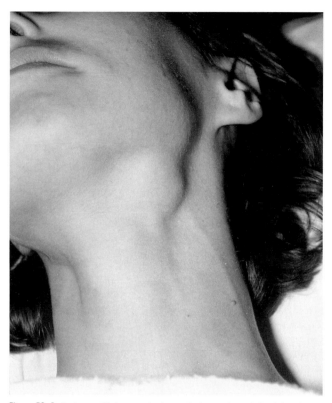

Figure 53–1. Patient with large calculus and obstruction of the left submandibular gland.

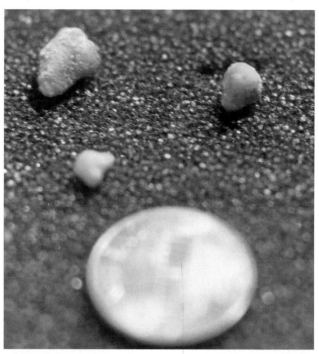

Figure 53–3. Photograph of three separate submandibular stones with a penny for size comparison.

tated (mucoprotein complexes), and then radial or lamellar microliths are produced in 25% of patients. Histologically, chronic obstruction with duct ectasia, squamous metaplasia, and ductular proliferation are seen. Later, there occurs atrophy of the secretory epithelium, periductal fibrosis, and lymphocytic, histiocytic, and plasma cell infiltrates.[7]

Sialectasis has also been reported in patients with AIDS, who may develop recurrent bouts of sialadenitis. Patients with AIDS may also develop multiple lymphoepithelial cysts within the parotid glands, which become infected[7, 14, 15] (Figs. 53–4 and 53–5).

In xerostomia, the decreased salivary secretions and stasis may lead to recurrent infections, as previously described.[6, 7, 13]

CLINICAL MANIFESTATIONS

Mumps, the most prevalent viral infection of the salivary glands, has a prodrome of headache, myalgia, malaise, and mild fever. Patients then develop swelling of one parotid gland, followed by swelling of the other gland in 75% of cases. The boggy swelling of the parotid may be associated

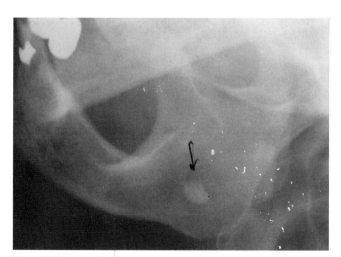

Figure 53–2. Lateral oblique radiograph of the mandible showing large submandibular calculus.

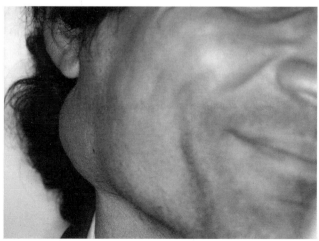

Figure 53–4. An AIDS patient with a right parotid lymphoepithelial cyst.

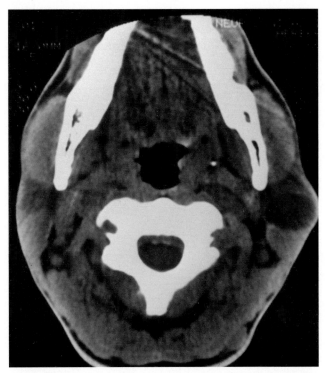

Figure 53–5. CT scan showing the lymphoepithelial cyst of the parotid.

the glands appear normal. Sialochemistry generally reveals the sodium content of the glands to be increased. The disease usually produces ductal ectasis and mucous inspissation but appears to reverse by puberty, usually leaving perfectly normal glands in adulthood.[6, 7, 13]

Tuberculosis of the salivary glands is a rare cause of salivary enlargement and tenderness. This disorder usually begins with intraglandular and periglandular lymph node enlargement of the parotid. Invasion of the salivary parenchyma is unusual. Unless calcifications are seen on x-ray, the diagnosis is difficult to make. Syphilis and gonorrhea may both cause inflammation of the parotid glands, producing bilateral, painless swelling of the glands. The diagnosis is made by serology or fine needle aspiration. Actinomycosis also may cause salivary gland inflammation but usually affects the minor salivary glands. The organisms enter through the salivary ducts or penetrate the gland parenchyma to produce granulomas.[7, 16–18]

Sjögren's syndrome also produces a picture of recurrent salivary swelling. In 1933, Sjögren, a Swedish ophthalmologist, described patients with xerophthalmia and keratoconjunctivitis who also had decreased salivary secretions. The patients were mostly older women who presented with parotid swelling and dry mouth, with many also having rheumatoid arthritis (Fig. 53–7).

The syndrome was therefore defined as a triad of keratoconjunctivitis sicca, xerostomia, and rheumatoid arthritis or other connective tissue disorder. Primary Sjögren's syndrome usually involves only the lacrimal and salivary glands, whereas secondary Sjögren's syndrome also includes systemic autoimmune disease, such as systemic lupus erythematosus, scleroderma, polymyositis, and periarteritis nodosa. Other systemic diseases associated with the syndrome are macrocytic anemia, pancreatitis, diabetes mellitus, Hashimoto's thyroiditis, and non-Hodgkin's lymphoma.[7, 13]

The disorder most typically occurs in patients aged 50 to 60 years. In 75% of the patients, serum antibodies against cytoplasmic antigens of salivary duct epithelium are present (anti-Sjögren's antibodies A and B). Bilateral parotid swell-

with eyelid swelling, edema of the external auditory canal, and trismus. The parotid swelling and symptoms last 1–2 weeks. During this time, the other salivary glands may become inflamed. Infection produces lifetime immunity.[6, 7]

Cytomegalovirus (CMV) has a clinical course that varies according to the patient's age. In prenatal infections, the virus passes the placenta and has been implicated in mental retardation and a number of malformations and dysfunctions. In the adult population, CMV infection produces symptoms like those of infectious mononucleosis, with fever, hepatosplenomegaly, jaundice, lymphadenopathy, leukopenia, and thrombocytopenia. CMV has been implicated in the production of salivary inclusion disease. The virus has also been associated with hepatitis, myocarditis, polyradiculitis, Guillain-Barré syndrome, and atypical bronchopneumonia.[6, 7, 14]

Patients with coxsackievirus infections, in addition to the parotitis, typically also have gingivitis and pharyngitis. Patients with infectious mononucleosis also may have salivary gland involvement, with extensive interstitial tissue infiltrates of monocytes and lymphocytes present.[7]

In acute bacterial sialadenitis, patients have salivary gland enlargement, tenderness, a metallic taste in the mouth, pain while eating, and also regional lymphadenitis. Thick, purulent material can be massaged from the gland[6, 7] (Fig. 53–6).

In chronic recurrent bacterial sialadenitis, there is usually a history of decreased saliva as well as tenderness and glandular enlargement while eating. During the acute phase of the infection, swelling, tenderness, fever, and thick purulent secretions are present.[6, 7, 13]

Another form of chronic sialadenitis is that found in children. Both parotid glands may be involved, with acute episodes lasting days to weeks, interspersed with a quiescent period of weeks to months. During the symptom-free period,

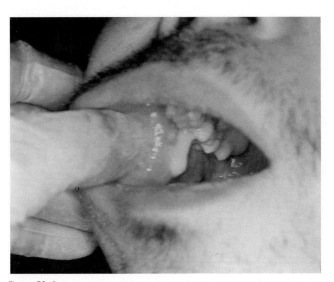

Figure 53–6. Pus emerging from Stenson's duct in a patient with acute bacterial sialadenitis.

increased IgM, enzyme-linked immunosorbent assay, an increased complement-binding reaction, a positive immunofluorescence test, virus in saliva, urine, or blood, and the histologic finding of giant cells with typical nuclear and cytoplasmic inclusion bodies.[6, 7, 14]

In acute bacterial sialadenitis, the diagnosis is usually made by culture, generally isolating staphylococci, streptococci, or *E. coli*. Generally, the patients have an elevated erythrocyte sedimentation rate and leukocytosis. In chronic cases, patients have a measurable decrease in salivary flow. Sialochemistry reveals increased lactoferrin, IgA, IgM, IgG, albumin, and sodium, and a decreased phosphate due to the breakdown of glandular tissue and subsequent leakage of these products into the saliva. There may also be high levels of lysozyme and myeloperoxidase, which are thought to be related to the inflammatory process in the acini.[6, 7]

Radiographic studies are useful in determining the nature of salivary ductal obstruction. Posteroanterior and lateral skull films may show parotid stones, and submental occlusal films are ideal for discovering submandibular duct stones. About 20% of submandibular calculi and 40% of parotid calculi are radiolucent (Fig. 53–8). If sialoliths cannot be identified on routine radiographs, then sialography can be utilized. The contraindications for sialography are acute inflammation of the gland and a history of sensitivity to the contrast material. Once the dye is introduced into the gland,

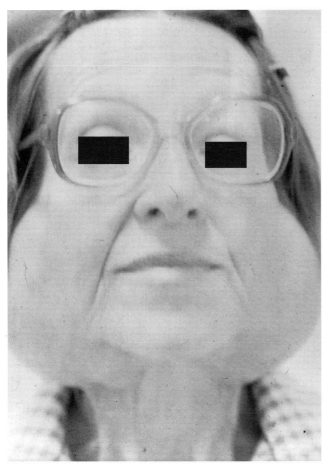

Figure 53–7. A patient with Sjögren's syndrome with bilateral large parotid swelling and xerostomia.

ing is typical, with submandibular swelling less common. Tenderness of the glands is uncommon.[7]

The salivary parenchyma may often become secondarily infected in relation to salivary stasis, producing a clinical picture resembling that of chronic recurrent sialadenitis. The sialographic changes also resemble those found in recurrent sialadenitis, ranging from early sialectasis to cystic degeneration of the parenchyma.[7]

DIAGNOSIS

The diagnosis of viral sialadenitis is made by identifying the virus in the blood or urine and by demonstrating the specific viral antigens. In mumps, the S, V, and hemagglutinin antigens may be found. Also present are leukopenia and increased serum amylase (salivary isoamylase). The complement-binding reaction and antibody titer are generally elevated fourfold. Histologically, there is interstitial inflammation, with infiltrates of lymphocytes and plasma cells in the periductal and periacinar tissue. This may lead to dissolution of the serous acini and vacuolation of the ductal epithelium. Electron microscopy shows dissolution of the endoplasmic reticulum and the secretory granules, with viral particles appearing as small inclusion bodies.[6, 7]

In CMV infection, the diagnosis is made by finding an

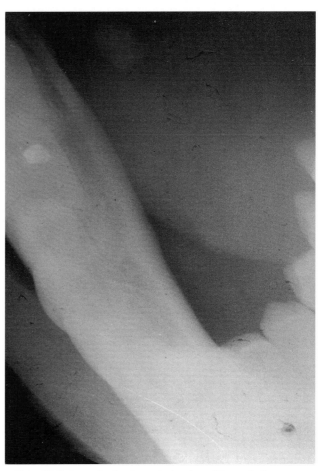

Figure 53–8. An occlusal radiograph showing a Wharton's duct stone.

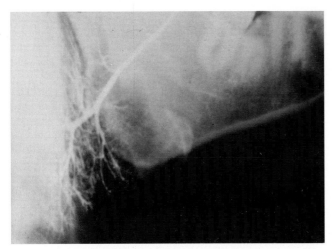

Figure 53–9. A normal parotid sialogram.

the ductal pattern and the parenchyma can be studied. Strictures and calculi are readily identified. Calcaterra and colleagues[19] have shown a false-positive rate of 20% for malignancy when sialography is used to evaluate either intrinsic or extrinsic mass lesions. The degree of filling and emptying can be assessed with postinjection films[6, 7, 13, 20] (Figs. 53–9 and 53–10).

Sialography in chronic cases may show varying degrees of ductal ectasia, a sausage link–like pattern in the ductal system, and pooling at the hilum (Figs. 53–11 to 53–13). Classification of sialectasia is based on the sialographic pattern. The earliest finding is called the pruned tree or tree in winter pattern, wherein the ducts are stretched and tapered and decreased in number, with nonfilling of the acini. The next stage is termed punctate sialectasis, in which peripheral ducts display dilations less than 1 mm and the intraglandular ductal system is stretched and tapered (see Fig. 53–12). The third stage is termed globular sialectasis, in which dilations of 1 or 2 mm are encountered, the ducts may be irregular or nonvisualized, and the radiograph has a mulberry pattern or fruit-laden tree appearance (see Fig. 53–13). The fourth stage is cavitary sialectasis (Fig. 53–14), in which there is

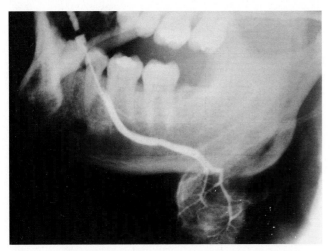

Figure 53–10. A normal submandibular sialogram.

coalescence of globules, forming cystic dilations. The final stage is destructive sialectasis, in which there is a bizarre pattern of pooling.[6, 7, 13, 20]

Some lesions are not well defined with these techniques, and other adjunctive studies may be necessary. Computed tomography (CT) scanning is particularly useful in the delineation of deep lobe parotid lesions. Som and Biller[21] reported the use of CT scanning with contrast sialography for this purpose. The CT scan gives an accurate assessment of the extent of disease and whether or not violation of the fascial compartments has occurred (Fig. 53–15). Magnetic resonance imaging does not show stones but demonstrates abscess formation, areas of inflammation, and tumors well.

Radionuclide scans are also helpful in diagnosing salivary gland disease. Gates[22] and Noyek and colleagues[23] have shown that salivary glands have greater vascularity than surrounding tissue, with the nuclide excreted into the saliva after the vascular phase (excretory phase). The lateral views are most useful. At the end of the excretory phase, evaluation of the gland is made by performing scans at 1, 15, 30, and 60 minutes. Cold areas (decreased uptake) with smooth margins generally represent benign lesions. Malignant cold nodules often have irregular margins. Hot lesions (increased uptake) are either Warthin's tumor or oncocytoma.

Ultrasound scanning has also been found to be helpful to differentiate cystic from solid lesions and to localize abscess cavities. Noyek and colleagues,[23] however, caution that cystic lesions and lymphomas can have the same ultrasound pattern.[24, 25]

Needle aspiration has been very successful in determining whether fluid or purulent material is present in a cavity and for sampling tissue for cytologic examination. Because this is cytologic analysis and not tissue block study, the tissue architecture cannot be reviewed, and errors can occur. For example, specimen containing groups of duct-type cells and psammoma bodies is suggestive of adenocarcinoma; however, psammoma bodies also occur in normal, inflamed, irradiated, and neoplastic conditions.[26]

In establishing the diagnosis of tuberculosis, skin testing is essential. In addition, needle biopsy of the enlarged gland may show granulomas consisting of epithelioid cells, lymphocytes, and Langhans's giant cells. In the more advanced cases, there may be significant necrosis.[7, 16, 17]

In patients suspected of having Sjögren's syndrome, the salivary parenchyma may often become secondarily infected because of salivary stasis, with the clinical picture resembling that of chronic recurrent sialadenitis. The sialographic changes are also similar to those found in recurrent sialadenitis. However, if the saliva is collected and tested, sialochemistry shows increases in sodium, chloride, IgA, IgG, lactoferrin, and albumin often accompanied by a decrease in phosphate.[7]

The histology of the gland shows atrophy, interstitial lymphocytic infiltration, and myoepithelial islands. With early lesions, there are periductal changes with focal invasion of the acini. With progression, there is increased parenchymal infiltration and atrophy with metaplasia of the ductal epithelium and proliferation of the myoepithelial cells.[7]

In patients with Sjögren's syndrome, there is a marked increase in IgG-containing plasma cells; in contrast, patients with chronic parotitis without autoimmune disease have a

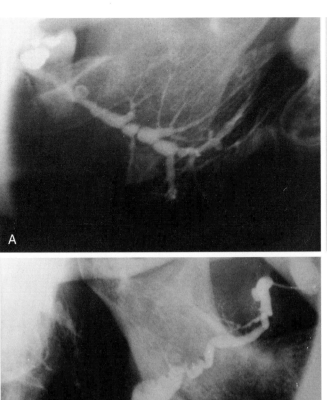

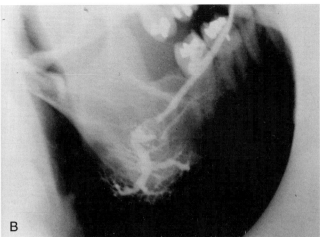

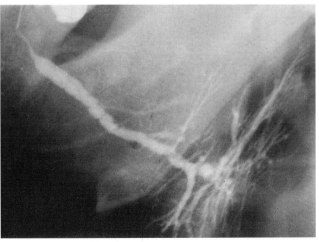

Figure 53–11. *A, B, C.* Sialograms of patients with chronic sialadenitis showing sausage link–like patterns and massive duct dilation.

marked increase in IgA plasma cells. A few plasma cells in the islands of myoepithelial cells surrounded by lymphocytes are found in patients with Sjögren's syndrome, which is not seen in chronic sialadenitis. There is evidence of hyperactivity of B cells in Sjögren's syndrome, with a polyclonal hypergammaglobulinemia and non–organ-specific antibodies. The minor salivary glands are found to be inflamed with ductal ectasia, lymphocytic infiltration, marked sclerosis, and atrophy of the acini and rare myoepithelial cells present.[7]

TREATMENT

The treatment of viral sialadenitis is essentially symptomatic. In mumps, occasionally gamma globulin is given to try to

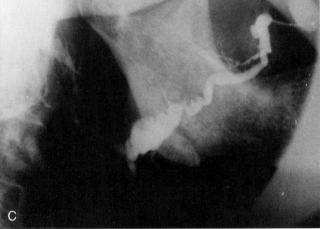

Figure 53–12. Sialogram showing punctate sialectasis.

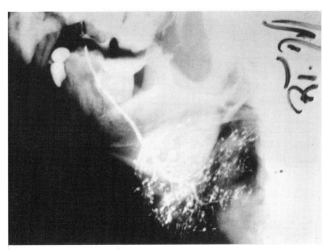

Figure 53–13. Sialogram showing the "mulberry pattern."

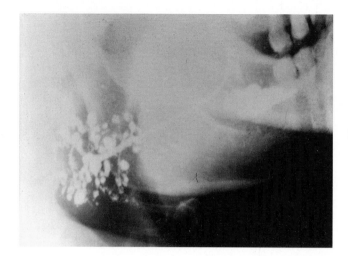

Figure 53–14. Sialogram showing "cavitary sialectasis."

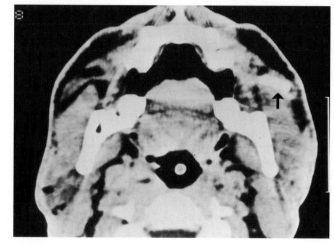

Figure 53–15. CT scan of the parotid showing a stone in Stenson's duct *(arrow)*.

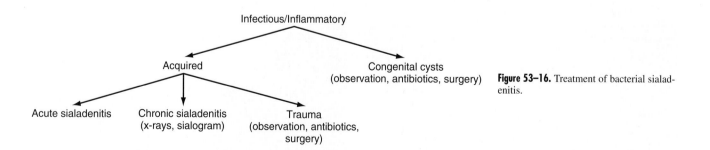

Figure 53–16. Treatment of bacterial sialadenitis.

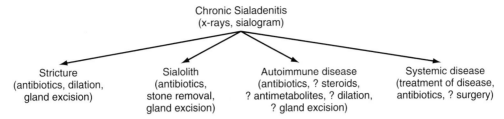

Figure 53–17. Treatment of chronic bacterial sialadenitis.

prevent orchitis in adults. Steroids may also be given to patients with orchitis or central nervous system involvement.[6, 7]

The treatment of acute bacterial sialadenitis is to give fluids, sialogogues to stimulate secretion, antibiotics, and gland massage. Some experts have suggested the use of trypsin inactivator factor to limit parenchymal damage. Incision and drainage may be necessary if the gland fails to drain via the ductal structure within 24–48 hours or if there is evidence of abscess formation. Needle aspiration or CT-guided needle aspiration has been used in medically unstable patients who cannot undergo formal incision and drainage.[6, 7]

In the chronic forms of bacterial sialadenitis, the initial treatment is the same as for the acute disorder. Treatment in these cases should also address the question of obstruction (tumor, stricture, stone). If an obstruction is discovered, therapy should be directed at it. Other measures, such as ductal dilation, removal of stone, duct ligation, irradiation of the gland, tympanic neurectomy, and gland excision, have all been reported, and their uses are related to the severity of the disease and the medical status of the patient (Figs. 53–16 and 53–17).[7]

In cases of stricture, simple dilation may be useful. In others, repair and stenting or bypass of the duct is performed. If the stricture cannot be bypassed, repaired, or enlarged, the gland may require excision.[7]

In cases in which an abscess has formed, drainage is necessary. Drainage of a parotid abscess is accomplished through a standard parotidectomy incision with an opening of the glandular capsule parallel to the course of the facial nerve. Multiple drains should be placed. Further dissection into the parapharyngeal space should be carried out if there is clinical or radiographic evidence of parapharyngeal space involvement.[6, 7]

In chronic recurrent sialadenitis in children, the therapy should be as conservative as possible and given for as long as possible, because in most cases the disease reverses at puberty. If the disease is uncontrollable, other measures, such as those used in adults, may be taken.[6, 7]

In tuberculosis of the salivary glands, the treatment is generally medical; however, if the gland becomes abscessed, surgery becomes necessary.[7, 16, 17]

In the patients with Sjögren's syndrome, the treatment is relatively unsatisfactory because of the progressive destruction of the lacrimal and salivary glands. Symptomatic treatment with methylcellulose tears and saliva is used for the dryness. If there are chronic recurrent infections, patients are treated similarly to those with chronic sialadenitis. Surgery should be reserved for recurrent parotitis uncontrolled by antibiotics and gland massage.[7]

COMPLICATIONS

In viral sialadenitis, the virus may also affect other organ systems. The major side effects of mumps are pancreatitis, meningitis, orchitis, and deafness. Orchitis has a rate of sterility of 10%–30% in males over the age of puberty. The ovaries are rarely involved. The virus also can cause a meningoencephalitis with cranial nerve injuries, particularly of cranial nerve VIII, resulting in deafness. Fortunately, the deafness is usually unilateral. In CMV infections, prolonged immunosuppression may be produced. The infection decreases the function of leukocytes, lymphocytes, and macrophages. There may also be a viral latency, with the splenic B lymphocytes or cells of the salivary gland acting as a reservoir for virus.[7]

Bacterial sialadenitis may produce abscesses when the infection penetrates the glandular fascia. In rare cases, facial paresis or paralysis may develop. In cases of tuberculosis, fistula formation into the overlying skin may occur.[6, 7]

In patients who have Sjögren's syndrome, systemic autoimmune diseases often develop. These disorders have been listed in the previous section.

PREVENTION

Mumps and its sequelae may be avoided with vaccination. Some of the other viral syndromes, such as CMV and coxsackievirus infection, do not currently have vaccinations. Bacterial infections can sometimes be avoided by the prevention of dehydration or the use of medications leading to ductal stasis. Early identification of obstruction in chronic cases prevents severe and irreversible glandular damage and the necessity of gland removal.[6, 7]

References

1. Stuchell RN, Blitzer A, Mandel ID: Medical management of non-neoplastic salivary gland disease. Otol Clin North Am 1984; 17: 697–703.
2. Zollner EJ, Klepsch DM, Zahn RK, Knepper R: Deoxyribonucleases in human parotid saliva. Enzyme 1974; 19: 60.
3. Seifert G, Miehlke A, Haubrich J, Chilla R: Physiology and biochemistry. In: Diseases of the Salivary Glands. New York: Thieme Medical Publishers, 1986, pp 27–43.
4. Seifert G, Miehlke A, Haubrich J, Chilla R: Topographic anatomy. In: Diseases of the Salivary Glands. New York: Thieme Medical Publishers, 1986, pp 1–6.
5. Seifert G, Miehlke A, Haubrich J, Chilla R: Histology and ultrastructure. In: Diseases of the Salivary Glands. New York: Thieme Medical Publishers, 1986, pp 7–23.

6. Rice DH: Diseases of the salivary glands—non-neoplastic. In: Bailey BJ (ed): Head and Neck Surgery—Otolaryngology. Philadelphia: JB Lippincott, 1993, pp 475–484.

7. Seifert G, Miehlke A, Haubrich J, Chilla R: Sialoadenitis. In: Diseases of the Salivary Glands. New York: Thieme Medical Publishers, 1986, pp 110–163.

8. Miyazawa K, Mikami T, Miasaka K, Aonuma S: Experimental models of acute and chronic sialadenitis in the guinea pig. Jpn J Pharmacol 1992; 59: 405–411.

9. Vissink A, Kalicharan D, S-Gravenmade EJ, et al.: Acute irradiation effects on morphology and function of rat submandibular glands. J Oral Pathol Med 1991; 20: 449–456.

10. Sorresso DJ, Mehta JB: Sialoadenitis: A rare but well-recognized complication of iodinated glycerol. Ann Otol Rhinol Laryngol 1995; 104: 162–163.

11. Mandel L, Fatehi J: Minor salivary gland sialolithiasis: Review and case report. N Y State Dent J 1992; 58: 31–33.

12. Cummins M, Dardick I, Brown D, Burford-Mason A: Obstructive sialoadenitis: A rat model. J Otolaryngol 1994; 23: 50–56.

13. Blitzer A: Inflammatory and obstructive disorders of the salivary glands. J Dent Res 1987; 66: 675–679.

14. Wax TD, Layfield LJ, Zaleski S, et al.: Cytomegalovirus sialoadenitis in patients with the acquired immunodeficiency syndrome: A potential diagnostic pitfall with fine-needle aspiration cytology. Diagn Cytopathol 1994; 10: 169–172.

15. Lamey PJ, Felix D, Nolan A: Sialectasis and HIV infection. Dento-Maxillo-Facial Radiology 1993; 22: 159–160.

16. Batsakis JG: Granulomatous sialadenitis. Ann Otol Rhinol Laryngol 1991; 100: 166–169.

17. Ataman M, Sozeri B, Ozcelik T, Gedikoglu G: Tuberculosis of the parotid salivary gland. Auris Nasus Larynx 1992; 19: 271–273.

18. O'Connell JE, George MK, Speculand B, Pahor AL: Mycobacterial infection of the parotid gland: An unusual cause of parotid swelling. J Laryngol Otol 1993; 107: 561–564.

19. Calcaterra TC, Hemenway WG, Hansen GC, Hanafee WN: The value of sialography in the diagnosis of parotid tumors. Arch Otolaryngol 1977; 103: 727–729.

20. Shimizu M, Uoshiura K, Kands S: Radiological and histological analysis of the structural changes in the rat parotid gland following release of Stenson's duct obstruction. Dento-Maxillo-Facial Radiology 1994; 23: 197–205.

21. Som PM, Biller HF: The combined CT sialogram. Radiology 1980; 135: 387–390.

22. Gates GA: Sialography and scanning of the salivary glands. Otol Clin North Am 1977; 10: 379–390.

23. Noyek A, Zizmor J, Musumeci R: The radiographic diagnosis of tumors of the salivary glands. J Otolaryngol 1977; 103: 727.

24. Bruneton JN, Mourou MY: Ultrasound in salivary gland disease. ORL J Otorhinolaryngol Relat Spec 1993; 55: 284–289.

25. Cvetinovic M, Jovic N, Mijatovic D: Evaluation of ultrasound in the diagnosis of pathologic processes in the parotid gland. J Oral Maxillo-facial Surg 1991; 49: 147–150.

26. Fierson HF, Fechner RE: Chronic sialadenitis with psammoma bodies mimicking neoplasia in a fine-needle aspiration from the submandibular gland. Am J Clin Pathol 1991; 95: 884–888.

Anthony W. Chow

Orofacial Infections

▼

The clinical spectrum of skin and mucous membrane infections of the face and oral cavity is quite diverse. Such infections may be localized and indolent or invasive and life-threatening. Virtually all infectious agents can present on the face or intraorally. Although bacterial and fungal infections of the skin and oral mucosa usually result from direct inoculation of opportunistic pathogens from the external or resident microflora, viral infections of the skin and oral mucosa generally arise by hematogenous dissemination or reactivation of a latent infection. In this chapter, the more common soft tissue infections of the face and oral mucosa are discussed. Odontogenic orofacial infections, cervicofacial actinomycosis, and deep neck space infections are described elsewhere.

ANATOMIC CONSIDERATIONS

The Maxillofacial Skin

The skin is a major organ, complete with epithelial, vascular, lymphoid, and neuronal tissues as well as specialized appendages. It maintains body temperature and hydration while acting as a barrier to microbial invasion. It consists of two layers, the *epidermis,* derived from the ectoderm, and the *dermis,* derived from the mesoderm (Fig. 54–1). The epidermis comprises four types of cell layers: stratum corneum, stratum granulosum, stratum spinosum, and the basal layer. The stratum corneum, the topmost layer, contains a continually regenerating zone of closely packed, keratin-producing squamous cells. The stratum granulosa cells in the next layer contain keratohyalin granules, which are closely involved with the process of keratinization and later migrate to form the stratum corneum. The stratum spinosum, adjacent to the basal layer, contains cells that are polyhedral and share prominent intercellular attachments known as desmosomes (Fig. 54–2). As these cells migrate toward the surface, they begin to flatten and assemble keratohyalin granules. The basal layer consists of a single row of germinal cells resting on the dermis. The mitotic rate of the basal cells determines the turnover rate of the stratum corneum. The dermis can be separated into the papillary and reticular regions, both of which consist primarily of collagen fibers. The dermis in the maxillofacial region contains several specialized appendages, including hair follicles, sweat glands, and sebaceous glands, which may descend into the superficial fascia. The sebaceous gland is part of the pilosebaceous apparatus, which empties through a duct into the hair follicle. Although located primarily in the dermis, the hair follicles are lined by epidermal cells.

The epidermis is devoid of blood vessels, nerves, and lymphatics and is, therefore, relatively removed from cellular and humoral host defenses, especially in the more superficial region. The arterial supply to the skin arises from a flat plexus of vessels located in the superficial fascia near its junction with the dermis. Smooth muscle cells in the precapillary arterioles function to control blood perfusion of the skin, thereby helping to regulate skin temperature. Venules and lymphatics accompany the arteries. Lymphatics in the dermis contain no valves, whereas those in the superficial fascia contain a few valves.[1]

The Oral Mucosa

The oral mucous membrane also consists of two layers: the epithelium (ectodermal origin), and the lamina propria (mesodermal origin). The composition of the epithelial layer of the oral mucosa is very similar to that of the epidermis of the skin and also comprises four cellular layers: stratum corneum, stratum granulosum, stratum spinosum (or prickle cell layer), and the basal layer. However, in contrast to that of the skin, the epithelium of the oral mucosa shows considerable variations in the extent of the keratinization process, depending on the precise location of the mucosa. Mucous membranes that contain fully keratinized epithelium typically overly the hard palate, the dorsal surface of the tongue, and parts of the gingivae. Nonkeratinized or partially keratinized epithelium is confined to the buccal mucosa, the floor of the mouth, and the ventral surface of the tongue.

In the lamina propria and the submucosa are scattered cells of the leukocyte series, and various mucous and sebaceous glands of the oral cavity. These are widely variable in distribution, with the mucous glands being most common in the mucosa of the lips and posterior palate, whereas the sebaceous glands are most concentrated in the buccal mucosa. The submucosal layer contains blood vessels, fat, and fibrous tissue, which vary according to the precise location within the oral cavity.[2]

Diseases of the oral mucosa often result from breakdown or abnormality of the epithelium. Typical epithelial lesions include hyperkeratosis (increased thickness of the keratin layer), acanthosis (increased thickness of the prickle cell layer with or without associated hyperkeratosis), atrophy (thinning of the epithelium, often associated with incomplete keratinization), and acantholysis (loss of the intercellular attachments in the prickle cell layer leading to separation of the cells). An atrophic epithelium may readily become ulcerated following minor trauma, whereas acantholytic lesions may lead to intraepithelial blisters owing to collection of

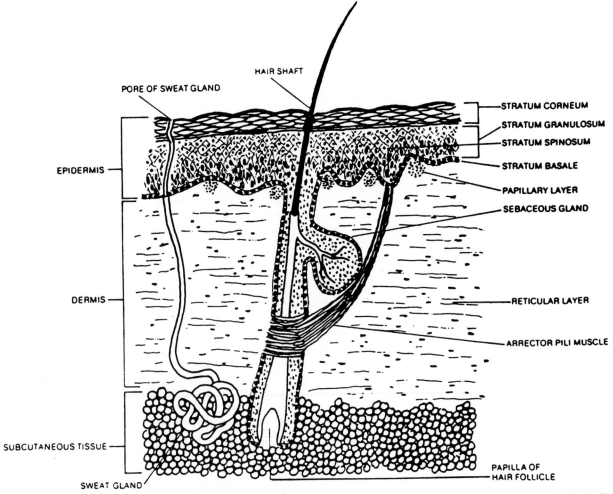

HAIR SHAFT

PORE OF SWEAT GLAND

STRATUM CORNEUM
STRATUM GRANULOSUM
STRATUM SPINOSUM
STRATUM BASALE
PAPILLARY LAYER
SEBACEOUS GLAND

EPIDERMIS

DERMIS

RETICULAR LAYER

ARRECTOR PILI MUSCLE

SUBCUTANEOUS TISSUE

PAPILLA OF
HAIR FOLLICLE

SWEAT GLAND

Figure 54–1. Anatomic structures of the skin. (From Thadepalli H, Mandal AK: Anatomic Basis of Infectious Disease, 1st ed. Springfield, Illinois: Charles C Thomas, Publisher, 1984.)

edema fluid in or between the prickle cells. Bullous lesions may develop with collection of edema fluid between the epithelium and the lamina propria in the region of the basal complex.

PATHOGENESIS

Intact skin is extraordinarily resistant to invasion by microbes. The stratum corneum, by virtue of constant desquamation and renewal, acts as the principal barrier to bacterial invasion. In addition, the sweat glands secrete a hypotonic saline solution that slightly acidifies the skin (pH approximately 5.5) and assists in its antimicrobial activities. The sebaceous glands also produce sebum, a mixture of lipids that are inhibitory to various bacteria, including both streptococci and staphylococci but not propionibacteria, the principal cause of acne. Other local host defense mechanisms of the skin depend on its degree of vascularity. Thus, the major factors predisposing to orofacial skin and soft tissue infections are related to minor traumatic or ischemic injury that causes a breakdown in the integrity of the epidermis. Even when these conditions are met, a relatively high bacte-

rial inoculum is required to initiate a soft tissue infection. The presence of foreign bodies such as dirt, grease, and suture material dramatically lowers the inoculum size necessary to induce infection.[1]

In addition to the intact epithelium, the oral mucosa has a number of other host defenses against microbial invasion. First, the normal indigenous oral flora provides a strong mucosal defense against colonization and infection by potential pathogens (colonization resistance).[3] Second, the constant flow of saliva contains a variety of nonspecific antimicrobial systems such as lysozyme, lactoferrin, β-lysin, and lactoperoxidase.[3] Various salivary glycoproteins and histidine-rich polypeptides have also been reported to inhibit different bacteria and fungi and to prevent microbial attachment to the oral epithelium by competitive binding to cellular receptors or clumping of microorganisms. A reduction in saliva volume also has significant effects on the oral environment and predisposes to microbial invasion. In addition to these nonspecific host defenses, specific humoral and cellular immune mechanisms are important. Microorganism-specific antibodies are present in saliva, with secretory immunoglobulin A (IgA) as the predominant immunoglobulin.[4] Salivary antibodies may also affect the oral flora by aggre-

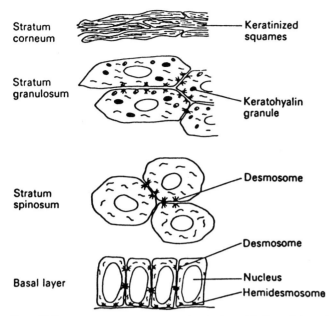

Figure 54–2. Diagram of cell layers in the keratinzing epithelium of the oral mucosa. (From Tyldesley WR: Oral Medicine, 1st ed. Oxford: Oxford University Press, 1981. By permission of Oxford University Press.)

gating organisms and preventing their attachment to the mucosal epithelium. Cell-mediated immunity is particularly important against intracellular pathogens such as viruses, fungi, and certain bacteria. In addition, various phagocytic cells, such as lymphocytes, granulocytes, and macrophages, appear important. These cells are abundant in the lamina propria and presumably contribute to the removal of foreign matter that has breached the epithelial barrier.

CLINICAL SYNDROMES

Pyogenic Infections of the Face and Neck

Impetigo

Impetigo is a primary superficial infection of the skin that is confined to the epidermis and is characterized by multiple lesions with little or no systemic toxicity. *Streptococcus pyogenes* accounts for the majority of cases, primarily among preschool children in warm and humid climates. Poverty, crowding, and poor personal hygiene are other contributing factors. The early lesions are vesiculopustular in appearance and are associated with localized lymphadenopathy. These lesions progress rapidly to crusting, which is characteristically thick and adherent to the underlying skin. A variant of streptococcal pyoderma that extends through the epidermis of the skin and presents as ulcerated lesions is known as ecthyma. A well-recognized complication of streptococcal impetigo is immune complex acute glomerulonephritis.[5] Although *Staphylococcus aureus* is often coisolated with *S. pyogenes* from impetiginous lesions, *S. aureus* can be the sole cause of impetigo in approximately 10 per cent of cases. Staphylococcal impetigo is clinically distinguished from streptococcal impetigo by the presence of large bullous lesions that rupture, leaving thin and nonpurulent crusts overlying the involved skin. Localized lymphadenopathy is not a prominent finding. This form of impetigo is more often seen in newborns and younger children.

Folliculitis and Furunculosis

Folliculitis is an inflammatory process localized to the hair follicles and resulting from pore obstruction. *S. aureus* is the most common bacterial cause. The lesions appear as small or pinhead-sized, erythematous papules that may progress to form pustules. A deeper infection may lead to the development of a furuncle, or boil, which is a localized abscess of the follicle with some destruction of its walls. A carbuncle forms when a group of furuncles coalesce into a large abscess. Midfacial furuncles have a potential risk of developing cavernous sinus thrombosis owing to extensive communications between the facial veins and the orbital venous plexuses. Recurrent furunculosis is more prone to develop in patients with obesity, diabetes mellitus, corticosteroid therapy, and defects in neutrophil function.

A pruritic form of folliculitis associated with exposure to contaminated whirlpools and hot tubs is caused by *Pseudomonas aeruginosa*. Characteristically, the skin lesions involve the buttocks, trunk, and other immersed areas of the body, less commonly the face and neck.

Folliculitis is a relatively self-limiting condition and generally does not need specific antimicrobial therapy. Furunculosis and carbuncles should be treated with systemic antibiotics mainly directed at *S. aureus*. Carbuncles usually require surgical drainage as well.

Erysipelas

Erysipelas is an inflammatory process involving primarily the superficial layers of the skin, including the dermis. The lesion has a distinctive fiery-red appearance and is indurated with a raised and sharply demarcated margin. Typically, there is a bilateral or "butterfly" distribution across the bridge of the nose. Erysipelas is classically caused by *S. pyogenes* but can occasionally be caused by other organisms, such as *Streptococcus pneumoniae*[6] and *Haemophilus influenzae*.[7] As with other pyogenic streptococcal skin infections, the lesions tend to spread rapidly. The patient may appear quite toxic, with fever, chills, and malaise. Lymphadenopathy and lymphangitis is usually present. As the lesions resolve, there is often desquamation of the skin overlying the involved area. Antibiotic treatment directed at *S. pyogenes* should be continued for 10–14 days.

Cellulitis

Cellulitis is an acute infection of the skin extending deep into subcutaneous tissues underlying the dermis. It can result either by inoculation of organisms through an open wound, by contiguous spread of infection from a more superficial source, or by hematogenous seeding. The involved tissue is erythematous, warm, edematous, and tender. In contrast to erysipelas, the margins of the lesion in cellulitis are nonelevated and poorly defined. The patient usually demonstrates constitutional signs of illness, such as fever, chills, and malaise.

In adolescents and adults, *S. pyogenes* is the most common etiologic agent of cellulitis in the maxillofacial region, which usually results from minor wounds and punctures. Once established, the infection progresses rapidly via the involved lymphatics, causing destruction of the superficial layers of the skin that may progress to streptococcal gangrene. Treatment generally requires surgical débridement of gangrenous skin, incision and drainage of the underlying tissue and fascial planes, as well as appropriate systemic antibiotics. *S. aureus* can also induce a cellulitis or pyoderma, but in contrast to streptococcal cellulitis, the infection usually arises from a furuncle and tends to be more slowly progressive.

In children, cellulitis in the maxillofacial region is most commonly caused by *H. influenzae* and *S. pneumoniae*. Bacteremia is frequently present, and the child appears toxic. *H. influenzae* cellulitis is particularly common in children less than 2 years of age, and the infected site may take on a bluish or purplish hue. Periorbital cellulitis is also more common in children and is generally preceded by trauma, sinusitis, otitis media, or other upper respiratory tract infections.[8, 9] There is diffuse swelling of the eyelid that may spread across the nasal bridge. Additional manifestations include conjunctival edema, proptosis, limitation of ocular motility, and decreased vision. Antibiotic treatment should be directed at staphylococci, streptococci, and *H. influenzae*, the most common pathogens in this entity.

Synergistic Necrotizing Cellulitis and Necrotizing Fasciitis

Synergistic necrotizing cellulitis is a rapidly progressive infection involving the subcutaneous tissues and superficial fascia. In the area of the face and neck, it more commonly results as a complication of an odontogenic "space" infection, but occasionally it can occur following minor trauma or a postoperative wound infection. The initial lesion is a reddish-brown bleb accompanied by local tenderness. However, the superficial appearance often belies the widespread destruction of the deeper tissues. There is extensive gangrene of the subcutaneous tissue with gelatinous fat necrosis of the superficial fascia. There is often a copious, brown, watery, and foul discharge ("dishwater pus"). Gram's-staining of the exudate reveals mixed organisms, and cultures usually demonstrate a polymicrobial infection involving both aerobic and anaerobic organisms, primarily *Peptostreptococcus, Bacteroides, Fusobacterium,* and Enterobacteriaceae. Treatment is primarily by surgical débridement of necrotic tissues, incision and drainage of tunneling dishwater pus, and broad-spectrum systemic antibiotics.[10]

Necrotizing fasciitis is an aggressive infection characterized by severe gangrene of the skin and of the superficial and deep fascia. The majority of cases involving the neck are either posttraumatic, postsurgical, or odontogenic in nature.[11, 12] Often, the patient has underlying ischemic small-vessel disease or diabetes mellitus. Although *S. pyogenes* and *S. aureus* can both produce this syndrome with or without a toxic shock–like presentation, most cases are polymicrobial in etiology, commonly involving anaerobic and/or aerobic gram-positive cocci and gram-negative bacilli. Once clinically apparent, the infection spreads rapidly within hours. Pain is a prominent finding initially, usually at the site of trauma or surgery. The area becomes edematous, warm, and erythematous, and rapidly develops a tense, shiny appearance that later changes to a dark, dusky discoloration. Bullous formation may occur, and the underlying skin becomes necrotic and may slough because of frank gangrene. Subcutaneous emphysema (crepitus) is present in up to 25% of cases.[13] As the necrosis progresses, the pain may actually decrease or abate completely, leaving local anaesthesia due to destruction of the cutaneous nerves in the subcutaneous tissues. Systemic toxicity with sepsis syndrome is a common presentation, and hypotension or shock may develop owing to sequestration of large volumes of fluid in the necrotic fascial spaces. Treatment requires aggressive surgical excision, incision, and drainage, as well as systemic broad-spectrum antibiotics.[14]

Infections of the Oral Mucosa

Acute Herpetic Gingivostomatitis

This condition, caused by the initial or primary infection with herpes simplex virus, occurs most commonly in children 2–5 years of age, although it can also be seen in adults. The initial symptoms are sore throat, enlarged submandibular lymph nodes, and a burning sensation of the oral mucosa. This is rapidly followed by a vesicular eruption of the oral mucosa, which soon becomes ulcerated. The mucosal ulcers may be small at first but often coalesce into large shallow lesions with serpiginous borders, becoming covered by a fibrinous, yellowish, firmly adherent membrane. The ulcer is very painful, and the patient is febrile and has considerable difficulty talking, eating, and swallowing. The microbiologic diagnosis is confirmed by a positive Tzanck smear (prepared from scrapings of the ulcer base that demonstrate the presence of multinucleated giant cells with intranuclear inclusions) and by immunofluorescence staining or virus isolation. Treatment requires topical analgesics and systemic antiviral agents (acyclovir, vidarabine, or foscarnet).[15]

Aphthous Stomatitis

Aphthous ulcers, among the most common causes of recurrent oral lesions,[4] must be distinguished from other conditions such as herpes simplex virus and coxsackie virus infections, agranulocytosis, and Behçet's disease. The etiology of aphthous ulcers remains uncertain, although a number of infectious agents, including viruses, have been implicated. The most prevailing hypothesis suggests that the mechanisms for mucosal ulceration is autoimmune in nature.[4]

Three major clinical variants are recognized: (1) minor aphthous ulcers, (2) major aphthous ulcers, and (3) herpetiform aphthous ulcers. Minor aphthous ulcers appear as a number of small ulcers on the buccal and labial mucosa, the floor of the mouth, or the tongue. The palatal soft tissues, pharynx, and tonsillar fauces are rarely involved. A prodromal stage is usually present. The ulcers appear gray-yellow, often with a raised and erythematous margin, and are exquisitely painful. Lymph node enlargement is seen only with secondary bacterial infection. The course of ulceration varies from a few days to several weeks, and is followed by spontaneous healing. Major aphthous ulcers are more protracted and last up to several months. All areas of the oral cavity, including the soft palate and tonsillar areas, may be involved. Prolonged periods of remission may be followed by intervals of intense ulcer activity.

Herpetiform aphthous ulcers are small and multiple, and they characteristically affect the lateral margins and tips of the tongue. The ulcers are gray with a delineating erythematous border and are extremely painful, making eating and speaking difficult. Despite the name of this variant, there is little clinical resemblance to an acute herpetic gingivostomatitis. Although intranuclear inclusions have been demonstrated in herpetiform aphthous ulcers, there is no evidence to suggest that these inclusions bear any relationship to the presence of viruses. Treatment is primarily symptomatic, with antiseptic mouthwashes and local anesthetic lozenges or gels. Topical or systemic steroids may be beneficial in selected individuals with extensive disease.

Herpangina and Hand, Foot, and Mouth Disease

Herpangina is an acute infection of the oropharynx that is caused by type A coxsackieviruses and affects mostly young children. The onset is sudden with relatively severe systemic reactions, including fever, sore throat, dysphagia, vomiting, and abdominal pains. Small grayish papules and vesicles surrounded by red areolas develop on the tonsillar fauces, soft palate, uvula, tongue, and oropharynx; these rarely occur on the buccal mucosa or periodontium. The disease is usually self-limiting and lasts 3–4 days, followed by complete recovery. Treatment consists of symptomatic measures only.

Hand, foot, and mouth disease is also caused by type A coxsackieviruses and affects primarily young children. It is characterized by the development of a maculopapular rash on the hands and soles of the feet, which may vesiculate. Maculopapular and vesicular lesions may also develop on the cheeks, hard and soft palate, tongue, oropharynx, tonsillar fauces, and buccal mucosa. This disease is self-limiting and lasts only several days, followed by complete recovery.

Gangrenous Stomatitis or Noma

Also known as cancrum oris, gangrenous stomatitis is an acute, fulminating and gangrenous infection of the oral and facial tissues. It usually occurs in the presence of severe debilitation and malnutrition, and children are most often affected. The earliest lesion is a small, painful, red spot or vesicle on the attached gingiva in the premolar or molar region of the mandible. A necrotic ulcer rapidly develops and undermines the deeper tissue. Painful cellulitis of the lips and cheeks is observed as the lesion extends outward in a conelike fashion. Within a short period, sloughing of necrotic soft tissues occurs, exposing the underlying bone, teeth, and deeper tissues. Fusospirochetal organisms such as *Treponema vincentii* and *Fusobacterium nucleatum* are consistently cultured from the lesions. *Prevotella melaninogenica* may also be present. Specimens obtained by biopsy from the advancing lesion show a mat of predominantly gram-negative threadlike bacteria that cannot be positively identified.[16] Thus, this lesion bears some resemblance to

acute necrotizing ulcerative gingivitis but appears to be more focal and destructive, involving deeper tissues beyond the gingiva. Treatment requires high doses of intravenous penicillin. Every effort should be made to correct the severe dehydration and underlying malnutrition and debility. Loose teeth and sequestra may be removed, but saucerization should be avoided. Healing is by secondary intention. Serious mutilation and facial deformity may require subsequent cosmetic surgery.

Mucositis in the Severely Immunocompromised Patient

Much of what is known about the management of oromucosal infections has been ascertained from cancer patients being treated with radiotherapy, chemotherapy, or bone marrow transplantation[17–19] and from patients with AIDS.[15, 20] The underlying mechanism of infection in these patients appears to be a breakdown of the mucosal epithelium that leads to mucositis, secondary bacterial or fungal infection, or reactivation of a latent viral infection. Oral candidiasis, herpes simplex, varicella-zoster, and cytomegalovirus infections are the most common manifestations. Mucositis that complicates radiation or chemotherapy most commonly involves the nonkeratinized oral epithelium, including the buccal and labial mucosa, soft palate, oropharynx, floor of the mouth, and ventral and lateral surfaces of the tongue. Ulceration and pseudomembrane formation are evident usually 4–7 days after the initiation of chemotherapy, when the rate of destruction of the basal epithelium exceeds that of proliferation of new cells. The clinical manifestations may be quite variable. The lesions often have a protracted duration and may not be associated with an inflammatory reaction, thereby masking the usual signs and symptoms of infection. Pain or tenderness may be the only abnormal finding.

Because the etiologic agents of infection cannot be readily predicted on clinical grounds alone in such patients, specific microbiologic diagnosis by culture, histopathology, or antigen detection techniques is critical for appropriate treatment. Topical as well as systemic antimicrobial agents may be indicated, along with antiseptic (e.g., chlorhexidine) and anesthetic (e.g., benzydamine, viscous lidocaine) applications.[21] Frequent saline rinses may reduce mucosal irritation, remove thickened secretions or debris, and increase moisture in the mouth. Coating agents such as milk of magnesia or aluminum hydroxide gel (Amphojel) have been useful for symptomatic relief of painful oral lesions. Topical or oral cytoprotective agents (e.g., sucralfate) and nonsteroidal anti-inflammatory analgesics (e.g., benzydamine and salicylates) may provide additional benefit. Meticulous oral and dental hygiene, effective management of xerostomia, selective suppression of oropharyngeal microbial colonization, and early control of reactivation by latent viral infections appear to be the critical steps in preventing and reducing the overall morbidity of oromucosal infections in the severely immunocompromised.[17]

Miscellaneous Infections

Tinea Barbae

Tinea barbae is a dermatophytic infection of the beard hair. It can be caused by different dermatophytes, but *Trichophyton verrucosum* and *Trichophyton mentagrophytes* account for the majority of cases. Typically, involvement is mild, with circinate and scaly lesions. Occasionally, a more severe form may occur as marked inflammation associated with follicular pustule formation and hair loss. Treatment requires oral griseofulvin (10 mg/kg/day), which is usually administered over several weeks.

Scabies and Pediculosis

Human scabies is a highly contagious infestation caused by the itch mite, *Sarcoptes scabiei.* The scabies mite is an obligate parasite that burrows into, resides in, and reproduces in human skin. Typically, there is intense itching with erythematous papules and excoriations. In infants and small children, the face and scalp as well as the trunk and extremities are often involved. Chronic infestations may lead to the development of pruritic, reddish brown nodules. These lesions are thought to be a manifestation of delayed hypersensitivity to retained mite products and may take weeks or months to resolve after adequate therapy. Treatment is with topical applications of 1% lindane. However, the major drawback of lindane is potential neurotoxicity caused by systemic absorption of the drug, because effective treatment requires that the medication be left on the skin for 8–12 hours.[22] Permethrin 5% cream is a safer alternative for children, because it is poorly absorbed by the skin and is less likely to have systemic side effects.[22] This treatment is usually repeated in 1 week.

Pediculosis capitis is caused by the human louse, *Pediculus humanus capitis.* Adult head lice and nits are localized primarily in the temporal and occipital areas of the scalp. The major complaint is severe pruritus of the scalp. Scratching may lead to excoriations and secondary bacterial infection, with weeping and crusting of the scalp and tender occipital and cervical lymphadenopathy. Head lice is highly contagious and may be transferred by close personal contact, and possibly by the sharing of hats, combs, and brushes. Treatment is similar to that for scabies.[23]

Infected Embryologic Cysts

Three distinct embryologic abnormalities can manifest as infections in the neck: (1) cystic hygroma or lymphangioma, (2) pharyngeal and bronchial cleft cysts, and (3) thyroglossal duct cysts.[24] Cystic hygroma is associated with a diffuse tumor mass usually evident within the first 2 years of life. It commonly involves the lower aspect of the neck but can appear anywhere in the cervical region. It is probably an abnormal development of lymphatic vessels from the jugular lymphatic sacs. Sudden enlargement by infection or hemorrhage into a lymphangioma may cause obstruction of the upper airways. Pharyngeal cleft cysts usually manifest in childhood as fistulas or masses just posterior to the angle of the mandible along the anterior border of the sternocleidomastoid muscle. The mass can fluctuate in size, and enlargement can be associated with an upper respiratory infection.

Thyroglossal duct cysts originate from the foramen cecum of the tongue and descend through the body of the hyoid bone into the anterior portion of the neck. Any residual secretory lining may give rise to a thyroglossal duct cyst that

is midline in location. It can cause respiratory obstruction or fistula formation if secondarily infected. Treatment of these congenital abnormalities during secondary bacterial infection requires broad-spectrum antibiotics. Definitive surgical excision to prevent recurrence should be performed after complete resolution of the acute process.

Cat-Scratch Disease and Oculoglandular Syndrome

Cat-scratch disease in the immunocompetent host is a self-limiting illness characterized by fever, malaise, inflammation of solitary lymph nodes, and development of a papule at the site of a cat scratch. Molecular studies have identified the organism *Bartonella* (formerly *Rochalimaea*) *henselae* as the major causative agent of cat-scratch disease as well as the related syndrome of bacillary angiomatosis, which is primarily seen in patients with AIDS.[25] This organism has been isolated directly from affected lymph nodes or identified by DNA amplification of biopsy specimens using polymerase chain reaction techniques. In addition, epidemiologic studies have found that one fourth to two fifths of apparently healthy cats in three locations in the United States have evidence of asymptomatic bacteremia due to this organism.[25]

The characteristic finding in cat-scratch disease in a child or young adult is a single, tender lymph node in the region draining the site of a cat scratch, often involving the cervical or preauricular nodes. The lesion at the site of inoculation may persist for several weeks after the initial injury. The enlarged lymph node is variable in size. Pain is not a prominent feature, but low-grade fever, headache, and malaise are usually present. Untreated, the disease usually resolves spontaneously within 2 months. Less commonly, acute encephalopathy or Parinaud's oculoglandular syndrome may occur. In the latter disorder, a single palpebral conjunctival granulomatous lesion is found. Preauricular lymphadenopathy, conjunctivitis, and fever are the cardinal manifestations.[26] Because the disease is usually self-limited in immunocompetent hosts, no specific antimicrobial therapy is required for the vast majority of patients. However, in severely ill or immunocompromised patients, antibiotic treatment with doxycycline or a macrolide is indicated.[27] Fluctuant lymph nodes should be aspirated.

Animal and Human Bites

Approximately 80% of animal bites are inflicted by dogs and 15% by cats. Bites from wild or laboratory animals are rare. Infection following animal bites is relatively uncommon (estimated to range from 5%–15% of bite wounds).[28] However, because the consequence of infection from a bite wound to the face, head, or neck is potentially serious, empirical antibiotic therapy is recommended. Streptococci and staphylococci as well as anaerobes are the main isolates from bite wounds inflicted by dogs. *Pasteurella multocida* is isolated in more than 50% of cat bites. Empiric antibiotic therapy should be directed at these organisms. Penicillin is the antibiotic of choice. Cefoxitin or ceftizoxime is appropriate for penicillin-allergic patients. *P. multocida* is resistant to clindamycin and erythromycin.

Human bites are more serious and become infected more easily than animal bites. Streptococci, *Eikenella corrodens,* and *S. aureus* are the most prevalent facultative organisms, and *Bacteroides* and *Peptostreptococcus* are the most common anaerobic isolates. Penicillin-resistant gram-negative rods are uncommon. Penicillin or amoxicillin-clavulanate is the recommended treatment.

DIAGNOSTIC APPROACHES

Because many orofacial infections originate from the oral cavity and are polymicrobial in nature, care must be taken during specimen collection to avoid contamination by the resident oral flora. Aerobic and anaerobic blood cultures should always be obtained. In selected patients with pyogenic infections of the face and neck, particularly compromised hosts, needle aspiration of the spreading edge of the skin lesion (using a tuberculin syringe containing 0.5 mL nonbactericidal saline and a 23-gauge hypodermic needle) is a worthwhile procedure. Even though Gram's stain and culture of needle aspirates have yielded the causative organism in only 10% of adults with cellulitis,[29, 30] prospective studies in children have reported positive cultures in more than 50% of cases.[31] Furthermore, because determination of the microbial cause of skin and soft tissue infections in the immunocompromised host is often unpredictable when based on clinical information alone, any procedure that would facilitate specific diagnosis and guide empirical antimicrobial therapy in these seriously ill patients is worthwhile. Multiple-needle aspiration or biopsy is also particularly useful for the microbiologic and histopathologic diagnosis of necrotizing soft tissue infections. Punch biopsy of the skin for histopathologic examination with special stains is invaluable for the investigation of chronic or granulomatous lesions.

For ulcerative oromucosal lesions, scrapings from the ulcer base should be obtained for Gram's stain, potassium hydroxide and Tzanck's preparations, and cytologic examination. Cultures for bacterial, fungal, mycobacterial, and viral pathogens should be obtained when appropriate. Punch biopsy is also valuable for the investigation of chronic mucosal lesions and for the diagnosis of malignant or premalignant conditions. Immunofluorescence staining for antigen detection can also be performed for herpes simplex and varicella-zoster as well as papilloma viruses and other pathogens. Identification of potential pathogens by DNA amplification and hybridization techniques is a powerful tool that is increasingly being utilized for suspected infections that are culture-negative.

THERAPEUTIC CONSIDERATIONS

Antimicrobial therapy of orofacial nonodontogenic infections should be guided by the clinical history, careful physical examination, and associated or underlying medical conditions. Results of culture and susceptibility data, although important for establishing the etiologic diagnosis and antibiotic resistance profiles, are often not available in orofacial infections. Thus, particularly in severely ill or immunocompromised patients, the initial choice of antimicrobial therapy is often empirical and designed to cover the most likely pathogens with broad-spectrum agents. Because the etiologic agents in nonodontogenic orofacial infections are remarkably diverse, every effort should be made to narrow down the differential diagnosis by pursuing a judicious but aggressive plan of investigation. In the immunocompetent host with a clinical impression of a pyogenic infection, the initial empirical therapy may consist of either penicillin, nafcillin, or clindamycin. A first- or second-generation cephalosporin (e.g., cefazolin, cefamandole, or cefuroxime) is another alternative. Ulcerative gingival lesions should be treated with either penicillin, clindamycin, or metronidazole. In the immunocompromised host, particularly if the patient is neutropenic, broad-spectrum antibiotics directed against *S. aureus,* gram-negative bacilli, streptococcus, and anaerobes should be considered. The initial empirical regimen may include ceftizoxime, cefotaxime, imipenem, or piperacillin-tazobactam, each plus or minus either nafcillin or vancomycin. Subsequent antimicrobial therapy should be tailored according to the initial clinical response as well as subsequent laboratory findings.

References

1. Hupp JR: In: Topazian RG, Goldberg MH (eds): Oral and Maxillofacial Infections, 2nd ed. Philadelphia: WB Saunders, 1987, pp 254–271.
2. Tyldesley WR: Principles and therapy. In: Oral Medicine. Oxford: Oxford University Press, 1981, pp 1–23.
3. Roscoe DL, Chow AW: Normal flora and mucosal immunity of the head and neck. Infect Dis Clin North Am 1988; 2: 1–19.
4. Tyldesley WR: Infections of the oral mucosa. In: Oral Medicine. Oxford: Oxford University Press, 1981, pp 24–48.
5. Wannamaker LW: Differences between streptococcal infections of the throat and of the skin. N Engl J Med 1970; 282: 78–85.
6. Milstein P, Gleckman R: Pneumococcal erysipelas: A unique case in an adult. Am J Med 1975; 59: 293–296.
7. Sokol RJ, Bowden RA: An erysipelas-like scalp cellulitis due to *Haemophilus influenzae* type b. J Pediatr 1980; 96: 60–61.
8. Weiss A, Friendly D, Eglin K, et al.: Bacterial periorbital and orbital cellulitis in childhood. Ophthalmology 1983; 90: 195.
9. Lessner A, Stern GA: Preseptal and orbital cellulitis. Infect Dis Clin North Am 1992; 6: 933.
10. Zeitoun IM, Dhanarajani PJ: Cervical cellulitis and mediastinitis caused by odontogenic infections: Report of two cases and review of literature. J Oral Maxillofac Surg 1995; 53: 203–208.
11. Valko PC, Barrett SM, Campbell JP: Odontogenic cervical necrotizing fasciitis. Ann Emerg Med 1990; 19: 568–571.
12. Roser SM, Chow AW, Brady FA: Necrotizing fasciitis. J Oral Surg 1977; 35: 730–732.
13. Krespi YP, Lawson W, Blaugrund SM, Biller HF: Massive necrotizing infections of the neck. Head Neck Surg 1981; 3: 475–481.
14. Chow AW: Life-threatening infections of the head and neck. Clin Infect Dis 1992; 14: 991–1004.
15. Safrin S, Crumpacker C, Chatis P, et al.: A controlled trial comparing foscarnet with vidarabine for acyclovir-resistant mucocutaneous herpes simplex in the acquired immunodeficiency syndrome. N Engl J Med 1991; 325: 551.
16. Topazian RG: Uncommon infections of the oral and maxillofacial regions. In: Topazian RG, Goldberg MH, eds. Oral and Maxillofacial Infections, 2nd ed. Philadelphia: WB Saunders, 1987, pp 317–338.
17. Epstein JB: Infection prevention in bone marrow transplantation and radiation. NCI Monogr 1990; 9: 73–85.
18. Nikoskelainen J: Oral infections related to radiation and immunosuppressive therapy. J Clin Periodontol 1990; 17: 504–507.
19. Heimdahl A, Nord CE: Oral infections in immunocompromised patients. J Clin Periodontol 1990; 17: 501–503.
20. Lee PL, Kiviat N, Truelove EL, et al.: Oral manifestations in patients with AIDS or AIDS-related disorders. J Dent Res 1987; 66: 183.
21. Epstein JB: The painful mouth—mucositis, gingivitis and stomatitis. Infect Dis Clin North Am 1988; 2: 183–202.

22. Amer M, El-Gharib I: Permethrin versus crotamiton and lindane in the treatment of scabies. Int J Dermatol 1992; 31: 357–358.

23. Leslie TA, Goldsmith PC, Dowd PM: Fungal and parasitic skin infestations: An update in treatment. Curr Opin Infect Dis 1993; 6: 658–667.

24. Brook I: The swollen neck—cervical lymphadenitis, parotitis, thyroiditis and infected cysts. Infect Dis Clin North Am 1988; 2: 221–236.

25. Koehler JE, Glaser CA, Tappero JW: *Rochalimaea henselae* infection: A new zoonosis with the domestic cat as reservoir. JAMA 1994; 271: 531–535.

26. Jawad ASM, Amen AAA: Cat-scratch disease presenting as the oculoglandular syndrome of Parinaud: A report of two cases. Postgrad Med J 1990; 66: 467–468.

27. Margileth AM: Antibiotic therapy for cat-scratch disease: Clinical study of therapeutic outcome in 268 patients and a review of the literature. Pediatr Infect Dis J 1992; 11: 474–478.

28. Weber DJ, Hansen AR: Infections resulting from animal bites. Infect Dis Clin North Am 1991; 5: 663.

29. Newell PM, Norden CW: Value of needle aspiration in bacteriologic diagnosis of cellulitis in adults. J Clin Microbiol 1988; 26: 401–404.

30. Hook EW, Hooton TM, Horton CA, et al.: Microbiologic evaluation of cutaneous cellulitis in adults. Arch Intern Med 1986; 146: 295–297.

31. Fleisher G, Ludwig S, Campos J: Cellulitis: Bacterial etiology, clinical features, and laboratory findings. J Pediatr 1980; 97: 591–593.

Anthony W. Chow

CHAPTER FIFTY-FIVE

Odontogenic Infections

Dental caries and periodontal disease are the most common afflictions of the tooth. These infectious diseases cause considerable pain and discomfort and ultimately loss of the tooth. Apart from local effects, these infections may extend beyond natural barriers and result in complications that can vary in severity from the excruciating pain of acute pulpitis to life-threatening infections of the deep fascial spaces of the head and neck. The infected tooth is also associated with various important systemic manifestations, such as fever of undetermined origin, bacteremic seeding to heart valves and prosthetic devices, and an increased risk for coronary heart disease.[1] Improved anaerobic culture techniques and microbial taxonomy have greatly advanced our knowledge of the pathogenesis and microbial specificity of these common infections. A thorough understanding of the anatomic considerations and salient clinical features is essential for early recognition and effective treatment of these infections and their complications.

ANATOMIC CONSIDERATIONS

Structure of the Tooth

In humans, there are two sets of teeth, the deciduous (milk or baby) teeth and the permanent teeth. The deciduous teeth, which number 20 in all, erupt at approximately 6 months to 2 years of age and are shed between 6 and 12 years of age. These are gradually replaced by 32 permanent teeth, consisting in each halfjaw of 2 incisors, 1 canine, 2 premolars, and, in adults, 3 molars. Each tooth has a visible crown that projects above the *gingiva* (gum), with one or more roots that extend into the alveolar bone of the maxilla or mandible (Fig. 55–1). The crown and root meet at the neck of the tooth. The tooth forms a peg and socket joint with the alveolar bone and is held in place by the periodontal membrane that allows slight movement of the tooth. The hard tissues of the tooth are dentin, enamel, and cementum, whereas the soft tissues are the pulp, the periodontal membrane, and the gingiva.

The pulp filling the core of the tooth, composed of fibroblasts and connective tissue, is supplied by blood vessels and nerves entering the pulp cavity through the apical foramen. At the periphery of the pulp is a layer of odontoblasts. Odontoblastic processes extend through the dentin in small canals called dentinal tubules. It is the odontoblasts with their processes that lay down dentin, which forms the bulk of the tooth. Dentin is similar to bone but is harder because of a greater calcium content.

Covering the crown of the tooth is enamel, which is the hardest material of the body, being 99% inorganic. The ultrastructure of enamel reveals units called enamel rods or prisms, which are embedded in a matrix. Both the rods and the interprismatic matrix are composed of apatite crystals. Enamel is laid down by ameloblasts, which form a membrane called the enamel cuticle on the surface of the unerupted tooth. With eruption of the tooth, the cuticle is worn off and lost.

Just as enamel covers the dentin in the crown, cementum covers dentin in the root of the tooth from the neck to the apex. It is structurally similar to bone, with cementocytes lying in lacunae and interconnected by canaliculi. The cementum anchors the tooth to the surrounding connective tissue by thick collagen bundles that run between the alveolar bone, through the periodontal tissue, and into cementum. These collagen bundles are known as Sharpey's fibers.

Finally, the gingiva surrounds each tooth like a collar and extends down over the crest of the alveolar bone to connect to the tooth just above the neck. The space formed between the tooth and the gingiva is the gingival crevice or recess.

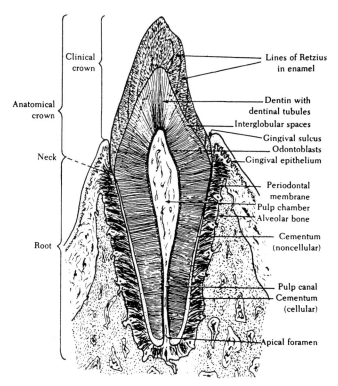

Figure 55–1. Structure of the tooth. (From Leeson CR, Leeson TS, Paparo AA: Textbook of Histology. Philadelphia, WB Saunders Co, 1985.)

Routes of Spread

Odontogenic infections originate from bacteria colonizing the surfaces of the tooth, called the *plaque*. Plaques located on tooth surfaces above the gingival margin (supragingival plaque) lead to dental caries that may invade the pulp (pulpitis or endodontic infection), and eventually perforate the alveolar bone (periapical abscess). Plaques located on tooth surfaces beneath the gingival margin (subgingival plaque) lead to periodontal infections (e.g., gingivitis, periodontitis, periodontal abscess, and pericoronitis) that may eventually penetrate the fascial spaces of the face and mouth (orofacial "space" infections) (Fig. 55–2).

Soft tissue infections of odontogenic origin tend to spread along planes of least resistance from the supporting structures of the affected tooth to various potential spaces in the vicinity. Accumulated pus, therefore, must perforate bone generally at the site where it is thinnest and weakest, before extending into the periapical areas or deeper fascial spaces. In the mandible, the bone is weakest, and perforation tends to occur on the lingual aspect in the region of the molar teeth and on the buccal aspect when more anterior teeth are involved.[2, 3] In the maxilla, the bone is weaker on the buccal aspect throughout and relatively thicker on the palatal aspect. If pus perforates through either the maxillary or mandibular buccal plate, it manifests intraorally if inside the attachment of the buccinator muscle to the maxilla or mandible, and extraorally if outside this muscle attachment (Fig. 55–3A).

Therefore, infection of the upper and lower molars, lower incisors, and lower canine teeth is often accompanied by extraoral manifestations. When a mandibular infection perforates lingually, it manifests in the sublingual space if the apices of the involved teeth lie above the attachment of the mylohyoid muscle (e.g., mandibular incisor, canines, premolars, and first molars) and in the submandibular space if they lie below the attachment of the muscle (e.g., the second and third molars) (Fig. 55–3B). Thus, these local anatomic barriers of bone, muscle, and fascia predetermine the routes of spread, extent, and clinical manifestations of many orofacial infections of odontogenic origin.

The clinically important "fascial spaces" around the face and oral cavity that are often involved in odontogenic infections are illustrated in Figure 55–4. These are potential spaces between layers of fascia that communicate with one another to varying extents. Infections involving the deep fascial spaces of the neck are described elsewhere (see Chapter 54).

PATHOGENESIS

Plaque formation plays a central role in both dental caries and periodontal infection. Apart from their anatomic localization on the tooth surface, various host and microbial factors influence plaque formation and their ability to cause dental caries or periodontal disease. Oral hygiene, diet, and

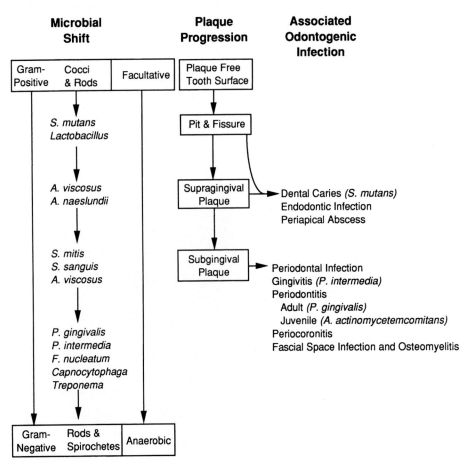

Figure 55–2. Microbial specificity in odontogenic infections. A unifying hypothesis demonstrating a microbial shift from a plaque-free tooth surface and progression to supragingival and subgingival organisms. (From Chow AW: Odontogenic infections. In: Schlossberg D: Infections of the Head and Neck. New York: Springer-Verlag, 1987, p 149.)

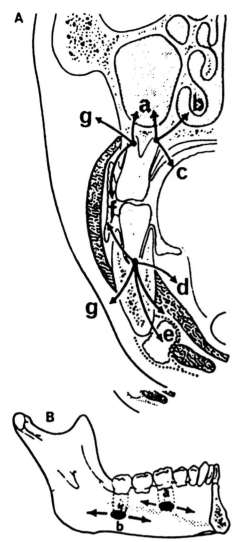

Figure 55–3. Routes of spread of odontogenic orofacial infections along planes of least resistance. *A,* Coronal section in the region of the first molar teeth: a, maxillary antrum; b, nasal cavity; c, palatal plate; d, sublingual space (above the mylohyoid muscle); e, submandibular space (below the mylohyoid muscle); f, intraoral presentation with infection spreading through the buccal plates inside the attachment of the buccinator muscle; g, extraoral presentation to buccal space with infection spreading through the buccal plates outside the attachment of the buccinator muscle. *B,* Lingual aspect of the mandible: a, apices of the involved tooth above the mylohyoid muscle, with spread of infection to the sublingual space; b, apices of involved tooth below the mylohyoid muscle, with spread of infection into the submandibular space. (Reproduced with permission from Chow AW, Roser SM, Brady FA: Orofacial odontogenic infections. Ann Intern Med 1978; 88: 392–402.)

genetic predisposition are particularly important determinants. In order for dental caries to develop, three factors need to be present: (1) a susceptible tooth surface (host factors), (2) acidogenic (acid-producing) and aciduric (able to grow at low pH) bacteria within a dental plaque (microbial factors), and (3) carbohydrates and simple sugars, which are acted upon by plaque bacteria to generate acids on the tooth surface, causing demineralization and tooth decay (dietary factors).[4] This, the most universally accepted acid-decalcification theory for dental caries, was originated by W.D. Miller[4] in 1882.

Unlike dental caries, diet does not appear to have a significant role in the pathogenesis of periodontal disease. More important is the presence of a periodontal microflora, which can penetrate the gingival epithelium and elicit an inflammatory host response that ultimately results in destruction of the periodontium.[5, 6]

Host Factors

The tooth has at least three intrinsic mechanisms protecting it from carious decay: (1) the cleansing action of the tongue and buccal membranes that act to remove food particles from the proximity of the tooth; (2) a constant flow of saliva of neutral pH that bathes the tooth, buffers and washes away bacterial acids, and supplies calcium and phosphate to remineralize and repair damaged tooth surfaces; and (3) the acquisition by the tooth of an acellular, structureless, bacteria-free coating known as the acquired pellicle, which is of salivary origin and acts as a surface barrier to most dietary and bacterial acids and to proteolytic substances.[7] However, with time, the acquired pellicle becomes colonized with bacteria and is replaced by the bacterial plaque. In addition to these protective mechanisms, the acts of tooth-brushing and flossing also serve to remove food particles and bacterial plaques adherent to the tooth surface. Hence, it is not surprising that carious lesions occur most often in areas inaccessible to the self-cleaning mechanisms of the mouth and in areas protected from the reaches of the toothbrush. In decreasing order of frequency, these are the pits and fissures of the occlusal (biting) surfaces of the molars and premolars, the interproximal areas (that is, between the teeth), and the gingival crevices, especially where there is poor oral hygiene and preexisting gingival disease.

Oral hygiene and increasing age are two major predisposing factors to periodontal disease. Other factors are hormonal status, with exacerbation of disease activity during puberty, menstruation, and pregnancy.[8] Diabetes causes a higher incidence of periodontal disease, particularly in juvenile diabetics. Finally, various genetic disorders are associated with an increased incidence of periodontal disease. In particular, patients with neutrophil defects (such as Chédiak-Higashi syndrome, agranulocytosis, cyclic neutropenia, and Down's syndrome) have a higher incidence of periodontal disease.[9–11]

Microbial Factors

The microbiota associated with odontogenic infections are complex and generally reflect the combined influence of the indigenous oral flora and the unique microbiota of the underlying conditions. In the healthy oral cavity, *Streptococcus, Peptostreptococcus, Veillonella,* and diphtheroids account for more than 80% of the total cultivable flora[12] (Table 55–1). Quantitative studies indicate that obligate anaerobes occur as much as eight times more often than facultative bacteria (see Chapter 22 for details).[13] Facultative gram-negative bacilli are uncommon in the healthy host but may be more prominent in seriously ill and hospitalized patients.[14, 15]

In addition, the oral cavity cannot be regarded as a single

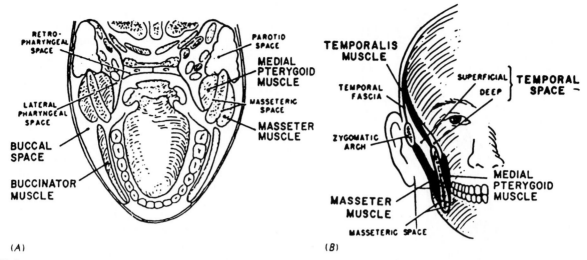

Figure 55–4. Fascial spaces around the mouth and face. *A,* Horizontal section at the level of the occlusal surface of the mandibular teeth. *B,* Frontal view of the face. (Reproduced with permission from Chow AW, Roser SM, Brady FA: Orofacial odontogenic infections. Ann Intern Med 1978; 88: 392–402.)

uniform environment. Although representative species of microorganisms can be isolated from most areas of the mouth, certain sites tend to favor colonization by specific organisms. For example, *Streptococcus salivarius* and *Veillonella* species have a predilection for the tongue and buccal mucosa and predominate before the eruption of teeth.[12] In contrast, *Streptococcus sanguis, Streptococcus mutans* as well as *Actinomyces viscosus* preferentially colonize the tooth surface, whereas *Fusobacterium,* pigmented *Prevotella,* and anaerobic spirochetes appear to be concentrated in the gingival crevice.[16, 17] Bacterial adherence and interaggregation, local environmental conditions such as oxygen tension and pH, as well as other host factors[12, 16] seem to govern these unique colonization patterns and to influence the composition of the oral flora.

The concept of microbial specificity of odontogenic infections has been appreciated only recently (see Fig. 55–2). In the case of dental caries, an etiologic association with *S. mutans* has been firmly established.[18, 19] *S. mutans* is the only organism consistently isolated from all decayed dental fissures and the only organism found in greater numbers in carious teeth than in noncarious teeth. The infectious and transmissible nature of this organism in dental caries has been further demonstrated in both experimental animals and longitudinal studies in humans.[20] Besides *S. mutans,* a streptococcus of importance is *S. sanguis,* which colonizes plaque early, probably as a result of its ability to attach to enamel. Owing to its inability to grow under acid conditions, counts of this bacteria drop off as the plaque matures. *Streptococcus mitis* is capable of storing carbohydrates and thus generating acid after dietary carbohydrate is no longer available as a substrate. *S. salivarius* can also produce caries-like lesions in vitro.

Similarly, in gingivitis and periodontitis, a unique and specific bacterial composition of the subgingival plaque has been identified.[5, 11] In the healthy periodontium, the microflora is sparse and consists mainly of gram-positive organisms such as *S. sanguis* and *Actinomyces* species. In the presence of gingivitis, the predominant subgingival flora shifts to a greater proportion of anaerobic gram-negative bacilli, with *Prevotella intermedia* being the predominant isolate.[21–23] In well-established periodontitis, the flora further increases in complexity, with a preponderance of anaerobic gram-negative bacilli and motile organisms, and with *Por-*

Table 55–1. PREDOMINANT CULTIVABLE FLORA FROM VARIOUS SITES OF THE ORAL CAVITY

Group	Predominant Genus or Family	Total Viable Count (Mean %)			
		Tongue	Saliva	Gingival Crevice	Dental Plaque
Anaerobes (10^{11} CFU/g)[1]					
Gram + cocci	*Peptostreptococcus*	4.2	13.0	7.4	13.0
Gram − cocci	*Veillonella*	16.0	15.9	10.7	6.0
Gram + rods	*Actinomyces, Eubacterium, Lactobacillus, Leptotrichia*	7.4	4.8	20.2	18.0
Gram − rods	*Fusobacterium, Bacteroides, Prevotella, Porphyromonas*	8.2	4.8	16.1	10.0
Aerobes (10^{10} CFU/g)[1]					
Gram + cocci	*Streptococcus*	44.8	46.2	28.8	28.0
Gram − cocci	*Moraxella*	3.4	1.2	0.4	0.4
Gram + rods	*Lactobacillus, Corynebacterium*	13.0	11.8	15.3	24.0
Gram − rods	Enterobacteriaceae	3.2	2.3	1.2	Not done

Modified from Chow AW, Roser SM, Brady FA: Orofacial odontogenic infections. Ann Intern Med 1978; 88: 392–402.
[1]Total viable colony-forming units per gram net weight.

Table 55–2. ISOLATES FROM 31 PATIENTS WITH ODONTOGENIC OROFACIAL INFECTIONS

Isolates	Periapical Abscess (n = 4)	"Space" Infection (n = 14)¹	Mandibular Osteomyelitis (n = 13)	Total No. (%) (n = 31)
Aerobes exclusively	0	1	0	1 (3)
Anaerobes exclusively	1	8	4	13 (42)
Mixed aerobes and anaerobes	3	4	9	16 (52)
Predominant isolates				
Streptococcus	3	3	8	14 (45)
Bacteroides/Prevotella	4	7	10	21 (68)
B. fragilis	0	0	3	3 (10)
P. melaninogenicus	1	6	8	15 (48)
Fusobacterium	0	4	3	7 (23)
Peptostreptococcus	2	8	6	16 (52)
Veillonella	0	1	2	3 (10)
Actinomyces	0	0	4	4 (13)
Lactobacillus	2	1	0	3 (10)
Eubacterium	0	2	2	4 (13)
Mean no. isolates per specimen	4.7	3.2	4.6	4.0

Reproduced with permission from Chow AW, Roser SM, Brady FA: Orofacial odontogenic infections. Ann Intern Med 1978; 88: 392–402.
¹One aspirate was sterile.

phyromonas gingivalis being the predominant isolate. In juvenile periodontitis, a clinical variant seen primarily in adolescents, the subgingival plaque mainly consists of saccharolytic organisms, with *Actinobacillus actinomycetemcomitans* and *Capnocytophaga* species as the most common identifiable isolates.[24] *P. gingivalis* is rarely found in this condition.

In suppurative odontogenic infections such as periapical abscess or fascial space infections, a polymicrobial flora is usually present, with *Fusobacterium nucleatum,* pigmented *Prevotella, Peptostreptococcus, Actinomyces,* and *Streptococcus* species being the most predominant isolates[25–27] (Table 55–2). Except in selected patients with serious underlying illnesses, facultative gram-negative bacilli and *Staphylococcus aureus* are uncommonly isolated.[16, 28–30]

Dietary Factors

From the preceding discussion, it is clear that diet is a major factor in dental caries. Ingestion of carbohydrates, especially monosaccharides and disaccharides, predisposes an individual to dental caries, as witnessed not only in animal studies but also in epidemiologic surveys in humans.[12] It is not so much the quantity of carbohydrates but the duration and frequency of exposure in the oral cavity that are important. In particular, soft carbohydrates that stick to teeth and in between teeth are particularly cariogenic. A modification of dietary habits is clearly important in the control of dental caries.

CLINICAL SYNDROMES

Odontogenic infections originate in either the dentoalveolar structures, the periodontium, or the pericoronal tissues (Fig. 55–5). Dental caries and pulpal infection are by far the most common.

Dentoalveolar Infections

Dental Caries

It is estimated that more than 95% of the population in the United States have experienced caries at some time and that

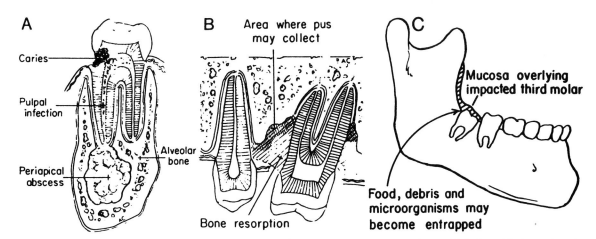

Figure 55–5. Odontogenic infections. *A,* Dental caries, pulpal infection, and periapical abscess. *B,* Periodontal infection with destruction of supporting structures. *C,* Pericoronal infection overlying impacted tooth. (Reproduced with permission from Chow AW, Roser SM, Brady FA: Orofacial odontogenic infections. Ann Intern Med 1978; 88: 392–402.)

there are 500 million unfilled cavities in the country in any given year.[7] Caries most commonly involves the occlusal (biting) surfaces of the posterior teeth, where the deep grooves and fissures are located. Next in frequency are the interproximal surfaces, where neighboring teeth come into contact, and the necks of the teeth at the gum margin (which is a more common location for caries in older people).

Because the infection must spread through highly calcified tissues (enamel and dentin), the carious process spreads very slowly. The earliest findings are the presence of pits and fissures, which gradually develop discoloration or staining due to demineralization of enamel and dentin. Further destruction eventually leads to collapse of the overlying enamel, which becomes unsupported. Caries located on interproximal surfaces are particularly difficult to detect clinically; routine radiographic examination by passing x-rays through the contact areas (bite-wing radiographs) is essential and demonstrates a radiolucent area. Dental caries, if untreated, is progressive until the pulp is infected and the crown destroyed. Since there are no cells or vascular elements in enamel or dentin except for the secondary odontoblasts lying on the pulpal surface of dentin, the diseased area is incapable of healing and replacement.

Distinction is often made between active and quiescent phases of the caries attack. Active or acute caries is a rapid process typified by a light yellow discoloration that may easily involve the dental pulp before the tooth has had a chance to protect itself; this is more commonly seen in young children. Chronic, or arrested, caries has a dark brown discoloration, which represents the formation of a calcified barrier owing to remineralization with inorganic ions from saliva while the microorganisms are metabolically quiescent. Rampant caries is characterized by a very rapid and burrowing process of sudden onset and is not uncommon in infants who indulge in prolonged sucking of a comforter bottle containing sweetened juices or milk and sugar. In the vast majority of cases, however, the carious process is asymptomatic and progresses silently until the infection has invaded deeply enough to cause pulpal reaction.

Pulpitis and Periapical Abscess

Infection of the pulp can occur in one of three ways: (1) through a defect in the enamel and dentin, such as might occur from extension of a carious lesion, traumatic fracture of the tooth, or a dental procedure, (2) through the apical foramen or lateral canals (e.g., from a periodontal pocket or an adjacent tooth with periapical abscess), or (3) through hematogenous seeding of pulp that has been irritated mechanically. Once the pulp is inflamed and infected, the pressure inside this rigid and unyielding space builds quickly and is transmitted to the blood vessels entering the pulp cavity through the apical foramen, causing ischemia and necrosis of the pulp tissue. Pus may egress from a cavity in the crown if one exists. More often, the pus extrudes apically, and if the periodontal tissue is also infected, an acute periapical periodontitis is said to occur and may result in extrusion of the tooth. Alternately, the infected material may erode out of the apical foramen into the surrounding tissue, resulting in a periapical or alveolar abscess. The accumulating pus causes loss of bone and tissue and may extend to

involve other teeth. A more serious complication is lateral extension of the abscesses into the planes of least resistance with resultant deep fascial space involvement (see Chapters 54 and 56).[31] However, perhaps the most common occurrences are a spontaneous resolution and the development of a low-grade infection.

The dominant symptom of an early acute pulpitis is severe pain elicited by thermal changes, especially cold drinks. In addition, the involved tooth may be sensitive to palpation and percussion. As disease progresses, the pain becomes continuous and severe, with greater intensity when the patient is lying down. A more indolent form of pulpitis is chronic pulpitis, in which the inflammation is low grade with partial drainage of the infected material. Symptoms are characterized by a mild dull intermittent pain that is not altered by thermal changes.

Periodontal Infections

Diseases of the periodontium are extremely common in man, with 97%–100% of the population having some type of periodontal affliction by 45 years of age.[32, 33] Of these, approximately half have extensive periodontal tissue destruction. In the United States, between 20 and 30 million adults have lost all of their teeth, half of these because of periodontal disease and the other half because of caries.[4] Before age 35, caries are the main cause of tooth loss, but after this age, periodontal disease becomes the main cause.

Periodontal disease is mainly a disease of the connective tissue that supports the tooth. The periodontium consists of alveolar bone that surrounds the root of the tooth, the periodontal membrane, and the gingiva. Periodontal disease can be classified into gingivitis and periodontitis. The main complication of periodontal disease is tooth loss, although local and systemic spread of infection can occur, leading to periodontal abscess and deep fascial space infections.

Gingivitis

The most common periodontal disease in childhood, gingivitis has a peak incidence in adolescence. It can range from mild to severe. Clinically, there is swelling and bluish purple discoloration of the gingiva with a tendency for bleeding after eating or brushing. There is usually no pain, but a mild fetor oris may be noticed. A variant is acute necrotizing ulcerative gingivitis, also known as Vincent's disease or trench mouth. The patient typically experiences sudden onset of pain in the gingiva, and the tissue appears eroded with superficial grayish pseudomembranes. There is halitosis and altered taste sensation in addition to fever, malaise, and lymphadenopathy. The pathogenesis of this disorder is poorly understood, except that it occurs in the setting of acute gingivitis in association with some stressful event. Treatment with local débridement, oxidizing agents such as hydrogen peroxide, and a systemic antibiotic such as penicillin or metronidazole should bring relief within 24 hours.[34]

Periodontitis and Periodontal Abscess

Chronic adult periodontitis is characterized by gingival inflammation accompanied by loss of supportive connective tissue. There is loss of alveolar bone as well as the periodontal ligamentous attachments of the cementum, with an apical migration of the junctional epithelium, leading to a deepening of the gingival sulcus with "pocket" formation around the tooth. The destructive process is slow and probably results from years of dental neglect and chronic gingivitis. Plaque and calculi are abundant both supragingivally and subgingivally, and frank pus may be present in the periodontal pockets. Rapidly progressive periodontitis is a variant in adults in whom the process of tissue loss is accelerated. In juvenile periodontitis, or periodontosis in adolescents, there is rapid vertical bone loss often localized to the molars, although other teeth may be involved. Plaque is usually minimal and calculi are not seen. The etiology of this rare condition is not known, although neutrophil dysfunction has been reported in these otherwise healthy patients.[34] Periodontal abscess may be focal or diffuse and presents as a red, fluctuant swelling of the gingiva that is extremely tender to palpation. Such abscesses always communicate with a periodontal pocket from which pus can be readily expressed after probing. Treatment is surgical and aimed at drainage of loculated pus.

Pericoronitis

Pericoronitis is an acute localized infection caused by trapping of food particles and microorganisms under the gum flaps of a partially erupted tooth or an impacted wisdom tooth. In adolescents and adults, the infection involves the wisdom teeth, whereas in children, it occurs during eruption of the permanent teeth. Prominent symptoms include pain and limitation of movement on opening the jaw, discomfort on mastication and swallowing, and facial swelling. Clinically, the pericoronal tissues are erythematous and swollen, and digital pressure can often express exudate from the infected flap. The masticator spaces are often involved, so the disorder may manifest as trismus. Localized painful lymphadenopathy may be noted, and the breath is usually foul. Treatment involves gentle débridement and irrigation under the tissue flap. If there is cellulitis with abscess formation or extension of infection into the fascial planes, treatment may consist of incision and drainage with tooth extraction in addition to administration of antibiotics.

COMPLICATIONS

Suppurative odontogenic infections may extend to potential fascial spaces in the orofacial area or deep in the head and neck. The latter (described in detail elsewhere) is often life-threatening.[2] Table 55–3 compares the salient clinical features of these space infections. In addition, odontogenic infections may spread contiguously to cause osteomyelitis of the jaws or hematogenously to produce systemic illness.

Orofacial Space Infections

Orofacial space infections, located in the more superficial potential spaces of the face and oral cavity, may involve the buccal, canine, masticator, submental, and infratemporal spaces. They serve as important clues to the precise location of the underlying infected tooth (Table 55–3). If unrecognized and untreated, these infections are potentially serious, because they may spread contiguously into the deeper fascial spaces of the head and neck, such as the submandibular, lateral pharyngeal, and retropharyngeal spaces, or into the carotid sheath (see Chapters 54 and 56).

Table 55–3. COMPARATIVE FEATURES OF ODONTOGENIC DEEP FASCIAL SPACE INFECTIONS OF THE HEAD AND NECK

Space Infections	Usual Site of Origin	Clinical Features				
		Pain	Trismus	Swelling	Dysphagia	Dyspnea
Masticator						
Masseteric and pterygoid	Molars (especially third)	Present	Prominent	May not be evident (deep)	Absent	Absent
Temporal	Posterior maxillary molars	Present	None	Face, orbit (late)	Absent	Absent
Buccal	Bicuspids, molars	Minimal	Minimal	Cheek (marked)	Absent	Absent
Canine	Maxillary canines, incisors	Moderate	None	Upper lip, canine fossa	Absent	Absent
Infratemporal	Posterior maxillary molars	Present	None	Face, orbit (late)	Occasional	Occasional
Submental	Mandibular incisors	Moderate	None	Chin (firm)	Absent	Absent
Parotid	Masseteric spaces	Intense	None	Angle of jaw (marked)	Absent	Absent
Submandibular	2nd, 3rd mandibular molars	Present	Minimal	Submandibular	Absent	Absent
Sublingual	Mandibular incisors	Present	Minimal	Floor of mouth (tender)	Present if bilateral	Present if bilateral
Lateral pharyngeal						
Anterior	Masticator spaces	Intense	Prominent	Angle of jaw	Present	Occasional
Posterior	Masticator spaces	Minimal	Minimal	Posterior pharynx	Present	Severe
Retropharyngeal (and danger)	Lateral pharyngeal space, distant via lymphatics	Present	Minimal	Posterior pharynx (midline)	Present	Present
Pretracheal	Retropharyngeal space, anterior esophagus	Present	None	Hypopharynx	Present	Severe

From Megran DW, Scheifele DW, Chow AW: Odontogenic infections. Pediatr Infect Dis J 1984; 3(3): 257–265.

Buccal and Submental Spaces

As noted previously, infections arising from mandibular or maxillary bicuspid and molar teeth tend to extend in a lateral or buccal direction. The relation of the root apices to the origins of the buccinator muscle determines whether infection will exit intraorally into the buccal vestibule or extraorally into the buccal space (see Fig. 55–3). Infection of the buccal space is readily diagnosed because of marked cheek swelling with minimal trismus and systemic symptoms. There is a great tendency to resolution with antibiotic therapy alone. Drainage, if required, is superficial and should be performed extraorally. Involvement of a mandibular incisor can perforate below the mentalis muscle and manifest as a submental space infection. The chin appears grossly swollen and is firm and erythematous. Surgical drainage is best accomplished percutaneously.

Masticator Spaces

The masticator spaces are the masseteric, pterygoid, and temporal spaces, all of which are well differentiated but intercommunicate with one another as well as with the buccal, submandibular, and lateral pharyngeal spaces (see Fig. 55–4). Infection of the masticator spaces occurs most frequently from molar teeth, particularly the third molars (wisdom teeth). Clinically, the hallmarks of masticator space infection are trismus and pain in the area of the body or ramus of the mandible. Swelling may not be a prominent finding, especially in the masseteric compartment, because infection exists deep to large muscle masses that obscure or prevent clinically apparent swelling. When present, swelling tends to be brawny and indurated, suggesting the possibility of cervicofacial actinomycosis or mandibular osteomyelitis. Infection of the deep temporal space usually originates from involvement of the posterior maxillary molar teeth. Very little external swelling is observed early in the course; if present, it usually affects the preauricular region and an area over the zygomatic arch. As infection progresses, the cheek, eyelids, and whole side of the face may be involved. Infection may extend directly into the orbit via the inferior orbital fissure and produce proptosis, optic neuritis, and abducens nerve palsy.

Canine and Infratemporal Spaces

Involvement of the maxillary incisors and canines may result in a canine space infection, which manifests as dramatic swelling of the upper lip, canine fossa, and frequently the periorbital tissues. Pain is usually moderate, and systemic signs are minimal. Occasionally, a purulent maxillary sinusitis may result from direct extension of infection into the adjoining antrum. Treatment consists of antibiotics and drainage, which can be accomplished intraorally. The infratemporal space is bounded medially by the lateral plate of the pterygoid process and the pharynx, posteriorly by the parotid gland, anteriorly by the maxilla, and superiorly by the roof of the infratemporal fossa, adjacent to which is the inferior orbital fissure. Primary infections of the infratemporal fossa usually originate from involvement of the posterior maxillary molar teeth, particularly the third molar. Not un-commonly, infection in this space results from an injection of local anesthetic in this area for a dental restoration. Clinically, marked trismus and pain are present, but very little swelling is observed early in the course. Late manifestations are similar to those of temporal space infections, including extension into the orbit through the inferior orbital fissure. In addition, if the infection extends internally, it can involve an area close to the lateral pharyngeal wall, resulting in dysphagia. As is the case in other areas of the face and neck, infections of the infratemporal fossa tend to localize, and treatment includes antibiotics and surgical drainage.

Osteomyelitis of the Jaws

The mandible is much more susceptible to osteomyelitis than the maxilla, mainly because the cortical plates of the former are thin and its medullary tissues are relatively poor in vascular supply. Nevertheless, osteomyelitis secondary to odontogenic infection is relatively uncommon. When it does occur, there is usually a predisposing condition such as compound fracture, irradiation, diabetes mellitus, or steroid therapy. With initiation of infection, the intramedullary pressure markedly increases, further compromising blood supply and leading to bone necrosis. Pus travels through the haversian and perforating canals, accumulates beneath the periosteum, and elevates it from the cortex. If pus continues to accumulate, the periosteum is eventually penetrated, and mucosal or cutaneous abscesses and fistulas may develop. As the inflammatory process becomes more chronic, granulation tissue is formed. Spicules of necrotic and nonviable bone may become either totally isolated (sequestrum) or encased in a sheath of new bone (involucrum). Severe mandibular pain is a common symptom and may be accompanied by anesthesia or hypesthesia on the affected side. In protracted cases, mandibular trismus may develop. A clinical variant is Garré's chronic sclerosing osteomyelitis, or proliferative periostitis. Clinically, this disorder is characterized by a localized, hard, nontender swelling over the mandible. Actinomycosis and radiation necrosis are two common causes of this form of osteomyelitis of the jaws.[35]

ODONTOGENIC MANIFESTATIONS AS SYSTEMIC ILLNESS

Studies have demonstrated that the teeth are frequently a source of bacteremia. Such infections are known to follow almost all types of dental manipulations, including rocking of the tooth, periodontal scaling, endodontic treatment, gingival message, tooth extraction, and even tooth-brushing, flossing, and chewing hard candy.[34] In most instances, the bacteremia is transient and inconsequential, but in patients with periodontal disease, the bacteremia tends to be more common and is an important cause of endocarditis on either native or prosthetic heart valves.[36] Hematogenous seeding leading to infection of other prosthetic devices, such as total hip replacements, is also well documented after dental procedures.[4] Despite this, the cost-effectiveness of prophylactic antibiotics during dental procedures, although frequently used in clinical practice, has remained a controversial issue.[36]

Dental infections can also be a cause of cryptic fever.[4] Extensive investigations of such patients often reveal little except for periodontal disease and abscess formation. Prompt defervescence of fevers has followed dental extraction and débridement of infected periodontal tissue. A careful examination for an odontogenic cause of fever should be included in the assessment of every patient presenting with fever of undetermined origin.

Finally, epidemiologic surveys have suggested that dental infections may predispose to a higher risk of coronary heart disease.[1] A large case-control study and a later 14-year follow-up of 9760 individuals have both indicated that periodontitis may be associated with an increased risk of coronary heart disease. Preliminary results suggest that the severity of dental infections correlates with the extent of coronary atheromatosis. The cause-effect relationship and precise mechanism behind this intriguing association remain to be determined. It appears that such an association with vascular disease may not be unique for dental infections, however, because septicemic patients with or without endocarditis have also been shown to have an increased risk of stroke, and patients with *Chlamydia pneumoniae* respiratory infections also appear to have an increased risk of acute myocardial infarction.[37]

DIAGNOSTIC APPROACHES

Specimen Collection and Processing

It is imperative that the normal resident oral flora be excluded during specimen collection in order that culture results can be appropriately interpreted. For closed space infections, needle aspiration of loculated pus by an extraoral approach is desirable, and specimens should be transported immediately to the laboratory under anaerobic conditions. For intraoral lesions, direct microscopic examination of stained smears often provides more useful information than culture results from surface swabs. Gram's stain and acid-fast stains for bacteria and potassium hydroxide preparations for fungi should be routinely performed. Tissue specimens examined for typical histopathology and presence of microbial antigens by immunofluorescence are particularly useful in suspected mycobacterial, fungal, and viral infections. In chronic osteomyelitis, soft tissue swelling and draining fistulas are frequently present. Aspirates from the adjacent soft tissue swellings may be valuable, but cultures from the sinus tracts may be misleading, because sinus tracts are often colonized by organisms that do not reflect what is actually occurring within the infected bone. Bone biopsies for histopathology and culture are often required for definitive diagnosis.

Imaging Techniques

Ultrasonography, radionuclide scanning, computed tomography (CT), and magnetic resonance imaging are particularly useful for localization of deep fascial space infections of the head and neck.[31, 38] A lateral radiograph of the neck may demonstrate compression or deviation of the tracheal air column, or the presence of gas within necrotic soft tissues. In retropharyngeal infections, lateral radiographs of the cervical spine or CT scanning can help determine whether the infection is in the retropharyngeal space or the prevertebral space. The former suggests an odontogenic source, whereas the latter suggests involvement of the cervical spine. Technetium bone scanning, used in combination with gallium- or indium-labeled white blood cells, is particularly useful for the diagnosis of acute or chronic osteomyelitis and for the differentiation of infection or trauma from malignancy.

THERAPEUTIC CONSIDERATIONS

Dental Caries and Periodontitis

For both caries prevention and treatment of periodontitis, the clinical goal must continue to be control of the supragingival and subgingival plaques. With the emerging concept of microbial specificity in these infections, the prospect of specific antimicrobial therapy appears increasingly promising.[21, 39–42] The successful treatment of acute necrotizing ulcerative gingivitis with metronidazole monotherapy has been well documented. In localized juvenile periodontitis, systemic tetracycline therapy directed against *A. actinomycetemcomitans* and combined with local periodontal treatment has yielded excellent results. Unfortunately, tetracycline resistance among periodontal pathogens has been increasingly recognized.[43] For advanced periodontitis, several double-blind studies have indicated that systemic metronidazole[41] or doxycycline[44] plus mechanical débridement of the root surfaces is effective.

Several topical agents appear to have cariostatic effects in humans. By far the most effective is fluoride, which complexes with the apatite crystals in dentin and promotes remineralization of the carious lesions. Topical chlorhexidine is another useful anticariogenic agent that is retained on the oral surfaces for prolonged periods and acts as a cationic detergent against a wide range of bacteria.[4] Among the antibiotics, although both penicillin and tetracycline have cariostatic effects in animal models, only topical application of vancomycin has been shown to reduce dental caries with some degree of success in human studies.[7]

Suppurative Odontogenic Infections

The most important therapeutic modality for pyogenic odontogenic infections is surgical drainage and removal of necrotic tissue. Potentially involved fascial spaces should be carefully examined, and incision and drainage performed at the optimal time. Premature incision into a poorly localized cellulitis can disrupt the normal physiologic barriers and cause further extension of infection. Needle aspiration by the extraoral route can be particularly helpful both for microbiologic sampling and evacuation of pus. Extraction of infected teeth and endodontic treatments with root-filling may be the definitive approach in some instances.

Antibiotic therapy is important in halting local spread

of infection and preventing hematogenous dissemination. Antimicrobial agents are generally indicated if fever and regional lymphadenitis are present. Immunocompromised patients are at particular risk for unhalted and spreading orofacial infections, and empiric antimicrobial therapy in these patients is usually warranted.

The initial choice of antibiotic regimens requires not so much the results of bacterial culture and sensitivity as knowledge of the indigenous organisms that colonize the teeth, gums, and mucous membranes. By far most of these organisms, both anaerobes and aerobes, are sensitive to penicillin.[21, 45, 46] Thus, penicillin monotherapy in doses appropriate for the severity of infection remains a good choice. However, the problem of beta-lactamase production among certain oral anaerobes, particularly pigmented *Prevotella* species and *F. nucleatum,* has been increasingly recognized,[47, 48] and treatment failures with penicillin in odontogenic infections due to such beta-lactamase–producing strains have been well documented.[49] Thus, in patients with life-threatening deep fascial space infections and in those who have had an unfavorable or delayed response to penicillin, alternative therapy with a broader spectrum against both anaerobes and aerobes should be considered. Ambulatory patients with less serious odontogenic infections may be treated with amoxicillin with or without a beta-lactamase inhibitor, or with either penicillin or ciprofloxacin in combination with metronidazole. Penicillin-allergic patients may be treated with clindamycin, cefoxitin, or ceftizoxime. Erythromycin and tetracycline are not recommended because of increasing resistance among some strains of streptococci. Metronidazole, although highly active against anaerobic gram-negative bacilli and spirochetes, is only moderately active against anaerobic cocci and is not active against aerobes, including streptococci. Except in acute necrotizing gingivitis and advanced periodontitis, metronidazole should not be used as a single agent in odontogenic infections. In the compromised host, such as the patient with leukemia and severe neutropenia following chemotherapy, it is prudent to cover for aerobic gram-negative bacilli as well, and agents with broad-spectrum activity against both aerobes and anaerobes are desirable (Table 55–4).

Osteomyelitis

Treatment of osteomyelitis of the jaws is complicated by the presence of teeth and persistent exposure to the oral environment. Antibiotic therapy needs to be prolonged, often weeks to months. Because mixed anaerobes and aerobes, including *Streptococcus* species, *Peptostreptococcus* species, *Bacteroides* species, *Prevotella* species, and *Actinomyces* species, are the predominant isolates (Table 55–2), clindamycin is an excellent choice for the treatment of odontogenic osteomyelitis. Penicillin plus metronidazole is an alternative. Ciprofloxacin is not indicated unless *S. aureus* or gram-negative bacilli are isolated. Adjuvant therapy with hyperbaric oxygen may prove beneficial in hastening the healing process, particularly for the chronic sclerosing variety.[35] Surgical management, including sequestrectomy, saucerization, decortication, and closed-wound suction irrigation, may occasionally be necessary. Rarely, in advanced cases, the entire segment of the infected jaw may have to be resected.

PREVENTION

Meticulous dental hygiene, fluoridation of water supplies, and modification of food habits (particularly less between-meal use of sugar-containing foods that are retained on tooth surfaces) are currently the best measures for reducing the accumulation of dental plaque and preventing caries.[19] Although preliminary studies of active and passive immunization with *S. mutans* vaccines appear promising,[50–53] the efficacy and safety of this approach for the general population remain to be determined.

References

1. Mattila KJ: Dental infections as a risk factor for acute myocardial infarction. Eur Heart J 1993; 14(suppl K): 51–53.
2. Chow AW: Infections of the oral cavity, neck and head. In: Mandell GL, Bennett JE, Dolin R (eds): Principles and Practice of Infectious Diseases, 4th ed. New York: Churchill-Livingstone, 1995, pp 593–606.
3. Thadepalli H, Mandal AK: Anatomic basis of head and neck infections. Infect Dis Clin North Am 1988; 2: 21–34.
4. Kureishi K, Chow AW: The tender tooth—dentoalveolar, pericoronal, and periodontal infections. Infect Dis Clin North Am 1988; 2:163–182.
5. Loesche WJ: Bacterial mediators in periodontal disease. Clin Infect Dis 1993; 16(suppl 4): S203.
6. Newman MG: Anaerobic oral and dental infection. Rev Infect Dis 1984; 6(suppl 1): S107–S114.
7. Schachtele CF: Dental caries. In: Schuster GS (ed): Oral Microbiology and Infectious Disease. Baltimore: Williams & Wilkins, 1983, pp 197–233.
8. Gusberti FA, Mombelli A, Lang NP, Minder CE: Changes in subgingival microbiota during puberty: A 4-year longitudinal study. J Clin Periodontol 1990; 17: 685–692.
9. Cianciola LJ, Genco RJ, Patters MR, et al: Defective polymorphonuclear leukocyte function in human periodontal disease. Nature 1977; 265: 445.
10. Van Dyke TE, Horoszewicz HU, Cianciola LJ, Genco RJ: Neutrophil chemotaxis dysfunction in human periodontitis. Infect Immun 1980; 27: 124–132.
11. Choi JI, Nakagawa T, Yamada S, et al.: Clinical, microbiological and immunological studies on recurrent periodontal disease. J Clin Periodontol 1990; 17: 426–434.
12. Schuster GS, Burnett GW: The microbiology of oral and maxillofacial infections. In: Topacian RG, Goldberg MH (eds): Management of Infections of the Oral and Maxillofacial Regions, 2nd ed. Philadelphia: WB Saunders, 1987, pp 33–71.
13. Sutter VL: Anaerobes as normal oral flora. Rev Infect Dis 1984; 6: S62–S66.
14. Valenti WM, Trudell RB, Bentley DW: Factors predisposing to oropha-

Table 55–4. EMPIRIC ANTIBIOTIC REGIMENS FOR ODONTOGENIC SOFT TISSUE INFECTIONS

Normal host
    Penicillin G, 1–4 million units IV every 4–6h
    Ampicillin-sulbactam, 1.5–3 g IV every 6h
    Clindamycin, 600 mg IV every 6–8h
    Cefoxitin, 1–2 g IV every 6h
    Cefotetan, 2 g IV every 12h
    Ceftizoxime, 1–2 g IV every 8–12h
Compromised host (one of the following ± an aminoglycoside)
    Ceftizoxime, 2 g IV every 8h
    Cefotaxime, 2 g IV every 6h
    Piperacillin-tazobactam, 3 g IV every 4h
    Imipenem/cilastatin, 500 mg IV every 6h

ryngeal colonization with gram-negative bacilli in the aged. N Engl J Med 1978; 298: 1108.

15. Rosenthal S, Tager IB: Relevance of gram-negative rods in the normal pharyngeal flora. Ann Intern Med 1975; 83: 355.

16. Hardie J: Microbial flora of the oral cavity. In: Schuster GS (ed): Oral Microbiology and Infectious Disease. Baltimore: Williams & Wilkins, 1983, pp 162–196.

17. Ogawa T, Kusumoto Y, Hamada S, et al: *Bacteroides gingivalis*–specific serum IgG and IgA subclass antibodies in periodontal diseases. Clin Exp Immunol 1990; 82: 318–325.

18. Loesche WJ: Role of *Streptococcus mutans* in human dental decay. Microbiol Rev 1986; 50: 353.

19. Shaw JH: Causes and control of dental caries. N Engl J Med 1987; 317: 996–1004.

20. Hamada S, Slade HD: Biology, immunology and cariogenicity of *Streptococcus mutans*. Microbiol Rev 1991; 44: 331.

21. Tanner A, Stillman N: Oral and dental infections with anaerobic bacteria: Clinical features, predominant pathogens, and treatment. Clin Infect Dis 1993; 16(suppl 4): S304.

22. Moore WEC, Holdeman LV, Smibert RM, et al.: Bacteriology of severe periodontitis in young adult humans. Infect Immun 1982; 38: 1137–1148.

23. Moore WEC, Holdeman LV, Cato EP, et al: Bacteriology of moderate (chronic) periodontitis in mature adult humans. Infect Immun 1983; 42: 510–515.

24. Slots J, Feik D, Rams TE: *Actinobacillus actinomycetemcomitans* and *Bacteroides intermedius* in human periodontitis—age relationship and mutual association. J Clin Periodontol 1990; 17: 659–662.

25. Chow AW, Roser SM, Brady FA: Orofacial odontogenic infections. Ann Intern Med 1978; 88: 392.

26. Brook I: Isolation of capsulate anerobic bacteria from orofacial abscesses. J Med Microbiol 1986; 22: 171–174.

27. Lewis MAO, MacFarlane TW, McGowan DA: Quantitative bacteriology of acute dento-alveolar abscesses. J Med Microbiol 1986; 21: 101–104.

28. Berkowitz R, McIlveen L, Obeid G: Pediatric odontogenic infections. Adv Pediatr Infect Dis 1993; 8: 131–144.

29. Heimdahl A, Nord CE: Oral infections in immunocompromised patients. J Clin Periodontol 1990; 17: 501–503.

30. Busch DF, Kureshi LA, Sutter VL, Finegold SM: Susceptibility of respiratory tract anaerobes to orally administered penicillins and cephalosporins. Antimicrob Agents Chemother 1976; 10: 713.

31. Chow AW: Life-threatening infections of the head and neck. Clin Infect Dis 1992; 14: 991–1004.

32. Epstein JB, Stevenson-Moore PB: Benzydamine hydrochloride in prevention and management of pain in oral mucositis associated with radiation therapy. Oral Surg 1986; 62: 145–148.

33. Haug RH, Picard U, Indresano AT: Diagnosis and treatment of the retropharyngeal abscess in adults. Br J Oral Max Surg 1990; 28: 34–38.

34. Patters MR: Periodontal disease. In: Schuster GS (ed): Oral Microbiol-

ogy and Infectious Disease. Baltimore: Williams & Wilkins, 1983, pp 234–264.

35. Topazian RG: Osteomyelitis of the jaws. In: Topazian RG, Goldberg MH (eds): Oral and Maxillofacial Infections, 2nd ed. Philadelphia: WB Saunders, 1987, pp 204–238.

36. Hall G, Hedstrom SA, Heimdahl A, Nord CE: Prophylactic administration of penicillins for endocarditis does not reduce the incidence of postextraction bacteremia. Clin Infect Dis 1993; 17: 188–194.

37. Grayston JT: Infections caused by *Chlamydia pneumoniae* strain TWAR. Clin Infect Dis 1992; 15: 757–763.

38. Salit IE: Diagnostic approaches to head and neck infections. Infect Dis Clin North Am 1988; 2: 35–55.

39. Cattabriga M, Di Murro C, Paolantonio M: General considerations in the treatment of periodontal disease: Infection control, medications, and wound healing. Curr Opin Dent 1991; 1: 66–73.

40. Slots J, Rams TE: Antibiotics in periodontal therapy—advantages and disadvantages. J Clin Periodontol 1991; 17: 479–493.

41. Loesche WJ: Rationale for the use of antimicrobial agents in periodontal disease. Int J Technol Assess Health Care 1990; 6: 403.

42. Socransky SS, Haffajee AD: Effect of therapy on periodontal infections. J Periodontol 1993; 64: 754–759.

43. Olsvik B, Tenover FC: Tetracycline resistance in periodontal pathogens. Clin Infect Dis 1993; 16(suppl 4): S310.

44. Wholey MH, Bruwer AJ, Baker HL: The lateral roentgenogram of the neck. Radiology 1958; 71: 350.

45. Hammert W: Odontogenic infections: Management and treatment. J Okla Dent Assoc 1993; 84: 32–34.

46. Gill Y, Scully C: Orofacial odontogenic infections: Review of microbiology and current treatment. Oral Surg Oral Med Oral Pathol 1990; 70: 155–158.

47. Brook I: Beta-lactamase producing bacteria in head and neck infection. Laryngoscope 1988; 98: 428–431.

48. Brook I: Infections caused by β-lactamase-producing *Fusobacterium* spp in children. Ped Infect Dis 1993; 12: 532–533.

49. Heimdahl A, von Konow L, Nord CE: Isolation of β-lactamase producing *Bacteroides* strains associated with clinical failures with penicillin treatment of human orofacial infections. Arch Oral Biol 1980; 25: 687.

50. Russell RRB, Johnson NW: The prospects of vaccination against dental caries. Br Dent J 1987; 162: 29.

51. Gregory RL, Filler SJ: Protective secretory immunoglobulin A antibodies in humans following oral immunization with *Streptococcus mutans*. Infect Immun 1987; 55: 2409–2415.

52. Michalek SM, Gregory RL, Harmon CC, et al.: Protection of gnotobiotic rats against dental caries by passive immunization with bovine milk antibodies to *Streptococcus mutans*. Infect Immun 1987; 55: 2341–2347.

53. Jackson S, Mestecky J, Childers NK, Michalek SM: Liposomes containing anti-idiotypic antibodies: An oral vaccine to induce protective secretory immune responses specific for pathogens of mucosal surfaces. Infect Immun 1990; 58: 1932–1936.

Paul W. Gidley
Charles M. Stiernberg

CHAPTER FIFTY-SIX

Deep Neck Space Infections

▼

Life-threatening infections of the fascial spaces of the neck continue to occur despite the wide use of antibiotics. The emergence of virulent, antibiotic-resistant organisms may account for the continued appearance of these grave infections. The infections follow along the fascial planes of the neck. The fascial planes create potential spaces in the neck when infected. The ability to treat and cure these infections depends on an understanding of the anatomy of the neck's fascial planes and spaces, the pathogenesis and bacteriology of such infections, and vigilance on the part of the treating physician to prevent potential complications.

FASCIAL PLANES AND POTENTIAL SPACES

The fascial layers of the neck are divided into a superficial layer and a deep layer. The superficial layer of fascia envelops the platysma muscle in the neck and continues in the face to cover the mimetic muscles. This layer of fascia does not form a boundary for a potential space and thus has little clinical significance with respect to these infections.

Much more importantly, however, the deep layers of cervical fascia are divided into three layers below the hyoid and do form potential spaces (Fig. 56–1). The superficial layer of deep cervical fascia has its origin at the spinal processes of the vertebral column, then encircles the neck by enveloping the trapezius muscles and the sternocleidomastoid muscles. Between the sternocleidomastoid muscles, this superficial layer of deep fascia splits to pass anterior and posterior to the sternum, forming the suprasternal space of Burns, which usually contains the anterior jugular veins and a lymph node.[1] This layer is attached at the hyoid bone.

Above the level of the hyoid, the superficial layer of deep cervical fascia splits to envelop the submandibular gland and the mandible (Fig. 56–2). It covers the superficial muscles of the floor of the mouth (the anterior digastric and mylohyoid muscles), forming the floor of a potential space between the muscles and the fascia. At the mandible, the outer layer covers the masseter up to the zygomatic arch as masseteric fascia. The inner layer follows the medial surface of the internal (medial) pterygoid muscle up to the skull base. Superiorly, between the sternocleidomastoid and the angle of the mandible, the superficial layer of deep cervical fascia continues upward to cover the parotid gland up to the zygomatic arch.

The middle layer of deep cervical fascia, or visceral layer of fascia, surrounds the infrahyoid strap muscles, larynx, esophagus, and thyroid gland. This layer passes into the upper mediastinum, where it fuses with the fibrous pericardium.[1] Above the level of the hyoid, this layer of fascia

continues to cover the pharynx posteriorly and buccinator superiorly and thus is called buccopharyngeal fascia.

The deep layer of deep cervical fascia, or prevertebral layer of fascia, envelops the vertebral muscles. It takes origin from the spinal process to surround the vertebral muscles. Posteriorly, this layer is immediately deep to the trapezius muscles and the superficial layer of deep cervical fascia. The spinal accessory nerve and lymph nodes lie between the superficial layer of deep cervical fascia and the prevertebral fascia. More anteriorly, the deep layer of cervical fascia surrounds the nerves of the brachial plexus, the subclavian vessels, and the scalene muscles before passing anterior to the vertebral column. Along the subclavian vessels and brachial plexus, this fascia is continued as the axillary sheath. It is densely adherent to the underlying muscles, which helps to prevent spread of infection along its sheath.

The deep cervical fascia splits at the transverse processes to form two layers, an anterior or alar layer and a posterior or prevertebral layer (Figs. 56–1 and 56–3). This important anterior layer allows the pharynx-larynx to slide as a unit over the prevertebral muscles during the act of deglutition. However, a potential space called the danger space is thus formed; this space extends as far inferiorly as the diaphragm.

All three layers of deep cervical fascia come together to create the carotid sheath, which envelops the carotid artery, the internal jugular vein, and the vagus nerve.

The potential spaces thus created are perhaps best examined with respect to the hyoid, which is the key surgical landmark of the neck during a drainage procedure. The potential space that is below the hyoid is the visceral space. Those that are above the hyoid are the parapharyngeal and submandibular/sublingual spaces. The spaces that run the length of the neck are the retropharyngeal space, the danger space, and the prevertebral space.

The visceral space or compartment contains the thyroid gland, trachea, and esophagus. This space is surrounded by the pretracheal fascia. Infections within this compartment can be transmitted into the upper mediastinum to the level of the arch of the aorta or to about the level of the fourth thoracic vertebra. At the level below the thyroid gland, this compartment is divided into an anterior or pretracheal space and a posterior or retrovisceral space by fascia that extends laterally from the pretracheal fascia to the prevertebral fascia. Thus, the retrovisceral space is actually a continuation of the retropharyngeal space.

The retropharyngeal space is bounded anteriorly by the visceral fascia, laterally by the carotid sheath, and posteriorly by the prevertebral fascia. This space extends from the skull base superiorly and ends in the mediastinum, running posteriorly to the viscera of the mediastinum. The retrovis-

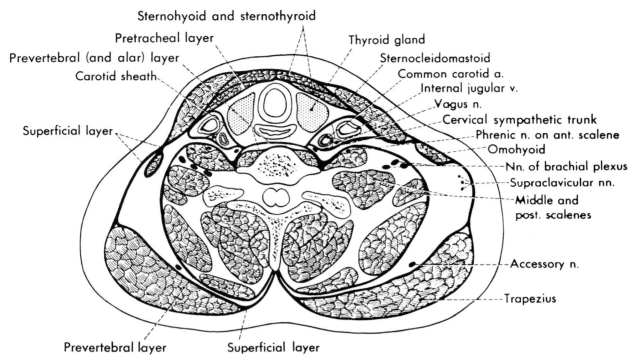

Figure 56-1. Deep layers of cervical fascia below the level of the hyoid.

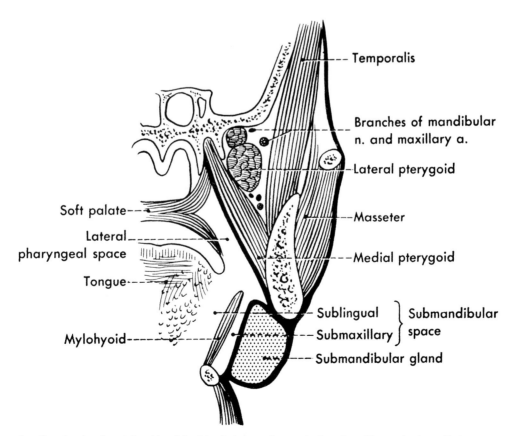

Figure 56-2. Coronal section showing the relationship of the lateral pharyngeal space to the submaxillary and submandibular spaces and the mandible. Notice that the superficial layer of deep cervical fascia splits to surround the submandibular gland, the mandible, and the muscles of mastication.

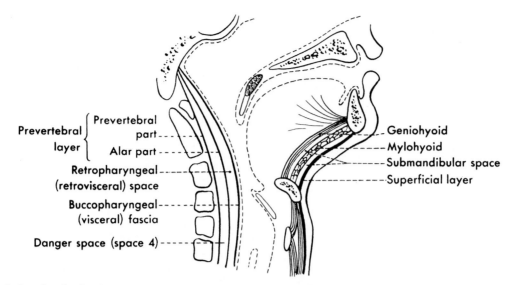

Figure 56–3. Sagittal section showing the retropharyngeal, danger, and prevertebral spaces. Notice also that the superficial layer forms the floor of the submandibular space.

ceral space extends to about the level of the fourth thoracic vertebra, where the space is obliterated by fusion of the pretracheal fascia and prevertebral fascia.

The danger area, as discussed previously, is created by the two layers of the anterior prevertebral fascia and lies behind the retropharyngeal or retrovisceral space. This layer runs along the length of the vertebral column from the skull base to the diaphragm.

The prevertebral space is a potential space between the prevertebral layer of fascia and the underlying vertebral muscles. It lies posterior to the danger space, although both may become involved by serious infections. The fascia extends along the entire length of the vertebral column; however, given the dense attachment of the fascia to the muscles, infections are limited in their ability to spread.

The spaces above the hyoid are the parapharyngeal and submandibular/sublingual spaces. The parapharyngeal space (also called the lateral pharyngeal space or pterygomaxillary space) is a conical potential space with its wide portion at the skull base and tapering to end at the hyoid. It is bounded anteriorly by the pterygomandibular raphe at the junction of the buccinator and superior constrictor muscles, laterally by the mandible, the parotid gland, and pterygoid muscles, and medially by the buccopharyngeal fascia on the lateral surface of the superior constrictor muscles (Fig. 56–4).[2] Posteriorly, it extends to the prevertebral fascia and communicates with the retropharyngeal space.

This space is divided by the styloid process into an anterior muscular compartment closely related to the tonsillar fossa and a posterior neurovascular compartment. The anterior or prestyloid compartment contains fat, muscle, lymph nodes, and connective tissue. The posterior or poststyloid compartment contains cranial nerves IX through XII and the carotid sheath.

The submandibular space includes the sublingual space above the mylohyoid and the submaxillary space below it. These spaces may be considered as a single unit because of their free communication posteriorly and their clinical behavior.[3] The entire space is bounded anteriorly and later-ally by the mandible, superiorly by the mucosa of the floor of the mouth, and inferiorly by the superficial layer of deep cervical fascia (see Fig. 56–3). This dense fibrous layer of deep cervical fascia prevents swelling inferiorly and forces the floor of the mouth and tongue to protrude superiorly and posteriorly into the airway.

The parotid space is formed by a split in the superficial layer of deep cervical fascia around the parotid gland and mandible. Connective tissue septa strongly attach the super-

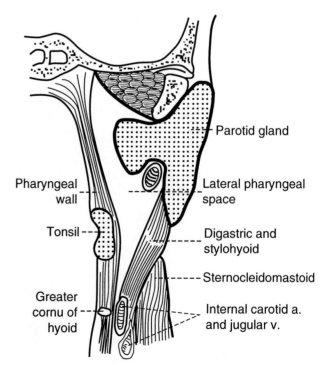

Figure 56–4. The parapharyngeal space as seen in a sagittal section. Notice that this space is an inverted cone that communicates medially with the pharynx, laterally with the parotid, superiorly with the skull base, and anteroinferiorly with the submandibular triangle, tapering at the level of the hyoid.

ficial fascia to the gland without an anatomic space between the two. The parotid space communicates directly with the parapharyngeal space, because the deep layer of cervical fascia is lacking on the upper inner surface of the parotid gland itself.

RETROPHARYNGEAL ABSCESS

Retropharyngeal abscess is the most common deep neck abscess found in the head and neck in children, with 96% occurring in children younger than 6 years and 50% in those 6–12 months of age.[4] Lymph nodes that lie in the retropharyngeal space may be seeded with bacteria from infected sites in the nose, paranasal sinuses, and pharynx.[5] These nodes tend to atrophy with age, accounting for the pediatric predominance of this disease. Alternatively, however, infection in this space may be due to direct trauma resulting from penetration of the posterior wall of the pharynx, such as with endoscopy or intubation, vertebral fractures, foreign bodies, or dental infections. As the infection progresses, the abscess may exceed the capacity of this space and may spill into either the parapharyngeal space laterally or the mediastinum inferiorly.

Classically, children may present with fever, irritability, difficulty breathing or swallowing, drooling, cervical adenopathy, or neck stiffness.[6] The posterior wall may appear swollen; however, children may not allow an adequate examination, and palpation may result in spontaneous rupture of the abscess or a bitten examiner's finger.

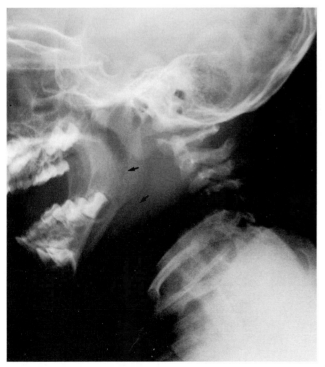

Figure 56–5. Lateral neck radiograph showing extensive prevertebral soft tissue swelling *(arrows)* consistent with a retropharyngeal abscess. This swelling measured 22 mm at the level of C2 and 16 mm at the level of C6. Notice also the loss of cervical lordosis. An external approach was used to drain this abscess.

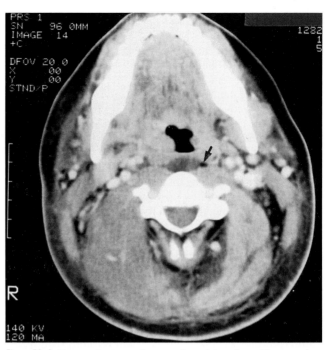

Figure 56–6. Computed tomography scan of an adult patient with a retropharyngeal abscess. Notice hypodense area and gas *(arrow)* in the retropharyngeal space.

Clinically, these patients may appear to have epiglottitis, meningitis, severe croup, or peritonsillar abscess. Diagnosis is aided by radiographic imaging studies (Fig. 56–5). Wholey and colleagues[7] studied more than 400 lateral neck films and recorded the average soft tissue thickness at C2 and C6. For both children and adults, the normal thickness at C2 is less than 7 mm. The soft tissue thickness at C6 is less than 14 mm for children and less than 22 mm for adults.[7] Lateral neck films must be taken in a true lateral position and with full inspiration. The differential diagnosis for prevertebral soft tissue swelling includes retropharyngeal abscess, inflammation, tumor (cystic hygroma, hemangioma, neuroblastoma), bleeding or hematoma, cervical spine trauma, nonopaque foreign body, and retropharyngeal thyroid. In addition to swelling, air or air-fluid levels, loss of cervical lordosis, vertebral fracture, or suspected osteomyelitis may be present, giving another sign of the infective process.[8] Computed tomography (CT), if available, may help to differentiate abscess (Fig. 56–6). If a retropharyngeal abscess is suspected, a chest radiograph should be performed to evaluate for mediastinal involvement.[9]

Treatment for retropharyngeal abscess demands hospitalization, intravenous antibiotics, and close monitoring of the airway. Antibiotics should be effective against the most likely pathogens. Up to 65% of patients have received antibiotics for the infection of the ear, nose, or throat prior to the development of retropharyngeal abscess. The most common organisms are alpha-hemolytic streptococcus, *Staphylococcus aureus, Bacteroides, Fusobacterium,* and *Peptostreptococcus.*[10] Brook[11] studied 14 patients with retropharyngeal abscess and found anaerobes in all of them. In those patients, he found almost six isolates per patient. Aerobes were mixed with anaerobes in 86% of the patients.[11] Beta-lactamase production has been found for *Bacteroides* and *Staphylococcus*.

Surgical therapy is necessary in patients with airway compromise, failure of antibiotic therapy or progression of disease, or demonstration of pus on CT. Usually, small abscesses can be drained through the mouth, whereas a larger abscess may require an external approach. For small abscesses, with an endotracheal tube in place to protect the airway, the patient is placed in the Rose position to prevent aspiration of pus. An incision is placed in the posterior pharyngeal wall and opened bluntly with a hemostat.[12] Once opened and irrigated, the abscess cavity is left to granulate, and a drain is not used.

For larger infections, especially with spread to the lateral pharyngeal space, an external approach is used for better exposure and drainage. The major vascular structures and nerves in this space and the possibility of their displacement by abscess necessitate a lateral neck incision for adequate visualization and vascular control. An incision parallel to the anterior border of the sternocleidomastoid or a horizontal submandibular incision with a vertical limb allows good access to this space. The abscess is opened between the carotid sheath, which lies laterally, and the constrictor muscles, which lie medially. If the abscess has extended down into the neck, the dissection is extended down along the carotid sheath to the sternum, exposing the trachea and esophagus. A drain is left in the wound to be advanced and removed as the patient improves.

SUBMANDIBULAR ABSCESS AND LUDWIG'S ANGINA

The term submandibular space was coined by Grodinsky and Holyoke[13] in 1938. The key to this space is the mylohyoid muscle. By reason of its slanted attachment to the mandible, the mylohyoid determines which space will be affected first according to the tooth of origin. The apices of the second and third mandibular molars are below the muscle attachment, leading to submaxillary space infection, whereas the apex of the first molar is above the mylohyoid, causing sublingual space infection.[6] Spread of infection from a tooth is through the relatively thin lingual cortex of the mandible.

The sublingual and submandibular spaces are continuous around the posterior edge of the mylohyoid. The submandibular space also communicates with the parapharyngeal space through the buccopharyngeal gap created by the styloglossus muscle as it pierces between the superior and middle constrictors to insert on the tongue.

Most infections of the submandibular space are odontogenic (70%–85%). However, lacerations of the floor of the mouth, mandible fractures, foreign bodies, mandibular tumors, lingual cancers, sialadenitis, lymphadenitis, and inferior alveolar nerve blocks have all been reported as causes of submandibular space infections (Figs. 56–7 and 56–8).

Ludwig's angina is a special type of submandibular space infection. There is cellulitis, not abscess, of the submandibular space, which (1) never involves only one space and usually is bilateral, (2) produces gangrene with serosanguineous, putrid infiltration but very little or no frank pus, (3) involves connective tissue, fascia, and muscle but not the

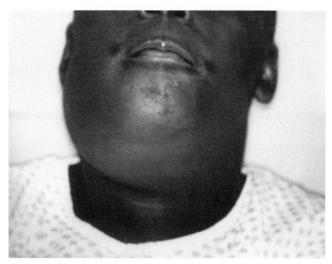

Figure 56–7. Frontal view of a young patient with extensive submandibular swelling. Compare with the computed tomography scan in Figure 56–8.

glandular structures, and (4) is spread by continuity and not by lymphatics.[14] The strong fibers of the superficial layer of deep cervical fascia limit external swelling; the floor of the mouth is readily distensible, resulting in massive swelling and displacement of tongue posteriorly into hypopharynx, superiorly against the palate, and anteriorly out of the mouth.

Patients with Ludwig's angina present with tachypnea, dyspnea, and stridor, which herald the onset of respiratory obstruction. Respiratory obstruction often occurs with alarming rapidity. These infections are rarely fluctuant and may progress rapidly over a few hours. Patients may have a

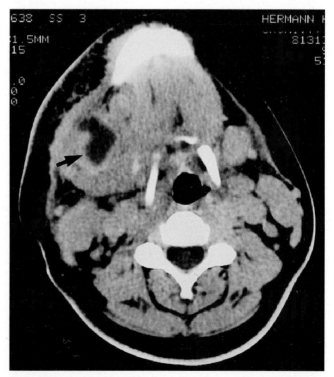

Figure 56–8. Computed tomography scan of the patient in Figure 56–7 showing a submandibular abscess. Notice the extensive soft tissue swelling.

muffled or "hot potato" voice with tender, woody swelling in the neck. Trismus is usually absent.

Airway control is foremost in the treatment of Ludwig's angina, followed by intravenous antibiotics and timely surgical drainage. Patients who are not in respiratory distress may be monitored closely with tracheostomy tray at bedside in an intensive care setting. Blind nasal intubation may precipitate obstruction or inadvertent rupture of associated parapharyngeal or retropharyngeal abscesses and should be avoided.[15] Tracheostomy is the best form of airway control.

The basic principle in surgery for Ludwig's angina is the release of tension in addition to adequate drainage. The causes of the tension in this area are the strong suprahyoid fascia and the mylohyoid muscle; therefore, these two structures must be divided to produce the best results.[14]

The usual organisms involved are aerobic *Streptococcus, Staphylococcus, Bacteroides,* and *Peptostreptococcus.* The anaerobes work synergistically with the aerobes to produce tissue necrosis, gas formation, and foul odor.[2] *Staphylococcus* and gram-negative rods should be considered if the patient is diabetic or alcoholic.[6] Given the rise in rates of organisms that produce a beta-lactamase, penicillin may not be the best choice. Ampicillin/sulbactam or clindamycin may be a better alternative.[5, 6] In 1943, Ludwig's angina had a mortality rate of 54%; the rate is now 0%–4%.[6]

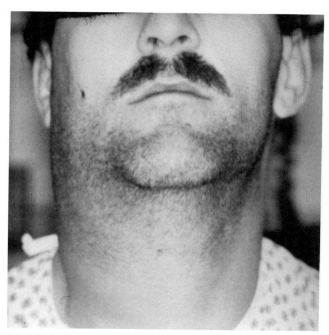

Figure 56–9. Frontal view of a patient with a right parapharyngeal abscess. Notice that the swelling extends from the angle of the mandible to about the level of the hyoid.

PARAPHARYNGEAL SPACE INFECTIONS

A cone-shaped, lateral neck space, the parapharyngeal space has its base on the skull base and its apex at the hyoid bone. It is one of the most common sites for suppuration in the head and neck. The portals of entry are the pharynx, the tonsils and adenoids, the teeth, the parotid gland, and the lymph glands that drain the nose and pharynx. Every peritonsillar abscess has the potential to become a parapharyngeal space abscess. Middle ear infections may cause a parapharyngeal space infection by breaking through the bone on the inner aspect of the mastoid tip in the region of the digastric ridge (incisura mastoidea) and form a Bezold's abscess. In up to 50% of patients with parapharyngeal space infection, a source cannot be identified. Parotid, submandibular, masticator, and retropharyngeal spaces communicate with the lateral pharyngeal space.

Signs and symptoms of infection in this space depend upon which of two compartments is involved. With infection limited to the anterior or prestyloid compartment, the internal pterygoid muscle is irritated, and marked trismus occurs. Induration along the angle of the jaw is also present (Fig. 56–9). The lateral pharyngeal wall and the tonsil are pushed medially, as with a peritonsillar abscess.

With infections of the posterior or poststyloid compartment, the muscles of mastication are not involved, and neither trismus nor tonsillar prolapse occurs. Rather, the neurovascular structures of this compartment are likely to be involved with deficits of cranial nerves IX through XII, or Horner's syndrome occurs from involvement of the cervical sympathetics. Sepsis from jugular vein thrombosis or hemorrhage from the carotid artery rupture may also be a sign of a poststyloid space infection.

Treatment involves hospitalization, intravenous antibiotics after appropriate cultures are taken, and incision and drainage of the abscess. Location and extent of disease can be determined with a CT scan (Fig. 56–10).

The parapharyngeal space should never be drained through an intraoral approach, for two reasons: (1) poor drainage and (2) more importantly, no control over the vessels through an intraoral incision. Either an incision parallel to the anterior border of the sternocleidomastoid muscle or a submandibular incision parallel to relaxed skin tension lines provides excellent access to these infections. The constant palpable nature of the hyoid bone serves as an excellent landmark in this swollen, fibrotic, and infected field. Blunt dissection to the level of the submandibular gland opens the superficial layer of deep cervical fascia. Using a finger or hemostat to bluntly dissect around the submandibular gland opens up the parapharyngeal space. The dissecting finger can then open up all loculations up to the level of the styloid process.

Additionally, the carotid artery should be palpated and located. According to Mosher, the key structure of the neck is the carotid sheath, "the Lincoln Highway of the neck."[16] Finding the carotid sheath enables all areas of pus to be found, because all three layers of fascia contribute to the carotid sheath.

Once the abscess cavity has been fully opened, cultured, and irrigated, a drain is left in the cavity to be advanced as the patient improves.

As in the other spaces, the likely organisms are *Streptococcus, Staphylococcus, Bacteroides, Peptostreptococcus,* and *Fusobacterium.* Treatment should include antibiotics effective against these organisms and should be modified according to the results of Gram's stain and culture. The presence of organisms on Gram's stain but lack of growth

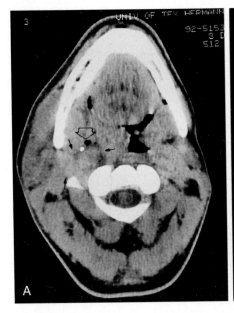
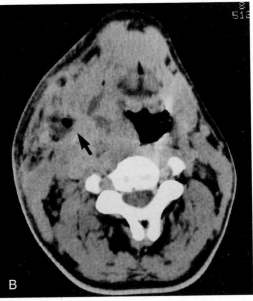

Figure 56–10. Computed tomography scan of the patient in Figure 56–9. *A,* At the level of the styloid tip, a large, enhanced area in the parapharyngeal space *(surrounded by arrows)* associated with soft tissue gas *(open arrow)* is displacing the tonsil medially. *B,* At the level of the tongue base, the abscess *(large arrow)* can be seen with its soft tissue gas, effacing the normal tissue planes. Notice the deviation of the airway in relation to the vertebral body.

on routine culture (or even anaerobic medium) weighs heavily in favor of anaerobes.

PAROTID SPACE INFECTIONS

The parotid space is formed from a split in the superficial layer of deep cervical fascia around the parotid gland and its associated lymph nodes, facial nerve, external carotid artery, and posterior facial vein. Infections readily pass into the parapharyngeal space, which lies just deep to the parotid gland. It is this relationship to the parapharyngeal space and thence to the danger space and the posterior mediastinum that makes some cases of parotitis so dangerous.

Acute suppurative parotitis is rare. Parotid abscesses may occur in patients with a history of chronic parotitis, parotid stone, or with the lymphoepithelial lesion of Sjögren's syndrome. Symptoms include marked swelling of the angle of the jaw without associated trismus or pharyngeal swelling (Figs. 56–11 and 56–12).

Treatment for early, small abscesses in the parotid consists of a small incision over the pointing, prominent portion of the abscess through skin alone in a cosmetically acceptable location (pretragal, ear lobe,). Blunt dissection is then carried out in the direction of the facial nerve.

PRETRACHEAL SPACE INFECTIONS

The anatomic boundaries for the pretracheal space are the attachments of pretracheal fascia to the hyoid superiorly and extending into the superior mediastinum to the level of the fourth thoracic vertebra and arch of the aorta. This space includes the infrahyoid strap muscles, larynx, trachea, thyroid, and the upper esophagus.

Infections of the pretracheal space are primarily due to trauma such as foreign body or instrumentation. The space may become secondarily infected from either the parapharyngeal or the retropharyngeal space.

The clinical signs and symptoms are related to the functions of the organs of this space. The symptoms include dysphagia, odynophagia, hoarseness, and dyspnea. On examination, patients may have unilateral swelling of the hypopharynx, neck swelling, or crepitus.

Time from injury to diagnosis and institution of therapy is closely linked with mortality. Infections of the pretracheal space may be associated with severe, progressive edema of

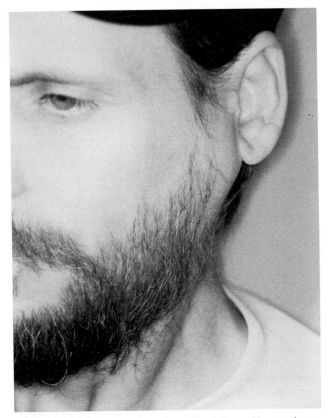

Figure 56–11. Oblique view of a patient with a left parotid space abscess.

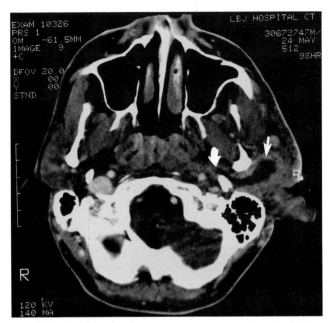

Figure 56–12. Computed tomography scan of the patient in Figure 56–11. An extensive abscess *(arrow)* is present that extends into the deep lobe past the styloid process *(curved arrow)* and that required further drainage after an inadequate procedure under local anesthetic.

the larynx. Additionally, these infections may spread to the mediastinum and account for approximately 8% of mediastinitis due to craniocervical origin. Affected patients are also at risk for developing pneumonia and other pulmonary complications.

Treatment is similar to that for retropharyngeal and parapharyngeal space infections.

COMPLICATIONS

Septic Jugular Vein Thrombosis

Septic internal jugular vein thrombosis (IJVT) is the most common vascular complication of deep neck space infection. Clinically, it is characterized by shaking chills, spiking fevers, prostration, tenderness, and swelling at the angle of the mandible or along the sternocleidomastoid muscle. IJVT may produce sepsis, bacteremia, circulating septic thrombi with distant infection, purulent meningitis, lateral sinus thrombosis, or pulmonary embolism.[17, 18] The rate of pulmonary embolism may be as high as 5%.[19] The rate of occurrence may be especially high in intravenous drug abusers, in whom the most common organism is *Staphylococcus* (72%), followed by beta-hemolytic *Streptococcus*.

IJVT can be diagnosed with CT, ultrasound, or magnetic resonance imaging (MRI). On CT, the thrombus appears as low density in the lumen, a sharply defined dense vessel wall from inflammation and engorgement of the vasa vasorum, enlargement of the thrombosed vein, and soft tissue swelling around the thrombosed vein.[20] MRI is perhaps more helpful at diagnosing IJVT. On MR images, the thrombus appears as an area of bright, intraluminal signal in sharp contrast to the lack of signal from the corresponding site in the unin-

volved contralateral vein.[21] The disadvantages of MRI and MR angiography are the long scanning times, potential for claustrophobia, high costs, and lack of availability. Venography is usually not required.

Treatment involves antibiotics determined by blood culture results, with wound culture results as a second choice. Anticoagulant therapy is controversial, although some studies recommend anticoagulation because of the high risk for pulmonary embolism. If antibiotics and anticoagulants are unsuccessful, then ligation and excision of the vein must be undertaken. If the thrombosed segment is well localized, drainage can be achieved and the affected jugular vein ligated, at the clavicular end first to lessen the chance of air or clot emboli. The infected segment should then be removed. In the preantibiotic period, the mortality rate was as high as 90%, but now IJVT occurs only rarely.[18]

Carotid Artery Rupture

Carotid artery rupture (CAR) was first reported by Liston in 1843,[22] and it still represents a grave complication of deep neck space infections, with a mortality rate between 20% and 40%. CAR has four cardinal signs: (1) recurrent small hemorrhages (which occur in arterial injuries more than vein injuries), (2) protracted clinical course (7–14 days), (3) hematoma of the surrounding tissues, and (4) shock.[17] CAR may also be preceded by persistent peritonsillar swelling after abscess resolution, ipsilateral Horner's syndrome, palsies in cranial nerves IX to XII, and ear hemorrhages. Ear hemorrhages occur primarily in the cartilaginous canal, where the fissures of Santorini spread the infection. A tenuous blood supply and unyielding canal wall make this area prone to erosion, unlike the pharyngeal wall, which has an excellent blood supply and is readily distensible. If blood clots are found upon exploration or drainage of an abscess, one should expect a hemorrhage.[22]

In 1933, Salinger and Pearlman[22a] reported on 227 cases of hemorrhage secondary to deep neck abscess. Sixty-two percent of patients had bleeding from the internal carotid artery, 13% from the common carotid, and 25% from the external carotid. Of the 73 patients who were treated with ligation, 64% survived. This situation demands aggressive treatment consisting of gaining proximal control of the common carotid artery. Distal control may not be available in this difficult and infected field. Infection also prevents reestablishment of vascular flow by patch or replacement graft.[23]

Mediastinitis

Mediastinitis most commonly occurs from esophageal disruption or tracheal injury; however, the spread of infection along fascial planes may produce this situation as well.[24] It is diagnosed on the basis of increasing chest pain, dyspnea, widening of the mediastinum on chest radiograph, or pneumomediastinum. CT is a useful adjunct to diagnose this infection (Fig. 56–13).

A transcervical approach can be used for early infections limited to the mediastinum above T4 or the tracheal bifurca-

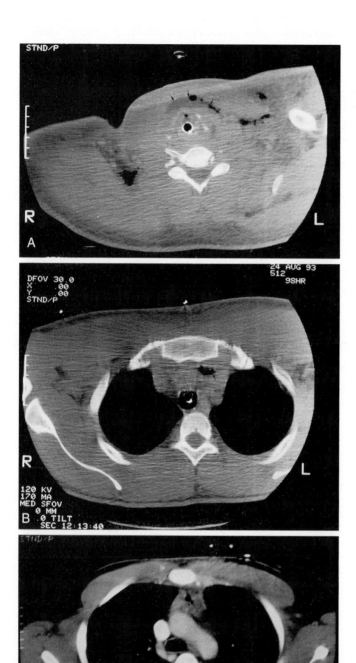

Figure 56–13. A series of computed tomography scan slices showing an odontogenic abscess and gas *(arrows)* that have tracked down into the mediastinum. *A,* Level of the true vocal cords; *B,* level of the manubrium; and *C,* level of the aortic arch.

tion. Tracheostomy is often not advisable, because it would be located in the center of an infected field. Intrathoracic infection requires tube thoracostomy or open-chest drainage. Median sternotomy should be avoided, since it could possibly expose the bone to serious infection.

CONCLUSIONS

Deep neck space abscesses are a common clinical problem that requires prompt diagnosis and treatment with special regard to the airway. Successful diagnosis and treatment depend on a well-founded understanding of the anatomy of the fascial planes of the neck. The organisms that typically cause these infections are those common to the upper respiratory tract, with anaerobes being slightly more prevalent. Complications from advanced illness may be devastating, prolonging hospitalization and producing significant morbidity and mortality.

References

1. Hollinshead W: Anatomy for Surgeons, vol 1: Head and Neck, 3rd ed. Philadelphia: Harper & Row, 1982.
2. Dyzak W, Zide M: Diagnosis and treatment of lateral pharyngeal space infections. J Oral Maxillofac Surg 1984; 42: 243–249.
3. Kaplan H, Eichel B: Deep neck infections. In: English G (ed): Otolaryngology. Philadelphia: JB Lippincott, 1992, pp 1–35.
4. Barratt G, Koopman C, Coulthard S: Retropharyngeal abscess—a ten year experience. Laryngoscope 1984; 94: 455–463.
5. Johnson J: Abscesses and deep space infections of the head and neck. Infect Dis Clin North Am 1992; 6: 705–717.
6. Blomquist I, Bayer A: Life-threatening deep fascial space infections of the head and neck. Infect Dis Clin North Am 1988; 2: 237–264.
7. Wholey M, Bruwer A, Baker H: The lateral roentgenogram of the neck. Radiology 1958; 71: 350–356.
8. Witt D, Craven D, McCabe W: Bacterial infections in adult patients with the acquired immune deficiency syndrome (AIDS) and AIDS-related complex. Am J Med 1987; 82: 900–906.
9. Seid A, Dunbar J, Cotton R: Retropharyngeal abscesses in children revisited. Laryngoscope 1979; 89: 1717–1724.
10. Thompson J, Cohen S, Reddix P: Retropharyngeal abscess in children: A retrospective and historical analysis. Laryngoscope 1988; 98: 589–592.
11. Brook I: Microbiology of retropharyngeal abscesses in children. Am J Dis Child 1987; 141: 202–204.
12. Levitt G: Cervical fascia and deep neck infections. Otolaryngol Clin North Am 1976; 9: 703–716.
13. Grodinsky M, Holyoke E: The fasciae and fascial spaces of the head, neck, and adjacent regions. Am J Anat 1938; 63: 367–408.
14. Patterson H, Kelly J, Strome M: Ludwig's angina: An update. Laryngoscope 1982; 92: 370–378.
15. Allen D, Loughnan T, Ord R: A re-evaluation of the role of tracheostomy in Ludwig's angina. J Oral Maxillofac Surg 1985; 43: 436–439.
16. Mosher H: The submaxillary fossa approach to deep pus in the neck. Trans Am Acad Ophthalmol Otolaryngol 1929; 34: 19–36.
17. Alexander DW, Leonard JR, Trail ML: Vascular complications of deep neck abscesses. Laryngoscope 1967; 77: 361–370.
18. Bartlett J, Gorbach S: Anaerobic infections of the head and neck. Otolaryngol Clin North Am 1976; 9: 655–678.
19. Chowdhury K, Bloom J, Black M, et al.: Spontaneous and nonspontaneous internal jugular vein thrombosis. Head Neck 1990; 12: 168–173.
20. Patel S, Brennan J: Diagnosis of internal jugular vein thrombosis by computed tomography. J Comput Assist Tomogr 1981; 5: 197–200.
21. Braun I, Hoffman J, Malko J, et al.: Jugular venous thrombosis: MRI imaging. Radiology 1985; 157: 357–360.
22. Langenbrunner D, Dejani S: Pharyngomaxillary space abscess with carotid artery erosion. Arch Otolaryngol 1971; 94: 447–457.
22a. Salinger S, Pearlman S: Hemorrhage from pharyngeal and peritonsillar abscesses. Arch Otolaryngol 1933; 18: 464–509.
23. Rabuzzi D, Johnson J: Diagnosis and management of deep neck infections. Presented at SIPac. AAO. 1978.
24. Snow N, Lucas A, Grau M, et al.: Purulent mediastinal abscess secondary to Ludwig's angina. Arch Otolaryngol 1983; 109: 53–55.

CHAPTER FIFTY-SEVEN

James D. Kellner
Elaine E. L. Wang

Cervical Lymphadenitis

▼

Palpable lymph nodes are a typical finding in children after the neonatal period.[1] At any time, most healthy children have several small (<0.5 cm) lymph nodes palpable in the cervical, axillary, or inguinal regions.[2] Enlargement of one or more regional nodes or generalized lymph node enlargement usually occurs with infections. Enlarged lymph nodes may be nontender (lymphadenopathy), tender and perhaps red and warm (lymphadenitis), or tender, red, warm, and fluctuant (suppurative lymphadenitis). Cervical lymphadenitis occurs ubiquitously in children worldwide.[1, 3] It is most often acute and caused by viral infections with regional or generalized lymph node involvement. Suppurative lymphadenitis is most commonly caused by pyogenic bacteria, particularly group A beta-hemolytic streptococcus (GABHS) or *Staphylococcus aureus.* Subacute or chronic cervical lymphadenitis is relatively common and also most likely caused by viruses, with other characteristic causes such as cat-scratch disease, mycobacteria (*Mycobacterium tuberculosis* and atypical mycobacteria), and toxoplasmosis.[1, 3, 4] All other causes of lymphadenitis are uncommon or rare.

ANATOMY

There are many lymph nodes in the head and neck region (Fig 57–1), and several nodes or groups of nodes may be palpable when enlarged. The submandibular and deep cervical nodes receive most of the lymphatic drainage of the head and neck; these nodes are involved in more than 80% of cervical adenitis.[3] Nodes that are clinically important and readily palpable if enlarged are listed in Table 57–1.[3–5]

EPIDEMIOLOGY AND ETIOLOGY

Many infectious agents can cause cervical lymphadenitis. The mode of spread is usually person to person, as occurs with viruses, GABHS, and *M. tuberculosis.*[1] Other common bacterial pathogens may also be normal inhabitants of the upper respiratory passages or skin, and acute person-to-person transmission does not occur. Another source of infection may be contact with animals, such as with cat-scratch disease or toxoplasmosis after contact with a cat.[1, 3, 6]

Viruses

The most common causes of cervical lymphadenitis are summarized in Table 57–2. Seasonal respiratory viruses,

including parainfluenza virus, respiratory syncytial virus, and common cold viruses, cause acute cervical lymphadenitis in association with features of upper respiratory tract infection.[7a] Adenovirus infections may cause influenza-like symptoms or conjunctivitis.[7b] Enterovirus infections are seasonal (summer and fall) and may cause many systemic features or an exanthem.[7c] Herpes simplex virus (HSV) infections typically cause gingivostomatitis in association with cervical lymphadenitis.[7c] Human herpesvirus–6 (HHV-6), the agent known to cause roseola infantum, commonly causes acute cervical lymphadenitis.[8] Epstein-Barr virus (EBV) and cytomegalovirus (CMV) cause cervical and generalized lymphadenopathy in association with characteristic features of mononucleosis.[7d] These illnesses all have acute features that may persist for weeks. Human immunodeficiency virus (HIV) can cause cervical and generalized lymphadenitis at the time of initial infection.[9, 10] This may be followed by a chronic lymphadenopathy.[11] Viral infections are unlikely to cause suppurative adenitis.[1, 3]

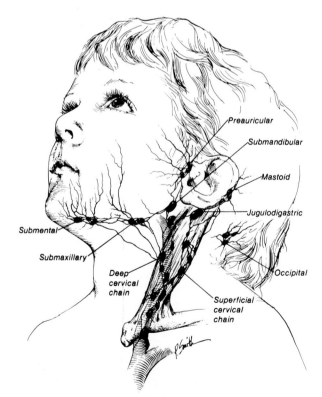

Figure 57–1. Cervical lymph nodes. (From Butler KM, Baker CJ: Cervical lymphadenitis. In: Feigin RD, Cherry JD [eds]: Textbook of Pediatric Infectious Diseases, 3rd ed. Philadelphia: WB Saunders Co, 1992, p 221.)

Table 57–1. CLINICALLY IMPORTANT AND READILY PALPABLE CERVICAL LYMPH NODES

Nodes	Location	Receive Drainage From	Drain To
Occipital	Proximal trapezius between occiput and mastoid process	Occipital scalp, superficial upper posterior neck	Deep cervicals
Postauricular (mastoid)	On mastoid process behind pinna	Parietal and temporal scalp, external auditory meatus, posterior pinna	Superficial cervicals
Preauricular (superficial parotid)	In front of tragus	Lateral eyelids, conjunctivae, temporal scalp, external auditory meatus, anterior pinna	Superficial cervicals
Jugulodigastric (tonsillar) and other upper deep cervical	At angle of jaw, below posterior digastric muscle	Palatine tonsils, tongue, pharynx	Lower deep cervicals
Superficial cervical	External surface of sternocleidomastoid muscle	Superficial tissues of neck, mastoid and preauricular nodes, submandibular nodes and glands	Deep cervicals
Submandibular (submaxillary)	Within submandibular fascial compartment, adjacent to salivary glands	Lateral lower lip, upper lip, nose, cheeks, medial eyelids, forehead, posterior mouth, gums, teeth, tongue, buccal and submental nodes	Superficial and deep cervicals
Submental	Between digastric muscles below myohyoid	Anterior tongue, central lower lip, floor of mouth, chin	Submandibular, deep cervicals
Lower deep cervical	Deep to sternocleidomastoid muscle below omohyoid muscle	Upper deep cervical nodes, back of scalp and neck, axillary nodes, skin of arm and pectoral region	Jugular lymphatic trunks, thoracic duct (on left), subclavian vein (on right)

Group A Beta-Hemolytic Streptococcus and *Staphylococcus aureus*

GABHS and *S. aureus* cause 53%–89% of cases of acute unilateral cervical lymphadenitis in children.[3] These two pathogens commonly cause suppuration. Older studies found that GABHS was the predominant pathogen, whereas later studies have found *S. aureus* to be more common, especially in young infants.[12] Both organisms colonize the upper respiratory tract prior to causing disease, GABHS in the nasopharynx and *S. aureus* in the anterior nares.[3] GABHS causes primary lymphadenitis, but *S. aureus* can cause primary disease as well as be a secondary invader after a viral or

GABHS infection.[3] Evidence for the latter scenario comes from data showing positive cultures growing *S. aureus* only in children who have serum evidence of an acute response to GABHS.[13]

Other Bacteria

Anaerobic bacteria, originating from the oral flora and associated with dental caries or gum disease, may cause acute suppurative lymphadenitis. Anaerobes known to cause lymphadenitis include *Bacteroides* species, *Peptococcus* species, *Peptostreptococcus* species, *Propionibacterium acnes*,

Table 57–2. COMMON INFECTIONS WITH CERVICAL LYMPHADENITIS

	Course of Disease		Lymph Node Involvement			
			Cervical Nodes			
Infection or Microorganism	Acute	Subacute or Chronic	Single or Unilateral	Bilateral	Suppuration	Generalized Adenopathy
Viruses						
Respiratory viruses	+			+		±
Adenovirus	+			+		+
Enterovirus	+			+		+
Cytomegalovirus	+	+		+		+
Epstein-Barr virus	+	+		+		+
Herpes simplex virus	+			+		
Human herpesvirus–6	+			+		
Human immunodeficiency virus	+	+		+		+
Bacteria						
Group A beta-hemolytic streptococcus	+		+	±	+	
Staphylococcus aureus	+		+		+	
Mycobacterium tuberculosis		+	+	±	+	±
Atypical *Mycobacterium* species		+	+		+	
Cat-scratch (*Bartonella henselae*)		+	+		±	
Anaerobic bacteria	+		+	±	±	
Protozoa						
Toxoplasmosis (*Toxoplasma gondii*)	+	+		+		+

+, usual feature; ±, occasional feature; blank, rare feature or never occurs.

and *Fusobacterium nucleatum*.[12] Anaerobic cultures require special laboratory techniques, and steps to detect them may not always be performed. The overall role of anaerobes, whether found singly or in mixed infections, has not been adequately determined.

Group B streptococcus causes sepsis with or without meningitis in newborns. It also causes a variety of focal infections. Rarely, it has been described as causing regional cervical lymphadenopathy with fever, submandibular cellulitis, and bacteremia in young infants.[14]

Mycobacteria

Atypical mycobacteria and *M. tuberculosis* are the most common causes of chronic, unilateral, suppurative cervical lymphadenitis (see Chapter 23). The most common species are *Mycobacterium avium-intracellulare, Mycobacterium chelonei, Mycobacterium scrofulaceum,* and *Mycobacterium malmoense*.[15–17]

M. tuberculosis lymphadenitis occurs after lymphatic or hematogenous spread from a primary pulmonary focus.[18] The reported coexistence of apparent pulmonary disease has varied widely, from 5% to 70%.[18] Tuberculous lymphadenitis is the most common extrathoracic manifestation of tuberculosis.[18] Atypical mycobacteria may be cultured from the mouths of healthy children.[1] Lymphadenitis due to these organisms is thought to arise from local invasion rather than systemic spread.[12] In developed countries, granulomatous cervical adenitis is most often caused by atypical mycobacteria.[15, 17, 19] The distinction between *M. tuberculosis* and atypical mycobacteria can usually be made from clinical features and response to the tuberculin skin test, as discussed later.

Cat-Scratch Disease

Cat-scratch disease is seasonal, with peaks in late autumn and winter.[20] Although this disease was initially reported as more common in children, a later report found that 43% of cases occurred in persons older than 20 years.[20] About 90%

of patients have a history of recent cat exposure (usually kittens).[20] Axillary lymphadenopathy is most common, followed by cervical involvement.[20] The pleomorphic, curved, gram-negative bacillus *Bartonella* (formerly *Rochalimaea*) *henselae* is now thought to be the predominant cause of the disease.[21] Antibodies to *B. henselae* have been found in 84% of patients, compared with only 3.6% of healthy controls.[20] This fastidious organism has been cultured from lymph nodes of patients with the disease and has been identified with polymerase chain reaction (PCR) and immunocytochemical labeling techniques. It has also been cultured from the blood of cats and amplified by PCR in fleas obtained from cats associated with human disease.[22]

Toxoplasmosis

Toxoplasma gondii is a ubiquitous protozoan that causes asymptomatic disease or chronic regional or generalized lymphadenopathy with or without a mononucleosis-like illness in immunocompetent older children and adults.[23] Immunocompromised patients, particularly those with HIV, often develop central nervous system disease, whereas multisystem congenital infection can occur in newborns of mothers who had primary disease during pregnancy.[23] The definitive host is the cat, and transmission of oocysts typically occurs from exposure to feces from acutely infected cats. Transmission can also occur from handling or ingesting undercooked meat or unpasteurized milk containing bradyzoites in tissue cysts. Rarely, transmission of tachyzoites or tissue cysts can occur with solid organ transplant or blood transfusion.

Other Infections

Many other microorganisms may cause cervical lymphadenitis. Uncommon diseases that commonly cause cervical lymphadenitis are listed in Table 57–3. Other diseases that uncommonly cause cervical lymphadenitis are listed in Table 57–4. For all of these conditions, characteristic clinical or laboratory features, apart from lymphadenopathy, are usually present, and a specific diagnosis can be made.

Table 57–3. UNCOMMON INFECTIONS WITH COMMON CERVICAL LYMPHADENITIS

Infection or Microorganism	Course of Disease		Lymph Node Involvement	
	Acute	Subacute or Chronic	Suppuration of Cervical Nodes	Generalized Adenopathy
Brucellosis (*Brucella* species)	+	+		+
Dengue fever (Dengue viruses)	+			+
Diphtheria (*Corynebacterium diphtheriae*)	+			
Group B streptococcus (*Streptococcus agalactiae*)	+			
Human herpesvirus–7	+			
Lyme disease (*Borrelia burgdorferi*)	+	+		+
Measles virus	+			+
Mumps virus	+			
Plague (*Yersinia pestis*)	+		+	+
Rat-bite fever (*Spirillum minus*)	+			+
Rubella virus	+			+
Secondary syphilis (*Treponema pallidum*)	+			+
Trypanosomiasis (*Trypanosoma* species)	+			+

+, usual feature; ±, occasional feature; blank, rare feature or never occurs.

Table 57–4. INFECTIONS WITH UNCOMMON CERVICAL LYMPHADENITIS

Infection or Microorganism	Course of Disease		Lymph Node Involvement	
	Acute	Subacute or Chronic	Suppuration of Cervical Nodes	Generalized Adenopathy
Actinomycosis (*Actinomyces* species)		+	±	
Anthrax (*Bacillus anthracis*)		+		+
Aspergillus species	+		±	
Candida species	+		±	
Coccidiomycosis (*Coccidioides immitis*)	+		±	
Enterobacteriaceae	+		±	
Leptospirosis (*Leptospira* species)	+			+
Nocardia species		+		
Pasteurella multocida	+			
Scrub typhus (*Rickettsia tsutsugamushi*)	+			+
Sporotrichosis (*Sporothrix schenckii*)		+		
Tularemia (*Francisella tularensis*)	+			+
Typhoid fever (*Salmonella typhi*)	+			+

+, usual feature; ±, occasional feature; blank, rare feature or never occurs.

PATHOLOGY

Lymph nodes are an integral part of the peripheral lymphoid system. They are encapsulated structures supplied with blood and lymphatic flow (Fig. 57–2).[24] Their functional cells include B lymphocytes, T lymphocytes, plasma cells, antigen-presenting cells, and macrophages.[25] Lymph nodes have three principal, interrelated functions.[24, 25] First, the macrophages remove particulate antigens, including microorganisms, as part of the nonspecific immune response. The other two functions are storage and proliferation of B lymphocytes and antibody production, and storage and proliferation of T lymphocytes. These last two functions are part of the adaptive immune response to produce antigen-specific humoral and cellular immunity.

Lymphadenopathy (lymph node enlargement) occurs when (1) intrinsic lymph node cells proliferate in response to infectious or inflammatory stimuli and/or (2) extrinsic leukocytes or neoplastic cells infiltrate and cause enlargement.[1] Lymphadenitis (lymph node inflammation) occurs as the result of edema with cellular infiltration and hyperplasia.[26, 27] Suppuration may occur. One or more nodes may be affected with cervical lymphadenitis, and there may be generalized lymph node involvement. The process is usually infectious, and it may be acute or chronic.

Acute cervical lymphadenitis most commonly occurs dur-

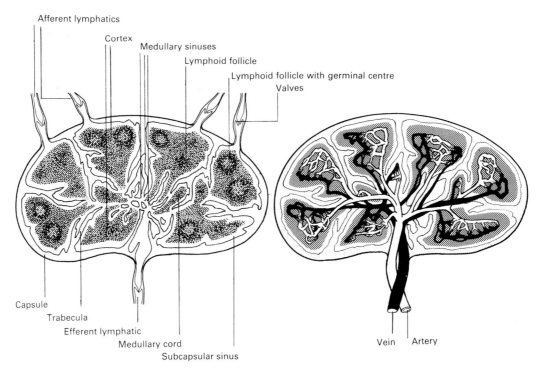

Figure 57–2. Lymph node anatomy. (From Wheater PR, Burkitt HG, Daniels VG: Functional Histology, 2nd ed. Edinburgh: Churchill-Livingstone, 1987, p 167.)

ing the response to direct drainage of microorganisms.[1, 3] The organism originates from the upper respiratory tract, mouth, or skin. Clinically evident infection at these sites of invasion may be present. Generalized lymphadenopathy occurs during the response to a systemic challenge to the immune system, typically a viral infection. In this case, the enlargement of individual lymph nodes occurs in response to circulating inflammatory mediators and leukocytes and/or to hematogenously spread microorganisms. Nonspecific or characteristic histopathologic patterns of lymphadenitis may occur (Table 57–5).[1, 3, 26, 27]

CLINICAL FEATURES

The clinical features of cervical lymphadenitis are diverse (see Tables 57–2 to 57–4). In addition to knowledge of the most likely infectious agents, consideration of several characteristic factors helps to determine the cause in each case. These factors are (1) duration of symptoms (acute, subacute, or chronic), (2) number of nodes involved (single, unilateral, regional, or generalized), (3) characteristics of enlarged lymph node(s) (lymphadenopathy, lymphadenitis, or suppurative lymphadenitis), (4) associated head and neck disease (oropharyngeal, dental, skin) or systemic disease, (5) specific risk exposure(s) (known contact with another case, unvaccinated, travel, animal), and (6) patient age.[1, 3, 6, 12]

Duration of Symptoms

Most patients present with acute symptoms of 1 or 2 days' duration. A subacute (more than 1 week of symptoms) or chronic (more than 3 weeks of symptoms) presentation is suggestive of viruses such as CMV, EBV, and HIV.[7] Mycobacteria, cat-scratch disease, toxoplasmosis, and some uncommon bacteria all can manifest as subacute or chronic symptoms.[7, 20]

Number of Nodes Involved

Many infections cause regional or generalized adenopathy. Thus, involvement of multiple lymph nodes is not a specific

finding. Common infections causing single or unilateral lymph node enlargement are discussed here.

Group A Beta-Hemolytic Streptococcus and *S. aureus*

The most common causes of acute, unilateral cervical lymphadenitis are GABHS and *S. aureus*.[1, 3, 12] There is no accurate way to determine on a clinical basis whether lymphadenitis is caused by either of the two organisms. *S. aureus* lymphadenitis may be more likely to suppurate, have slower resolution, and have a longer duration of symptoms prior to presentation. GABHS may be suspected if there is antecedent impetigo or, in young infants, the "streptococcus" syndrome, with coryza, low-grade fever, nasal discharge, and excoriation of the nares, as well as vomiting and anorexia.[1] Toxin-mediated invasive GABHS disease has only rarely been associated with cervicofacial disease.[28] Seventy percent to 80% of cases due to either organism occur in patients between the ages of 1 and 4 years. Both organisms most commonly cause primary involvement of a submandibular node (50%–60%), followed by involvement of upper cervical nodes (25%–30%) and, less commonly, by submental, occipital, and lower cervical nodes.[3] Approximately one fourth to one third of cases have suppuration, and 86% of these do so within 2 weeks of the onset of symptoms. Systemic symptoms and signs are uncommon unless there is cellulitis, a clinically apparent metastatic focus, or bacteremia. Antecedent upper respiratory symptoms occur in 40%. Lymphadenopathy elsewhere occurs in about a third of cases, although hepatosplenomegaly is rare.

Mycobacteria

The most common causes of subacute or chronic, unilateral cervical lymphadenitis are atypical mycobacteria and *M. tuberculosis*. The distinction between *M. tuberculosis* and atypical mycobacteria can usually be made from clinical features and response to the tuberculin skin test. All mycobacteria can cause suppurative lymphadenitis with spontaneous purulent drainage from the node. Systemic symptoms are usually absent, and the involved node, although fluctuant, is only mildly tender, with little other sign of inflammation.[3] However, children with *M. tuberculosis* are more likely to be at least 5 years old, to have bilateral cervical node

Table 57–5. PATHOLOGIC PATTERNS WITH INFECTIOUS CERVICAL LYMPHADENITIS

Pattern of Inflammation	Description	Example
Acute nonspecific	Prominent lymphoid follicles, with large germinal centers; macrophages may contain particulate debris Neutrophilic infiltrate Suppurative necrosis may occur	Pyogenic bacteria
Follicular hyperplasia	Enlarged germinal centers with mantle of normal B lymphocytes Centers contain activated B lymphocytes and macrophages	Viral Early human immunodeficiency virus
Interfollicular (paracortical) lymphoid hyperplasia	Enlarged paracortex, with activated T lymphocytes Mixed cellular infiltrate wtih macrophages and sometimes eosinophils	Viral
Mixed pattern	Elements of follicular, interfollicular, and nonspecific inflammation	Toxoplasmosis
Granulomatous with caseating necrosis	Aggregation of macrophages that are transformed into epithelium-like cells surrounded by collar of lymphocytes and plasma cells Central caseous necrosis may occur	Mycobacteria
Granulomatous without caseating necrosis	Follicular hyperplasia followed by formation of scattered stellate granulomas with necrosis and microabscesses	Cat-scratch disease

involvement or even generalized lymphadenopathy, to have a history of exposure to tuberculosis, and to reside in an urban setting.[15, 18, 19] Pulmonary disease has been reported in 5%–70% of patients with *M. tuberculosis* cervical adenitis but in only 0%–2% of patients with atypical mycobacteria.[3, 18] Finally, the tuberculin skin test (five tuberculin units of purified protein derivative [PPD]) often produces a small reaction (5–15 mm) in children with atypical mycobacteria, but virtually never more than 15 mm, as would be expected in patients with *M. tuberculosis*.[3, 17]

Cat-Scratch Disease

In many patients, a primary skin lesion (papule, pustule, or vesicle) occurs after 7–14 days at the site of innoculation.[22] One to two weeks later, tender lymphadenitis develops. A single node is involved in about half of cases, with regional or multiple site involvement in the remainder.[20] The diagnosis is usually made after about 1 week of lymph node enlargement, and the node(s) remain enlarged for 2–4 months, with a range up to 2 years, with no treatment.[22] Suppuration occurs in about 10% of cases. Fever occurs in about a third of cases, with other systemic features in 10%–15%, including anorexia, headache, weight loss, and splenomegaly. Rare manifestations include oculoglandular disease, encephalopathy, radiculitis, neuroretinitis, hepatic granulomas, and osteomyelitis.[22]

Characteristics of Enlarged Nodes

The distinction between enlarged, nontender nodes (lymphadenopathy) and tender, more distinctly inflamed enlarged nodes is nonspecific. However, as discussed previously and noted in the tables in this chapter, some infections are more likely to cause suppurative lymphadenitis with formation of a fluctuant node, which may spontaneously rupture or yield pus on aspiration. The most common causes of suppurative cervical lymphadenitis are shown in Table 57–3.

Associated Head and Neck Disease or Systemic Disease

Cervical lymphadenitis often develops secondary to another local condition. Exudative tonsillitis would suggest GABHS, whereas nonspecific nasopharyngitis would suggest viruses. Dental caries and gum disease are associated with anaerobic oral bacteria, including *Actinomyces* species. Gingivostomatitis occurs with HSV or enteroviruses. Oral thrush in an immunocompromised patient may precede fungal lymphadenitis. Impetigo, skin abrasions, or lacerations can be associated with GABHS and/or *S. aureus*. The presence of a single papule, vesicle, or pustule in the head or neck skin would suggest cat-scratch disease. An exanthem could occur with many viruses, but a maculopapular exanthem erupting soon after the defervescence of fever of several days' duration in a young infant would specifically suggest HHV-6.[8] Conjunctivitis can occur with viruses such as adenovirus and enteroviruses and also with cat-scratch disease.

Many infections that can cause cervical lymphadenitis have specific or nonspecific systemic symptoms and signs. The variety of these features is beyond the scope of this chapter.

Specific Risk Exposures

Most microorganisms causing cervical lymphadenitis are spread acutely from person to person. Some bacteria, such as *S. aureus* and atypical mycobacteria, may be part of the normal flora of the upper respiratory passages and may be carried asymptomatically for some time before causing disease.[3] Many infections are seasonal, and knowledge of the usual time of occurrence of infections helps in diagnosis.

Patients with underlying diseases may have unique predispositions to some infections. For example, persons with HIV infection may have acute or chronic lymphadenopathy directly caused by HIV.[9, 11] Alternatively, they may have CMV, *M. avium-intracellulare*, tuberculosis, or syphilis.[22, 29] Patients with immunodeficiency related to malignancies may have cervical lymphadenitis caused by fungi. Patients who are immunosuppressed after solid organ transplantation may have cervical and generalized lymphadenopathy related to CMV or EBV.

Cervical lymphadenitis may occur after exposure to animals, including arthropods.[1, 3] The most common are cat-scratch disease and toxoplasmosis with cat exposure. Toxoplasmosis may also result from ingestion of undercooked meats or unpasteurized milk as well as from blood transfusions and solid organ transplants. Other animal exposures to consider in determining the etiology of cervical lymphadenitis are domestic livestock and their products (brucellosis, leptospirosis, anthrax), dogs and cats (*Pasteurella* species, leptospirosis), and rats (rat bite fever, leptospirosis).[1, 3] Arthropod exposures to consider include mosquitos (dengue fever), ticks (Lyme disease, tularemia), rat fleas (plague), chiggers (scrub typhus), and kissing bugs (trypanosomiasis).[1, 3]

A history of recent travel may be of importance. Infections that are rarely or never acquired in the United States or Canada include brucellosis, dengue fever, plague, scrub typhus, trypanosomiasis, and typhoid fever.[7]

Age

Patient age is a nonspecific factor for many causes of lymphadenitis. However, some infections do characteristically present at certain ages. In neonates, the most common cause of acute unilateral lymphadenitis is *S. aureus*.[1] Group B streptococcus causes the uncommon "cellulitis-adenitis" syndrome with acute regional cervical lymphadenitis.[14]

During infancy, bacterial lymphadenitis is uncommon, and viral causes with acute regional and generalized lymph node involvement are most common. HHV-6, the agent known to cause roseola infantum, occurs at an average age of about 7 months. Cervical lymphadenopathy occurs in about 30% of cases. Other characteristic features are fever, maculopapular rash on the face and/or trunk after subsidence of the fever ("slapped cheeks"), diarrhea, cough, enanthem, and eyelid swelling.[8]

During the preschool age (1–4 years), viruses remain common. Acute unilateral adenitis caused by GABHS and *S. aureus* occurs most commonly from ages 1–4 years (70%–80% of all cases are caused by these bacteria). Atypical mycobacteria, causing subacute or chronic adenitis, most commonly occur in this age group.[3, 12]

In children of school age (5–18 years), viruses become less common, although EBV, the cause of infectious mononucleosis with generalized acute and subacute lymphadenopathy, becomes common. Other infections that commonly occur in this age group are *M. tuberculosis*, cat-scratch disease, anaerobic bacteria, and toxoplasmosis.[3, 6]

DIFFERENTIAL DIAGNOSIS

Lymph Node Disorders

The differential diagnosis of cervical lymphadenitis includes other conditions that can affect cervical lymph nodes, as well as other neck masses (Table 57–6). The most important noninfectious lymph node disorders to consider are neoplasms. Hodgkin's and non-Hodgkin's lymphomas are the most common, followed by neuroblastoma.[3, 16, 30] Leukemia and metastatic carcinoma occur rarely. In these conditions, lymphadenopathy is single or regional, is usually located in the posterior cervical region, is nontender, and manifests subacutely. Collagen vascular disorders such as juvenile rheumatoid arthritis and systemic lupus erythematosus may manifest as generalized lymphadenopathy as part of multisystem involvement.[3] Regional or generalized lymphadenopathy with or without systemic features of serum sickness has been reported with phenytoin therapy.[31] Other causes of serum sickness may produce lymphadenopathy. The syndrome of periodic fever associated with aphthous stomatitis, pharyngitis, and cervical adenitis (FAPA syndrome) has been described in children.[32] Symptoms are present for more than

1 year and may recur for up to 15 years. This condition is of uncertain etiology.

Cervical lymphadenopathy may also be caused by inflammatory disorders that are possibly infectious conditions. For example, Kawasaki disease is diagnosed as the presence of at least five of the following features: fever, rash, nonpurulent conjunctivitis, mucositis, extremity changes, and cervical lymphadenopathy ≥1.5 cm.[33] Most cases occur in children younger than 4 years. There is usually a single anterior cervical node involved, which may be mildly tender and erythematous but not fluctuant. Lymph node involvement occurs in 50%–75% of cases, may be bilateral, and rarely may cause massive neck swelling. An infectious etiology has long been postulated for Kawasaki disease, which has many features of a bacterial toxin superantigen–mediated disease. Microorganisms that have been implicated include toxin-producing *S. aureus* and parvovirus B19.[34]

Kikuchi's disease, first described in Japan in 1972, usually occurs in the third decade of life, predominantly in women, and consists of regional cervical lymphadenopathy, often associated with fever, antecedent flu-like symptoms, and leukopenia.[35] Generalized lymphadenopathy and hepatosplenomegaly are occasionally noted. The pathologic features include interfollicular hyperplasia with necrosis. The disease is self-limited with a subacute presentation and a course lasting several months. Resolution may be hastened by the excision of an involved node. An infectious etiology is thought most likely.

Other Neck Masses

Numerous neck masses apart from lymph nodes may enlarge and mimic adenopathy. Thyroid neoplasms are rare in children and usually can be distinguished from lymph nodes by their midline position. Congenital anomalies are the most common and can usually be distinguished by location and chronic symptoms; however, they may enlarge rapidly if they are secondarily infected.[3, 36] Thyroglossal duct cysts can occur anywhere in the midline of the neck above the thyroid, and they move when the tongue is protruded. Branchial cleft cysts and sinuses can develop from remnants of the embryonic cervical sinus, second pharyngeal pouch, or second branchial groove, most commonly the last. They are typically positioned at the upper anterior border of the sternocleidomastoid muscle. A skin dimple may be obvious, but secondary infection can produce an inflammatory mass that may have a draining sinus tract.

Cystic hygromas develop from isolated portions of the jugular lymph sac or mesenteric tissue that failed to establish connections with the main lymphatic channels. They usually arise in the lower third of the neck posterior to the sternocleidomastoid muscle. They form soft compressible masses and are often present at birth. They may increase in size with an upper respiratory infection owing to increased lymph flow. They may also become secondarily infected. Parotid inflammation can occur with viral infections such as mumps or parainfluenza virus, or with suppurative bacterial infections. The parotid can also enlarge with tumors. Parotid masses are usually distinguished from lymph nodes on the

Table 57–6. DIFFERENTIAL DIAGNOSIS OF CERVICAL LYMPHADENITIS

Lymph node disorders	
Kawasaki disease	
Neoplasms	Lymphoma (Hodgkin's and non-Hodgkin's), neuroblastoma, metastatic carcinoma
Collagen vascular disorders	Juvenile rheumatoid arthritis, systemic lupus erythematosus
Drugs	Phenytoin
Periodic fever with aphthous stomatitis, pharyngitis, and cervical adenitis (FAPA syndrome)	
Kikuchi's disease	
Other cervical masses	
Congenital	Branchial cleft cyst, thyroglossal duct cyst, cystic hygroma, epidermoid cyst
Parotid	Parotitis (viral or bacterial), tumor
Sternocleidomastoid	Hematoma, tumor
Other soft tissue	Actinomycosis

basis of the characteristic position of the parotid about the angle of the mandible, and by its larger size.

Sternocleidomastoid tumors or hematomas can mimic adenopathy because of their proximity to the superficial and deep cervical nodes, which run superficial and deep to the muscle. Such masses can usually be distinguished from nodes by their immobility. Cervicofacial actinomycosis causes chronic granulomatous suppurative infections. The *Actinomyces* species usually invade soft tissue via carious teeth.[37] Established infections spread slowly in a contiguous manner, across tissue planes. Lymphatic involvement is uncommon, although the characteristic swelling may be indistinguishable from an enlarged lymph node. The presentation is typically chronic, with a painless mass at the angle of the mandible; however, the mass may occur anywhere in the head and neck region. A sinus tract often develops.

DIAGNOSIS

The diagnostic evaluation of a patient with neck swelling has two primary purposes. First, the diagnosis of infectious cervical adenitis must be confirmed or ruled out, and second, the etiologic infectious agent may need to be identified to guide therapy and prognosis.

The history and physical examination often provide enough information to make a diagnosis of the probable etiology of cervical lymphadenitis. Factors to determine from the history are patient age, duration of symptoms, known infectious contacts, recent travel, animal exposure or ingestion of undercooked meats or unpasteurized milk, and underlying diseases. The physical examination should determine the following factors: location and characteristics of the enlarged lymph node(s); signs of inflammation in addition to swelling, including tenderness, erythema, and warmth; evidence of fluctuation; associated head and neck disease; and systemic features, including fever, generalized lymphadenopathy, rash, and hepatosplenomegaly.

There are three characteristic clinical presentations with cervical lymphadenopathy, as follows:

- An acute illness of several days' duration or less, at any age, with enlargement of numerous cervical nodes with or without generalized lymphadenopathy, and associated with features suggestive of an upper respiratory or systemic infection in a patient who is mildly unwell, is almost certainly caused by a virus. In most cases, no laboratory investigations are necessary either to confirm the diagnosis or to guide therapy.

- An acute illness, in a patient between 1 and 4 years of age, with enlargement of a single node that is tender, warm, and erythematous, in association with fever, tonsillitis, or impetigo but no dental abnormality, is likely caused by GABHS or *S. aureus*. If there is no fluctuation, overlying cellulitis, or systemic toxicity suggesting bacteremia or generalized disease, no laboratory investigations are necessary prior to a trial of therapy for 48–72 hours.

- A subacute or chronic illness, in a patient of any age after infancy, with enlargement of one or several unilateral, well-localized, nontender cervical nodes suggests a myco-

bacterial infection, cat-scratch disease, toxoplasmosis, or a malignancy. Less commonly, if there is a history of dental disease, travel, or animal exposure (including insects), an infection such as actinomycosis, brucellosis, or Lyme disease should be considered. In this case, an etiologic diagnosis is imperative.

Direct Diagnostic Tests

Needle aspiration, excisional biopsy, and incision and drainage are the procedures of choice for direct diagnosis of cervical adenitis.[1] With each procedure, the minimal microbiologic studies should include Gram's stain, acid-fast bacteria stain, and cultures for aerobic and anaerobic bacteria. If the clinical presentation is subacute or chronic or suggests etiologies other than pyogenic bacteria, investigations to consider include special stains for viruses (Giemsa), fungi, and *B. henselae* (Warthin-Starry silver stain). Cultures for mycobacteria, viruses, fungi, and *B. henselae* should also be performed. If an excisional biopsy is performed, histopathologic processing should include studies to determine the pattern of inflammation, which may be specific for a microorganism (see Table 57–5), and studies to detect a malignancy.

The child who presents with acute unilateral cervical lymphadenitis and has marked overlying cellulitis, is systemically unwell at presentation, or fails to show response to initial empirical antibiotic therapy after 24–48 hours should undergo needle aspiration to determine etiology. If the patient has a fluctuant node at presentation or after a trial of therapy, needle aspiration, incision and drainage, or excision should be performed for both diagnosis and therapy.

The patient who presents with subacute or chronic enlargement of one or several cervical nodes should have an excisional biopsy as a diagnostic procedure. If the diagnosis of atypical mycobacteria infection is made, the excisional biopsy is also the definitive therapeutic procedure.

Indirect Diagnostic Tests

Numerous indirect tests may support a specific diagnosis with cervical lymphadenitis. Throat cultures for bacteria (particularly GABHS) and viruses can be performed. Aspirates of dental abscesses or other head and neck abscesses help to identify other bacteria. Immunofluorescent studies for respiratory viruses can be performed on nasopharyngeal aspirates. Swabs of oral ulcers can be examined by electron microscopy, immunofluorescence, or viral culture to look for HSV. Blood cultures should be performed in patients who have fever and signs of systemic disease.

Serology may help determine acute or persistent infections. Paired serum specimens, collected at least 2 weeks apart, can be tested for total antibody or, if available, immunoglobulin G (IgG) and IgM antibodies. The presence of IgM antibodies and/or a fourfold rise in total titer over time usually indicates an acute infection. Serology is of particular importance to diagnose cat-scratch disease, toxoplasmosis, Lyme disease, syphilis, brucellosis, and viruses such as CMV, EBV, HHV-6, HIV, measles, mumps, and rubella.

Indirect serologic evidence of acute GABHS disease may be obtained by measuring the antibody response to extracellular products, i.e., antistreptolysin O titer. Other blood investigations that may be helpful to determine the nature of systemic disease include complete blood count, erythrocyte sedimentation rate, C-reactive protein, and liver function tests.

Skin testing to detect a delayed hypersensitivity reaction is most useful in the diagnosis of tuberculosis. The PPD test for tuberculosis may also react in individuals with atypical mycobacteria infections; however, the amount of reaction seldom exceeds 15 mm of induration, as discussed previously. Skin testing is no longer routinely available for the diagnosis of cat-scratch disease.

Some radiologic procedures may be helpful. A chest radiograph may show intrathoracic adenopathy or lung disease suggestive of tuberculosis or an anterior mediastinal mass suggestive of a malignancy. Ultrasound or computed tomography (CT) of the neck is not commonly performed but may be helpful to detect suppuration in a deep node not readily palpable on physical examination. Ultrasound or CT examination of the abdomen is useful to detect intraabdominal lymph nodes or to measure accurately liver and spleen enlargement, which is suggestive of generalized processes.

THERAPY

Treatment with antibiotics or surgery is necessary for acute pyogenic cervical lymphadenitis as well as for subacute and chronic disease caused by mycobacteria. Therapy may be considered for cat-scratch disease and toxoplasmosis. Treatment of other, uncommon causes of cervical lymphadenitis is guided by the knowledge of the specific etiology in each case.

The management of pyogenic cervical lymphadenitis is summarized in Table 57–7.[38] Other antimicrobials apart from those listed may be used. The suggested antimicrobials provide a choice between beta-lactams and alternatives, with consideration of agents with appropriate spectrums of activity (yet not too broad a spectrum) and reasonable cost. The decision whether to perform an initial needle aspiration for diagnosis or relief of symptoms depends on the severity of symptoms at presentation and the strength of desire to prove the etiology. Once antimicrobials have been provided for 48 hours or more, the likelihood of obtaining a positive culture from subsequent aspiration or incision and drainage diminishes considerably. Similarly, the decision to provide initial therapy with oral or intravenous antimicrobials depends on the severity of presenting clinical features. If the decision is made to start oral therapy (as is most often the case), it is imperative to ensure that appropriate medical follow-up will take place during the first 3 days of treatment. The total duration of antimicrobial therapy generally is 10–14 days, regardless of whether a surgical procedure is performed.[1, 3] Lymph node enlargement may persist for many weeks after antimicrobials are given; however, after a course of antibiotics, the involved lymph nodes are very likely sterile, and the persistent enlargement is a reflection of the resolution of local inflammatory response.[3]

Table 57–7. MANAGEMENT OF CERVICAL LYMPHADENITIS

Type and Severity	Management
Acute pyogenic	
Presumed group A beta-hemolytic streptococci or *Staphylococcus aureus* (GABHS)	
Moderate to severe systemic features, markedly enlarged node(s) with overlying cellulitis	Needle aspiration and
	IV cloxacillin, 200 mg/kg/day q6h (max 12 g/day), *or*
	IV cefazolin, 150 mg/kg/day q8h (max 6 g/day), *or*
	IV clindamycin, 40 mg/kg/day q6h (max 1.8 g/day), *or*
	IV vancomycin, 60 mg/kg/day q6h (max 4 g/day)
Mild systemic features, moderately enlarged node(s), no overlying cellulitis	PO cloxacillin, 100 mg/kg/day qid (max 4 g/day), *or*
	PO cephalexin, 50 mg/kg/day qid (max 4 g/day), *or*
	PO clindamycin, 30 mg/kg/day qid (max 2 g/day), *or*
	PO erythromycin, 40 mg/kg/day qid (max 2 g/day)
Suppuration at presentation or after trial of antibiotic therapy	Incision and drainage and IV antibiotics as above
Proven GABHS after aspiration or incision and drainage	IV penicillin G, 200,000 U/kg/day qid (max 20 MU/day), *or*
	PO penicillin VK, 50 mg/kg/day qid (max 3 g/day), *or*
	IV cefazolin *or* PO cephalexin *or* PO erythromycin
Proven *S. aureus* after aspiration or incision and drainage	IV or PO cloxacillin *or* IV cefazolin *or* PO cephalexin *or* IV or PO clindamycin *or* IV vancomycin
Presumed anaerobic infection	
Moderate to severe systemic features, markedly enlarged node(s) with overlying cellulitis	Needle aspiration and IV penicillin G *or* IV clindamycin
Mild systemic features, moderately enlarged node(s), no overlying cellulitis	PO penicillin V *or* PO clindamycin
Suppuration at presentation or after trial of antibiotic therapy	Incision and drainage and IV antibiotics as above
Mycobacteria infections	
Atypical mycobacteria	Surgical excision is curative and preferred
	Use of antimicrobials guided by sensitivity testing for specific organism
Mycobacterium tuberculosis	Isoniazid, 10 mg/kg/day OD (max 300 mg) × 6 months, *and*
	Rifampin, 20 mg/kg/day OD (max 600 mg) × 6 months, *and*
	Pyrazinamide, 25 mg/kg/day OD (max 2 g) × 2 months

Supportive measures in the therapy of pyogenic lymphadenitis include provision of analgesics and antipyretics. For pyogenic adenitis, periodic application of warm, moist dressings may hasten the localization of an abscess. Once an abscess has formed, incision and drainage of the node are necessary.

The treatment of choice for atypical mycobacterial adenitis is excision of the affected node(s). Excision is curative, with a low risk of recurrence.[17] In contrast, antituberculous therapy for 6 months is necessary for tuberculous adenitis.[39] This is because tuberculous adenitis is an extrapulmonary manifestation of tuberculosis, and medical therapy is necessary to maximize the systemic killing of *M. tuberculosis*.

Drug therapy is not necessary for most cases of cat-scratch disease, because symptoms are mild and spontaneous resolution occurs regardless of whether antimicrobials are provided. In patients in whom fever is persistent and systemic features are prominent (neurologic, hepatic, or musculoskeletal), it may be worthwhile to try a course of antimicrobial therapy. Agents that may be successful are ciprofloxacin, erythromycin, trimethoprim/sulfamethoxazole, and gentamicin for 1–2 weeks.[21, 40]

Toxoplasmosis in the immunocompetent host rarely requires treatment. However, in cases in which there is persistent lymphadenitis with fever and abdominal pain associated with elevation of liver enzymes, a course of therapy may be warranted.[23]

COMPLICATIONS

Local complications have been rare since the advent of antibiotics. The most common complication of cervical adenitis is suppuration with abscess formation. Spontaneous drainage through the skin may occur. Suppuration most commonly occurs with bacterial adenitis (see Table 57–2). Uncommon bacteria or fungi can also cause suppuration (see Tables 57–3 and 57–4). Chronic sinus tracts may form after mycobacteria infections. Local cellulitis and bacteremia may occur acutely with GABHS and *S. aureus* infections.

Very rarely, at a time distant from the acute course, a recurrence of pyogenic adenitis may occur. Such an event should prompt investigations to look for an undetected focus of untreated infection (i.e., osteomyelitis, endocarditis) or an underlying disorder that would predispose a patient to recurrent infections (i.e., chronic granulomatous disease).

The inflammatory process with cervical lymphadenitis occasionally causes acute torticollis.[41] Rarely, vascular complications such as internal jugular vein thrombosis, septic embolization, carotid artery rupture, mediastinal abscess, and purulent pericarditis may occur.[1]

References

1. Chesney PJ: Cervical adenopathy. Pediatr Rev 1994; 15: 276–284.
2. Herzog LW: Prevalence of lymphadenopathy of the head and neck in infants and children. Clin Pediatr 1983; 22: 485–487.
3. Butler KM, Baker CJ: Cervical lymphadenitis. In: Feigin RD, Cherry JD (eds): Textbook of Pediatric Infectious Diseases, vol 1, 3rd ed. Philadelphia: WB Saunders Co, 1992, pp 220–230.
4. Marcy SM: Cervical adenitis. Pediatr Infect Dis J 1985; 4: S23–S27.
5. Jeghers M, Clark SL Jr, Templeton AC: Lymphadenopathy and disorders of the lymphatics. In: Blacklow RS (ed): MacBryde's Signs and Symptoms: Applied Pathologic Physiology and Clinical Interpretation, 6th ed. Philadelphia: JB Lippincott Co, 1983, pp 467–534.
6. Swartz MN: Lymphadenitis and lymphangitis. In: Mandell GL, Bennett JE, Dolin R (eds): Principles and Practice of Infectious Diseases, vol 1. New York: Churchill-Livingstone, 1995, pp 936–944.
7a. Cherry JD: Pharyngitis (pharyngitis, tonsillitis, tonsillopharyngitis, and nasopharyngitis). In: Feigin RD, Cherry JD (eds): Textbook of Pediatric Infectious Diseases, vol 1, 3rd ed. Philadelphia: WB Saunders, 1992, pp 159–161.
7b. Cherry JD: Adenoviral infections. In: Feigin RD, Cherry JD (eds): Textbook of Pediatric Infectious Diseases, vol 2, 3rd ed. Philadelphia: WB Saunders, 1992, pp 1670–1687.
7c. Kohl S: Postnatal herpes simplex virus infections. In: Feigin RD, Cherry JD (eds): Textbook of Pediatric Infectious Diseases, vol 2, 3rd ed. Philadelphia: WB Saunders, 1992, pp 1558–1583.
7d. Sumaya CV: Epstein-Barr virus. In: Feigin RD, Cherry JD (eds): Textbook of Pediatric Infectious Diseases, vol 2, 3rd ed. Philadelphia: WB Saunders, 1992, pp 1547–1557.
8. Asano Y, Yoshikawa T, Suga S, et al.: Clinical features of infants with primary human herpesvirus 6 infection (exanthem subitum, roseola infantum). Pediatrics 1994; 93: 104–108.
9. Kinloch de Loës S, deSaussure P, Saurat J-H, et al.: Symptomatic primary infection due to human immunodeficiency virus type 1: Review of 31 cases. Clin Infect Dis 1993; 17: 59.
10. Clark SJ, Saag MS, Decker WD, et al.: High titers of cytopathic virus in plasma of patients with symptomatic primary HIV-1 infection. N Engl J Med 1991; 324: 954.
11. Pantaleo G, Graziosi C, Fauci AS: The immunopathogenesis of human immunodeficiency virus infection. N Engl J Med 1993; 328: 327.
12. Bodenstein L, Altman RP: Cervical lymphadenitis in infants and children. Semin Pediatr Surg 1994; 3: 134–141.
13. Yamauchi T, Ferrieri P, Anthony BF: The aetiology of acute cervical adenitis in children: Serological and bacteriological studies. J Med Microbiol 1980; 13: 37–43.
14. Baker CJ: Group B streptococcal cellulitis-adenitis in infants. Am J Dis Child 1982; 136: 631–633.
15. Benjamin DR: Granulomatous lymphadenitis in children. Arch Pathol Lab Med 1987; 111: 750–753.
16. Torsiglieri AJ, Tom LWC, Ross AJ, et al.: Pediatric neck masses: Guidelines for evaluation. Int J Pediatr Otorhinolaryngol 1988; 16: 199–210.
17. White MP, Bangash H, Goel KM, Jenkins PA: Non-tuberculous mycobacterial lymphadenitis. Arch Dis Child 1986; 61: 368–371.
18. Hopewell PC: Overview of clinical tuberculosis. In: Bloom BR (ed): Tuberculosis: Pathogenesis, Protection and Control. Washington, DC: American Society for Microbiology Press, 1994, pp 25–46.
19. Gill MJ, Fanning EA, Chomyc S: Childhood lymphadenitis in a harsh northern climate due to atypical mycobacteria. Scand J Infect Dis 1987; 19: 77–83.
20. Zangwill KM, Hamilton DH, Perkins BA, et al.: Cat scratch disease in Connecticut: Epidemiology, risk factors and evaluation of a new diagnostic test. N Engl J Med 1993; 329: 8–13.
21. Adal KA, Cockerell CJ, Petri WA: Cat scratch disease, bacillary angiomatosis, and other infections due to *Rochalimaea*. N Engl J Med 1994; 330: 1509–1515.
22. Fischer GW: Cat scratch disease. In: Mandell GL, Bennett JE, Dolin R (eds): Principles and Practice of Infectious Diseases, vol 1, 4th ed. New York: Churchill-Livingstone, 1995, pp 1310–1312.).
23. Wilson CB, Remington JS: Toxoplasmosis. In: Feigin RD, Cherry JD (eds): Textbook of Pediatric Infectious Diseases, vol 2, 3rd ed. Philadelphia: WB Saunders, 1992, pp 2057–2069.
24. Wheater PR, Burkitt HG, Daniels VG: Immune system. In: Functional Histology: A Text and Colour Atlas. Edinburgh: Churchill-Livingstone, 1987, pp 161–177.
25. Roitt IM, Brostoff J, Male DK: The lymphoid system. In: Immunology. St Louis: CV Mosby, 1993, pp 3.1–3.12.
26. Bonner H, Erslev AJ: The blood and lymphoid organs. In: Rubin E, Farber JL (eds): Essential Pathology, 2nd ed. Philadelphia: JB Lippincott, 1995, pp 551–594.
27. Cotran RS, Kumar V, Robbins SL: Diseases of white cells, lymph nodes, and spleen. In: Schoen FJ (ed): Robbins Pathologic Basis of Disease, 5th ed. Philadelphia: WB Saunders, 1994, pp 629–672.

28. Demers B, Simor AE, Vellend H, et al.: Severe invasive group A streptococcal infections in Ontario, Canada. Clin Infect Dis 1993; 16: 792–800.

29. Heller H, Fromowitz F, Fuhrer J: Luetic cervical adenitis in patients with human immunodeficiency virus type 1 infection. Arch Otolaryngol Head Neck Surg 1992; 118: 757–758.

30. Chua CL: The value of cervical lymph node biopsy: A surgical audit. Aust N Z J Surg 1986; 56: 335–339.

31. Butler JJ: Non-neoplastic lesions of lymph nodes of man to be differentiated from lymphomas. Natl Cancer Inst Monogr 1969; 32: 233–249.

32. Feder HM: Cimetidine treatment for periodic fever associated with aphthous stomatitis, pharyngitis and cervical adenitis. Pediatr Infect Dis J 1992; 11: 318–321.

33. Nadel S, Levin M: Kawasaki disease. Curr Opin Pediatr 1993; 5: 29–34.

34. Leung DYM, Meissner HC, Fulton DR, et al.: Toxic shock syndrome toxin-secreting *Staphylococcus aureus* in Kawasaki syndrome. Lancet 1993; 342: 1385–1388.

35. Tsang WYW, Chan JKC, Ng CS: Kikuchi's lymphadenitis: A morphologic analysis of 75 cases with special reference to unusual features. Am J Surg Pathol 1994; 18: 219–231.

36. Moore KL: The branchial apparatus. In: The Developing Human. Philadelphia: WB Saunders, 1977, pp 156–187.

37. Russo TA: Agents of actinomycosis. In: Mandell GL, Bennett JE, Dolin R (eds): Principles and Practice of Infectious Diseases, vol 2. New York: Churchill-Livingstone, 1995, pp 2280–2288.

38. Kowalczyk A, Smith J (eds): The 1994 Formulary of Drugs, 13th ed. Toronto: The Hospital for Sick Children, 1994.

39. Committee on Infectious Diseases: Tuberculosis. In: Peter G, Halsey NA, Marcuse EK, Pickering LK (eds): 1994 Red Book: Report of the Committee on Infectious Diseases, 23rd ed. Elk Grove Village, Illinois: American Academy of Pediatrics, 1994, pp 480–500.

40. Margileth AM: Antibiotic therapy for cat-scratch disease: Clinical study of therapeutic outcome in 268 patients and a review of the literature. Pediatr Infect Dis J 1992; 11: 474–478.

41. Bredenkamp JK, Maceri DR: Inflammatory torticollis in children. Arch Otolaryngol 1990; 116: 310–313.

Stephen A. Berger

Thyroid Infections

Infectious diseases of the thyroid gland are potentially life threatening, albeit rare. Indeed, standard textbooks of endocrinology and infectious diseases devote only a paragraph or two to these conditions.[1, 2] With the exception of a 1983 review article, the relevant literature consists largely of individual case reports and small series on bacterial,[3–115] actinomycotic,[116–121] gummatous,[122–126] mycobacterial,[127–149] fungal,[150–179] Pneumocystis,[180–191] and parasitic[192–212] infections.

HISTORY

Bacterial Infection

Bauchet published the first case report of "suppurative thyroiditis" in 1857,[213] and by 1911 Robertson had collected 96 cases from the world literature.[4] In 1928, Burhans summarized more than 200 reports of "acute thyroiditis" and added 80 of his own.[5] In retrospect, much of the early literature assumed that "acute thyroiditis" was primarily infectious in origin.[9–13, 214–228] Cases in which bacteriologic study of thyroid tissue was normal were thought to be infections in the early stages of development.[12]

During the 1920s it was believed that 60% of thyroiditis cases became suppurative[11, 12] and that the appearance of pus increases the mortality from thyroiditis to levels of 20%–25%.[11, 13, 217]

Tuberculous Thyroiditis

In 1861 Rokitansky stated that tuberculosis never involves the thyroid gland.[228] The first case report of tuberculous thyroiditis was published the following year,[229] but some authors suggest that the disease had been documented as early as 1847.[136] In 1893 thyroidal tuberculosis was first diagnosed antemortem,[133] and in 1894 the first tuberculous abscess of the gland was reported.[138]

Syphilis

In 1928 Henry examined the theory that myxedema is due to syphilis and is hereditary and added that one in three cases of Basedow's disease is due to syphilis.[230] Indeed, since spirochetes were first described in thyroid tissue in 1908, a wide variety of thyroid disorders have been ascribed to Treponema infection.[124]

In 1878 a relationship between hypothyroidism and congenital syphilis was first hypothesized, and by 1929 a number of authorities felt that pediatric endocrine disease was primarily syphilitic in origin.[231] It was said that syphilis serologic testing was positive in 12% of hypothyroid children.[232] In addition, Menninger was able to identify 40 cases of thyroid dysfunction due to acquired syphilis,[231] and others reported that as much as 50% of secondary syphilis in women was associated with painful thyroid swelling.[124, 233, 234]

By 1932 34 instances of hyperthyroidism due to congenital syphilis had also been reported,[124, 235] and goiter associated with positive syphilis serology was said to respond favorably to antisyphilis therapy (which often included iodides).[126, 234] Gummas of the thyroid gland were first described in 1879.[233] Seventeen thyroidal gummas were reviewed in 1907 (of which only five had histologic evidence for diagnosis)[236]; by 1918 23 cases had been published.[125]

Parasitic Diseases

Thirty-one cases of thyroidal echinococcosis had been published by 1915,[198] but only sporadic reports have appeared in recent years.

ANATOMY, FUNCTION, AND DEVELOPMENT

The thyroid is a highly vascular gland consisting of two lobes connected by an isthmus. The proximity of the trachea, parathyroid glands, esophagus, recurrent laryngeal nerve, and vital blood vessels underlines the significance of infection in the thyroid gland. In addition to its normal position in the anterior neck, accessory tissue may be found in the tongue, mediastinum, or other structures. Lingual thyroid tissue is a remnant of the embryonal median tubular diverticulum, which grows downward and bifurcates to form the adult thyroid. Remnants of this tube may persist in the form of a thyroglossal duct. Contiguous fistulae arising from the pyriform laryngeal sinuses may extend to the thyroid capsule or parenchyma and serve as foci for infection. These structures extend from fossae in the laryngeal inlet, bounded by the aryepiglottic folds, thyroid membrane, and thyroid cartilage.[237] In rare instances, pyriform sinus fistulae actually facilitate spontaneous drainage of the abscess cavity.[89]

In addition to their importance in metabolism, thyroid hormones mediate the systemic response to infectious diseases.[238, 239] The rarity of thyroid infection has been ascribed to the unique anatomic isolation of the gland and its rich system of drainage for blood and lymph. High concentrations of iodine-containing chemicals may also exert a local antibacterial effect.[5, 233]

PATHOPHYSIOLOGY

Bacterial Infection

In 1931, Womack and Cole found that inoculation of staphylococci or streptococci into the carotid arteries of dogs failed to produce thyroid infection.[240] Infection via a lymphatic route has been suggested by some authors[5]; others favor the possibility of hematogenous infection.[17, 18]

The most common determinant of thyroid infection is preexisting thyroid disease.[4, 11] In such cases, infection generally involves only the previously diseased area of thyroid. Suppurative thyroiditis may also originate from a patent thyroglossal fistula[5, 6, 20–22] or ruptured thymic[95] or branchial cleft cyst,[241] perforation of the esophagus by a foreign body[22] or malignancy,[90, 109] a postoperative stitch sinus,[242] or extension from surrounding cervical tissues.[23] Nevertheless, the gland appears relatively resistant to direct inoculation of bacteria. Thus, although wound infection follows 0.3%–2.4% of thyroid operations,[243] postoperative infection of the gland itself has not been described.

More than 65 cases of thyroid abscess have resulted from infection through a pyriform sinus fistula, all reported since 1980.[83, 86, 89, 92, 97, 100, 105, 109, 111, 237, 244–250] Although bilateral infections have been reported, virtually all such cases involve the left lobe (the reason for this is not known).[246] In many cases such infections are localized to the parathyroid space.[97] Recurring infection through pyriform sinus fistulae is particularly common (89%[102]) among children with thyroid abscess.[86, 92, 102, 237, 251]

Tuberculosis and Aspergillosis

The pathogenesis of thyroid tuberculosis is ill-understood, but most cases appear to be associated with disseminated infection.[128] Seven percent of miliary tuberculosis cases are associated with multiple thyroidal granulomas.[127, 133] Other pathologic forms include goiter with caseation, cold abscess, chronic fibrosing thyroiditis, gumma-like lesions,[252] and, least common, acute abscess.[132] Women are affected most often.[122] *Aspergillus* is thought to infect the thyroid hematogenously, perhaps as emboli originating from infected pulmonary veins.[153] Focal abscesses, patchy hemorrhagic lesions due to vascular invasion, or diffuse necrotizing thyroiditis is seen.[253] Some cases have occurred following thyroid adenomas or Hashimoto's thyroiditis.[166, 253]

Systemic Infections

A variety of nonthyroidal infections may affect the thyroid gland. For example, chronic mucocutaneous candidiasis and other congenital syndromes[254] are associated with hypothyroidism, as are rare instances of acquired *Candida* folliculitis.[255] Excessive exposure to x-rays in the course of tuberculosis may induce thyroid tumors,[256] whereas iodine 131 therapy may promote tinea corporis of the overlying skin.[257] Anti-infective agents can alter thyroid function and laboratory results of tests for thyroid hormones: antiseptics containing iodine,[258–260] iodoquinol, potassium iodide, clio-quinol,[261] interferon alpha-α (used in chronic viral hepatitis),[262, 263] cotrimoxazole,[264] and fluconazole.[265] Drugs used in the treatment of thyroid disease (e.g., methimazole) may induce agranulocytosis, with resulting systemic infection.[266, 267]

Infection may affect thyroid function without overt invasion of the gland.[268–270] Autoimmune thyroiditis is associated with a variety of viruses and bacteria (most notably *Yersinia enterocolitica*).[271–276] Human T-lymphotrophic virus type 1 (HTLV-1) or a related retrovirus[277] may play a role in the development of antithyroid antibody,[278] Hashimoto's thyroiditis,[279, 280] Graves's disease, or Graves's disease–associated uveitis.[281, 282] The better-known retrovirus human immunodeficiency virus (HIV) appears to have little effect on thyroid function in all but advanced cases of AIDS.[283–289] Altered thyroid function in these patients should alert the physician to the possibility of concurrent thyroid malignancy[290]; opportunistic infection of the thyroid, pituitary, or hypothalamus by infectious agents[167, 168, 180, 184, 186, 291–295]; or Kaposi's sarcoma.[296] Low serum levels of tri-iodothyronine (T$_3$) carry a poor prognosis for those with *Pneumocystis carinii* pneumonia.[297]

Cytokines generated during severe infection (notably interleukin-6) may interfere with the normal thyroid reaction to stress,[298] either directly or through effects on the pituitary gland.[299, 300] In general, infection is associated with a reduction in thyroid-stimulating hormone (TSH) secretion, thyroid-binding globulin (TBG)–binding activity, and serum levels of thyroxine (T$_4$) and free T$_3$.[268]

MICROBIOLOGY

Bacteria

Bacteria were seen in gram-stained pus from 89.5% of thyroid abscesses and were cultured in 92%. Blood cultures were positive in 40%, and seven papers describe drainage of sterile pus.

The pathogens identified most frequently were staphylococci (principally *Staphylococcus aureus*), which were found in 33% of culture-positive specimens. Aerobes or facultative organisms alone were isolated from 83.9% and were mixed with anaerobic bacteria in 3.6%. At least 16 reports described a foul or putrid infection, associated with aerobic bacteria or sterile pus. Seven cases of anaerobic thyroiditis followed infections that did not involve the thyroid gland, including postabortal septicemia, urinary tract infection, subphrenic abscess, pilonidal abscess, and perforation of the esophagus. In five instances gas was seen on cervical radiographs prior to drainage; in one, a colon carcinoma was diagnosed subsequent to drainage of a thyroid abscess caused by *Clostridium septicum*.[48] An association of this species with bowel cancer subsequently was described.[301] No other relationship was apparent between bacteria species and clinical presentation or prognosis.

As of 1903 18 different bacterial species had been isolated from infected thyroid tissue.[11] The most common ones were those associated with typhoid fever, puerperal sepsis (presumed streptococci), and pneumococcal pneumonia. Eight cases of thyroidal gas gangrene were reported before 1911.[4]

By 1927 the most frequent isolates were staphylococci, streptococci, and *"Bacillus coli" (Escherichia coli).*[66]

Although *Salmonella* thyroiditis no longer is common, 16 cases of thyroidal typhoid had been reported before 1925,[12] and 40 cases of *Salmonella* thyroiditis by 1951.[31] One study described 40 instances of thyroiditis in 73 patients who had typhoid fever.[11] Thyroidal *Salmonella* infections have continued to be reported in recent years.[92–94, 96, 99, 251, 302, 303]

Other unusual pathogens have included *Brucella melitensis,*[304] *Eikenella corrodens,*[101, 112, 114, 305] *Capnocytophaga ochracea,*[105] *Clostridium perfringens,*[113] *Fusobacterium* species,[102] and *Actinobacillus actinomycetemcomitans.*[33]

Mycobacteria and *Actinomyces*

As early as 1908 it was observed that only 3 of 103 specimens of "tuberculous" thyroid tissue contained identifiable mycobacteria, and 6 additional ones were associated with viable bacteria at distant sites only (lung, bone, neck).[306] A review published in 1926 could cite only three reports of bacteriologically proven tuberculous thyroiditis in the world literature.[307] Using such criteria, 26 cases of mycobacterial thyroiditis were identified in the English language literature since 1900 (24 due to *Mycobacterium tuberculosis,* and one each due to *Mycobacterium chelonei* and *Mycobacterium intracellulare*). Four of the cases reviewed were characterized by sterile caseating thyroid granulomas in patients with pulmonary or miliary tuberculosis[128, 143] or mediastinal lymphadenitis.[149] Interestingly, both patients with atypical mycobacteriosis were 4-year-old girls, and both were treated successfully with drainage and antituberculosis medications.[61, 139]

Biopsy-proven actinomycotic thyroiditis was first reported in 1931.[121] The patient was treated successfully with injections of potassium iodide and novocaine. Two of the five additional cases of localized or disseminated actinomycosis involving the thyroid gland affected agricultural workers.[118, 119] Two additional patients initially were thought to have thyroid malignancy.[116, 119]

Fungi and Parasites

Of 42 instances of fungal thyroiditis 29 were due to *Aspergillus* species, three to *Coccidioides immitis,* two to *Candida,*[164, 177] two to *Cryptococcus neoformans,*[168, 169] one to *Histoplasma capsulatum,*[171] one to mixed *Aspergillus* and *Candida* organisms,[172] and one each to *Scedosporium inflatum,*[173] *Cunninghamella bertholletiae,*[175] *Trichosporon capitatum,*[179] and *Allescheria boydii.*[165] The thyroid is occasionally involved in echinococcosis, disseminated strongyloidiasis,[203] and cysticercosis.[194]

Agents of Reactive Thyroiditis

Thyroiditis and thyroid dysfunction have been associated with several viruses: measles,[308] rubella,[309–311] influenza,[312] adenovirus,[313, 314] echovirus,[312] mumps,[315] cytomegalovirus (acquired[316] and congenital[317]), St. Louis encephalitis,[318] and infectious mononucleosis.[319–321] Most cases of subacute (DeQuervain's) thyroiditis occur during the summer and follow a prodrome of upper respiratory inflammation. The condition is often heralded by malaise, myalgia, and fatigue, and thyroid biopsy reveals infiltration by lymphocytes and giant cells.[1, 322] Although rising serologic titers to a variety of viruses have been documented, viral inclusions have not been demonstrated in thyroid tissue.[1]

A viral cause has also been proposed for malignant thyroid lymphoma,[323] and various case reports have implicated malaria,[315] Q fever,[324] streptococcal toxins,[315] psittacosis,[325] cat-scratch disease,[326] infection by *Mycoplasma,*[327] and other common bacteria,[328] African trypanosomiasis,[201, 202] paracoccidioidomycosis,[329] and malacoplakia[330] in thyroid dysfunction.

EPIDEMIOLOGY

Bacterial Infection

Thyroid abscesses accounted for 0.1%–0.72% of thyroid operations reviewed between 1931 and 1955.[5, 7, 8] Using strict criteria for infection, Hawbaker[14] and Horine[15] identified a total of 144 cases of suppurative thyroiditis in the world literature before 1933, 24 of which had occurred during the two decades immediately preceding publication of their papers.

Virtually all *noninfectious* thyroid diseases are more common in women than in men. Since infection rarely occurs in a normal gland, women with preexisting thyroid disease constitute the group most likely to develop thyroid infection.[5, 11, 18, 25] The fact that most infections involve the left lobe may reflect the anatomy of the pyriform sinuses and the proximity of this lobe to the esophagus.

Acute bacterial infections of the thyroid have been described in patients ranging in age from 7 weeks[237] to 80 years. The mean age among adults was 32.8 years (30.6 years for males and 35.1 for females). The world literature from 1906–1973 includes 35 cases of suppurative thyroiditis in children.[49] Although earlier reviews stressed a peak incidence between ages 20 and 40 years,[5, 24] only 28% of cases fell into this age group. Women account for 53%–65% of reported patients.[4, 5, 24]

Tuberculous Thyroiditis

Thyroidal tuberculosis was described in 0.1% of 20,758 tissue specimens examined at the Mayo Clinic[306] but in only 2 of 74,393 specimens examined elsewhere.[127] A third study claimed that tuberculous tissue was found in 21 of 2114 partial thyroidectomies.[331] Seventy-three such cases had been reported before 1926,[134] and by 1934 225 had been reported (including 27 tuberculous abscesses).[137] Klassen and Curtis reviewed 130 instances of tuberculous thyroid abscess reported before 1945.[136] In retrospect, the majority of such diagnoses were based solely on the finding of lymphocytic infiltration or granulomas.[228, 229, 307, 332–337]

Fungal and Parasitic Infections

Thirty-one instances of fungal thyroiditis had been identified in the world literature as of 1981. From 1951 to 1971, 53 patients with disseminated aspergillosis were identified at Memorial Sloan-Kettering Hospital[156, 162]; 6 of them had thyroid infection. Other investigators have found infection of the thyroid in 20%–36% of such patients.[158, 166, 253] Immune deficiency may also predispose to thyroid infection by *P. carinii;* at least 13 such cases have been documented.[176, 180, 183, 187, 188, 190]

Echinococcosis was reported to involve the thyroid gland in 1 of 112 patients seen in Iran[338] and 3 of 296 in Iraq[195]; the thyroid was not involved in any of 596 cases of echinococcosis reported in the United States between 1822 and 1965.[338]

CLINICAL MANIFESTATIONS

Concurrent and Predisposing Illness

Sixty-one percent of adults with bacterial infection had a history of thyroid disease: 35% goiters or "enlargement," 8.8% adenomas, 7.0% nodular goiters, 5.3% miscellaneous lesions (cancer, thyroiditis, thyroid nodule), and 16.2% unspecified disease. Such disorders were slightly more common among female patients than males (70% versus 53%, respectively) and had been present for periods ranging from 2 to 24 years before the onset of infection. Infection was generally localized to the diseased lobe or nodule. An association between infection and preexisting tumor is also characteristic of pituitary abscess.[339]

In some cases, infection was preceded by pyelonephritis,[11, 44] gastroenteritis,[94] prostatitis,[11, 44, 68] brain abscess,[23] esophageal perforation by fish or chicken bones,[22] ulcerative glossitis,[70] otitis,[16] mastoiditis,[23] intestinal vascular compromise,[38] pleuropulmonary infection,[16, 38, 54] postpartum sepsis,[35] pilonidal[98] or subphrenic abscess,[14] erysipelas,[46] dental infection,[144] regional cancer,[32] or abnormal cervical fistula.[5, 6, 8, 19–21] The most commonly implicated nidus for infection was a previous regional infection or pharyngitis.[102] In one instance, suppurative thyroiditis followed diphtheria.[4]

Most fungal infections, including 86% of those due to *Aspergillus* organisms, were associated with generalized dissemination and immune compromise: leukemia,[170, 172–175, 177, 179] AIDS,[167, 168] and diabetes mellitus.[169, 171] Virtually all *P. carinii* infections have occurred in patients with AIDS, usually in the setting of pentamidine prophylaxis (which presumably achieves therapeutic levels in lung tissue but not in thyroid and other organs).[180] Interestingly, one of the first reported cases was associated with thymic alymphoplasia in the pre-AIDS era.[190]

Symptoms (Table 58–1)

The duration of symptoms before the diagnosis of acute bacterial infection ranged from 1 to 180 days (mean 18 days). Most acute bacterial infections were characterized by fever, pain, tenderness, and dysphagia. Absence of fever

Table 58–1. CLINICAL CHARACTERISTICS OF INFECTIOUS THYROIDITIS

	Bacterial Infection	Tuberculous Infection
Number	262	26
Male-female ratio	1.25:1	1:1
Age		
Mean	32.8 years	36.2 years
Range	7 weeks–81 years	41 days–79 years
Diseased lobe (%)*		
Right	14.9	34.6
Left	57.5	26.9
Isthmus	4.4	7.7
Bilateral	21.5	7.7
Unspecified	1.7	23.1
Signs/symptoms (%)		
Pain	99.2	50.0
Tenderness	94.0	71.4
Fever	92.0	50.0
Dysphagia	91.0	62.5
Erythema	82.0	40.0
Dysphonia	82.0	75.0
Local warmth	70.0	0

*Percentage of patients for whom information is recorded.

was not related to age, sex, symptoms, bacterial species, or survival. Other clinical and bacteriologic variables were not associated with specific locations. Dysphonia and stridor[85] were previously ascribed to compression of local structures, including the recurrent laryngeal nerve.[18]

The classic presentation of pain, swelling, hoarseness, and dysphagia was stressed as early as 1903.[11] Subsequently, fluctuance was reported in 38.8% of cases; however, it is possible that additional cases of nonfluctuant thyroiditis were noninfectious in origin.[16] Rarely, thyroid abscess may present as a pulsatile mass.[107] Two additional signs, reported in 1917, were ascribed to pressure on neck muscles: limitation of cervical extension and involuntary depression of the chin on swallowing.[52]

Concurrent pharyngitis or pharyngeal pain was present in 69% of bacterial thyroiditis cases and in all but one of the cases associated with group A streptococci. The incidences of fever, dysphonia, dysphagia, and dermal erythema in this series were higher than those described previously[5]; this might reflect differences in inclusion criteria.

Symptoms among patients with tuberculous thyroiditis had been present for a mean interval of 105 days before diagnosis (range, 2 weeks to 1 year); this is in sharp contrast to the mean of 18 days' duration for patients with acute bacterial thyroiditis. Fever, pain, and tenderness are less common in tuberculous infection than in suppurative thyroiditis (see Table 58–1).[3]

Physical Findings

In most cases infection was either limited to the left thyroid lobe or bilateral. Isolated left lobe infection was identified in 43% of female patients and 28% of males. Tenderness, dermal erythema, and local warmth were more often seen with bacterial infection and less often with tuberculous thyroiditis.

Thyroid gummas were not associated with fever, pain,

pharyngitis, erythema, or local heat, but symptoms of compression were common. Patients with thyroid echinococcosis ranged in age from 6 months to 40 years; however, most were young adults. Chandra and Prakash state that females are affected twice as often as males.[192] The lesions are chronic (1.5 months–35 years), and abdominal calcifications or eosinophilia was documented in only four patients. In fact, thyroidal echinococcosis is often diagnosed as "goiter" before excision.

P. carinii thyroid infection has no specific clinical features. Most patients have presented with diffuse, tender "goiter"[180] in the setting of AIDS.

Differential Diagnosis

The differential diagnosis of thyroid pain and swelling includes malignancy, intracystic hemorrhage, and subacute thyroiditis.[148, 314, 340–343] Rare instances of painful Hashimoto's thyroiditis have also been described.[344] Some features of hyperthyroidism may mimic local or systemic infection,[345] whereas painless infected lesions may simulate thyroid carcinoma.[100, 146, 207] Both thyroid tuberculosis and subacute thyroiditis may present as "fever of unknown origin."[346, 347]

Histologic changes suggestive of tuberculosis are found in several unrelated conditions, including thyroid sarcoidosis,[348] granulomatous syphilis,[125] "parenchymatous giant cell granulomas,"[349] Hashimoto's thyroiditis ("hyperthyroid tuberculous thyroiditis"),[336] carcinoma,[143] and simple invagination of thyroid epithelial nests.[350] Although some authors believe that the histologic changes are sufficiently characteristic of this disease, most now require bacteriologic confirmation.[351]

Review of six thyroid gummas reported in the English-language literature since 1900 suggests that this entity may mimic other slow-growing lesions of the gland.[122]

DIAGNOSIS

Laboratory Findings

Leukocytosis exceeding 10,000 cells per microliter was present in 73% of patients at the time of diagnosis. Anaerobic infection, "foul pus," or a thyroid air-fluid level was present in most patients who did not exhibit leukocytosis; however, a normal leukocyte count apparently was not related to prognosis, as all such patients survived.

Thyroid function studies were normal during 75% of infection episodes. In 21.4%, at least one test result suggested hyperthyroidism, whereas 3.6% demonstrated depression of serum protein-bound iodine (PBI) concentration. Older papers reported elevation of the basal metabolic rate during 92% of episodes and depression in 8%. The serum concentrations of T_3, T_4, and TSH were normal in 80%, 88%, and 92.3%, respectively. Some 58% of the patients were characterized as clinically hypothyroid during the course of thyroiditis, and the remaining 42% appeared to be euthyroid. Thyroid uptake of iodine 131 was elevated in 11.5% of cases, depressed in 42.3%, and normal in 46.2%.

Several patients with thyroidal *P. carinii* infection have been characterized as hypothyroid[180, 183]; however, the underlying disease (AIDS) may have affected thyroid function in some instances. In one case, hyperthyroidism was the presenting manifestation of extrapulmonary *Pneumocystis* infection.[185]

These data are difficult to assess, since preexisting thyroid disease had been present in most cases and baseline studies were not recorded. When present, a chemical abnormality may reflect a nonspecific reaction of the thyroid to the stress of infection rather than damage to the gland itself; nevertheless, some authors have suggested a direct role for thyroid necrosis in the elevation of PBI concentration.[43]

Aspiration and fine needle aspiration may be helpful in establishing an etiologic diagnosis[145, 146, 168–170, 180, 182, 183]; however, rarely, this procedure may *cause* infection.[352]

Imaging

Plain roentgenograms are not helpful in establishing an infectious cause for acute thyroiditis, with the occasional exception of gas-forming infection or calcification (related to *Echinococcus* cysts—and rarely *Pneumocystis* infection[181]). Computed tomography offers more precise mapping of the infectious lesion.[353–355] Barium swallow is extremely helpful in demonstrating pyriform sinus fistulae.[86, 97] Using microlaryngoscopy a probe may then be inserted into the fistula to facilitate subsequent removal.[92, 111, 248]

Radionuclide scans of the thyroid are both sensitive and reliable in the evaluation of infectious thyroiditis. Ninety percent of patients for whom information was recorded were found to have a "cold area" in the infected thyroid lobe, which in most instances resolved following therapy. All of 60 pediatric cases were characterized by a positive scan.[102] Ultrasonography has been used to define cystic lesions[107, 356, 357] and rule out the possibility of contiguous cervical abscess.[358] Technetium 99 is useful in demonstrating functional thyroid tissue[97] and distinguishing acute from subacute inflammation.[106] Although gallium 67 accumulates in both the abscess and surrounding inflammatory tissue,[170, 177, 359] such scans may not distinguish between tumor and infection.[360] Indium 111 has also been used to pinpoint infectious lesions.[361]

TREATMENT

Although there was no significant difference in course of illness or survival among patients treated for bacterial thyroiditis with drainage or antimicrobial agents, it would seem prudent to drain any collections thoroughly and administer antimicrobial agents directed against identified or suspected pathogens.

COMPLICATIONS

Residua of infection were unusual and included vocal cord paralysis,[18] transitory hypothyroidism (occasionally requiring replacement therapy),[24, 42, 45] myxedema,[81] progression to pericarditis,[26] disruption of regional sympathetic nerves,[18] recurrence of as many as 12 episodes,[21, 74, 97] and rheumatic fever (following streptococcal thyroiditis).[362]

Death from bacterial thyroiditis has been ascribed to pneumonia,[69] tracheal obstruction[16] or perforation,[75] metastatic infection,[5] concurrent sepsis (postabortal or osteomyelitic),[35] rupture of a thyroid abscess,[16, 35, 62] and mediastinitis due to infection of intrathoracic thyroid tissue.[50, 363] In other instances, death immediately followed either tracheostomy or incision and drainage of the thyroid.[11, 16]

Residua are rarely noted following tuberculous thyroiditis; however, recurrent laryngeal paralysis has been described.[130] Rare instances of ulceration,[123] myxedema,[233] and pressure on local structures[123] have been attributed to thyroid gummas. Complications of thyroid echinococcosis have included suffocation, vocal cord paralysis, hemorrhage, and tracheal perforation.[192]

PROGNOSIS

The reported mortality rate for cases of bacterial infection was 9%. Most deaths occurred in patients who were not treated for the infection. In two instances, intrathoracic pain and cough had apparently misdirected diagnostic efforts.[57] Fatal cases did not differ from others with respect to patient age or sex, bacteriology, duration of infection before therapy, or clinical presentation.

Mortality from infections covered by this review is somewhat lower than that quoted during the preantibiotic era (11.4%–25%).[4, 5, 11, 13] Although these differences may be related to the subsequent availability of antimicrobial agents, case selection, and definition of infection, certain complications described previously were not encountered in the English-language literature (e.g., esophageal rupture and internal jugular phlebitis).

Three of the four fatal cases of tuberculous thyroiditis were ascribed to miliary tuberculosis,[128, 137, 147] one following resection of infected thyroid tissue.[128] The fourth patient had received no antituberculosis medication, and thyroid tuberculosis was first discovered at autopsy.[127] No fatal cases of thyroid echinococcosis were identified among the cases reviewed; however, other authors have described two deaths from suffocation and a surgical mortality rate of 1 in 30 patients.[193]

PREVENTION

The common association of bacterial thyroiditis with pyriform sinus fistula suggests that a barium swallow study be performed in all patients, particularly children and persons with recurrent infection. Since thyroiditis due to *Aspergillus* is often first diagnosed at autopsy in cases of disseminated infection, it would seen prudent to examine the gland carefully in all patients with aspergillosis and to perform imaging studies if possible.

References

1. Larsen PR, Ingbar SH: The thyroid gland. In: Wilson JD, Foster DW (eds): Williams Textbook of Endocrinology, 8th ed. Philadelphia: WB Saunders, 1992, pp 478–480.
2. Chow AW: Infections of the oral cavity, neck and head. In: Mandell GL, Bennett JE, Dolin R (eds): Mandell, Douglas and Bennett's Principles and Practice of Infectious Diseases, 4th ed. New York: Churchill Livingstone 1995, p 604.
3. Berger SA, Zonszein J, Villamena P, et al.: Infectious diseases of the thyroid gland. Rev Infect Dis 1983; 5: 108–122.
4. Robertson WS: Acute inflammation of the thyroid gland. Lancet 1911; 1: 930–931.
5. Burhans EC: Acute thyroiditis. A study of sixty-seven cases. Surg Gynecol Obstet 1928; 47: 478–488.
6. Mann CH: Thyroid abscess in a 3½-year-old child. Arch Otolaryngol 1977; 103: 299–300.
7. Henderson J: Abscess of the thyroid. A discussion and report of four cases. Am J Surg 1935; 29: 36–41.
8. Hendrick JW: Diagnosis and management of thyroiditis. JAMA 1957; 164: 127–133.
9. Beilby GE: Acute thyroiditis. NY State J Med 1919; 19: 224–227.
10. Derbyshire JW, Gray PA Jr: Acute suppurative thyroiditis—report of a case. US Navy Med Bull 1944; 42: 419–420.
11. McArthur LL: Acute suppurative thyroiditis. Chicago Med Rec 1903; 25: 99–105.
12. Mora JM: Acute thyroiditis. Am J Med Sci 1929; 178: 99–105.
13. Stein OJ: Acute inflammation of the thyroid gland. Laryngoscope 1912; 22: 1020–1025.
14. Hawbaker EL: Thyroid abscess. Am Surgeon 1931; 37: 290–292.
15. Horine CF: Suppurative thyroiditis. Bull School Med Univ Maryland 1933; 18: 8–11.
16. Cochrane RC, Novack SJG: Acute thyroiditis with report of ten cases. N Engl J Med 1934; 210: 935–942.
17. Abe K, Taguchi T, Okuno A, et al.: Acute suppurative thyroiditis in children. J Pediatr 1979; 94: 912–914.
18. Gaafar H, El-Garem F: Acute thyroiditis with gas formation. J Laryngol Otol 1975; 89: 323–327.
19. Bussman YC, Wong ML, Bell MJ, et al.: Suppurative thyroiditis with gas formation due to mixed anaerobic infection [letter]. J Pediatr 1977; 90: 321–322.
20. Shaw A: Acute suppurative thyroiditis [letter]. Am J Dis Child 1979; 133: 757.
21. Takai SI, Miyauchi A, Matsuzuka F, et al.: Internal fistula as a route of infection in acute suppurative thyroiditis. Lancet 1979; i: 751–752.
22. Jemerin EE, Aronoff JS: Foreign body in thyroid following perforation of esophagus. Surgery 1949; 25: 52–59.
23. Higbee D: Acute thyroiditis in relation to deep infections of the neck. Ann Otol Rhinol Laryngol 1943; 52: 620–627.
24. Adler ME, Jordan G, Walter RM Jr: Acute suppurative thyroiditis. Diagnostic, metabolic and therapeutic observations. West J Med 1978; 128: 165–168.
25. Abe K, Taguchi T, Okuno A, et al.: Recurrent acute suppurative thyroiditis. Am J Dis Child 1978; 132: 990–991.
26. Alsever RN, Stiver HG, Dinerman N, et al.: *Hemophilus influenzae* pericarditis and empyema with thyroiditis in an adult. JAMA 1974; 230: 1426–1427.
27. Altemeier WA: Acute pyogenic thyroiditis. Arch Surg 1950; 61: 76–85.
28. Altemeier WA: Symposium on thyroiditis. Transactions of the American Goiter Association. 1951, pp 242–249.
29. Backer M: Masked abscess in colloid goiter—a case report. Connecticut State Med J 1944; 8: 298–300.
30. Bonney GW: A case of acute inflammation of the thyroid gland. Lancet 1911; 11: 155.
31. Brenizer AG Jr: Suppurative strumitis caused by *Salmonella typhosa*. Ann Surg 1951; 133: 247–252.
32. Brooks V: Suppurative soft tissue infection of the head and neck. West Indian Med J 1963; 12: 200–210.
33. Burgher LW, Loomis GW, Ware F: Systemic infection due to *Actinobacillus actinomycetemcomitans*. Am J Clin Pathol 1973; 60: 412–415.
34. Carpenter G: A case of acute primary thyroiditis in an infant. Reports of the Society for the Study of Diseases in Children 1902; 3: 157–158.
35. Cleland JP: Purulent infiltration in and around the thyroid gland. Med J Aust 1927; 1: 790–791.
36. Coope R: Acute suppurative thyroiditis. Lancet 1936; 1: 1172–1173.
37. Deaver JB, Burden VG: Suppurative thyroiditis. Surg Clin North Am 1929; 9: 1017–1020.
38. Edwards CR: Acute infection of the thyroid gland. JAMA 1921; 76: 637–639.

39. Ford RV, Sanders DY, Myers RT: Thyroid abscess in a 14-month-old child. J Pediatr Surg 1973; 8: 943–944.
40. Gilman PK: Acute suppurative thyroiditis. Calif State J Med 1921; 19: 294–295.
41. Greenberg D: Metastatic abscesses of the thyroid associated with hyperthyroidism: Report of a case following repeated attacks of sore throat. JAMA 1920; 74: 165–166.
42. Greenfield J, Curtis GM: Acute suppurative thyroiditis during childhood. Am J Dis Child 1939; 58: 837–846.
43. Hagan AD, Goffinet J, Davis JW: Acute streptococcal thyroiditis. JAMA 1967; 202: 842–843.
44. Haines WD: Suppurating thyroid. Lancet Clinics 1915; 113: 559–560.
45. Himsworth RL, Kark AE: Studies on a case of suppurative thyroiditis. Acta Endocrinol 1977; 85: 55–63.
46. Moore AH: Abscess of the thyroid gland. JAMA 1933; 101: 122.
47. Jackson AS, Gilman LC: Thyroiditis. Am J Surg 1954; 88: 891–895.
48. Joffe N, Schamroth L: Gas-forming infection of the thyroid gland. Clin Radiol 1966; 17: 95–96.
49. Kirkland RT, Kirkland JL, Rosenberg HS, et al.: Solitary thyroid nodules in 30 children and report of a child with thyroid abscess. Pediatrics 1973; 51: 85–90.
50. Kirschbaum JD, Rosenblum AH: Suppurative intrathoracic thyroiditis. Arch Surg 1938; 36: 867–873.
51. Kohler PO, Floyd WL, Wynn J: Indications for thyroid needle biopsy: Suppurative thyroiditis. South Med J 1966; 59: 182–184.
52. Lahey FH: Thyroid abscess (with mention of two new signs of this condition). Boston Med Surg J 1917; 176: 94–95.
53. Lambert MJ III, Johns ME, Mentzer R: Acute suppurative thyroiditis. Am Surg 1980; 46: 461–463.
54. Lane WM: Acute suppurative thyroiditis: Presentation of two cases. J Natl Med Assoc 1934; 26: 63–65.
55. Meara FS, MacGregor RS: A case of acute suppurative thyroiditis, with pressure symptoms relieved by intubation. Arch Pediatr 1906; 23: 591–594.
56. Montgomery GH: Acute thyroiditis processing to suppuration. J Med Assoc Ala 1961; 30: 497–499.
57. Moore AH: Abscess of the thyroid gland. JAMA 1933; 101: 122.
58. Mora JM: Acute suppurative thyroiditis in children. Am J Dis Child 1930; 40: 500–502.
59. Olambiwonnu NO, Penny R, Frasier SD: Thyroid abscess in childhood [letter]. Pediatrics 1973; 52: 465–467.
60. Oliech JS: Case report of pyogenic thyroiditis at Kenyatta National Hospital. E Afr Med J 1979; 56: 40–41.
61. Olin R, LeBien WE, Leigh JE: Acute suppurative thyroiditis. Report of two cases including one caused by *Mycobacterium intracellulare* (Battey bacillus). Minn Med 1973; 56: 586–588.
62. Porter MF: Old nodular goiter surrounding trachea, posterior to carotid with the isthmus posterior to the esophagus: Report of a case with sudden death from acute abscess. Arch Surg 1929; 19: 466–470.
63. Prioleau WH: The treatment of abscess of the thyroid gland causing tracheal obstruction. Surgery 1943; 14: 871–875.
64. Reece MW: Thyroid abscess. Br J Surg 1955; 43: 218–220.
65. Richie JL: Acute suppurative thyroiditis in a child. Am J Dis Child 1959; 97: 493–494.
66. Rogers L: Suppurative thyroiditis. A report of two cases. Lancet 1927; i: 868–869.
67. Roth H: Acute suppurative thyroiditis. Am J Med Sci 1904; 127: 101–104.
68. Saksouk F, Salti IS: Acute suppurative thyroiditis caused by *Escherichia coli*. Br Med J 1977; 2: 23–24.
69. Sallick MA: Suppurative thyroiditis with *Streptococcus viridans* bacteremia: Recovery following surgical drainage. J Mount Sinai Hosp NY 1942; 9: 26–28.
70. Schriver LH: Suppurative thyroiditis. J Med 1927; 8: 253–255.
71. Secord ER: A case of acute primary thyroiditis. Can Lancet 1902; 36: 365–369.
72. Sharma RK, Rapkin RH: Acute suppurative thyroiditis caused by *Bacteroides melaninogenicus*. JAMA 1974; 229: 1470.
73. Stock FE: Abscess of the thyroid gland. Report on two cases. Lancet 1944; 1: 789–790.
74. Szego PL, Levy RP: Recurrent acute suppurative thyroiditis. Can Med Assoc J 1970; 103: 631–633.
75. Theisen CF: A case of suppurative thyroiditis with perforation of the trachea. Trans Am Laryngol Assoc 1914; 36: 240–244.
76. Van Heerden JA, O'Connell P: Acute suppurative thyroiditis due to *Salmonella enteritidis*. Vet Admin Med Monthly 1971; 98: 556–557.
77. Warren CPW, Mason BJ: *Clostridium septicum* infection of the thyroid gland. Postgrad Med J 1970; 46: 586–588.
78. Weeks LM: A case of erysipelas terminating in acute thyroiditis. Br Med J 1920; 2: 476–477.
79. Weinstein ML: Acute suppurative thyroiditis with report of one case. Illinois Med J 1933; 63: 275–278.
80. Weissel M, Wolf A, Linkesch W: Acute suppurative thyroiditis caused by *Pseudomonas aeruginosa* [letter]. Br Med J 1977; 2: 580.
81. Wilcox MB: A case of suppurative destruction of the thyroid with resulting myxedema. Nebraska State Med J 1925; 10: 100–101.
82. Wilkins AG: Suppurative goitre. Br Med J 1904; 2: 1005.
83. Jeng LB, Lin JD, Chen MF: Acute suppurative thyroiditis: A ten-year review in a Taiwanese hospital. Scand J Infect Dis 1994; 26: 297–300.
84. Hsu CY, Kao CH, Wang SJ: Multinodular goitre with a huge infected cyst. Clin Nucl Med 1994; 19: 455–456.
85. Desmukh HG, Verma A, Siegel LB, et al.: Stridor, the presenting symptom of thyroid abscess [letter]. Postgrad Med J 1994; 70: 847.
86. Onishi H, Wataki K, Sasaki N, et al.: Clinical study of 15 children with acute suppurative thyroiditis. Nippon Naibunpi Gakkai Zasshi 1994; 70: 529–535.
87. Handberg J, Kirkegaard BD: Acute suppurative thyroiditis. Ugeskr Laeger 1993; 155: 4095–4096.
88. Ohno Y, Ilo K, Imamura M, et al.: A case of acute suppurative thyroiditis associated with thyroid papillary carcinoma. Nippon Naibunpi Gakkai Zasshi 1993; 69: 1003–1012.
89. Pantaleoni M, Velardo A, Smerieri A, et al.: Acute suppurative thyroiditis in a patient with prior subacute thyroiditis. Minerva Endocrinol 1992; 17: 133–136.
90. Premawardhana LD, Vora JP, Scanlon MF: Suppurative thyroiditis with oesophageal carcinoma. Postgrad Med J 1992; 68: 592–593.
91. Echevarria Villegas MP, Franco Vicario R, Solano Lopez D, et al.: Acute suppurative thyroiditis and *Klebsiella pneumoniae* sepsis. A case report and review of the literature. Rev Clin Esp 1992; 190: 458–459.
92. Skuza K, Rapaport R, Fieldman R, et al.: Recurrent acute suppurative thyroiditis. J Otolaryngol 1991; 20: 126–129.
93. Igler C, Zahn T, Muller D: Thyroid abscess caused by *Salmonella enteritidis*. Dtsch Med Wochenschr 1991; 116: 695–698.
94. Gudipati S, Westblom TU: Salmonellosis initially seen as a thyroid abscess. Head Neck 1991; 13: 153–155.
95. Ozaki O, Sugimoto T, Suzuki A, et al.: Cervical thymic cyst as a cause of acute suppurative thyroiditis. Jpn J Surg 1990; 20: 593–596.
96. Nmadu PT: Infective thyroiditis in northern Nigeria: A fifteen-year study. East Afr Med J 1989; 66: 748–751.
97. Miyauchi A, Matsazuka F, Kuma K, et al.: Piriform sinus fistula: An underlying abnormality common in patients with acute suppurative thyroiditis. World J Surg 1990; 14: 400–405.
98. Quin JD, Gray HW, Baxter JN, et al.: Thyroid abscess complicating subacute thyroiditis: A consequence of therapy? Clin Endocrinol Oxf 1992; 37: 570–571.
99. Chiovato L, Canale G, Maccherini D, et al.: *Salmonella brandenburg*: A novel cause of acute suppurative thyroiditis. Acta Endocrinol Copenh 1993; 128: 439–442.
100. Yamashita J, Ogawa M, Yamashita S, et al.: Acute suppurative thyroiditis in an asymptomatic woman: An atypical presentation simulating thyroid carcinoma. Clin Endocrinol Oxf 1994; 40: 145–149.
101. Queen JS, Clegg HW, Council JC, et al.: Acute suppurative thyroiditis caused by *Eikenella corrodens*. J Pediatr Surg 1988; 23: 359–361.
102. Rich EJ, Mendelman PM: Acute suppurative thyroiditis in pediatric patients. Pediatr Infect Dis J 1987; 6: 936–940.
103. Smeal WE, Schenfeld LA, Caroff RJ: Acute suppurative thyroiditis in a 3-year-old boy. Postgrad Med 1986; 80: 105–107.
104. Evengard B, Julander I: Suppurative *Staphylococcus aureus* thyroiditis. Scand J Infect Dis 1986; 18: 483–485.
105. Goudreau E, Comtois R, Bayardelle P, et al.: *Capnocytophaga ochracea* and group F beta-hemolytic streptococcus suppurative thyroiditis. J Otolaryngol 1986; 15: 59–61.
106. Elias AN, Kyaw T, Winikoff J, et al.: Acute suppurative thyroiditis. J Otolaryngol 1985; 14: 17–19.
107. Baker SR, van Merwyk AJ, Singh A: Abscess of the thyroid gland presenting as a pulsatile mass. Med J Aust 1985; 143: 253–254.

108. Tovi F, Gatot A, Bar Ziv J, et al.: Recurrent suppurative thyroiditis due to fourth branchial pouch sinus. Int J Pediatr Otorhinolaryngol 1985; 9: 89–96.

109. Walfish PG, Chan JY, Ing HD, et al.: Esophageal carcinoma masquerading as recurrent acute suppurative thyroiditis. Arch Intern Med 1985; 145: 346–347.

110. Reichling JJ, Rose DN, Mendelson MH, et al.: Acute suppurative thyroiditis caused by *Serratia marcescens*. J Infect Dis 1984; 149: 281.

111. Hirata A, Saito S, Tsuchida Y, et al.: Surgical management of piriform sinus fistula. Am Surg 1984; 50: 454–457.

112. Vichyanond P, Howard CP, Olson LC: *Eikenella corrodens* as a cause of thyroid abscess. Am J Dis Child 1983; 137: 971–973.

113. Gigot JF, Mannell A: Acute emphysematous thyroiditis. Br J Surg 1983; 70: 256–258.

114. Appelbaum PC, Cohen IT: Thyroid abscess associated with *Eikenella corrodens* in a 7-year-old child. Clin Pediatr Phila 1982; 21: 241–242.

115. Donato JO: Acute suppurative thyroiditis: Report of two cases. Int Surg 1972; 57: 750–752.

116. Diaconescu MR, Costinescu V, Simon L, et al.: Thyroid actinomycosis (actinobacteriosis). Rev Med Chir Soc Med Nat Iasi 1993; 97: 231–233.

117. Bertrand E, Tarnowska-Dziduszko E, Cichy S: Generalized form of cerebral actinomycosis. Neuropatol Pol 1989; 27: 237–243.

118. Arfeen S, Boast MT, Large DM: Unilateral thyroid swelling due to actinomycosis. Postgrad Med J 1986; 62: 847–848.

119. Dan M, Garcia A, von Westarp C: Primary actinomycosis of the thyroid mimicking carcinoma. J Otolaryngol 1984; 13: 109–112.

120. Leers WD, Dussault J, Mullens JE, et al.: Suppurative thyroiditis: Unusual case caused by *Actinomyces naeslundi*. Can Med Assoc J 1969; 101: 714–718.

121. McQuay RW: Actinomycosis. Can Med Assoc J 1931; 25: 694–695.

122. Barber AH: Gumma of the thyroid. Lancet 1947; 1: 791.

123. Davis BF: Syphilis of the thyroid. Arch Intern Med 1910; 5: 47–60.

124. Netherton EN: Syphilis and thyroid disease with special reference to hyperthyroidism. Am J Syphilis 1932; 16: 479–510.

125. Senear FE: Gummatous syphilis of the thyroid gland. Am J Med Sci 1918; 155: 691–703.

126. Williams C, Steinberg B: Gumma of the thyroid. Surg Gynecol Obstet 1924; 38: 781–783.

127. Barnes P, Weatherstone R: Tuberculosis of the thyroid: Two case reports. Br J Dis Chest 1979; 73: 187–191.

128. Corner EM: Primary and secondary local tuberculosis of the thyroid gland. Trans Clin Soc London 1904; 37: 112–114.

129. Crompton GK, Cameron SJ: Tuberculosis of the thyroid gland mimicking carcinoma. Tubercle 1969; 50: 16–64.

130. Emery P: Tuberculous abscess of the thyroid with recurrent laryngeal nerve palsy: A case report and review of the literature. J Laryngol Otol 1980; 94: 553–558.

131. Goldfarb H, Schifrin D, Graig FA: Thyroiditis caused by tuberculous abscess of the thyroid gland. Am J Med 1965; 38: 825–828.

132. Gutman LT, Handwerger S, Zwadyk P, et al.: Thyroiditis due to *Mycobacterium chelonei*. Am Rev Respir Dis 1974; 110: 807–809.

133. Johnson AG, Phillips ME, Thomas RJS: Acute tuberculous abscess of the thyroid gland. Br J Surg 1973; 60: 668–669.

134. Jones JB: Tuberculosis of the thyroid gland. Am J Surg 1928; 7: 629–632.

135. Keynes G: Tuberculosis of the thyroid gland. Lancet 1938; ii: 1357–1358.

136. Klassen KP, Curtis GM: Tuberculous abscess of the thyroid gland. Surgery 1945; 17: 552–559.

137. Lindsay LM, Mead CI: Tuberculosis of the thyroid gland with report of a case in a child aged three. Can Med Assoc J 1934; 30: 373–377.

138. Postlehwait RW, Berg P Jr: Tuberculous abscess of the thyroid gland. Arch Surg 1944; 48: 429–437.

139. Rodgers BM, Wolfe W, Detmer DE: Atypical mycobacterial infection of the thyroid gland. J Pediatr Surg 1975; 10: 827–829.

140. Smith LW, Leech JV: Tuberculosis of the thyroid gland. Surg Clin North Am 1928; 8: 185–194.

141. Stubbins WM, Guthrie RF: Tuberculosis abscess of thyroid gland. Southern Surgeon 1948; 14: 351–357.

142. Viranuvatti V, Viseshakul B, Chainuvat T, et al.: Dysphagia due to tuberculosis of thyroid: A case report. J Med Assoc Thai 1980; 63: 291–295.

143. Wang Y, Sabow LT, Dee WF: [131]I study of thyroid tuberculosis mimicking thyroid carcinoma. CRC Crit Rev Radiol Sci 1972; 3: 101–103.

144. Young TO: Inflammatory disease of the thyroid gland. Minn Med 1940; 23: 105–111.

145. Winkler S, Wiesinger E, Graninger W: Extrapulmonary tuberculosis with paravertebral abscess formation and thyroid involvement. Infection 1994; 22: 420–422.

146. Magboo ML, Clark OH: Primary tuberculous thyroid abscess mimicking carcinoma diagnosed by fine needle aspiration biopsy. West J Med 1990; 153: 657–659.

147. Kang GH, Chi JG: Congenital tuberculosis—report of an autopsy case. J Korean Med Sci 1990; 5: 59–64.

148. Sachs MK, Dickenson G, Amazon K: Tuberculous adenitis of the thyroid mimicking subacute thyroiditis. Am J Med 1988; 85: 573–575.

149. Liote HA, Spaulding C, Bazelly B, et al.: Thyroid tuberculosis associated with mediastinal lymphadenitis. Tubercle 1987; 68: 229–231.

150. Allan GW, Andersen DH: Generalized aspergillosis in an infant 18 days of age. Pediatrics 1960; 26: 432–440.

151. Berry CZ, Goldberg LC, Shepard WL: Systemic lupus erythematosus complicated by coccidioidomycosis. JAMA 1968; 206: 1083–1085.

152. Fraumeni JF Jr, Fear RE: Purulent pericarditis in aspergillosis. Ann Intern Med 1962; 57: 823–828.

153. Grcevic N, Matthews WF: Pathologic changes in acute disseminated aspergillosis. Am J Clin Pathol 1959; 32: 536–551.

154. Grekin RH, Cawley EP, Zheutlin B: Generalized aspergillosis. Arch Pathol 1950; 49: 387–392.

155. Halazun JF, Anast CS, Lukens JN: Thyrotoxicosis associated with *Aspergillus* thyroiditis in chronic granulomatous disease. J Pediatr 1972; 80: 106–108.

156. Hutter RVP, Lieberman PH, Collins HS: Aspergillosis in a cancer hospital. Cancer 1964; 17: 747–756.

157. Keane WM, Potsic WP, Perloss LJ, et al.: *Aspergillus* thyroiditis. Otolaryngology 1978; 86: 761–765.

158. Khoo TK, Sugai K, Leong TK: Disseminated aspergillosis. Am J Clin Pathol 1966; 45: 697–703.

159. Lisbona R, Lacouciere Y, Rosenthall L: Aspergillomatous abscesses of the brain and thyroid. J Nucl Med 1973; 14: 541–542.

160. Loeb JM, Livermore BM, Wofwy D: Coccidioidomycosis of the thyroid. Ann Intern Med 1979; 91: 409–411.

161. Luke JL, Bolande RP, Gross S: Generalized aspergillosis and *Aspergillus* endocarditis in infancy. Pediatrics 1963; 31: 115–122.

162. Myer RD, Young LS, Armstrong D, et al.: Aspergillosis complicating neoplastic disease. Am J Med 1973; 54: 6–15.

163. Murray HW, Moore JO, Luff RD: Disseminated aspergillosis in a renal transplant patient: Diagnostic difficulties reemphasized. Johns Hopkins Med J 1975; 137: 235–237.

164. Robinson MF, Forgan-Smith WR, Craswell PW: *Candida* thyroiditis—treated with 5-fluorocytosine. Aust NZ J Med 1975; 5: 472–474.

165. Rosen F, Deck JHN, Rewcastle NB: *Allescheria boydii*—unique systemic dissemination to thyroid and brain. Can Med Assoc J 1965; 93: 1125–1127.

166. Winzelberg GG, Gore J, Yu D, et al.: *Aspergillus flavus* as a cause of thyroiditis in an immunosuppressed host. Johns Hopkins Med J 1979; 144: 90–93.

167. Barbera JR, Forns MC, Capdevila JA, et al.: Disseminated aspergillosis in patients with acquired immunodeficiency syndrome. Med Clin Barc 1994; 103: 101–104.

168. Kaw YT, Brunnemer C: Initial diagnosis of disseminated cryptococcosis and acquired immunodeficiency syndrome by fine needle aspiration of the thyroid. A case report. Acta Cytol 1994; 38: 427–430.

169. Vaidya KP, Lomvardias S: Cryptococcal thyroiditis: Report of a case diagnosed by fine-needle aspiration cytology. Diagn Cytopathol 1991; 7: 415–416.

170. Gahdhi RT, Tollin SR, Seely EW: Diagnosis of *Candida* thyroiditis by fine needle aspiration. J Infect 1994; 28: 77–81.

171. Chan KS, Looi LM, Chan SP: Disseminated histoplasmosis mimicking miliary tuberculosis: A case report. Malays J Pathol 1993; 15: 155–158.

172. Ramos-Fernandez V, Prieto-Rodriguez M, Paradis-Alos A, et al.: An-

gio-invasive disseminated aspergillosis: Autopsy diagnosis in leukemic patients. Ann Med Interna 1993; 10: 337–340.

173. Marin J, Sanz MA, Sanz GF, et al.: Disseminated *Scedosporium inflatum* infection in a patient with acute myeloblastic leukemia. Eur J Clin Microbiol Infect Dis 1991; 10: 759–761.

174. Kalina PH, Campbell RJ: *Aspergillus terreus* endophthalmitis in a patient with chronic lymphocytic leukemia. Arch Opthalmol 1991; 109: 102–103.

175. Chiba N, Miki R: Zygomycosis caused by *Cunninghamella bertholletiae*. Rinsho Byori 1990; 38: 1219–1295.

176. Amin MB, Abrash MP, Mezger E, et al.: Systemic dissemination of *Pneumocystis carinii* in a patient with acquired immunodeficiency syndrome. Henry Ford Hosp Med J 1990; 38: 68–71.

177. Bach MC, Blattner S: Occult Candida thyroid abscess diagnosed by gallium-67 scanning. Clin Nucl Med 1990; 15: 395–396.

178. Tan KK, Sugai K, Leong TK: Disseminated aspergillosis. Am J Clin Pathol 1966; 45: 687–701.

179. Ito T, Ishikawa Y, Fujii R, et al.: Disseminated *Trichosporon capitatum* infection in a patient with acute leukemia. Cancer 1988; 61: 585–588.

180. Guttler R, Singer PA, Axline SG, et al.: *Pneumocystis carinii* thyroiditis. Report of three cases and review of the literature. Arch Intern Med 1993; 153: 393–396.

181. McCarty M, Coker R, Claydoin E: Case report: Disseminated *Pneumocystis carinii* infection in a patient with the acquired immune deficiency syndrome causing thyroid gland calcification and hypothyroidism. Clin Radiol 1992; 43: 209–210.

182. Walts AE, Pitchon HE: *Pneumocystis carinii* in FNA of the thyroid. Diagn Cytopathol 1991; 7: 615–617.

183. Spitzer RD, Chan JC, Marks JB, et al.: Case report: Hypothyroidism due to *Pneumocystis carinii* thyroiditis in a patient with acquired immunodeficiency syndrome. Am J Med Sci 1991; 302: 98–100.

184. Ragni MV, Dekker A, DeRubertis FR, et al.: *Pneumocystis carinii* infection presenting as necrotizing thyroiditis and hypothyroidism. Am J Clin Pathol 1991; 95: 489–493.

185. Battan R, Mariuz P, Raviglione MC, et al.: *Pneumocystis carinii* infection of the thyroid in a hypothyroid patient with AIDS: Diagnosis by fine needle aspiration biopsy. J Clin Endocrinol Metab 1991; 72: 724–726.

186. Drucker DJ, Bailey D, Rotstein L: Thyroiditis as the presenting manifestation of disseminated extrapulmonary *Pneumocystis carinii* infection. J Clin Endocrinol Metab 1990; 71: 1663–1665.

187. Matsuda S, Urata Y, Shiota T, et al.: Disseminated infection of *Pneumocystis carinii* in a patient with the acquired immunodeficiency syndrome. Virchows Arch [A] 1989; 414: 523–527.

188. Gallant JE, Enriquez RE, Cohen KL, et al.: *Pneumocystis carinii* thyroiditis. Am J Med 1988; 84: 303–306.

189. Radio SJ, Hansen S, Goldsmith J, et al.: Immunohistochemistry of *Pneumocystis carinii* infection. Mod Pathol 1990; 3: 462–469.

190. Rahimi SA: Disseminated *Pneumocystis carinii* in thymic alymphoplasia. Arch Pathol 1974; 97: 162–165.

191. Pilon VA, Echol RM, Celo JS, et al.: Disseminated *Pneumocystis carinii* infection in AIDS (letter). N Engl J Med 1987; 316: 1410–1411.

192. Chandra T, Prakash A: A case of hydatid cyst of thyroid. Br J Surg 1965; 52: 235–237.

193. Coppleson VM: Hydatid cyst of the left lobe of the thyroid. Aust NZ J Surg 1948; 18: 144.

194. Leelachaikul P, Chuahirun S: Cysticercosis of the thyroid gland in severe cerebral cysticercosis. Report of a case. J Med Assoc Thai 1977; 60: 405–410.

195. Majumdar P, Ghosh DP: Hydatid cyst of the thyroid. Indian J Surg 1970; 32: 496–499.

196. Misgar MS, Mir MA, Narboo T, et al.: Primary *Echinococcus* cyst of the thyroid gland. Int Surg 1977; 62: 600.

197. Porges SB: A case of hydatid disease of the thyroid gland. Med J Aust 1971; 1: 641–642.

198. Reddy DG, Thangavelu M: Hydatid cyst—thyroid. Indian J Surg 1946; 8: 49–50.

199. Shaw HW: A case of hydatid disease of the thyroid gland. Med J Aust 1946; 2: 413–414.

200. Skalkeas GD, Sechas MN: Echinococcosis of the thyroid gland. Report of two cases. JAMA 1967; 200: 178–179.

201. Reincke M, Allolio B, Petzke F, et al.: Thyroid dysfunction in African trypanosomiasis: A possible role for inflammatory cytokines. Clin Endocrinol Oxf 1993; 39: 455–461.

202. Boersma A, Hublart M, Boutignon F, et al.: Alterations in thyroid function in patients with *Trypanosoma brucei gambiense* infection. Trans R Soc Trop Med Hyg 1989; 83: 208–209.

203. Miller SE: Helminthic infections in the acquired immunodeficiency syndrome. J Electron Microsc Tech 1988; 8: 133–135.

204. Chetty R, Crowe P, Cant P: An unusual thyroid cyst. A case report. S Afr J Surg 1991; 29: 158–159.

205. Ben Attia M, Sayed S, Houissa T: Hydatid cyst in the thyroid in children. 3 cases. Tunis Med 1991; 69: 55–60.

206. de Moura LS, da Silva CP: Thyroid hydatid disease in an 8-year-old girl. J Pediatr Surg 1991; 26: 216.

207. van Rensburg PS, Joubert IS, Nel CJ: Primary echinococcus cyst of the thyroid. A case report. S Afr J Surg 1990; 28: 157–158.

208. Touhami M, Moumen M: Hydatidosis of the cervicofacial glands. Apropos of 6 cases. J Chir Paris 1990; 127: 220–222.

209. Sharma AK, Sarda AK: Hydatid disease of the thyroid gland—(a case report). J Postgrad Med 1989; 35: 230–231.

210. Audoin J, Cenac A, Ceveloux M, et al.: Hydatid cyst of the thyroid. Apropos of a case in the Republic of Niger. Bull Soc Pathol Exot Filiales 1988; 81: 360–364.

211. Dotzenrath C, Burringt KF, Goretzki PE: Echinococcus cyst of the thyroid gland. A case report. Chirurg 1988; 59: 106–107.

212. Burrig KF, Dotzenrath C, Borchard F: Echinococcus cysticus of the thyroid gland. Pathologe 1988; 9: 59–61.

213. Bauchet LJ: De la thyroidite (goitre aigu) et du goitre enflamme (goitre chronique enflamme). Gaz Hebel Med Chir 1857; 4: 19–23.

214. Alderfer HH, David JB: Acute thyroiditis. J Indiana State Med Assoc 1954; 47: 606–613.

215. Armstrong GL: Acute thyroiditis (letter). JAMA 1911; 56: 289.

216. Bowles AJ: Thyroiditis. Northwest Med 1944; 43: 224–227.

217. Clute HM, Smith LW: Acute thyroiditis. Surg Gynecol Obstet 1927; 44: 23–29.

218. Hazard JB: Thyroiditis: A review. Am J Clin Pathol 1955; 25: 289–298.

219. Jelks E: Acute thyroiditis. J Fla Med Assoc 1945; 31: 419–421.

220. Jensen VW: Syphilitic ophthalmic goiter. J Mich State Med Soc 1928; 27: 273–274.

221. Jones KH: A case of acute thyroiditis. Br Med J 1909; 1: 1064.

222. Kast E, Dannenberg T: Acute non-suppurative thyroiditis. Permanente Found Med Bull 1945; 3: 142–144.

223. Lamb DS: Case of acute thyroiditis. Wash Med Ann 1907; 6: 243.

224. Scheinberg D: Acute thyroiditis treated with penicillin. J Tenn Med Assoc 1946; 39: 132–133.

225. Sherris CA: A case of recurrent acute thyroiditis. Guy's Hosp Gazette 1916; 30: 35.

226. Thorburn IB: Acute thyroiditis following teeth extraction. Br Med J 1934; 1: 428.

227. Voorhees IW: A case of acute thyroiditis. Med Rec NY 1914; 86: 883.

228. Budd SW, Williams C: Tuberculosis of the thyroid gland. JAMA 1929; 92: 1741–1744.

229. Dinsmore RS: Tuberculosis of the thyroid gland. Surg Clin North Am 1935; 15: 885–891.

230. Henry CE: Syphilis of the thyroid gland. Am J Syphilis 1928; 12: 322–324.

231. Menninger WC: Congenital syphilis of the thyroid gland. Am J Syphilis 1929; 13: 164–179.

232. Gordon MB: The incidence of syphilis in hypothyroidism and myxedema in children. NY Med J 1922; 115: 350–352.

233. Thompson L: Syphilis of the thyroid. Am J Syphilis 1917; 1: 179–191.

234. Storck JA: Syphilis of the thyroid. New Orleans Med Surg J 1917; 70: 414–417.

235. Clark O: Exophthalmic goiter as a clinical manifestation of hereditary syphilis. JAMA 1914; 63: 1951.

236. Davis BF: Gumma of the thyroid. Trans Chicago Pathol Soc 1907–1909; 7: 273–274.

237. DeLozier HL, Sofferman RA: Pyriform sinus fistula: An unusual cause of recurrent retropharyngeal abscess and cellulitis. Ann Otol Rhinol Laryngol 1986; 95: 377–382.

238. Schoenfeld PS, Myers JW, LaRocque JC: Suppression of cell-mediated immunity in hypothyroidism. South Med J 1995; 88: 347–349.

239. Wolach B, Lebanon B, Jedeikin A, et al.: Neutrophil chemotaxis, random migration, and adherence in patients with hyperthyroidism. Acta Endocrinol Copenh 1989; 121: 817–820.

240. Womack NA, Cole WH: Normal and pathologic repair in the thyroid gland. Arch Surg 1931; 23: 466–476.

241. Montgomery GL, Ballantine TV, Kleiman MB, et al.: Ruptured branchial cleft cyst presenting as acute thyroid infection. Clin Pediatr Phila 1982; 21: 380–383.

242. Vesely DL, Angtuaco EJ, Boyd CM: Sinus tract in the neck: A rare complication of subtotal thyroidectomy for Graves' disease. J Med 1986; 17: 253–261.

243. Colcock BP, King ML: The mortality and morbidity of thyroid surgery. Surg Gynecol Obstet 1962; 114: 131–136.

244. Szabo SM, Allen DB: Thyroiditis. Differentiation of acute suppurative and subacute. Case report and review of the literature. Clin Pediatr Phila 1989; 28: 171–174.

245. Lucaya J, Berdon WE, Enriquez G, et al.: Congenital pyriform sinus fistula: A cause of acute left-sided suppurative thyroiditis and neck abscess in children. Pediatr Radiol 1990; 21: 27–29.

246. Rossiter JL, Topf P: Acute suppurative thyroiditis with bilateral piriform sinus fistulae. Otolaryngol Head Neck Surg 1991; 105: 625–628.

247. Park BW, Park CS: Pyriform sinus fistula. Yonsei Med J 1993; 34: 386–390.

248. Makino S, Tsuchida Y, Yoshioka H, et al.: The endoscopic and surgical management of pyriform sinus fistulae in infants and children. J Pediatr Surg 1986; 21: 398–401.

249. Taylor WE Jr, Myer CM 3rd, Hays LL, et al.: Acute suppurative thyroiditis in children. Laryngoscope 1982; 92: 1269–1273.

250. Taguchi T, Okuno A, Fujita K, et al.: Etiologic factors in acute suppurative thyroiditis. J Infect Dis 1982; 146: 447.

251. Walter RM Jr, McMonagle JR: *Salmonella* thyroiditis, apathetic thyrotoxicosis, and follicular carcinoma in a Laotian woman. Cancer 1982; 50: 2493–2495.

252. Guillaume P: Etiology and pathogenesis of tertiary syphilis of the thyroid gland. Med J Recorder 1925; 121: 159–160.

253. Young RC, Bennett JE, Vogel CL, et al.: Aspergillosis. The spectrum of the disease in 98 patients. Medicine 1970; 49: 147–173.

254. Powell BR, Buist NR, Stenzel P: An X-linked syndrome of diarrhea, polyendocrinopathy, and fatal infection in infancy. J Pediatr 1982; 100: 731–737.

255. Dekio S, Imaoka C, Jidoi J: *Candida* folliculitis associated with hypothyroidism [letter]. Br J Dermatol 1987; 117: 663–664.

256. Kaplan MM, Boice JD Jr, Ames DB, et al.: Thyroid, parathyroid, and salivary gland evaluations in patients exposed to multiple fluoroscopic examinations during tuberculosis therapy: A pilot study. J Clin Endocrinol Metab 1988; 66: 376–382.

257. Moreno AJ, Harshorne MF, Yedinak MA, et al.: Tinea corporis overlying the thyroid gland after radioiodine (131I) treatment of Graves' disease. Cutis 1986; 37: 271–273.

258. Smerdely P, Lim A, Boyages SC, et al.: Topical iodine-containing antiseptics and neonatal hypothyroidism in very low birthweight infants. Lancet 1989; ii: 661–664.

259. Ryan CA, Hallgren RA, Finer NN: The use of povidone iodine in neonatal bowel surgery. J Pediatr Surg 1987; 22: 317–319.

260. Zellner PR, Bugyi S: Povidone iodine in the treatment of burn patients. J Hosp Infect 1985; 6(suppl A): 139–146.

261. Safran M, Paul TL, Roti E, et al.: Environmental factors affecting autoimmune thyroid disease. Endocrinol Metab Clin North Am 1987; 16: 327–342.

262. Marcellin P, Benhamou JP: Treatment of chronic viral hepatitis. Baillieres Clin Gastroenterol 1994; 8: 233–253.

263. Saracco G, Touscoz A, Durazzo M, et al.: Autoantibodies and response to alpha-interferon in patients with chronic viral hepatitis. J Hepatol 1990; 11: 339–343.

264. Smellie JM, Bantock HM, Thompson BD: Co-trimoxazole and the thyroid (letter). Lancet 1982; ii: 96.

265. Davenport MH, Crook D, Wynn V, et al.: Metabolic effects of low-dose fluconazole in healthy female users and non-users of contraceptives. Br J Clin Pharmacol 1989; 27: 851–859.

266. Meyer-Gessner M, Benker G, Lederbogen S, et al.: Antithyroid drug-induced agranulocytosis: Clinical experience with ten patients treated at one institution and review of the literature. J Endocrinol Invest 1994; 17: 29–36.

267. Hou GL, Tsai CC: Oral manifestations of agranulocytosis associated with methimazole therapy. J Periodontol 1988; 59: 244–248.

268. Cavalieri RR: The effects of nonthyroid disease and drugs on thyroid function tests. Med Clin North Am 1991; 75: 27–39.

269. Meinhold H, Gramm HJ, Meissner W, et al.: Elevated serum diiodotyrosine in severe infections and sepsis: DIT, a possible new marker of leukocyte activity. J Clin Endocrinol Metab 1991; 72: 945–953.

270. Fallon JJ Jr, Yelovich RM, Green PJ: Euthyroid sick syndrome. Association with urosepsis in an elderly man. Postgrad Med 1984; 75: 117–121.

271. Toivanen P, Toivanen A: Does *Yersinia* induce autoimmunity? Int Arch Allergy Immunol 1994; 104: 107–111.

272. Eguchi K, Matsuoka N, Nagataki S: Cellular immunity to autoimmune thyroid disease. Baillieres Clin Endocrinol Metab 1995; 9: 71–94.

273. Wolf MW, Misaki T, Bech K, et al.: Immunoglobulins of patients recovering from *Yersinia enterocolitica* infections exhibit Graves' disease–like activity in human thyroid membranes. Thyroid 1991; 1: 315–320.

274. Arscott P, Rosen ED, Koenig RJ, et al.: Immunoreactivity to *Yersinia enterocolitica* antigens in patients with autoimmune thyroid disease. J Clin Endocrinol Metab 1992; 75: 295–300.

275. Volpe R: A perspective on human autoimmune thyroid disease: Is there an abnormality of the target cell which predisposes to the disorder? Autoimmunity 1992; 13: 3–9.

276. Tomer Y, Davies TF: Infection, thyroid disease and autoimmunity. Endocr Rev 1993; 14: 107–120.

277. Ciampolillo A, Marini V, Mirakian R, et al.: Retrovirus-like sequences in Graves' disease: Implications for human autoimmunity. Lancet 1989; i: 1096–1100.

278. Mizokami T, Okamura K, Ikenoue H, et al.: A high prevalence of T-lymphotropic virus type I carriers in patients with antithyroid antibodies. Thyroid 1994; 4: 415–419.

279. Kawai H, Inui T, Kashiwagi S, et al.: HTLV-I infection in patients with autoimmune thyroiditis (Hashimoto's thyroiditis). J Med Virol 1992; 38: 138–141.

280. Kawai H, Kashiwagi S, Inui T, et al.: HTLV-I–associated myelopathy (HAM/TSP) with Hashimoto's thyroiditis. Tokushima J Exp Med 1991; 38: 99–102.

281. Yamaguchi K, Mochizuki M, Watanabe T, et al.: Human T lymphotrophic virus type 1 uveitis after Graves' disease. Br J Ophthalmol 1994; 78: 163–166.

282. Increased prevalence of non-secretors in patients with Graves' disease: Evidence for an infective aetiology? Br Med J Clin Res Ed 1988; 296: 1162.

283. Blethen SL, Nachman S, Chasalow FI: Thyroid function in children with perinatally acquired antibodies to human immunodeficiency virus. J Pediatr Endocrinol 1994; 7: 201–204.

284. Olivieri A, Sorcini M, Battisti P, et al.: Thyroid hypofunction related with the progression of human immunodeficiency virus infection. J Endocrinol Invest 1993; 16: 407–413.

285. Lambert M, Zech F, De Nayer P, et al.: Elevation of serum thyroxine-binding globulin (but not of cortisol-binding globulin and sex hormone–binding globulin) associated with the progression of human immunodeficiency virus infection. Am J Med 1990; 89: 748–751.

286. Dobs AS, Dempsey MA, Ladenson PW, et al.: Endocrine disorders in men infected with human immunodeficiency virus. Am J Med 1988; 84: 611–616.

287. LoPresti JS, Fried JC, Spencer CA, et al.: Unique alterations of thyroid hormone indices in the acquired immunodeficiency syndrome. Ann Intern Med 1989; 110: 970–975.

288. Merenich JA, McDermott MT, Asp AA, et al.: Evidence of endocrine involvement early in the course of human immunodeficiency virus infection. J Clin Endocrinol Metab 1990; 70: 563–565.

289. Schwartz LJ, St Louis Y, Wu R, et al.: Endocrine function in children with human immunodeficiency virus infection. Am J Dis Child 1991; 145: 330–333.

290. Manfardini S, Vaccher E, Pizzocaro G, et al.: Unusual malignant tumors in 49 patients with HIV infection. AIDS 1989; 3: 449–452.

291. Lambert M: Thyroid dysfunction in HIV infection. Baillieres Clin Endocrinol Metab 1994; 8: 825–835.

292. Aron DC: Endocrine complications of the acquired immunodeficiency syndrome. Arch Intern Med 1989; 149: 330–333.

293. Marks JB: Endocrine manifestations of human immunodeficiency virus (HIV) infection. Am J Med Sci 1991; 302: 110–117.

294. Merenich JA: Hypothalamic and pituitary function in AIDS. Baillieres Clin Endocrinol Metab 1994; 8: 757–767.

295. Donovan DS Jr, Dluhy RG: Status of endocrine disease with HIV infection. Curr Ther Endocrinol Metab 1994; 5: 190–194.

296. Mollison LC, Mijch A, McBride G, et al.: Hypothyroidism due to destruction of the thyroid by Kaposi's sarcoma. Rev Infect Dis 1991; 13: 826–827.

297. Fried JC, LoPresti JS, Micon M, et al.: Serum triiodothyronine values. Prognostic indicators of acute mortality due to *Pneumocystis carinii* pneumonia associated with the acquired immunodeficiency syndrome. Arch Intern Med 1990; 150: 406–409.

298. Hashimoto H, Igarashi N, Yachie A, et al.: The relationship between serum levels of interleukin-6 and thyroid hormone in children with acute respiratory infection. J Clin Endocrinol Metab 1994; 78: 288–291.

299. Scarborough DE: Cytokine modulation of pituitary hormone secretion. Ann NY Acad Sci 1990; 594: 169–187.

300. Hermus RM, Sweep CG, van der Meer MJ, et al.: Continuous infusion of interleukin-1 beta induces a nonthyroidal illness syndrome in the rat. Endocrinology 1992; 131: 2139–2146.

301. Koransky JR, Stargel MD, Dowell VR Jr: *Clostridium septicum* bacteremia. Its clinical significance. Am J Med 1979; 66: 63–66.

302. Lalitha MK, John R: Unusual manifestations of salmonellosis—a surgical problem. Q J Med 1994; 87: 301–309.

303. Zimmermann CW, Lingenfelser T, Melms A, et al.: Abscess of the thyroid gland caused by *Salmonella enteritidis* in immunosuppressive treatment of generalized myasthenia gravis with thymoma. Nervenarzt 1990; 61: 626–628.

304. von Graevenitz A, Colla F: Thyroiditis due to *Brucella melitensis*—report of two cases. Infection 1990; 18: 179–180.

305. Cheng AF, Man DW, French GL: Thyroid abscess caused by *Eikenella corrodens*. J Infect 1988; 16: 181–185.

306. Rankin FW, Graham AS: Tuberculosis of the thyroid gland. Ann Surg 1932; 96: 625–648.

307. Coller FA, Huggins CB: Tuberculosis of the thyroid gland: A review of the literature and report of five new cases. Ann Surg 1926; 84: 804–820.

308. Candel S: Acute nonspecific thyroiditis following measles—report of a case. US Navy Med Bull 1946; 46: 1109–1113.

309. Nakamura S, Kosaka J, Sugimoto M, et al.: Silent thyroiditis following rubella. Endocrinol Jpn 1990; 37: 79–85.

310. Freij BJ, South MA, Sever JL: Maternal rubella and the congenital rubella syndrome. Clin Perinatol 1988; 15: 247–257.

311. Clarke WL, Shaver KA, Bright GM, et al.: Autoimmunity in congenital rubella syndrome. J Pediatr 1984; 104: 370–373.

312. Volpe R, Row VV, Ezrin C: Circulating viral and thyroid antibodies in subacute thyroiditis. J Clin Endocrin 1967; 27: 1275–1284.

313. Swann NH: Acute thyroiditis. Five cases associated with adenovirus infection. Metabolism 1964; 13: 908–910.

314. Geva T, Theodor R: Atypical presentation of subacute thyroiditis. Arch Dis Child 1988; 63: 845–846.

315. Greene JN: Subacute thyroiditis. Am J Med 1971; 51: 97–108.

316. Tashiro T, Goto Y, Shigeno H, et al.: A clinicopathological study on cytomegalovirus infection. Kansenshogaku Zasshi 1989; 63: 1171–1177.

317. Lo SK, Ip KW, Chan PK, et al.: Congenital infection by human cytomegalovirus with a 65bp deletion in the morphological transforming region II. Arch Virol 1993; 129: 295–299.

318. Goldman AJ, Bochna AJ, Becker FO: St. Louis encephalitis and subacute thyroiditis [letter]. Ann Intern Med 1977; 87: 250.

319. Fennell JS, Tomkin GH: Sub-acute thyroiditis and hepatitis in a case of infectious mononucleosis. Postgrad Med J 1978; 54: 351–352.

320. Mosonyi L: Thyroiditis letter. Br Med J 1960; 1: 1132.

321. Coyle PV, Wyatt D, Connolly JH, et al.: Epstein-Barr virus infection and thyroid dysfunction [letter]. Lancet 1989; i: 899.

322. Volpe R: The management of subacute (DeQuervain's) thyroiditis. Thyroid 1993; 3: 253–255.

323. Matsubayashi S, Tamai H, Morita T, et al.: Malignant lymphoma of the thyroid and Epstein-Barr virus. Endocrinol Jpn 1989; 36: 343–348.

324. Somlo F, Kovalik M: Acute thyroiditis in a patient with Q fever. Can Med Assoc J 1966; 95: 1091–1093.

325. Schofield PM, Keal EE: Subacute thyroiditis associated with *Chlamydia psittaci* infection. Postgrad Med J 1986; 62: 33–34.

326. Shumway M, Davis PL: Cat-scratch thyroiditis treated with thyrotropic hormone. J Clin Endocrinol 1954; 14: 742–743.

327. Sack J, Zilberstein D, Barile MF, et al.: Binding of thyrotropin to selected *Mycoplasma* species: Detection of serum antibodies against a specific *Mycoplasma* membrane antigen in patients with autoimmune thyroid disease. J Endocrinol Infect 1989; 12: 77–86.

328. Valtonen VV, Ruutu P, Varis K, et al.: Serological evidence for the role of bacterial infections in the pathogenesis of thyroid diseases. Acta Med Scand 1986; 219: 105–111.

329. Kiy Y, Machado JM, Mendes RP, et al.: Paracoccidioidomycosis in the region of Botucatu (state of Sao Paulo, Brazil). Evaluation of serum thyroxine (T_4) and triiodothyronine (T_3) levels and of the response to thyrotropin releasing hormone (TRH). Mycopathologia 1988; 103: 3–9.

330. Katoh R, Ishizaki T, Tomichi N, et al.: Malacoplakia of the thyroid gland. Am J Clin Pathol 1989; 92: 813–820.

331. Levitt T: The status of lymphadenoid goitre, Hashimoto's and Riedel's diseases. Ann R Coll Surg Engl 1952; 10: 369–404.

332. Dean JR, Hall EM: Tuberculosis of the thyroid gland. Am J Surg 1934; 25: 347–350.

333. Hare HF, Simpson HN: Tuberculosis of the thyroid gland: Report of two cases. Lahey Clin Bull 1941; 2: 123–126.

334. Kipp HA: Tuberculosis of the thyroid gland. Pa Med J 1929; 32: 496–497.

335. Mosimann RE: Tuberculosis of the thyroid. Surg Gynecol Obstet 1917; 24: 680–693.

336. Phillips JR, Waldron GW: Non-caseous tuberculosis of the thyroid gland (report of a case). Am J Surg 1939; 44: 643–645.

337. Tinker MB: Surgery in tuberculosis of thyroid. Southwest Med 1934; 18: 62–63.

338. Bonakdarpour A: *Echinococcus* disease. Report of 112 cases from Iran and a review of 611 cases from the United States. Am J Roentgenol 1967; 99: 660–667.

339. Berger SA, Edberg SC, David G: Infectious disease in the sella turcica. Rev Infect Dis 1986; 5: 747–755.

340. Brook I: The swollen neck. Cervical lymphadenitis, parotitis, thyroiditis, and infected cysts. Infect Dis Clin North Am 1988; 2: 221–236.

341. Hamburger JI: The various presentations of thyroiditis. Diagnostic considerations. Ann Intern Med 1986; 104: 219–224.

342. Hay ID: Thyroiditis: A clinical update. Mayo Clin Proc 1985; 60: 836–843.

343. Woolf PD: Thyroiditis. Med Clin North Am 1985; 69: 1035–1048.

344. Tauveron I, Aumaitre O, Marcheix JC, et al.: Painful chronic thyroiditis. A rare cause of thyroid pain. Ann Endocrinol Paris 1994; 54: 359–361.

345. Becker CB, Trock DH: Thyrotoxicosis resembles Lyme disease [letter]. Ann Intern Med 1991; 114: 914–915.

346. Garg SK, Ganapathy V, Bandhopadhya PK, et al.: Pyrexia of unknown origin as a rare presentation of tuberculous thyroiditis. Indian J Chest Dis Allied Sci 1987; 29: 52–55.

347. Gelfand JA, Wolff SM: Fever of unknown origin. In: Mandell GL, Bennett JE, Dolin R (eds): Mandel, Douglas and Bennett's Principles and Practice of Infectious Diseases, 4th ed. New York: Churchill Livingstone, 1995, p 545.

348. Birchall G: Sarcoidosis and thyroiditis. Br J Clin Pract 1966; 20: 586–587.

349. Pino Sacca F: Caratteri istologici distinivi, fra tiroidite subacuta parenchimatosa e tubercolosi della tiroide. Minerva Med 1949; 1: 334–341.

350. German WM: Granulomas in struma fibrosa of thyroid. West J Surg Obstet Gynecol 1941; 49: 120–131.

351. Van Ravenswaay A, Van Ravenswaay AC: Tuberculosis of the thyroid—case report and a review of the literature. Am J Surg 1933; 19: 128–136.

352. Isenberg SF: Thyroid abscess resulting from fine-needle aspiration. Otolaryngol Head Neck Surg 1994; 111: 832–833.

353. Bernard PJ, Som PM, Urken ML, et al.: The CT findings of acute thyroiditis and acute suppurative thyroiditis. Otolaryngol Head Neck Surg 1988; 99: 489–493.

354. Vibhakar SD, Eckhauser C, Bellon EM: Computed tomography of the nasopharynx and neck. J Comput Tomogr 1983; 7: 259–265.

355. Rauschkolb EK, Keen SJ, Patel S: High-dose computed tomography in the evaluation of low attenuation lesions in the neck. J Comput Tomogr 1983; 7: 159–166.

356. Barki Y: Ultrasonographic evaluation of neck masses—sonographic patterns in differential diagnosis. Isr J Med Sci 1992; 28: 212–216.

357. Conrad C: Ultrasonography of the thyroid. An intracystic carcinoma and mouse typhoid induced abscess. A report of two cases. Eur J Radiol 1985; 5: 218–220.

358. Kleinmann RE, Vagenakis AG, Abreau G, et al.: Anterior neck abscess masquerading as acute suppurative thyroiditis. J Nucl Med 1979; 29: 1051–1052.

359. Kawanaka M, Sugimoto Y, Suehiro M, et al.: Thyroid imaging in a

typical case of acute suppurative thyroiditis with abscess formation due to infection from a persistent thyroglossal duct. Ann Nucl Med 1994; 8: 159–162.

360. Pretorius D, Taylor A Jr: The role of nuclear scanning in head and neck surgery. Head Neck Surg 1982; 4: 427–432.

361. Barton GM, Shoup WB, Bennett WG, et al.: Combined *Escherichia coli* and *Staphylococcus aureus* thyroid abscess in an asymptomatic man. Am J Med Sci 1988; 295: 133–136.

362. Sultany GL, Kahaleh MB: Acute rheumatic fever after thyroid abscess in an adult. South Med J 1983; 76: 810–812.

363. Karadeniz A, Hacihanefioglu U: Abscess formation in an intrathoracic goitre. Thorax 1982; 37: 556–557.

Linden T. Hu
Mark S. Klempner

CHAPTER FIFTY-NINE

Lyme Disease

▼

Lyme disease is a disseminated infection caused by a tick-borne spirochete, *Borrelia burgdorferi*. It is the most common vector-borne disease in the United States. There were 13,084 cases reported from 44 states in 1994.[1] The actual incidence of Lyme disease in the United States is unknown but surely exceeds this number many-fold because of underreporting. Patients with early neurologic involvement may present with symptoms localizing to the head and neck. Physicians should be aware of the ear, nose, and throat (ENT) manifestations of Lyme disease in order to facilitate diagnosis and treatment of these patients.

HISTORY

The first description of erythema migrans, the characteristic skin rash of early Lyme disease, was made by Afzelius[2] in 1909. Although Afzelius suspected that erythema migrans lesions were related to tick bites, Lipshitz was the first to associate the bite of *Ixodes ricinus* ticks with erythema migrans.[3] In the 1940s, European investigators found that erythema migrans was linked to neurologic syndromes, including acute meningitis, lymphocytic meningopolyneuritis (Bannwarth's syndrome), and progressive encephalomyelitis.[4] By the 1950s, the efficacy of penicillin and tetracycline in the treatment of Bannwarth's syndrome was known.[5]

The first case of erythema migrans in the United States was reported in 1970 by Scrimenti[6] in Wisconsin. The syndrome received its current name when, in 1975, Steere and colleagues[7] investigated an unusual clustering of juvenile rheumatoid arthritis in Old Lyme, Connecticut. Although the predominant symptom in these patients was arthritis, it was quickly realized that many of them had erythema migrans lesions and that the syndrome could also affect multiple organ systems—especially the heart and nervous system. By 1982, Willy Burgdorfer and colleagues[3] had isolated a new species of *Borrelia, Borrelia burgdorferi,* as the causative organism.[8]

CAUSATIVE ORGANISM

Borrelia burgdorferi sensu latu are in the family Spirochaetaceae. Within this family are three genuses that cause human disease: *Borrelia, Leptospira,* and *Treponema.* Three distinct genomic groups of *Borrelia* cause Lyme disease: *B. burgdorferi sensu stricto, Borrelia garinii,* and *Borrelia afzelii. B. garinii* and *B. afzelii* are the predominant strains in Europe. *B. burgdorferi sensu stricto* has been the only strain isolated in North America.

B. burgdorferi are coiled, spiral bacteria that measure 20–30 μm by 0.2–0.3 μm, making them the longest and the narrowest of the *Borrelia* species. They are best visualized by phase-contrast or dark-field microscopy. They stain gramnegative, and can be seen with silver, Giemsa, or acridine orange stain or by immunohistochemical techniques; however, identification in stained tissue section is difficult.[9, 10] *B. burgdorferi* are microaerophilic and grow best at 33° C in a liquid medium called Barbour-Stoenner-Kelly medium.[11] The doubling time for *B. burgdorferi* is quite long (8–24 hours, compared with less than 30 minutes for *Escherichia coli*), making it difficult to use cultures to diagnose Lyme disease.

EPIDEMIOLOGY

The epidemiology of Lyme disease in humans is closely tied with the geographic distribution and life cycle of its vector. *Ixodes* ticks are hard-bodied ticks commonly found in areas of high humidity, such as along coastal areas, rivers, and lake shores. Several different species of *Ixodes* ticks have been found to carry *B. burgdorferi: Ixodes scapularis* (formerly *Ixodes dammini*) in the northeastern and midwestern United States, *Ixodes pacificus* in the western United States, *Ixodes ricinus* in Europe, and *Ixodes persulcatus* in Asia. Lyme disease has been reported infrequently in areas not inhabited by *Ixodes* ticks; other ticks, such as *Amblyomma americanum* as well as mosquitoes and deer flies have been implicated in rare cases of Lyme disease outside the distribution of *Ixodes* ticks.

Although transovarial infection of ticks with *B. burgdorferi* can occur, less than 1% of ticks are thought to be infected this way.[12] The major route of transmission to ticks is horizontal, through feeding on infected animals. *Ixodes* ticks feed once during each stage of their three-stage life cycle (Fig. 59–1). Each tick stage has a preferred host: larvae favoring small rodents such as the white-footed mouse; nymphs favoring white-footed mice, but also larger mammals such as raccoons and squirrels; and adults favoring large mammals such as the white-tailed deer. All stages of ticks have been found to feed on humans. The larvae feed during the late summer. Nymphs typically feed during the succeeding spring and early summer—infecting animals that the next generation of larvae will feed on in the late summer. Adult *Ixodes* ticks feed in the autumn and early winter. The infection rate among ticks varies seasonally and by geographic region, but adult ticks tend to have the highest infection rates. In the United States, the white-footed mouse and the white-tailed deer are probably the most important animal reservoirs of *B. burgdorferi*.[13]

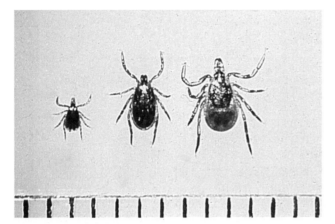

Figure 59–1. Nymph, adult male and adult female (left to right) *Ixodes scapularis* on a millimeter scale.

The spirochetes are usually limited to the midgut of the ticks. Transmission to animals is thought to occur through the tick saliva or through regurgitation of midgut contents during feeding. Studies suggest that transmission of the spirochetes may not occur efficiently before 24–48 hours of tick attachment.[14] However, ticks that have been allowed to feed partially prior to attachment to an uninfected host transmit *B. burgdorferi* efficiently after less than 1 day of attachment, suggesting that the act of feeding or some component in the blood may play a role in transmission of the spirochete.[15]

CLINICAL MANIFESTATIONS

General

The clinical manifestations of Lyme disease have traditionally been divided into stages paralleling the stages of syphilis: an acute phase, with localized and disseminated stages, and a chronic phase. Although it is convenient to discuss Lyme disease as occurring in stages, it is important to note that dissemination often occurs very early and patients frequently present with later-stage symptoms without having noted localized disease.[16, 17] In addition, as more is being discovered about borrelial infections, it appears that some of the pathophysiologic changes in acute and chronic disseminated disease may be the same; thus, the differences between acute and chronic disease may be more quantitative than qualitative.

Acute Localized Disease

The hallmark of acute localized Lyme disease is the development of an erythema migrans skin lesion at the site of the tick bite. Erythema migrans is characteristically an expanding annular lesion with central clearing; however, variations include lesions that are scaling, vesicular, purpuric, or homogeneous (Fig. 59–2). The lesions are usually painless; slight localized pruritus may be noted. Erythema migrans may be located on any part of the body; the most common

sites are the thigh, back, groin, and axilla. Probably because of their height, children commonly present with facial erythema migrans. The interval between a tick bite and development of erythema migrans ranges from 3 to 32 days with a median of 7 days. Without treatment, erythema migrans usually clears spontaneously within weeks to months; rarely, erythema migrans can persist for longer than 1 year.[17, 18] In untreated or inadequately treated disease, erythema migrans can relapse. Patients treated successfully early in the course of erythema migrans are not protected against reinfection and can develop new lesions.

Acute disease may be accompanied by nonspecific constitutional symptoms, such as fatigue, headache, chills and lymphadenopathy. Despite lesions that can reach large sizes (>15 cm), patients with erythema migrans are not "toxic-appearing." Borrelial lymphocytoma, which is a dense lymphocytic infiltrate in the dermis or subcutaneous tissue, may occur at the site of the tick bite concurrent with erythema migrans. Lymphocytomas have also been reported at distant sites during the disseminated portion of the disease.[19]

Acute Disseminated Disease

Acute, disseminated Lyme borreliosis is the result of the spread of *B. burgdorferi* from the site of the tick bite to distant organs. The time from the tick bite to dissemination is variable but can be quite early in the disease. Spread to distant skin sites is common, with multiple erythema migrans lesions being reported within days in up to 50% of cases.[17] Other organs commonly affected are the joints, heart, and nervous system. European investigators have reported greater prominence of neurologic symptoms (radicular pain, meningitis, myelitis), whereas American investigators have described a preponderance of rheumatologic symptoms. There are some data to suggest that these differences may be due to differences in the infecting strain. Arthritis is particularly prominent in patients infected with *B. burgdorferi sensu stricto;* meningopolyneuritis appears to be related to infections with *B. garinii;* and acrodermatitis atrophicans is most common with *B. afzelii* infections.[20] However, despite these differences, the disease remains largely similar in Europe and the United States.

Many patients with Lyme disease complain of migratory arthralgias and myalgias without any specific joint swelling. Left untreated, more than 50% of patients develop an inflammatory monoarticular or oligoarticular arthritis. The arthritis most typically affects the large joints, especially the knees. Attacks of arthritis can last from less than 1 week to several months and may recur after long symptom-free periods.[21, 22]

The neurologic symptoms of acute Lyme disease span a wide spectrum from mild headaches to meningitis. Headaches and neck stiffness are quite common, with, respectively, 64% and 48% of patients with erythema migrans reporting these symptoms in one series.[17] Over weeks to months, around 15% of untreated patients develop focal neurologic signs or symptoms, including meningitis, cranial neuropathies, encephalitis, myelitis, Argyll Robertson pupil, and papilledema.[23, 24] Neurologic manifestations with specific ENT implications are discussed later.

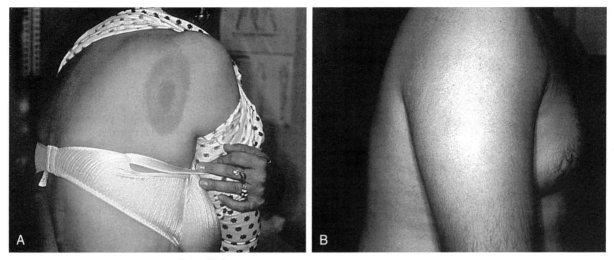

Figure 59-2. *A* and *B,* Examples of erthyema migrans lesions.

Acute cardiac manifestations of Lyme disease are less common than either rheumatologic or neurologic involvement—being seen in ~8%–10% of patients with early disseminated Lyme disease.[25] Clinical symptoms of cardiac involvement include fatigue, syncope, shortness of breath, and, rarely, chest pain. Up to 90% of patients with cardiac symptoms develop some degree of atrioventricular block; the block is usually temporary, with a median duration of less than 1 week. Mild myocarditis or pericarditis is seen in up to 65% of patients with cardiac involvement.

Chronic Disseminated Disease

Unlike the acute manifestations of Lyme disease, signs and symptoms of chronic Lyme disease are often not fully reversible with treatment. Approximately 10% of patients with acute arthritis go on to develop a chronic arthritis, characterized by erosion of bone and cartilage. The synovium is usually markedly inflamed with a heavy infiltration of mononuclear cells. Pathologically, endarteritis obliterans of small vessels is characteristic. Synovectomy may provide some relief for patients with intractable pain.[22]

The chronic neurologic manifestations of Lyme disease can involve both the central and peripheral nervous systems. The most common abnormality is a subacute encephalopathy affecting memory, mood, or sleep.[26, 27] Myelitis, localized encephalitis, and cerebellar ataxia have been reported but are uncommon. Cerebrospinal fluid (CSF) may show a persistent monocytic pleocytosis. Peripheral nervous system disease is most frequently manifested as paresthesias or hyperesthesias. Peripheral neuritis is not related to the area of the original tick bite or erythema migrans lesion and is often asymmetric, resembling polyneuritis multiplex. Untreated, symptoms may progress to spastic paraparesis or may involve bowel or bladder function; at this point, treatment may not fully reverse the symptoms.[28] Electrophysiologic studies of affected patients reveal axonal damage without isolated demyelinization.[29] On histologic examination, there is axonal injury with perivascular infiltration of lymphocytes and plasmocytes surrounding epineural blood vessels.[30]

Acrodermatitis atrophicans is a chronic skin condition of Lyme borreliosis seen almost exclusively in European patients—primarily women and the elderly. Acrodermatitis atrophicans develops years after the original infection, and *B. burgdorferi* have been recovered from lesions as long as 10 years after their onset. The lesions are violaceous with a doughy consistency; they are usually seen on the distal extremities, sparing the face, palms and soles. The lesions may be multicentric and can involve the area of the primary erythema migrans lesion. Allowed to progress, the lesions can become sclerotic or atrophic and resemble localized scleroderma or lichen sclerosis atrophicans.

B. burgdorferi can rarely involve the eye.[31] Keratitis, episcleritis, and inflammations of the posterior eye such as neuroretinitis, choroiditis, retinal vasculitis, optic neuritis, and vitreitis have all been reported, mostly in late-stage Lyme disease.[32–35] Response to therapy has generally been poor.[31]

ENT Considerations

Table 59–1 tabulates the head and neck symptoms noted by 266 patients with Lyme disease presenting to a clinic in Westchester County, New York.[36] Sore throat, headaches, and tinnitus are common but nonspecific signs seen during the early disseminated phase of the illness. The most characteristic head and neck sign affecting patients with Lyme disease is facial nerve palsy (Fig. 59–3). Facial palsies are reported in 40%–50% of Lyme disease patients with neurologic involvement, and in endemic areas, Lyme disease is the most common cause of facial palsies in children.[37, 38]

Facial nerve palsy occurs early in the course of Lyme disease. In the largest series to date, Clark and colleagues[43] found that 85 of 101 patients (84%) with facial palsy secondary to Lyme borreliosis had erythema migrans lesions and that, in 81% of these, palsy developed within 4 weeks of the onset of rash. In 3 patients, the palsy preceded the rash. Erythema migrans lesions involving the face were reported in 7 of 8 patients who subsequently developed facial nerve paralysis secondary to Lyme disease in Southampton, England.[39] The high frequency of this finding has not been noted in other series of adult patients. However, erythema

Table 59–1. HEAD AND NECK SYMPTOMS IN PATIENTS WITH LYME DISEASE

Symptom	No. of Patients (Total 266)	Percentage of Patients
Headache	149	56.0
Neck pain	112	42.1
Stiff neck	94	35.3
Throat pain	71	26.7
Dizziness	69	25.9
Cervical adenopathy	22	8.3
Facial paresthesia	17	6.4
Temporomandibular joint pain	14	5.3
Otalgia	14	5.3
Tinnitus	14	5.3
Hoarseness	13	4.9
Facial muscle spasm	13	4.9
Change in vision	13	4.9
Facial weakness	12	4.5
Aural fullness	11	4.1
Facial pain	9	3.4
Dysphagia	6	2.2
Facial hypesthesia	5	1.9
Hearing loss	4	1.5
Facial swelling	4	1.5
Decreased taste	4	1.5

From Moscatello AL, Worden AL, Nadelman RB, et al.: Otolaryngologic aspects of Lyme disease. Laryngoscope 1991: 101: 592–595.

migrans lesions involving the face have been commonly noted in children. In a series of 16 children with facial palsy from Lyme disease, either erythema migrans or a tick bite in the facial region was found in 9. The frequency of facial palsy also appears to be higher in children with Lyme disease than in adults.[37]

Two mechanisms have been proposed for facial nerve paralysis by *B. burgdorferi*: (1) damage of the cranial nerve in the subarachnoid space by meningitis or (2) a mononeuritis multiplex affecting the nerve's peripheral portion.[28] Most commonly, the nerve is affected distal to the branching

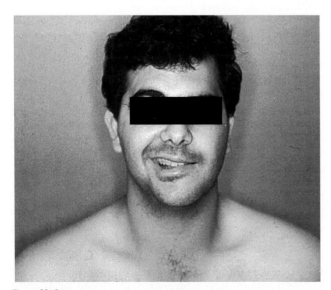

Figure 59–3. Facial nerve palsy in a patient with Lyme disease. (Reprinted by permission of the New England Journal of Medicine, Klempner MS, 327, 1788, 1992. Copyright 1992. Massachusetts Medical Society. All rights reserved.)

of the chorda tympani.[24] There is mounting evidence to suggest that facial nerve paralysis secondary to injury to the cranial nerve roots in the subarachnoid space occurs rarely or not at all.[28–30, 40, 41]

The facial nerve palsy is usually not complete. Of 20 patients from Switzerland, only 1 had 100% degeneration.[38] In 11 patients presenting to ENT clinics, the greatest facial nerve degeneration noted by topographic mapping was 69%.[42] Notably, bilateral involvement of the facial nerve is common in Lyme facial palsies, with up to 30% of patients showing bilateral weakness.[24, 38]

Facial weakness is often preceded or accompanied by numbness or tingling on the affected side; however, typically, no sensory abnormality can be demonstrated.[24] Temporomandibular joint pain is also frequently reported.[24, 43]

Recovery from facial palsy is usually complete. Of 122 patients with facial nerve palsy due to Lyme disease, 105 recovered completely, 16 had near complete recovery, and only 1 patient was left with a significant residual. Median time to recovery in these patients was 26 days (range 1–270 days). Bilateral facial palsy appears to be associated with a poorer prognosis, including higher incidence of incomplete and/or late recovery. The single patient in this study with significant residual had bilateral palsy, and of the 16 patients with near recovery, 8 had bilateral paralysis. Of the 12 patients who took longer than 3 months to recover, 4 had bilateral involvement.[43] Bilateral facial paralysis is also associated with an increased incidence of clinical meningoencephalitis and CSF pleocytosis.[44]

Although the facial nerve is, by far, the most commonly affected cranial nerve, Lyme disease has been reported to affect many other cranial nerves. In Pachner and Steere's[24] series of 38 patients with Lyme meningitis, one patient developed a 6th nerve palsy with an ipsilateral seventh nerve palsy; two patients had loss of taste with 9th and 10th nerve palsies, and one patient had hearing changes without hyperacusis.[24] In a series of 15 ENT patients with Lyme disease, Diehl and Holtmann[45] reported four patients with sudden hearing loss, three with tinnitus, and one with vestibular neuronitis. Hearing loss is usually total, and recovery of hearing is unusual. Tinnitus may also persist despite treatment.[45] Vertigo indistinguishable from acute vestibular neuronitis has been ascribed to Lyme borreliosis in up to 4% of patients presenting with otologic symptoms in Finland.[46] Paralysis of the recurrent laryngeal nerve causing vocal cord paralysis, odynophagia, and dysphagia have rarely been reported.[47, 48] Chronic Lyme disease can be related to irreversible cranial nerve palsies. Olivier and colleagues[49] reported a patient with undiagnosed Lyme disease who presented with diploplia, dysphonia, and problems with deglutition. The patient subsequently developed bilateral lesions of cranial nerve XII, paralysis of the tongue and soft palate, and partial paralysis of the frontalis muscle—none of which was reversed with treatment.[49]

DIFFERENTIAL DIAGNOSIS

Like syphilis, Lyme borreliosis is a spirochetal disease that can mimic many other infectious and noninfectious conditions. The differential diagnosis for each of the common symptoms of Lyme disease is long.

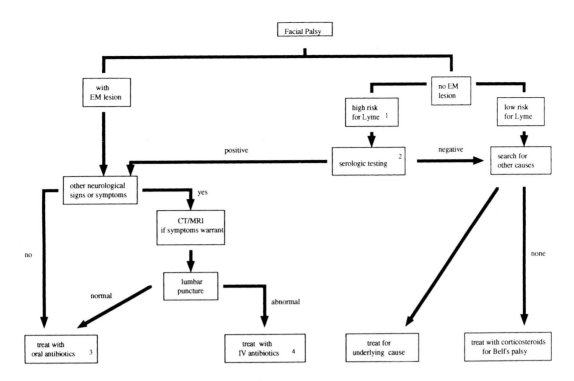

1
high risk patients include those patients in Lyme endemic areas who have manifestations of Lyme disease, history of tick bite, constitutional symptoms, bilateral facial palsy or children

2
serological testing with paired acute and convalescing specimens and/or serial testing with ELISA and Western blot

3
doxycycline 100 mg bid or amoxicillin 500 mg qid for 21 days are first line choices

4
penicillin G 5 million units qid or ceftriaxone 2 gm/day for 3-4 weeks are first line choices

Figure 59–4. Strategy for work-up of facial palsy in an endemic region for Lyme disease.

The differential diagnosis for facial palsy comprises both localized and systemic diseases (Fig. 59–4). Localized conditions causing facial palsy include temporal bone fractures, acoustic neuromas, suppuration or tumor of the middle ear and disorders of the parotid gland; systemic diseases causing facial palsy include leukemia, sarcoidosis, tuberculosis, Guillain-Barré syndrome, and multiple sclerosis. Of these, only sarcoidosis, Guillain-Barré, tuberculosis, and Lyme disease commonly cause bilateral facial palsy.

The most common diagnosis given to patients with facial nerve paralysis is Bell's (idiopathic) palsy. Bell's palsy accounts for 50%–75% of all diagnoses of facial palsy.[50, 51] In endemic regions, Lyme borreliosis may account for up to one quarter of cases ascribed to Bell's palsy.[52] Bell's palsy and Lyme facial palsy are equally distributed among the sexes and cause similar degrees of paralysis. Patients with paralysis secondary to Lyme disease tend to be younger and to have a better prognosis for recovery than patients with Bell's palsy.[43]

The prevalence of Lyme borreliosis among patients with isolated facial palsy without additional clinical manifestations of Lyme disease is low. When the clinical criteria history of tick bite, bilateral facial palsy, or symptoms related to Lyme borreliosis (erythema migrans, radiculoneuropathy, headache, fever, and arthritis) were used to exclude patients with Lyme disease, none of 69 patients given the diagnosis of Bell's palsy subsequently were found to have Lyme disease in a Lyme-endemic region.[53] Therefore, we believe it unnecessary to pursue the diagnosis of Lyme disease in a patient with facial palsy unless there are other manifestations of Lyme disease, constitutional symptoms, or the patient is in a high-risk group for Lyme disease (e.g., bilateral facial palsy, children in an endemic area with onset of palsy from May to September).

DIAGNOSIS

Imaging Studies

Magnetic resonance imaging (MRI), computed tomography (CT), and ultrasonography have limited utility in the diagnosis of Lyme disease. In patients with neurologic disease, MRI can show multiple, subcortical white matter lesions. The lesions are nonspecific and can be seen in almost any region of the brain, although there may be a slight predilection for the frontal and parietal lobes.[54–57] Lesions enhance with contrast with both MRI and CT. MRI is probably more sensitive than CT for identifying lesions due to Lyme disease. Resolution of lesions with therapy has not been extensively studied, but in case reports, lesions often persisted despite clinical improvement.[26, 58]

Gadolinium-enhanced MRI in patients with Lyme facial palsy can show increased signal intensity at the level of the geniculate ganglion and the fundus of the internal auditory canal.[59, 60] Minor enhancement of the nerve in the region of the fundus has been described in patients with Bell's palsy;

however, this does not occur to the same intensity as in patients with Lyme disease.[61, 62]

Ultrasound has been proposed as a method for diagnosing nonpalpable lymph node enlargement in patients with Lyme facial palsy. Facial nerve lymphatics are located within the nerve along the vasa nervorum and drain in parallel with the long blood vessels of the facial nerve trunk located in the connective tissue of the bony facial canal. In a series of 10 patients with unilateral facial nerve paralysis thought to be secondary to Lyme disease, all were shown to have nonpalpable lymph node enlargement within the parotid gland. Lymph nodes ranged in size 4–7 mm and were most commonly situated around the stylomastoid foramen. Ultrasonography of the contralateral (unaffected) parotid gland did not show any lymph node enlargement, and parotid lymph node enlargement has not been reported in patients with Bell's palsy.[62]

Laboratory Studies

Recovery of an organism from infected tissue or fluid is the gold standard of diagnosis for most bacterial diseases. Although *B. burgdorferi* has been cultured in Barbour-Stoenner-Kelly media from skin, cerebrospinal fluid, blood, and joints, the success rate is low.[63–66] Yields are highest in patients with acute disease. Cultures from erythema migrans lesions have higher yields than from other sites and are positive in 6%–45% of patients.[65] *B. burgdorferi* cannot be recovered from patients who have received even one dose of an antibiotic.

Visualization of the organism on histologic sections is also difficult. *B. burgdorferi* can be identified in sections stained with acridine orange, Dieterle, or Warthin-Starry stains or by dark-field microscopy. Identification of *Borrelia* is specific for disease, but because of low numbers of organisms at most sites, absence of *Borrelia* on histopathologic section does not rule out Lyme borreliosis.

The difficulties with culture and histologic identification of *B. burgdorferi* has led to a reliance on serodiagnosis for Lyme disease. The currently available serologic tests include indirect enzyme-linked immunosorbent assay (ELISA), indirect immunofluorescence assay (IFA), antibody capture enzyme immunoassay (EIA), and Western blot analysis.[67–69] These tests utilize whole, fixed bacteria or crude fractions of sonicated organisms; recombinant borrelial proteins are available and may eventually replace whole or sonicated bacteria in some of these tests.

The initial immune response in patients with Lyme disease is T-cell mediated. Assessments of the cellular immune response to *B. burgdorferi* have been studied, but their usefulness in clinical settings is limited by a high false-positive rate and the technical difficulty of performing the tests.[70, 71] The B-cell response develops more slowly; only 30%–40% of patients are seropositive at the time of their erythema migrans lesions.[69, 72] Detectable immunoglobulin (Ig) M responses usually develop 3–4 weeks after infection, peak at 6–8 weeks, and then gradually decline.[10, 73, 74] The early antibody response is primarily directed against a 41-kD flagellar antigen that is shared with other borrelia and treponemes.[74, 75] Antibodies to other more specific antigens

develop over time—with some developing quite late in the course. For example, the IgM response to the 34-kD outer-surface protein B may not develop for months. It is unclear why this occurs; it has been proposed that the spirochete may express different antigens during the course of infection, but this theory has not been substantiated. Regardless of the cause, even late antibody responses follow the typical pattern of IgM preceding IgG and IgA. This complicates the use of IgM antibody to diagnose acute disease, because IgM may be present concurrently with IgG late in the disease.[76] IgG and IgA responses usually develop in the second month after *B. burgdorferi* infection, and approximately 90% of patients have detectable IgG antibody to *B. burgdorferi* 4–6 weeks after infection. Antibiotic therapy early in the course of Lyme disease can abort the development of a diagnostic antibody response. If antibiotics are given after the development of a mature humoral response, antibody levels gradually fall—with >50% of patients having a negative IgG ELISA after 5 years. However, some patients have continued to have positive IgG ELISA for longer than 10 years.[76]

The use of serologic tests has been hampered by lack of standardization and interlaboratory variation—resulting in both false-positive and false-negative tests. Currently, each laboratory establishes its own criteria for positive and negative test results. Cross-reaction of antibodies to *B. burgdorferi* with other pathogenic and nonpathogenic spirochetes is a significant problem. Many laboratories use negative cutoffs of between 1:64 and 1:256 for IFA and absorbancies of greater than 3 standard deviations above the mean of healthy controls for ELISA. The sensitivity and specificity of the IgM ELISA in early Lyme disease are in the range of 40% and 94%, respectively and for the IgG ELISA, sensitivity and specificity are approximately 90% and 70%, respectively.[69] Patients with rheumatoid arthritis and systemic lupus erythematosus may have falsely positive ELISAs secondary to cross-reacting antibodies; Western blot analysis for borrelial proteins is negative in these patients. Because Lyme disease is not usually a rapidly progressing disease requiring immediate treatment, serologic testing of paired samples obtained 4–6 weeks apart may help to distinguish acute, ongoing infection from distant infection in patients whose clinical histories are questionable for Lyme disease.

To balance sensitivity and specificity in Western blot analysis, some experts recommend that at least 2 of the 8 most common IgM bands (sensitivity 40%, specificity 94%) or 5 of the 10 most common IgG bands (sensitivity 83%, specificity 95%) be present for a specimen to be considered positive.[69] As with the strategy of serologic testing for human immunodeficiency virus, the Centers for Disease Control and Prevention (CDC) now recommend the use of the more specific Western blot analysis to confirm the more sensitive but less specific ELISA.

In patients with suspected Lyme neuroborreliosis, the measurement of intrathecal antibody may be a useful adjunct. A ratio of CSF to serum antibody greater than 1 suggests intrathecal production of antibody and is highly specific for neuroborreliosis. Using a cutoff ratio of 1.3:1.0, Halperin and colleagues[27] obtained a specificity of 100% and a sensitivity of 53% in diagnosing neuroborreliosis in patients with lymphocytic mentingitis; when they used a cutoff of 0.9:1.0, the sensitivity improved to 87% and the specificity decreased to 93%.[27] In chronic neuroborreliosis, the specificity of CSF antibodies has ranged from 50% to 100%. False-positive results do occur in patients with neurosyphilis. Patients with only peripheral nervous system involvement do not produce intrathecal antibodies. European patients with neuroborreliosis have higher CSF-to-serum IgG antibody ratios to *B. burgdorferi* than American patients. Also, 20%–25% of European patients with Lyme neuroborreliosis have positive CSF antibodies to *B. burgdorferi* without positive serum antibodies; this does not appear to occur in American patients.[27, 77–79]

The term seronegative Lyme disease has been applied to a syndrome seen in patients living in *B. burgdorferi* endemic areas who have chronic pain or fatigue and negative *B. burgdorferi* serology results. In reality, the chronic symptoms of Lyme disease are closely related to the immune response in patients. Although it is true that patients treated early in the course of Lyme disease may not develop antibodies to *B. burgdorferi,* their clinical symptoms are also attenuated or aborted with treatment. Rarely, patients who have been treated early in the course of disease may continue to have a treatable infection in a protected site, such as the central nervous system (CNS), without developing systemic antibodies.[16] Measurement of intrathecal antibody in these patients may be helpful.[27] In general, clinicians should search for other diagnoses in patients with chronic symptoms and negative Lyme disease serologies.

The use of polymerase chain reaction (PCR) in diagnosing Lyme disease remains investigational. PCR has been used successfully to identify borrelial DNA in blood, CSF, urine, skin, and synovial fluid samples.[80–83] Although the specificity of CSF PCR for Lyme neuroborreliosis is close to 100%, the sensitivity, to date, has been disappointing (10%–50%).[81, 84] The detection of *B. burgdorferi* DNA by PCR after antibiotic treatment disappears rapidly (<20 days) in murine models.[85] If human studies confirm this finding, PCR may eventually have a role in monitoring the efficacy of antibiotic treatment in patients with Lyme disease.

Antitreponemal tests such as the fluorescent treponemal antibody absorption test (FTA-ABS) may be positive in Lyme disease. However, unlike in syphilis, the Venereal Disease Research Laboratory Test (VDRL) and rapid plasmin reagin test (RPR) are negative. Other nonspecific laboratory abnormalities seen in Lyme borreliosis include a mildly elevated erythrocyte sedimentation rate (ESR), mildly increased liver transaminases, and elevated white blood cell counts.[17] Tests for rheumatoid factor or antinuclear antibodies are usually negative. CSF in patients with Lyme meningitis usually reveals a lymphocytic pleocytosis.[86]

TREATMENT

There are few randomized, prospective studies comparing the efficacy of different treatment regimens for Lyme disease. In vitro, the tetracyclines and beta-lactam antibiotics have good activity against *B. burgdorferi.* Acute localized disease responds well to either amoxicillin, 500 mg four times daily (with or without probenecid) or doxycycline, 100 mg twice daily given for 21 days. Doxycycline has several advantages over amoxicillin: (1) it is better absorbed orally;

(2) it has better penetration into the cerebrospinal fluid; and (3) it is active against human granulocytic ehrlichiosis (which is transmitted by *Ixodes* ticks and may cause coinfection) and rickettsial diseases (which may sometimes be confused with Lyme disease). Erythromycin, 250 mg four times daily, or cefuroxime axetil, 500 mg twice daily, is an alternative for the penicillin-allergic patient or for children and pregnant women who cannot receive tetracyclines.[87–91] *B. burgdorferi* are resistant to rifampin, ciprofloxacin, and aminoglycosides.[87, 92] Failure of therapy for local infections has been reported and may be related to unrecognized dissemination to the CNS or to resistant bacteria. High-level resistance to penicillin has been noted in some strains of *B. burgdorferi.*[87, 88]

Treatment for disseminated disease usually requires intravenous antibiotics. Possible exceptions to this rule are patients with isolated facial nerve palsy, mild cardiac disease, or dermatologic signs only (multiple erythema migrans lesions or acrodermatitis chronicum atrophicans). Penicillin G, 5 million units four times daily and ceftriaxone, 2 gm per day, are the most widely used intravenous antibiotics for disseminated Lyme borreliosis. There are some limited data suggesting that ceftriaxone may be more effective than penicillin.[93, 94] Therapy may be accompanied by the development of Jarisch-Herxheimer reactions within 24 hours of initiation in up to 15% of patients with disseminated disease.

The success of antibiotic treatment for chronic symptoms of Lyme borreliosis is variable. Although acute meningitis and meningoencephalitis usually respond well to antibiotics, failure rates of up to 50% have been reported for patients with severe neurologic signs. Complete recovery in patients with chronic arthritis, acrodermatitis atrophicans, or peripheral neuropathy is rare.[23, 26, 95–97]

Resolution of facial palsy occurs independent of antibiotic therapy. Corticosteroids also do not seem to affect the course of Lyme facial palsy.[43]

PREVENTION

Two vaccines for Lyme disease are currently in development. One utilizes recombinant outer surface A lipoprotein (osp A) of *B. burgdorferi;* the other uses a recombinant bacille Calmette-Guérin (BCG) expressing osp A as an intranasal delivery system. Both vaccines have been shown to be immunogenic in humans.[98, 99] Antibody against osp A confers protection from infection in animal models.[100]

Avoidance of tick bites remains the mainstay of Lyme disease prevention. Simple measures such as tucking trousers into socks and inspection for ticks after possible exposures reduce the risk of Lyme disease. Use of chemical repellants on clothing, such as *N,N*-diethylmetoluamide (DEET) and permethrin, also increases protection.

Reduction of host availability as a means to control Lyme disease is difficult. Near-total elimination of deer in Great Island, Cape Cod, Massachusetts, resulted in marked decreases in *Ixodes* ticks and Lyme disease transmission; however, less drastic decreases in deer population were not shown to have any effect.[101] Similarly, broad scale rodent control is unlikely to be a feasible strategy in controlling tick populations.

The use of tick parasites and predators to reduce tick numbers has not been extensively studied. The tick predator *Hunterellus hookeri,* an encyrtid wasp, lays its eggs in the *Ixodes* larvae. These eggs hatch from the bloodfed nymphal tick, killing the tick in the process. Ticks parasitized by the wasp are only rarely infected with *B. burgdorferi,* possibly owing to preferential wasp oviposition in the tick midgut. Unfortunately, in American locations where wasp parasitism of *Ixodes* ticks is high, the risk of Lyme disease has remained high.[102]

The issue of prophylactic antibiotic use in patients bitten by ticks is an area of ongoing debate. Cost-benefit analysis concluded that prophylactic treatment would be cost-effective if the risk of infection in a given area was greater than or equal to 3.6%.[103] However, in a later study conducted around Lyme, Connecticut, where one third of the ticks are infected with *B. burgdorferi,* the risk of development of Lyme disease in placebo-treated patients was only 1.2% after a recognized tick bite.[104] Prophylactic antibiotics are not indicated for patients who have ticks attached for less than 24 hours. If prophylactic antibiotics are used, a 10-day course of amoxicillin or doxycyline is sufficient. Topical prophylaxis with tetracycline or beta-lactam antibiotics in a dimethyl sulfoxide carrier applied to the site of a tick bite was effective in preventing *B. burgdorferi* infection in mice bitten by infected ticks.[105] There is currently no evidence to recommend this treatment in humans.

References

1. Lyme Disease—United States, 1994. MMWR 1995; 44: 459–462.
2. Afzelius A: Verhandlungen der dermatologischen Gesellschaft zu Stockholm. Arch Dermatol Syphilol 1910; 101: 104.
3. Burgdorfer W: Discovery of the Lyme disease spirochete: A historical review. Zentralbl Bakteriol Mikrobiol Hyg 1986; 263: 7.
4. Bannwarth A: Zur klinik und pathogenese der "chronischen lymphocytaren meningitis." Arch Psychiatr Nervenkr 1944; 117: 161–185.
5. Hollstrom E: Penicillin treatment of erythema chronicum migrans Afzelius. Acta Derm Venereol 1958; 38: 285
6. Scrimenti RJ: Erythema chronicum migrans. Arch Dermatol 1970; 236: 859–860.
7. Steere AC, Malawista SE, Snydman DR, et al.: Lyme arthritis: An epidemic of oligoarticular arthritis in children and adults in three Connecticut communities. Arthritis Rheum 1977; 20: 7–17.
8. Burgdorfer W, Hayes SF, Benach JL, et al.: Lyme disease: A tickborne spirochetosis? Science 1982; 216: 1317–1319.
9. De Koning J, Bosma RB, Hoogkamp-Korstanje JA: Demonstration of spirochaetes in patients with Lyme disease with a modified silver stain. J Med Microbiol 1987; 23: 261–267.
10. Barbour AG: Immunochemical analysis of Lyme disease spirochetes. Yale J Biol Med 1984; 57: 581–586.
11. Barbour AG: Isolation and cultivation of Lyme disease spirochetes. Yale J Biol Med 1984; 57: 521–525.
12. Benach JL, Coleman JL, Skinner RA, et al.: Adult *Ixodes dammini* on rabbits: A hypothesis for the development and transmission of *Borrelia burgdorferi.* J Infect Dis 1987; 155: 1300–1306.
13. Bosler EM, Coleman J, Benach JL, et al.: Natural distribution of the *Ixodes dammini* spirochete. Science 1983; 220: 321–322.
14. Piesman J, Mather TN, Sinsky RJ: Duration of attachment and *Borrelia burgdorferi* transmission. J Clin Microbiol 1987; 25: 557.
15. Shih CM, Spielman A: Accelerated transmission of Lyme disease spirochetes by partically fed vector ticks. J Clin Microbiol 1993; 31: 2878–2781.
16. Stiernstedt G, Gustafsson R, Karlsson M, et al.: Clinical manifestations and diagnosis of neuroborreliosis. Ann N Y Acad Sci 1988; 539: 46–55.
17. Steere AC, Craft JE, Hutchinson GJ, et al.: The early clinical manifestations of Lyme disease. Ann Intern Med 1983; 99: 76–82.
18. Berger B: Erythema chronicum migrans of Lyme disease. Arch Dermatol 1984; 120: 1017–1021.
19. Asbrink E, Hovmark A: Early and late cutaneous manifestations in *Ixodes*-borne borreliosis. Ann N Y Acad Sci 1988; 539: 4–15.
20. Dressler F, Ackermann R, Steere AC: Antibody responses to the three genomic groups of *Borrelia burgdorferi* in European Lyme borreliosis. J Infect Dis 1994; 169: 313–318.
21. Steere AC, Malawista SE, Hardin JA, et al.: Erythema chronicum migrans and Lyme arthritis: The enlarging clinical spectrum. Ann Intern Med 1977; 86: 685–698.
22. Steere AC, Schoen RT, Taylor E: The clinical evolution of Lyme arthritis. Ann Intern Med 1987; 107: 725–731.
23. Reik L, Steere AC, Bartenhagen NH, et al.: Neurologic abnormalities of Lyme disease. Medicine 1979; 58: 281–294.
24. Pachner AR, Steere AC: The triad of neurologic manifestations of Lyme disease. Neurology 1985; 35: 47–53.
25. Steere AC, Batsford WP, Weinber M, et al.: Lyme carditis: Cardiac abnormalities of Lyme disease. Ann Intern Med 1980; 93: 8–16.
26. Logigian EL, Kaplan RF, Steere AC: Chronic neurologic manifestations of Lyme disease. N Engl J Med 1990; 323: 1438–1444.
27. Halperin JJ, Volkman DJ, Wu P: Central nervous system abnormalities in Lyme neuroborreliosis. Neurology 1991; 41: 1571–1582.
28. Halperin JJ, Luft BJ, Volkman DJ, et al.: Lyme neuroborreliosis: Peripheral nervous system manifestations. Brain 1990; 113: 1207–1221.
29. Logigian EL, Steere AC: Clinical and electrophysical findings in chronic neuropathy of Lyme disease. Neurology 1992; 42: 303–311.
30. Vallat JM, Leboutet MJ, Loubet A, et al.: Tick bite neuropathy: An analysis of nerve biopsies from seven cases. Neurology (N Y) 1984; 34(suppl): 146.
31. Karma A, Seppala I, Mikkila H, et al.: Diagnosis and clinical characteristics of ocular Lyme borreliosis. Am J Ophthalmol 1995; 119: 127–135.
32. Flach AJ, Lavoie PE: Episcleritis, conjunctivitis, and keratitis as ocular manifestations of Lyme disease. Ophthalmology 1990; 97: 973–975.
33. Wu G, Lincoff H, Ellsworth RM, et al.: Optic disc edema and Lyme disease. Ann Ophthalmol 1986; 18: 252–255.
34. Baum J, Barza M, Weinstein P, et al.: Bilateral keratitis as a manifestation of Lyme disease. Am J Ophthalmol 1988; 105: 75–77.
35. Bialasiewicz AA, Ruprecht KW, Naumann GOH, et al.: Bilateral diffuse choroiditis and exudative retinal detachments with evidence of Lyme disease. Am J Ophthalmol 1988; 105: 419–420.
36. Moscatello AL, Worden DL, Nadelman RB, et al.: Otolaryngologic aspects of Lyme disease. Laryngoscope 1991; 101: 592–595.
37. Christen HJ, Bartlau N, Hanefeld F, et al.: Peripheral facial palsy in childhood—Lyme borreliosis to be suspected unless proven otherwise. Acta Paediatr Scand 1990; 79: 1219–1224.
38. Hanny PE, Hauselmann HJ: Die Lyme-krqande sicht des neurologen. Schweiz Med Wochenschr 1987; 117: 901–915.
39. Markby DP: Lyme disease facial palsy: Differentiation from Bell's palsy. Br Med J 1989; 299: 605–606.
40. Halperin JJ, Little BW, Coyle PK, et al.: Lyme disease: Cause of a treatable peripheral neuropathy. Neurology 1987; 37: 1700–1706.
41. Vallat JM, Hugon J, Lubeau M, et al.: Tick bite meningoradiculoneuritis. Neurology 1987; 37: 749–753.
42. Lesser THJ, Dort JC, Simmen DPB: Ear, nose and throat manifestations of Lyme disease. J Laryngol Otol 1990; 104: 301–304.
43. Clark JR, Carlson RD, Sasaki CT, et al.: Facial paralysis in Lyme disease. Laryngoscope 1985; 95: 1341–1345.
44. Morgan M, Nathwani D: Facial palsy and infection: The unfolding story. Clin Infect Dis 1991; 14: 263–271.
45. Diehl GE, Holtmann S: Die Lyme—Borreliose und ihre Bedeutung fur den HNO-Arzt. Laryngol Rhinol Otol 1989; 68: 81–89.
46. Ishizaki H, Pyykko I, Nozue M: Neuroborreliosis in the etiology of vestibular neuronitis. Acta Otolaryngol (Stockh) 1993; 503: 67–69.
47. Schroeter V, Belz GG, Blenk H. Paralysis of recurrent laryngeal nerve in Lyme disease. Lancet 1988; 8622: 1245.
48. Lacau St. Guily J, Ferroir JP, et al.: Deglutition disorders in Lyme disease with severe neurological involvement. Presse Med 1993; 22: 421–424.
49. Olivier R, Godfroid E, Heintz R, et al.: Lyme borreliosis in a patient with severe multiple cranial neuropathy. Clin Infect Dis 1995; 20: 200.

50. Devriese PP, Schumacher T, Scheide A, et al.: Incidence, prognosis and recovery of Bell's palsy: A survey of about 1000 patients (1974–1983). Clin Otolaryngol 1990; 15: 15–27.

51. Adour KK: Current concepts in neurology, diagnosis and management of facial palsy. N Engl J Med 1982; 307: 348–351.

52. Halperin JJ, Golightly M: Lyme borreliosis in Bell's palsy. Neurology 1992; 42: 1268–1270.

53. Kuiper H, Devriese PP, de Jongh BM, et al.: Absence of Lyme borreliosis among patients with presumed Bell's palsy. Arch Neurol 1992; 49: 940–943.

54. Reik L, Smith L, Khan A, et al.: Demyelinating encephalopathy in Lyme disease. Neurology 1985; 235: 267–269.

55. Bonatti GP, Huber R, Gostner P, et al.: Computer tomographisches und MR-tomogrisches bild. Fortschr Geb Rontgenstr Nuklearmed Erganzungsband 1986; 147: 97–98.

56. Krohler J, Kasper J, Kern U, et al.: Borrelia encephalomyelitis [letter]. Lancet 1986; 2: 35.

57. Belman AL, Coyle PK, Roque C, et al.: MRI findings in children infected by Borrelia burgdorferi. Pediatr Neurol 1992; 8: 428–431.

58. Fernandez RE, Rothberg M, Ferencz G, et al.: Lyme disease of the CNS: MRI imaging findings in 14 cases. Am J Neuroradiol 1990; 11: 479–481.

59. Nelson JA, Wolf MD, Yuh WTC, et al.: Cranial nerve involvement with Lyme borreliosis demonstrated by magnetic resonance imaging. Neurology 1992; 42: 671–673.

60. Halperin JJ, Luft BJ, Anand AK, et al.: Lyme neuroborreliosis: Central nervous system manifestations. Neurology 1989; 39: 753–759.

61. Tien R, Dillon WP, Jackler RH: Contrast-enhanced MR imaging of the facial nerve in 11 patients with Bell's palsy. Am J Neuroradiol 1990; 11: 735–741.

62. Mann WJ, Amedee RG, Schreiber J: Ultrasonography for the diagnosis of Lyme disease in cases of acute facial paralysis. Laryngoscope 1992; 102: 525–527.

63. Snydman DR, Schenkein D, Berardi VP, et al.: Borrelia burgdorferi in joint fluid in chronic Lyme arthritis. Ann Intern Med 1986; 104: 798–800.

64. Rawlings JA, Fournier PV, Teltow GA: Isolation of Borrelia spirochetes from patients in Texas. J Clin Microbiol 1987; 25: 1148–1150.

65. Steere AC, Grodzicki RL, Craft JE, et al.: Recovery of Lyme disease spirochetes from patients. Yale J Biol Med 1984; 57: 557–560.

66. Benach JL, Bosler EM, Hanrahan JP, et al.: Spirochetes isolated from the blood of two patients with Lyme disease. N Engl J Med 1983; 308: 740–742.

67. Magnarelli LA, Meegan JM, Anderson JF, et al.: Comparison of an indirect fluorescent antibody test with an enzyme-linked immunosorbent assay for serological studies of Lyme disease. J Clin Microbiol 1984; 20: 181.

68. Russell H, Sampson JS, Schmid GP, et al.: Enzyme linked immunosorbent assay and indirect immunofluorescence assay for Lyme disease. J Infect Dis 1984; 149: 465.

69. Dressler F, Whalen JA, Reinhardt BN, et al.: Western blotting in the serodiagnosis of Lyme disease. J Infect Dis 1993; 167: 392–400.

70. Dattwyler RJ, Volkman DJ, Halperin JJ, et al.: Specific immune responses in Lyme borreliosis: Characterization of T cell and B cell response to Borrelia burgdorferi. Ann N Y Acad Sci 1988; 539: 93–102.

71. Dressler F, Yoshinari NH, Steere AC: The T-cell proliferative assay in the diagnosis of Lyme disease. Ann Intern Med 1991; 115: 533–539.

72. Shrestha M, Grodzicki RL, Steere AC: Diagnosing early Lyme disease. Am J Med 1985; 78: 235–240.

73. Craft JE, Fischer D, Shimamoto GT, et al.: Antigens of Borrelia burgdorferi recognized during Lyme disease: Appearance of a new immunoglobulin in response and expansion of the immunoglobulin G response late in the illness. J Clin Invest 1986; 78: 934–939.

74. Barbour AG, Burgdorfer W, Grunwaldt E, et al.: Antibodies of patients with Lyme disease to components of the Ixodes dammini spirochete. J Clin Invest 1983; 72: 504–515.

75. Coleman JL, Benach JL: Isolation of antigenic components from the Lyme disease spirochete: Their role in early diagnosis. J Infect Dis 1987; 155: 756–765.

76. Hammers-Berggren S, Lebech AM, Karlsson M, et al.: Serological follow-up after treatment of patients with erythema migrans and neuroborreliosis. J Clin Microbiol 1994; 32: 1519–1525.

77. Steere AC, Berardi VP, Weeks KE, et al.: Evaluation of the intrathecal antibody response to Borrelia burgdorferi as a diagnostic test for Lyme neuroborreliosis. J Infect Dis 1990; 161: 1203–1209.

78. Kaiser R, Rasiah C, Gassmann G, et al.: Intrathecal antibody synthesis in Lyme neuroborreliosis: Use of recombinant p41 and 14kDa flagellin fragment in ELISA. J Med Microbiol 1993; 39: 290–297.

79. Hansen K, Cruz M, Link H: Oligoclonal Borrelia burgdorferi–specific IgG antibodies in cerebrospinal fluid in neuroborreliosis. J Infect Dis 1990; 161: 1194–1202.

80. Nocton JJ, Dressler F, Rutledge BJ, et al.: Detection of Borrelia burgdorferi DNA by polymerase chain reaction in synovial fluid from patients with Lyme arthritis. N Engl J Med 1994; 330: 229–234.

81. Lebech AM, Hansen K: Detection of Borrelia burgdorferi in urine samples and cerebrospinal fluid samples from patients with early and late Lyme neuroborreliosis by the polymerase chain reaction. J Clin Microbiol 1992; 30: 1646–1653.

82. Schwartz I, Wormser GP, Schwartz JJ, et al.: Diagnosis of early Lyme disease by polymerase chain reaction amplification and culture of skin biopsies from erythema migrans lesions. J Clin Microbiol 1992; 30: 3082–3088.

83. Goodman JL, Jurkovich P, Kramber JM, et al.: Molecular detection of persistent Borrelia burgdorferi in the urine of patients with active Lyme disease. Infect Immun 1991; 59: 269–278.

84. Pachner AR, Delaney E: The polymerase chain reaction in the diagnosis of Lyme neuroborreliosis. Ann Neurol 1993; 34: 544–550.

85. Malawista WE, Barthold SW, Persing DH: Fate of Borrelia burgdorferi DNA in tissues of infected mice after antibiotic treatment. J Infect Dis 1994; 170: 1312–1316.

86. Maida E, Kristoferitsch W, Spiel G: Cerebrospinal fluid changes in Garin-Bujadoux-Bannwarth meningoradiculitis. Nervenarzt 1986; 57: 149–152.

87. Johnson RC, Kodner C, Russell M: In vitro and in vivo susceptibilities of the Lyme disease spirochete, Borrelia burgdorferi, to four antimicrobial agents. Antimicrob Agents Chemother 1987; 31: 164–167.

88. Preac-Mursic V, Wilske B, Schierz G, et al.: Comparative antimicrobial activity of the new macrolides against Borrelia burgdorferi. Eur J Clin Microbiol Infect Dis 1989; 8: 651–653.

89. Dattwyler RJ, Volkman DJ, Conaty SM, et al.: Amoxicillin plus probenecid versus doxycyline for treatment of erythema migrans borreliosis. Lancet 1990; 336: 1404–1406.

90. Massarotti EM, Luger SW, Rahn DW, et al.: Treatment of early Lyme disease. Am J Med 1992; 92: 396–403.

91. Nadelman RB, Luger SW, Frank E, et al.: Comparison of cefuroxime axetil and doxycycline in the treatment of early Lyme disease. Ann Intern Med 1992; 117: 273–280.

92. Dever LL, Jorgensen JH, Barbour AG: In vitro antimicrobial susceptibility testing of Borrelia burgdorferi: A microdilution MIC method and time-kill studies. J Clin Microbiol 1992; 30: 2692–2697.

93. Dattwyler RJ, Halperin JJ, Pass H, et al.: Ceftriaxone as effective therapy in refractory Lyme disease. J Infect Dis 1987; 155: 1322–1325.

94. Dattwyler RJ, Halperin JJ, Volkman DJ, et al.: Treatment of late Lyme borreliosis—randomized comparison of ceftriaxone and penicillin. Lancet 1988; 1: 1191–1194.

95. Kristoferitsch W, Sluga E, Graf M, et al.: Neuropathy associated with acrodermatitis chronica atrophicans: Clinical and morphological features. Ann N Y Acad Sci 1988; 539: 35–45.

96. Kampner AL, Anderson J: Reversible bladder denervation in acute polyradiculitis. Scand J Urol Nephrol 1982; 16: 291.

97. Steere AC, Green J, Schoen RT, et al.: Successful parenteral penicillin therapy of established Lyme disease. N Engl J Med 1985; 312: 869–874.

98. Langermann S, Palaszynski S, Sadziene A, et al.: Systemic and mucosal immunity induced by BCG vector expressing outer-surface protein A of Borrelia burgdorferi. Nature 1994; 372: 552–555.

99. Keller D, Koster FT, Marks DH, et al.: Safety and immunogenicity of a recombinant outer surface protein A Lyme vaccine. JAMA 1994; 271: 1764–1768.

100. Fikrig E, Barthold SW, Kantor FS, et al.: Protection of mice against the Lyme disease agent by immunizing with recombinant Osp A. Science 1990; 250: 553–556.

101. Wilson ML, Levine JF, Spielman A: Effect of deer reduction on abundance of the deer tick (Ixodes dammini). Yale J Biol Med 1984; 57: 697–705.

102. Jaenson TG, Fish D, Ginsberg HS, et al.: Methods for control of

tick vectors of Lyme borreliosis. Scand J Infect Dis Suppl 1994; 77: 151–157.

103. Magid D, Schwartz B, Craft J, et al.: Prevention of Lyme disease after tick bites: A cost-effectiveness analysis. N Engl J Med 1992; 327: 534–541.

104. Shapiro ED, Gerber MA, Holabird NB, et al.: A controlled trial of antimicrobial prophylaxis for Lyme disease after deer-tick bites. N Engl J Med 1992; 327: 1769–1773.

105. Shih CM, Spielman A: Topical prophylaxis for Lyme disease after tick bite in a rodent model. J Infect Dis 1993; 168: 1042–1045.

David F. Bennhoff

CHAPTER SIXTY

Actinomycosis

▼

Actinomycosis is a subacute and chronic cellulitic invasion of soft tissues. It is caused by various bacterial species of the Actinomycetes group, which gain tissue entry by way of a mucosal break. Actinomycosis begins as an inflammatory soft tissue mass, which can enlarge into an abscess-like swelling with penetration of the overlying skin and development of weeping fistulae.

HISTORY

Actinomycosis is a very old human disease, possibly existing as early as the third century.[1] Prior to the antibiotic era, it was a common illness and was easily recognized clinically; however, the microbiology of the etiologic organisms was not fully clarified until the 1940s. The cervicofacial disease typically began as a localized swelling in the face or neck. Regional spread led to bony involvement. Surgical excision of sinus tracts, drainage of abscess cavities, removal of bulky infected masses, and curettage of osteomyelitic and bony lesions were all used.[2] Therapeutic outcome was variable, however, and even if healing occurred, sequelae and complications were common. The disease often became lifelong and death was not unusual. With the advent of sulfa and then penicillin, the incidence and morbidity of actinomycosis declined. This led to a general lack of familiarity with the disease, eventually resulting in delayed diagnoses.

Human actinomycosis was first described in the medical literature in 1857,[3] although similar disease in cattle had been described in 1826.[2] Analysis of bovine lesions in 1877 resulted in discovery of a fungus-like organism with radiating filaments, which caused the disease to be named actinomycosis or "ray fungus condition."[3, 4] Within a year of this landmark discovery, Israel isolated an *Actinomyces* species from sulfur granules in a human patient.[5] He further described the human form of the disease and discovered that *Actinomyces* did not survive outside of its mammalian hosts and was not found exogenously in plants or soil.[5, 6] The species he discovered was subsequently named *Actinomyces israelii* in his honor. In 1940 Erikson showed that *Actinomyces bovis* and *A. israelii* were distinct etiologic agents for the bovine and human diseases, respectively.[7] Although other *Actinomyces* species have been identified in human disease,[8, 9] *A. bovis* does not normally cause illness in humans.[3, 10]

MICROBIOLOGY

The etiologic agents for actinomycosis are bacteria. However, because the *Actinomyces* organisms resembled fungi in appearance and because the disease mimicked a slowly progressive mycotic illness, the misconception arose that actinomycosis was a fungal disease.[3] In the past some investigators placed them in an intermediate status between fungi and bacteria.[11, 12]

The species causing actinomycosis are members of the bacterial order Actinomycetales (synonym "Actinomycetes"), which is divided into numerous families (Table 60–1). The pathogens of primary medical interest are the family Actinomycetaceae (including the three genera that cause actinomycosis in humans and animals), the family Nocardiaceae (including the two genera and several species that cause nocardiosis and several cutaneous diseases), and the two families containing the genera (*Actinomadura* and *Streptomyces*) in which are found species causing actinomycotic mycetoma.[3] The Mycobacteriaceae family is another member of this order and includes the agents for tuberculosis, leprosy, and atypical mycobacteriosis (Table 60–1).

The three genera causing actinomycosis *(Actinomyces, Propionibacterium,* and *Bifidobacterium)* are anaerobic or microaerophilic, and they are not acid-fast. Their mycelial-like colony breaks up into bacillary or coccoid elements. These features distinguish the organisms causing actinomycosis from the organisms in the other related families.[3]

Absence of a nuclear membrane places *Actinomyces*

Table 60–1. PARTIAL TAXONOMY OF THE PATHOGENIC ACTINOMYCETES

Superkingdom: Prokaryotae
Kingdom: Monera
Phylum: Schizomycota
Class: Eubacter
Order: Actinomycetales
Family: Actinomycetaceae
Genus: Actinomyces
Species: *israelii, viscosus, naeslundii, odontolyticus, meyerii, bovis, suis, hordeovulnaris, keratolyticus*
Genus: *Propionibacterium*
Species: *propionica*
Genus: *Bifidobacterium*
Species: *dentium*

Family: Nocardiaceae
Genus: *Nocardia*

Family: Maduramycetaceae
Genus: *Actinomadura*

Family: Streptomycetaceae
Genus: *Streptomyces*

Family: Dermatophilaceae
Genus: *Dermatophilus*

Family: Mycobacteriaceae
Genus: *Mycobacterium*

among the higher prokaryotic bacteria.[3] The lack of chitin and glutans,[9] plus the presence of muramic acid in the cell walls and the absence of mitochondria,[3] is a distinct bacterial feature. The branching filaments of *Actinomyces* are distinctly narrower than the similar branching filaments of fungi. *Actinomyces* reproduces by bacterial fission rather than by sporogenic or filamentous budding as do fungi.[3] Unlike *Actinomyces*, true fungi have a plant body.[13] Finally, growth of all *Actinomyces* species is impaired by antibacterial agents but not by antifungal agents.[3] Ribonucleic acid sequencing analysis has now confirmed their phylogenetic position within bacterial classification.[14]

Although *A. israelii* is the causative bacteria for most cases of human actinomycosis, six other species have been implicated as occasional etiologic agents. An example of this is *Propionibacterium propionica*. Formerly called *Arachnia propionica*, this interesting variant was originally classified as *Actinomyces propionicus*,[15] but based on certain differences in metabolism it was given its own family.[3] It is otherwise essentially identical to *A. israelii*.[8] *Actinomyces viscosus*, *Actinomyces naeslundii*, *Actinomyces odontolyticus*, *Actinomyces meyerii*,[16, 17] and *Bifidobacterium dentium*, formerly *Actinomyces eriksonii*,[3] are the other proven agents in human actinomycosis. They all cause a clinical illness indistinguishable from that due to *A. israelii*.[3, 9, 10, 15]

All species of *Actinomyces* are normal commensal inhabitants of the oral and buccal cavities in humans and certain other mammals.[3] Their relationship is not classified as symbiotic because there is no mutual benefit achieved. They are not true parasites because they normally cause no harm to the host. However, they assume a parasitic role when infection with inflammatory tissue response is initiated. Like *Mycobacterium tuberculosis*, they survive phagocytosis by host cells, and in this role they are defined as facultative intracellular parasites.[11] The *Actinomyces* organisms are not found outside of their hosts,[11] probably because they do not thrive at a temperature less than 30° C.[18]

ASSOCIATED BACTERIA

Cultures from lesions of actinomycosis typically reveal a variety of accompanying bacteria, including anaerobic streptococci, fusiform bacilli, *Haemophilus* species, and gram-negative bacilli. These bacteria apparently interact synergistically, perhaps helping to establish an anaerobic medium or otherwise somehow enhancing the conditions that encourage *Actinomyces* to thrive and expand.[19] These accompanying bacteria are found in the closed tissue lesions of actinomycosis, as well as in the open fistulous forms of the illness, and therefore they are not likely due to coincidental contamination or secondary infection. The most common bacterium found in association with actinomycosis is appropriately named *Actinobacillus actinomycetemcomitans*,[2] which is another oral commensal and is frequently found in the cervicofacial form of the disease.[15, 20]

Identification of these accompanying bacteria often obscured the true etiology of actinomycosis in the past, and it is still a problem in diagnosis today. The presence of a *Streptomyces* organism found in actinomycotic lesional material in 1890 led to the assumption that it was the causative agent for actinomycosis. Because this contaminating organism was also found in straw, actinomycosis was thought for many years to be an occupational hazard of farmers.[3, 9]

The presence of these associated bacteria appears to be fundamental to the development of clinical actinomycosis because of the minimal pathogenicity of the *Actinomyces* species by themselves.[3, 21] The selection of an antibiotic that is effective in eliminating the associated bacteria may also eliminate conditions that promote *Actinomyces* growth.[3, 9, 22, 22a] Thus, it is perhaps appropriate to think of actinomycosis as a polymicrobial infection.

EPIDEMIOLOGY

Actinomyces species are found in the oral cavity and are isolated readily from tonsillar crypts, interdental sulci, periodontal membranes, and saliva. Poor oral hygiene and dental caries appear to be primary predisposing conditions for developing the illness. Cope stated that the disease was at one time so common and easy to diagnose that it "existed wherever there was a microscope and a laboratory."[23] Widespread use of antibiotics has markedly decreased the incidence of this disease so that it is now seen only infrequently in people. However, in dairy cattle and stud bulls, actinomycosis is still commonly seen as "lumpy jaw."[2] Interestingly, it is not seen in feed lot steers who receive antibiotics in their grain.[24]

The incidence of human actinomycosis has declined in the United States. Weese and Smith found one case per 12,000 admissions in the 1930s and then one case per 21,000 admissions in the 1950s.[25, 26] Bennhoff found only one case per 63,000 admissions in the 1970s.[26] However, actinomycosis is still a problem in less developed nations and in Third World countries.[3] Poor oral hygiene, increased dental disease, and less accessible medical care are important contributors to this Third World pattern. Actinomycosis is also found in greater frequency in inner city populations of the United States.[26] Nevertheless, actinomycosis affects all socioeconomic levels and all races and is not limited to any one segment of the population.[25–29]

Interestingly, there has always been a male-to-female predominance in a ratio of approximately 3:1.[23, 25, 28, 30–32] It has been postulated that this sexual predilection derives from the greater likelihood for facial and oral trauma in males.[26] The incidence of the disease is increased in persons from ages 30 to 60[26, 28, 30, 31] but is very rare in children.[33, 34] This may be due to the lower incidence of periodontal disease in the young and the old.[26]

Contrary to past belief, there is no predilection for actinomycosis in rural communities,[25] among farmers,[3] or in individuals who chew straw or grass.[35] Also there is no recorded instance of contagion from person to person or from cattle to person.[6, 29] Limited outbreaks within cattle herds have been traced to cattle that ate hay containing thorns that punctured the oral mucosa.[24]

Although gingival inflammation is the usual portal of entry, there have been reports of direct inoculation, including otherwise normal eruption of a molar tooth,[31] routine dental extraction, and open injury to the oral mucosa.[13] Actinomycosis of the skin has resulted from a human bite[3, 13] and a cow's bite *(A. bovis)*.[3] Cellulitis of the knuckles[13] and osteomyelitis of the hand[36] have followed fistfights in which the teeth were struck. Many minor dental infections may actually be due to actinomycosis,[11, 37, 38] but they are cured by empirical antibiotic administration.

Actinomycosis is not an "opportunistic" infection. For example, actinomycosis does not occur in immunosuppressed patients despite speculation to the contrary.[33, 39] Although it has been reported on occasion in patients receiving corticosteroids[25] and in patients infected by the human immunodeficiency virus,[40–43] these few instances appear to be coincidental. Actinomycosis is difficult to produce in laboratory animals, and then only limited lesions are formed, suggesting that the organism is relatively avirulent.[21, 44]

CLINICAL MANIFESTATIONS

The cervicofacial disease presents with a mass in the lower face or upper neck, especially common along the inferior mandibular border.[9] Initially it is painless, discrete, and semisoft. After a short time, the mass may become more diffuse and painful with mild discoloration and swelling of the overlying skin. The infection spreads by direct extension as a burrowing low-grade inflammatory mass, without regard for anatomic tissue planes or for lymphatic channels.[3] Proteolytic enzyme production by *Actinomyces* may play a role in this expanding lesion.[45] The locally enlarging mass can mimic a neoplasm[9, 13, 46] (Figs. 60–1 and 60–2). Lymphatic spread is very uncommon and usually occurs only in later stages of the disease. Regional adenopathy is therefore typically absent. Hematogenous spread is very rare and occurs only in advanced forms of the cervicofacial disease when the mandibular cortex is eroded and organisms reach the marrow cavity.[3]

A notable clinical clue is recurrent fluctuation in the size of the mass coinciding with the administration and discontinuation of antibiotics; such a pattern of fluctuating size should raise the index of suspicion for actinomycosis. The mass commonly develops a nodular, "wooden," brawny character that ultimately degenerates centrally and softens into a semi–abscess-like fullness.[9] Incision into such a lesion is reminiscent of cutting into the meaty core of a coconut. As the margins of the burrowing expanding lesion extend, skin may be penetrated, and weeping fistulous sites may arise.[3] These classic sinus tracts may be multiple and open and close spontaneously (Fig. 60–3). Discomfort is common, but severe pain is not typical. Trismus may occur and is more likely due to the mass effect than inflammation.[3]

If the disease is not treated, the facial bones may become involved. Extension to the marrow space of the mandible may lead to metastatic infection with widespread dissemination.[25] Death due to intracranial involvement has occurred in some of these cases. Other presentation sites in the head and neck have included the tongue,[23, 46, 47] cheek,[25, 48] palate,[25] periodontal membrane,[11] periapical cyst,[37, 38] temporomandibular joint,[49] paranasal sinus,[25, 50] lacrimal canaliculus,[25, 51, 52]

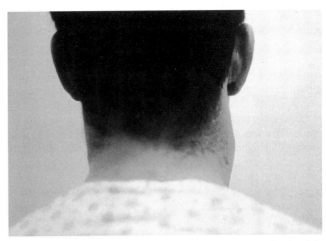

Figure 60–2. A rear view of the same patient; the fullness in the right cervical area is more obvious.

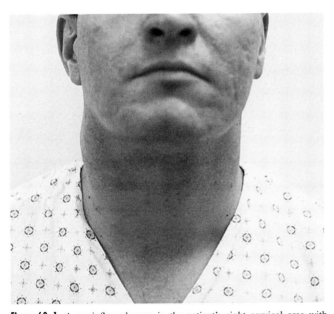

Figure 60–1. A noninflamed mass in the patient's right cervical area with cervicofacial actinomycosis.

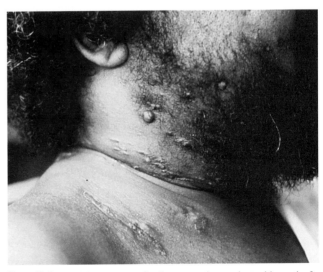

Figure 60–3. Multiple cutaneous fistulous tracts in a patient with cervicofacial actinomycosis.

lacrimal gland,[31] parotid gland,[25] orbit,[53] scalp,[25] ear and mastoid,[54] thyroglossal cyst,[55] branchial cyst,[56] thyroid gland,[57] hypopharynx,[31] and larynx.[58–62] Also, actinomycosis has mimicked a cholesteatoma in the middle ear[63] and has complicated osteoradionecrosis of the mandible following radiation therapy.[64] Curiously, a primary localized tonsil lesion itself has never been reported even though *Actinomyces* is commonly found existing in crypts of tonsils both in clinical bacteriologic studies and in ordinary laboratory examinations following routine tonsillectomy procedures. It has been speculated that the presence of *Actinomyces* may be a contributing factor in cases of noninfectious tonsillar hypertrophy associated with obstructive clinical symptoms.[65]

The cervicofacial form is the most common presentation of actinomycosis, occurring in 55% of cases. Tracheobronchial aspiration from the oral cavity leads to the pulmonothoracic presentation in 15% of cases. Gastrointestinal ingestion of the organism leads to the abdominopelvic form in approximately 20% of cases.[25] Other various manifestations include a pelvic form associated with intrauterine contraceptive devices.[66–68]

DIFFERENTIAL DIAGNOSIS

On initial encounter, the tissue mass is easily mistaken for a benign salivary tumor, an inflammatory node, or a branchial cyst with or without infection. Later, it may mimic a deep fascial space infection or an expanding malignancy. The mass can also appear as any other chronic deep-seated granulomatous disease, including tuberculosis, atypical mycobacteriosis, blastomycosis, coccidioidomycosis, nocardiosis, glanders, tularemia, bacterial osteomyelitis, syphilitic gumma, and sarcoidosis.[3, 29, 39]

PATHOLOGY

Grossly, in the very early actinomycotic lesion, there is a localized cellulitic reaction associated with swelling, but with less vascularity than expected with other forms of bacterial cellulitis. As the infection spreads, inflammatory changes with modest edema and occasional suppuration follow. Later, a chronic granulomatous lesion develops, often with central breakdown and a resultant abscess-like mass. Brawny induration may accompany this, but true fibrosis is not typical and is usually associated with healing. The classic thick peripheral zone of a well-established lesion is dense, collagenous, and remarkably avascular. There is a combination of seropurulent and granulomatous involvement centrally. The eventual development of fistulae results in a watery, semipurulent exudate. Visible within this exudative fluid, or within the center of the semiabscess itself, can often be found the classic macroscopic sulfur granules. These are actually tiny aggregated colonies of the organism, which may achieve 1–2 mm in size. These granules are typically yellowish-white, firm, grainy, and may be spheroid or lobulated. Cellular debris clings to the colonies and may harbor other microorganisms.[3]

Microscopically, the sulfur granule is an adherent mass of neutrophils fixed to club-shaped filaments, which in turn

extend in a raylike fashion forming a "rosette." The rosette may measure from fewer than 100 to more than 300 μm, most being within that range. The coccoid and bacillary bodies of *Actinomyces* can be seen within this rosette.[3] This central aggregate is surrounded by a wall of lymphocytes, plasma cells, epithelioid cells, and histiocytes. In the periphery, the granulation tissue mixed with lipoid cells contributes to the yellowish cast, which originally gave rise to the name "sulfur" granule. Occasional giant cells may be seen.

In a fresh preparation the clubbed filaments may be seen without staining after moistening and crushing the grains between slides. Examination with low power reveals a zone of central opacification with a surrounding clear area occupied by gelatinous debris. A Gram's stain of the granule demonstrates the radiating gram-positive filaments and also the scattered coccoid and bacillary bodies. The granules also color easily with a hematoxylin and eosin preparation (Figs. 60–4 and 60–5). The central core of the rosette appears basophilic, and the peripheral shafts of the club take up eosin.[3] Methenamine silver stains are useful because even older filaments take up the stain.[35] Periodic acid–Schiff and other fungal stains can be of value in uncertain situations because they do not stain *Actinomyces*.[3]

DIAGNOSIS

Definitive diagnosis requires isolation of the organism. However, a positve *Actinomyces* culture is found in less than 50% of cases. If actinomycosis is being considered, discontinuation of all antibiotics for 10 days, followed by fine needle aspiration, with anaerobic transportation to the laboratory, increases the culture success rate.[69] A large bore needle biopsy may be required, or even an open biopsy may be necessary to obtain tissue for culture or to search for the typical granules.[35]

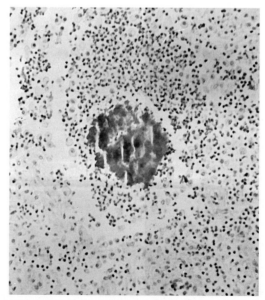

Figure 60–4. A sulfur granule stained with hematoxylin and eosin. The granule appears as a pink amorphous mass located within an abscess (×100).

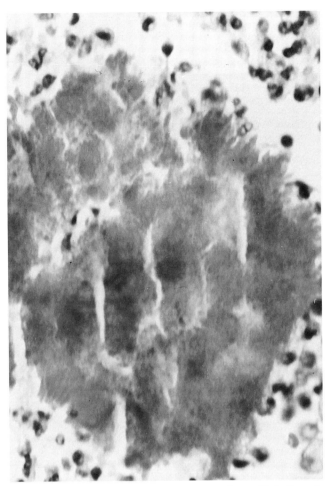

Figure 60–5. Close-up of the sulfur granule in Figure 60–4. Note the neutrophils surrounding the granule (×400).

Culture technique requires washing the grains, or sulfur granules, in sterile saline to remove associated bacteria. Inoculation in brain-heart agar or blood agar in an anaerobic media, with 5% carbon dioxide atmosphere at 37° C is necessary. Simultaneous aerobic incubation can identify other associated bacteria. Growth after 2–4 days yields loose branching filaments or white irregular specks like tiny grains of sand. At 4–6 days, colonies develop into an opaque white or cream-colored mass of spider-like filaments. These are often organized into a small irregular molar tooth-like shape. An opaque, white, heaped-up, rough colony usually stands out even in the face of abundant other bacterial growth. Isolation in glucose infusion broth with anaerobic incubation results in crumb-like or cauliflower-like growth. *A. israelii* may be subcultured into a thioglycollate broth where it grows more slowly into a hard fuzzy-edged granule. The other individual *Actinomyces* species can be further differentiated by various biochemical and microbiologic features.[3, 7]

Even when proper techniques are employed, a positive culture can be thwarted in several ways. Prior clinical use of antibiotic treatment in a patient can suppress subsequent laboratory growth of the organism even with proper media and conditions, or the extreme microaerophilic or anaerobic environment necessary for successful culture of the organism

may not be met.[9] The frequent overgrowth of associated bacteria can sometimes obscure proper identification of *Actinomyces*. Also, actinomycotic filaments show true branching, which may be mistaken for fungi. Therefore, when submitting material from lesions of uncertain etiology, it is advisable to request culture studies for actinomycosis specifically, along with the routine requests for aerobic and anaerobic organisms, acid-fast bacilli, and fungi.

In the absence of a positive culture of an *Actinomyces* species, a strong, presumptive diagnosis may be made on other grounds. Identification of the bacterium *A. actinomycetemcomitans* should raise the index of suspicion for actinomycosis, especially if it is isolated in the context of a compatible clinical situation.[2, 3]

The discovery of sulfur granules is virtually diagnostic, although they may be hard to find. In one study, only one sulfur granule was found in 26% of the 181 cases of actinomycosis reviewed.[30] Sliding purulent material down the wall of a test tube or a slide may be helpful in picking out the granules grossly as they adhere to the glass. Microscopically, they may be seen with a hematoxylin and eosin stain[35, 58] (Fig. 60–4). However, other microbes may obscure the granules, and then only persistent examination will yield success.

Although actinomycosis is the disease most commonly associated with the finding of sulfur granules, similar but not identical grains can occasionally be found in other illnesses. Nocardiosis, which produces a morphologically similar granule,[3] is the most common example.[30, 39] Myerowitz stated, however, that those instances are so rare that the presence of sulfur granules "virtually guarantees" the diagnosis of actinomycosis.[70] Furthermore, nocardiosis granules are almost always acid-fast,[3, 15] but the granules of actinomycosis never are.[3, 9, 69] Other conditions may occasionally demonstrate sulfur granule–like manifestation as a host response to foreign material. This response is known as the Splendore-Hoeppli phenomenon, which may be seen as a response to suture material, helminths, fungi, and also other bacteria, especially staphylococci, in which case the term botryomycosis is used.[71] This type of granule is different morphologically and is therefore distinguished from the *Actinomyces* sulfur granules.[69]

The isolation of *Actinomyces* from routine sputum culture, which is subject to oral contamination, has no diagnostic significance.[11, 13] *Actinomyces* and sulfur granules can be found routinely in the crypts of tonsils[72] or salivary duct calculi,[11] and this discovery also has no clinical significance.

There are no serologic tests or skin tests currently available for screening purposes. Serology is impractical for diagnosis as a result of cross-precipitating antibodies that form in other illnesses, especially tuberculosis.[73] However, typing of species can be performed by using a fluorescein isothiocyanate antiserum. This technique can even identify more than one *Actinomyces* species in a single granule.[74]

Imaging studies may reveal the extent of disease but offer no specific diagnostic clues. Maxillary periostitis and mandibular osteomyelitis can be seen occasionally on x-ray.[3] Cervicovertebral involvement has also been reported. Computed tomography scanning may demonstrate an ill-defined mass in the neck with obliteration of anatomic tissue planes and areas of soft tissue destruction.[75]

TREATMENT

Antibacterial agents are the mainstay of therapy. Surgery has become less important but might be indicated when grossly necrotic material requires evacuation or densely collagenous tissue must be resected.[2, 76] These procedures may be beneficial as they reduce the volume of anaerobic tissue in which *Actinomyces* thrives. Most antibiotics are effective in varying degrees against *Actinomyces*. Penicillin remains the agent of choice. Doses of penicillin G from 18 to 24 million units per day intravenously in six divided doses is the generally accepted initial therapy in more advanced cases. This high dose is necessary to penetrate the avascular fibrous walls of the lesion and to reach the core of the sulfur granules.[18, 77] In less severe cervicofacial presentations, several days to 2 weeks of intravenous penicillin can be administered until response is seen. Subsequent oral penicillin V 250 to 500 mg orally four times a day for 3 to 12 months is generally curative. Administration of oral penicillin should be continued until at least 6 weeks after the facial or neck lesion is fully resolved.[12] The cervicofacial form of the disease carries a very good prognosis when treated with antibiotics alone, especially when it is diagnosed early before extensive induration or bone involvement occurs. The occasional failure of treatment should stimulate a search for an undrained abscess[18] as acquired antibiotic resistance has not yet been demonstrated in actinomycosis.[78]

Alternative antibiotics are available. Tetracyclines are useful in the penicillin-allergic patient.[79] The tetracycline analogues, minocycline and doxycycline, have been favored because of their longer half-life with twice daily dosing. Erythromycin is acceptable,[9] although gastrointestinal side effects may be a limiting factor. The clinical efficacy of the newer macrolides remains to be evaluated, although *A. meyerii* was sensitive to clarithromycin and azithromycin in vitro.[80] Clindamycin has been used successfully for initial intravenous therapy and subsequent maintenance oral therapy, as well as for prolonged oral administration alone.[61, 81-83] Imipenem was successful in a complicated case of combined abdominal and thoracic disease.[84] Rifampin is highly active in vitro,[78, 85] and excellent results have been reported for disease in the neck[26] and the lung.[86] Sulfonamides,[39] chloramphenicol,[13] streptomycin,[18] vancomycin,[2] isoniazid,[87] and lincomycin[88] have also been reported with varying success. Cephalothin[89] and cephaloridine[90] have been effective, but cephalexin shows weak activity in vitro.[79] Ampicillin is active in vitro,[79] and amoxicillin has been effective clinically.[91]

References

1. Molto JE: Differential diagnosis of rib lesions: A case study from Middle Woodland Southern Ontario, circa 230 A.D. Am J Phys Anthropol 1990; 83: 437–439.
2. Richtsmeier WJ, Johns ME: Actinomycosis of the Head and Neck. Crit Rev Clin Lab Sci 1979; 11: 175–202.
3. Rippon JW: Medical Mycology: The Pathogenic Fungi and the Pathogenic Actinomycetes, 3rd ed. Philadelphia: WB Saunders Co., 1988, pp 15, 52, 61, 64.
4. Bollinger O: Ueber eine neue Pilzkrankheit beim Rinde. Centralbl Med Wissensch 1877; 15: 481.
5. Israel J: Neue Beobachtungen auf dem Gebiete der Mykosen des Menschen. Arch für Pathol Anat Physiol 1878; 74: 15.
6. Delacretz J, Grigoriu D, Ducel G: Medical Mycology (Atlas). Hans Huber, 1976, pp 149–151.
7. Erikson D: Pathogenic anaerobic organisms of the *Actinomyces* group. Br Med Res Council (Special Report Series) 1940; 240: 1–63.
8. Brock DW, Georg LK, Brown JM, et al.: Actinomycosis caused by *Arachnia proprionica*: Report of 11 cases. Am J Clin Pathol 1973; 59: 66–77.
9. Russo TA: Agents of actinomycosis. In: Mandell G, Bennett J, Dolin R (eds.): Principles and Practice of Infectious Diseases, 4th ed. New York: Churchill-Livingstone, 1995, pp 2280–2288.
10. Georg LK: The agents of human actinomycosis. In: Balows A (ed): Anaerobic Bacterial Role in Disease. Springfield, Illinois: Charles C Thomas, 1974, pp 237–250.
11. Youmans GP, Paterson PY, Sommers HM: The Biologic and Clinical Basis of Infectious Disease, 2nd ed. Philadelphia: WB Saunders Co., 1980, pp 13, 21, 285–299.
12. Emmons CW, Binford CA, Utz JP, Kown-Chung KJ: Medical Mycology, 3rd ed. Philadelphia: Lea and Febiger, 1977, pp 14, 29, 87, 89–102.
13. Dubos R, Hirsch J (eds): Bacterial and Mycotic Infections of Man, 4th ed. Philadelphia: JB Lippincott Co., 1965, pp 329–341, 490, 825.
14. Stackebrandt E, Charfreitag O: Partial 16S rRNA primary structure of five *Actinomyces* species: Phylogenetic implication. J Gen Microbiol 1990; 136: 137–143.
15. Smego RA Jr: Actinomycosis. In: Hoeprich PD, Jordan MC, Ronald AR (eds): Infectious Diseases, 5th ed. Philadelphia: JB Lippincott Co., 1994, pp 493–497.
16. Marty H, Wust J: Disseminated actinomycosis caused by *Actinomyces meyeri*. Infection 1989; 17: 154–155.
17. Lentino JR, Allen JE, Stachowski M: Hematogenous dissemination of thoracic actinomycosis due to *Actinomyces meyeri*. Pediatr Infect Dis 1985; 4: 698–699.
18. Peabody JW, Seabury JH: Actinomycosis and nocardiosis: A review of basic differences in therapy. Am J Med 1960; 28: 99–115.
19. Wangensteen OH: The role of surgery in the treatment of actinomycosis. Ann Surg 1936; 104: 752–770.
20. McGowan JE Jr, Steinberg JP: Other gram-negative bacilli. In: Mandell GL, Bennett JE, Dolan R (eds): Principles and Practice of Infectious Diseases, 4th ed. New York: Churchill Livingstone, 1995, pp 2106–2107.
21. Brown JR, von Lichtenberg F: Experimental actinomycosis in mice: A study of pathogenesis. Arch Pathol 1970; 90: 391–402.
22. Holm P: Some investigations into the penicillin sensitivity of human pathogenic Actinomycetes and some comments on penicillin treatment of actinomycosis. Acta Pathol Microbiol Scand 1948; 23: 376–404.
22a. Schall KP, Beaman BL: Clinical significance of Actinomycetes. In: Goodfellow M, Modarski M, Williams ST (eds): The Biology of the Actinomycetes. New York: Academic Press, 1983, pp 389–424.
23. Cope Z: Actinomycosis. London: Oxford University Press, 1938.
24. Midla Lowell T, D.V.M. Telephone communication, May 15, 1995.
25. Weese WC, Smith IM: A study of 57 cases of actinomycosis over a 36-year period. Arch Intern Med 1975; 135: 1562–1568.
26. Bennhoff DF: Actinomycosis: Diagnostic and therapeutic considerations and a review of 32 cases. Laryngoscope 1984; 94: 1198–1217.
27. Eastridge CE, Prather JR, Hughes FA Jr, et al.: Actinomycosis: A 24-year experience. South Med J 1972; 65: 839–843.
28. Harvey JC, Cantrell JR, Fisher AM: Actinomycosis: Its recognition and treatment. Ann Intern Med 1957; 46: 868–885.
29. Peabody JW, Seabury JH: Actinomycosis and nocardiosis. J Chron Dis 1957; 5: 374–403.
30. Brown JR: Human actinomycosis: A study of 181 subjects. Hum Pathol 1973; 4: 319–330.
31. Davis MIJ: Analysis of 46 cases of actinomycosis with special reference to etiology. Am J Surg 1941; 52: 447–457.
32. Spilsbury BW, Johnstone FRC: The clinical course of actinomycotic infections: A report of 14 cases. Can J Surg 1962; 5: 33–48.
33. Stanley TV: Deep actinomycosis in childhood. Acta Pediatr Scand 1980; 69: 173–176.
34. Friduss M, Maceri D: Cervicofacial actinomycosis in children. Henry Ford Hosp Med J 1990; 38: 28–32.
35. Everts EC: Cervico-facial actinomycosis. Arch Otolaryngol 1970; 92: 468–474.
36. Blinkhorn R, Strimbu V, Effrond D, et al.: "Punch" actinomycosis

causing osteomyelitis of the hand. Arch Intern Med 1988; 148: 2668–2670.

37. Kerr D, Ash M, Millard HD: Oral Diagnosis, 4th ed. St. Louis: CV Mosby, 1974, pp 305–307.
38. Weir J, Buck W: Periapical actinomycosis: Report of a case and review of the literature. Oral Surg 1982; 54: 36–40.
39. Graybill JR, Silverman BD: Sulfur granules: Second thoughts. Arch Intern Med 1969; 123: 430–432.
40. Yeager BA, Hoxie J, Weisman RA, et al.: Actinomycosis in the acquired immunodeficiency syndrome–related compex. Arch Otolaryngol Head Neck Surg 1986; 112: 1293–1295.
41. Watkins KV, Richmond AS, Langstein IM: Nonhealing extraction site due to *Actinomyces naeslundii* in patient with AIDS. Oral Surg Oral Med Oral Pathol 1991; 71: 675–677.
42. Kingdom TT, Tami TA: Actinomycosis of the nasal septum in a patient infected with the human immunodeficiency virus. Arch Otolaryngol Head Neck Surg 1994; 111: 130–133.
43. Klapholz A, Talavera W, Rorat E, et al.: Pulmonary actinomycosis in a patient with HIV infection. Mt Sinai J Med 1989; 56: 300–303.
44. Jordan H, Kelly D, Heeley J: Enhancement of experimental actinomycosis in mice by *Eikenella corrodens*. Infect Immun 1984; 46: 367–377.
45. Varkey B, Landis FB, Tang RB, et al.: Thoracic actinomycosis: Dissemination to skin, subcutaneous tissue, and muscle. Arch Intern Med 1974; 134: 689–693.
46. Sodager R, Kohout E: Actinomycosis of the tongue as a pseudo-tumor. Laryngoscope 1972; 82: 2149–2152.
47. Becker DG, McKinney CD, Huhn JF, Reibel JF: Pathologic Quiz Case. Arch Otolaryngol Head Neck Surg 1992; 118: 1356, 1359–1360.
48. Chuong R, Goldberg M: CPC, case 60: Preauricular mass. J Oral Maxillofac Surg 1986; 44: 214–217.
49. Bradley P: Actinomycosis of the temporomandibular joint. Br J Oral Surg 1971; 9: 54–56.
50. Per-Lee JH, Clairmont AA, et al.: Actinomycosis masquerading as depression headache: Case report and management review of sinus actinomycosis. Laryngoscope 1974; 84: 1149–1158.
51. Smith R, Henderson P: Actinomycotic cannaliculitis. Aust N Z J Ophthalmol 1980; 8: 75–79.
52. Pine L, Hardin H, Turner L, et al.: Actinomycotic lacrimal cannaliculitis: a report of two cases with a review of the characteristics which identify the causal organism, *Actinomyces israelii*. Am J Ophthalmol 1960; 49: 1278–1288.
53. Roussel T, Olson R, Rice T, et al.: Chronic postoperative endophthalmitis associated with *Actinomyces* species. Arch Ophthalmol 1991; 109: 60–62.
54. Miglets AW, Branson D: *Arachnia propionica (Actinomyces propionicus)* as an unusual agent in tympanomastoiditis. Arch Otolaryngol 1983; 109: 410–412.
55. Cobb R, Ross H: Actinomycosis in a persistent thyroglossal duct. Br J Surg 1986; 73: 751.
56. Adeniyi-Jones C, Minielly JA, Matthews WR, et al.: *Actinomyces viscosus* in a branchial cyst. Am J Clin Pathol 1973; 60: 711–713.
57. Arfeen S, Boast M, Large D: Unilateral thyroid swelling due to actinomycosis. Postgrad Med J 1986; 62: 847–848.
58. Brandenburg JH, Finch WW, Kirkham WR: Actinomycosis of the larynx and pharynx. Ann Otol Rhinol Laryngol 1978; 86: 739–742.
59. Jackson C, Jackson CL: The Larynx and its Diseases. Philadelphia: WB Saunders Co., 1937, pp 225–227.
60. Thomson Sir SC, Negus VE: Diseases of the Nose and Throat. London: Cassel, 1948, p 566.
61. Nelson EG, Tybor AG: Actinomycosis of the larynx. Ear Nose Throat J 1992; 71: 356–358.
62. Tsuji D, Fukuda H, Kawasaki Y, et al.: Actinomycosis of the larynx. Auris Nasus Larynx 1991; 18: 79–85.
63. Shelton C, Brackman D: Actinomycosis otitis media. Arch Otolaryngol Head Neck Surg 1988; 114: 88–89.
64. Happonen RP, Viander M, Pelliniemi L, et al.: *Actinomyces israelii* in osteoradionecrosis of the jaws. Oral Surg 1983; 55: 580–588.
65. Pransky SM, Feldman JI, Kearns DB, et al.: Actinomycosis in obstructive tonsillar hypertrophy and recurrent tonsillitis. Arch Otolaryngol Head Neck Surg 1991; 117: 883–885.
66. de la Monte SM, Gupta PK, White CL III: Systemic *Actinomyces* infection. JAMA 1982; 248: 1876–1877.
67. Duguid H, Duncan I, Parratt D, Traynor R: Actinomyces and intrauterine devices. JAMA 1982; 248: 1579–1580.
68. Valicenti JF Jr, Pappas AA, Graber CD, et al.: Detection and prevalence of IUD-associated *Actinomyces* colonization and related morbidity. JAMA 1982; 247: 1149–1152.
69. Pollock PG, Koontz FP, Viner TF, et al.: Cervicofacial actinomycosis: Rapid diagnosis by thin-needle aspiration. Arch Otolaryngol 1978; 104: 491–494.
70. Myerowitz RL: The Pathology of Opportunistic Infections, 1st ed. New York: Raven Press, 1983, pp 24, 41.
71. Heffner JE, Harley RA: Thoracic actinomycosis. Semin Respir Med 1992; 13: 234–241.
72. Slack JM: The source of infection in actinomycosis. J Bacteriol 1942; 43: 193–209.
73. Lerner PI: Serologic screening for actinomycosis. In: Balows A (ed): Anaerobic Bacterial Role in Disease. Springfield, Illinois: Charles C Thomas, 1974, pp 571–584.
74. Hotchi M, Schwarz J: Characterization of actinomycotic granules by architecture and staining methods. Arch Pathol 1972; 93: 392–400.
75. Silverman PM, Farmer JC, Korobkin M, et al.: CT diagnosis of actinomycosis of the neck. J Comput Assist Tomogr 1984; 8: 793–794.
76. Tomm KE, Raleigh JW, Guinn GA: Thoracic Actinomycosis. Am J Surg 1972; 124: 46–48.
77. Nichols DR, Herral WE: Penicillin in the treatment of actinomycosis. J Lab Clin Med 1948; 33: 521–525.
78. Lerner PI: Susceptibility of pathogenic actinomycetes to antimicrobial compounds. Antimicrob Agents Chemother 1974; 5: 302–309.
79. Wehrle PF, Top FH (eds): Communicable and Infectious Diseases, 9th ed. St Louis: CV Mosby, 1981, pp 109–113, 494, 499.
80. Spangler SK, Jacobs MR, Appelbaum PC: Susceptibilities of 201 anaerobes to erythromycin, azithromycin, clarithromycin and roxithromycin by oxyrase agar dilution and E test methodologies. J Clin Microbiol 1995; 33: 1366–1367.
81. Lee-Chiong TL Jr, Horowitz BL, Perazella MA, Brackett JW: Thoracic actinomycosis: Forgotten but not gone. J Respir Dis 1994; 15: 1062–1072.
82. Rose HD, Rytel MW: Actinomycosis treated with clindamycin. JAMA 1972; 221: 1052.
83. deVries J, Bentley KC: Clindamycin in the treatment of cervicofacial actinomycosis. Int J Clin Pharmacol 1974; 9: 46–48.
84. Edelmann M, Cullman W, Nowak KH, et al.: Treatment of abdominothoracic actinomycosis with imipenem. Eur J Clin Microbiol 1987; 6: 194–195.
85. Weinstein L, Fields BN: Seminars in Infectious Disease. New York: Stratton, 1978, vol 1: pp 97–121; vol 2: pp 1–27.
86. King JW, White MC: Pulmonary actinomycosis: Rapid improvement with isoniazid and rifampin. Arch Intern Med 1981; 141: 1234–1235.
87. McVay LV, Sprunt DH: Treatment of actinomycosis with isoniazid. JAMA 1953; 153: 95–98.
88. Mohr JA, Rhoades ER, Muchmore HG: Actinomycosis treated with lincomycin. JAMA 1970; 212: 2260–2262.
89. Caldwell JL: Actinomycosis treated with cephalothin. South Med J 1971; 64: 947–950.
90. Bhatti S: Cervico-facial actinomycosis in pregnancy. Br Dent J 1989; 166: 83–85.
91. Martin MV: The use of oral amoxicillin for the treatment of actinomycosis: a clinical and in vitro study. Br Dent J 1984; 156: 252–254.

SECTION V

SPECIAL PROBLEMS IN OTOLARYNGOLOGY

Joseph P. Lynch, III

CHAPTER SIXTY-ONE

Nosocomial Pneumonia

▼

Hospital-acquired pneumonia (nosocomial pneumonia) occurs in 0.5%–2% of hospitalized patients and has been associated with mortality rates of 30%–70%.[1-3] Nosocomial pneumonia extends the duration and costs of hospitalization,[2] and annual costs for treatment in the United States exceed $2 billion.[1] One third to one half of nosocomial pneumonias occur in patients in intensive care units.[2, 3] The prevalence of nosocomial pneumonia approaches 10%–20% in critically ill, intubated patients in postsurgical or respiratory intensive care units.[1-3] The dominant mechanism by which nosocomial pneumonia occurs is aspiration of pharyngeal or gastric contents into the lower respiratory tract,[1, 4-7] although additional mechanisms exist.[1, 6, 8-10] Diverse strategies to reduce the incidence of nosocomial pneumonia have been advocated,[6, 9, 11-13] but morbidity and mortality remain high. The high mortality rates reflect several factors, including highly virulent pathogens, increasing antimicrobial resistance, serious preexisting diseases, and impairments in host defenses.[1-3, 14-17] Prompt, effective antibiotic therapy is essential to reduce mortality and morbidity associated with nosocomial pneumonia. In this chapter, before discussing specific therapeutic approaches, the pathogenetic mechanisms, clinical features, epidemiology, and microbiology of nosocomial pneumonia are reviewed.

PATHOGENESIS

Both host and environment factors contribute to the high prevalence of nosocomial pneumonia. Risk factors predisposing to nosocomial pneumonia include severe underlying disease, debilitation, advanced age, prolonged hospitalization, complicated upper abdominal or thoracic surgery, malnutrition, impaired mental status, and preexisting pulmonary disease.[1, 3, 6, 18] Iatrogenic factors implicated in the pathogenesis include excessive sedation; invasive devices; nasogastric, endotracheal, nasotracheal, and tracheostomy tubes; and prolonged mechanical ventilatory support.[1, 3, 6] Reintubation is also an independent risk factor.[5] Aspiration of oropharyngeal and gastric contents is a major mechanism contributing to the pathogenesis of nosocomial pneumonia.[1-3, 5, 6] Endotracheal tubes prevent vocal cord closure, may be coated with a bacterial biofilm, and may inoculate contaminated upper airway secretions directly to the lower respiratory tract.[6] Contaminated secretions accumulating above the inflated endotracheal tube may serve as a reservoir for lower respiratory tract inoculation and infection.[5, 19] The gastrointestinal tract is an important reservoir for pathogenic enteric gram-negative bacteria.[1, 4, 6, 7, 20] Once gastric colonization has occurred, nasogastric tubes may facilitate migration of flora

into the tracheobronchial tree.[1, 6, 20] Histamine 2 antagonists or antacids may increase gastric colonization with enteric gram-negative bacteria and the rate of nosocomial pneumonia.[1, 20] Sucralfate does not promote gastric colonization and is preferred for prophylaxis of stress ulceration in critically ill patients in intensive care units (ICUs).[1, 20] Selective gastrointestinal tract decontamination, using topical nonabsorbable antibiotics (often combined with a brief course of parenteral antibiotics), may reduce bacterial colonization of the gastrointestinal tract and secondary infections in critically ill patients.[11, 21, 22] However, several prospective randomized trials of selective gastrointestinal tract decontamination in mechanically ventilated patients in ICUs have failed to show any reduction in mortality.[11, 13, 21, 22] Because selective gastrointestinal tract decontamination adds significantly to the costs of medical care and has the potential to facilitate antimicrobial resistance, the author sees no current role for its use. More importantly, colonization of the lower respiratory tract may occur without antecedent colonization of the gastrointestinal tract.[4, 7, 23, 24] For *Pseudomonas aeruginosa* and *Enterobacter* species, colonization of the trachea or oropharynx appears to be the dominant mode of transmission to the lower respiratory tract.[24] By contrast, for some species (e.g., *Klebsiella, Enterococcus faecalis*) colonization of the gastrointestinal tract usually precedes lower respiratory tract colonization.[24] Species-dependent differences in the initial site of colonization suggest that strategies designed to reduce gastrointestinal colonization may not significantly affect lower respiratory tract infections with *P. aeruginosa* and other selected pathogens. Alternative preventive strategies designed to reduce oropharyngeal or tracheal colonization may be more appropriate.[9] In addition to colonization of the upper airway, trachea, and gastrointestinal tract, additional mechanisms of endemic and epidemic nosocomial pneumonia exist.[6, 8-10, 12] Nosocomial pneumonia may occur via contaminated ventilator tubing, pharmaceuticals or nebulizer solutions, transmission by medical personnel or patient-to-patient transfer, faulty infection control practices, and hematogenous spread from distant foci of infection.[6, 8-10, 12] Strict compliance with handwashing and isolation of patients with highly resistant strains may reduce epidemic spread.[9, 12]

DIAGNOSIS

The diagnosis of nosocomial pneumonia may be difficult, as clinical and radiographic findings overlap with those of other entities.[2, 19, 25] Most physicians rely upon the following clinical criteria to substantiate the diagnosis of pneumonia: new or progressive pulmonary infiltrates on chest radiograph, fever, leukocytosis, and purulent tracheobronchial secretions.[26] Unfortunately, these clinical criteria do not reliably discriminate pneumonia from noninfectious causes of infiltrates.[2, 5, 19, 25, 27] Fever and leukocytosis, the hallmark of bacterial infection, may be lacking in up to 25% of patients with nosocomial pneumonia, particularly in the aged or in patients with impaired host defenses. Purulent tracheobronchial secretions are common in patients on prolonged mechanical ventilatory support, even in the absence of pneumonia.[2, 19, 27]

Chest radiographic findings of nosocomial pneumonia are nonspecific. Patchy bronchopneumonic infiltrates or diffuse interstitial markings are most commonly observed, and they may be mistaken for congestive heart failure or fluid overload. The presence of cavitation or dense lobar pneumonia with consolidation strongly suggests an infectious etiology but is infrequently seen in nosocomial pneumonia. More importantly, pulmonary infiltrates may be observed in diverse noninfectious causes (e.g., atelectasis, congestive heart failure, pulmonary embolism, adult respiratory distress syndrome, and hemorrhage).[2, 19] Nonpulmonary causes of fever (e.g., extrapulmonary sources of infections, thrombophlebitis, pancreatitis, atelectasis, and drug fever) have been identified in more than 40% of mechanically ventilated patients with *suspected* pneumonia in some series.[19, 25] A myriad of postoperative infections (e.g., skin and soft tissue, wounds, urinary tract, bacteremias, intravascular catheter infections, cholecystitis, and sinusitis) may erroneously be ascribed to pneumonia.[19]

Perhaps of greatest interest to the otolaryngologist is the frequent presence of sinusitis in critically ill, mechanically ventilated patients (discussed in Chapter 41).[28, 29] Infectious maxillary sinusitis occurs in at least 10%–30% of mechanically ventilated postsurgical or trauma patients, and it is an important risk factor for nosocomial pneumonia.[28, 29] Nasal endotracheal or gastric tubes may obstruct the nares and sinus ostia, thus predisposing to sinusitis.[29] The incidence of sinusitis is lower with oral endotracheal or gastric tubes.[29] High concentrations of bacteria in sinuses may lead to colonization and infection of the oropharynx, trachea, and lung parenchyma.[29] Seeding of distant foci may result in bronchopneumonia, empyema, intracranial infections, or septicemia.[29] Sinusitis developing in critically ill patients is often not suspected, as classic symptoms of facial pain, headache, and purulent nasal discharge may be absent.[29] Plain sinus radiographs are insensitive in diagnosing sinusitis; thin-section computed tomography (CT) scans are preferred.[19, 29] The incidence of sinusitis may be striking among patients requiring prolonged mechanical ventilatory support, particularly when sensitive diagnostic techniques are applied. In a recent prospective study of 162 patients ventilated for more than 7 days, 133 (75%) had maxillary sinusitis on CT scans.[29] Bronchopneumonia developed in 67% of these 133 patients. The organisms isolated from sinus aspirates mirrored those obtained by bronchoalveolar lavage (BAL) in patients with nosocomial pneumonia.[29] Transnasal drainage of infected sinuses, and local instillation of antibiotics and saline lavage, may be efficacious for localized sinusitis.[29] Parenteral antibiotics are warranted for severe sinusitis.[29] A more extensive discussion of the differential diagnosis and approach to nonpulmonary causes of fever and pulmonary

infiltrates is available for review.[19] Before discussing an approach to therapy of nosocomial pneumonia, the epidemiology and salient pathogens are reviewed.

EPIDEMIOLOGY

Enteric gram-negative bacteria account for 70%–85% of nosocomial pneumonia; gram-positive cocci (primarily *Staphylococcus aureus*) have been implicated in 15%–40% of nosocomial pneumonia, usually admixed with enteric gram-negative bacteria.[1, 2, 14, 30–35] Twenty percent to forty percent of nosocomial pneumonia is polymicrobial.[2, 14, 30, 33] *P. aeruginosa* is the single most important cause of nosocomial pneumonia, accounting for 15%–20% of cases.[1, 2, 14, 33, 36] Seven percent to twelve percent of nosocomial pneumonia is due to *Enterobacter* species (e.g., *E. cloacae* and *E. aerogenes*); *Klebsiella* species, *Escherichia coli*, *Haemophilus influenzae*, and *Acinetobacter* species each account for 3%–7% of cases.[2, 14, 15, 30, 32, 34, 37] Myriad other enteric gram-negative bacteria are rare causes of nosocomial pneumonia (e.g., *Citrobacter, Proteus* species, *Providencia, Serratia marcescens*, and *Stenotrophomonas maltophilia*).[2, 14, 30, 32, 34, 38] Anaerobes have infrequently been ascribed as a cause of nosocomial pneumonia[2, 14, 32, 34] but this is controversial.[1] The frequency of nosocomial pneumonia due to *Legionella* species is highly variable.[39–44] Endemic and epidemic outbreaks of nosocomial pneumonia due to respiratory viruses, fungi, *Pneumocystis carinii*, and *Mycobacteria* have been described, but they are beyond the scope of this chapter.

SPECIFIC PATHOGENS

Pseudomonas aeruginosa

P. aeruginosa accounts for 15%–20% of nosocomial pneumonias, with even higher rates (up to 40%) among mechanically ventilated patients in ICUs.[2, 14, 18, 32, 36] *P. aeruginosa* is ubiquitous in hospital environments and can thrive in distilled water, sinks, ventilator tubing, plants, and other environmental sources.[36] Colonization of the upper respiratory tract and trachea occurs commonly in mechanically ventilated and intubated patients and may be facilitated by prior antibiotic use.[2, 18, 32, 36] In one study, *P. aeruginosa* was implicated in 40% of ventilator-associated pneumonias (VAPs) in patients who had received prior antibiotics but in only 5% of VAP in antibiotic-naive patients.[32]

Chest radiographic features of *P. aeruginosa* pneumonia are nonspecific, but cavitation, multilobar involvement, and nodular infiltrates are frequent.[36] *P. aeruginosa* produces a variety of exotoxins, proteases, and hemolysins that may cause necrosis, microabscess formation, and destruction of vascular walls.[36] Mortality from *P. aeruginosa* pneumonia is high (>50%), which reflects not only the virulence of the organism but also the debilitated state of infected patients.[2, 32, 36] Clinical and microbiologic failures, antimicrobial resistance, or relapses are noted in one third or more of patients.[14, 36, 45–47] Given the high mortality rate and proclivity for relapse associated with *P. aeruginosa* pneumonia, monotherapy is inadequate.[14, 36, 45, 47, 48] The author recommends combining a beta-lactam active against *P. aeruginosa* (e.g., antipseudomonal penicillin, ceftazidime, or imipenem/cilastatin) with an aminoglycoside. Other treatment options include ciprofloxacin combined with an aminoglycoside, aztreonam, or an antipseudomonal penicillin.[14] A 14–21 day course of therapy is recommended.

Enterobacteriaceae

Klebsiella pneumoniae and *E. coli,* within the class Enterobacteriaceae, each account for 4%–8% of nosocomial pneumonias.[2, 14, 27, 49] These pathogens are usually highly susceptible to second- or third-generation cephalosporins, extended spectrum penicillins with beta-lactamase inhibitors, imipenem/cilastatin, and fluoroquinolones.[14, 15] Monotherapy with one of these agents is usually adequate. Highly resistant *K. pneumoniae* displaying extended spectrum beta-lactamases[50, 51] and *E. coli* exhibiting high-grade resistance to quinolones[52] have been described. However, in most centers, high-grade resistance is unusual. By contrast, other species within the class Enterobacteriaceae (e.g., *Enterobacter, Serratia, Providencia,* and *Citrobacter freundii*) may possess inducible beta-lactamases and may have or acquire resistance to cephalosporins and antipseudomonal penicillins.[14, 53] Most isolates are susceptible to fluoroquinolones or imipenem/cilastatin,[54–56] but resistance to these antimicrobials may be increasing.[45, 57] *Enterobacter* species is the prototype for an organism that possesses inducible beta-lactamases and is discussed in the following section.

Enterobacter species

Within the past decade, *Enterobacter* species have assumed increasing importance as a cause of nosocomial pneumonia.[15, 30, 32, 34, 37] *Enterobacter* species were implicated in 7%–12% of nosocomial pneumonias in recent series.[30, 32, 34, 37] The emergence of *Enterobacter* species is in part due to selection pressure from heavy use of third-generation cephalosporins.[15, 16, 53] *Enterobacter* species are usually resistant to first- and second-generation cephalosporins, and up to 40% are resistant to third-generation cephalosporins.[16, 17, 53, 58] Antimicrobial resistance (by inducible, chromosomally mediated beta-lactamases) may emerge rapidly during antibiotic therapy.[15–17, 53] Cephalosporins should not be used to treat pneumonia due to *Enterobacter* species (regardless of in vitro susceptibility results).[14, 53] Fluoroquinolones or trimethoprim/sulfamethoxazole are highly effective, even as monotherapy.[14, 45] Antipseudomonal penicillins, aztreonam, or imipenem/cilastatin may be adequate for beta-lactamase-negative strains.[14, 45, 53] Combining an aminoglycoside with one of the preceding agents in severe *Enterobacter* pneumonia is reasonable[14, 45, 53] but has not been shown to improve outcome.[59]

Haemophilus influenzae

H. influenzae has been implicated in 3%–8% of nosocomial pneumonias in most series[2, 30] but in up to 22% in others.[31, 35, 37] *H. influenzae* is a frequent commensal in patients with chronic obstructive lung disease, the elderly, and in healthy hosts and may be an important cause of nosocomial pneumonia early in the hospital course in antibiotic-naive patients.[31, 32, 35, 37] However, other enteric gram-negative bacteria usually replace *H. influenzae* as part of respiratory tract flora within the first few hospital days. *H. influenzae* is also easily eradicated by most antibiotics. Thus, *H. influenzae* is a rare cause of nosocomial pneumonia among critically ill patients with prolonged hospital stays, particularly those who have recently received antibiotics.[32, 35, 37] Pneumonia due to *H. influenzae* can be treated with a second- or third-generation cephalosporin, ampicillin/sulbactam, or a fluoroquinolone.[2, 14, 15, 30, 32, 38]

Acinetobacter species

Acinetobacter species (*Acinetobacter calcoaceticus* or *baumannii*), aerobic gram-negative coccobacilli, are usually resistant to multiple antibiotics and may emerge by selection pressure in critically ill, debilitated patients.[2, 30, 32, 38] *Acinetobacter* species are rare causes of nosocomial pneumonia encountered outside of ICUs, but they have been implicated in 5–15% of pneumonias in critically ill, mechanically ventilated patients in recent series.[2, 30, 32, 38] Mortality associated with *Acinetobacter* pneumonia may exceed 50%.[2, 38] Risk factors for acquisition of *Acinetobacter* species include prolonged hospitalization, mechanical ventilatory support, residence in an ICU, invasive devices, and prior antibiotics.[38] Contaminated environmental reservoirs (e.g., respiratory therapy equipment, mattresses, dialysis baths, hands of medical personnel) may be sources of infection and colonization.[38] Strict infection control measures are important to limit endemic and epidemic spread. Treatment and eradication of *Acinetobacter* species is difficult, as most isolates are resistant to cephalosporins and aminoglycosides.[38] Activity of the antipseudomonal penicillins, trimethoprim/sulfamethoxazole, and fluoroquinolones is variable.[38] The choice of therapy should be determined by in vitro susceptibilities. For empirical therapy, imipenem/cilastatin is usually the drug of choice,[38] but resistance may develop with monotherapy.[51]

Staphylococcus aureus

S. aureus (coagulase-positive staphylococci) is the second most common cause of nosocomial pneumonia, accounting for 15%–30% of cases.[2, 12, 30, 33, 60] Fifteen to forty percent of nosocomial isolates of *S. aureus* are methicillin-resistant.[12, 61, 62] Risk factors associated with colonization or infection with *S. aureus* include recent neurosurgery, head trauma, indwelling lines, diabetes mellitus, burns, renal failure, and corticosteroids.[33] Acquisition of methicillin-resistant *S. aureus* (MRSA) is enhanced by prior use of beta-lactam antibiotics,[12, 33] prior nasal carriage, or transmission from medical personnel.[12] Selection pressure imposed by prior antibiotics is critically important. In a study of VAP caused by *S. aureus,* all 11 patients with MRSA had received prior antibiotics.[33] By contrast, only 8 of 38 (21%) with methicillin-susceptible strains (MSSA) had previously received antibiotics.[33] The prognosis of *S. aureus* pneumonia due to MRSA is worse than that for MSSA,[33] but the severity and extent of coexisting illnesses are important determinants of outcome.[12, 32, 33, 63] Mortality rates for pneumonia due to methicillin-susceptible *S. aureus* have generally been below 5% in patients without severe comorbidities[32, 33] but may exceed 40% in debilitated patients with serious coexisting illnesses[12, 63] or with MRSA.[33] Optimal treatment of *S. aureus* pneumonia depends upon whether other pathogens are present concomitantly. Concomitant infection with *P. aeruginosa* is common with MRSA, but rare with MSSA.[33] For monomicrobial pneumonia due to MSSA, antistaphylococcal penicillins (e.g., nafcillin and oxacillin) or cefazolin may be adequate. When polymicrobial infections are a consideration, broader-spectrum antibiotics with activity against enteric gram-negative bacteria and anaerobes are warranted (e.g., piperacillin/tazobactam, ticarcillin/clavulanate, and imipenem/cilastatin). For methicillin-resistant strains (MRSA), intravenous vancomycin is indicated, as MRSA is predictably resistant to all beta-lactam antibiotics.[61, 62] Liberal use of vancomycin for less rigorous indications should be discouraged, as this may promote antimicrobial resistance.[64] Patients experiencing severe adverse effects from vancomycin may be treated with trimethoprim/sulfamethoxazole, clindamycin, or a fluoroquinolone, but susceptibility to these antimicrobials is variable.[61, 62]

Other Gram-Positive Cocci

Coagulase-negative *Staphylococcus (S. epidermidis)* has been implicated in fewer than 3% of nosocomial pneumonias and is often observed admixed with other pathogens.[2, 14, 30, 34, 49] Up to 75% of *S. epidermidis* organisms are methicillin-resistant.[61, 62] Because nosocomial pneumonia due to *S. epidermidis* is usually polymicrobial, specific therapy against *S. epidermidis* is usually not necessary. Streptococci (e.g., *S. pneumoniae*, group A and B streptococci) have been isolated in culture in 3%–22% of nosocomial pneumoniaes[30–32, 35, 37] but are often admixed with other potential pathogens. Streptococci are part of normal oral flora and may cause nosocomial pneumonia early in the hospital course (first 3 days) but are rarely implicated in nosocomial pneumonias in critically ill patients requiring prolonged hospitalization.[2, 31, 35] When streptococci are recovered as the predominant or sole organism, antibiotics should cover these isolates. However, as other pathogens frequently coexist, narrow-spectrum agents (e.g., penicillin and ampicillin) may not be adequate. Extended-spectrum penicillins with beta-lactamase inhibitors (e.g., ampicillin/sulbactam, ticarcillin/clavulanate, and piperacillin/tazobactam) have excellent activity against streptococci as well as enteric gram-negative bacteria and are useful in this setting.[65, 66] Imipenem/cilastatin is highly active but far more expensive.[67] Ceftazidime and ciprofloxacin have only modest activity against streptococci and are less desirable.[54]

Legionella

Nosocomial pneumonia due to *Legionella* species may occur in endemic and epidemic settings.[39–43] Legionellae thrive in warm water and may contaminate hospital water supplies.[39–43] Nosocomial legionellosis may occur when legionellae are transmitted to the lower respiratory tract via aspiration or aerosolization.[39, 41, 44] The prevalence of nosocomial legionellosis ranges from 0–30% and is dependent upon local and geographic factors influencing the water distribution systems.[39–42, 44] Case fatality rates may be as high as 47%.[39, 40] Risk factors for acquisition of legionellae include serious underlying disease,[40, 44] corticosteroid or immunosuppressive therapy,[39, 40, 44] nasogastric tubes,[39, 43] renal failure,[40] and contaminated tap water disseminated by humidifiers, nebulizers, and feeding tubes.[41, 44] The diagnosis of legionellosis is often missed unless specialized surveillance measures are in place. Specialized testing for legionellae may identify cases, even in hospitals where nosocomial legionellosis had not previously been recognized.[40, 42, 44] A prospective study identified 36 cases of *Legionella* pneumonia among 300 episodes of nosocomial pneumonia over 5 years.[40] *Legionella* species were implicated in 30% of postoperative pneumonias in patients with head and neck cancer in one study.[39, 41, 42] This extraordinarily high incidence likely reflects the propensity for patients with extensive head and neck tumors to aspirate. Laryngectomized patients did not develop legionellosis.

Clinical features of pneumonia due to *Legionella* species are indistinguishable from other nosocomial pneumonias. However, *Legionella* species should be suspected when pneumonia progresses despite therapy with beta-lactam or aminoglycoside antibiotics (which lack significant activity against *Legionella*). Direct fluorescent antibody (DFA) stains can identify legionellae quickly in respiratory secretions but sensitivity is only 25%–65%.[39, 41] Cultures using specialized media are positive in 30%–90% of cases but require 3–5 days to grow the organisms.[39, 41] Bronchoscopy with bronchoalveolar lavage may be useful when sputum is nondiagnostic. Urinary antigen assays are sensitive, rapid, and relatively inexpensive but only detect *Legionella* serogroup 1.[68] Serologies (fourfold titer rise or a single titer >1:128 to antibodies against *Legionella* species) are useful for epidemiologic studies but have no immediate value in individual patients.[44] Because of the difficulty in establishing a timely diagnosis of legionellosis, treatment is often initiated empirically for suspected cases. Intravenous erythromycin (1 g every 6 hours) was once the treatment of choice for legionellosis.[44] However, the newer oral macrolides (e.g., clarithromycin and azithromycin) and fluoroquinolones (e.g., ciprofloxacin and ofloxacin) have excellent activity against legionellae and will likely displace erythromycin as the drugs of choice. Rifampin (600 mg every 12 hours) may confer synergy and should be added for fulminant cases.

ROLE OF SPUTUM OR BRONCHOSCOPIC CULTURES IN GUIDING THERAPY

Unfortunately, sputum smears and cultures are of limited value in the management of nosocomial pneumonia.[2, 27, 49, 69, 70] Sputum Gram's stains may demonstrate a predominant organism but provide no information regarding antibiotic susceptibilities. Conventional (nonquantitative) sputum cultures are sensitive (>80%) but nonspecific (<30%).[2, 27, 49, 69, 70]

Sputum cultures cannot discriminate colonization from true infection. Fiberoptic bronchoscopy using a protected brush or bronchoalveolar lavage and quantitative cultures is the best technique to discriminate pneumonia from noninfectious etiologies.[2, 5, 27, 29, 49, 71] The presence of more than 10^3 organisms/mL in a protected brush specimen or more than 10^4 by bronchoalveolar lavage (BAL) are highly predictive of pneumonia (sensitivity approximately 70%–91%; specificity exceeds 88%).[2, 5, 27, 29, 71] Lower colony counts make infection unlikely, but false-negatives may occur among patients recently receiving antibiotics.[2, 27, 49, 69, 72] Stains of cytocentrifuged BAL specimens (Gram's stains, Diff-Quik) may allow rapid characterization of predominant organism(s).[19, 49] The presence of more than 5% intracellular organisms within phagocytes has a sensitivity and specificity of approximately 90% for pneumonia.[49, 71] Despite these impressive data, bronchoscopy is invasive and expensive, and its role in the management of nosocomial pneumonia is controversial.[49, 69, 70] Less invasive nonbronchoscopic techniques using plugged or protected catheters and quantitative cultures are promising, but their application is limited to ventilated patients.[19, 34, 73] Nonbronchoscopic "mini-BAL," using commercially available catheters passed through the endotracheal tube, has been comparable to protected brush or BAL.[34, 73]

Quantitative cultures of sputum or endotracheal aspirates (using 10^6 organisms/mL as the threshhold) have been at least as sensitive as protected brush (55–82%) with acceptable specificity (>80%).[69, 71, 72] These quantitative techniques are superior to conventional sputum cultures but are logistically more complex and add expense and burden to the clinical laboratories. These various techniques are promising, but they have not yet been shown to influence mortality.[2, 19, 70] Their role needs to be better defined in studies that assess clinical outcomes and cost-effectiveness. Bronchoscopy has the potential to worsen gas exchange and precipitate respiratory failure in nonintubated patients with marginal pulmonary reserve, and the author is reluctant to perform routine bronchoscopy in this setting. Currently, the author reserves bronchoscopy (to include protected brush or BAL and quantitative cultures) for the following indications: VAPs; progressive nosocomial pneumonia in nonventilated patients failing antibiotics; and nosocomial pneumonia in immunocompromised hosts at risk for nonbacterial opportunists. For most nosocomial pneumonias in nonventilated patients, the author obtains an initial Gram's stain and culture of sputum. Only Gram's stains showing greater than 25 leukocytes and fewer than 10 epithelial cells per low-power field are accepted for culture.[19, 26] Numerous neutrophils and intracellular organisms suggest true infection is present.[49] Sputum results rarely influence initial therapy but may guide subsequent therapy once cultures and susceptibility results are available. Because up to 40% of nosocomial pneumonias are polymicrobial, the author is reluctant to use narrow-spectrum agents, even when a dominant pathogen has been isolated. At a minimum, antimicrobial therapy should cover the predominant pathogen(s) or those displaying a high level of virulence or antimicrobial resistance (e.g., *P. aeruginosa*). Surgical (open or thoracoscopic) lung biopsies are rarely warranted for the diagnosis of nosocomial pneumonia. Transtracheal and needle aspiration are dangerous and have no role.

INFLUENCE OF ANTIMICROBIAL RESISTANCE ON ANTIBIOTIC STRATEGIES

Initial treatment strategies for nosocomial pneumonia (while awaiting cultures) are empirical and should take into account the likely pathogen, severity of pneumonia, comorbidities, risk factors for highly resistant pathogens (e.g., residence in an ICU, mechanical ventilatory support, and recent antibiotics), and antimicrobial resistance patterns within the institution (or individual units).[14–17] Antimicrobial resistance in nosocomial settings has increased at an alarming rate, primarily due to selection pressure from antibiotic use.[14, 15, 46, 50, 52, 58, 74] This trend is most evident in ICUs or large teaching hospitals.[15–17, 38, 51, 58, 75] Beta-lactamase production is the most common mechanism of resistance; additional mechanisms confer resistance to vancomycin, aminoglycosides, carbapenems, fluoroquinolones, and multiple classes of antibiotics.[14–17, 46, 51] Antimicrobial resistance may develop when single classes of antibiotics are used extensively or the ratio of the concentration of the antimicrobial to the minimal inhibitory concentration of the infecting organisms is inadequate.[57, 75] Resistance trends observed with particular classes of antibiotics are discussed in the sections on individual antibiotics. One of the most compelling reasons to consider combination therapy for serious nosocomial pneumonia is to limit the potential for emergence of antimicrobial resistance,[14, 15, 46, 58] even though studies confirming that this strategy reduces resistance are lacking.[59]

SELECTION OF ANTIBIOTICS FOR NOSOCOMIAL PNEUMONIA

Optimal antibiotic strategies for empirical therapy of nosocomial pneumonia are controversial.[14, 59, 76] For mild to moderate nosocomial pneumonia in patients not critically ill, *P. aeruginosa* or highly resistant organisms are unlikely and monotherapy with a third-generation cephalosporin (e.g., cefotaxime or ceftriaxone), ampicillin/sulbactam, or a fluoroquinolone may be adequate. First- and second-generation cephalosporins have a relatively narrow spectrum and are less desirable (unless a susceptible organism has been identified). When risk factors for *P. aeruginosa* exist (e.g., residence in an ICU, recent antibiotic use, and serious comorbidity), the author initiates therapy with a broad-spectrum antipseudomonal beta-lactam (e.g., ceftazidime, piperacillin/tazobactam, ticarcillin/clavulanate, or imipenem/cilastatin) combined with an aminoglycoside. This approach may achieve synergistic killing and may reduce the potential for antimicrobial resistance.[14, 15] If contraindications to an aminoglycoside exist, monotherapy with ceftazidime, imipenem/cilastatin, or ciprofloxacin may be used. Some investigators advocate monotherapy with a broad-spectrum antipseudomonal agent as initial therapy for nosocomial pneumonia, even in ICU patients.[59] Aminoglycosides or vancomycin can be added later if *P. aeruginosa*, MRSA, or resistant pathogens are isolated.[59] The pros and cons of monotherapy or combination therapy for nosocomial pneumonia in the ICU have been reviewed.[14, 59] Antibiotic strategies for beta-lactam–allergic patients include a fluoroquinolone (preferably ciprofloxacin because of its enhanced activity against *P. aeruginosa*),[54, 55] alone or combined with clindamycin or metronidazole; aztreonam plus clindamycin, metronidazole, or vancomycin[14, 77]; or trimethoprim/sulfamethoxazole (alone or combined with an aminoglycoside). The use of broad-spectrum or combination therapies is expensive, and therapy should be modified to a narrow-spectrum, less expensive antibiotic if a specific pathogen has been substantiated.

SPECIFIC ANTIBIOTICS

Third-Generation Cephalosporins

Monotherapy with a broad-spectrum beta-lactam (e.g., third-generation cephalosporin or imipenem/cilastatin) is appealing because aminoglycoside toxicity can be avoided. Arbo and Snydman analyzed 15 randomized trials, evaluating monotherapy in 1324 patients with nosocomial pneumonia.[59] Favorable responses were observed in 48%–100% of patients with monotherapy; differences between respective regimens were minor.[59] Six randomized trials noted similar rates of clinical responses and antimicrobial resistance with monotherapy with a third-generation cephalosporin or combination therapy.[59] Ceftazidime monotherapy was comparable to ciprofloxacin in four randomized trials (success rates in 96 of 108 [88%] patients).[14] Data from these various studies should be interpreted with caution, as patients with rapidly progressive illness or resistant pathogens were often excluded and the proportion of patients receiving mechanical ventilatory support was low.[59] A multicenter trial randomized 297 patients with nosocomial pneumonia to ceftazidime monotherapy or combination therapy with ceftriaxone/tobramycin.[78] Response rates were similar with both regimens (73% and 65%, respectively).[78] Surprisingly, both regimens were effective, even when *P. aeruginosa* was isolated (70%–89% responses, respectively).[78] Despite these favorable results, the widespread use of ceftazidime monotherapy has been associated with increases in *Enterobacter* species producing inducible beta-lactamases,[53] increases in extended-spectrum beta-lactamases among Enterobacteriaceae,[50, 51] and multidrug-resistant *P. aeruginosa*.[75] Data from 144 U.S. hospitals in the National Nosocomial Infections Surveillance System from 1987 to 1991 noted a linear increase in ceftazidime-resistant isolates of *Enterobacter* species and *K. pneumoniae*.[58] From 1990 to 1991, 39% of *Enterobacter* species, 3.6% of *K. pneumoniae*, and 9.1% of *P. aeruginosa* isolates were resistant to ceftazidime.[58] Surprisingly, ceftazidime resistance did not increase among *P. aeruginosa* isolates, whereas resistance to imipenem increased considerably during this time.[46] In some centers, the prevalence of ceftazidime-resistant isolates is striking.[50, 51, 58] In one hospital, the proportion of *K. pneumoniae* resistant to ceftazidime increased from 1%–40% within 3 years.[58] These resistance trends are troubling[50, 51, 53, 58, 75] and cast doubt on the adequacy of monotherapy for severe nosocomial pneumonia, particularly in ICUs.

Extended-Spectrum Penicillins with Beta-lactamase Inhibitors

Extended-spectrum penicillins with beta-lactamase inhibitors (e.g., ampicillin/sulbactam, ticarcillin/clavulanate, and piperacillin/tazobactam) may be used to treat nosocomial pneumonia.[14, 65] Extended-spectrum penicillins are less likely than cephalosporins to induce beta-lactamases; substituting these agents for cephalosporins may result in a decline of beta-lactamase–producing organisms.[14, 53] Ampicillin/sulbactam lacks activity against *P. aeruginosa* and other enteric gram-negative bacteria that may be encountered in nosocomial settings and is of limited utility as empirical therapy for severe nosocomial pneumonia.[15] However, ampicillin/sulbactam may have a role for nosocomial pneumonia due to susceptible organisms. Ticarcillin/clavulanate or piperacillin/tazobactam have broad-spectrum activity against an array of enteric gram-negative bacteria (including *P. aeruginosa*), many gram-positive cocci, and anaerobes and may be used to treat severe nosocomial pneumonia.[65, 66] In this context, combination therapy with an aminoglycoside is advised.[14] Data comparing ticarcillin/clavulanate with other broad-spectrum antimicrobials are limited, but cure rates appear comparable to third-generation cephalosporins.[14] Piperacillin/tazobactam, introduced for clinical use in the United States in 1994, has been highly effective for serious infections (including pneumonias) in both immunocompetent and immunosuppressed hosts,[66, 79, 80] but data in nosocomial pneumonia are limited. In a randomized trial, piperacillin/tazobactam was superior to ticarcillin/clavulanate for community-acquired pneumonia.[80] Piperacillin/tazobactam (4.5 g every 6 hours) plus amikacin was superior to ceftazidime (2 g every 8 hours) plus amikacin in a randomized study of 706 neutropenic patients with fever.[79] Among patients with lower respiratory tract infections, 19 of 24 responded to piperacillin/tazobactam/amikacin (compared with 9 of 24 responses with ceftazidime/amikacin).[79] Lower dosages of piperacillin/tazobactam (3.75 g every 6 hours) are not adequate for *P. aeruginosa* pneumonia.[15] Because of its broad-spectrum activity,[79] piperacillin/tazobactam is an attractive new agent, but additional studies are required to define its role for nosocomial pneumonia.

Imipenem/Cilastatin

Imipenem/cilastatin, the first of the carbapenem class of antimicrobials, has exceptionally broad antimicrobial activity against both gram-positive and gram-negative bacteria and resists degradation by many beta-lactamases capable of hydrolyzing penicillins or cephalosporins.[67, 77] In prospective randomized trials of severe nosocomial pneumonia, favorable responses were noted in 56%–84% of patients with imipenem/cilastatin monotherapy.[45, 81, 82] These response rates were comparable to that for ceftazidime[81] but slightly less effective than that for ciprofloxacin.[45, 47] A high rate of treatment failure, persistence of the organism, clinical relapse, or emergence of antimicrobial resistance has been noted when imipenem/cilastatin is used alone for pneumonia due to *P. aeruginosa*.[45, 47, 81] In theory, combining imipenem/

cilastatin with an aminoglycoside may confer synergy and limit the development of resistance.[14] However, in a randomized trial, the addition of an aminoglycoside (netilmycin) to imipenem/cilastatin did not improve rates of response, superinfections, or emergence of resistance compared with that for imipenem/cilastatin alone.[82] Imipenem should not be combined with other beta-lactams because antagonism may occur.[67, 77] Compared with other beta-lactams, imipenem/cilastatin is expensive and more toxic (principally causing nausea and vomiting, but rarely seizures).[14, 51, 67] More importantly, overzealous use of imipenem may predispose to development of resistance or superinfections with *S. maltophilia, P. cepacea, P. aeruginosa, Acinetobacter* species, or MRSA, which are often resistant to most beta-lactams.[14, 51, 67, 83] Resistance to imipenem may occur via chromosomally mediated beta-lactamases, carbapenemases, changes in permeability, or changes in penicillin-binding affinity.[14, 16, 46, 84] Imipenem/cilastatin should not be used as "routine" treatment for nosocomial pneumonia but may be ideal in patients who have recently received or failed broad-spectrum beta-lactam antibiotics or when extended-spectrum beta-lactamases are suspected.[14, 67]

Aztreonam

Aztreonam, a monobactam within the beta-lactam class of antibiotic, has outstanding activity against enteric gram-negative bacteria (including most strains of *P. aeruginosa*) but lacks activity against anaerobes or gram-positive cocci.[77, 85] Monotherapy with aztreonam is highly effective for infections due to enteric gram-negative bacteria, but aztreonam has been associated with a high rate of colonization or superinfections due to gram-positive cocci.[77, 85] Because of its narrow spectrum, aztreonam has limited application as therapy for nosocomial pneumonia. Aztreonam may be used to treat nosocomial pneumonia in patients allergic to beta-lactams, but it should be combined with an agent with gram-positive activity (e.g., antistaphylococcal penicillin, clindamycin, or vancomycin).[14, 77]

Fluoroquinolones

Fluoroquinolones (e.g., ciprofloxacin and ofloxacin) have outstanding activity against enteric gram-negative bacteria; activity against gram-positive cocci and anaerobes is modest.[54, 55, 83] The fluoroquinolones are well absorbed (65% for ciprofloxacin, 97% for ofloxacin) and may be used as "step-down therapy" following initial parenteral antibiotic therapy.[54, 83, 86] Compared with ofloxacin, ciprofloxacin has superior activity against *P. aeruginosa* but is less active against streptococci.[55, 83] The fluoroquinolones are not affected by beta-lactamases and may be active against isolates resistant to beta-lactams.[54, 55] Ciprofloxacin monotherapy (200 mg twice daily) was comparable to ceftazidime in several randomized studies of community-, nursing home-, or hospital-acquired pneumonia (97% response rate).[14] In a study of 47 patients with gram-negative pneumonia, ciprofloxacin monotherapy was curative in 63%, even though nearly half had failed prior antibiotic therapy.[87] Ciprofloxacin (400 mg

every 8 hours) was superior to imipenem/cilastatin (1 g every 8 hours) in a multicenter, randomized trial of severe nosocomial pneumonia (favorable responses in 69% and 59%, respectively).[45] However, several studies have noted a high failure rate and development of resistance when ciprofloxacin was used alone for *P. aeruginosa*.[14, 45-47, 54, 87] Higher doses of ciprofloxacin (400 mg every 8 hours) may be necessary for organisms with marginal minimal inhibitory concentrations (MICs).[14, 88] Ofloxacin has been associated with high cure rates in community-acquired pneumonia[83, 86] and infections in immunocompromised hosts[89] but data evaluating this agent in nosocomial pneumonia are limited. Ofloxacin may be the ideal agent for infections due to Enterobacteriaceae and many other enteric gram-negative bacteria but is less active than ciprofloxacin against *P. aeruginosa*.[55] Because of their excellent bioavailability, fluoroquinolones may be substituted for parenteral agents (including beta-lactams) after an initial response (provided the isolates are susceptible and the gastrointestinal tract is functioning). This approach may markedly reduce hospital costs and shorten length of stay.[83, 86] Unfortunately, antimicrobial resistance to the fluoroquinolones may develop rapidly and may pose obstacles to the future efficacy of these agents.[52, 90] Fluoroquinolone resistance has increased dramatically to *P. aeruginosa* and *S. aureus*.[57, 90] Although fewer than 4% of Enterobacteriaceae (and only 1.6% of *E. coli*) are resistant to fluoroquinolones in the United States,[57] studies citing a high (37%) prevalence of quinolone-resistant *E. coli* among neutropenic patients receiving prophylactic norfloxacin[52] are of interest. Liberal use of fluoroquinolones may promote resistant isolates, which may also be resistant to beta-lactams or other antibiotic classes.[14, 52, 55, 57, 83] Thus, fluoroquinolones should not be used indiscriminately for infections that can be treated with beta-lactams.

Vancomycin

Vancomycin has a narrow spectrum and has significant potential toxicity.[91] Vancomycin is the drug of choice for methicillin-resistant staphylococci[12, 33, 62] but has often been used for less rigorous indications (e.g., prophylaxis and empirical treatment of nosocomial infections without culture evidence for staphylococci).[92, 93] The use of vancomycin in the United States has skyrocketed in the past decade, a trend that may facilitate resistance. At one major university hospital, the use of parenteral vancomycin rose 161-fold from 1978 to 1992,[92] only one third of which was for culture-proven infections.[93] Liberal use of vancomycin has been associated with dramatic increases in vancomycin-resistant enterococci (VRE).[64, 74] From 1989 through 1993, nosocomial enterococcal infections reported to the National Nosocomial Infections Surveillance System increased from 0.3% to 7.9%, with even greater increases in ICUs.[64] Risk factors for acquisition of VRE include serious underlying disease or debilitation, immunosuppression, residence in an ICU, prolonged hospital stay, and prior therapy with vancomycin or multiple antimicrobials.[64, 74] Strict hospital infection control measures and epidemiologic surveillance are required to limit spread of VRE. Although enterococci rarely cause nosocomial pneumonia, these resistance trends are worrisome, as vancomycin-resistance genes present in VRE theoretically may be transferred to other gram-positive cocci (including *S. aureus*).[64] In order to prevent and limit the spread of vancomycin resistance in nosocomial settings, the author agrees with Centers for Disease Control and Prevention guidelines that reserve vancomycin for serious infections caused by gram-positive cocci resistant to beta-lactam antibiotics or in patients allergic to beta-lactams.[64] Vancomycin may also be initiated empirically for severe nosocomial pneumonia failing broad-spectrum agents when gram-positive cocci are identified on Gram's stains (pending results of cultures and susceptibilities).[18]

Aminoglycoside Antibiotics

Despite their potential toxicity, aminoglycoside antibiotics continue to have a role for severe nosocomial pneumonia. Aminoglycosides are not adequate as monotherapy for pneumonia, but combining an aminoglycoside with a beta-lactam may achieve synergistic killing and expand the antimicrobial spectrum.[14, 15] Synergy may be an important determinant of outcome for highly virulent organisms (e.g., *P. aeruginosa, Acinetobacter* species, *Serratia,* and *S. maltophilia*).[14, 15] Although the role of aminoglycosides for nosocomial pneumonia remains controversial,[59] several studies in people support an adjunctive role for aminoglycosides for *P. aeruginosa* and probably for other enteric gram-negative bacteria.[14, 15] Peak serum antiglycoside levels greater than 6 μg/mL have been associated with improved outcome for gram-negative pneumonia.[14] In a nonrandomized study of *P. aeruginosa* bacteremia, mortality with the combination of an aminoglycoside and an antipseudomonal beta-lactam was 27% compared with 47% mortality with an antipseudomonal beta-lactam alone.[48] The survival advantage with combination therapy was even greater among patients with pneumonia or in an ICU.[48] A prospective randomized trial in neutropenic patients with fever, malignancy, and gram-negative bacteremia noted an enhanced response rate and survival with ceftazidime plus 9 days of amikacin as compared with ceftazidime plus short-course (3 days) amikacin.[94] Several studies have noted high failure rates for pneumonias due to *P. aeruginosa* with monotherapy, even when the organisms were susceptible.[15, 45, 47, 54, 81] The synergistic killing achieved with the adjunctive use of an aminoglycoside may be important for pathogens with high virulence and high MICs (e.g., *P. aeruginosa* and *Acinetobacter* species) but is probably not necessary for more susceptible, less virulent organisms (e.g., *E. coli* and *Klebsiella* species). Theoretically, the use of combinations of antibiotics that act by different mechanisms may limit the development of antimicrobial resistance,[14] but this has not been consistent in clinical studies.[59] Toxicity associated with aminoglycosides may be minimized as long as appropriate dosing and monitoring are carried out. Recent strategies employing once-daily tobramycin or gentamicin (4 to 5 mg/kg) have been as effective and no more toxic than more frequent dosing regimens and may be cost-effective.[36, 79, 95, 96] Aerosolized or topical endotracheal aminoglycosides have been used but are of unproven value.

Other Antibiotic Combinations

Other antibiotic combinations may have a role in selected patients. Optimal combinations are those that achieve synergistic killing or expand the spectrum of activity. In this context, combining a fluoroquinolone with a beta-lactam antibiotic is attractive because synergy may be achieved against some isolates.[14, 88] By contrast, combining a fluoroquinolone with an aminoglycoside usually is indifferent or at best additive.[54] The author does not advocate combining two beta-lactam agents because synergy is usually not achieved and both agents may be degraded by beta-lactamases.[14] For beta-lactam–allergic patients, possible strategies include a fluoroquinolone or aztreonam (for enteric gramnegative bacteria) combined with clindamycin or metronidazole (to cover gram-positives and anaerobes).

Duration of Antibiotic Therapy

Studies assessing optimal duration of antibiotic therapy have not been performed. However, given the high mortality rate associated with nosocomial pneumonia, a minimum of 10–14 days of therapy is advised.[14] A more prolonged course (up to 21 days) may be required when adverse prognostic factors are present (e.g., persistent respiratory failure, multilobar involvement, isolation of *P. aeruginosa*, slow resolution, granulocytopenia, immunosuppression, or serious comorbidities). Converting to an oral agent after an initial 5–7 days of parenteral therapy may be adequate (provided the organism(s) are susceptible) and may achieve substantial cost savings.[54, 86, 89]

References

1. Craven DE, Steger KA: Epidemiology of nosocomial pneumonia: New perspectives on an old disease. Chest 1995; 108 (suppl): 1S–16S.
2. Fagon JY, Chastre J, Hance AJ, et al.: Nosocomial pneumonia in ventilated patients: A cohort study evaluating attributable mortality and hospital stay. Am J Med 1993; 94: 281–288.
3. Joshi N, Localio AR, Hamory BH: A predictive risk index for nosocomial pneumonia in the intensive care unit. Am J Med 1992; 93: 135–142.
4. Torres A, El-Ebiary M, Gonzales J, et al.: Gastric and pharyngeal flora in nosocomial pneumonia acquired during mechanical ventilation. Am Rev Respir Dis 1993; 148: 352–357.
5. Torres A, Gatell JM, Aznar E, et al.: Re-intubation increases the risk of nosocomial pneumonia in patients needing mechanical ventilation. Am J Respir Crit Care Med 1995; 152: 137–141.
6. George DL: Epidemiology of nosocomial pneumonia in intensive care unit patients. Clin Chest Med 1995; 16: 29–44.
7. Palmer LB, Conelan SV, Fox G, et al.: Gastric flora in chronically mechanically ventilated patients: Relationship to upper and lower airway colonization. Am J Respir Crit Care Med 1995; 151: 1063–1067.
8. Hamill RJ, Houston ED, Georghiou PR, et al.: An outbreak of *Burkholderia* (formerly *Pseudomonas*) *cepacia* respiratory tract colonization and infection associated with nebulized albuterol therapy. Ann Intern Med 1995; 122: 762–766.
9. Centers for Disease Control and Prevention: Draft guidelines for prevention of nosocomial pneumonia. Federal Register 1994; 59: 4980–5021.
10. Dreyfuss D, Djedaini K, Gros I, et al.: Mechanical ventilation with heated humidifiers or heat and moisture exchangers: Effects on patient colonization and incidence of nosocomial pneumonia. Am J Respir Crit Care Med 1995; 151: 986–992.

11. Duncan RA, Steger KA, Craven DE: Selective decontamination of the digestive tract: Risks outweigh benefits for intensive care unit patients. Semin Respir Infect 1993; 8: 308–324.

12. Iwahara T, Ichiyama S, Nada T, Shimokata K, Nakashima N: Clinical and epidemiologic investigations of nosocomial pulmonary infections caused by methicillin-resistant *Staphylococcus aureus*. Chest 1994; 105: 826–846.

13. Wiener J, Itokazu G, Nathan C, et al.: A randomized, double-blind, placebo-controlled trial of selective digestive decontamination in a medical-surgical intensive care unit. Clin Infect Dis 1995; 20: 861–867.

14. Lynch JP III: Combination antibiotic therapy is appropriate for nosocomial pneumonia in the intensive care unit. Semin Respir Infect 1993; 8: 268–284.

15. Lynch JP III, Watts CM: Nosocomial pneumonia in the ICU: Current treatment strategies: The pros and cons of monotherapy versus combination regimens. J Crit Illness 1995; 10: 332–353.

16. Grayson ML, Eliopoulos GM: Antimicrobial resistance in the intensive care unit. Semin Respir Infect 1990; 5: 204–214.

17. Pierson CL, Friedman BA: Comparison of susceptibility to beta-lactam antimicrobial agents among bacteria isolated from intensive care units. Diagn Microbiol Infect Dis 1992; 15: 19S–30S.

18. Rello J, Ausina V, Ricart M, Puzo C: Risk factors for infection by *Pseudomonas aeruginosa* in patients with ventilator-associated pneumonia. Intensive Care Med 1994; 20: 193–198.

19. Meduri GU: Diagnosis and differential diagnosis of ventilator-associated pneumonia. Clin Chest Med 1995; 16: 61–93.

20. Driks MR, Craven DE, Celli BR, et al.: Nosocomial pneumonia in intubated patients given sucralfate as compared with antacids of histamine type 2 blockers. N Engl J Med 1987; 317: 1376–1382.

21. Selective Decontamination of the Digestive Tract Trialists' Collaborative Group: Meta-analysis of randomized, controlled trials of selective decontamination of the digestive tract. BMJ 1993; 307: 525–532.

22. Verhoef J, Verhage EAE, Visser MR: A decade of experience with selective decontamination of the digestive tract as prophylaxis for infections in patients in the intensive care unit: What have we learned? Clin Infect Dis 1993; 17: 1047–1054.

23. Cade JF, McOwat E, Siganporia R, et al.: Uncertain relevance of gastric colonization in the seriously ill. Intensive Care Med 1992; 18: 210–217.

24. Bonten MJM, Gaillard CA, van Tiel FH, et al.: The stomach is not a source of colonization of the upper respiratory tract and pneumonia in ICU patients. Chest 1994; 105: 878–884.

25. Fagon J, Chastre J, Hance A, et al.: Evaluation of clinical judgment in the identification and treatment of nosocomial pneumonia in ventilated patients. Chest 1992; 103: 547–553.

26. Pingleton SK, Fagon JY, Leeper KV: Patient selection for clinical investigation of ventilator-associated pneumonia: Criteria for evaluating diagnostic techniques. Chest 1992; 102 (suppl): 553S–556S.

27. Chastre J, Fagon JV, Bornet-Lesco M, et al.: Evaluation of bronchoscopic techniques for the diagnosis of nosocomial pneumonia. Am J Respir Crit Care Med 1995; 152: 231–240.

28. Holzapfel L, Chevret S, Madinier G, et al.: Influence of long-term oro- or nasotracheal intubation on nosocomial maxillary sinusitis and pneumonia: Results of a prospective, randomized, clinical trial. Crit Care Med 1993; 21: 1132–1138.

29. Rouby JJ, Laurent P, Gosnach M, et al.: Risk factors and clinical relevance of nosocomial maxillary sinusitis in the critically ill. Am J Respir Crit Care Med 1994; 150: 776–783.

30. Maloney SA, Jarvis WR: Epidemic nosocomial pneumonia in the intensive care unit. Clin Chest Med 1995; 16: 209–224.

31. Prod-hom G, Leuenberger P, Koerfer J, et al.: Nosocomial pneumonia in mechanically ventilated patients receiving antacid, ranitidine, or sucralfate as prophylaxis for stress ulcer: A randomized controlled trial. Ann Intern Med 1994; 120: 653–662.

32. Rello J, Ausina V, Ricart M, et al.: Impact of previous antimicrobial therapy on the etiology and outcome of ventilator-associated pneumonia. Chest 1993; 104: 1230–1235.

33. Rello J, Torres A, Ricart M, et al.: ventilator-associated pneumonias by *Staphylococcus aureus*: Comparison of methicillin-resistant and methicillin-sensitive episodes. Am J Respir Crit Care Med 1994; 150: 1545–1550.

34. Rouby JJ, de Lassale EM, Poete P, Nicholas MH: Nosocomial pneumonia in the critically ill: Histologic and bacteriologic aspects. Am Rev Respir Dis 1992; 146: 1059–1066.

35. Schleupner CJ, Cobb DK: A study of the etiologies and treatment of nosocomial pneumonia in a community-based teaching hospital. Infect Control Hosp Epidemiol 1992; 13: 515–525.

36. Dunn M, Wunderink RG: Ventilator-associated pneumonia caused by *Pseudomonas* infection. Clin Chest Med 1995; 16: 95–110.

37. Rello J, Ricart M, Ausina V, et al.: Pneumonia due to *Haemophilus influenzae* among mechanically ventilated patients: Incidence, outcome, and risk factors. Chest 1992; 102: 1562–1565.

38. Lortholary O, Fagon JY, Hoi AB, et al.: Nosocomial acquisition of multiresistant *Acinetobacter baumanii*: Risk factors and prognosis. Clin Infect Dis 1995; 20: 790–796.

39. Blatt SP, Parkinson MD, Pace E, et al.: Nosocomial Legionnaire's Disease: Aspiration as a primary mode of transmission. Am J Med 1993; 95: 16–22.

40. Carratala J, Gudiol F, Pallares R, et al.: Risk factors for nosocomial *Legionella pneumophila* pneumonia. Am J Respir Crit Care Med 1994; 149: 625–629.

41. Korvick JA, Yu VL, Fang GD: *Legionella* species as hospital-acquired respiratory pathogens. Semin Respir Infect 1987; 2: 34–47.

42. Johnson JT, Yu VL, Best M, et al.: Nosocomial legionellosis uncovered in surgical patients with head and neck cancer: Implications for epidemiologic reservoir and mode of transmission. Lancet 1985; 2: 298–300.

43. Marrie TJ, Haldane D, MacDonald S, et al.: Control of endemic nosocomial Legionnaire's disease by using sterile potable water for high-risk patients. Epidemiol Infect 1991; 107: 591–605.

44. Yu VL: Could aspiration be the major mode of transmission for *Legionella*? Am J Med 1993; 95: 13–15.

45. Fink M, Snydman D, Niederman M, et al.: Treatment of severe pneumonia in hospitalized patients: Results of a multicenter, randomized, double-blind trial comparing intravenous ciprofloxacin with imipenem/cilastatin. Antimicrob Agents Chemother 1994; 38: 547–557.

46. Gaynes RP, Culver DH: Resistance to imipenem among selected gram-negative bacilli in the United States. Infect Control Hosp Epidemiol 1992; 13: 10–14.

47. Lode H, Wiley R, Höffken G, et al.: Prospective randomized controlled study of ciprofloxacin versus imipenem/cilastatin in severe clinical infections. Antimicrob Agents Chemother 1987; 31: 1491–1496.

48. Hilf M, Yu VL, Sharp JA, et al.: Antibiotic therapy for *Pseudomonas aeruginosa* bacteremia: Outcome correlations in a prospective study of 200 patients. Am J Med 1989; 87: 540–546.

49. Chastre J, Fagon JV: Invasive diagnostic testing should be routinely used to manage ventilated patients with suspected pneumonia. Am J Respir Crit Care Med 1994; 150: 570–574.

50. Bradford PA, Cherubin CE, Idemyor V, et al.: Multiply resistant *Klebsiella pneumoniae* strains from two Chicago hospitals: Identification of the extended-spectrum TEM-12 and TEM-10 ceftazidime-hydrolyzing beta-lactamases in a single isolate. Antimicrob Agents Chemother 1994; 38: 761–766.

51. Meyer KS, Urban C, Eagan JA, et al.: Nosocomial outbreak of *Klebsiella* infection resistant to late-generation cephalosporins. Ann Intern Med 1993; 119: 353–358.

52. Carratala J, Fernandez-Sevilla A, Tubau F, et al.: Emergence of quinolone-resistant *Escherichia coli* bacteremia in neutropenic patients with cancer who have received prophylactic norfloxacin. Clin Infect Dis 1995; 20: 557–560.

53. Chow JW, Fine MJ, Shlaes DM, et al.: *Enterobacter* bacteremia: Clinical features and emergence of antibiotic resistance during therapy. Ann Intern Med 1991; 115: 585–590.

54. Hooper DC, Wolfson JS: Fluoroquinolone antimicrobial agents. N Engl J Med 1991; 324: 383–394.

55. Jones RN, Reller B, Rosati LA, et al.: Ofloxacin, a new broad-spectrum fluoroquinolone: Results from a multicenter, national, comparative activity surveillance study. Diagn Microbiol Infect Dis 1992; 15: 425–434.

56. Thornsberry C: Susceptibility of clinical bacterial isolates to ciprofloxacin in the United States. Infection 1994; 22 (suppl 2): S80–S89.

57. Ball P: Editorial response: Is resistant *Escherichia coli* bacteremia an inevitable outcome for neutropenic patients receiving a fluoroquinolone as prophylaxis? Clin Infect Dis 1995; 20: 561–563.

58. Burwen DR, Banerjee SN, Gaynes RP, et al.: Ceftazidime resistance among selected nosocomial gram-negative bacilli in the United States. J Infect Dis 1994; 170: 1622–1625.

59. Arbo MDJ, Snydman DR: Monotherapy is appropriate for nosocomial pneumonia in the intensive care unit. Semin Respir Infect 1993; 8: 259–267.

60. Al-Ujayli, Nafziger DA, Saravolatz L: Pneumonia due to *Staphylococcus aureus* infection. Clin Chest Med 1995; 16: 111–121.

61. Panlilio AL, Culver DH, Gaynes RP, et al.: Methicillin-resistant *Staphylococcus aureus* in U.S. hospitals, 1975–1991. Infect Control Hosp Epidemiol 1992; 13: 582–586.

62. Mulligan ME, Murray-Leuisure KA, Ribenr BS, et al.: Methicillin-resistant *Staphylococcus aureus*: A consensus review of the microbiology, pathogenesis, and epidemiology with implications for prevention and management. Am J Med 1993; 94: 313–328.

63. Musher DM, Lamm N, Darouiche RO, et al.: The current spectrum of *Staphylococcus aureus* infection in a tertiary care hospital. Medicine (Baltimore) 1994; 73: 186–208.

64. Centers for Disease Control and Prevention, Department of Health and Human Services: Preventing the spread of vancomycin resistance. Federal Register 1994; 59: 25758–25763.

65. Rolinson GN: Evolution of beta-lactamase inhibitors. Rev Infect Dis 1991; 13 (suppl 9): S727–S732.

66. Mouton Y, Leroy O, Beuscart C, et al.: Efficacy, safety, and tolerance of parenteral piperacillin/tazobactam in the treatment of lower respiratory tract infections. J Antimicrob Chemother 1993; 31 (suppl A): 87–96.

67. Buckley MM, Brogden RN, Barradell LB, Goa KL: Imipenem/cilastatin: A reappraisal of its antibacterial activity, pharmacokinetic properties, and therapeutic efficacy. Drugs 1992; 44: 408–444.

68. Plouffe JF, File TM Jr, Breiman RF, et al.: Re-evaluation of the definition of Legionnaire's disease: Use of the urine antigen assay. Clin Infect Dis 1995; 20: 1286–1291.

69. Marquette CH, Copin MC, Wallet F, et al.: Diagnostic tests for pneumonia in ventilated patients: Prospective evaluation of diagnostic accuracy using histology as a gold standard. Am J Respir Crit Care Med 1995; 151: 1878–1888.

70. Niederman MS, Torres A, Summer W: Invasive diagnostic testing is not needed routinely to manage suspected ventilator-associated pneumonia. Am J Respir Crit Care Med 1994; 150: 565–570.

71. Jourdain B, Novara A, Joly-Guillou ML, et al.: Role of quantitative cultures of endotracheal aspirates in the diagnosis of nosocomial pneumonia. Am J Respir Crit Care Med 1995; 152: 241–246.

72. Marquette C, Georges H, Wallet P, et al.: Diagnostic efficiency of endotracheal aspirates for the diagnosis of ventilator-associated pneumonia. Am Rev Respir Dis 1993; 148: 138–144.

73. Kollef MH, Bock KR, Richards RD, Hearns ML: The safety and diagnostic accuracy of minibronchoalveolar lavage in patients with suspected ventilator-associated pneumonia. Ann Intern Med 1995; 122: 743–748.

74. Edmond MB, Ober JF, Weinbaum DL, et al.: Vancomycin-resistant *Enterococcus faecium* bacteremia: Risk factors for infection. Clin Infect Dis 1995; 20: 1126–1133.

75. Richard P, Le Floch R, Chamox C, et al.: *Pseudomonas aeruginosa* outbreak in a burn unit: Role of antimicrobials in the emergence of multiply resistant strains. J Infect Dis 1994; 170: 377–383.

76. Mandell LA, Niederman MS: The Canadian Hospital Acquired Pneumonia Consensus Group: Initial antimicrobial treatment of hospital-acquired pneumonia in adults: a conference report. Can J Infect Dis 1993; 4: 317–321.

77. Sobel JD: Imipenem and aztreonam. Infect Dis Clin North Am 1989; 3: 613–624.

78. Rubinstein E, Lode H, Grassi C, et al.: Ceftazidime monotherapy vs. ceftriaxone/tobramycin for serious hospital-acquired gram-negative infections. Clin Infect Dis 1995; 20: 1217–1228.

79. Cometta A, Zinner S, de Bock R, Calandra T, et al.: Piperacillin-tazobactam plus amikacin versus ceftazidime plus amikacin as empiric therapy for fever in granulocytopenic patients with cancer. Antimicrob Agents Chemother 1995; 39: 445–452.

80. Schlaes DM, Baughman R, Boylen CT, et al.: Piperacillin/tazobactam compared to ticarcillin/clavulanate in community-acquired bacterial lower respiratory tract infection. J Antimicrob Chemother 1994; 34: 565–577.

81. Norrby SR, Finch RG, Glauser M, et al.: Monotherapy in serious hospital-acquired infections: A clinical trial of ceftazidime versus imipenem/cilastatin. Antimicrob Agents Chemother 1993; 31: 927–937.

82. Cometta A, Baumgartner JD, Lew D, et al.: Prospective, randomized comparison of imipenem monotherapy with imipenem plus netilmicin for treatment of severe infections in non-neutropenic patients. Antimicrob Agents Chemother 1994; 38: 1309–1313.

83. Sanders WE, Morris JF, Alessi PK, et al.: Oral ofloxacin for the treatment of acute bacterial pneumonia: Use of a nontraditional protocol to compare experimental therapy with usual care in a multicenter clinical trial. Am J Med 1991; 91: 261–266.

84. Livermore DM: Carbapenemases. J Antimicrob Chemother 1992; 29: 609–613.

85. Cook JL: Gram-negative bacillary pneumonia in the nosocomial setting: Role of aztreonam. Am J Med 1990; 88 (suppl 3C): 34S–37S.

86. Gentry LO, Rodriguez-Gomez G, Kohler RB, et al.: Parenteral followed by oral ofloxacin for nosocomial pneumonia and community-acquired pneumonia requiring hospitalization. Am Rev Respir Dis 1992; 145: 31–35.

87. Peloquin CA, Cumbo TJ, Nix DE, et al.: Intravenous ciprofloxacin in patients with nosocomial lower respiratory tract infections: Impact of plasma concentrations, organism MIC, and clinical condition on bacterial eradication. Arch Intern Med 1989; 149: 2269–2273.

88. Forrest A, Nix DE, Ballow CH, et al.: Pharmacodynamics of intravenous ciprofloxacin in seriously ill patients. Antimicrob Agents Chemother 1993; 37: 1073–1081.

89. Malik IA, Khan WA, Karim M, et al.: Feasibility of outpatient management of fever in cancer patients with low-risk neutropenia: Results of a prospective, randomized trial. Am J Med 1995; 98: 224–231.

90. Dalhoff A: Quinolone resistance in *Pseudomonas aeruginosa* and *Staphylococcus aureus*: Development during therapy and clinical significance. Infection 1994; 22 (suppl 2): S111–S121.

91. Wilhelm MP: Vancomycin. Mayo Clin Proc 1991; 66: 1165–1170.

92. Pallares R, Dick R, Wenzel RP, et al.: Trends in antimicrobial utilization at a tertiary teaching hospital during a 15-year period (1978–1992). Infect Control Hosp Epidemiol 1993; 14: 376–382.

93. Ena J, Dick RW, Jones RN, Wenzel RP: The epidemiology of intravenous vancomycin usage in a university hospital: A 10-year study. JAMA 1993; 269: 598–602.

94. EORTC International Antimicrobial Therapy Cooperative Group: Ceftazidime combined with a short or long course of amikacin for empirical therapy of gram-negative bacteremia in cancer patients with granulocytopenia. N Engl J Med 1987; 317: 1692–1698.

95. Bates RD, Nahata MC: Once-daily administration of aminoglycosides. Ann Pharmacother 1994; 28: 757–766.

96. Prins JM, Buller HR, Kuijper EDJ, et al.: Once versus thrice daily gentamicin in patients with serious infections. Lancet 1993; 341: 335–339.

Jonas T. Johnson
Randal S. Weber

CHAPTER SIXTY-TWO

Management of Postoperative Head and Neck Wound Infections

▼

Postsurgical wound infection is a major source of morbidity and mortality in the United States. It is estimated that approximately 4% of surgical patients develop postoperative infection. Calculation of the relative risk of postoperative wound infection requires a complex equation that considers the nature and magnitude of the surgical insult, a patient's resistance to infection, and the virulence and size of the bacterial inoculum.

The risk of postoperative wound infection varies according to the surgical procedure. Clean procedures in which exposure to a bacterial inoculum is prevented through routine surgical sterile technique are associated with risk of postoperative infection in less than 5% of the cases.[1] For example, postoperative infection rates among patients undergoing a thyroidectomy or removal of a cervical mass should be 1% or less. Similarly, patients undergoing removal of salivary gland tumors in which there does not exist evidence of preoperative infection have a risk of postoperative wound infection less than 5%. The risk of wound infection in patients undergoing radical neck dissection in which the wound is not exposed to pharyngeal secretions is 0%–9%.[2]

Contamination of the surgical wound by oropharyngeal secretions greatly increases the risk of postoperative wound infection. In these circumstances, the infection rate may reach 87% if perioperative antibiotics are not administered.[3] The incidence of perioperative infections can be reduced significantly (3%–20%) through the administration of prophylactic antibiotics.[3–5]

The magnitude of the surgical procedure does correlate with the relative risk of postoperative infection. Patients being treated for advanced stage tumors are more likely to have wound infection when compared with a cohort group of patients with small tumors. This may be reflective of patients' immune function, nutritional status, duration of surgery, or the complexity of the repair. All of these factors are interrelated and play a potentially important role in determining risk.

Johnson and colleagues reported a series of 109 patients undergoing major head and neck surgical resection for whom flaps were required for repair.[6] Overall infection rate was 22% in spite of antibiotic prophylaxis. Weber and colleagues noted an infection rate of 38% associated with flap reconstruction in major head and neck surgical procedures.[7] In this series, the incidence of postoperative wound infection increased among patients with advanced disease who also required allogeneic blood transfusions.

Postoperative wound infection is associated with increased morbidity and greatly inflated health-care costs. Infections may delay the administration of postoperative radiotherapy in a timely fashion, increasing a patient's risk of tumor recurrence. Mandell-Brown and colleagues estimated that hospitalization averaged an extra 14 days for patients suffering postoperative wound infection.[8] The overwhelming majority of patients who incur postoperative wound infection were receiving antibiotic prophylaxis at the time of diagnosis. This underscores the frequent observation that successful accomplishment of the surgical procedure reflects careful coordination of a wide variety of events indicative of the health-care team's skill and vigilance. When preventive measures fail, early recognition and treatment may limit the morbidity of postoperative sepsis, resulting in more rapid convalescence with reduced morbidity and ultimately a better functional and cosmetic result.

DIAGNOSIS

Wound infection developing postoperatively is diagnosed based upon the treatment team's adequate understanding of the pathophysiology of wound healing. Erythema, edema, and induration are normal sequelae of head and neck surgical procedures. The magnitude and location of these cutaneous changes are reflective of the shape of the cervical incisions employed and vary widely among patients. For instance, the commonly used apron flap results in venous and lymphatic obstruction to the superiorly based flap. This invariably causes flap edema, erythema, and induration. Patients with fair complexions usually demonstrate more erythema than patients with darker skin pigmentation.

Similarly, low-grade fever (38.5°C) and leukocytosis (12,500 white blood cells/mm[3]) are commonly encountered on the first postoperative day following major head and neck surgery. These findings may be secondary to pulmonary atelectasis and aspiration and cannot be used to accurately gauge the status of the wound.

The sine qua non of wound infection is the development of a purulent collection under the cervical skin flap. A scale for defining postoperative wound infection has been developed (Table 62–1). Varying amounts of erythema, edema, and induration, which describe grades I, II, and III, are not indicative of wound infection. Grade IV and grade V wounds should be diagnosed as infected. The timing of onset of purulence in the wound may provide clues to the cause of the infection. Purulent drainage before the fifth

Table 62–1. SCHEME TO GRADE WOUNDS

Grade	Finding
I	Normal skin healing
II	Less than 1 cm of erythema along incision
III	Diffuse skin erythema
IV	Purulent drainage
V	Mucocutaneous fistula

postoperative day most often represents persistent salivary contamination of the cervical viscera due to a breakdown of or failure to ever have achieved a watertight closure of the mucosal surfaces. In a series of 212 patients, of whom 43 developed grade IV or V wounds, the median interval from surgery to the diagnosis of wound infection was 8 days (range 1–12 days).[7]

When physical findings are equivocal, analysis of the effluent from the cervical drains may be helpful in determining the presence of infection. Attempts to correlate cultures obtained from neck drains, however, have been disappointing in predicting the development of wound sepsis. Becker reports that 100% of drain effluence grew aerobic bacteria.[9] However, infection developed in only 13% of patients. The presence of saliva characterized as clear fluid with bubbles in the drain effluent may be interpreted as indication of a salivary leak (fistula). Serious wound breakdown in these circumstances may be prevented through maintenance of drain patency until the salivary fistula ceases. In unusual circumstances, when a large breakdown of the pharyngeal closure occurs, the drain may actually present itself in the hypopharynx. Salivary drainage, understandably enough, never ceases spontaneously. However, the drain can be advanced and removed once the cervical flap has had an opportunity to heal to the deep tissues of the neck. In normal circumstances, this takes 10–12 days, after which the drain can be safely advanced and removed.

A contrast pharyngogram may be used to identify sinus tracts or fistulas in suspicious cases. An alternative approach is to offer the patient colored fluid to drink; the presence of the colored fluid on the cervical skin or dressing is an indication of fistula.

LABORATORY EVALUATION

The overwhelming majority of infections developing in head and neck wounds are polymicrobial in nature. Two to as many as a dozen different organisms may be identified from a single culture specimen. Pathogenicity of a single organism may be difficult or impossible to identify.[10]

In a placebo-controlled clinical trial, the authors identified bacteremia in three patients randomized to the placebo arm of the study.[11] In each case, the bacterium identified in the blood was an anaerobe that was simultaneously identified in the wound effluent. This confirmed that oropharyngeal anaerobes play an important role in the pathogenesis of wound infection. Rubin and colleagues noted that *Candida* was identified in wounds of 48% of patients developing wound infection.[10] None of these patients were treated with antimycotic agents, and all of the wounds healed unevent-

fully. This suggested that *Candida* was only colonizing the wound in these circumstances. When the purulent collection is identified and drained from a cervical wound, a specimen should be obtained for aerobic and anaerobic culture and sensitivity testing as well as a Gram's stain. This is especially important for patients who develop signs of systemic sepsis or who fail to respond to early intervention. If sepsis is noted as characterized by fever, tachycardia, and leukocytosis, blood cultures should be obtained.

TREATMENT

Early diagnosis of wound sepsis is imperative to prevent further tissue necrosis. Bacterial endotoxins and salivary enzymes result in flap autolysis and exposure of vital structures. If saliva or ingested material is noted in the cervical drain, it is imperative that the drain patency be maintained. The importance of stopping all oral intake is debatable. Certainly, solid foods should not be offered because contamination of the cervical viscera by food seems imprudent. Administration of clear liquids by mouth probably has minimal deleterious effect and may actually serve to irrigate and dilute the bacteria present.

Soiling of the tracheobronchial tree through aspiration via a tracheostomy or laryngectomy stoma must be prevented. Use of a cuffed tracheotomy tube and bulky absorbent dressing may aid in preventing aspiration.

A patient's protein and caloric needs must be maintained during the convalescent period. This is most commonly accomplished through the use of enteral feeding through a tube. The highest incidence of sepsis associated with total parental nutrition is observed in patients with head and neck wound infections. Accordingly, insertion of a central line may be imprudent in the case of a head and neck infection.

When a purulent collection is undrained or if it is draining into a location that compromises the trachea, efforts should be made to establish drainage more laterally in the neck. This may occasionally be accomplished at the bedside through removal of selected sutures. Principles of managing an infected wound include wide drainage and débridement of devitalized tissue. Opening the wound removes the anaerobic environment that favors the proliferation of these organisms. Placement of catheters for frequent wound irrigation facilitates removal of accumulated pus and oropharyngeal secretions. Most patients benefit from a return to the operating room, where proper drainage can be accomplished under anesthesia. The surgeon can irrigate the wound carefully and place the new drainage catheter in a site ideally suited to help reduce the potential for aspiration.

Exposure of the carotid artery in the cervical wound due to wound infection represents a potential surgical emergency. Desiccation of the carotid artery may result in rupture with neurologic injury or death. Early intervention to cover the exposed carotid with well-vascularized soft tissue and concurrent diversion of the salivary stream must be the goal of surgery. The most commonly used intervention for an exposed carotid artery is a pectoralis muscle or myocutaneous flap.

Fulminant infection in the postoperative wound may be associated with small-vessel thrombosis, tissue necrosis, and major wound breakdown. This sequence of events is most commonly observed in patients who have previously received a full course of radiation therapy to the soft tissues of the neck and in patients with immune compromise, such as diabetics. In these circumstances, healing by secondary intention may not occur, and further surgery may be required for reconstruction. It is prudent to postpone reconstructive surgery until the full extent of tissue necrosis has been properly identified. Exposure of the carotid artery in these circumstances remains, however, an emergency. Flap coverage with vascularized muscle such as the pectoralis major is appropriate to intervene while waiting for the wound to fully declare itself.

Use of antibiotics during the evolution of a postoperative wound infection is appropriate for patients with evidence of cellulitis or sepsis. The fundamental treatment of wound infection is incision and drainage of any purulent material. When drainage has been properly established, the benefit of continued antibiotic administration becomes somewhat more contentious.

Selection of antibiotics for patients with postoperative wound infections should be guided by the findings of the Gram's stain, wound culture, and sensitivity. The antimicrobial agent used for preoperative prophylaxis should be avoided in treating a postoperative wound infection. The organisms encountered in a postoperative infection are nosocomial and likely to be resistant to the prophylactic agent. Many of these infections are polymicrobial and therefore require broad-spectrum antibiotics. Because of the delay in receiving microbiologic results, initial therapy must be empirical; organisms targeted for therapy should include gram-positive and gram-negative aerobes and anaerobes. A broad-spectrum drug combination, such as ticarcillin and clavulanic acid or ampicillin-sulbactam, is a reasonable choice for initial therapy. These antibiotics have beta-lactamase inhibitor activity and target staphylococcus and streptococcus species and aerobic gram-positive and gram-negative organisms and anaerobes. For the patient allergic to penicillin, a combination of an aminoglycoside and clindamycin provides broad-spectrum coverage. In some institutions where methicillin-resistant *Staphylococcus aureus* is frequently encountered, the addition of vancomycin should be considered.

Once the sensitivity of the infecting organisms is known, the therapy can be altered as needed. Antibiotic therapy is only one aspect of the overall management, which also includes aggressive nutritional supplementation, wide drainage of the wound, and débridement of devitalized tissue. When there is no further purulent exudate draining from the wound and the cellulitis has resolved, the antibiotics may be discontinued. In general, 1 week of therapeutic antibiotics is adequate, but the duration should be guided by the clinical course of the wound.

Irrigation of the infected wound with antimicrobial agents is an adjuvant treatment that has unproven merit. However, reduction in the number of colonizing organisms is an appealing approach to control of postoperative wound infection.

References

1. Johnson JT, Wagner RL: Infection following uncontaminated head and neck surgery. Arch Otolaryngol 1987; 113: 368–369.
2. Carrau RL, Byzakis J, Wagner RL, Johnson JT: Role of prophylactic antibiotics in uncontaminated neck dissections. Arch Otolaryngol Head Neck Surg 1991; 117: 194–195.
3. Becker GD, Parell GJ: Cefazolin prophylaxis in head and neck cancer surgery. Ann Otol Rhinol Laryngol 1979; 88: 183–186.
4. Johnson JT: Antibiotics for contaminated surgery. In: Johnson JT (ed): Antibiotic Therapy in Head and Neck Surgery. New York: Marcel Dekker, Inc., 1987; pp 51–91.
5. Johnson JT, Yu VL, Myers EN, Wagner RL: An assessment of the need for gram-negative bacterial coverage in antibiotic prophylaxis for oncological head and neck surgery. J Infect Dis 1987; 155: 331–333.
6. Johnson JT, Schuller DE, Gluckman JL, et al.: Antibiotic prophylaxis in high-risk head and neck surgery: One-day v five-day therapy. Otolaryngol Head Neck Surg 1986; 95: 554–557.
7. Weber RS, Raad I, Frankenthaler R, et al.: Ampicillin-sulbactam vs clindamycin in head and neck oncologic surgery: The need for gram-negative coverage. Arch Otolaryngol Head Neck Surg 1992; 118: 1159–1163.
8. Mandell-Brown MM, Johnson JT, Wagner RL: Cost effectiveness of prophylactic antibiotics in head and neck surgery. Otolaryngol Head Neck Surg 1984; 92: 520–523.
9. Becker GD, Welch WD: Quantitative bacteriology of closed-suction wound drainage in contaminated surgery. Laryngoscope 1990; 100: 403–406.
10. Rubin J, Johnson JT, Wagner RL, Yu VL: Bacteriology analysis of wound infection following major head and neck surgery. Arch Otolaryngol Head Neck Surg 1988; 114: 969–972.
11. Johnson JT, Myers EN, Thearle PB, et al.: Antimicrobial prophylaxis for contaminated head and neck surgery. Laryngoscope 1984; 94: 46–51.

Stuart Johnson
Dale N. Gerding

CHAPTER SIXTY-THREE

Nosocomial Diarrhea

▼

ETIOLOGY

Diarrhea is a common complication of hospitalization and is frequently associated with antimicrobial administration. Although the etiologic agent and pathogenic mechanisms responsible for most of these diarrheal episodes are unknown, *Clostridium difficile* is the most commonly known infectious cause of nosocomial diarrhea in adults and is responsible for 15%–25% of all cases of antibiotic-associated diarrhea.[1–3] Other agents implicated in antibiotic-associated diarrhea include *Salmonella*, enterotoxin-producing *Clostridium perfringens*, and *Candida albicans*, although the data implicating these latter two agents are limited.[1]

Salmonella has several epidemiologic similarities to *Clostridium difficile* in regard to both antimicrobial therapy and hospitalization as risk factors for infection. Data from volunteer studies indicate that ingestion of a moderately large inoculum (10^6 to 10^9 organisms) is necessary to cause disease by *Salmonella*. Administration of antibiotics, however, decreases the required inoculum 10^4-fold, presumably by altering the colonization resistance afforded by normal gut bacterial flora.[4] Epidemiologic investigations of community outbreaks have shown that recent exposure to antimicrobials significantly increases the risk of infection with *Salmonella*, regardless of the susceptibility pattern of the organism.[5] Outbreaks of *Salmonella* infection also occur in patients in hospitals where antimicrobial exposure also confers a risk.[6] Hospital acquisition may result from food-borne transmission and from cross infection as a result of person-to-person or fomite transmission.[7]

Nosocomial viral enteritis has also been documented in pediatric wards and in bone marrow transplant patients. Rotavirus is a major cause of diarrhea in children worldwide, and a distinct seasonality is seen in temperate climates, with most infections occurring in the winter months.[8] In addition to causing dehydration diarrheal illness in the community, rotavirus is also responsible for nosocomial outbreaks in pediatric wards; rotavirus was the second most common nosocomial pathogen in one study of a large pediatric hospital during a 12-month period.[9] Adenovirus, rotavirus, and coxsackievirus are also responsible for nosocomial diarrhea in bone marrow transplant recipients.[10]

Although *Salmonella* and, less often, other enteric pathogens are occasionally responsible for hospital-associated outbreaks, two large studies of 3 years' and 18 months' duration at an academic teaching hospital and a community hospital have demonstrated that testing for pathogens other than *C. difficile* in nosocomial diarrhea in adult patients is not efficacious.[11, 12] Cultures for routine enteric pathogens and examination of stools for ova and parasites in this setting are not indicated unless a patient has a profound state of immune deficiency such as occurs in advanced human immunodeficiency virus infection or bone marrow transplantation. *C. difficile* diarrhea may occur either as an endemic or as an epidemic nosocomial infection in different hospitals and may be endemic or epidemic in the same institution at different times.[13] *C. difficile* infection should be the prime diagnostic consideration in any patient who develops diarrhea or fever, leukocytosis, and abdominal symptoms without diarrhea following surgery, including ear, nose, and throat procedures.[14]

CLOSTRIDIUM DIFFICILE DIARRHEA

Pathogenesis

C. difficile is a unique enteric pathogen in regard to risk factors and clinical setting. The nearly universal history of prior antimicrobial exposure in patients with *C. difficile* diarrhea implies that colonization immunity afforded by normal colonic bacterial flora is a critical barrier for this anaerobic bacteria to overcome. *C. difficile* diarrhea has occurred following the administration of short courses of antimicrobials given for surgical prophylaxis,[15] but more often it follows therapeutic administration of antimicrobials.[2] *C. difficile* diarrhea is commonly precipitated by clindamycin, cephalosporins, and ampicillin, whereas vancomycin, metronidazole, and aminoglycosides are infrequently implicated. Although *C. difficile* has been postulated to be present in the normal human colonic flora in low numbers and proliferate or overgrow the other flora under the pressure of antimicrobial therapy, careful epidemiologic studies with discriminating organism-typing methods have shown that nearly all *C. difficile* infections are exogenously acquired, with the major reservoir being hospitals.[16–18]

Enteric pathogens are usually classified by the type of virulence mechanism and the intestinal location of the disease. Secretory diarrheal pathogens, such as *Vibrio cholerae*, elaborate enterotoxins that cause marked fluid secretion at the level of the small intestine but little mucosal damage. Inflammatory pathogens, such as *Shigella*, usually infect the colon, are typically invasive, and are suspected when white and red blood cells are detected in stool specimens. *C. difficile*, however, has features of both secretory and inflammatory diarrheal syndromes. The pathologic findings are limited to the colon, and the lesions of pseudomembranous colitis, one manifestation of *C. difficile* disease, stop at the iliocecal junction.[19] In contrast to *Shigella*, however, *C.*

difficile is not invasive, and fecal leukocytes are found in less than 40% of cases of associated disease.[20, 21]

C. difficile produces two large, single-peptide toxins: toxin A, a potent enterotoxin, and toxin B, a potent cytotoxin.[22] Although measurement of cytotoxicity (primarily the effect of toxin B) in stool specimens is used to diagnose *C. difficile* diarrhea, experimental evidence implicates toxin A as the critical virulence factor in the initiation of the disease.[22] Toxin A causes extensive mucosal damage with hemorrhagic fluid response by a mechanism entirely different than that initiated by the cholera enterotoxin.[23] The receptor for toxin A involves a trisaccharide moiety, Galα1-3Galβ1-4GlcNAc,[24] which is present on antigens within the brush border of human and hamster intestinal epithelium.[25] Subsequent toxic cellular events are only partially understood but involve marked cytoskeletal disruption.[26] The genes for both toxins A and B are coregulated and show a considerable amount of homology, but they are distinguished by a series of 38 contiguous repeating sequences on the 3' end of the toxin A gene.[27] These repeating sequences code for toxin A epitopes involved in binding to the toxin receptor and may explain the different effects of toxins A and B.[28] *C. difficile* strains either produce both toxins A and B or produce neither toxin; the latter strains are considered to be avirulent.

Clinical Manifestations

Infection with *C. difficile* may present as a mild diarrhea that resolves once the offending antimicrobial therapy is discontinued or, more often, persists and worsens if appropriate treatment is not initiated. The spectrum of disease ranges from asymptomatic colonization to nonspecific colitis, pseudomembranous colitis (PMC), and toxic megacolon. In hospital settings where *C. difficile* diarrhea is recognized, asymptomatic colonization is two to five times more common than clinical disease.[16, 17] These colonized patients are not at increased risk for subsequent illness,[16] and treatment is not advised.[29] Symptoms of *C. difficile* diarrhea may consist of only a few loose stools per day or multiple, large-volume, watery stools and signs of dehydration.[30] Stools may have mucus or evidence of occult blood but are rarely associated with visible blood.[2] In addition, a distinct fecal odor is often recognized by personnel caring for these patients. Abdominal pain, ileus, fever, and leukocytosis occur in 22%, 21%, 28%, and 50% of cases, respectively.[2]

Despite successful treatment, clinical recurrence of *C. difficile* diarrhea may follow in up to 20% of treated cases and may result from either relapse with the same strain or reinfection with a new strain.[31] Recurrences predictably respond to retreatment with the original anticlostridial therapy, but a small number of patients have multiple clinical relapses.

The presence of PMC usually implies more severe disease. The pseudomembranous intestinal lesions associated with *C. difficile* have a characteristic gross and histologic appearance[19] (Fig. 63–1). Early in the disease, small (1– 2 mm), raised, yellowish-white plaques may enlarge and coalesce.[32] Although PMC can be visualized by the sigmoidoscope in 90% of cases, some patients have disease limited to the

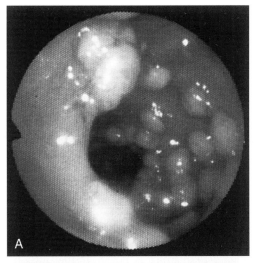

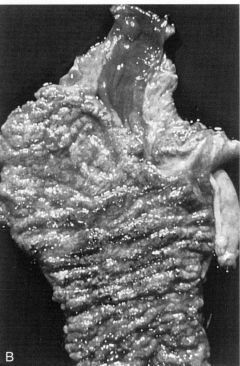

Figure 63–1. *A*, Endoscopic view of pseudomembranous colitis demonstrating round, elevated, yellow-white plaques that are adherent to the mucosa. *B*, Postmortem specimen of the cecum and ileum of a different patient demonstrating confluent pseudomembranes in the cecum with an abrupt demarcation at the ileocecal valve. (From Gerding DN, Gebhard RL, Sumner HW, Peterson LR: Pathology and diagnosis of *Clostridium difficile* disease. In: Rolfe RD, Finegold SM (eds): *Clostridium difficile*: Its Role in Intestinal Disease. San Diego: Academic Press, Inc., 1988.)

right colon, and the presentation may mimic appendicitis or Crohn's disease.[33, 34]

Toxic megacolon is a serious complication of *C. difficile* infection, with a high mortality rate that may require surgical intervention.[34, 35] It is important to recognize that this severe manifestation may not be associated with diarrhea, and the diagnosis is often missed or significantly delayed.[36] This complication is often seen following surgery for a nonabdominal condition (e.g., thoracotomy and hip surgery) in which the patient has prolonged ileus with leukocytosis, fever, abdominal distention, and pain.[36]

Other, rare manifestations associated with *C. difficile* include splenic abscess, bacteremia, wound infections, osteomyelitis, pleuritis, peritonitis, and urogenital tract infections.[37] Reactive arthritis has also been noted in association with *C. difficile* infection, similar to other enteric infections.[38]

Diagnosis

Laboratory tests used to diagnose *C. difficile* diarrhea are based on the detection of either the organism or its toxins in stool. Interpretation of any of these tests must first take into account the clinical setting, particularly in light of the high frequency of asymptomatic carriers in hospital settings where *C. difficile* diarrhea is noted. Testing for *C. difficile* diarrhea or its toxins should be done in patients who have received antimicrobials and who develop significant diarrhea (≥3 unformed or watery stools per day for ≥2 days) or ileus with signs of toxicity. A positive result from any of these tests may be considered presumptive evidence of *C. difficile* diarrhea. *C. difficile* diarrhea may occur during antimicrobial administration or several weeks after discontinuation of the antimicrobial.[39]

Detection of stool specimen cytoxicity in cell culture assay that is neutralized by appropriate antisera is the most specific laboratory test available for *C. difficile* diarrhea.[40] Sensitivity of the cell cytotoxin assay has ranged from 67%–100%.[40] Despite its relative insensitivity, stool testing for cytotoxin remains the "gold standard" against which newer *C. difficile* laboratory tests have been evaluated. Because of the slow turnaround time and the reluctance of many laboratories to use cell culture systems, a variety of enzyme immunoassays have been developed to detect toxin A and toxin B. These tests use monoclonal and polyclonal antibodies to detect *C. difficile* toxins and have a somewhat lower sensitivity (63%–85%) than cell cytotoxin assay but are reasonably specific.[41]

Tests that detect *C. difficile* in stool specimens include culture, the latex agglutination test, and polymerase chain reaction (PCR). Stool culture of *C. difficile* on selective media (cycloserine-cefoxitin-fructose-agar) is the most sensitive test for *C. difficile* diarrhea.[41] The major criticism of culture as a diagnostic test for *C. difficile* diarrhea is that it lacks specificity when compared with the cytotoxin assay. As a result, patients with diarrhea may be found to have a stool culture positive for *C. difficile* but a normal toxin test. The majority of such patients have a toxigenic strain of *C. difficile* present in the stool despite the normal stool cytotoxin assay.[42] The authors believe that most of these patients deserve a trial of therapy; failure to do so in one study was associated with increased morbidity and mortality.[43]

The latex agglutination test is a commercially available stool test that was originally thought to detect toxin A but was subsequently shown to detect a different *C. difficile* protein, glutamate dehydrogenase.[44] The test is rapid, simple to use, and relatively inexpensive, but it is lacking in both sensitivity and specificity and should be considered a suboptimal test, particularly when used alone.[41] The use of PCR

to detect *C. difficile* in stools is still an experimental procedure but one that, with the selection of appropriate primers, can potentially be used to detect toxigenic and nontoxigenic strains of *C. difficile*.[45]

In addition to the laboratory tests, endoscopy can be used to make a rapid, indirect diagnosis of *C. difficile* disease by the demonstration of PMC (see Fig. 63–1). Flexible sigmoidoscopy allows visualization of the distal 60 cm of the colon, and the diagnosis can be made by direct visualization or by biopsy if the lesions are small.[32] The major deficiency of endoscopy is that it is highly insensitive, with pseudomembranes detected in only 51% of cases.[2] However, visualization of PMC by endoscopy can avert exploratory abdominal surgery in critically ill patients in whom *C. difficile* disease mimics an acute abdomen.

Testing of stools for occult blood and fecal leukocytes and examination by Gram's stain for gram-positive bacilli are not helpful in the diagnosis of *C. difficile* diarrhea because of low sensitivity and low specificity.[20, 21]

Treatment

Before initiating specific treatment for *C. difficile* diarrhea, it should be remembered that the symptoms resolve spontaneously in up to 23% of patients once the offending antimicrobial agent is discontinued.[46] On the other hand, treatment need not be delayed in more seriously ill patients and can be started empirically once the specimen has been sent for testing. Vancomycin and metronidazole are the two agents that have been used most extensively for treatment of *C. difficile* diarrhea. Oral vancomycin was the first treatment shown effective for *C. difficile* diarrhea, and even at lower dosages (125 mg four times daily) fecal drug levels several logs higher than the minimum inhibitory concentration for the organism are easily achieved.[47] Unlike vancomycin, metronidazole is highly absorbed, and fecal drug levels are much lower than those achieved with oral vancomycin. Despite this theoretical drawback, metronidazole has been shown to be highly effective in the treatment of *C. difficile* diarrhea and is considerably less expensive.[13, 46] Accepted regimens are shown in Table 63–1. Other agents that have

Table 63–1. RECOMMENDED THERAPY FOR *Clostridium difficile* DIARRHEA AND COLITIS

Agent	Dose	Comments
Metronidazole	250 mg orally four times daily for 10 days	Least expensive
Vancomycin	125 mg orally four times daily for 10 days	Potential risk of vancomycin-resistant enterococci*
Vancomycin	500 mg rectally every 6 hours, plus	Empirical therapy for severe ileus†
Vancomycin	500 mg via nasogastric tube every 6 hours, plus	
Metronidazole	500 mg intravenously every 6 hours	

*Hospital Infection Control Practices Advisory Committee recommendations for preventing the spread of vancomycin resistance.[48]

†Six of eight patients with severe ileus survived after treatment with this regimen.[13]

been shown effective include teicoplanin, bacitracin, and fusidic acid.

Therapy for *C. difficile* diarrhea should be given orally. However, in patients with ileus several other administration methods have been used empirically. Fecal drug levels have been achieved with intravenous metronidazole, but not vancomycin, and intravenous metronidazole has anecdotal evidence to support its use in this manner.[49] In severely ill patients with ileus, the authors have advocated a regimen of vancomycin administered by retention enema and by nasogastric tube (using the intravenous vancomycin formulation) with metronidazole given intravenously.[13] As with invasive diarrheal syndromes, antimotility drugs such as phenoxylate-atropine (Lomotil) should be avoided in the treatment of *C. difficile* diarrhea as these agents have been implicated in the development of complications such as toxic megacolon.[35] Surgical treatment of toxic megacolon due to *C. difficile* may be required. Efficacy has been difficult to assess in this relatively uncommon but highly lethal complication, and subtotal colectomy with sparing of the rectal stump appears to be the preferred surgical option.[34, 35]

References

1. Bartlett JG: Antibiotic-associated diarrhea. Clin Infect Dis 1992; 15: 573–581.
2. Gerding DN, Olson MM, Peterson LR, et al.: *Clostridium difficile*-associated diarrhea and colitis in adults: A prospective case-controlled epidemiologic study. Arch Intern Med 1986; 146: 95–100.
3. McFarland LV, Mulligan ME, Kwok RYY, Stamm WE: Nosocomial acquisition of *Clostridium difficile* infection. N Engl J Med 1989; 320: 204–210.
4. Bonhoff M, Miller CP, Martin WR: Resistance of the mouse's intestinal tract to experimental salmonella infection. J Exp Med 1964; 120: 805–813.
5. Pavia AT, Shipman LD, Wells JG, et al.: Epidemiologic evidence that prior antimicrobial exposure decreases resistance to infection by antimicrobial-sensitive *Salmonella*. J Infect Dis 1990; 161: 255–260.
6. Robins-Browne RM, Rowe B, Ramsaroop R, et al.: A hospital outbreak of multiresistant *Salmonella typhimurium* belonging to phage type 193. J Infect Dis 1983; 147: 210–216.
7. Joseph CA, Palmer SR: Outbreaks of salmonella infection in hospitals in England and Wales 1978–87. BMJ 1989; 298: 1161–1164.
8. LeBaron CW, Lew J, Glass RI, et al.: Annual rotavirus epidemic patterns in North America. JAMA 1990; 264: 983–988.
9. Welliver RC, McLaughlin S: Unique epidemiology of nosocomial infection in a children's hospital. Am J Dis Child 1984; 138: 131–135.
10. Yolken RH, Bishop CA, Townsend TR, et al.: Infectious gastroenteritis in bone-marrow transplant recipients. N Engl J Med 1982; 306: 1009–1012.
11. Yannelli B, Gurevich I, Schoch PE, Cunha BA: Yield of stool cultures, ova and parasite tests, and *Clostridium difficile* determinations in nosocomial diarrheas. Am J Infect Control 1988; 16: 246–249.
12. Siegel DL, Edelstein PH, Nachamkin I: Inappropriate testing for diarrheal diseases in the hospital. JAMA 1990; 263: 979–982.
13. Olson MM, Shanholtzer CJ, Lee JT Jr, Gerding DN: Ten years of prospective *Clostridium difficile*-associated disease surveillance and treatment at the Minneapolis VA Medical Center, 1982–1991. Infect Control Hosp Epidemiol 1994; 15: 371–381.
14. Griebie M, Adams GL: *Clostridium difficile* colitis following head and neck surgery. Arch Otolaryngol 1985; 111: 550–553.
15. Yee J, Dixon CM, McLean APH, Meakins JL: *Clostridium difficile* disease in a department of surgery: The significance of prophylactic antibiotics. Arch Surg 1991; 126: 241–246.
16. Johnson S, Clabots CR, Linn FV, et al.: Nosocomial *Clostridium difficile* colonization and disease. Lancet 1990; 336: 97–100.

17. McFarland LV, Mulligan M, Kwok RYY, Stamm WE: Nosocomial acquisition of *Clostridium difficile* infection. N Engl J Med 1989; 320: 204–210.
18. Clabots CR, Johnson S, Olson MM, et al.: Acquisition of *Clostridium difficile* by hospitalized patients: Evidence for colonized new admissions as a source of infection. J Infect Dis 1992; 166: 561–567.
19. Gerding DN, Gebhard RL, Sumner HW, Peterson LR: Pathology and diagnosis of *Clostridium difficile* disease. In: Rolfe RD, Finegold SM (eds): *Clostridium difficile*: Its Role in Intestinal Disease. San Diego: Academic Press, Inc., 1988.
20. Shanholtzer CJ, Peterson LR, Olson MM, et al.: Prospective study of Gram-stained stool smears in diagnosis of *Clostridium difficile* colitis. J Clin Microbiol 1983; 17: 906–908.
21. Marx CE, Morris A, Wilson ML, Reller LB: Fecal leukocytes in stool specimens submitted for *Clostridium difficile* toxin assay. Diagn Microbiol Infect Dis 1993; 16: 313–315.
22. Lyerly DM, Saum KE, MacDonald DK, Wilkins TD: Effects of *Clostridium difficile* toxins given intragastrically to animals. Infect Immun 1985; 47: 349–352.
23. Lima AAM, Lyerly DM, Wilkins TD, et al.: Effects of *Clostridium difficile* toxins A and B in rabbit small and large intestine in vivo and on cultured cells in vitro. Infect Immun 1988; 56: 582–588.
24. Krivan HC, Clark GF, Smith DF, Wilkins TD: Cell surface binding site for *Clostridium difficile* enterotoxin: Evidence for a glycoconjugate containing the sequence Galα1-3Galβ1-4G1cNAc. Infect Immun 1986; 53: 573–581.
25. Tucker KD, Wilkins TD: Toxin A of *Clostridium difficile* binds to the human carbohydrate antigens I, X, and Y. Infect Immun 1991; 59: 73–78.
26. Hecht G, Pothoulakis C, LaMont JT, Madara JL: *Clostridium difficile* toxin A perturbs cytoskeletal structure and junction permeability in cultured human epithelial monolayers. J Clin Invest 1988; 82: 1516–1524.
27. Dove CH, Wang S-Z, Price SB, et al.: Molecular characterization of the *Clostridium difficile* toxin A gene. Infect Immun 1990; 58: 480–488.
28. Frey SM, Wilkins TD: Localization of two epitopes recognized by the monoclonal antibody PCG-4 on *Clostridium difficile* toxin A. Infect Immun 1992; 60: 2488–2492.
29. Johnson S, Homann SR, Bettin KM, et al.: Treatment of asymptomatic *Clostridium difficile* carriers (fecal excretors) with vancomycin or metronidazole: A randomized, placebo-controlled trial. Ann Intern Med 1992; 117: 297–302.
30. Bartlett JG: *Clostridium difficile*: Clinical considerations. Rev Infect Dis 1990; 12 (suppl 2): S243–S251.
31. Johnson S, Adelmann A, Clabots CR, et al.: Recurrences of *Clostridium difficile* diarrhea not caused by the original infecting organism. J Infect Dis 1989; 159: 340–343.
32. Gebhard RL, Gerding DN, Olson MM, et al.: Clinical and endoscopic findings in patients early in the course of *Clostridium difficile*-associated pseudomembranous colitis. Am J Med 1985; 78: 45–48.
33. Tedesco FJ, Corless JK, Brownstein RE: Rectal sparing in antibiotic-associated pseudomembranous colitis: A prospective study. Gastroenterology 1982; 83: 1259–1260.
34. Morris JB, Zollinger RM Jr, Stellato TA: Role of surgery in antibiotic-associated pseudomembranous enterocolitis. Am J Surg 1990; 160: 535–539.
35. Cone JB, Wetzel W: Toxic megacolon secondary to pseudomembranous colitis. Dis Colon Rectum 1982; 25: 478–482.
36. Burke GW, Wilson ME, Mehrez IO: Absence of diarrhea in toxic megacolon complicating *Clostridium difficile* pseudomembranous colitis. Am J Gastroenterol 1988; 83: 304–307.
37. Levett PN: *Clostridium difficile* in habitats other than the human gastrointestinal tract. J Infect 1986; 12: 253–263.
38. Lofgren RP, Tadlock LM, Soltis RD: Acute oligoarthritis associated with *Clostridium difficile* pseudomembranous colitis. Arch Intern Med 1984; 144: 617–619.
39. Tedesco FJ, Barton RW, Alpers DH: Clindamycin-associated colitis: A prospective study. Ann Intern Med 1974; 81: 429–433.
40. Peterson LR, Kelly PJ: The role of the clinical microbiology laboratory in the management of *Clostridium difficile*-associated diarrhea. Infect Dis Clin North Am 1993; 7: 277–293.
41. Gerding DN, Johnson S, Peterson LR, et al.: Society for Healthcare Epidemiology of America position paper on *Clostridium difficile*-asso-

ciated diarrhea and colitis. Infect Control Hosp Epidemiol 1995; 16: 459–477.

42. Clabots CR, Johnson S, Olson MM, et al.: *Clostridium difficile*-associated diarrhea diagnosis in patients with positive stool culture and negative stool cytotoxin assays. Program and abstracts, 33rd Interscience Conference on Antimicrobial Agents and Chemotherapy, October 17–20, 1993, New Orleans, Abstract #1567.

43. Lashner BA, Todorczuk J, Sahm DF, Hanauer SB: *Clostridium difficile* culture-positive toxin-negative diarrhea. Am J Gastroenterol 1986: 81: 940–943.

44. Lyerly DM, Barroso LA, Wilkins TD: Identification of the latex test-reactive protein of *Clostridium difficile* as glutamate dehydrogenase. J Clin Microbiol 1991; 29: 2639–2642.

45. Gumerlock PH, Tang YJ, Weiss JB, et al.: Specific detection of toxigenic strains of *Clostridium difficile* in stool specimens. J Clin Microbiol 1993; 31: 507–511.

46. Teasley DG, Olson MM, Gebhard RL, et al.: Prospective randomized trial of metronidazole versus vancomycin for *Clostridium difficile*-associated diarrhea and colitis. Lancet 1983; 2: 1043–1046.

47. Fekety R, Silva J, Kauffman C, et al.: Treatment of antibiotic-associated *Clostridium difficile* colitis with oral vancomycin: Comparison of two dosage regimens. Am J Med 1989; 86: 15–19.

48. Hospital Infection Control Practices Advisory Committee (HICPAC): Recommendations for preventing the spread of vancomycin resistance. Infect Control Hosp Epidemiol 1995; 16: 105–113.

49. Kleinfeld DI, Sharpe RJ, Donta ST: Parenteral therapy for antibiotic-associated and pseudomembranous colitis. J Infect Dis 1988; 157: 389.

Thomas A. Tami
Steven Gold
Nina Singh

CHAPTER SIXTY-FOUR

AIDS in Otolaryngology

▼

By all accounts, AIDS has become the most important public health problem of our time. From its first identification in the early 1980s, the epidemic has swept through the United States at a lightning pace and has become a devastating global problem. Although sub-Saharan Africa is frequently cited as the geographic area where AIDS has had its greatest influence, the rapid spread of the human immunodeficiency virus (HIV) in southeast Asia poses an even greater global threat. In northern Thailand, for example, recent blood screening surveys have detected an HIV seropositive rate of approximately 12% among young, otherwise healthy military recruits.[1] The continued rapid spread of this fatal disease will affect both the socioeconomic and the medical and public health policymaking of these countries, as well as that of the rest of the world well into the twenty-first century. In the United States alone, more than 440,000 cases of AIDS had been reported to the Centers for Disease Control and Prevention (CDC) through December 1994, and it is estimated that well over one million persons (or nearly 1 in 200) are currently infected with HIV. If past trends can predict the future, these staggering numbers will continue to grow. Because ear, nose, and throat problems are common in this population, otolaryngologists will be called upon increasingly to assist in the medical diagnosis and management of these patients. Infectious manifestations in the head and neck are the primary emphasis of this chapter.

HUMAN IMMUNODEFICIENCY VIRUS (HIV)

HIV is a retrovirus that, like other retroviruses, has an outer cell membrane (a bilipid layer containing the surface and transmembrane proteins gp120 and gp41, respectively). When the virus enters the blood stream, it attaches to host cell CD4 surface receptors. Whereas CD4 receptors are present on numerous cells, they predominate on CD4 lymphocytes (helper T lymphocytes). It is probably the gp120 surface protein that has the highest affinity for these surface receptors and that allows the HIV cell membrane to fuse with that of the host. Following cell membrane fusion, the contents of the retrovirus, which include the single-stranded viral ribonucleic acid (RNA) and the enzyme reverse transcriptase, are introduced into the host cell. Under the influence of reverse transcriptase, a DNA copy of the viral RNA is produced. This viral DNA migrates to the host cell nucleus to become integrated into the host cell chromosomal DNA to become a provirus.

In its proviral form, the viral DNA replicates with the host DNA. At some point the viral genome recruits the transcriptional machinery of the host cell and begins virus

production. Viral proteins as well as RNA copies of the viral DNA are assembled within the host cell, and new HIV particles are produced and released. The host cell is destroyed, and viral particles are available to infect other cells, thus completing the viral cell cycle (Fig. 64–1).

This life cycle of the HIV virus is typical of retroviruses. What separates retroviral infection from other more classic viral infections is the existence of a provirus form of the virus. As a provirus, the retrovirus is an integral part of the genome of the host cell and, as such, can be destroyed only by destroying the host cell itself. Because treatment strategies must account for this unusual life cycle, successful treatment protocols of this viral disease have been difficult to establish.

The Clinical Course of HIV Infection

Following primary HIV infection a prolonged period (usually 6–10 years) of clinical latency follows. Although asymptomatic, the infection during this period is not truly latent as viral kinetic studies have demonstrated continued high-level replication. The progressive CD4+ lymphocyte depletion is primarily a consequence of destruction, not of lack of production of these cells; an estimated 1.8 billion CD4 cells are destroyed per day.[2] The lymphoid organs are the major reservoirs and sites of viral replication.

In 50%–70% of patients with primary HIV infection, an acute mononucleosis-like syndrome develops approximately 3–6 weeks after initial infection. Because this syndrome precedes the development of host antibodies against HIV (seroconversion), early recognition is very important. Acutely infected patients who are HIV-seronegative by current antibody screening tests can be extremely infectious[3] (Fig. 64–2).

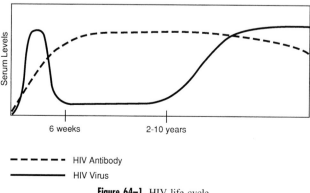

Figure 64–1. HIV life cycle.

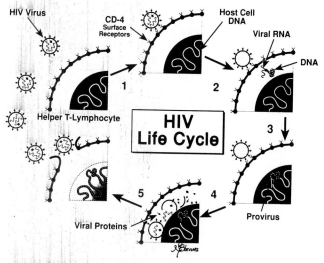

Figure 64–2. Typical pattern of HIV infection. Serum viral levels are very high and HIV antibody levels undetectable during the first weeks of infection. Antibody levels remain high while viral levels fall during a period of controlled infection. Viral levels rise again when clinical manifestations of AIDS appear.

Opportunistic infections in HIV-infected patients are responsible for 90% of the deaths. The predisposition to infection from various opportunistic pathogens varies with the extent of immunosuppression. Therefore, knowledge of patients' CD4+ lymphocyte count is crucial in evaluating the opportunistic infection and the likely causative pathogen. Tuberculosis, mucosal candidiasis, and varicella-zoster virus may occur in patients with a CD4 count greater than 200/mm³. *Pneumocystis carinii* infections usually occur in patients with a CD4 count less than 200/mm³, *Cryptococcus neoformans* and *Toxoplasma gondii* infections in patients with a CD4 count less than 100/mm³, and cytomegalovirus and *Mycobacterium avium-intracellulare* infections in patients with a CD4 count less than 50/mm³. The frequency and characteristics of opportunistic infections in patients with AIDS, however, have changed during the years. The remarkable efficacy of prophylactic therapy for *P. carinii* has resulted in a decrease in the incidence of such infections. The incidence of cytomegalovirus and *M. avium* complex infections, on the other hand, has increased, partially because of the increased life expectancy of HIV-infected patients with profound immunosuppression.

Medical Management of HIV Disease

A mainstay of treatment for HIV disease is antiretroviral therapy. A major challenge has been to develop a drug that is effective, safe, and affordable and that exhibits minimal toxicity. Unfortunately, no such drug currently exists. In 1985, however, 3'-azido-3'-deoxythymidine (AZT), also known as zidovudine, was shown to have in vitro activity against HIV-1. It received U.S. Food and Drug Administration (FDA) approval 2 years later when clinical trials showed some beneficial results. Didanosine (ddI), zalcitabine (ddC), stavudine (d4T), and lamivudine[4] are other antiretroviral agents that have received FDA approval. All these agents are nucleoside analogues that act by inhibiting the viral enzyme reverse transcriptase, which has been the primary target of most successful antiretroviral therapy. The principal problems with these drugs are their limited efficacy, toxicity, and lack of durable antiviral effect that is likely related to the development of viral resistance. HIV protease inhibitors are a relatively new class of drugs that represent a major advance in the management of HIV infection.[5–10] These drugs target the HIV protease, an enzyme that cleaves the polyproteins into functional protein products during the late stages of HIV replication. Saquinavir, indinavir, and ritonavir are the protease inhibitors currently approved by the FDA. These drugs are promising antiretroviral drugs based on the clinical and HIV surrogate marker data available to date. However, development of resistance is a major concern, especially if administered at suboptimal doses or when given as monotherapy.[10] Protease inhibitors should therefore always be administered in combination with nucleoside analogues for the treatment of HIV infection.

The most common side effect of AZT is bone marrow toxicity, although this has been less problematic with the 500–600 mg/day dosages of AZT that are currently used. Macrocytic anemia is very common, and both neutropenia and thrombocytopenia have been observed. Other common side effects are nausea, fatigue, and headaches. The main side effects of the other available nucleoside reverse transcriptance inhibitors (e.g., ddI, ddC, and d4T) include peripheral neuropathy, hyperamylasemia, and pancreatitis. The major toxicity of lamivudine is in bone-marrow suppression. Gastrointestinal symptoms (e.g., nausea and diarrhea) for saquinavir and ritonavir[6, 7]; elevated triglycerides and liver transaminase levels for ritonavir[5, 7]; and hyperbilirubinemia and nephrolithiasis for indinavir are the predominant side effects.[9]

HEAD AND NECK INFECTIOUS MANIFESTATIONS OF HIV

External Ear

The external ear is very susceptible to infectious conditions associated with HIV. Otitis externa is a common infectious otologic problem in this population. The frequent occurrence of this condition is probably related to chronic dermatitis of the external auditory canal. *Pseudomonas aeruginosa* is frequently isolated from patients with this condition. Appropriate management consists of frequent removal of debris from the external auditory canal along with otic drops containing antimicrobials and steroids (e.g., Cortisporin) 3 to 4 times daily. Rapid improvement with this regimen is usually seen.[11, 12] If more extensive soft tissue involvement is present, a systemic oral antibiotic such as ciprofloxin 500–750 mg twice daily for 14 days may be of added benefit.[12]

In the immunocompromised or diabetic patient, otitis externa occasionally progresses to skull base osteomyelitis. See Chapter 36 for an overview of necrotizing external otitis in AIDS. In most of these cases the pathogen is usually

Pseudomonas; rarely have other bacteria or fungi been implicated.[13] One series reported two cases of skull base osteomyelitis in AIDS patients caused by *Aspergillus fumigatus.* Both patients responded to therapy with amphotericin B followed by oral itraconazole 200 mg twice daily. In one patient, however, surgical débridement, including sacrifice of the involved facial nerve, was required.[14] Overall it still remains unclear whether the incidence of skull base osteomyelitis is higher in the AIDS population.

Polyps of the external auditory canal have been reported as manifestations of both *Pneumocystis* and tuberculous infections. With the increased use of aerosolized pentamidine as prophylaxis against *P. carinii,* the incidence of extrapulmonary *Pneumocystis* infection seems to have increased.[12] The diagnosis of *Pneumocystis* otitis can be made with a biopsy of the external auditory canal polyp, followed by light microscopy using Gomori's methenamine silver stain, or by electron microscopy.[15, 16] Subcutaneous cysts due to *P. carinii* can also occur in the external auditory canal. These cysts can enlarge to the point of occluding the external auditory canal.[17] Treatment of *Pneumocystis* otitis consists of trimethoprim/sulfamethoxazole for 2–6 weeks. Rapid resolution usually follows.

Mycobacterium tuberculosis infections of the middle ear can also present with an aural polyp extending into the external auditory canal. This presentation is frequently accompanied by a conductive hearing loss and clear otorrhea. Diagnosis usually requires a biopsy to demonstrate acid-fast organisms. Once a diagnosis is confirmed, appropriate medical therapy for *M. tuberculosis* usually results in rapid improvement.[12]

Any HIV-infected patient diagnosed with either *M. tuberculosis* or *P. carinii* infection of the ear should also be evaluated for concurrent pulmonary infection by these organisms.

Middle Ear

The most common otologic problems reported in HIV-infected patients are serous otitis media and recurrent acute otitis media. Both adult and pediatric AIDS patients are susceptible to otitis media predominantly as a result of eustachian tube dysfunction. In the pediatric patient this inherent problem coupled with diminished cell-mediated immunity predisposes HIV-infected children to middle ear infections.[18] In the adult, recurrent viral infections, adenoidal lymphoid hyperplasia, nasopharyngeal neoplasms, sinusitis, and immunoglobulin (Ig) E (IgE)-mediated atopic disease can all lead to poor eustachian tube function.[19]

Benign nasopharyngeal lymphoid hyperplasia is well recognized in AIDS and has been reported as a cause of nasal obstruction, hearing loss, and otitis media with effusion.[20] In many of these patients, adenoidectomy improves eustachian tube function. The authors usually reserve adenoidectomy for those cases in which the diagnosis of lymphoid hyperplasia is not clear (i.e., Kaposi's sarcoma or aggressive B-cell lymphoma) or symptoms cannot otherwise be easily relieved. Office myringotomy with tympanostomy tube placement usually provides symptomatic relief with minimal morbidity.[19]

The bacteriology of otitis media in AIDS patients is very similar to that in the non-AIDS population. *Streptococcus* and *Haemophilus influenzae* are the most common pathogens; however, *Pseudomonas* and *Staphylococcus* species must also be considered.[12] Unusual pathogens such as *P. carinii, M. tuberculosis, Nocardia asteroides,* and *Candida* have also been isolated from middle ear aspirates.[19, 12] Tuberculous otitis media is believed to result from hematogenous spread of tubercle bacilli from the lungs. A rare but documented complication of tuberculosis otitis in HIV is tuberculous meningitis.[21]

Treatment with standard antibiotic therapy consisting of amoxicillin or trimethoprim/sulfamethoxazole is usually adequate. Failure of medical therapy may be due to beta-lactamase–producing organisms or to unusual pathogens. If treatment with broader spectrum antibiotics (e.g., amoxicillin-clavulanate potassium) is unsuccessful, tympanocentesis with cultures including fungal, acid-fast, and routine bacteria should be performed.

Mastoiditis in HIV-infected patients has been reported by several authors.[19] The usual pathogens, such as *Streptococcus pneumoniae,* are the most common cause of mastoiditis in the AIDS population. Unusual cases of otomastoiditis caused by *Aspergillus* or *M. tuberculosis* in AIDS patients have been reported.[19, 22] To date, however, there is no evidence that chronic otitis media, cholesteatoma, intracranial complications, or other suppurative complications of otitis media occur more frequently in this population.[19, 12]

Inner Ear

Neurosensory hearing loss occurs in up to 50% of HIV-infected patients.[12, 19, 23] Possible causes for this loss include the direct effects of HIV infection on the central nervous system and auditory nerve, iatrogenic use of ototoxic medications, and opportunistic infections and/or neoplasia of the central nervous system.

The central hearing impairment observed in this disease probably results from direct HIV infection.[19] Auditory brain stem testing has demonstrated increased latencies consistent with a demyelinating disorder. This finding has been substantiated by tissue samples of patients demonstrating focal areas of demyelination secondary to HIV infection of glial cells and neurons of the brain stem.[23] Hearing loss often worsens with disease progression.[19]

Opportunistic infections of the central nervous system are also common in AIDS and may be associated with sensorineural hearing loss. Examples include cryptococcal meningitis, central nervous system toxoplasmosis, tuberculous meningitis, and bacterial and viral meningitis.[24] There is also evidence that hearing loss can arise from viral central nervous system pathogens in AIDS, including cytomegalovirus (CMV), herpes simplex virus (HSV), and herpes zoster virus.[25]

Syphilis is often a more severe disease when associated with AIDS. Otosyphilis can occur at any stage of HIV and should be suspected in all HIV-infected patients with otologic symptoms. Because otosyphilis often has an accelerated course in HIV-infected patients,[26] serologic testing should be routine in patients with neurosensory hearing loss.

Facial Nerve Palsy

Facial nerve palsy is more prevalent in HIV-infected patients. Reported causes of facial palsy in this population include central nervous system neoplasias; bacterial, viral, or parasitic central nervous system infections; herpes zoster oticus; progressive multifocal leukoencephalopathy; and AIDS encephalopathy.[19] According to one report, up to 7.2% of patients with HIV have either unilateral or bilateral facial nerve paralysis.[19] The most frequently identifiable cause was central nervous system toxoplasmosis, followed by AIDS encephalopathy and central nervous system lymphoma.

Idiopathic facial nerve palsy, or Bell's palsy, is still the most common reason for 7th-nerve palsy in the AIDS population. The relative increase in Bell's palsy in this population may be due to primary infection or reactivation of herpes simplex virus secondary to altered host immunity. In general, the outcome for these patients is excellent, with facial nerve function usually returning within 3 weeks to 3 months.[12, 19, 27] Standard treatment with acyclovir and corticosteroids is recommended; however, corticosteroid therapy may be contraindicated in the patient with opportunistic infection.

Radiculitis due to cytomegalovirus involving cranial nerves is a significant cause of facial nerve palsy in patients with advanced HIV; 23% of HIV-infected patients with cytomegalovirus ventriculo-encephalitis had facial nerve palsy.[28] Facial nerve palsy is usually part of a distinct clinical syndrome characterized by encephalitis associated with cranial nerve deficits (including ocular motor palsy), gaze-directed nystagmus, cerebrospinal fluid pleocytosis, hypoglycorrhachia, and progressive ventriculomegaly. Nearly 50% of patients with this syndrome had CMV diagnosed at other sites previously (most commonly retinitis), and all had CD4 counts less than 50/mm³. CMV ventriculo-encephalitis developed in some patients while receiving ganciclovir or foscarnet sodium as maintenance therapy for CMV retinitis; the role of combination therapy for this entity remains to be proved.

Herpes zoster opticus, or Ramsay Hunt syndrome, is also more common in HIV-infected patients. Management includes high-dose acyclovir (800 mg five times daily) and high-dose steroids, unless contraindicated. Symptoms tend to be more severe, post-herpetic neuralgia more common, and response to medical therapy less predictable.

Dermatologic Manifestations

Cutaneous abnormalities occur in nearly 100% of patients with HIV infection. Inflammatory, infectious, or neoplastic processes can all affect the skin and can occasionally be the initial presentation of this systemic disease.[29]

Staphylococcus aureus is the most common cutaneous and systemic bacterial pathogen in HIV-infected patients. The prevalence of nasal colonization in these patients is 50%, a rate twice that of non–HIV-infected individuals.[30] The frequent occurrence of breaks in the skin secondary to multiple needle sticks, dermatoses, and the presence of indwelling catheters provides a route of introduction of this pathogen. This, combined with a quantitative and qualitative neutropenia secondary to myelosuppressive medications, bone marrow infections, and the direct effects of HIV on neutrophils, leads to an increased incidence of cutaneous and systemic *S. aureus* as well as other bacterial infections.

The management of cutaneous *S. aureus* infections in HIV-infected patients is identical to that of HIV-seronegative patients; however, therapy must often be prolonged. Appropriate surgical drainage of any loculated collection and administration of oral antistaphylococcal antibiotics (i.e., dicloxacillin or cephalexin) are required. The addition of rifampin, 600 mg once daily for 5–10 days, is often helpful for recalcitrant cases. Antibacterial soaps and topical mupirocin are also effective adjuncts.

Bacillary angiomatosis is an infectious disease of the skin and viscera caused by *Bartonella henselae*.[30, 31] It is characterized by angiomatous lesions and is most commonly found in the setting of immunosuppression, especially in HIV disease. Skin lesions, most commonly elevated, friable, bright red, granulation tissue–like papules or, less commonly, subcutaneous nodules, are the most common initial presentation. As cutaneous lesions can be associated with visceral and/or bone marrow infection, suspicious lesions must be tested by biopsy. Treatment with erythromycin 500 mg orally four times daily (or, alternatively, doxycycline 100 mg twice daily) has been very effective. Lesions demonstrate significant involution by 4–7 days; complete resolution takes 3–4 weeks.[30]

As HIV infection progresses and the CD4 count decreases, the incidence and severity of viral and fungal skin infections increase. HSV is usually a self-limited disorder consisting of grouped vesicular eruptions followed by ulceration and healing within 2 weeks. As immune function diminishes, chronic, expansile, and extremely painful lesions can develop. Although mucocutaneous lesions are the most common manifestation of HSV, other mucosal surfaces of the upper aerodigestive tract, such as the tracheobronchial tree and esophagus, may be affected and can be associated with considerable morbidity.[30]

Treatment is usually effective with oral acyclovir, 200–800 mg five times daily; however, larger lesions may require intravenous therapy (5 mg/kg three times daily). Prophylactic treatment with 400 mg of oral acyclovir twice daily is helpful in patients with frequent recurrent infections.[12, 30]

Acyclovir-resistant herpesvirus strains are being identified more frequently, perhaps to the increased use of acyclovir prophylaxis. In these cases treatment with foscarnet sodium has usually proved effective.[12, 30, 31]

Varicella-zoster virus infection is also commonly observed early in the course of HIV infection. In fact, zoster infection may precede oral thrush and hairy leukoplakia by a year or more.[30] Vesicular lesions arise in a dermatomal pattern, most commonly on the hard or soft palate, lips, gingiva, or face.[12, 30, 32] Although infection is usually confined to a specific dermatomal distribution, viral dissemination can occur in the severely immune-compromised host.

Tzanck's smear or viral culture can be helpful in diagnosing this herpetic infection. Treatment with acyclovir and analgesics is appropriate in most cases. Dermatomal zoster may be treated with oral acyclovir (800 mg five times daily), whereas intravenous acyclovir (10 mg/kg three times daily) is recommended for disseminated disease. Foscarnet sodium can be used in acyclovir-resistant strains. Postlesional neuropathy manifested by severe pain and pruritus can be a prominent feature of this infection.[12, 32]

Molluscum contagiosum, caused by a pox virus, occurs in 10%–20% of AIDS patients.[4] As with the other viral infections, the lesions become more severe as the CD4 count decreases. Although these flesh-colored, hemispheric papules are typically 2–4 mm, they can grow extremely large, forming giant molluscum bodies requiring cryotherapy or excision.[30, 33]

Cutaneous fungal infection such as cryptococcosis and histoplasmosis has been reported in AIDS patients; however, these conditions are uncommon. Cryptococcus infection is very common in advanced HIV disease, and virtually all infections involve the central nervous system. Less than 5% of HIV-infected patients with cryptococcosis have skin lesions. The lesions are most commonly found in the head and neck region and often resemble those of molluscum contagiosum. Diagnosis is made with biopsy and culture. Because the presence of cutaneous cryptococcosis almost always indicates systemic disease, an appropriate work-up, especially to exclude central nervous system involvement, is indicated. Serum cryptococcal antigen is positive in virtually all cases of cryptococcosis.[30, 34] Once the diagnosis is established, amphotericin B with or without 5-flucytosine is the treatment of choice. Indefinite maintenance therapy with oral fluconazole is indicated after induction therapy with amphotericin.

Disseminated histoplasmosis is becoming more common as HIV penetrates histoplasma-endemic regions of the Midwest. More than 90% of the cases have occurred in patients with CD4 counts below 100/mm[3]. Approximately 10% of AIDS patients with disseminated histoplasmosis develop skin lesions. Unlike cryptococcosis, in which the cutaneous lesions are similar, there is no characteristic skin lesion associated with histoplasmosis. Because histopathologic evaluation of these skin lesions reveals granulomas, and methenamine silver staining reveals the organisms, a skin biopsy is essential for establishing this diagnosis.[30] Amphotericin B is usually effective in treating this infection.

Kaposi's sarcoma of the skin was a rare disorder before 1981. With the emergence of AIDS, Kaposi's sarcoma has become the most common neoplasm associated with HIV. Presently, 15%–20% of HIV-positive homosexual and bisexual men develop Kaposi's sarcoma during the course of HIV disease. In contrast, only 4% of HIV-positive heterosexual men develop Kaposi's sarcoma, and almost none of the population of HIV-infected hemophiliacs have developed this condition.[30, 34] This striking difference in prevalence rates has always raised the intriguing possibility that a second infectious agent other than HIV may be responsible for the occurrence of this tumor. Recent evidence suggests that a herpes-like virus may play a role in Kaposi's sarcoma. Genetic evidence of this virus has been identified in HIV-infected patients with Kaposi's sarcoma. The virus is not present in non–HIV-infected patients with Kaposi's sarcoma.[35]

Diagnosis of Kaposi's sarcoma is made by clinical appearance and biopsy. Biopsy is recommended in all cases as cutaneous pneumocystosis may mimic the lesions of Kaposi's sarcoma.[36] Therapy is aimed primarily at palliation as patients rarely die as a direct result of Kaposi's sarcoma.

Treatment is indicated for lesions that cause severe pain and disfigurement or that significantly impair function. Urgent intervention is indicated in the case of pending airway compromise. Systemic chemotherapy is indicated for rapidly progressive tumors or in the case of advanced, widespread disease. Low-dose adriamycin, bleomycin, and vincristine all have shown promising results.[33, 34] Interferon-α has not been effective in patients with Kaposi's sarcoma and a CD4 count less than 200/mm[3].

Local therapy can often control pain and improve function. Although low-dose radiation therapy is usually effective, its use is often limited by the severe mucositis that develops in patients with low CD4 counts. Intralesional vinblastine injection has proved to be a successful and reliable means of palliating small, discrete lesions. CO_2 laser and cryotherapy may also be effective for resecting Kaposi's sarcoma lesions.

Sinusitis

The prevalence of sinusitis in patients with AIDS is reported to be 10%–20% and as high as 68%. The clinical presentation in the HIV-seropositive patient is similar to that in noninfected patients.[37] Headache, facial and retro-orbital pain, and nasal congestion and purulent nasal discharge are common symptoms. Postnasal drainage of thick tenacious mucus is particularly troublesome, even in the absence of clinical sinusitis. Sinusitis occasionally presents as exacerbations of pulmonary disease, occult sources of fever, recurrent episodes of life-threatening sepsis, central nervous system involvement,[38] or as a trigger for the progressive weight loss seen in patients with the "AIDS wasting syndrome."[39]

Several factors account for the poor response to medical management observed in these patients. The most important of these is the gradual depletion of helper T lymphocytes (CD4 cells). As the CD4 count falls below 200 cells/mm[3], infection often becomes refractory to standard medical management. Another factor is the increased IgE-mediated allergic disease in this population due to the overproduction of IgE. As much as a twofold increase in allergic symptoms has been described in HIV-infected men (41% prevalence before infection compared with 87% after infection),[40] a finding that seems to correlate with the observed elevations of IgE levels found in this population.[41, 42] This allergic phenomenon undoubtedly contributes to sinonasal disease. Another factor that may be important is the altered mucus blanket that results in impaired mucociliary clearance in these patients.

The evaluation and management of acute sinusitis in HIV-infected patients are no different than for noninfected patients as signs and symptoms are similar in both groups. Because the posterior sinuses (sphenoid and posterior ethmoids) are more commonly involved in HIV-infected patients,[43] and these sinuses are poorly visualized on plain sinus radiographs, computed tomography (CT) scanning is the preferred method for imaging the sinuses in these patients.

Medical management should include appropriate antibiotics and aggressive decongestant therapy. Amoxicillin or sulfamethoxazole/trimethoprim can be used for primary therapy; however, amoxicillin with clavulanate (Augmentin) or an oral cephalosporin (cefuroxime axetil) may provide broader coverage. Oral antibiotics should be continued for 3 weeks. Because nasal secretions seem to be much thicker and more tenacious in these patients, high-dose guaifenesin (1200 mg every 12 hours) may also be effective.[44] If antihistamines are added, the newer second-generation antihistamines (terfenadine, astemizole, loratadine) are preferred owing to their low anticholinergic activity. In this case, concurrent medications (such as macrolide antibiotics and ketoconazole) are contraindicated so as to avoid the potential cardiac arrhythmias produced by combining these drugs.

As immune function diminishes, chronic sinusitis becomes a prominent feature.[45, 46] Although many unusual organisms have been reported,[47–55] the specific pathogens that cause HIV-related chronic sinusitis have not been well characterized. In non–HIV-infected patients, chronic sinusitis is often due to *S. aureus, S. pneumoniae, H. influenzae,* and anaerobic bacteria. In addition, *P. aeruginosa* has been implicated in up to 20% of patients with HIV-related chronic sinusitis.[43, 56] The combination of ciprofloxacin and clindamycin provides good empirical coverage until cultures can be obtained. Although antral puncture is a standard culture technique, endoscopically directed aspiration from the middle meatus or sphenoethmoid recess is an easy, noninvasive, and useful alternative.[57] Early culture is important in severely immunocompromised patients who are susceptible to infection with aggressive opportunistic organisms (Fig. 64–3).

The use of systemic decongestants, guaifenesin, and topical nasal steroids can help decrease chronic inflammation and facilitate mucociliary clearance. The use of topical nasal steroids has not been associated with local nasal infection with *Candida* or other opportunistic organisms in this population.

If symptoms persist despite maximal medical management, surgery should be considered. Although surgery often provides dramatic improvement for these patients, many patients continue to have persistent nasal symptoms.[58] Although surgical success tends to correlate with the severity of immunologic dysfunction, some patients with severely depressed CD4 counts respond surprisingly well to surgery. Even when a surgical "cure" is not achieved with endoscopic sinus surgery, quality of life is usually improved.

Neutropenia often results from HIV infection alone or may be due to the myelosuppressive effects of AZT and other antiretroviral agents. Neutropenic patients often have profound systemic symptoms (fevers, chills, myalgias, malaise) in the immediate postoperative period. The preoperative use of granulocyte colony–stimulating factor to boost the absolute neutrophil count is often effective in preventing these symptoms.

The risk of HIV or hepatitis exposure during endoscopic sinus surgery is quite small if caution is used. As ESS takes less than 3 hours, uses few sharp instruments, and requires a single operating surgeon, this surgery poses one of the lowest risks of bloodborne pathogen exposure of all procedures performed by otolaryngologists.[59]

Unlike bacterial sinusitis, which may occur at any time, fungal sinusitis in patients with HIV generally occurs when CD4 count is below 50/mm³ (see Chapter 43). *Pseudallescheria boydii, Schizophyllum commune, Rhizopus arrhizus, Candida* species, *Cryptococcus neoformans,* and *Alternaria* species have been documented in HIV-infected patients with sinusitis; however, nearly 81% of the fungal sinusitis in HIV patients is due to *Aspergillus* species.[60] Previously recognized risk factors (e.g., neutropenia and corticosteroid use) are present in the majority of HIV-infected patients with aspergillosis. Concomitant pulmonary involvement was present in only 17% of patients in one report.[61] Systemic antifungal therapy with amphotericin B and surgery is the treatment of choice, although outcome despite aggressive therapy has been uniformly fatal.[61]

ORAL, PHARYNGEAL, AND LARYNGEAL MANIFESTATIONS

Oral symptoms are very common in HIV disease. A wide spectrum of problems including infectious, neoplastic, inflammatory, and degenerative processes can affect this region. Because many of these same diseases also occur in the pharynx and larynx, the otolaryngologist will invariably be called upon when symptoms relating to the oral cavity and pharynx persist (Table 64–1).

Oral candidiasis or thrush is by far the most common oral manifestation of HIV disease. Thrush is often an early manifestation of otherwise asymptomatic HIV infection. The most common presentation is of creamy white plaques or pseudomembranes with underlying erosive, erythematous mucosal surfaces. An atrophic or erythematous form can also present as hyperemic and tender oral mucosa. A chronic hypertrophic form with thick, heaped-up, white plaques that will not scrape off is another variant of oral candidiasis. Angular cheilitis, a nonhealing, erythematous erosion at the oral commissure, is also often due to infection with *Candida* and can appear alone or in conjunction with other forms of candidiasis.[12, 32, 62, 63]

Diagnosis is based on clinical appearance and detection

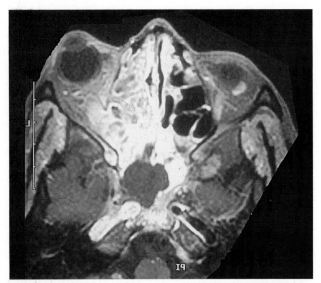

Figure 64–3. MRI demonstrating invasive aspergillus sinusitis in a patient with end stage AIDS. Note the significant orbital and intracranial involvement with thrombosis of the internal carotid artery.

Table 64–1. ORAL MANIFESTATIONS OF HIV DISEASE

Diagnosis	Presentation	Treatment	Complications
Candidiasis	Pseudomembranous plaques with underlying erythema or atrophic lesions with hyperemia	Topical versus systemic antifungals	Severe local symptoms; regional spread to esophagus or larynx
Hairy leukoplakia	Corrugated white thickening on the lateral tongue	None, except for superinfection	Uncommon
Aphthous ulcers	Usually single, may be multiple; major (2–4 cm) ulcers are common	Topical steroids in orabase, analgesics	Severe pain; potential for compromise of oral intake
Orolabial herpes	Raised vesicles and ulcerative lesions on an erythematous base	Oral acyclovir analgesics	Frequent recurrence, drug resistance
Kaposi's sarcoma	Flat or raised violaceous lesions most commonly on the palate	Intralesional or systemic chemotherapy, surgical or laser excision, radiation therapy	Severe pain, secondary infection, local complications (airway obstruction, dysphagia)
Gingival and periodontal disease	Loss of gingival and periodontal soft tissue	Aggressive oral hygiene, débridement, and antiseptic rinses	Sequestration and exposure of alveolar bone, loss of teeth

of hyphae and yeast on potassium hydroxide smears. Esophageal candidiasis should be considered when severe dysphagia, odynophagia, and retrosternal pain occur in the setting of oropharyngeal candidiasis. The work-up for *Candida* esophagitis requires radiographic contrast studies and, in some cases, esophagoscopy. Esophageal contrast studies usually demonstrate markedly irregular mucosal surfaces due to plaques and ulcers. Esophagoscopy can allow detection and biopsy of persistent lesions.

Laryngeal candidiasis usually presents with hoarseness, dysphagia, and occasionally with stridor. The diagnosis can usually be confirmed with fiberoptic laryngoscopy because typical white plaques or pseudomembranes can be seen. Patients who do not respond to antifungal therapy may require direct laryngoscopy with biopsies for culture and histopathologic evaluation.

Initial treatment of oropharyngeal candidiasis with topical agents such as nystatin or clotrimazole is often effective. In advanced HIV disease, in cases due to resistant *Candida* species, and in esophageal and laryngeal candidiasis, systemic antifungal therapy with fluconazole, and occasionally amphotericin B, is required.

Oral hairy leukoplakia is a white vertically corrugated lesion that commonly appears on the lateral surface of the tongue (Fig. 64–4). It can be found less commonly on the buccal mucosa, labial mucosa, floor of the mouth, soft palate, and oropharyngeal mucosa. The presence of hairy leukoplakia indicates severe immunocompromise and is associated with the progression to advanced-stage HIV disease. Although this condition is thought to be caused by the Epstein-Barr virus, treatment is usually not required because it is usually an asymptomatic condition. Lesions sometimes disappear when patients are placed on high-dose acyclovir for concomitant HSV infection.[63–65]

Recurrent aphthous ulcers are common in HIV-infected patients. The cause of these lesions is unknown; however, many factors, including altered cellular immunity, stress, and infectious agents, may play a role. Unlike the general population in which minor aphthous ulcers (0.5–1 cm) are common, HIV-infected patients often present with major aphthous ulcers (2–4 cm) that often result from the coalescence of many smaller lesions into larger ulcers that can occur anywhere in the oral cavity or pharynx. Although most

commonly found in the oral cavity, lesions can also be found on the tonsils, tonsillar pillars, and base of the tongue. The morbidity associated with major aphthous ulcers, most notably severe pain, odynophagia, and secondary infection, can lead to malnutrition, dehydration, and progression of the AIDS wasting syndrome.[12, 66]

Therapy for aphthous ulcers is symptomatic. First-line therapy with topical steroids such as fluocinonide ointment, triamcinolone ointment, or dexamethasone rinse is often effective. Secondary infection can often be treated with topical tetracycline or systemic oral clindamycin. Severe cases involving the pharynx and larynx associated with compromised oral intake require systemic steroids and intravenous antibiotics. Nutritional support with enteral feeding is also occasionally necessary.[12, 63, 66]

Oral ulcers or stomatitis has been reported in up to 5% of patients receiving the antiretroviral agent ddC.[67] This agent has also been associated with esophageal ulcers; the ulcerative disease is reversible upon discontinuation of therapy.

Severe gingivitis and periodontal disease are common in this population and often present in a more aggressive fashion than similar diseases in non–HIV-infected patients. Rapid progression from a mild gingivitis to an acute necrotizing process with severe pain, soft-tissue loss, bone exposure,

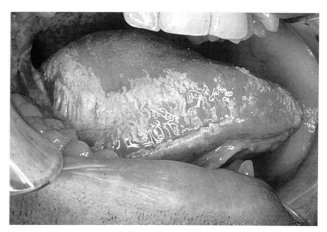

Figure 64–4. Hairy leukoplakia of lateral tongue is often confused with oral thrush or other oral infections.

and sequestration of alveolar bone is occasionally encountered. Initial symptoms often include erythema and edema at the gum line associated with mucosal friability. Bleeding from the gums can be associated with slight trauma or can even be spontaneous. As periodontal disease progresses, periodontal attachments loosen and pockets form between the affected teeth and alveolar bone. In acute necrotizing ulcerative gingivitis, ulcers appear at the tips of interdental papillae and along the gingival margin. Significant loss of the periodontal soft tissue can be associated with severe pain as necrotic bone along the gingival margin begins to sequestrate.[32, 63] Oral antibiotics targeted at anaerobic organisms (i.e., clindamycin or metronidazole) and topical irrigation with povidone-iodine (Betadine) and chlorhexidine gluconate (Peridex) should be initiated early.[32] Even with aggressive medical management, the periodontitis is often difficult to control.

Viral infections of the upper aerodigestive tract, especially those due to HSV, are also very common. Although orolabial HSV and anogenital HSV infections are most common, HSV esophagitis and laryngitis also can occur. Retrosternal pain associated with severe odynophagia is a sign of esophageal involvement, and hoarseness associated with these symptoms may signify laryngeal involvement. On examination or at endoscopy, typical discrete vesicles with underlying mucosal ulceration are usually encountered. Definitive diagnosis is via biopsy for histopathologic examination and viral culture. Appropriate therapy with acyclovir should be initiated early.

Cytomegalovirus (CMV) infection is the most common cause of serious opportunistic infections in HIV-infected individuals.[68, 69] The clinical presentation of CMV infection can take several forms, including retinitis, encephalitis, pneumonia, hepatitis, colitis, adrenalitis, and esophagitis. Significant disease involving the larynx and trachea, although rare, has also been described.[70–73] Not all patients with serologic or tissue cultures positive for CMV have clinical disease related to the infection. Additionally, as CMV can be cultured from respiratory or gastrointestinal secretions in healthy individuals, results of cultures must be interpreted carefully. Definitive diagnosis requires demonstration of intranuclear and cytoplasmic inclusion bodies on histopathologic evaluation.

Signs and symptoms of CMV infection of the larynx are usually nonspecific, such as hoarseness, odynophagia, fever, and nonproductive cough.[71, 72] Laryngoscopy usually reveals an ulcerative lesion with associated edema and erythema. Mass-like lesions due to CMV resembling tumors have also been observed.[74] CMV can also directly involve the recurrent laryngeal nerves without any evidence of mucosal lesions. Reports of vocal cord paralysis with no associated structural abnormalities have revealed CMV involvement of the recurrent laryngeal nerves.[70] This clinical diagnosis can be made with concomitant biopsy-proven CMV infection; however, confirmation requires a formal postmortem examination.

Necrotizing tracheitis has also been caused by CMV.[73] Patients present with nonspecific symptoms such as productive cough and subsequently with dyspnea. The potential for airway obstruction in these cases requires prompt diagnosis and serial bronchoscopy with débridement of intratracheal secretions.

Treatment for acute CMV with ganciclovir should be instituted once the diagnosis is established. Ganciclovir is an analogue of acyclovir with approximately 50 times greater activity against CMV.[75] Because it is available only as an intravenous preparation, long-term intravenous access is a necessary part of therapy. Ganciclovir is limited by its myelosuppressive toxicity in addition to the development of ganciclovir-resistant CMV strains. Foscarnet sodium, a good alternative therapy, has shown similar response rates without significant myelotoxicity.[75, 76]

In addition to *Candida* (see Chapter 23), *Cryptococcus* and *Aspergillus* infections have been described in the larynx and pharynx.[13, 77, 78] In one report of invasive *Cryptococcus* of the larynx, laryngoscopy revealed only an erythematous and edematous true vocal cord. As histopathologic examination should reveal the presence of this organism, definitive diagnosis requires tissue biopsy with histopathologic examination and culture. Treatment with amphotericin B should be effective. Invasive aspergillosis of the larynx has also been reported. Tissue biopsy and culture are very important in establishing the diagnosis, and treatment with amphotericin B followed by long-term itraconazole is recommended.

Acute bacterial epiglottitis has been reported in HIV-infected patients.[79] The presentation is similar to that of non–HIV-infected patients, with rapid progression of odynophagia, dysphagia, drooling, and respiratory distress; however, the clinical course seems to be more aggressive in HIV-infected patients. Flexible fiberoptic examination readily reveals the presence of epiglottitis. The causative organisms are usually *S. pneumoniae*, *S. aureus*, and *H. influenzae*.

Salivary Gland Disease

The major and minor salivary glands are often affected in patients with HIV disease. Xerostomia is a frequent complaint in these patients, and it is usually associated with a Sjögren's syndrome–like lymphocytic infiltration of the salivary glands.[80] Although this infiltration is usually not associated with a discernible change in appearance of the salivary glands, some patients, particularly children, may present with dramatic parotid enlargement.

Severe xerostomia can be associated with increased dental disease as well as problems with deglutition. In patients with this syndrome, meticulous attention to dental hygiene, with a focus on fluoride applications, is especially important. If poor swallowing becomes a major symptom, sialagogues such as sugarless lemon-flavored candies can help stimulate salivary production of the remaining glands. Oral hydration with frequent sips of water or one of the commercially available salivary substitutes can also be helpful.

Another frequent finding in adult HIV-infected patients is multiple benign lymphoepithelial cysts of the parotid glands (see Fig. 53–4). The precise cause of these cysts is unclear; however, they usually have no clinical significance. While generally asymptomatic, these cysts can become clinically bothersome if continued enlargement or secondary infection occurs. Radiographic imaging with CT scan or magnetic resonance imaging is usually sufficient to make the diagnosis as single and occasionally multiple cystic masses can be seen within the parotid gland. Multiple needle aspirations can often provide both cosmetic improvement as well as symptomatic relief; however, recurrence is generally the rule. Superficial parotidectomy provides a permanent solution, but this procedure can rarely be justified for this benign condition. Radiation therapy has also been used with some success; however, the severe local reaction experienced by some HIV-infected patients undergoing radiation therapy limits this therapeutic alternative.[81] One report employed tetracycline sclerosis following fluid aspiration with good long-term efficacy.[82] Given the low morbidity associated with this technique, this may prove to be the treatment of choice for these lesions.

Opportunistic infections in HIV-infected patients may also involve the salivary glands. Autopsy findings for the submandibular glands of 60 patients with AIDS revealed CMV as the most frequent pathogen.[82a] CMV infection was present in 17% (10/60) of the total cases and in 35% (9/26) of the cases with disseminated CMV; the submandibular gland was the sole site of CMV infection in one case. Despite the presence of characteristic CMV intranuclear and cytoplasmic inclusions in both acinar and ductal cells, no inflammatory cells were detected. *Pneumocystis carinii* was detected in 2% (1/60) of the patients. No mycobacterial or fungal pathogens were detected in the salivary glands, even though 18% of the patients had disseminated mycobacterial and 16% had disseminated fungal infections. The antifungal activity of saliva was proposed as a possible factor protecting against fungal salivary gland infection.

MYCOBACTERIAL INFECTIONS

The incidence of tuberculosis in HIV-infected patients continues to increase, with more and more infections involving extrapulmonary sites, most commonly the cervical nodes and bone marrow.[12, 83] See Chapter 23 for an overview. Many patients with tuberculous lymphadenitis exhibit minimal symptoms other than a persistent or enlarging neck mass. Typically these nodes are rubbery and painless, but up to 10% of patients present with pain and fluctuance, and 5% have draining sinuses.[84–86] Interestingly, only 16%–38% of patients with cervical tuberculosis present with systemic disease.[85] As a result, systemic or pulmonary signs cannot be relied on to suspect this diagnosis; tuberculosis must be included in the differential diagnosis of all patients with a neck mass.[86]

Cervical lymphadenitis is the most common head and neck site for a tuberculous infection; however, the larynx and the middle ear can also be involved. Rare cases of nasal, nasopharyngeal, oral, cervical spine, and pharyngeal infection have also been reported.[86–89]

Patients suspected of having tuberculosis should have a purified protein derivative (PPD) skin test along with several controls to detect anergy. Even in late stages of HIV disease, 20%–40% of patients with tuberculosis have a positive PPD. In HIV-infected patients, a skin reaction greater than 5 mm (not the usual 10 mm criterion) is considered positive.[90] A positive PPD skin test can result from nontuberculous mycobacterial infections because of the great extent of cross-reactivity to the tuberculosis antigen. These infections must be included in the differential diagnosis of a positive PPD.

If there is no skin reaction to the anergy panel, additional diagnostic tests may be needed to establish the diagnosis.

Although the "gold standard" for diagnosing tuberculosis is tissue biopsy and culture, fine needle aspiration biopsy can establish the diagnosis in most cases. Although the presence of acid-fast bacilli on cytologic smear is highly suggestive of a mycobacterial infection, definitive diagnosis requires a positive organism-specific culture that can take as long as 6–8 weeks. Empirical therapy should be started before definitive culture results in cases in which the cytopathology and clinical history suggest tuberculosis. If the diagnosis of tuberculosis cannot be established by fine needle aspiration biopsy and lymphadenopathy persists despite antimycobacterial therapy, open excisional biopsy is indicated.[86]

HIV-infected patients are susceptible to mycobacterial infections other than *M. tuberculosis*. In fact, *M. avium* complex (MAC) is the most common mycobacterial infection in HIV patients. Because most MAC infections present as disseminated disease in the late stages of AIDS and are generally resistant to standard antimycobacterial medications, infection with MAC must be differentiated from tuberculosis as it will affect long-term medical treatment.

OCCUPATIONAL EXPOSURE TO HIV

With the continued spread of HIV throughout the world, it has become impossible to practice medicine without being exposed to HIV-infected patients. As AIDS prevention is currently the only means of true protection from this virus, health-care workers must know and understand the modes of transmission of HIV and take all appropriate precautions to minimize risk of infection.

It is estimated that 40%–60% of all HIV-infected individuals will present with head and neck manifestations of the disease.[91] Thus, otolaryngologists have an inherent risk in their daily practice. According to CDC reports, however, despite thousands of job-related exposures to HIV-contaminated blood or body fluid, relatively few health-care workers have actually become seropositive for HIV.[92] Even though the risk of contracting HIV through an occupational exposure is less than 1%, the additive effects of a 30-year career must be considered.[93] An individual health-care worker's particular risk depends on a number of factors including the number of HIV-infected patients treated, the number and type of body fluid exposures, and the risk of infection with each exposure. For instance, the incidence of seroconverting after a hollow bore needle stick is 0.4%–0.5%.[94] Solid needles, like suture needles, scalpels, and metal wires, have a lower but very real incidence of infection. HIV seroconversion from mucous membrane exposure with HIV-infected blood has also been reported; however, this is a very rare means of transmission, and the precise risk of such an exposure has not yet been determined. Furthermore, the theoretical risk of infection from body fluids such as saliva, tears, nasal mucus, and gastrointestinal fluids has not been documented as real.[94]

Knowing that a real risk of exposure and possibly infection exists, health-care workers must minimize this risk by altering behavior. The best way to avoid contracting HIV from a patient is to treat every patient as potentially HIV-infected, a policy outlined in 1987 by the CDC and called "Universal Blood and Body Fluid Precautions"[95] (Table 64-2).

In addition to these basic universal precautions, specific techniques for office and operating room procedures should be modified. Double gloving allows for decreased exposure from inadvertent puncture. Studies have demonstrated both a decreased inner glove puncture rate and a decreased cutaneous exposure when using double gloves.[94, 96] Additionally, cut-resistant gloves are recommended for facial plastics and reconstructive surgery using wires, implants, and plates.[97] Although these gloves limit dexterity, they provide significantly more protection for these high-risk cases. In otolaryngology, high-risk cases include facial trauma with intermaxillary fixation and any case with operative time greater than 3 hours, especially when blood loss is greater than 250 mL (i.e., major head and neck surgery).[94, 97] Double gloving and, in some cases, using cut-resistant gloves are strongly recommended as important means of minimizing HIV exposure risk.

Sharp instruments, a necessary part of most surgical procedures, are the most common cause of inadvertent stick injuries. In order to reduce the risks from using sharp instruments, handling techniques must be changed. Most notably, recapping needles should be condemned as this is the single most common cause of needle stick injuries. Also, when using sharp instruments in the operating room, a no-pass technique should be adopted. Two individuals should never handle the same sharp object at the same time. This is accomplished by indirect passing of instruments between the surgeon and the scrub nurse by way of a Mayo stand, kidney basin, or magnetic field pad (Fig. 64-5). Finally, the surgeon should reconsider the use of sharp hook or rake retractors.

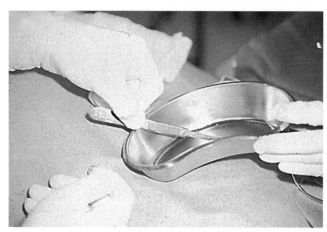

Figure 64-5. A "no-touch" technique for passing sharp instruments avoids inadvertent injury to operating room staff.

These provide a significant risk of inadvertent puncture to the surgical team and can safely and effectively be replaced with blunt retractors or non-traumatic tissue clamps. Appropriate protective eyewear is also an important part of personal protective attire in the operating room.

In the office, strict adherence to universal precautions must be maintained. Gloves and protective eyewear should be used for most head and neck examinations to prevent exposure to potentially contaminated secretions. All instruments required for each patient examination should be readily available on the instrument cabinet before starting. This prevents contamination of clean instruments by searching through drawers during an examination. Additionally, the use of disposable applicators for topical anesthetics and disposable ear specula eliminates the possibility of cross contamination.

All instruments must be sterilized and disinfected between uses according to Occupational Safety and Health Administration guidelines. After endoscopes and nasopharyngoscopes are cleaned of organic debris, they may be immersed in 2% glutaraldehyde solution for 20 minutes. Recently developed nasopharyngoscope sheaths provide an easier and faster method of ensuring sterility. Although the sheaths are more expensive than traditional sterilization, patient turnover time is decreased and expensive fiberoptic instruments do not have to soak in harsh chemicals.

As soon as a health-care worker is exposed to blood or body fluid, the exposed skin or wound should be decontaminated with soap and water and the incident clearly documented. When the possibility of HIV transmission exists, careful evaluation of the type and severity of the exposure should be assessed. If the patient's HIV status is unknown, informed consent should be obtained and the patient tested. The health-care worker should also obtain a baseline HIV test so that the status at the time of exposure is available. Periodic testing at 6 weeks, 3 months, and 6 months is recommended by the CDC.[98]

Postexposure chemoprophylaxis has been shown to have some possible benefits in animal models when started within 24 hours postexposure.[99] However, no scientific data supporting the efficacy of AZT for postexposure chemoprophylaxis in humans exist. Despite this, more than 40% of health-care

Table 64-2. UNIVERSAL PRECAUTIONS FOR THE OTOLARYNGOLOGIST

1. Gloves should be used during office examinations when contact with potentially contaminated oral, nasal, or laryngeal secretions is anticipated; double gloving during all surgical procedures is recommended. Thorough handwashing between all patient encounters is imperative.
2. Patient care should be avoided when exudative or weeping skin lesions or dermatitis is present.
3. Eye protection must be implemented whenever splashes may occur (laryngeal and oral office examination, endoscopy, other operating room procedures).
4. Gowns and masks should be used when contamination of clothing or substantial aerosolization of secretions is anticipated.
5. Have all examination instruments available on the table top prior to beginning a head and neck examination. This will prevent contamination of clean drawered instruments by the examiner's contaminated hands.
6. Prevent needle stick injury by properly disposing of all needles and syringes. Never recap or bend needles.
7. Carefully handle scalpels and other sharp instruments during surgical procedures. A "no touch" technique should be implemented for passing sharp instruments between the surgeon, assistant, and scrub nurse. Sharp instruments should be avoided whenever possible (e.g., staples and sharp hook retractors).
8. Properly dispose of all potentially contaminated office and surgical suite materials.
9. Thoroughly and carefully clean and disinfect all instruments between use according to the applicable OSHA requirements (e.g, laryngeal mirrors, nasal specula, and fiberoptic scopes).

workers elect to take AZT chemoprophylaxis.[98–100] Clearly, this is an area in which further research and investigation are required.

References

1. Nelson K, Celentano D, Suprasert S, Wright N: Risk factors for HIV infection among young adult men in northern Thailand. JAMA 1993; 270: 955–960.
2. Ho D, Neuman A, Perelson A, et al.: Rapid turnover of plasma virions and CD4 lymphocytes in HIV-1 infection. Nature 1995; 373: 123–126.
3. Crowe S, McGrath M: Acute HIV infection. In: Cohen P, Sande M, Volderding P (eds): The AIDS Knowledge Base: A Textbook on HIV Disease from the University of California, San Francisco, and the San Francisco General Hospital, 2nd ed. Boston: Little Brown and Company, 1994: Chap 4.2, pp 1–7.
4. Eron JJ, Benoit SL, Jemsek J, et al.: Treatment with lamivudine, zidovudine or both in HIV-positive patients with 200 to 500 CD4+ cells per cubic millimeter. N Engl J Med 1995; 333: 1662–1669.
5. Danner SA, Carr A, Leonard JM, et al.: A short-term study of the safety, pharmacokinetics, and efficacy of ritonavir, an inhibitor of HIV-1 protease. N Engl J Med 1995; 333: 1528–1533.
6. Collier AC, Combbs RW, Schoenfeld DA: Treatment of human immunodeficiency virus infection with saquinavir, zidovudine, and zalcitabine. N Engl J Med 1996; 334: 1011–1017.
7. Markowitz M, Saag M, Powderly WG, et al: A preliminary study of ritonavir, an inhibitor of HIV-1 protease, to treat HIV-1 infection. N Engl J Med 1995; 333: 1534–1539.
8. Gulick R, Mellors J, Havlir D, et al: Potent and sustained antiretroviral activity of indinavir in combination with zidovudine and lamivudine (abstract). Third Conference on Retroviruses and Opportunistic Infections. IDSA, NIH, and CDC, Washington, D.C., 28 January–1 February, 1996.
9. Massari F, Conant M, Mellors J, et al.: A phase II open-labeled, randomized study of the triple combination of indinavir, zidovudine, and didanosine versus indinavir alone and zidovudine/didanosine alone and zidovudine/didanosine in antiretroviral naive patients (abstract). Third Conference on Retroviruses and Opportunistic Infections. IDSA, NIH, and CDC, Washington, D.C., 28 January–1 February, 1996.
10. Bartlett JG: Protease inhibitors for HIV infection. Ann Intern Med 1996; 124: 1086–1088.
11. Morris M, Prasad S: Otologic disease in the acquired immunodeficiency syndrome. Ear Nose Throat J 1990; 69: 451–453.
12. Tami T, Lee K: Otolaryngologic manifestations of HIV disease. In: Cohen P, Sande M, Volderding P (eds): The AIDS Knowledge Base: A Textbook on HIV Disease from the University of California, San Francisco, and the San Francisco General Hospital, 2nd ed. Boston: Little Brown and Company, 1994: Chap 5.29, pp 1–25.
13. Menachof M, Jackler R: Otogenic skull base osteomyelitis caused by fungal infection. Otolaryngol Head Neck Surg 1990; 102: 285–289.
14. Reiss P, Hadderingh R, Schot L: Invasive external otitis caused by *Aspergillus fumigatus* in two patients with AIDS. AIDS 1991; 5: 605–606.
15. Smith M, Hirschfield L, Zahtz G, Siegal F: *Pneumocystis carinii* otitis media (letter). Am J Med 1988; 85: 745–746.
16. Gherman C, Ward R, Bassis M: *Pneumocystis carinii* otitis media and mastoiditis as the initial manifestation of the acquired immunodeficiency syndrome. Am J Med 1988; 85: 250–252.
17. Tami T, Lee K: SiPAC AIDS and the otolaryngologist. Alexandria, VA: Academy of Otolaryngology: Head and Neck Surgery Foundation, 1993.
18. Church J: Human immunodeficiency virus (HIV) infection at Children's Hospital in Los Angeles: Recurrent otitis media or chronic sinusitis as the presenting process in pediatric AIDS. Immunol Allergy 1987; 9: 25–32.
19. Lawani A, Sooy C: Otologic and neurotologic manifestations of acquired immunodeficiency syndrome. Otolaryngol Clin North Am 1992; 25: 1183–1197.
20. Stern J, Lin P, Lucente F: Benign nasopharyngeal masses and human immunodeficiency virus infection. Arch Otolaryngol Head Neck Surg 1990; 116: 206–208.
21. Gettler J, Casarona J: Tuberculous otitis media in an HIV-infected patient. Infect Dis Clin 1995; 4: 68–69.
22. Struss M, Fine E: Aspergillus otomastoiditis in acquired immunodeficiency syndrome. Am J Otol 1991; 12: 49–53.
23. Bankaitas A, Keith R: Audiologic changes associated with HIV infection. Ear Nose Throat J 1995; 74: 353–359.
24. Kohan D, Rothstein S, Cohen N: Otologic disease in patients with acquired immunodeficiency syndrome. Ann Otol Rhinol Laryngol 1988; 97: 636–640.
25. Wilson W. The relationship of the herpesvirus family to sudden hearing loss: A prospective clinical study and literature review. Laryngoscope 1986; 96: 870–877.
26. Smith M, Canalis R: Otologic manifestations of AIDS: The otosyphilis connection. Laryngoscope 1989; 99: 365–372.
27. Murr A, Benecke JE: Association of facial paralysis with HIV positivity. Am J Otol 1991; 12: 450–451.
28. Kalayjian R, Cohen M, Bonomo R, Flanigan T: Cytomegalovirus ventriculo-encephalitis in AIDS: A syndrome with distinct clinical and pathological features. Medicine 1993; 72: 67–77.
29. Cockerell C: Organ-specific manifestations of HIV infection: Update on cutaneous manifestations of HIV infection. AIDS 1993; 7: 213–218.
30. Berger T: Dermatologic findings in the head and neck in human immunodeficiency virus–infected persons. Otolaryngol Clin North Am 1992; 25: 1227–1247.
31. Meduri G, Stover D, Lee M: Pulmonary Kaposi's sarcoma in the acquired immunodeficiency syndrome. Am J Med 1986; 81: 11.
32. Dichtel W: Oral manifestations of human immunodeficiency virus infection. Otolaryngol Clin North Am 1992; 25: 1211–1226.
33. Gill P, Rarick M, McCutchen L: Systemic treatment of AIDS-related Kaposi's sarcoma: Results of a randomized trial. Am J Med 1991; 90: 427.
34. Berger T: Dermatologic manifestations of HIV infection. In: Cohen P, Sande M, Volderding P (eds): The AIDS Knowledge Base: A Textbook on HIV Disease from the University of California, San Francisco, and the San Francisco General Hospital, 2nd ed. Boston: Little Brown and Company, 1994; Chap 5.5, pp 1–31.
35. Moore PS, Chang Y. Detection of *Herpesvirus*-like DNA sequences in Kaposi's sarcoma in patients with and without HIV infection. N Engl J Med 1995; 332: 227–230.
36. Litwin M, Williams C: Cutaneous *Pneumocystis carinii* infection mimicking Kaposi's sarcoma. Ann Intern Med 1992; 117: 48–49.
37. Tami T, Wawrose S: Diseases of the nose and paranasal sinuses in the human immunodeficiency virus–infected population. Otolaryngol Clin N Am 1992; 25: 1199–1210.
38. Cheug S, Lee K, Imok C: Orbitocerebral complications of *Pseudomonas* sinusitis. Laryngoscope 1992; 102: 1385–1389.
39. Grunfeld C, Pang M, Shimizu L, et al.: Resting energy expenditure, caloric intake, and short-term weight change in human immunodeficiency virus infection and the acquired immunodeficiency syndrome. Am J Clin Nutr 1992; 55: 455–460.
40. Sample S, Chernoff D, Lenahan G: Elevated serum concentration of IgE antibodies to environmental antigens in HIV-seropositive male homosexuals. J Allergy Clin Immunol 1990; 86: 876–880.
41. Grieco M: Immunoglobulins and hypersensitivity on human immunodeficiency virus (HIV) infection. J Allergy Clin Immunol 1989; 84: 1–4.
42. Wright DN, Nelson RP Jr, Ledford DK, et al: Serum IgE and human immunodeficiency virus (HIV). J Allergy Clin Immunol 1988; 81: 216.
43. Godofsky E, Zinreich J, Armstrong M: Sinusitis in HIV-infected patients: A clinical and radiographic review. Am J Med 1992; 93: 163–170.
44. Wawrose S, Tami T, Amoils C: The role of guaifenesin in the treatment of sinonasal disease in patients infected with the human immunodeficiency virus (HIV). Laryngoscope 1992; 102: 1225–1228.
45. Armstrong M, McArthur J, Zinreich S: Radiographic imaging of sinusitis in HIV infection. Otolaryngol Head Neck Surg 1993; 108: 36–43.
46. Zurlo J: Sinusitis in HIV-1 infection. Am J Med 1992; 93: 157–162.
47. Wiest P, Wiese K, Jacobs M, et al.: *Alternaria* infection in a patient with acquired immunodeficiency syndrome: Case report and review of invasive *Alternaria* infections. Rev Infect Dis 1987; 9: 799–803.
48. Schlanger G, Lutwick L, Kurzman M: Sinusitis caused by *Legionella pneumophila:* A patient with the acquired immune deficiency syndrome. Am J Med 1984; 77: 957–960.

49. Carranza E, Rossitch E, Morris J: Isolated central nervous system aspergillosis in the acquired immunodeficiency syndrome. Clinical Neurol Neurosurg 1991; 93: 227–230.

50. Choi S, Lawson W, Buttone E: Cryptococcal sinusitis: A case report and review of literature. Otolaryngol Head Neck Surg 1988; 99: 414–418.

51. Colmenero C, Monur A, Valencia E, Castro A: Successfully treated *Candida* sinusitis in AIDS patients. J Craniomaxillofac Surg 1990; 18: 175–178.

52. Gonzales M, Gould E, Dickinson G, et al.: Acquired immunodeficiency syndrome associated with *Acanthamoeba* infection and other opportunistic organisms. Arch Pathol Lab Med 1986; 110: 749–751.

53. Brillhart T, Gath J, Piot D, et al.: Symptomatic cytomegaloviral rhinosinusitis in patients with AIDS (Abstract). In: Proceedings from the VIIth International Conference on AIDS. Florence: 1991: 227.

54. Sooy C: The impact of AIDS on otolaryngology: head and neck surgery. Otolaryngol Head Neck Surg 1987; 1: 1–28.

55. Blatt S, Lucey D, DeHoff D, Zellmer RB: Rhinocerebral zygomycosis in a patient with AIDS (letter). J Infect Dis 1991; 164: 215–216.

56. Tami T. The management of sinusitis in patients infected with the human immunodeficiency virus (HIV). Ear Nose Throat J 1995; 74: 360–363.

57. Poole M: Endoscopically guided vs. blind nasal cultures in sinusitis (Abstract). Otolaryngol Head Neck Surg 1992; 107: 272.

58. Blevins N, Lee K, Tami T: Endoscopic sinus surgery in patients infected with the human immunodeficiency virus (HIV) (Abstract). Otolaryngol Head Neck Surg 1992; 107: 274.

59. Benninger M, Gupta N, Gilmore K: Intraoperative infectious disease exposure to otolaryngology operating room personnel. Laryngoscope 1991; 101: 1276–1279.

60. Meyer R, Gaultier G, Yamashita J, et al.: Fungal sinusitis in patients with AIDS: Report of 4 cases and review of the literature. Medicine 1994; 73: 69–78.

61. Teh W, Matti B, Marisiddaiah H, Minamoto G: *Aspergillus* sinusitis in patients with AIDS: Report of 3 cases and review. Clin Infect Dis 1995; 21: 529–535.

62. Syrjanen S, Valle S, Antonen J: Oral candidal infection as a sign of HIV infection in homosexual men. Oral Surg Oral Med Oral Path 1988; 65: 36–40.

63. Greenspan D: Opportunistic infections of the mouth. In: Cohen P, Sande M, Volderding P (eds): The AIDS Knowledge Base: A Textbook on HIV Disease from the University of California, San Francisco, and the San Francisco General Hospital, 2nd ed. Boston: Little Brown and Company, 1994: Chap 5.2, pp 1–9.

64. Greenspan J, Greenspan D: Oral hairy leukoplakia: Diagnosis and management. Oral Surg Oral Med Oral Path 1989; 67: 396–403.

65. Resnick L, Herbst J, Ablashi D: Regression of oral hairy leukoplakia after orally administered acyclovir therapy. JAMA 1988; 259: 384–388.

66. Phelan J, Eisig S, Freedman P: Major aphthous-like ulcers in patients with AIDS. Oral Surg Oral Med Oral Path 1991; 71: 68–72.

67. Abrams D, Goldman A, Launer C, et al.: A comparative trial of didanosine or zalcitabine after treatment with zidovudine in patients with human immunodeficiency infection. N Engl J Med 1994; 330: 657–662.

68. Jacobson M, Mills J: Serious cytomegalovirus disease in patients with the acquired immunodeficiency syndrome (AIDS). Ann Intern Med 1988; 108: 585–594.

69. Welch K, Finkbeiner W, Alpers C: Autopsy findings in the acquired immune deficiency syndrome. JAMA 1984; 252: 1152–1159.

70. Small P, McPhaul L, Sooy C, et al.: Cytomegalovirus infection of the laryngeal nerve presenting as hoarseness in patients with acquired immunodeficiency syndrome. Am J Med 1989; 86: 108–110.

71. Marelli R, Biddinger P, Gluckman J. Cytomegalovirus infection of the larynx in the acquired immunodeficiency syndrome. Otolaryngol Head Neck Surg 1992; 106: 296–301.

72. Siegle R, Browning D, Schwartz D, Hudgins P: Cytomegalovirus laryngitis and probable malignant lymphoma of the larynx in a patient with acquired immunodeficiency syndrome. Arch Pathol Lab Med 1992; 116: 539–541.

73. Imoto E, Stein R, Shellito J, Curtis J: Central airway obstruction due to cytomegalovirus-inducing necrotizing tracheitis in a patient with AIDS. Am Rev Respir Dis 1990; 142: 884–886.

74. Tinelli M, Castelnuovo P, Panigazzi A, et al.: Mass lesiosn of the larynx due to cytomegalovirus infection in a patient infected with the human immunodeficiency virus. Clin Infect Dis 1995; 20: 726–727.

75. Tyms A, Taylor D, Parkin J: Cytomegalovirus and the acquired immunodeficiency syndrome. J Antimicrob Chemother 1989; 23: 89–105.

76. Jacobson M, Drew W, Feinberg J: Foscarnet therapy in the treatment of gancyclovir-resistant cytomegalovirus retinitis in patients with AIDS. J Infect Dis 1991; 163: 1348–1351.

77. Fairley C, Kent S, Street A: Invasive aspergillosis in AIDS. Aust N Z J Med 1991; 21: 747–749.

78. Browning D, Schwartz D, Jurado R: Cryptococcosis of the larynx in a patient with AIDS: An unusual cause of fungal laryngitis. South Med J 1992; 85: 762–764.

79. Rothstein S, Persky M, Edelman B: Epiglottitis in AIDS patients. Laryngoscope 1989; 99: 389–392.

80. Schiodt M, Dodd C, Greenspan D, et al.: Natural history of HIV-associated salivary gland disease. Oral Surg Oral Med Oral Path 1992; 74: 326–331.

81. Terry J, Loree T, Thomas M, Marti J: Major salivary gland lymphoepithelial lesions and the acquired immunodeficiency syndrome. Am J Surg 1991; 162: 324–329.

82. Echavez M, Lee K, Sooy C: Tetracycline sclerosis for treatment of benign lymphoepithelial cysts of the parotid gland in patients infected with human immunodeficiency virus. Laryngoscope 1994; 104: 1499–1502.

82a. Wagner RP, Tian H, McPherson MJ, et al: AIDS-associated infections in salivary glands: autopsy survey of 60 cases. Clin Infect Dis 1996; 22: 369–371.

83. CDC: Screening for tuberculosis and tuberculous infections in high-risk populations and the use of preventative therapy for tuberculosis. MMWR 1990; 39: 1–2.

84. Lee K, Tami T, Lalwani A: Contemporary management of cervical tuberculosis. Laryngoscope 1992; 102: 60–64.

85. Castro D, Hoover L, Castro DJ: Cervical mycobacterial lymphadenitis: Medical vs surgical management. Arch Otolaryngol 1985; 111: 816–819.

86. Lee K, Schecter G: Tuberculous infection of the head and neck. Ear Nose Throat J 1995; 74: 395–399.

87. Chopra R, Kerner M, Calcaterra T: Primary nasopharyngeal tuberculosis: A case report and review of this rare entity. Otolaryngol Head Neck Surg 1994; 111: 820–823.

88. Dimitrakopoulos I, Zoumoumis L, Lazaridis N: Primary tuberculosis of the oral cavity. Oral Surg Oral Med Oral Path 1991; 72: 712–715.

89. Bahadori R, Arjmand E, Goldberg A: Tuberculosis of the cervical spine. Otolaryngol Head Neck Surg 1994; 110: 595–597.

90. Department of Public Health: Tuberculosis in San Francisco, 1992. San Francisco Epidemiologic Bulletin 1993; 9: 1–4.

91. Davidson T, Stabile B: Acquired immunodeficiency syndrome precautions for otolaryngology head and neck surgery (commentary). Arch Otolaryngol Head Neck Surg 1991; 117: 1343–1344.

92. CDC: Surveillance for ocupationally acquired HIV infection-United States, 1981–1992. MMWR 1992; 4: 823–825.

93. Wagner B, Johnson J: OSHA standards for bloodborne pathogens: Strategies to increase compliance among otolaryngologists. Ear Nose Throat J 1995; 74: 348–352.

94. Murr A, Lee K: Universal precautions for the otolaryngologist: Techniques and equipment for minimizing exposure risk. Ear Nose Throat J 1995; 74: 338–346.

95. CDC: Recommendations for prevention of HIV transmission in health care settings. MMWR 1987; 36(2S).

96. Enders D, Jones TA, Morrisey M: The effectiveness of double gloving in otolaryngology. Clin Otolaryngol 1990; 15: 535–536.

97. Kelly K, Lee K, Tami T: Surgical glove perforation in otolaryngology: Prevention with cut-resistant gloves. Otolaryngol Head Neck Surg 1993; 108: 91–95.

98. CDC: Public health service statement on management of occupational exposure to human immunodeficiency virus, including considerations regarding zidovudine postexposure use. MMWR 1990; 39: 1–14.

99. Shih C, Kaneshima H, Rabin L: Postexposure prophylaxis with zidovudine suppresses human immunodeficiency virus type 1 infection in SCID-humice in a time-dependent manner. J Infect Dis 1991; 163: 625–627.

100. Gerberding J: Management of occupational exposures to blood-borne viruses. N Engl J Med 1995; 332: 444–451.

Peter Lees
Anne Davis

CHAPTER SIXTY-FIVE

Postoperative Meningitis

▼

Postoperative meningitis is a challenging disease: the symptoms may be atypical or insignificant early in the course and can, therefore, be misleading; treatment needs to begin before the results of microbiologic investigations are available. There is no simple way of monitoring success, and hence the duration of therapy is difficult to gauge and is colored by the fear of relapse. These factors together make a curable complication potentially life-threatening; this is all the more distressing because the original surgery is often relatively routine. Because of the close proximity of the middle ear, nasal cavities, and paranasal sinuses, surgery in these regions carries a small but significant risk of postoperative meningitis.

EAR, NOSE, AND THROAT PROCEDURES CLOSE TO THE DURA

All types of intracranial infection may occur following ear, nose, and throat (ENT) surgery close to the dura, although they are rare. The risk of postoperative meningitis or intracranial abscess is greater if surgery is performed for infective problems such as acute mastoiditis or obstructed sinusitis, but the incidence of these complications remains low.

Apart from a direct breach of the dura during ENT surgery, infection can travel through the pterygoid plexus of veins, which drains venous blood from the paranasal sinuses and the skin of the nose and mid-face to the intracranial cavity. This may rarely result in meningitis or cavernous sinus thrombosis.

Nasal Surgery

The cribriform plate is the closest area of connection between the nose and the anterior cranial fossa, and this plate has defects in many cases with approximation of the dura to the intranasal mucosa.

Meningitis can arise following purely intranasal surgery if infection is introduced through the cribriform plate. This may occur in rare cases following extensive submucosal resection of the septum or packing of the nose with breaching of the cribriform plate as well as in congenital defects such as a nasal encephalocele.

Paranasal Sinuses

The frontal, superior ethmoid and sphenoid paranasal sinuses are adjacent to the anterior and middle fossae of the intracranial cavity.

The surgery of these structures that is most likely to cause meningitis involves the ethmoid, frontal, and sphenoid sinuses. Intranasal ethmoidectomy is a procedure that is hazardous to the cribriform plate with risk of meningitis; it is now rarely performed. Surgery of the frontal sinus includes drainage procedures such as frontal trephining and frontoethmoidectomy. It is not uncommon to see a cerebrospinal fluid leak at transsphenoidal pituitary surgery; this is usually brief but gives rise to the potential for postoperative meningitis, which is a well-recognized complication. Even if these procedures do not directly breach the dura, there is a theoretical risk of infection entering the meninges via the pterygoid plexus of veins.

Ear Surgery

The normally developed mastoid has extensive air cells close to the middle fossa dura and the posterior fossa dura medial to the lateral sinus. Although there is a bony plate between these air cells and the dura, this is very thin and often has defects where the dura is directly adherent to the mastoid mucosa.

In patients in whom there has been enduring chronic middle ear disease, the mastoid may be poorly developed and sclerotic and, in these cases, the bony plates are thicker. There is also a direct communication between the subarachnoid space and the inner ear through the cochlear aqueduct; meningitis has been blamed on infection traveling through this route.

In open mastoid surgery the middle fossa dura is frequently exposed and cerebrospinal fluid (CSF) leak is a well-recognized complication of mastoid surgery of all types. In the presence of extensive infected respiratory mucosa in the mastoid and particularly in revision mastoid surgery, a breach of the dura may occur with CSF leak. Chronic CSF leaks through the ear may be associated with repeated meningitis and are frequently only evident because of CSF rhinorrhea due to CSF leaking down the eustachian tube. This is particularly so if the tympanic membrane is intact and the mastoid surgery has preserved the normal ear anatomy.

Major Skull Base Surgery

Otolaryngologic surgery of the skull base itself is rarely associated with dural exposure, but there is a theoretical risk of venous transmission of infection. This is more likely to cause intracranial abscess than meningitis.

Acoustic Neuroma Surgery

This is surgery in which the dura is deliberately opened through a translabyrinthine or other approach. Postoperatively, the risk of CSF leak is 2%–15%, but both this and the smaller risk of associated meningitis are decreasing with improvements in surgical techniques.

NORMAL FLORA AND COMMON INFECTING BACTERIA

The choice of antibiotic treatment in postoperative meningitis is empirical and based largely on covering the organisms that make up the normal flora of the ear, nose, and paranasal sinuses[1, 2] or, where surgery is for established infection, on knowledge of the common infecting organisms. Unfortunately there is a wide range of commensal bacteria found in the nose, nasopharynx, and ear, and early treatment has, therefore, to be broad-spectrum and cognizant of the potential for multiple organisms.

The anterior nares usually harbor diphtheroids, *Streptococcus viridans*, and *Staphylococcus epidermidis*. As much as 20%–50% of the normal population (and higher for hospitalized patients) carries *Staphylococcus aureus*. Less commonly, *Neisseria*, *Haemophilus*, *Streptococcus pneumoniae*, beta-hemolytic streptococci, and proteus species are present. The nasopharynx has a narrower spectrum including *Streptococcus viridans*, *Neisseria* species (not *Neisseria meningitidis*), *Haemophilus influenzae*, and *Streptococcus pneumoniae*, with beta-hemolytic streptococci and *N. meningitidis* occurring less frequently. The accessory nasal sinuses are relatively sterile.

Common infections of the sinuses involve *H. influenzae*, *S. pneumoniae*, and other nonhemolytic streptococci, *Neisseria* species, and anaerobic organisms, especially *Bacteroides* and *Corynebacterium*. In the frontal sinus, *Haemophilus* infections are less common, and occasionally *Staphylococcus aureus* and *Proteus mirabilis* occur.

The normal flora of the ear is similar to that of the skin and includes *S. epidermidis*, *S. aureus*, diphtheroids, and less commonly *Streptococcus viridans*, coliforms (especially *Proteus* species), and *Pseudomonas aeruginosa*.

Otitis externa is usually staphylococcal, streptococcal, fungal (especially *Candida* or *Aspergillus*), or caused by *P. aeruginosa* or *P. mirabilis*. It is common practice to treat this condition with topical antibiotics, which has created the problem of difficult infections caused by gentamicin-resistant *P. aeruginosa*.

Otitis media is often part of a viral upper respiratory tract infection, but bacterial superinfection is common. Infecting organisms are frequently *Streptococcus pyogenes*, *S. pneumoniae* and, in infants, *H. influenzae*. Mastoiditis has similar causative organisms, with the addition of anaerobes. Chronic otitis media is similar to otitis externa with a broad and often mixed range of organisms: streptococci, diphtheroids, *Pseudomonas*, coliforms (including *Escherichia coli*, *Klebsiella*, *Enterobacter*, and *Proteus* species), anaerobes, and fungi (*Candida* and *Aspergillus*).

DIAGNOSIS

The symptoms of postoperative meningitis are no different from those of primary meningitis, namely headache, neck stiffness, pyrexia, photophobia and, as the disease advances, decreasing level of consciousness. When the first four symptoms are present, the diagnosis is relatively easy to make, but in the early postoperative period, the diagnosis may be confounded by other surgical complications with similar symptomatology. Furthermore, the classic symptoms may not all be present or may be mild and seemingly insignificant.

DIFFERENTIAL DIAGNOSIS

Headache is relatively common after otologic and some nasal surgery, but it is usually brief, seldom persisting more than a few hours. Following a significant intraoperative CSF leak or when a protective postoperative lumbar drain is used, the patient may suffer low-pressure headaches and, although the relationship to posture is often helpful, they can be particularly severe and associated with photophobia. Following major skull base surgery, acoustic neuroma, and, less commonly, transsphenoidal pituitary surgery, intracranial complications can cause headache; these include raised intracranial pressure due to intracranial hematoma and obstructive or communicating hydrocephalus. Blood in the CSF incites a so-called chemical meningitis that, in addition to the headache, may also be associated with neck stiffness, photophobia, nausea, vomiting, and fever.[3]

Neck stiffness is not generally seen following uncomplicated ear and nasal surgery, with the exception of the short-term effects of suxamethonium, often used during anaesthesia, which can produce spasm in the neck muscles in the first few hours after surgery.

Photophobia has been mentioned in the context of both blood in the CSF and low intracranial pressure states. It is not uncommon in the first few hours after surgery, but beyond this, it should be regarded as suspicious.

Pyrexia is a common postoperative sign that can be due to infection in the operative site and a range of general postoperative complications, for example, deep venous thrombosis and chest infection.

Following mastoid surgery, not only can bacterial perichondritis of the pinna mimic many of the symptoms and signs of meningitis—the patients are often systemically sick with pyrexia and headache—but it can also be complicated by bacterial meningitis in rare cases.

Finally, after mastoid and sinus surgery, cerebral abscess can occur and can also coexist with either bacterial meningitis or a meningitic picture in the CSF. An undiagnosed cerebral abscess can be fatal and, therefore, a computed tomography (CT) or magnetic resonance (MR) scan should always be performed when this is a possibility. Lumbar puncture can have fatal complications in this condition and is, therefore, contraindicated.

The many differential diagnoses demonstrate the difficulties in making the clinical diagnosis of meningitis after ear and sinus surgery, especially at an early stage when signs and symptoms may be minor. If the syndrome of headache, neck stiffness, pyrexia, and photophobia is present, then meningitis must be excluded or treated blind if examination of the CSF is contraindicated. When the syndrome is incomplete, clinical judgment must prevail against the background that it is far safer to "overtreat" than to miss the diagnosis of meningitis.

INVESTIGATION

The mainstay of investigation is examination of the CSF. Following more straightforward surgery there should be few contraindications to performing lumbar puncture, but if raised intracranial pressure is suspected, an urgent CT (or MR) scan should be performed. Meningeal enhancement may be seen in meningitis, but this is not particularly helpful and, importantly, its absence does not exclude the diagnosis. After more major and especially skull base surgery, the situation is more complex as there may be raised intracranial pressure. Treatment of postoperative raised intracranial pressure is beyond the scope of this chapter, but lumbar puncture is usually contraindicated. If there is raised intracranial pressure and a CSF sample is needed, the only alternative is to tap the ventricle, but even this may be contraindicated if there is significant shift of the midline or if the ventricles are small. Inevitably there are occasions when it has to be accepted that laboratory confirmation of the diagnosis is of secondary importance to treatment and is not possible. This is not the situation in the majority of cases because microbiologic investigation of the CSF helps in the following ways:

1. It establishes the diagnosis *indirectly* by typical cytologic and biochemical patterns. This is particularly valuable early before culture results are available and later if culture is normal.

2. It establishes the nature of the organism by cytologic examination and later by the results of bacterial culture; antibiotic sensitivities are also very important for guiding therapy.

3. Follow-up examination, although used infrequently, can assess success of treatment by demonstrating a falling leukocyte count and sterile culture.

Following major skull base surgery or when a significant dural opening has occurred, the interpretation of CSF examination is more difficult: following such procedures (in the absence of postoperative infection) there are commonly changes in the CSF that overlap widely with those seen in bacterial meningitis. These changes of so-called aseptic meningitis include an often substantial rise in the white blood cell count, usually with a predominance of polymorphonuclear leukocytes.[4, 5]

TREATMENT

Once the diagnosis of meningitis is suspected, the patient must be treated urgently; although laboratory proof of the diagnosis is ideal, this must not delay the start of antimicrobial therapy. Successful treatment depends on the prompt administration of the appropriate antibiotic (single or multiple) in adequate dosage and for long enough to eradicate the infection; this is difficult and relies on clinical judgment and experience. Furthermore, the close involvement of the microbiologist experienced in the management of central nervous system sepsis is essential.

Postoperative meningitis is potentially life-threatening and, consequently, treatment must start prior to bacteriologic identification and antibiotic sensitivity results. The choice of antibiotic can be helped by the following factors:

1. Knowledge of the likely origin of the infection because the offending organism(s) is likely to be part of the normal flora.

2. When surgery is for established sepsis, there may already be culture and sensitivity results regarding the primary infection. When surgery is for chronic sepsis in a patient who has received many previous courses of antibiotics (topical or systemic), postoperative meningitis may be caused by multiply-resistant organisms; often, such organisms pose considerable therapeutic problems.

3. Morphologic examination of bacteria seen on CSF microscopy can help, but postoperative meningitis may be caused by multiple organisms, some of which may not be seen on microscopy.

The duration of treatment is usually empirical and based on clinical judgment. There are few methods available for the monitoring of success beyond observation of symptomatic improvement and the resolution of pyrexia, neither of which is particularly reliable; cessation of therapy too early can lead to relapse. Ideally, the CSF should be reexamined, but lumbar puncture is disliked by many patients and is rarely repeated; however, if in doubt, it should always be considered, especially if the fever does not resolve or the patient remains systemically unwell. It is therefore not possible to give precise guidelines regarding duration of therapy, but most would agree that the minimum course should be 7–10 days of intravenous antibiotics. If a switch to oral therapy is undertaken, the antibiotic chosen must cross the blood-brain barrier in adequate concentration; this rules out most drugs, with the exception of agents such as rifampicin, metronidazole, and chloramphenicol.

In postoperative meningitis, a wide range of organisms may be potential pathogens and, therefore, broad-spectrum antibiotic treatment is recommended at maximal doses to ensure penetration of the blood-brain barrier. Empirical therapy is necessary if the microorganism is unknown: a popular regimen consists of a third-generation cephalosporin combined with an antistaphylococcal agent. Cefotaxime and ceftriaxone are popular choices for the third-generation cephalosporin, but their coverage against *P. aeruginosa* is suboptimal. In clinical situations in which *P. aeruginosa* may be a potential pathogen—this includes prolonged hospitalization, prior receipt of broad-spectrum antibiotics, and isolation of *P. aeruginosa* from another body site—ceftazidime may be preferred because of its excellent antipseudomonal activity. To cover staphylococcal infection, nafcillin or oxacillin penetrates the blood-brain barrier readily. However, if methicillin-resistant *S. aureus* is a problem within the institution, vancomycin is preferred.

If anaerobic infection is strongly suspected, metronidazole, chloramphenicol, or beta-lactam agent/beta-lactam inhibitor agents (for example, ticarcillin-clavulanate, piperacillin-tazobactam) are antianaerobic antibiotics that penetrate the blood-brain barrier.

Clearly there are many other combinations of both antibiotics and infecting organisms. This account aims to guide the initial treatment before bacteriologic results are available. Beyond that, and in the difficult case, clinicians must work closely with microbiologists and consult specific texts.[6] Finally, there are a number of other neurologic complications, both infective (for example, intracranial abscess in its various forms) and non-infective (for example, epilepsy and cerebral infarction), that must be kept in mind and investigated as appropriate, usually in collaboration with the neuroradiologist and neurosurgeon or neurologist.

Because treatment usually starts before laboratory confirmation of infection, there are occasions when the diagnosis is questioned after treatment has started; in this circumstance it is only safe to stop a course of antibiotics if the CSF white blood cell count is not raised and culture is normal; this inevitably means a minimum course of 48 hours of treatment. In the early stages of meningitis, a normal white blood cell count can give a false sense of security.

MANAGEMENT OF CSF LEAKS

CSF leaks frequently settle spontaneously and generally do not result in meningitis unless prolonged; there is, however, no room for complacency, and in all such cases the potential for meningitis must be appreciated. Following acoustic neuroma surgery, a wait of 2–3 weeks is advisable prior to surgical repair, unless the leak is very major. Following ear and sinus surgery, the wait should be only a few days before surgical repair because the route of drainage is more direct and less likely to seal spontaneously.

TECHNIQUE FOR CLOSURE OF LEAKS

There are many approaches to and some controversy in the management of CSF leaks, a detailed description of which is beyond the scope of this chapter; comprehensive accounts of the various methods can be found in both ENT and skull base operative surgical texts. However, there are two basic principles. First, prevention is better than cure. When a CSF leak is seen at operation, rigorous dural closure should be performed and usually protected by lumbar spinal CSF drainage for up to 5 days. Second, the diagnosis of CSF leak must be confirmed. Although it is often clinically obvious, this is not always the case and there are biochemical (for example, beta-transferrin assay) and radiologic methods (radioisotope or contrast cisternography) to help. Following

nasal surgery there can often be a brisk and relatively clear nasal discharge that is not CSF and that settles spontaneously.

A proportion of established CSF leaks resolve spontaneously, but most surgeons advocate the use of lumbar CSF drainage for up to 5 days as initial treatment. Persistent or large leaks are unlikely to heal, and formal surgical repair is usually necessary, the precise technique depending on the site of the leak and surgeon preference. Repair can be performed extracranially in, for example, bony defects in the labyrinth; nasal endoscopic techniques are being used increasingly for leaks following sinus surgery. In refractory cases and especially leaks occurring through the cribriform plate, intracranial repair may be necessary.

Prophylactic antibiotics are often given to patients with CSF leaks, but this practice may be unnecessary and even harmful: in the case of posttraumatic CSF leak there is evidence that prophylactic antibiotics do not reduce the incidence of meningitis and may predispose to meningitis with antibiotic-resistant organisms that can be very difficult to treat.[2] Meningitis may even occur when the causative organism is sensitive to the antibiotic used for prophylaxis.

SUMMARY

The successful management of meningitis occurring after ear, nose, and throat surgery depends on early clinical suspicion and diagnosis, with prompt medical treatment using high-dose, broad-spectrum antibiotics that adequately cross the blood-brain barrier. In general, the initial management of coexistent CSF leaks should be conservative (using spinal drainage); surgical closure should be delayed until the meningitis has fully settled and is not necessary if the leak resolves with conservative treatment.

References

1. Noone P: Bacteriology in relation to otorhinolaryngology. In: Ballantyne J, Groves J, (eds): Scott Brown's Diseases of the Ear, Nose and Throat. London: Butterworths, 1979, vol. 1, pp 559–599.
2. Brown EM, de Louvois J, Bayston R, et al.: Antimicrobial prophylaxis in neurosurgery and after head injury. Lancet 1994; 334: 1547–1551.
3. Carmel PW, Fraser RAR, Stein BM: Aseptic meningitis following posterior fossa surgery in children. J Neurosurg 1974; 41: 44–48.
4. Ross D, Rosegay H, Pons V: Differentiation of aseptic and bacterial meningitis in postoperative neurosurgical patients. J Neurosurg 1988; 69: 669–674.
5. Kaufman BA, Tunkel AR, Pryor JC, et al.: Meningitis in the neurosurgical patient. Infect Dis Clin North Am 1990; 4: 677–701.
6. Roos KL, Tunkel AR, Scheld WM: Acute bacterial meningitis in children and adults. In: Scheld WM, Whitley RJ, Durack DT (eds): Infections of the Central Nervous System. New York: Raven Press Ltd, 1991, pp 335–409.

SECTION VI

ANTIBIOTIC PROPHYLAXIS FOR HEAD AND NECK SURGERY

Jonas T. Johnson

Principles of Antibiotic Prophylaxis

Nosocomial pneumonia and postoperative wound infection are the most important and leading causes of hospital-acquired infection. It is estimated that nosocomial wound infection costs $5 billion per year.[1] The real expense in terms of lost productivity, pain, and suffering cannot be calculated. Accordingly, strategies developed to prevent or reduce the occurrence of postoperative wound infection are critical to every surgeon.

Administration of antibiotics is associated with the potential for drug-related toxicities, contributes to the overall cost of hospitalization, and is partially responsible for the development of antibiotic-resistant organisms. It is estimated that 30% of the entire cost attributable to administration of hospitalized patients is for antibiotic prophylaxis.[2] The appropriate use of antibiotics may contribute to a reduced incidence of postoperative wound infection. The responsible use of these antibiotics helps contain the cost of medical care while limiting the potential for toxicity or emergence of antibiotic-resistant organisms.

RISK OF POSTOPERATIVE WOUND INFECTION

The Centers for Disease Control and Prevention have promulgated guidelines to be used in estimating the potential for the development of postoperative wound infections.[1, 3] These guidelines consider the preoperative condition at the operative site together with expected exposures during surgery. "Clean" surgical procedures (class I) are those in which no evidence of infection exists prior to surgery. An example is thyroidectomy. During the performance of the surgical procedure, sterile techniques are maintained, and the wound is not exposed to contaminated material. The wound is closed at the completion of the procedure. The estimated risk of postoperative wound sepsis is less than 5%. Current standards suggest that patients undergoing clean procedures do not benefit from the routine administration of antibiotic prophylaxis.

"Clean-contaminated" procedures (class II) exist when wound infection does not exist prior to surgery; however, the respiratory or gastrointestinal tract has been entered without gross spillage or with minor breaks in surgical technique in atraumatic wounds. Because of the nature of the procedure, the wound is, of necessity, contaminated by secretions, which contain microorganisms. For example, procedures performed in the nose and oral cavity may be contaminated during surgery. Postoperative wound infection varies with the surgical procedure, the inoculum, the virulence of the microorganisms, the adequacy of host defense mechanisms, and the length and magnitude of the operative procedure. Class II procedures are associated with an infection rate of less than 10%.[3]

The anterior nares and nose are normally colonized by bacteria. *Staphylococcus aureus* is encountered in the nose of 30%–50% of normal individuals.[4] Intranasal surgery may rarely be accompanied by simultaneous bacteremia.[4, 5] Nevertheless, prospective randomized clinical trials suggest that the risk of postoperative sinonasal infection is less than 5%.[6–8] Clinical studies performed to date have not demonstrated efficacy for the routine administration of antibiotic prophylaxis for routine sinonasal surgery. This is reflective of the low incidence of observed infections in patients receiving no antibiotic.

The middle ear and mastoid are considered normally sterile; however, in patients undergoing surgery for chronic otitis media, colonization by bacteria is observed. *Pseudomonas aeruginosa* is most commonly associated with chronic otitis media. In spite of the presence of this potential pathogen, efficacy of routine antibiotic prophylaxis has failed to show a benefit for patients undergoing routine otologic procedures such as tympanoplasty, tympanomastoidectomy, and mastoidectomy.[7–10]

"Contaminated" surgery (class III) describes a situation when there is gross spillage of contaminated materials into the surgical wound.

Prospective randomized placebo-controlled clinical trials have convincingly proved that patients undergoing major head and neck surgery in which the cervical viscera are grossly contaminated by oropharyngeal secretions do benefit from the administration of antibiotic prophylaxis. Infection rates as high as 87% have been reported in patients undergoing head and neck surgery randomized to clinical trials in which placebo (no antibiotic) was administered, in contrast to infection rates of 3%–17% in patients receiving prophylactic antibiotics.[11–14]

Normal oral flora contains approximately 1 to 10 million bacteria per milliliter of saliva[15] (see Chapter 22). The number of bacteria may increase in the face of poor dentition. Approximately 90% are anaerobic including *Bacteroides* species, *Peptostreptococcus*, and *Fusobacterium*. Aerobic bacteria constitute approximately 10% of oral bacteria; the majority are gram-positive cocci such as streptococci and staphylococci. Gram-negative aerobic organisms are rarely encountered as normal flora in the upper respiratory tract, except in patients having prolonged hospitalization and in those who have previously received radiation therapy to the oral cavity.

"Dirty contaminated" or infected surgery (class IV) occurs in patients who have evidence of infection preoperatively or in whom the tissues are exposed preoperatively to contamination (e.g., penetrating trauma). In these circumstances, a patient should be considered infected, and administration of antibiotics would be considered therapeutic. To call antibiotic usage in this situation "prophylactic" is a misnomer.

PREOPERATIVE PREPARATION

The development of postoperative wound infection cannot be attributed totally to the choice of a perioperative antimicrobial agent. Fundamental to our understanding of infectious disease is the recognition that infection reflects a dynamic interplay between host resistance and bacterial inoculum. The size of the inoculum sufficient to cause wound infection is related to virulence. A number of aspects of surgical care may significantly influence host resistance. This includes establishment of proper nutrition, correction of metabolic abnormalities, and elimination of potential sources of sepsis.

Before setting up a course of surgical therapy, a patient's nutritional needs should be assessed. Preoperative malnutrition correlates with the incidence of postoperative wound infection.[16] Efforts directed at reestablishment of proper nutrition and subsequent maintenance of protein-calorie requirements can contribute to a successful postoperative result.

Patients with systemic disorders benefit from maximizing therapeutic intervention prior to surgery. This includes control of diabetes mellitus; electrolyte disorders; and renal, hepatic, and circulatory disorders to maximize the potential for normal healing.

Performance of an elective surgical procedure in the face of existing infection is generally contraindicated. Dental sepsis is frequently encountered in patients presenting with carcinoma of the oral cavity. Preoperative dental restorations and/or extractions may be associated with improved postoperative healing with a reduced risk of wound infection. In the course of extracting infected carious teeth, huge numbers of organisms may be expelled into the secretions of the upper aerodigestive tract. In addition, a transient bacteremia may occur. Clayman and colleagues[17] found a significantly higher number of anaerobic isolates in wound infections in patients who underwent concomitant dental extractions at the time of resection of their upper aerodigestive tract cancer.[17] Among patients with periodontal disease, consideration should be given to extracting the teeth as a separate procedure or administering a therapeutic course of antibiotics.

INTRAOPERATIVE CONSIDERATIONS

Successful wound healing following a major surgical procedure is a measure of the surgeon's skill. It reflects careful handling of tissues and good judgment. Intraoperative he-

mostasis is critical because postoperative hematoma may result in compromised tissue perfusion and provides media for bacterial proliferation. Similarly, the wound must be carefully irrigated to remove debris. Prior to wound closure, suction drains must be placed to maximize the aspiration of serum, blood, or salivary leakage. Accordingly, the author advocates placement of drains in dependent portions of the neck and adjacent to suture lines. These drains must be tunneled through skin to effect an airtight seal and maintained patent during transportation of the patient. Wound repair must be performed meticulously to avoid salivary leakage and prevent necrosis. In experimental studies, only 10^5 bacteria per gram of tissue may be necessary to cause a wound infection; however, if a foreign body such as a mandibular prosthesis is present, only 10^2 bacteria are required to produce an infection.[18, 19]

POSTOPERATIVE CONSIDERATIONS

Care of the patient following surgery is critical for successful healing. Nutrition is maintained by the use of tube feeding. Metabolic status of the patient should be monitored and abnormalities corrected. Good tissue perfusion remains important. Patients should be normotensive. Circulation in the flaps must not be compromised by tight dressings, tracheal collars, and the like.

Careful maintenance of the suction drainage system is especially important following major head and neck surgery. Elimination of blood and serum from the potential dead spaces created by neck dissection promotes good wound healing. The patency of the drains must be assessed. Obstructed drains should be aspirated. Premature removal of drains may be associated with development of space collection and infection.

Nursing care complements surgery. Tracheotomy care, wound care, and early ambulation of patients contribute to complication-free recovery. In providing this care, however, the basic principle of hospital infection control (e.g., the prevention of cross infection between patients) must be adhered to through rigorous attention to such principles as hand washing and appropriate disposal of contaminated materials.

All aspects of postoperative care are the responsibility of the attending surgeon. Over-zealous or premature institution of tube feeding, which results in emesis, may have a disastrous effect on a pharyngeal suture line. Similarly, failure to recognize and appropriately treat organic brain syndrome or delirium tremens may be associated with premature removal of drains or disruption of suture lines. These preventable mishaps are the responsibility of the attending surgeon. Successful management requires careful coordination of all care activities.

ROUTE OF ANTIBIOTIC ADMINISTRATION

The most commonly employed routes of antibiotic administration are enteral (by mouth), parenteral, intramuscular, and topical. Routine administration of oral antibiotics for operative patients is impractical as absorption is slow and relatively unreliable. The parenteral route is most commonly chosen for antibiotic prophylaxis. The availability of venous access in patients undergoing surgery makes this the obvious route of choice.

Topical antibiotic administration may be appropriate in some circumstances. This is especially apparent in patients undergoing clean-contaminated surgical procedures in which the wound is continuously exposed to contaminated secretions. The concentration of topical antibiotics deliverable to the site of incision may be a hundred-fold higher than that delivered parenterally. Topical antibiotics have been shown to eradicate bacterial flora for up to 8 hours.[20-22] This creates a potential window of opportunity to perform the surgical procedure under "clean" conditions. Topical application of the same antibiotic solution resulted in near eradication of organisms in oropharyngeal secretions. In a series of 30 patients undergoing laryngectomy with neck dissection, Grandis and colleagues[22] reported an infection rate of 3% in patients receiving topical antibiotic prophylaxis only. Simultaneous use of parenteral and topical antibiotics may potentially result in a further reduction in the incidence of postoperative wound infection. Clinical trials are in progress to validate this hypothesis.

TIMING OF ANTIBIOTIC ADMINISTRATION

In an animal model Burke[23] demonstrated that there exists a window of maximum opportunity for the prevention of postoperative wound infection. Antibiotics are maximally effective when administered prior to contamination of the wound. The efficacy of antibiotic administration decreases with time. Antibiotics administered 3 or more hours after contamination are ineffective in preventing subsequent wound infection.

The relevance of timing in the administration of prophylactic antibiotics for prevention of surgical wound infections has been well established. Classen and colleagues[24] studied patients undergoing a variety of general surgical procedures. They found the risk of wound infection was reduced in patients receiving antibiotic 2-0 hours prior to surgery or 0-3 hours after surgery. Patients receiving antibiotics more than 2 hours before surgery or more than 3 hours after surgery experienced an increased risk of postoperative wound infection.

These observations have great practical importance in patients undergoing contaminated surgical procedures. When antibiotic administration is indicated, the antibiotics must be administered prior to the surgical procedure such that adequate concentrations of antibiotics are at the site of operation. Initiation of antibiotic prophylaxis 3 or more hours postoperatively is ineffective.

DURATION OF ANTIBIOTIC PROPHYLAXIS

It is generally agreed that therapeutic drug levels should be maintained throughout the entire duration of a surgical procedure. Extended procedures may require administration of a second dose. Timing is calculated based upon the half-life of the antibiotic used. Studies in general surgery,

cardiovascular surgery, gynecology, and urology demonstrate little advantage to patients receiving antibiotics for 24 hours when compared with patients receiving a single intraoperative dose.[24, 25] Prolonged administration of antibiotics after the first postoperative day has not been convincingly demonstrated to improve antibiotic efficacy.[26-29]

Extended administration of antibiotics for "prophylaxis" is, however, associated with increased expense and increased risk of toxicity and may be associated with the development of infection with resistant organisms. Attempts to prevent pneumonia in ventilator-dependent patients with multiple antibiotics have led to the emergence of antibiotic-resistant bacteria. The risk of *Clostridium difficile* enterocolitis is increased in patients receiving prolonged broad-spectrum antibiotics.

CHOICE OF ANTIBIOTICS

The drug chosen for prophylaxis should have a spectrum that includes microorganisms likely to be found at the operative site and the potential for antibiotic-related toxicity (Table 66-1). A variety of antibiotics have had demonstrated efficacy in prospective randomized clinical trials performed in patients undergoing major head and neck surgical procedures.[13, 30-32] Secretions of the upper aerodigestive tract are largely colonized by anaerobic bacteria and some gram-positive aerobes. Antibiotic-resistant patterns reflective at an institution are also important in selection of an antibiotic. For instance, the emerging prevalence of beta-lactamase–producing anaerobic bacteria at some institutions mandates that an antibiotic effective against these organisms is more likely to prevent postoperative wound infection in these same institutions.

Table 66-1. CHOOSING A DRUG FOR PROPHYLAXIS

Procedure	Antimicrobial Recommendation	Notes
Nasal surgery	None	
Otology	None	
Mandibular fracture	Cefazolin	Not needed if closed
Maxillary fracture	None	
Frontal sinus	Unclear	Not needed for isolated anterior wall
Oral surgery	Penicillin or erythromycin	
Orthognoptic surgery	None	
Thyroidectomy	None	
Salivary gland excision	None	
Radical neck dissection	Unclear	Assume no contamination
Laryngectomy	Cefazolin	Perioperative administration
Major oral cavity	Moxalactam	
Oropharyngeal	Clindamycin	Stop 24 hours after surgery
Hypopharyngeal resection	Cefoperazone	
	Cefotaxime	
	Ampicillin/sulbactam	
	Clindamycin/gentamicin	
	Clindamycin/amikacin	
	Ticarcillin/clavulanate	

DOSE AND INTERVAL CONSIDERATION

The dose of the antibiotic should be calculated to achieve concentrations severalfold higher than the minimal inhibitory concentrations (MICs) for potential pathogens after a single bolus infusion. Low doses may be inadequate in preventing wound infection. For example, in one study performed in patients undergoing major contaminated head and neck surgical procedures, 500 mg of cefazolin was administered every 8 hours[33]; infection was observed in 33% of patients. Another study administered cefazolin at the higher dose of 1 g every 8 hours[12]; infection rates of 16%–18% were reported. A third study administered cefazolin 2 g every 8 hours[30]; the infection rate was 9%. The peak serum and tissue concentrations of cefazolin at the lower doses may have been below the MICs for some frequently encountered organisms for major head and neck surgery.

Accelerated dosing is a potentially effective strategy for intraoperative administration of antibiotics for prophylaxis. Dosing recommendations for therapy based upon multiple sequential drug administration are for a prolonged period of time. Nadir (trough) serum concentrations, which occur between the first and second dose, may be inadequate for surgical prophylaxis. Shortening the interval between intravenous bolus administration of antibiotics may serve to maintain therapeutic levels of drug throughout the surgical procedure.

SIMULTANEOUS PARENTERAL AND TOPICAL ANTIBIOTIC USAGE

A potential for synergy exists when employing parenteral antibiotics simultaneously with the use of intraoperative antibiotic irrigation. Normal flora of the oral cavity contains 1 million to 10 million bacteria per milliliter. Intravenous administration of an antibiotic can prevent systemic infections and also ensure antibiotic concentrations within the tissue. Topical antibiotics may be more effective against organisms at the operative site. Combination of both routes of administration may be highly effective.

SPECIAL CONSIDERATIONS

Human Immunodeficiency Virus (HIV) Infections

HIV infection may be associated with a wide range of opportunistic infections. Antimicrobial prophylaxis for dental extraction in HIV-infected individuals was evaluated by Porter and colleagues.[34] Complications in HIV-infected individuals were similar to those encountered in a comparable HIV-negative patient population. These observations suggest there is little need for routine antimicrobial prophylaxis in HIV-infected patients undergoing dental extraction.

Artificial Joint

Bacteremia may result in sepsis of a prosthetic joint. Infection of a prosthesis may occur any time after placement.

Accordingly, surgeries on contaminated surfaces that may be associated with temporary bacteremia may increase the risk of joint infection in patients with prosthetic joints. Most orthopedic surgeons recommend routine antimicrobial prophylaxis for patients with artificial joints when undergoing a procedure known to produce a significant bacteremia.

Cardiac Prophylaxis

The American Heart Association recommends antimicrobial prophylaxis for endocarditis for surgical operations that involve the respiratory mucosa. Accordingly, patients with a history of rheumatic heart disease, patients with mitral valve prolapse, and patients with a history of prior cardiac valve surgery or valve disease should receive antimicrobial prophylaxis administered intravenously immediately prior to surgery followed by a second dose postoperatively (see Chapter 69).

References

1. Haley RW, Culver DH, Morgan WM, et al.: Identifying patients at high risk of surgical wound infection: A simple multivariate index of patient susceptibility and wound contamination. Am J Epidemiol 1985; 121: 206–215.
2. Shapiro M: Perioperative prophylactic use of antibiotics in surgery: Principles and practice. Infect Control Hosp Epidemiol 1982; 3: 38–40.
3. Garner J, Hughes JM, Davis B, et al.: CDC guideline for prevention of surgical wound infections, 1985. Infect Control Hosp Epidemiol 1986; 7: 193–200.
4. Silk KL, Ali MB, Cohen BJ, et al.: Absence of bacteremia during nasal septoplasty. Arch Otolaryngol Head Neck Surg 1991; 117: 54–55.
5. Slavin SA, Rees TD, Guy CL, Goldwyn RM: An investigation of bacteremia during rhinoplasty. Plast Reconstr Surg 1983; 71: 196–198.
6. Eschelman LT, Schleuning AJ, Brummett RE: Prophylactic antibiotics in otolaryngologic surgery: A double-blind study. Trans Am Acad Ophthamol Otolaryngol 1971; 75: 387–394.
7. Weimert TA, Yoder MG: Antibiotics and nasal surgery. Laryngoscope 1980; 90: 667–672.
8. Strong MS: Wound infection in otolaryngologic surgery and the inexpediency of antibiotic prophylaxis. Laryngoscope 1963; 73: 165–183.
9. Jackson CG: Antimicrobial prophylaxis in ear surgery. Laryngoscope 1988; 98: 1116–1123.
10. Donaldson JA, Snyder IS: Prophylactic chemotherapy in myringoplasty surgery. Laryngoscope 1966; 76: 1201–1214.
11. Piccart M, Klastersky J: Antimicrobial prophylaxis of infections in head and neck cancer surgery. Scand J Infect Dis 1983; 39: 92–96.
12. Becker GD, Parell GJ: Cefazolin prophylaxis in head and neck cancer surgery. Ann Otol 1979; 88: 183–186.
13. Johnson JT, Yu VL, Myers EN, Wagner RL: An assessment of the need for gram-negative bacterial coverage in antibiotic prophylaxis for oncological head and neck surgery. J Infect Dis 1987; 155: 331–333.
14. Johnson JT, Yu VL: Antibiotic use during major head and neck surgery. Ann Surg 1988; 207: 108–111.
15. Bartlett JG, Gorback SL: Anaerobic infections of the head and neck. Otolaryngol Clin North Am 1976; 9: 655–678.
16. Goodwin WJ, Torres J: The value of the prognostic nutritional index in the management of patients with advanced carcinoma of the head and neck. Head Neck Surg 1984; 6: 932–937.
17. Clayman GL, Raad II, Hankins PD, Weber RS: Bacteriologic profile of surgical infection after antibiotic prophylaxis. Head Neck 1993; 15: 526–531.
18. Elek SD: Experimental staphylococcal infections in the skin of man. Ann NY Acad Sci 1956; 65: 85–90.
19. Johnson JT: Antibiotics for contaminated surgery. In: Johnson JT (ed): Antibiotic Therapy in Head and Neck Surgery. New York: Marcel Dekker, Inc., 1987, pp 51–91.

20. Elledge ES, Whiddon RG, Fraker JY, Stambaugh KI: The effects of topical oral clindamycin antibiotic rinses on the bacterial content of saliva on healthy human subjects. Otolaryngol Head Neck Surg 1991; 105: 836–839.

21. Kirchner JC, Edberg SC, Sasaki CT: The use of topical oral antibiotics in head and neck prophylaxis: Is it justified? Laryngoscope 1988; 98: 26–29.

22. Grandis JR, Vickers RM, Rihs JD, et al.: The efficacy of topical antibiotic prophylaxis for contaminated head and neck surgery. Laryngoscope 1994; 104: 719–724.

23. Burke JF: Use of preventive antibiotics in clinical surgery. Am J Surg 1973; 39: 6–11.

24. Classen DC, Evans S, Pestontnik SL, et al.: The timing of prophylactic administration of antibiotics and the risk of surgical-wound infection. N Engl J Med 1992; 326: 281–286.

25. Stone HH, Hooper CA, Kolb LD, Geheber CE, Dawkins EJ: Antibiotic prophylaxis in gastric, biliary and colonic surgery. Ann Surg 1976; 184: 443–452.

26. Membelli G, Coppers L, Dor P, Klastersky J: Antibiotic prophylaxis in surgery for head and neck cancer: Comparative study of short and prolonged administration of carbenicillin. J Antimicrob Chemother 1981; 7: 665–671.

27. Fee WE, Glenn M, Haden C, Hopp ML: One day vs. two days of prophylactic antibiotics in patients undergoing major head and neck surgery. Laryngoscope 1984; 94: 612–614.

28. Johnson JT, Myers EN, Thearle PB, et al.: Antimicrobial prophylaxis for contaminated head and neck surgery. Laryngoscope 1994; 94: 46–51.

29. Johnson JT, Schuller DE, Silver F, et al.: Antibiotic prophylaxis in high-risk head and neck surgery: One-day or five-day therapy. Otolaryngol Head Neck Surg 1986; 95: 554–557.

30. Johnson JT, Yu VL, Myers EN, et al.: Cefazolin vs moxalactam? Arch Otolaryngol Head Neck Surg 1986; 112: 151–153.

31. Johnson JT, Yu VL, Myers EN, et al.: Efficacy of two third-generation cephalosporins in prophylaxis for head and neck surgery. Arch Otolaryngol 1984; 110: 224–227.

32. Weber RS, Raad I, Frankenthaler R, et al.: Ampicillin-sulbactam vs clindamycin in head and neck oncologic surgery: The need for gram-negative coverage. Arch Otolaryngol Head Neck Surg 1992; 118: 1159–1163.

33. Brand B, Johnson JT, Myers EN, et al.: Prophylactic perioperative antibiotics in contaminated head and neck surgery. Otolaryngol Head Neck Surg 1982; 90: 315–318.

34. Porter SR, Scully C, Luker J: Complications of dental surgery in persons with HIV disease. Oral Surg Oral Med Oral Pathol 1993; 75: 165–167.

CHAPTER SIXTY-SEVEN

Jonas T. Johnson
Randal S. Weber

Prophylaxis for Contaminated Head and Neck and Cranial Base Surgery

▼

Most major head and neck surgical procedures are accomplished in a surgical field contaminated by secretions from the upper aerodigestive tract. According to guidelines promulgated by the Centers for Disease Control and Prevention,[1] clean-contaminated operations are those in which no clinical evidence of infection exists prior to surgery, but due to the nature of the procedure undertaken, the wound is, of necessity, contaminated by secretions. The relative risk of postoperative wound infection cannot be precisely estimated; however, it is related to the magnitude of the surgical procedure performed, the relative size and virulence of the bacterial inoculum, and host defense mechanisms. A variety of investigators have reported prospective, randomized, placebo-controlled trials of antibiotic prophylaxis in patients undergoing head and neck surgery. The infection rates observed vary from 28% to 87% in the placebo groups, and infection rates of 3%–17% were observed in the patients receiving antibiotic prophylaxis.[2–9] Methodologic differences used by these investigators, such as entry criteria and definition of wound infection, probably account for the wide variation in incidence of postoperative wound infections. It is agreed that prophylactic administration of antibiotics in patients undergoing major contaminated head and neck surgical procedures is required.

Patients undergoing cranial base procedures represent a high-risk group. These operations frequently result in a large surgical defect contaminated by secretions of the upper aerodigestive tract. The risk of meningitis, brain abscess, and osteomyelitis is real. Carrau and colleagues[10] conducted a retrospective analysis of 95 patients undergoing clean-contaminated cranial base procedures during a 2-year period. All received perioperative antibiotics. The infection rate observed was 7%. An increased risk of infection was noted in patients receiving antibiotics for less than 24 hours.

ANTIBIOTICS AND TONSILLECTOMY

A number of studies have been conducted to investigate the efficacy of antibiotic therapy in eradicating tonsillitis in a effort to establish eligibility criteria for tonsillectomy. As chronic inflammation of the tonsils is associated with bacterial colonization of both the tonsillar core and surface, it seems likely that the morbidity of tonsillectomy may be reduced by the administration of antibiotics. There are only two prospective, randomized, placebo-controlled trials, however, that have addressed the impact of antibiotic therapy on recovery following tonsillectomy.[11, 12]

Both clinical trials examined the impact of the systemic administration of a postoperative course of antibiotics on recovery parameters (e.g., mouth odor, activity level, dietary intake, pain severity, and fever). The first study looked at ampicillin/amoxicillin in children and found that they were effective in minimizing postoperative symptoms and fever.[11] The next study examined the consequences of ticarcillin plus clavulanate/amoxicillin plus clavulanate in adults and reported that those patients who received antibiotics consistently fared better in the postoperative period, although there was essentially no incidence of fever in either antibiotic or placebo groups.[12] Extrapolating from the data on perioperative prophylaxis in contaminated head and neck surgery, especially the more recent results using topical antibiotics, it seems reasonable to expect that posttonsillectomy morbidity could be reduced by 24 hours of antibiotics given as a liquid whereby patients are instructed to swish, gargle, and swallow. In addition, the oropharyngeal bacteria may be reduced dramatically by irrigating the tonsillar fossae intraoperatively with an antibiotic–containing solution. Further clinical trials are needed to address these issues.

CLEAN HEAD AND NECK SURGERY

The role of perioperative antibiotics in head and neck surgery that is not contaminated by secretions is somewhat more controversial. Surgery on the salivary glands is potentially contaminated via the ductal communication with the oral cavity. Nevertheless, the incidence of wound infections observed in patients operated upon without antibiotic prophylaxis suggests that little is to be gained through the use of antimicrobials.[13] Thyroidectomy is rarely contaminated by oral pharyngeal secretions. Infection rates observed are less than 2%, and most investigators concur that there does not exist an indication for antibiotic prophylaxis.[13]

In a study of patients undergoing cervical lymphadenectomy (neck dissection) in which contamination was not encountered, the infection rate observed among patients administered antibiotics (N = 100) was 3%, in contrast to patients who received no prophylaxis, in whom the observed infection rate was 9% (N = 100).[14] These differences reported in a retrospective study did not achieve statistical significance (p>.05). However, the risk that a statistically significant difference was not observed based upon lack of power in this study was significant ($\beta = .5$). The risk of wound infection in patients undergoing clean neck dissection is somewhat higher than the incidence of infection in patients undergoing other clean cervical procedures. This may reflect the well-known relationship between infection rate and duration of surgery.

COST

Wound infections are the single largest group of postoperative infectious complications of surgery. Mandell-Brown and colleagues[15] estimated the dollar cost of a wound infection subsequent to major head and neck surgery. Wound infection was associated with an average increase in length of stay by 14.7 days. This resulted in more than $10,000 per patient added cost (1984 dollars). Associated costs such as lost work, pain, and suffering are conjectural at best.

Administration of perioperative antibiotics contributes to the cost of hospitalization and surgical care. This cost reflects preparation and administration as well as the purchase cost of the chosen antibiotic. When deciding upon the proper antibiotic for prophylaxis, cost is an important factor. The antibiotic must provide the proper spectrum of coverage and have low toxicity, and in most cases a single agent is preferred over the use of multiple antibiotic agents.

A hidden cost built into the decision to use perioperative antibiotics is the possible development of resistant strains of bacteria. With the introduction of new antimicrobials, new forms of drug resistance have emerged. This problem is exacerbated by the widespread use of prophylactic antibiotics.

CURRENT RECOMMENDATIONS

Bacteriologic Spectrum

For a prophylactic antibiotic to be successful in preventing a postoperative wound infection, the organisms contaminating the wound at the time of operation must be targeted. In clean-contaminated head and neck oncologic procedures, the skin flora (predominantly *Staphylococcus aureus*) and group A beta-hemolytic streptococcus must be considered. In addition, the commensal microorganisms of the upper aerodigestive tract, which are found in saliva, must also be targeted. In the oropharyngeal secretions, anaerobic organisms are 10 times more common than aerobic organisms. The bacterial counts are 10^8–10^9/mL. These organisms colonize the tongue, teeth, and dental crevices. Among the organisms in the saliva are anaerobic species such as *Bacteroides melaninogenicus* and *Fusobacterium* species. Gram-positive aerobic organisms such as alpha streptococci also are found. Therefore, the principal organisms that must be targeted are gram-positive aerobes and anaerobes.

Gram-negative aerobic organisms are not usually present in the saliva of normal individuals. The bacterial spectrum found in secretions of the upper aerodigestive tract is affected by the presence of a necrotic tumor and other comorbid conditions. For instance, although gram-negative aerobic organisms are not usually found in the secretions of healthy individuals, among patients with necrotic upper aerodigestive tract tumors, *Klebsiella, Pseudomonas*, and *Proteus* are often present.[16] Patients hospitalized for extended periods also become colonized with pathogenic aerobic gram-negative organisms. Unfortunately, there is little correlation between the results of preoperative cultures and those obtained from infected wounds.[17, 18] Nevertheless, most postoperative wound infections are polymicrobial, containing both aerobic and anaerobic pathogens. The use of antibiotics that are specific to anaerobic organisms has been shown to decrease the incidence of postoperative wound infection in head and neck oncologic procedures. Rubin and colleagues[19] conducted a retrospective analysis of bacteria isolated following wound infection in 23 of 354 patients who participated in a series of clinical trials while undergoing major contaminated head and neck surgery. The microbiology of these infections was characterized as polymicrobial in 96% of cases. Aerobic bacteria were identified in 91% of patients, and anaerobic bacteria were identified in 74%. The identification of fungi from 48% of wounds was interpreted as colonization because infections resolved without antifungal therapy.

Choice of Drug

Normal saliva contains up to 100 million bacteria per cubic centimeter, 90% of which are anaerobic.[20] In most circumstances, the presence of aerobic gram-negative organisms is not expected. Patients receiving prior irradiation therapy to the upper aerodigestive tract and patients with prolonged hospitalization may be found to be colonized by aerobic gram-negative bacilli. Similarly, the presence of tracheotomy in excess of 10 days is associated with an 85% risk of colonization by *Pseudomonas*. Accordingly, patients presenting with histories of prior tracheotomy, prolonged hospitalization, or prior irradiation therapy may represent a special-risk group.

Preoperative, intraoperative, and postoperative wound cultures are relatively unreliable in predicting the bacteriology of subsequent wound infection. Becker and colleagues[21] report that only 35% of preoperative cultures were reflective of subsequent pathogenicity. In a subsequent study, Becker and Welch[22] reported poor correlation between the bacteria identified in closed suctioned drainage systems and the development of wound infection. The presence of bacteria in the drains did not predict infection. The species of bacteria cultured from the drain did not correlate closely with bacteriology of wound infection.

A wide array of antibiotics currently available may be effective in prevention of wound infection. Johnson and colleagues[8] at the University of Pittsburgh performed a series of prospective randomized trials of antibiotic prophylaxis. Only patients undergoing a major oncologic head and neck surgery that required transcervical approach to the upper aerodigestive tract were enrolled. All patients' wounds were closed at the completion of the surgery. Prior to randomization, patients were stratified for factors known to predispose to infection, including prior exposure to radiation therapy, stage of disease (stage I or II versus stage III or IV), and reconstructive technique (primary closure versus flap reconstruction). Wound infection was explicitly defined as development of a purulent collection underneath the cervical skin flap or development of a mucocutaneous fistula. Wound infection rates were remarkably similar for all antibiotics evaluated (Table 67–1). The number of patients accrued to each arm of the study was insufficient to detect minimal differences between these various antibiotics.

Other investigators have reported a variety of other successful antibiotic regimens in preventing postoperative wound infection in patients undergoing major head and neck surgical procedures. Robbins and colleagues[23] in a prospective randomized study demonstrated the efficacy of a combination of cefazolin plus Flagyl. Weber and colleagues[24] reported efficacy of ampicillin/sulbactam, and Johnson and colleagues[25] demonstrated clindamycin alone was as effective as clindamycin plus gentamicin. In contrast, Gerard and colleagues[26] reported a reduction in postoperative wound infection in patients receiving clindamicin plus amikacin when compared with ticarcillin/clavulanic acid. Direct comparison between studies is often difficult because of methodologic differences in terms of study population, surgical techniques, and outcomes assessment. A variety of agents have been documented to be effective.

Route of Administration

Intravenous administration of antibiotics for patients having surgery is the standard of care. Peak blood levels are achieved within 3–5 minutes. Antibiotics should be administered just prior to the induction of anesthesia or shortly thereafter. A second dose of antibiotics may be required in patients undergoing surgery that is longer than 4 hours.

Topical Antibiotics in Contaminated Head and Neck Surgery

Antibiotic prophylaxis for contaminated head and neck surgery has traditionally been administered intravenously. Because the development of a postoperative wound infection likely results from intraoperative salivary contamination of the wound, the efficacy of parenteral prophylaxis depends on the penetration of the systemically delivered medication from the blood stream into the tissues. In addition, there is some incidence of hypersensitivity reactions associated with intravenously administered antibiotics. Two studies in normal healthy volunteers demonstrated the efficacy of a single

dose of clindamycin mouthwash in reducing quantitative aerobic and anaerobic bacteriology in the oral cavity for up to 4 hours.[27, 28] It seemed biologically plausible, therefore, that eliminating the bacteria in the salivary secretions with a noningested antibiotic mouthwash would prevent postoperative wound infection in patients undergoing contaminated head and neck surgery.

To test this hypothesis, the authors have designed and completed a series of studies. Initially, we cultured four oral cavity sites and saliva to identify four indicator organisms (two aerobic and two anaerobic) for subsequent bacteriology. We then compared the effect on oral cavity bacteriology of the same antibiotic (clindamycin) given as a topical mouthwash or parenterally and found that whereas intravenous clindamycin had virtually no effect on oral cavity microbiology, a single dose of the same antibiotic given as a mouthwash virtually eliminated the aerobic and anaerobic bacteria for up to 8 hours.[29] A feasibility study was then completed in which 10 patients undergoing total laryngectomy plus neck dissection received topical perioperative antibiotic prophylaxis alone (a single dose of clindamycin [1.5 g] as mouthwash before and after surgery and intraoperative irrigation with a clindamycin-containing solution [900 mg in 1 liter]). No patient developed a wound infection; however, there was an overgrowth of *Haemophilus* species (not *Haemophilus influenzae*) in the oral cavity on postoperative days 3 and 4.[29]

To address the issues of antibiotic spectra as well as duration of prophylaxis, we then conducted a prospective randomized clinical trial in which 20 patients undergoing laryngectomy with or without neck dissection received one of the following: (1) parenteral clindamycin for 1 day (900 mg on call to the operating room and three doses postoperatively with intraoperative irrigation using saline); (2) topical clindamycin for 1 day (clindamycin mouthwash [1.5 g] given as an elixir preoperatively; patients were instructed to swish, gargle, and expectorate but not swallow; surgical wounds were irrigated with 900 mg of clindamycin in 1 L of saline; postoperatively, a single dose of clindamycin mouthwash was given); (3) topical clindamycin for 5 days (equivalent to regimen (2), except patients received a postoperative mouthwash once a day for 5 days); or (4) topical amoxicillin plus clavulanate/ticarcillin plus clavulanate (3.76 g of amoxicillin plus 927.5 mg of clavulanate elixir given once preoperatively and once postoperatively as a mouthwash; intraoperatively, wounds were irrigated with 3.1 g of ticarcillin/clavulanate in 1 L of saline).[30] No patient had a wound infection in the immediate postoperative period. One patient who received 5 days of topical clindamycin developed pneumonia on postoperative day 2, was treated successfully with parenteral antibiotic therapy, and subsequently developed a pharyngocutaneous fistula on postoperative day 14. Despite having more bacteria (aerobic and anaerobic) in their oral cavities preoperatively (by chance), the patients who received topical amoxicillin plus clavulanate/ticarcillin plus clavulanate had fewer bacteria in their neck intraoperatively compared with the other three treatment groups. In addition, the mean decrease in oral cavity bacteria (preoperative versus postoperative) was also greatest in these five patients. Despite our small sample size, the superior bacteriologic efficacy seen in the topical amoxicillin plus clavulanate/ticar-

Table 67–1. HEAD AND NECK SURGERY: 24 HOURS' PROPHYLAXIS

Antibiotic	Dose	Infection Rate
Cefazolin[35]	2 g every 8 hours	9%
Moxalactam[35]	2 g every 8 hours	6%
Clindamycin[25]	600 mg every 8 hours	3%
Cefoperazone[8]	2 g every 8 hours	10%
Cefotaxime[8]	2 g every 8 hours	9%

cillin groups suggests that topical prophylaxis using an agent(s) with activity against gram-negative aerobic bacilli may be advantageous.

The cumulative results of these studies have implications for the general field of surgical prophylaxis, suggesting that optimal antimicrobial efficacy is achieved not only by providing adequate concentrations of antibiotic in the tissues at the time of surgery but also by reducing the bacterial contamination of the wound. Studies are under way to quantitate the benefit of the addition of topical antibiotic prophylaxis to a standard parenteral regimen in patients with unusually high rates of postoperative wound infection (e.g., those undergoing reconstruction of their surgical defects with a pedicled or free flap).

Duration of Antibiotic Administration

The optimal duration throughout which the surgical patient should receive antibiotic prophylaxis remains contentious in the field of head and neck surgery, this being a unique situation. There is general agreement in the fields of general surgery, thoracic surgery, gynecology, and urology that antibiotic prophylaxis limited to the perioperative period (e.g., during and shortly after surgery) is as effective as prolonged administration of antibiotics in the prevention of postoperative wound infection. Nevertheless, many head and neck surgeons continue to administer antibiotics for days following head and neck surgery.

Prospective randomized clinical trials of patients undergoing major contaminated head and neck surgery have failed to document increased benefit to patients receiving antibiotics beyond the first perioperative day.[2, 31, 32, 33] Johnson and colleagues[32] conducted a prospective multi-institutional randomized trial of patients having major head and neck surgical procedures in which flap reconstruction was required. Of 109 patients randomized into the study, 53 were given 1 day of prophylactic antibiotics, and 56 received 5 days of prophylaxis. Wound infection was encountered in 19% of patients receiving prophylaxis for 1 day and 26% of patients receiving prophylaxis for 5 days. This difference was not statistically significant (p>.05). Furthermore, it suggests that there is little reason to suspect that prolonged administration of antibiotics results in further reduction in wound infection.

Carrau and colleagues[10] reported a retrospective study of patients having cranial base surgical procedures. A placebo group was not used. The lowest rate of wound infection was noted in the group of patients receiving prophylaxis for 48 hours. No benefit was demonstrated for patients receiving antibiotics for longer than 48 hours.

SYSTEMIC INFECTION FOLLOWING MAJOR HEAD AND NECK SURGERY

Pneumonia represents an important source of septic complications following many of the procedures performed on the upper aerodigestive tract. Conservation laryngeal procedures as well as surgery on the oral pharynx and oral cavity compromise the physiology of swallowing, thereby promoting the potential for aspiration. Not surprisingly, the incidence of postoperative aspiration pneumonia is high in patients in whom the swallowing mechanism is compromised by surgery. This is in sharp contrast to patients having total laryngectomy, which, of course, affords aerodigestive separation. The group of patients having laryngectomy rarely experiences postoperative pneumonia.

Aspiration pneumonia cannot be prevented by the administration of antibiotics. Aspiration of contaminated secretions may result in sepsis of the tracheal bronchial tree. Intractable aspiration in the face of antibiotic administration almost invariably results in pneumonia due to an organism resistant to the antibiotic being used. Weber and colleagues[34] noted among patients undergoing clean-contaminated head and neck cancer surgery that 24 of 225 patients (10.7%) developed distant-site infections. The most common nonwound or distant site of infection among these patients was pneumonia or tracheobronchitis. A logistic regression analysis of 25 variables thought to correlate with the risk of postoperative pulmonary infections demonstrated that a greater than 70-pack-a-year smoking history or transfusion of allogeneic blood was significantly associated with infection risk. Among patients who were not heavy smokers and did not require blood transfusions, the risk of a pulmonary infection following ablative surgery was 4% compared with 58% for those with the other profile. The majority of infections were caused by gram-negative aerobic organisms.

Prevention of pulmonary complications in aspiration-prone patients is a complex and multifaceted challenge. Insertion of a cuffed tracheotomy tube may reduce the volume of aspiration while permitting the nursing staff to assist the patient in the evacuation of aspirated secretions. The fact that tracheotomy potentiates aspiration must be acknowledged. It is well recognized that tracheotomy serves to tether the larynx and, with splinting due to perioperative pain, may potentiate aspiration through inadequate laryngeal elevation on swallowing. Furthermore, tracheotomy compromises the efficiency of the cough in clearing aspirated material.

Ambulatory patients with an intact cough mechanism can ordinarily resist minimal amounts of aspiration. Pulmonary physiotherapy (blow bottles, cupping and clapping, and deep breathing) may contribute to a patient's capacity to further resist the potential deleterious effects of aspiration.

Intractable life-threatening aspiration in spite of cuffed tracheotomy and outstanding nursing and pulmonary care may be considered indication for surgical aerodigestive separation. Alternatives include a laryngeal plug, laryngotracheal separation, or laryngectomy.

References

1. Communicable Disease Center; Public Health Service; U.S. Department of Health, Education and Welfare: Tetanus Surveillance, Report No. 1, February 1, 1968.
2. Piccart M, Klastersky J: Antimicrobial prophylaxis of infection in head and neck cancer surgery. Scand J Infect Dis 1983; 39: 92–96.
3. Dor P, Klastersky J: Prophylactic antibiotics in oral, pharyngeal and laryngeal surgery for cancer: A double-blind study. Laryngoscope 1973; 83: 1992–1998.
4. Seagle MB, Duberstein LE, Gross CW, et al.: Efficacy of cefazolin as a prophylactic antibiotic in head and neck surgery. Otolaryngol 1978; 86: 568–572.
5. Eschelman LT, Schleuning AJ, Brummett RE: Prophylactic antibiotics

in otolaryngologic surgery: A double-blind study. Trans Am Acad Ophthamol Otolaryngol 1971; 75: 387–394.

6. Saginus R, Odell PF, Poliquin JF: Antibiotic prophylaxis in head and neck cancer surgery. J Otolaryngol 1988; 17: 78–80.

7. Raine CH, Bartzokas CA, Stell PM, et al.: Chemoprophylaxis in major head and neck surgery. J R Soc Med 1984; 77: 1006–1009.

8. Johnson JT, Yu VL, Myers EN, et al.: Efficacy of two third-generation cephalosporins in prophylaxis for head and neck surgery. Arch Otolaryngol 1984; 110: 224–227.

9. Becker GD, Parell GJ: Cefazolin prophylaxis in head and neck cancer surgery. Ann Otol Rhinol Laryngol 1979; 88: 183–186.

10. Carrau RL, Snyderman C, Janecka IP, et al.: Antibiotic prophylaxis in cranial base surgery. Head Neck 1991; 13: 311–317.

11. Telian SA, Handler SD, Fleisher GR, et al.: The effect of antibiotic therapy on recovery after tonsillectomy in children. Arch Otolaryngol Head Neck Surg 1986; 112: 610–615.

12. Grandis JR, Johnson JT, Vickers RM, et al.: The efficacy of perioperative antibiotic therapy on recovery following tonsillectomy in adults: Randomized double-blind placebo-controlled trial. Otolaryngol Head Neck Surg 1992; 106: 137–142.

13. Johnson JT, Wagner RL: Infection following uncontaminated head and neck surgery. Arch Otolaryngol 1987; 113: 368–369.

14. Carrau RL, Byzakis J, Wagner RL, Johnson JT: Role of prophylactic antibiotics in uncontaminated neck dissections. Arch Otolaryngol Head Neck Surg 1991; 117: 194–195.

15. Mandell-Brown M, Johnson JT, Wagner RL: Cost-effectiveness of prophylactic antibiotics in head and neck surgery. Otolaryngol Head Neck Surg 1984; 92: 520–523.

16. Johanson WG, Pierce AK, Sanford JP: Changing pharyngeal bacterial flora of hospitalized patients: Emergence of gram-negative bacilli. N Engl J Med 1969; 281: 1137–1140.

17. Becker GD, Parell GJ, Busch DF, et al.: Anaerobic and aerobic bacteriology in head and neck cancer surgery. Arch Otolaryngol 1978; 104: 591–594.

18. Suarez Nieto C, Martin R, Mendez JC, Prendes P: Comparative studies of two systems of prophylactic antibiotics in head and neck surgery. Clin Otolaryngol 1981; 6: 159–164.

19. Rubin J, Johnson JT, Wagner RL, Yu VL: Bacteriology analysis of wound infection following major head and neck surgery. Arch Otolaryngol Head Neck Surg 1988; 114: 969–972.

20. Bartlett JG, Gorbach SL: Anaerobic infections of the head and neck. Otolaryngol Clin North Am 1976; 9: 655–678.

21. Becker GD, Parell CJ, Busch DF, et al.: The non-value of preoperative and intraoperative cultures in predicting the bacteriology of subsequent wound infection in patients undergoing major head and neck cancer surgery. Laryngoscope 1980; 90: 1933–1940.

22. Becker GD, Welch WD: Quantitative bacteriology of closed-suction wound drainage in contaminated surgery. Laryngoscope 1990; 100: 403–406.

23. Robbins KT, Byers RM, Cole R, et al.: Wound prophylaxis with metronidazole in head and neck surgical oncology. Laryngoscope 1988; 98: 803–806.

24. Weber RS, Raad I, Frankenthaler R, et al.: Ampicillin-sulbactam vs clindamycin in head and neck oncologic surgery: The need for gram-negative coverage. Arch Otolaryngol Head Neck Surg 1992; 118: 1159–1163.

25. Johnson JT, Yu VL, Myers EN, Wagner RL: An assessment of the need for gram-negative bacterial coverage in antibiotic prophylaxis for oncological head and neck surgery. J Infect Dis 1987; 115: 331.

26. Gerard M, Meunier F, Dor P, et al.: Antimicrobial prophylaxis for major head and neck surgery in cancer patients. Antimicrob Agents Chemother 1988; 32: 1557–1559.

27. Grandis JR, Vickers RM, Rihs JD, et al.: The efficacy of topical antibiotics prophylaxis for contaminated head and neck surgery. Laryngoscope 1994; 104: 719–724.

28. Kirchner JC, Edberg SC, Sasaki CT: The use of topical oral antibiotics in head and neck prophylaxis: Is it justified? Laryngoscope 1988; 98: 26–29.

29. Elledge ES, Whidden RF, Fraker JT, et al.: The effects of topical oral clindamycin antibiotic rinses on the bacterial content of saliva on healthy human subjects. Otolaryngol Head Neck Surg 1991; 105: 836–839.

30. Grandis JR, Vickers RM, Rihs JD, et al.: Efficacy of topical amoxicillin plus clavulanate/ticarcillin plus clavulanate and clindamycin in contaminated head and neck surgery: Effect of antibiotic spectra and duration of therapy. J Infect Dis 1994; 170: 729–732.

31. Fee WR, Glenn M, Handen C, Hopp ML: One day vs two days of prophylactic antibiotics in patients undergoing major head and neck surgery. Laryngoscope 1984; 94: 612.

32. Johnson JT, Schuller DE, Gluckman JL, et al.: Antibiotic prophylaxis in high risk head and neck surgery: one-day vs five-day therapy. Otolaryngol Head Neck Surg 1986; 95: 554–557.

33. Johnson JT, Myers EN, Thearle PB, et al.: Antimicrobial prophylaxis for contaminated head and neck surgery. Laryngoscope 1984; 94: 46–51.

34. Weber RS, Hankins P, Rosenbaum B, Raad I: Nonwound infections following head and neck oncologic surgery. Laryngoscope 1993; 103: 22–27.

35. Johnson JT, Yu VL, Myers EN, et al.: Cefazolin vs. moxalactam? Arch Otolaryngol Head Neck Surg 1986; 112: 151–153.

J. Anon
M. Rontal
J. Bernstein

CHAPTER SIXTY-EIGHT

Prophylaxis for Sinonasal Surgery

▼

Infection following nasal and/or sinus surgery may have a direct effect on the outcome of the surgical procedure. In the case of septoplasty and rhinoplasty, postoperative infection may lead to cosmetic as well as functional complications. Infection following sinus surgery, although rare, could lead to intracranial or orbital disaster. There are many explanations presented for the use of prophylactic antibiotics. This chapter presents a view of the studied and scientific reasons that guide the decision to use these drugs.

IMMUNOLOGY AND MICROBIOLOGY OF THE NOSE, SINUSES, AND NASOPHARYNX

The bacterial flora of the nasal cavity and nasopharynx is controlled by a number of factors, including the local mucosal immune system and the microecologic interaction among the normal commensal organisms (including gram-positive bacteria such as *Streptococcus viridans*) and potential pathogens (nontypable *Haemophilus influenzae*, *Streptococcus pneumoniae*, and *Moraxella catarrhalis*).[1] In addition, nonimmunologic factors such as the mucociliary system, lysozyme, and lactoferrin are also extremely efficient in maintaining normal bacterial flora in the nose and nasopharynx.[2] The rhinologic surgeon must consider these nonspecific and specific mechanisms as well as constitutive and induced defense mechanisms that the nasal and nasopharyngeal mucosal barriers develop after encountering a bacterium.

This chapter presents an overview of the ecologic and immunologic control mechanisms of the upper respiratory tract flora. Table 68–1 summarizes some of the defense mechanisms of the mucosal surface of the nose that are available to the host in the maintenance of normal nasal and nasopharyngeal flora.

HOST DEFENSES AGAINST MUCOSAL COLONIZATION

Mucosal surfaces have several mechanisms that prevent bacterial colonization and penetration. Host mechanical defenses, including nonspecific mechanisms, serve as barriers that are effective against most bacteria. These mechanisms include the sweeping actions of the ciliated epithelium, which remove bacteria trapped in mucus and thereby decrease the interactions of the bacteria with host cell surfaces.

The resident flora, especially that in the upper respiratory tract (for example, *S. viridans*), plays a large role in inhibiting colonization by potential incoming pathogens as well as by potential pathogens that make up part of the normal flora in most healthy patients. Microbial antagonism or bacterial interference by the resident flora can work in several ways. For example, normal flora may prevent adherence by occupying the same receptor sites that pathogens adhere to, or competition for nutrients and production of antimicrobial metabolites by indigenous microorganisms may prevent establishment of potential pathogens in the nasal cavity and nasopharynx.

The host has a plethora of other defenses to protect mucosal surfaces. These include cellular defenses such as resident macrophages and polymorphonuclear leukocytes. In addition, several antibacterial substances are secreted by the host onto mucosal surfaces; these include secretory immunoglobulin A (IgA), lysozyme, lactoferrin, and other antimicrobial peptides.

Bacteria that succeed in reaching and adhering to mucosal cells have to cope with another characteristic feature of mucous membranes: the rapid turnover of mucosal cells. In fact, mucosal cells are among the most rapidly dividing populations of cells in the body and are constantly being produced and released from the membrane. This process is best understood, of course, in the intestine, where mucosal cells are born in depressions called crypts, move up the villi toward the lumen, and are released into the lumen as cells move up behind them and replace them. Bacteria that manage to attach themselves to mucosal cells are eventually expelled from the membrane as the cells are released; the bacteria must therefore be able to divide and reattach rapidly to remain at the site.

Table 68–1. DEFENSES AND MUCOSAL SURFACES

Site	Defenses	Functions
Mucosal surface	Mucin layer	Physical barrier Trap bacteria
Mucous layer	Lysozyme	Digests bacterial peptidoglycans
	Secretory IgA	Prevents bacterial attachment to mucosal cells; helps to trap bacteria in mucin
	Lactoferrin	Binds iron; prevents bacterial growth
	Lactoperoxidase	Kills bacteria by generating toxic superoxide radicals
Mucous membrane	Sloughing cells	Removes adherent bacteria
	Tight junctions	Prevents bacteria from invading between mucosal cells
Beneath mucosal membrane	Mucosa-associated tissue (adenoid)	Produces secretory IgA; phagocytic cells kill bacteria

Bacteria that do manage to colonize a surface of the nasal mucous membrane are prevented from passing through this membrane by tight junctions between the mucosal cells. These junctions, which are made by specialized proteins that connect adjacent cells, may even prevent water in small molecules from passing through them. Few, if any, bacteria are capable of disrupting these tight junctions and crossing the membrane.

Finally, perhaps the most important part of the local defense in the nasal cavity and nasopharynx is the mucus-associated lymphoid tissue, the presence of which is especially pronounced in the adenoidal tissue in the nasopharynx.

The cellular components and activities of the mucosa-associated lymphoid tissue in the nose and nasopharynx are illustrated in Figure 68–1. Briefly, the tonsil and adenoids are capable of producing J chain–positive B cells, which can seed the salivary glands, the lacrimal gland, and the nasal mucosa, or the middle ear when inflammation occurs there.[3]

The most important immunoglobulin produced by the nasal mucosa is secretory IgA, the primary function of which is to prevent adsorption of viruses and bacteria to epithelial surfaces by increasing the hydrophilicity of the bacterial organism.[4] Secretory IgA may also act as a blocking antibody in that it is anti-inflammatory and prevents fixation of complement and therefore influx of inflammatory cells such as neutrophils.

IgA-producing immunocytes represent about 70% of the cells around the seromucinous glands in the nasal mucosa.[5]

The overuse or misuse of antibiotics may compromise the normal microecology of the nasopharynx and nasal cavity by destroying the commensal organisms or the so-called normal flora such as *S. viridans*. A number of investigators have demonstrated that *S. viridans* is capable of inhibiting the colonization and proliferation of *Staphylococcus aureus*,[6] nontypable *Haemophilus influenzae*,[7] *S. pneumoniae*,[8] and beta-hemolytic streptococci.[9] Thus, *S. viridans* is capable of preventing the colonization and replication of those pathogens that are responsible for the development of sinusitis, otitis media, and lower respiratory tract infection such as chronic bronchitis and pneumonia.

The local immune mechanism provided by secretory IgA and the nonimmunologic defenses present in the nasal mucus, such as lactoferrin, lysozyme, and the normal mucociliary system, are quite capable of defending the nose and nasopharynx from potential pathogens. Furthermore, the specific local immune system represented by secretory IgA and secreted IgG are capable of neutralizing most toxins, viruses, and bacteria that might gain entry into the nasal cavity. Thus, the rhinologic surgeon must consider the normal host immune mechanisms prior to the use of antibiotics, which may not only alter the normal flora but may also lead to the emergence of potentially resistant bacteria, both in the host and in those in contact with the patient.

SEPTAL AND RHINOPLASTY SURGERY

A review of the literature shows that antibiotic prophylaxis is not necessary for routine septal and rhinoplasty surgery.

Strong[10] looked prospectively at 40 patients who underwent submucous resection or rhinoplasty. Prophylactic antibiotics were not used, and there were no postoperative infections.

Perioperative antibiotic prophylaxis for patients undergoing nasal surgery is probably unnecessary. Eschelman and colleagues[11] in a prospective randomized placebo-controlled study found that the incidence of postoperative infectious complications was similar in all study groups. Weimert and Yoder[12] analyzed 305 patients having septoplasty or septorhinoplasty. Five minor infections (1.6%) were encountered. A subsequent prospective randomized placebo-controlled trial showed no advantage for patients receiving antibiotic prophylaxis.

Fifty-two patients undergoing rhinoplasty (without septoplasty) were studied by Slavin and colleagues.[13] The organisms identified in preoperative nasal smears and their incidence were *Staphylococcus epidermidis*, 83%; *S. aureus*, 23%; *S. viridans*, 17%; and *Enterobacter*, 4%. None of the patients received perioperative antibiotics. Blood cultures drawn preoperatively, intraoperatively, and immediately postoperatively were evaluated. Only one postoperative culture grew *S. epidermidis*, and this was thought to represent contamination. There were no local or systemic infections. The authors thus questioned the use of perioperative antibiotics for rhinoplasty surgery.

In a follow-up to an earlier article, Krizek and colleagues[14] analyzed the results of a survey of 1718 plastic surgeons in the United States and Canada. They found that prophylactic antibiotics were almost always used during rhinoplasty by 25% of respondents. Rhinoplasty with a cartilage graft led to antibiotic use by 50%, and when alloplastic material was used, 74% almost always used prophylactic antibiotics. Interestingly, the authors reported that many of those surveyed said that their use of antibiotics was motivated by the medicolegal climate rather than by scientific justification.

Silk and colleagues[15] studied 50 patients who had septal surgery. Preoperative nasal swabs of these patients showed that 46% had *S. aureus*. During surgery, blood cultures were obtained, and there was no evidence of bacteremia. The authors concluded that there was no evidence to support the use of prophylactic antibiotics.

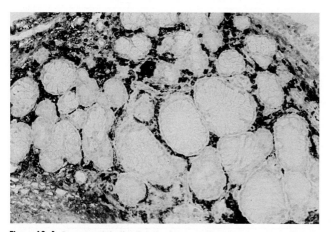

Figure 68–1. Immunoglobulin (Ig) A plasma cells are seen surrounding the seromucinous glands in the laminal propria of the inferior turbinate of the nose. IgG was not present in these areas. IgA is the predominant immunoglobulin in the nasal mucosa. Immunoperoxidase stain is ×200.

Yoder and Weimert[16] updated their previous work by studying 1040 patients who underwent septoplasty and/or rhinoplasty procedures. None of these patients received prophylactic antibiotics, and no topical surgical preparations were used. Only five patients developed minor postoperative infections (incidence: 0.5%).

To be sure, there are scattered reports in the literature of cases of infections associated with routine septal/rhinologic surgery, including septic cavernous sinus thrombosis,[17] staphylococcal endocarditis,[18] and staphylococcal spinal osteomyelitis.[19] As Cohen and colleagues[19] point out, however, there is no evidence that these infections can be prevented by perioperative antibiotics, and the general consensus remains that prophylactic antibiotics are not recommended for this type of surgery.

ENDOSCOPIC SINUS SURGERY

No studies could be found to support the use of antibiotics in surgery for chronic sinusitis.[20]

TOXIC SHOCK SYNDROME

First recognized in 1978, toxic shock syndrome (TSS) was initially thought to be associated only with women using superabsorbent tampons.[21] Subsequent reports found this syndrome in a variety of situations, including nasal surgery, and it is now well described in association with nasal procedures.

TSS, in its full presentation, is characterized by fever, rash, hypotension, desquamation, and multisystem organ involvement. The full presentation of TSS is not necessary to make a diagnosis. Table 68–2 shows the entire picture of this condition; according to the Centers for Disease Control and Prevention (CDC), four of the major criteria must be present and three of the minor findings.

Symptomatically, there appears to be a delay of 24–48 hours before the condition begins to manifest itself. The onset is usually characterized by sepsis, fever, nausea and vomiting, multiple organ involvement, hypotension, and a macular rash. Skin desquamation in sheets follows 1–2 weeks later.

Several reports have been published that associate TSS with nasal packing.[22] It was initially thought that the packing had to be porous (e.g., gauze packing),[23] but the condition has been reported with latex-covered packing,[24] with nonporous nasal splints, and with tight and loose packing.[20] TSS has also been reported after functional endoscopic surgery in which only light packing was used. In addition, TSS has been found without the presence of packing—after submandibular gland excision,[25] breast surgery,[26] lipectomy,[27] and burns. It has also been associated with influenza.

The incidence of TSS was as high as 16 per 100,000 in the mid-1980s but has now dropped to less than 1 per 100,000.

The one factor that underlies all these situations is the presence of *S. aureus* that produces the toxic shock syndrome toxin 1 enterotoxin.[28] It is the preformed toxin that produces the syndrome and not necessarily the actual infection with this organism. *S. aureus* may be colonizing only

Table 68–2. CDC CRITERIA FOR TOXIC SHOCK SYNDROME

The Following Must Be Present:

Fever:	>38.9° C
Rash:	Diffuse macular erythroderma
Desquamation:	1–2 weeks after onset of illness, particularly of palms and soles
Hypotension:	Systolic blood pressure <90 mm Hg for adults or below fifth percentile by age for children under 16 years. Orthostatic drop in diastolic blood pressure >15 mm Hg from lying to sitting, orthostatic syncope, or orthostatic dizziness.

Three or More of the Following Must Be Present:

Gastrointestinal:	Vomiting or diarrhea at onset of illness
Muscular:	Severe myalgia or creatine phosphatase level at least twice upper limit of normal
Mucous membranes:	Vaginal, oropharyngeal, or conjunctival hyperemia
Renal:	Blood urea nitrogen or creatinine at least twice upper limit of normal or urinary sediment with pyuria in absence of urinary trace infection
Hepatic:	Total bilirubin, aspartate aminotransferase, or alanine aminotransferase at least twice upper limit of normal
Hematologic:	Platelets <100,000
Central nervous system:	Disorientation or alteration in consciousness without focal neurologic signs when fever and hypotension are absent
Serology:	Negative serologic tests for Rocky Mountain spotted fever, leptospirosis, and measles

From Abram AC, Bellian KT, Giles WJ, et al: Toxic shock syndrome after functional sinus surgery: An all-or-none phenomenon. Laryngoscope 1994; 104: 927–931.

the mucous membranes of the nose, with the toxin entering through disturbed mucous membranes.[20] There may be only minimal signs of inflammation; thus, in all patients suspected of having toxic shock syndrome the surgical site should be cultured.

Thirty-five percent of the general population with rhinosinusitis are carriers of *S. aureus*. Health-care workers are well recognized as carriers—50% of physicians, 70% of nurses, and 90% of hospital attendants. In one study, 30% of patients electing to have nasal surgery were carriers, and 40% of those tested positive for the toxin producing *Staphylococcus*.[29] Approximately 7% of the population carry the toxin producing *S. aureus*. Individuals who are chronic carriers of the toxin producing *S. aureus* appear to produce an antibody to the toxin (TSA).[30] In a burn unit, a nurse who appeared to have transmitted the organism to three patients had a low titer of TSA during the transmission period, but when her TSA titer rose, there were no further cases.[31]

The treatment[20, 21] consists of the rapid removal of any obstruction to the clearance of the nasal cavities (packs, splints, or implants) and thorough cleansing of the nose or nasal cavities. Antistaphylococcal antibiotics that are active against penicillinase-producing forms are necessary. Corticosteroids are useful if given early. Support of the hypotensive symptoms and multiorgan manifestations is given. As antibody to the toxin is rare in most patients, gamma globulin may be used for severely ill patients. This syndrome usually resolves with only occasional sequelae. There is a reported 7% prevalence of death due to multiple-organ failure.

It appears that there is no prophylaxis for this condition.[31]

A systemic antibiotic does not seem appropriate. Indeed, a study of prophylaxis for toxic shock by the administration of systemic antibiotics was shown not to prevent TSS. The only antistaphylococcal antibiotic that enters the nasal mucus is rifampin.[20] Topical antibiotics have been tried with mixed results.[31] It is interesting that polymyxin binds the toxin; thus, theoretically, use of this antibiotic on any packing would be helpful. Derkay and colleagues[32] has shown that soaking the packing material in cephalosporin antibiotic reduces the bacteria in the packing and is conjectured to decrease the incidence of TSS. Other local antibiotics on the packing material are also advantageous (e.g., water-miscible 2% mupirocin).

There is no scientifically proven means of preventing TSS. It is these authors' opinion that some measures make sense. Thorough preoperative cleaning of the nasal vestibule is essential to remove colonizing bacteria. Postoperatively, early removal of packing is logical. As the organism colonizes the mucus blanket of the nose, washing of the area with saline appears to decrease the presence of toxin-producing bacteria.

CEREBROSPINAL FLUID RHINORRHEA

Cerebrospinal fluid (CSF) rhinorrhea may be spontaneous or traumatic. Traumatic CSF rhinorrhea is easier to diagnose, as a great amount of suspicion is maintained by the treating physician. Spontaneous CSF leaks may not be diagnosed until after the patient has actually had meningitis. The repair of a CSF fistula may be performed through either an intracranial or, preferably, an extracranial approach, most recently using the sinus endoscope.

The use of prophylactic antibiotics as part of the treatment regimen for this disorder is controversial. MacGee and colleagues[33] reviewed the charts for 58 posttraumatic CSF leaks. Twenty-three of these patients had CSF rhinorrhea, and 35 had CSF otorrhea. The data showed no significant difference between the patients treated with prophylactic antibiotics and the group that did not receive antibiotics.

The topic of prophylactic antibiotics for basilar skull fractures was addressed in a prospective study of 129 patients by Ignelzi and Vanderark.[34] The CSF rhinorrhea group consisted of 8 treated and 10 untreated patients. None of the patients treated with antibiotics developed infection, but three of the patients with CSF rhinorrhea on antibiotics developed a central nervous system infection. This study showed that prophylactic antibiotics do not favorably alter a patient's course of recovery and, indeed, use of antibiotics may actually lead to more serious infection by resistant organisms.

In a study of 168 basilar skull fractures, Dagi and colleagues[35] identified 18 patients with CSF rhinorrhea. Thirteen of these patients had received prophylactic antibiotics and had no infectious sequelae, whereas two of the five patients not treated developed meningitis. The authors felt that prophylactic antibiotics for CSF rhinorrhea "may prove to be effective" but that the number of patients with CSF fistula was too small to make a judgment regarding the role of antibiotics.

Stankiewicz[36] reported on the endoscopic management of

CSF rhinorrhea in eight patients. All patients had successful surgery. Antibiotics were not used, and the author cautioned that antibiotics are not needed and that their indiscriminate use may actually be harmful.

A retrospective study of 215 patients by Eljamel[37] revealed that 106 had received prophylactic antibiotics and 109 had not. Eljamel's data supported the findings from his literature review: that prophylactic antibiotics do not prevent meningitis in either the early or late phases of a CSF leak. Eljamel also pointed out that antibiotics affect the normal microflora of the nasopharynx and that more resistant organisms may be selected out.

De Louvis and colleagues[38] discussed that even though meningitis after head injury with accompanying CSF leak occurs in 11%–25% of patients (mainly as a result of pneumococcal infection) prophylactic antibiotics are not recommended. These authors feel that the use of prophylactic antibiotics may lead to the growth of resistant organisms. They concluded that these patients should be closely monitored for developing signs of meningitis.

Many reports on the repair of CSF rhinorrhea indicate that controversy exists, but the reports do not address the question in a scientific manner. In general, most of the modern studies that do address this subject show that antibiotics do not play a major role in reducing the risk of meningitis.

References

1. Bernstein JM, Altaie S, Dryja D, et al.: Bacterial interference in nasopharyngeal flora of otitis-prone and non-otitis prone children. Acta Otorhinolaryngol Belg 1994; 48: 1–9.
2. Brandtzaeg P: Immune functions of human nasal mucosa and tonsils in health and disease. In: Bienstock J (ed): Immunology of the Lung and Respiratory Tract. New York: McGraw Hill, 1984, pp 28–95.
3. Nadal D, Soh N, Schlapfer AE, et al.: Distribution characteristics of immunoglobulin secreting cells in adenoids: Relationship to age and disease, Int J Pediatr Otolaryngol 1992; 24: 121–130.
4. van Oss CJ, Gillman CF, Neumann AW: Phagocytic Engulfment and Cell Adhesiveness as Cellular Surface Phenomenon. New York: Marcell Dekker, Inc., 1975.
5. Brandtzaeg P: Humoral immune response patterns of human mucosae: Induction and relation to bacterial respiratory tract infections. J Infect Dis 1992; 165: S165–S176.
6. Shinefield HR, Ribble JC, Boris M, Eichenwald HF: Bacterial interference in the *Staphylococci*. In: Cohen JO (ed): The Staphylococci. New York: Wiley Interscience, 1972, p 503.
7. Bernstein JM, Faden HF, Dryja DM, Wactawski-Wende J: Microecology of the nasopharyngeal bacterial flora in otitis-prone and non–otitis-prone children. Acta Otolaryngol (Stock)Supp 1992; 112: 1–7.
8. Johanson WG, Blackstock R, Pierce AK, Sanford JP: The role of bacterial antagonism in pneumococcal colonization of the human pharynx, J Lab Clin Med 1970; 75: 946–952.
9. Sanders EF: Bacterial interference: Its occurrence among the respiratory tract flora and characterization of inhibition of group A streptococci by viridans streptococci. J Infect Dis 1969; 120: 698–707.
10. Strong MS: Wound infection in otolaryngic surgery and the inexpediency of antibiotic prophylaxis. Laryngoscope 1963; 73: 165–184.
11. Eschelman LT, Schleuning AJ, Brummett RE: Prophylactic antibiotics in otolaryngologic surgery: A double-blind study. Trans Am Acad Ophthalmol Otolaryngol 1971; 75: 387–394.
12. Weimert TA, Yoder MG: Antibiotics and nasal surgery. Laryngoscopy 1980; 90: 667–671.
13. Slavin SA, Rees TD, Guy CL, Goldwyn RM: An investigation of bacteremia during rhinoplasty. Plast Reconstr Surg 1983; 71: 196–198.
14. Krizek TJ, Gottlieb LJ, Koss N, Robson MC: The use of prophylactic

antibacterials in plastic surgery: A 1980s update. Plast Reconstr Surg 1985; 76: 953–963.

15. Silk KL, Ali MB, Cohen BJ, et al.: Absence of bacteremia during nasal septoplasty Arch Otolaryngol Head Neck Surg 1991; 117: 54–55.

16. Yoder MG, Weimert TA: Antibiotics and topical surgical preparation solution in septal surgery. Otolaryngol Head Neck Surg 1992; 106: 243–244.

17. Casaubon JN, Dion MA, Larbrisseau A: Septic cavernous sinus thrombosis after rhinoplasty. Plast Reconstr Surg 1977; 59: 119–123.

18. Coursey DL: Staphylococcal endocarditis following septorhinoplasty. Arch Otolaryngol 1974; 99: 454–455.

19. Cohen BJ, Johnson JD, Raff MJ: Septoplasty complicated by staphylococcal spinal osteomyelitis. Arch Intern Med 1985; 145: 556–557.

20. Abram AC, Bellian KT, Giles WJ, Gross CW: Toxic shock syndrome after functional sinus surgery: An all-or-none phenomenon. Laryngoscope 1994; 104: 927–931.

21. Schlievert PM, MacDonald KC: Toxic shock syndrome. In: Gorback SL, Bartlett JC, Blacklow NR (eds): Infectious Disease. Philadelphia: WB Saunders Co., 1990, pp 889–894.

22. Huang IT, Podkomorska D, Murphy MN, Hoffer I: Toxic shock syndrome following septoplasty and partial turbinectomy, J Otolaryngol 1986; 15: 310–312.

23. Allen ST, Liland JB, Nichols CG, Glew RH: Toxic shock syndrome associated with use of latex nasal packing. Arch Intern Med 1990; 150: 2587–2588.

24. Wagner R, Toback JM: Toxic shock syndrome following septoplasty using plastic septal splints. Laryngoscope 1986; 96: 609–610.

25. Fornadley JA, Gomaz PJ, Crane RT, Rickman LS: Toxic shock syndrome following submandibular gland excision. Head Neck 1990; 12: 66–68.

26. Tobin G, Shaw RC, Goodpasture HC: Toxic shock syndrome following breast and nasal surgery. Plast Reconstr Surg 1987; 80: 111–114.

27. Rhee CA, Smith RJ, Jackson IT: Toxic shock syndrome associated with suction assisted lipectomy. Aesthetic Plast Surg 1994; 18: 161–163.

28. Cone LA, Woodard DR, Byrd RG, et al.: *Staphylococcus aureus* nasal carriage in patients with rhinosinusitis. Laryngoscope 1991; 101: 733–737.

29. Arnow PM, Chou T, Weil D, et al.: Spread of a toxic shock syndrome associated strain of *Staphylococcus aureus* and measurement of antibodies to staphylococcal enterotoxin F. J Infect Dis 1984; 149: 103–107.

30. Chow AW, Wong CK, MacFarlane AM, Bartlett KH: Toxic shock syndrome: Clinical and laboratory findings in 30 patients. Can Med Assoc J 1984; 130: 425–430.

31. Ritz HL, Kirkland JJ, Bond GG, et al.: Association of high levels of serum antibody to staphylococcal toxic shock antigen with nasal carriage of toxic shock antigen-producing strains of *Staphylococcus aureus*. Infect Immun 1984; 43: 954–958.

32. Derkay CS, Hirsch BE, Johnston JT, Wagner RL: Posterior packing: Are intravenous antibiotics really necessary? Arch Otolaryngol 1989; 115: 439–441.

33. MacGee EE, Cauthen JC, Brackett CE: Meningitis following acute traumatic cerebrospinal fluid fistula. J Neurosurg 1970; 33: 312–316.

34. Ignelzi RJ, Vanderark GD: Analysis of the treatment of basilar skull fractures with and without antibiotics. J Neurosurg 1975; 43: 721–726.

35. Dagi TF, Meyer FB, Poletti CA: The incidence and prevention of meningitis after basilar skull fracture. Am J Emerg Med 1983; 3: 295–298.

36. Stankiewicz JA: Cerebrospinal fluid fistula and endoscopic sinus surgery. Laryngoscope 1991; 101: 250–256.

37. Eljamel MS: Antibiotic prophylaxis in unrepaired CSF fistulae. Br J Neurosurg 1993; 7: 501–505.

38. de Louvis J, Brown EM, Bayston R: Antimicrobial prophylaxis in neurosurgery and after head injury. Lancet 1994; 344: 1547–1551.

CHAPTER SIXTY-NINE   Matthew E. Levison

Prophylaxis for Bacterial Endocarditis

▼

Infective endocarditis is a uniformly fatal disease if untreated and still carries considerable morbidity and mortality even when treated appropriately. The American Heart Association (AHA) has published recommendations for its prevention by antimicrobial prophylaxis; the most recent revision of these guidelines appeared in 1990.[1] Because of the low incidence of infective endocarditis following a medical or dental procedure, there has been no prospective controlled trial proving the effectiveness of antimicrobial prophylaxis. Therefore, the AHA recommendations should be taken only as guidelines that must be individualized for each specific clinical situation. Nevertheless, prevention of endocarditis clearly represents the accepted standard of practice, and all practicing physicians should be knowledgeable about these guidelines and their underlying concepts and assumptions.

The following sequence of events is thought to result in endocarditis:[2]

1. Certain types of congenital or acquired heart disease result in a high-velocity jet stream from a high- to low-pressure chamber or across a narrowed orifice, which leads to turbulent blood flow distal to the pressure gradient, and thereby to damage to the valvular and endocardial endothelium in a predictable pattern distal to the pressure gradient.

2. Platelets deposit on the surface of the damaged endothelium, degranulate, and stimulate local deposition of fibrin. As a result of this process, a sterile thrombus is formed on the endothelial surface, the so-called nonbacterial thrombotic endocarditis.

3. Nonbacterial thrombotic endocarditis is the point of attachment and subsequent proliferation for certain microorganisms, once these microorganisms have gained access to the circulation.

4. Trauma to mucosal surfaces that are normally laden with microorganisms releases these organisms into the blood stream, and some of these organisms are capable of causing infective endocarditis.

Prevention of endocarditis requires the following:

1. Identifying patients with predisposing cardiac lesions and assigning relative risk of endocarditis to the cardiac lesion.

2. Identifying procedures likely to cause bacteremia.

3. Determining organisms likely to be found in the blood stream and their likely antimicrobial susceptibilities.

4. Reducing the frequency and intensity of the bacteremia by appropriately timed administration of antimicrobial agents.

5. Reducing the adherence and proliferation of organisms on the damaged endothelium.

IDENTIFYING PATIENTS WITH PREDISPOSING CARDIAC LESIONS

Preexisting cardiac lesions that are believed to promote the formation of nonbacterial thrombotic endocarditis can be identified in about two thirds of patients with infective endocarditis. The level of risk varies with the nature of the underlying cardiac lesion and can be determined by the incidence of endocarditis in the population of people having the particular cardiac lesion.[3] Risk can be also assessed by the frequency with which the cardiac lesion occurs in a large series of patients with endocarditis as compared with the general population. Although precise data are lacking for all cardiac lesions, cardiac lesions can be divided into those that place patients at risk of endocarditis and those that do not (Table 69–1[1]).

Antimicrobial prophylaxis is recommended for those cardiac lesions that place patients at risk of endocarditis, espe-

Table 69–1. CARDIAC CONDITIONS

Endocarditis Prophylaxis Recommended

Prosthetic cardiac valves, including bioprosthetic and homograft valves
Previous bacterial endocarditis, even in the absence of heart disease
Most congenital cardiac malformations
Rheumatic and other acquired valvular dysfunction, even after valvular surgery
Hypertrophic cardiomyopathy
Mitral valve prolapse with valvular regurgitation

Endocarditis Prophylaxis Not Recommended

Isolated secundum atrial septal defect
Surgical repair without residua beyond 6 months of secundum atrial septal defect, ventricular septal defect, or patent ductus arteriosus
Previous coronary artery bypass graft surgery
Mitral valve prolapse without valvular regurgitation*
Physiologic, functional, or innocent heart murmurs
Previous Kawasaki disease without valvular dysfunction
Previous rheumatic fever without valvular dysfunction
Cardiac pacemakers and implanted defibrillators

From Dajani AS, Bisno AL, Kyung JC, et al.: Prevention of bacterial endocarditis: Recommendations by the American Heart Association. JAMA 1990; 264: 2919–2922. Copyright 1990, American Medical Association.
This table lists selective conditions but is not meant to be all-inclusive.
*Individuals who have a mitral valve prolapse associated with thickening and/or redundancy of the valve leaflets may be at increased risk for bacterial endocarditis, particularly men who are 45 years of age or older.

cially prosthetic cardiac valves, prior endocarditis, or surgically constructed systemic-pulmonary shunts or conduits. Prosthetic cardiac valves are the major risk factor for endocarditis. Mechanical prosthetic cardiac valves probably have about the same risk as bioprostheses (e.g., porcine heterografts). Risk probably does not vary by site of prosthetic valve replacement, but it is greatest during the first few postoperative months. Endocarditis that occurs during this early postoperative period probably results from contamination during the intraoperative and perioperative period. Prior native valve endocarditis also poses a significant risk for subsequent episodes of endocarditis as a consequence of both the continued presence of the risk factors that contributed to the initial episode (e.g., intravenous drug use or periodontitis) plus the additional risk posed by the damage to the valve sustained in the initial episode of endocarditis. Rheumatic heart disease is another risk factor for endocarditis, with an incidence rate only slightly lower than that of prosthetic valves. Most uncorrected congenital abnormalities of the heart and great vessels are also high risk factors. As a general rule, cardiac lesions not associated with turbulent blood flow, such as cardiac lesions in a relatively low pressure system (e.g., on the right side of the heart) or abnormal flow through a wide orifice (e.g., secundum type of atrial septal defect), are less likely to be complicated by endocarditis. Although the AHA does not recommend preventive antibiotic therapy for patients who have no residual hemodynamic abnormalities more than 6 months after surgical correction of their congenital defect, surgical correction of the congenital defects, such as a ventricular septal defect, lowers but does not eliminate risk.

Because of its high prevalence in the population, estimated to be 2%–21%, mitral valve prolapse is the most frequent lesion predisposing to endocarditis. Men with mitral valve prolapse who are older than 45 years are at relatively greater risk. However, the absolute risk for endocarditis among patients with mitral valve prolapse and an audible murmur of mitral insufficiency is considerably lower than that of other cardiac abnormalities, and indeed mitral valve prolapse without mitral insufficiency poses a minimal risk. Echocardiography has identified mitral valve thickening and redundancy as a risk for endocarditis. Use of echocardiography to detect the presence of these findings or mitral valvular insufficiency in the absence of an audible murmur is not cost-effective or convenient, so that in everyday practice the decision for prophylaxis with mitral valve prolapse has relied on detection of an audible systolic murmur. Kaye and Abrutyn[4] have recommended that for a holosystolic murmur prophylaxis be given; for either spontaneous or evoked late systolic murmur, prophylaxis is optional; and for no murmur, prophylaxis is not given. Similarly, degenerative valvular lesions in elderly patients are common in the general population and in patients with endocarditis. Prophylaxis is given if there is clinical or echocardiographic (if available) evidence of significant valvular dysfunction. Other cardiac lesions that rarely predispose to endocarditis are shown in Table 69–1.[1] Endocarditis can occur on structurally normal native valves in 25% or more of patients. In these patients, endocarditis is more likely to be nosocomial, caused by more virulent organisms such as *Staphylococcus aureus,* or the patient is more likely to be an intravenous drug user.

CIRCUMSTANCES LEADING TO TRANSIENT BACTEREMIA

Transient bacteremia is a common event and occurs as a consequence of trauma to skin or mucosal surfaces that are normally laden with an endogenous flora. Mucosal sites that have a dense endogenous flora include the gingival crevice, oropharynx, terminal ileum and colon, and distal urethra and vagina. The bacteremia is characterized by a low number of organisms/mL of blood (usually <10 colony-forming U/mL) and very short duration (15–30 minutes). The intensity of the bacteremia is related directly to the magnitude of the trauma, the density of the microbial flora, and the presence of inflammation or infection at the site of skin or mucosal injury. Minor trauma to the gingival crevice as routine as that resulting from brushing teeth or chewing hard candy causes bacteremia that usually is asymptomatic because of the small numbers of relatively avirulent organisms involved. However, the cumulative risk of these transient episodes of low-grade bacteremia probably accounts in large part for the 75% of patients with viridans streptococcal endocarditis who fail to recall any medical or dental procedure that preceded the onset of their endocarditis.

Antimicrobial prophylaxis is feasible only if the occurrence of bacteremia is predictable. Indeed, dental procedures that are extensive enough to be associated with bleeding (e.g., dental extractions and periodontal care) cause bacteremia in up to 90% of patients.[5] A history of medical and dental procedures known to predispose to transient bacteremia is obtained in about 25% of patients with viridans streptococcal endocarditis, and dental extraction is the most frequent procedure temporally associated with nonenterococcal endocarditis. Similarly, certain ear, nose, and throat procedures (Table 69–2[1]) also predictably result in low-grade bacteremia, and endocarditis has been reported to be temporally related to these procedures, although a causal relationship cannot be proved in any particular case. These procedures include tonsillectomy, adenoidectomy, surgical

Table 69–2. DENTAL OR SURGICAL PROCEDURES

Endocarditis Prophylaxis Recommended

Dental procedures known to induce gingival or mucosal bleeding, including professional cleaning
Tonsillectomy and/or adenoidectomy
Surgical operations that involve respiratory mucosa
Bronchoscopy with a rigid bronchoscope

Endocarditis Prophylaxis Not Recommended*

Dental procedures not likely to induce gingival bleeding, such as simple adjustment of orthodontic appliances or fillings above the gum line
Injection of local intraoral anesthetic (except intraligamentary injections)
Shedding of primary teeth
Tympanostomy tube insertion
Endotracheal intubation
Bronchoscopy with a flexible bronchoscope, with or without biopsy

From Dajani AS, Bisno AL, Kyung JC, et al.: Prevention of bacterial endocarditis: Recommendations by the American Heart Association. JAMA 1990; 264: 2919–2922. Copyright 1990, American Medical Association.
    This table lists selected procedures but is not meant to be all-inclusive.
    *In patients who have prosthetic heart valves, a previous history of endocarditis, or surgically constructed systemic pulmonary shunts or conduits, physicians may choose to administer prophylactic antibiotics even for low-risk procedures that involve the lower respiratory, genitourinary, or gastrointestinal tracts.

procedures involving the respiratory mucosa, and bronchoscopy with a rigid bronchoscope.

INFECTING MICROORGANISMS

Trauma to the skin or mucosal surfaces that harbor a prolific endogenous flora releases into the blood stream many different microbial species. The array of microorganisms entering the circulation varies with the unique endogenous microflora at the particular traumatized site. Staphylococci and diphtheroids are characteristic for the skin; oral anaerobes and viridans streptococci for the oropharyngeal mucosa; colonic anaerobes, enteric aerobic gram-negative bacilli, and enterococci for the lower intestinal mucosa; and enteric aerobic gram-negative bacilli and enterococci for the genitourinary tract. However, only a few of these species, most commonly oral viridans streptococci, staphylococci, and enterococci, are capable of causing endocarditis. The frequency with which a particular organism will cause endocarditis depends on the frequency with which the organism can gain access to the circulation and its ability to survive in the blood stream; ability to adhere to the components of nonbacterial thrombotic endocarditis, exposed subendothelial structures, or the endothelial surface itself; and ability to proliferate on the endothelial surface. Trauma to the oropharyngeal and upper respiratory tract mucosa produces viridans streptococcal bacteremia. About 50% of cases of endocarditis are caused by viridans streptococci, and this organism has predictable antibiotic susceptibility patterns.

REDUCING THE FREQUENCY OF BACTEREMIA

When a surgical procedure is anticipated, giving patients appropriately timed therapy directed at viridans streptococci has been shown to decrease the frequency and intensity of

Table 69–3. RECOMMENDED STANDARD PROPHYLACTIC REGIMEN FOR DENTAL, ORAL, OR UPPER RESPIRATORY TRACT PROCEDURES IN PATIENTS WHO ARE AT RISK*

Drug	Dosing Regimen†
	Standard Regimen
Amoxicillin	3.0 g orally 1 h before procedure, then 1.5 g 6 h after initial dose
	Amoxicillin/Penicillin-Allergic Patients
Erythromycin	Erythromycin ethylsuccinate, 800 mg, or erythromycin stearate, 1.0 g orally 2 h before procedure, then half the dose 6 h after initial dose
or	
Clindamycin	300 mg orally 1 h before procedure and 150 mg 6 h after initial dose

From Dajani AS, Bisno AL, Kyung JC, et al.: Prevention of bacterial endocarditis: Recommendations by the American Heart Association. JAMA 1990; 264: 2919–2922. Copyright 1990, American Medical Association.

*Includes those with prosthetic heart valves and other high-risk patients.

†Initial pediatric doses are as follows: amoxicillin, 50 mg/kg; erythromycin ethylsuccinate or erythromycin stearate, 20 mg/kg; and clindamycin, 10 mg/kg. Follow-up doses should be one half the initial dose. Total pediatric dose should not exceed total adult dose. The following weight ranges may also be used for the initial pediatric dose of amoxicillin: <15 kg, 750 mg; 15 to 30 kg, 1500 mg; and >30 kg, 3000 mg (full adult dose).

the bacteremia immediately after dental procedures and is assumed to decrease the risk of endocarditis. This latter assumption has been supported by studies in experimental animal models. Data from these animal models suggest that antimicrobial prophylaxis may be effectively administered within 2 hours following the procedure. Antibiotics administered more than 4 hours after the procedure are likely to be of no prophylactic benefit. In one clinical retrospective study,[6] in which 533 patients with cardiac valvular prostheses, the highest-risk group, underwent 677 dental or surgical procedures, 6 cases of endocarditis developed in 229 patients who received no antimicrobial prophylaxis within 14 days of the procedure, as compared with no cases in 304 patients who did (p = .04). Two case-control studies have been done, one showing the efficacy of antimicrobial prophylaxis, the other not.[7, 8] Additional methods to reduce the frequency of bacteremia in patients known to be at increased risk of endocarditis include minimizing the invasiveness of procedures, choosing an endodontic procedure that does not extend beyond the root canal rather than dental extraction if possible, use of gentle oral rinsing for 1–2 minutes before the dental procedure with chlorhexidine, and aggressively treating local foci of infection prior to the anticipated surgery. Sustained or frequent, repeated use of chlorhexidine is not indicated as this may select for resistant microorganisms.

PREVENTING DEVELOPMENT OF VEGETATION

Once adherent to the endothelial surface, the microorganisms stimulate further deposition of platelets and fibrin on their surface. Within this secluded focus, the buried microorganisms then begin multiplying as rapidly as they would in broth cultures, apparently uninhibited by host defenses (i.e., phagocytes, antibody, and complement) to reach maximally dense populations of 10^{8-11} colony-forming units/g of vegetation. More than 90% of the microorganisms in these established vegetations are metabolically inactive and nongrowing (in a phase least susceptible to the bactericidal effects of beta-lactam and aminoglycoside antibiotics). In animal models, giving an appropriately timed single dose of an antibiotic may prevent experimental endocarditis by inhibition of bacterial adherence to the endothelial surface as well as inhibition of multiplication of bacteria once they adhere to the valve.

ANTIBIOTIC REGIMENS FOR DENTAL AND RESPIRATORY TRACT PROPHYLAXIS

Tables 69–3 and 69–4[1] list the antibiotic regimens recommended for dental and respiratory tract procedures. Amoxicillin has replaced penicillin V as the standard oral agent for prophylaxis in all patients undergoing dental, oral, and upper respiratory tract procedures at intermediate or high risk of endocarditis. Amoxicillin is as active as penicillin V in vitro against viridans streptococci and achieves higher serum levels for equivalent doses; the serum protein binding is lower, the serum half-life is longer, and the resulting serum bactericidal activity is greater than that of penicillin V. Note should be made of a second dose of half the amount 6 hours

Table 69–4. ALTERNATE PROPHYLACTIC REGIMENS FOR DENTAL, ORAL, OR UPPER RESPIRATORY TRACT PROCEDURES IN PATIENTS WHO ARE AT RISK

Drug	Dosing Regimen*
Patients Unable to Take Oral Medications	
Ampicillin	Intravenous or intramuscular administration of ampicillin, 2.0 g 30 min before procedure; then intravenous or intramuscular administration of ampicillin, 1.0 g, or oral administration of amoxicillin, 1.5 g 6 h after initial dose
Ampicillin/Amoxicillin/Penicillin-Allergic Patients Unable to Take Oral Medications	
Clindamycin	Intravenous administration of 300 mg 30 min before procedure and an intravenous or oral administration of 150 mg 6 h after initial dose
Patients Considered High Risk and Not Candidates for Standard Regimen	
Ampicillin, gentamicin, and amoxicillin	Intravenous or intramuscular administration of ampicillin, 2.0 g, plus gentamicin, 1.5 mg/kg (not to exceed 80 mg), 30 min before procedure; followed by amoxicillin, 1.5 g, orally 6 h after initial dose; alternatively, the parenteral regimen may be repeated 8 h after initial dose
Ampicillin/Amoxicillin/Penicillin-Allergic Patients Considered High Risk	
Vancomycin	Intravenous administration of 1.0 g over 1 h, starting 1 h before procedure; no repeated dose necessary

From Dajani AS, Bisno AL, Kyung JC, et al.: Prevention of bacterial endocarditis: Recommendations by the American Heart Association. JAMA 1990; 264: 2919–2922. Copyright 1990, American Medical Association.

*Initial pediatric doses are as follows: ampicillin, 50 mg/kg; clindamycin, 10 mg/kg; gentamicin, 2.0 mg/kg; and vancomycin, 20 mg/kg. Follow-up doses should be one half the initial dose. Total pediatric dose should not exceed total adult dose. No initial dose is recommended in this table for amoxicillin (25 mg/kg is the follow-up dose).

after the initial dose. For penicillin-allergic patients, either clindamycin or erythromycin is recommended. Erythromycin is frequently poorly tolerated because of gastrointestinal side effects. Parenteral regimens are recommended for patients who cannot take oral agents and are an option for high-risk patients (e.g., patients with prosthetic cardiac valves).

SUMMARY

The effect of endocarditis prophylaxis with antimicrobial agents has been estimated to be modest, i.e., fewer than 10% of all cases are preventable by prophylaxis.[4] For example, only about half of cases have recognizable predisposing cardiac lesions, most cases do not follow an invasive procedure, and only about two thirds of cases are due to microorganisms (viridans streptococci and enterococci) against which prophylactic regimens are directed. Indeed, transient low-grade bacteremias that occur many times a day associated with activities of everyday life, such as brushing teeth, eating a steak, or chewing on hard candy, probably account

for most of these nonprocedure-associated and nonpreventable cases of endocarditis. However, in those patients (1) who are known to have a risky cardiac lesion (Table 69–1); (2) who are to undergo a procedure that is likely to induce bacteremia (Table 69–2); (3) in whom the bacteremia is due to microorganisms having predictable susceptibility to antibiotics; and (4) for whom the indicated antimicrobial agents have minimal inconvenience, toxicity, and cost, the AHA has made the recommendations shown in Table 69–3 and Table 69–4. Additional preventive measures are to minimize invasive procedures, avoid use of intravascular catheters (a major predisposing event for prosthetic valve endocarditis), treat focal infections aggressively, and maintain good dental hygiene in patients at increased risk for endocarditis.

It is important to recognize that recommendations for the prevention of endocarditis have been revised about every 7 years since originally issued by the AHA in 1977. The next revision is expected in 1997. Because the formulation of these recommendations is an evolving process, the AHA recommendations are not meant to be rigid rules. Indeed, the Endocarditis Working Party of the British Society for Antimicrobial Chemotherapy has a different set of recommendations, although similar in many ways to the AHA recommendations.[9] As with each previous revision, the new AHA recommendations are expected to simplify and improve the antimicrobial regimens, focus more clearly the cardiac conditions, and decrease the number of procedures for which prophylaxis is recommended. Moreover, because of the recent emergence of penicillin-resistance among viridans streptococci under the selective pressure of antibiotic usage, reliance on nonantibiotic means of prophylaxis for low-risk procedures, such as gentle oral rinsing for 1–2 minutes with chlorhexidine solution immediately before a dental procedure, will be encouraged.

References

1. Dajani AS, Bisno AL, Kyung JC, et al.: Prevention of bacterial endocarditis: Recommendations by the American Heart Association. JAMA 1990; 264: 2919–2922.
2. Levison ME: Infective endocarditis. In: Bennett JG, Plum F (eds): Cecil Textbook of Medicine, 20th ed. Philadelphia: WB Saunders Co., 1995.
3. Steckelberg JM, Wilson WR: Risk factors for infective endocarditis. Infect Dis Clin North Am 1993; 7: 9–19.
4. Kaye D, Abrutyn E: Prevention of bacterial endocarditis: 1991. Ann Intern Med 1991; 114: 803–804.
5. Durack DT: Prevention of infective endocarditis. N Engl J Med 1995; 332: 38–44.
6. Horstkotte D, Rosin H, Friedrichs W, Loogen F: Contribution for choosing the optimal prophylaxis of bacterial endocarditis. Eur Heart J 1987; 8(Suppl J): 379–381.
7. Imperiale TF, Horwitz RI: Does prophylaxis prevent postdental infective endocarditis? A controlled evaluation of protective efficacy. Am J Med 1990; 88: 131–136.
8. van der Meer JTM, van Wijk W, Thompson J, et al.: Efficacy of antibiotic prophylaxis for prevention of native-valve endocarditis. Lancet 1992; 339: 135–139.
9. Simmons NA: Recommdndations for endocarditis prophylaxis. J Antimicrob Chemother 1993; 31: 437–438.

C. Gary Jackson
Ian S. Storper

CHAPTER SEVENTY

Antibiotic Prophylaxis in Otology and Neurotology

▼

The benefit of prophylactic antibiotics in otologic and neuro-tologic surgery has been debated ever since the concept was proposed by Gaudin and colleagues in 1938.[1] Despite almost six decades of medical progress, neurotologic surgeons continue to seek enhanced surgical success and the minimization of surgical complications under the protective umbrella of antimicrobial prophylaxis. Antimicrobial prophylaxis is abused by many surgeons. This abuse will continue as long as postoperative wound infections compromise outcome.

Contradictory and inconclusive neurotologic literature proposes a dilemma for the clinician seeking established guidelines—there are none. The consensus established for prophylaxis in head and neck surgery, as well as for general surgery, does not exist for the neurotologist. Lack of consensus breeds abuse of prophylaxis: Kass and Townsend[2] estimated that 40% of all administered antibiotics were prescribed as prophylaxis for surgical procedures. Tally and Gorbach[3] acknowledged an "accusation of reckless poly-pharmacy." Excessive use in the absence of clinically proven benefits continues. The dearth of scholarly investigations featuring well-controlled, statistically significant data continues to be perpetuated by medicolegal obstacles to trial design and execution.

Chodak and Plant[4] reviewed the literature in English written on this subject during the years 1960–1976. Of 131 articles reporting clinical trials for antimicrobial prophylaxis in surgery, only 24 met the criteria for being appropriately designed. Berger and associates[5] similarly performed a review of 157 clinical investigations summarizing more than 100,000 operations. They found that 64% of authors considered prophylactic antibiotics useful and 36% did not. In addition, adherence to the prophylaxis guidelines defined in the earlier portion of the study did not influence infection rates in the later portion of the studies. These observations were echoed by other authors.[4, 6–11] Alternately, Guglielmo and colleagues[12] observed that of 150 well-done trials prior to 1983, 80% demonstrated a significant advantage from the use of prophylactic antibiotics.

In 1970, the Committee on Trauma of the National Research Council recommended categorizing wounds into "clean, clean-contaminated, and dirty."[13] Kaiser,[14] however, noted the wide variability within each category of infection rates and stressed the need for "risk factors" in investigations for the stratification of populations.

There are other obstacles to the generation of useful data. Ethical considerations have continued to impede the design and execution of valuable clinical trials in a clinical popula-tion in which even a single infection complication could be disastrous. Furthermore, in otologic and neurotologic cases, in which infection rates are customarily low, sample size must be commensurately high (more than 1000 patients) to identify statistically significant reductions in infection rates.[15] With the dispersion of patients among larger numbers of practitioners, the achievement of high-grade data is increasingly unlikely.[15] The concept that a postoperative infection complication could have been prevented medicolegally compels the indiscriminate use of prophylactic antibiotics.

The question of the value of prophylactic antibiotics has become magnified for otolaryngologists. Strong[16] stated that antibiotic prophylaxis is more commonly employed in oto-laryngology than in any other field of surgery. Numerous rigorous studies have documented the efficacy of prophylactic antibiotics for head and neck surgical procedures.[17–22] A general misconception has emerged that the success of many procedures in otolaryngology (head and neck surgery) can be attributed to the use of prophylactic antibiotics. But like otolaryngologists, ear surgeons erratically and indiscriminately use prophylactic antibiotics in non-standardized protocols to achieve improved otologic outcomes. These practices are not based on conclusive data and may be erroneous.[9, 15, 16, 23]

As so much controversy continues to exist about the value of prophylactic antibiotics in otology and neurotology, it is the purpose of this chapter to discuss modern concepts of this therapy and to offer suggestions for the relevant use of antimicrobials based on the valid neurotologic literature.

BASIC CONSIDERATIONS

A host tissue responds to the presence of bacterial invasion by the now well-defined mechanisms of inflammation. If the inoculum is small, the degrees of corresponding inflammation correlate well and are often subclinical. As host defense mechanisms are overwhelmed by more significant degrees of inoculation, tissues are invaded and the process of infection ensues, usually with clinically obvious and systemic manifestations. Infection severity often occurs in degrees. Before the development of wound infection, bacteria must either be present endogenously or be introduced exogenously. The factors that control virulence (attachment, invasion, and toxicity) and host resistance (humoral and cellular) are incompletely understood.[14]

Aseptic technique is critical to control inoculation and to

prevent proliferation of infection. Asepsis is augmented by skilled, attentive surgical technique in the prevention of wound infection. The intent of antimicrobial prophylaxis is (controversially) to augment host mechanisms to the end of prevention of infection; bacterial inoculation is conceded rather than avoided. The host-inoculum-antibiotic interaction is complex and poorly understood. Current concepts are reviewed next.

Contamination Versus Infection

It has been estimated that up to 90% of clean surgical wounds are contaminated by potentially pathogenic bacteria at the time of closure.[13–17, 24–33] It is also apparent that colonization of a wound by these bacteria does not necessarily result in a wound infection.[13]

In normal circumstances, surgical infection is unusual with inocula of less than 10^5 organisms.[15, 16, 32] Host defense mechanisms may lessen this number.[34] Nevertheless, the presence of bacterial contamination in a wound closure is not without consequence. Wound infections were more likely to occur in incisions cultured as colonized, compared with those that were sterile.[25, 30] Polk and Lopez-Mayor[33] showed that the incidence of wound infection correlated with the density of organisms at the time of wound closure. This study classically defined the aim of antibiotic prophylaxis: "to saturate tissues with antibiotic, to augment host defense mechanisms at the time of bacterial invasion, decreasing the size of the inoculum in the process."[15]

Timing of Antibiotic Administration

Although there is very little literature specific for otology and neurotology, there is a large general body of literature concerning timing of prophylactic antibiotic administration. The timing differs from that for therapeutic administration, which is guided by culture and sensitivity data. Prophylactic therapy is directed at infection *before* it occurs pre-, post-, or intraoperatively.[15]

Before 1960, antibiotics were usually administered postoperatively, and no real benefit was demonstrated.[14, 15, 31, 35–42] The importance of proper timing of therapy was established later.[43] Burke[44] recognized the critical period during which the efficacy of antibiotic prophylaxis is maximized as being present in tissue when bacteria arrive.[44] Miles and associates[45] noted a 4-hour period postinoculation during which maximum inhibition is achieved with prophylactic antibiotics. Antibiotic prophylactic effect is maximized if administered prior to incision.[46–53] The parenteral route is most efficacious. Administration can occur in the operating room. Repeated doses beyond 24 hours postoperatively will likely have no effect.[14, 15, 54–63]

Bacteriology

The bacteriology of the ear has been well studied.[15] A review of the potential pathogens is essential for the selection of appropriate antibiotics.

For the transcanal and stapes surgeons, knowledge of the bacteriology of the external auditory canal (EAC) is important. The predominant organisms in the EAC are commensal skin flora, notably *Staphylococcus epidermidis*[64–70] and *Corynebacterium* species.[71] Linthicum[72] found growth in 90% of 200 external auditory canals cultured prior to stapedectomy, with *Staphylococcus aureus* in 85%. Commensal skin flora was not different between the sexes nor was it affected by seasonal variation; cerumen did not inhibit bacterial growth.[71] The presence of actual pathogens is rare.[66–70]

The middle ear is normally sterile.[64] The bacteriology of chronic otitis media with and without cholesteatoma presupposes a contaminated operative site and has received much attention.[15] Up to 255 different organisms have been cultured from these ears.[73] The most commonly isolated include *Pseudomonas, Staphylococcus,* and *Proteus* species.[9, 17, 73–82] In more than 90% of isolates, there is more than one organism present.[15] Anaerobes are commonly identified in the presence of aerobic bacteria.[73–78] The most commonly isolated anaerobes are *Bacteroides* and *Peptostreptococcus* species. The frequency of anaerobic isolation has been suggested to be greater in the presence of cholesteatoma,[9, 15, 73–77] where it has been estimated to be approximately 70%; without cholesteatoma, it has been estimated to be 30%–50%.

Like the middle ear, the cerebellopontine angle is sterile. Neurotologic approaches to the intracranial contents often involve transgression of the mastoid and ear. Bacterial colonization of these structures should be considered when planning surgical prophylaxis.

OTHER FACTORS

There is no substitute for asepsis; no combination of prophylactic antibiotics can be expected to provide coverage for faulty technique. Prolonged duration of operation has been suggested as enhancing the risk of postoperative infection. Duration of operation was not found to correlate significantly with the development of a postoperative infection in a variety of otologic procedures.[83] The decision to use prophylactic antibiotics should not be made on the duration of operation.

ANTIBIOTIC CHOICE FOR PROPHYLAXIS

Otologic Surgery

These basic considerations represent important criteria necessary for planning antimicrobial prophylaxis. The presence of microorganisms does not constitute an infection; instead, it constitutes contamination.[83] Furthermore, common infecting organisms may not represent the common contaminants found on culture. The best regimen of prophylaxis should not be directed against *all* possible offending organisms; rather, it should be directed against the most common infecting ones.[83, 84, 85]

Most operations that are performed by otologists are clean operations. Chronic otitis media with or without cholesteatoma is considered contaminated. A typical clean middle ear surgery is the stapedectomy. While the external auditory canal is contaminated, the actual operative site, the middle ear, is clean. The external auditory canal can be prepared preoperatively. Infections are rare postoperatively.[17, 64–66, 83, 86] Any number of verified poststapedectomy infections with disastrous consequences, including labyrinthitis, hearing loss, and meningitis, have been reported.[87–93] Although staphylococcal infecting organisms predominate, no consistent bacteriology emerges. A randomized, blinded study of prophylactic antibiotics in 4000 diverse ear surgeries failed to show any benefit from the use of prophylactic antibiotics in this population.[15]

The presence of purulent otorrhea presupposes a contaminated operative site. Contaminating organisms, however, are incompletely represented in postoperative infections. In-depth analyses of postoperative infections are scarce for this population.[9, 17, 22, 77, 79] Wound infections are commonly gram-positive and usually staphylococcal. *Pseudomonas* and anaerobic infections are rare.[83] The most common cause of postoperative infection is technical; i.e., failure to remove all diseased mastoid cells.[94] Whether or not to perform surgery on actively draining ears is controversial. Glasscock and colleagues,[95] Smyth,[96] and Lee and Schuknecht[97] believe postoperative outcome has little to do with the preoperative status of the ear. Cultured flora of otorrhea is generally resistant to most nonototoxic antibiotics; prophylaxis is neither appealing nor effective.[15, 83] Paparella and Kim,[98] however, administered prophylaxis from 1 week before to 10 days after surgery on the draining ear.

Fitzgerald[9] noted a 2% prevalence of life-threatening complications from mastoid surgery without prophylactic antibiotics. In these cases, there was "significant dural damage." He, therefore, concluded that chloramphenicol with metronidazole or cefotaxime would be appropriate if there is a significant dural dehiscence. More recently, cephalosporin coverage has been recommended.

The role of antibiotic prophylaxis in mastoid surgery has been unclear. The single statistically valid study of 4000 patients concluded that prophylaxis is not recommended.[15, 83] Details of this study are presented in the appendix.

There are, however, instances in which prophylaxis is appropriate. When, with a reasonable amount of statistical certainty, a set of circumstances exists in which the development of an infection complication is likely, antimicrobial prophylaxis is indicated.

Surgery for chronic otitis media is an operation in a contaminated field. The violation of an adjacent clean anatomic site, such as the central nervous system, in this circumstance risks, with a reasonable statistical amount of certainty, a serious infection complication with potentially disastrous consequences. Whether the chronic ear is actively discharging or not appears relatively irrelevant.

The unanticipated violation of the anatomic integrity of the labyrinth warrants antibiotic prophylaxis against severe consequences of labyrinthitis. An antibiotic with adequate cerebrospinal fluid (CSF) penetration is an appropriate choice. Clinical situations include the following:

- Stapes subluxation, footplate fracture, or perilymph fistula in the course of chronic otitis media surgery;

- Round window violation; and

- Unplanned disruption of a labyrinthine fistula caused by cholesteatoma.

CSF leakage in this contaminated environment risks equal infection consequence. Clinical situations could include the following:

- Unplanned interruption of dura;

- (Sub)arachnoid cyst or brain herniation;

- CSF leak through proximal facial nerve dissection; and

- Cochlear aqueduct disruption.

An acknowledged serious violation of sterile technique warrants prophylaxis (for example a surgeon being informed, at the conclusion of an elective ear case, that the instruments employed were thought not to be sterile).

Neurotologic Surgery

Generally, the epidemiology of postoperative neurotologic infections mirrors that of clean otologic procedures.[83] One important difference, however, is that postoperative neurotologic infection could have disastrous consequences. Several erudite and technical reports of operative techniques and outcome describe acoustic and glomus tumor surgery; few address postoperative infection. The neurosurgical literature, however, emphasizes infection rates of 0.7%–5.7%.[99] Reports reliably suggest rates in the 1% range but as high as 10%.[35, 100–105] The predominant organism appears to be *S. aureus*.[105–107] Some neurosurgical studies deserve mention for historical significance, although their design was retrospective.

The work of Malis[108] represents the standard against which neurosurgeons compare their infection data. On the basis of the sensitivity characteristics of pathogens isolated during a 5-year period, a single dose of gentamicin IM, vancomycin IV, and streptomycin 50 mg in each liter of irrigating saline regimen was established in single-dose format and administered intraoperatively. Of 1732 cases, no postsurgical infections were identified. This work was updated by Savitz and Katz[109] to 4000 cases without a primary infection. This work has not been reproducible.[83] Geraghty and Feely,[110] in a controlled study, did improve infection rates using this regimen from 3.5% to 0.5%.

Savitz and Katz[109] reviewed 2000 consecutive cases employing cephalosporin administered at incision and at closure in conjunction with wound irrigation with 50 cc of saline and 50,000 units of bacitracin. Patients with indwelling foreign bodies were also given methicillin and oxacillin until suture removal. No primary wound infections occurred. Lack of a control population in this study is a flaw; nevertheless, postoperative infection was completely eradicated, making it a noteworthy study.

More recently, Kartush and associates[111] examined the use of bacitracin irrigation in neurotologic surgery. In a study of 236 patients, bacitracin irrigation was found to decrease the prevalence of wound infection from 9% to 2%, of CSF leak from 12% to 5%, and of all complications from 22% to 9%. These results were all statistically significant. The use of intravenous antibiotics alone did not significantly decrease the incidence of complications. Complication rates were significantly decreased when bacitracin wound irrigations were used alone. Although this study was not blinded, it does suggest that the prophylactic use of bacitracin irrigation, 50,000 units in 200 mL normal saline, could significantly lower the complication rates in neurotologic surgery. Until the performance of this study, there were no data suggesting a statistically significant improvement from any method of antibiotic prophylaxis in neurotologic surgery.

CONCLUSION

The only study in the otologic literature[15] that carries statistical strength claims prophylactic antibiotic administration in otologic as well as neurotologic cases, for the antibiotic protocol investigated, has no effect on postoperative infection or on surgical outcome. The issue of antibiotic irrigation as efficacious prophylaxis remains open. The statistical power of the data that are valid[15] precludes the imposition of any medicolegal standard that might assert that failure to use prophylaxis constitutes (neuro)otologic negligence. This study was presented in 1988. More recent, rigid guidelines for antimicrobial prophylaxis in ear surgery do not exist.

....

A P P E N D I X   F O R   C H A P T E R   S E V E N T Y[15]

I. Methods
  A. Analyzing the principles of antimicrobial prophylaxis and surveying the preferences of eight prominent otologists, the following prophylaxis protocol was chosen:
    1. Surgery for clean middle ear and chronic otitis media: cephalothin/cefazolin.
    2. Neurotology: oxacillin.
  B. Administration protocol
    1. Antibiotics intramuscularly with preoperative medications.
    2. Antibiotics intravenously just prior to incision.
    3. Antibiotics intravenously or intramuscularly 24 hours every 6 hours postoperative period.
  C. Penicillin allergy
    1. Immediate and/or severe penicillin reaction precluded cephalosporin administration and oxacillin.
    2. Vancomycin was substituted.
  D. Special considerations
    1. Patients having received any antibiotic for any reason within 7 days pre- or postsurgery were excluded.
    2. All cases were surgically prepared identically.
    3. No antibiotics were used in irrigation fluids.
  E. Infection status
    1. All neurotology is clean.
    2. Chronic ears.
      a. Dry: clean-contaminated
      b. Discharging: contaminated
  F. Prospectively and consequently patients assigned "antibiotic" or "no antibiotic" status according to computer-generated randomization.
    1. Done by staff other than surgeon.
    2. Operative surgeon blinded.
    3. Postoperative status checked:
      a. Infection was recorded at any time it occurred up to 3 weeks.
      b. Study interval: 3 weeks.
  G. Age
    1. Age 12 or younger: "pediatric."
    2. Age 13 or older: "adult."
  H. Operation duration
    1. Short: less than 1 hour.
    2. Intermediate: 1–3 hours.
    3. Long: more than 3 hours.
  I. Statistics
    1. The relationship of antibiotic administration and postsurgical infection was principal association of interest.
      a. Pearson chi-square test employed.
      b. Goodman and Kruskal tau test supplemented data analysis.
    2. Covariates
      a. Patient age: Age.
      b. Operative precondition: Precondition.
      c. Operation duration: Optime.
      d. Covariates possibly could influence the relationship of ANTIBIOTIC and POSTINFECTION. This was assessed by assessing any changes in the ANTIBIOTIC vs POSTINFECTION relationship when controlling for a third variable.
      e. Tests
        I. General Log-Linear Model
        II. Likelihood Ratio Test
    3. Data management statistical software
      a. BMDP (1987)
      b. SAS (Version 5.16)
II. Case Material
  A. July 1980–July 1987
    1. 4000 patients: prospective/consecutive.
    2. 3481 qualified for study.
      a. 519 (12.9%) disqualified for stipulated reasons.
    3. Preoperative patient data: Table 70–1.
    4. Clinical population data: Table 70–2.
    5. Operative procedures: Table 70–3.
III. Results
  A. Primary associations
    1. Effect of antibiotic prophylaxis on the population: Table 70–4.
    2. Effect of antibiotic on graft take rate: Table 70–5.

Text continued on page 616

Table 70–1. PREOPERATIVE PATIENT DATA

	Frequency	Percent	Cumulative Frequency	Cumulative Percent
Age				
Child	488	14.9	488	14.9
Adult	2793	85.1	3281	100.0
Unspecified	200			
Sex				
Male	1369	46.9	1369	46.9
Female	1553	53.1	2992	100.0
Unspecified	559			
Antibiotic				
Administered	1749	50.2	1749	50.2
None	1732	49.8	3481	100.0

N = 3481

Table 70–2. CLINICAL POPULATION DATA

	Frequency	Percent	Cumulative Frequency	Cumulative Percent
Optime				
Short	1418	46.0	1418	46.0
Intermediate	1141	37.0	2559	83.0
Long	523	17.0	3082	100.0
Unspecified	399			
Precondition				
Uninfected	3017	89.1	3017	89.1
Discharge	370	10.9	3387	100.0
Unspecified	94			
Perforation				
None	2183	65.0	2183	65.0
Present	1174	35.0	3357	100.0
Unspecified	124			

N = 3481

Table 70–3. OPERATIVE PROCEDURES

Procedure	Frequency	Percent	Cumulative Frequency	Cumulative Percent
Tymp w/o mastoid	497	14.7	497	14.7
Tymp w/ mastoid	553	16.3	1050	31.0
Tymp 2nd stage	182	5.4	1232	36.4
Mod radical	215	6.4	1447	42.8
Radical	11	0.3	1458	43.1
Stapedectomy	341	10.1	1799	53.2
Shunt	260	7.7	2059	60.9
Labyrinthectomy	70	2.1	2129	62.9
MFVNS/SOVNS	45	1.3	2174	64.3
CPA tumor	431	12.7	2065	77.0
Skull base tumor	51	1.5	2656	78.5
Simple FND	21	0.6	2677	79.1
Total FND	34	1.0	2711	80.1
Facial hypoglossal	28	0.8	2739	81.0
Tymp w/wo	40	1.2	2779	82.1
Other	604	17.9	3383	100.0
Unspecified	98			

N = 3481
MFVNS/SOVNS = middle fossa vestibular nerve section/suboccipital vestibular nerve section; FND = facial nerve decompression.

Table 70–4. ANTIBIOTIC VERSUS POSTINFECTION

Antibiotic	None	Percent	Postinfection Wound	Percent	Canal	Percent	Total	Percent
Administered	1644	94.0	25	1.4	80	4.6	1749	100
None	1632	94.2	30	1.7	70	4.0	1732	100
Total	3276	94.1	55	1.6	150	4.3	3481	100

Statistic	Value	df
Pearson chi square	1.082	2*

Statistic	Value	ASE
Tau asymmetric	0.000	0.000

*p>.05
df = degrees of freedom
ASE = asymptotic standard error. When multiplied by 2 and added to or subtracted from the statistic, the resulting range would not include 0 for the statistic to be significant.

Table 70–5. ANTIBIOTIC VERSUS GRAFT TAKE

Antibiotic	Graft Failure	Percent	Graft Take	Percent	Total	Percent
Administered	13	1.2	1105	98.8	1118	100
None	15	1.5	1003	98.5	1018	100

Statistic	Value	df
Pearson chi square	0.398	1*

Statistic	Value	ASE
Tau asymmetric	0.000	0.001

*p>.05

Table 70–6. ANTIBIOTIC VERSUS POSTINFECTION FOR THE VARIABLE AGE

Antibiotic	Pediatric Postinfection None	Percent	Wound	Percent	Canal	Percent	Total	Percent	Adult Postinfection None	Percent	Wound	Percent	Canal	Percent	Total	Percent
Administered	166	91.7	2	1.1	13	7.2	181	100	1398	94.4	23	1.6	60	4.1	1481	100
None	288	93.8	5	1.6	14	4.6	307	100	1237	94.3	24	1.8	51	3.9	1312	100
Total	454	93.0	7	1.4	27	5.5	488	100	2635	94.3	47	1.7	111	4.0	2793	100

Statistic	Value	df
Pearson chi square	1.687	2*

Statistic	Value	ASE
Tau asymmetric	0.002	0.004

Statistic	Value	df
Pearson chi square	0.364	2*

Statistic	Value	ASE
Tau asymmetric	0.000	0.000

Cochran-Mantel-Haenzel Statistics	Value	df
General association	0.981	2*

*p>.05

Table 70–7. ANTIBIOTIC VERSUS POSTINFECTION FOR THE VARIABLE PRECONDITION

Antibiotic	Preinfected Postinfection								Uninfected Postinfection							
	None	Percent	Wound	Percent	Canal	Percent	Total	Percent	None	Percent	Wound	Percent	Canal	Percent	Total	Percent
Administered	154	83.2	7	3.8	24	13.0	185	100	1440	95.4	18	1.2	52	3.4	1510	100
None	152	82.2	12	6.5	21	11.4	185	100	1445	95.9	15	1.0	47	3.1	1507	100
Total	306	82.7	19	5.1	45	12.2	370	100	2885	95.6	33	1.1	99	3.3	3017	100

Preinfected Postinfection

Statistic	Value	df
Pearson chi square	1.529	2*

Statistic	Value	ASE
Tau asymmetric	0.001	0.001

Uninfected Postinfection

Statistic	Value	df
Pearson chi square	0.531	2*

Statistic	Value	ASE
Tau asymmetric	0.000	0.000

Cochran-Mantel-Haenzel Statistics	Value	df
General association	0.528	2*

*p>.05

Table 70–8A. ANTIBIOTIC VERSUS POSTINFECTION FOR VARIABLE OPTIME (SHORT)

Antibiotic	None	Percent	Wound	Percent	Canal	Percent	Total	Percent
				Postinfection				
Administered	639	95.1	6	0.9	27	4.0	672	100
None	712	95.4	7	0.9	27	3.6	746	100
Total	1351	95.3	13	0.9	54	3.8	1418	100

Statistic	Value	df
Pearson chi square	0.160	2*

Statistic	Value	ASE
Tau asymmetric	0.000	0.000

*p>.05

Table 70–8B. ANTIBIOTIC VERSUS POSTINFECTION FOR VARIABLE OPTIME (INTERMEDIATE)

Antibiotic	None	Percent	Wound	Percent	Canal	Percent	Total	Percent
				Postinfection				
Administered	572	90.8	12	1.9	46	7.3	630	100
None	462	90.4	13	2.5	36	7.0	511	100
Total	1034	90.6	25	2.2	82	7.2	1141	100

Statistic	Value	df
Pearson chi square	0.557	2*

Statistic	Value	ASE
Tau asymmetric	0.000	0.000

*p>.05

Table 70–8C. ANTIBIOTIC VERSUS POSTINFECTION FOR VARIABLE OPTIME (LONG)

Antibiotic	None	Percent	Wound	Percent	Canal	Percent	Total	Percent
				Postinfection				
Administered	266	97.8	6	2.2	0	0.0	272	100
None	243	96.8	7	2.8	1	0.4	251	100
Total	509	97.3	13	2.5	1	0.2	523	100

Statistic	Value	df
Pearson chi square	1.275	2*

Statistic	Value	ASE
Tau asymmetric	0.001	0.002

Cochran-Mantel-Haenzel Statistics (Tables 70–8A, 70–8B, 70–8C)	Value	df
General association	0.666	2*

*p>.05

Table 70–9. GRAFT TAKE VERSUS POSTINFECTION

| | Postinfection | | | | | | | |
	None	*Percent*	*Wound*	*Percent*	*Canal*	*Percent*	*Total*	*Percent*
Graft failure	13	50.0	4	15.9	9	34.6	26	100
Graft take	1968	93.3	24	1.1	117	5.5	2109	100
Total	1981	92.8	28	1.3	126	5.9	2135	100

Statistic	Value	df
Pearson chi square	81.712	2*

Statistic	Value	ASE
Tau asymmetric	0.026	0.012

*p>.05

Table 70–10. OPERATIVE PRECONDITION VERSUS POSTINFECTION

| | Postinfection | | | | | | | |
Precondition	*None*	*Percent*	*Wound*	*Percent*	*Canal*	*Percent*	*Total*	*Percent*
Preinfection	308	82.8	19	5.1	45	12.1	372	100
Uninfected	2906	95.7	33	1.1	99	3.3	3038	100
Total	3214	94.3	52	1.5	144	4.2	3410	100

Statistic	Value	df
Pearson chi square	102.262	2*

Statistic	Value	ASE
Tau asymmetric	0.023	0.007

*p>.05

B. Covariates
   1. Patient age: Table 70–6.
   2. Preoperation condition of ear: Table 70–7.
   3. Operation duration: Tables 70–8 A, B, C.
C. Secondary associations
   1. Association between infection rate and graft take: Table 70–9.
   2. Preoperative condition of the ear associated with postoperative infection: Table 70–10.
D. Miscellaneous
   1. Of 1749 cases of antimicrobial prophylaxis, two antibiotic minor complications noted.
IV. Conclusions
   A. For this protocol, no statistically significant influence on postoperative infection rate as an effect of antimicrobial prophylaxis was identified.
      1. This observation was consistent when addressing operation duration, patient age, and operative precondition.
   B. Intuitively, it is expected that preinfected ears would have higher incidence of postinfection.
      1. True.
      2. Antibiotics did not affect this.
   C. Intuitively, postinfection resulted in lower graft take rate.

      1. True.
      2. Antibiotics did not affect this.
D. Overwhelming safety of antibiotics of this protocol was noted.
E. High statistical significance of this data produces otologic guidelines:
   1. Prophylactic antibiotics are harmless but also useless.
   2. Medicolegal imposition of a standard that suggests negligence by not using prophylactic antibiotics is precluded.

References

1. Gaudin HJ, Zide HA, Thompson GJ: Use of sulfanilamide after transurethral prostatectomy. JAMA 1938; 110: 1887.
2. Kass EH, Townsend T: The role of controlled clinical observation in defining standards of antibiotic usage. In: McCabe WR, Finland M (eds): Contemporary Standards for Antimicrobial Usage. Mt. Kisco, New York: Futura Publishing Co., 1977, pp 19–27.
3. Tally F, Gorbach S: Antibiotics in surgery. Adv Surg 1975; 9: 41.
4. Chodak GW, Plant ME: Use of asystemic antibiotics for prophylaxis in surgery. Arch Surg 1977; 112: 326–334.
5. Berger SA, Nagar H, Weitzman S: Prophylactic antibiotics in surgical procedures. Surg Gynecol Obstet 1978; 146: 469–475.

6. Byar DB, Simon RM, Friedwald WT, et al.: Randomized clinical trials: Perspectives on some recent ideas. N Engl J Med 1976; 295: 74.
7. Ingelfinger JA, Goldman P: The serum digitalis concentration. N Engl J Med 1976; 294: 867.
8. Mahon WA, Daniel EE: A method for the assessment of reports of drug trials. Can Med Assoc J 1964; 90: 55.
9. Fitzgerald DC: Use of prophylactic antibiotics in otologic and neurotologic surgery. Am J Otol 1985; 6: 121–125.
10. Depiro JT, Record KE, Schanzenback KS, et al.: Antimicrobial prophylaxis in surgery, Part 1. Am J Hosp Pharm 1981; 38: 320.
11. Depiro JT: Antimicrobial prophylaxis in surgery, Part 2. Am J Hosp Pharm 1981; 38: 487.
12. Guglielmo BJ, Hohn DC, Koo PJ, et al.: Antibiotic prophylaxis in surgical procedures: A critical analysis of the literature. Arch Surg 1983; 118: 943–955.
13. Committee on Trauma, Division of Medical Sciences, Academy of Sciences, National Research Council: Postoperative wound infections: The influence of UV irradiation of the operating room and of various other factors. Ann Surg 1964; 160(suppl 2): 1–92.
14. Kaiser AB: Antimicrobial prophylaxis in surgery. N Engl J Med 1986; 315: 1129–1138.
15. Jackson CG: Antimicrobial prophylaxis in ear surgery. Laryngoscope 1988; 98: 1116–1122.
16. Strong SM: Wound infections in otolaryngologic surgery and the inexpediency of antibiotic prophylaxis. Laryngoscope 1963; 73: 165–184.
17. Robbins KT, Favrot S, Hanna D, et al.: Risk of wound infection in patients with head and neck cancer. Head Neck 1990; 12: 143–148.
18. Piccart M, Dor P, Klastersky J: Antimicrobial prophylaxis of infections in head and neck cancer surgery. Scand J Infect Dis 1983; (suppl 39): 92–96.
19. Johnson JT, Yu VL, Myers EN, et al.: Efficacy of two third-generation cephalosporins in prophylaxis for head and neck surgery. Arch Otolaryngol 1984; 110: 224–227.
20. Dor P, Klastersky J: Prophylactic antibiotics in oral, pharyngeal, and laryngeal surgery for cancer: A double-blind study. Laryngoscope 1973; 83: 1992–1998.
21. Johnson JT, Myers EN, Thearle PB, et al.: Antimicrobial prophylaxis for contaminated head and neck surgery. Laryngoscope 1984; 94: 46–51.
22. Eschelman LT, Schleuning AJ II, Brummett RE: Prophylactic antibiotics in otolaryngologic surgery: A double-blind study. Trans Am Acad Oththalmol Otolaryngol 1971; 75: 387–394.
23. Parnes SM: The use of prophylactic antibiotics in otology. In: Johnson JT (ed): Antibiotic Therapy in Head and Neck Surgery. New York: Marcel Dekker, Inc, 1987, pp 13–20.
24. Balch RE: Neurosurgical wound infections complicating neurosurgical procedures. J Neurosurg 1967; 26: 41–45.
25. Davidson AIG, Clark C, Smith G: Postoperative wound infection: A computer analysis. Br J Surg 1971; 58: 333–337.
26. Culbertson WR, Altemeier WA, Gonzales LL, et al: Studies on the epidemiology of postoperative infection of clean operative wounds. Ann Surg 1961; 154: 599–610.
27. Howe CW, Marston AT: A study on sources of postoperative staphylococcal infection. Surg Gynecol Obstet 1962; 115: 266–275.
28. Burke JF: Identification of the sources of staphylococci contaminating the surgical wound during operation. Ann Surg 1963; 158: 898–904.
29. Meleney FL: Treatise on Surgical Infections. New York: Oxford Medical Publications, 1948, p 713.
30. Hunt EL: Some further observations on contamination of operative wounds by air-borne bacteria. N Engl J Med 1933; 209: 931–933.
31. Howe CW: Postoperative wound infections due to *Staphylococcus aureus*. N Engl J Med 1954; 251: 411–417.
32. Elek SD: Experimental staphylococcal infections in the skin of man. Ann NY Acad Sci 1956; 65: 85–90.
33. Polk HC, Lopez-Mayor JF: Postoperative wound infection: A prospective study of determinant factors and prevention. Surgery 1969; 66: 97–103.
34. Burke JF: Use of preventative antibiotics in clinical surgery. Am Surg 1973; 39: 6–11.
35. Velghe L, Dereymaeker A, Voorde H Vande: L'Ecourillon du champ operatoire en neurochirurgie: Analyse d'un millier de controles. Acta Neurochir 1964; 11: 686–693.
36. McKittrick LS, Wheelock FC Jr: The routine use of antibiotics in elective abdominal surgery. Surg Gynecol Obstet 1954; 99: 376–377.
37. Pulaski EJ: Discriminate antibiotic prophylaxis in elective surgery. Surg Gynecol Obstet 1959; 108: 385–388.
38. Sanchez-Ubeda R, Fernand E, Rousselot LM: Complication rate in general surgical cases: The value of penicillin and streptomycin as postoperative prophylaxis—A study of 511 cases. N Engl J Med 1958; 259: 1045–1050.
39. Johnstone FRC: An assessment of prophylactic antibiotics in general surgery. Surg Gynecol Obstet 1958; 116: 1–10.
40. Finland M: Antibacterial agents: Uses and abuses in treatment and prophylaxis. RI Med J 1960; 43: 499–520.
41. Appleton DM, Waisbren BA: The prophylactic use of chloramphenicol in transurethral resections of the prostate Gland. J Urol 1956; 75: 304.
42. Tachdjian MO, Compere EL: Postoperative wound infection in orthopedic surgery: Evaluation of prophylactic antibiotics. J Internat Coll Surg 1957; 28: 797.
43. Hawes EL: Prevention of wound infection by the injection of nontoxic antibacterial substances. Ann Surg 1946; 124: 268–276.
44. Burke JF: The effective period of preventative antibiotic action in experimental incisions and dermal lesions. Surgery 1961; 50: 161–168.
45. Miles AA, Miles EM, Burke J: The value and duration of defense reactions of the skin to the preliminary lodgement of bacteria. Br J Exp Pathol 1957; 38: 79.
46. Burke JF: Preoperative antibiotics. Surg Clin North Am 1963; 43: 665–676.
47. Alexander JW, McGloin JJ, Altemeirr WA: Penicillin prophylaxis in experimental wound infections. Surg Forum 1960; 11: 299–300.
48. Poth EJ, Miller TE, Dunlap W: The protection of contaminated deep wounds against infection by intraperitoneal neomycin solutions. Am J Surg 1961; 101: 766–768.
49. Shapiro M, Shimon D, Freud U, et al.: A decisive period in the antibiotic prophylaxis of cutaneous lesions caused by *Bacteroides fragilis* in guinea pigs. J Infect Dis 1980; 141: 532.
50. Bartlett JG: Experimental aspects of intra-abdominal abscess. Am J Med 1984; 76: 91–98.
51. Polk HC Jr, Miles AA: The decisive period in primary infections of muscle by *E. coli*. Br J Exp Pathol 1973; 54: 99.
52. Bernard HR, Cole WR: The prophylaxis of surgical infection: The effect of prophylactic antimicrobial drugs in the incidence of infection following potentially contaminated wounds. Surgery 1966; 56: 151.
53. Stone HH, Hooper CA, Kolb LD, et al.: Antibiotic prophylaxis in gastric, biliary, and colonic surgery. Ann Surg 1976; 184: 443.
54. Fullen WD, Hunt J, Altemeier WA: Prophylactic antibiotics in penetrating wounds of the abdomen. J Trauma 1972; 12: 282–289.
55. Alexander JW, Alexander NS: The influence of route of administration on wound fluid concentration of prophylactic antibiotics J Trauma 1976; 16: 488–495.
56. Burdon DW: Principles of antimicrobial prophylaxis. World J Surg 1982; 6: 262–267.
57. Kaiser AB: Effective and creative surveillance and reporting of surgical wound infections. Infect Control Hosp Epidemiol 1982; 3: 41–43.
58. Goldmann DA, Hopkins CC, Karchmer AW, et al.: Cephalothin prophylaxis in cardiac valve surgery: A prospective double-blind comparison of two-day and six-day Regimens. J Thoracic Cardiovasc Surg 1977; 73: 470–479.
59. Kaiser AB, Herrington JL Jr, Jacobs JK, et al.: Cefoxitin vs erythromycin, neomycin and cefazolin in colorectal operations: Importance of the duration of the surgical procedure. Ann Surg 1983; 198: 525–530.
60. Antimicrobial prophylaxis for surgery. Medical Lett Drugs Ther 1981; 23: 77–80.
61. Nelsen CL, Green TG, Porter RA, et al.: One-day vs seven-days of preventive antibiotic therapy in orthopedic surgery. Clin Orthoped 1983; 176: 258–263.
62. Conte JE, Cohen SN, Roe BB: Antibiotic prophylaxis and cardiac surgery: A prospective double-blind comparison of single-dose vs multiple-dose regimens. Ann Intern Med 1972; 76: 943–949.
63. Stone HH, Harvey BB, Kalb LD, et al: Prophylactic and preventive antibiotic therapy: Timing, duration, and economics. Ann Surg 1979; 189: 691–699.
64. Leonard JR: Prophylactic antibiotics in human stapedectomy. Laryngoscope 1967; 77: 663–680.
65. Moon CN Jr, Wallenborn WM, Bobbitt OB: Bacterial flora of the external auditory canal before and after preoperative preparation. South Med J 1965; 58: 285–288.
66. Singer DE, Freeman E, Haffert WR, et al.: Otitis externa: Bacteriological and mycological studies. Ann Otol 1952; 61: 317–330.

67. Haley LD: Etiology of otomycosis: Bacterial flora of the ear. Arch Otolaryngol 1950; 52: 208–223.
68. Saunders WH, Ray JW: Preoperative preparation of the ear canal. Arch Otolaryngol 1965; 81: 564–565.
69. Hardy AV, Mitchell RB, Schreiber M, et al.: Bacteriological studies of otitis externa, 1951, 1952, 1953. Laryngoscope 1954; 64: 1020.
70. Donaldson SA, Snyder IS: Prophylactic chemotherapy in myringoplasty surgery. Laryngoscope 1966; 76: 1201–1214.
71. Perry ET, Nichols AC: Studies of the growth of bacteria in the human ear canal. J Invest Dermatol 1956; 27: 165–170.
72. Linthicum FH: Bacteria and stapedectomy. Arch Otolaryngol 1964; 80: 489–495.
73. Karma P, Jokipii AM, Ojala K, et al.: Bacteriology of the chronically discharging middle ear. Acta Otolaryngol 1978; 86: 110–114.
74. Harker LA, Koontz FP: Bacteriology of cholesteatoma: Clinical significance. Trans Am Acad Ophthal Otolaryngol 1977; 84: 683–686.
75. Brook I: Aerobic and anaerobic bacteriology of cholesteatoma. Laryngoscope 1981; 91: 250–253.
76. Sugita R, Kawamura S, Ichikawa G, et al.: Studies on anaerobic bacteria in chronic otitis media. Laryngoscope 1981; 91: 816–821.
77. Winerman I, Segal S, Man A: Effectiveness of prophylactic antibiotic treatment in mastoid surgery. Am J Otol 1981; 3: 65–67.
78. Jokipii AM, Karma P, Ojapa K: Anaerobic bacteria in chronic otitis media. Arch Otolaryngol 1977; 103: 278–280.
79. Bagger-Sjoback DE, Mendel L, Nord CE: The role of prophylactic antibiotics in middle ear surgery. Am J Otol 1987; 8: 519–523.
80. Palva T, Karja J, Palva A, et al.: Bacteria in the chronic ear: Pre- and post-operative evaluation. Pract Otorhinolaryngol 1969; 31: 30–45.
81. Deka R, Kacker SK: Chronic otitis media: A clinical and bacteriological study. Eye, Ear, Nose and Throat Monthly 1975; 54: 198–201.
82. Kenna M, Bluestone CD, Reilly JS, et al.: Medical management of chronic suppurative otitis media without cholesteatoma in children. Laryngoscope 1986; 96: 146–151.
83. Jackson CG. Antimicrobial prophylaxis in ear surgery. Thesis to the Triological Society, 1987, pp 1–51.
84. Antimicrobial Prophylaxis for Surgery. Medical Lett 1983; 25: 113–116.
85. Weinstein L: The misuse and use of antimicrobial agents. Chicago Med 1962; 65: 9–16.
86. Causse JB: Etiology and therapy of cochlear hydrops following stapedectomy. Am J Otol 1980; 1: 221–224.
87. Wright WK, Marmesh PJ: Anti-infection measures in stapes surgery. Arch Otolaryngol 1965; 81: 566–569.
88. Wolff O: Untoward sequelae eleven months following stapedectomy. Ann Otol Rhinol Laryngol 1964; 73: 297.
89. Sheehy JL, House HP: Causes of failure in stapes surgery. Laryngoscope 1962; 72: 10.
90. Shea JJ Jr: Complications of the stapedectomy operation. Ann Otol Rhinol Laryngol 1963; 72: 1109.
91. Rutledge LJ, Lewis ML, Sanabria F: Fatal meningitis related to stapes operation. Arch Otolaryngol 1963; 78: 263.
92. House HP: Early and late complications of stapes surgery. Arch Otolaryngol 1963; 78: 606.
93. Gristwood RE: Acute otitis media following the stapedectomy operation. J Laryngol Otol 1966; 80: 312–317.
94. Nadol JB Jr: Causes of failure of mastoidectomy for chronic otitis media. Laryngoscope 1985; 95: 410–413.
95. Glasscock ME III, Jackson CG, Nissen AJ, Schwaber MK: Postauricular undersurface tympanic membrane grafting: A followup report. Laryngoscope 1982; 92: 718–727.
96. Smyth GDL: Outline of surgical management in chronic ear disease. Otolaryngol Clin North Am 1972; 5: 59–77.
97. Lee KJ, Schuknecht HF: Results of tympanoplasty and mastoidectomy at the Massachusetts Eye and Ear Infirmary. Laryngoscope 1971; 81: 529–543.
98. Paparella WM, Kim CS: Mastoidectomy update. Laryngoscope 1977; 87: 1977–1989.
99. Woodhall B, Neil RG, Dratz HM: Ultraviolet irradiation as an adjunct to the control of postoperative neurosurgical infection. Ann Surg 1949; 129: 820–825.
100. Cruse PJE, Foord R: A 5-year prospective study of 23,649 surgical wounds. Arch Surg 1973; 107: 206–210.
101. Quartley GRC, Polyzoidis K: Intraoperative antibiotic prophylaxis in neurosurgery: A clinical study. Neurosurg 1981; 8: 669–671.
102. Haines SJ, Goodman ML: Antibiotic prophylaxis of postoperative neurosurgical wound infection. J Neurosurg 1982; 103–105.
103. Wright L: A survey of possible etiologic agents in postoperative craniotomy infections. J Neurosurg 1955; 25: 125–132.
104. Balch RE: Wound infections complicating neurosurgical procedures. J Neurosurg 1956; 26: 41–45.
105. Thornton GF, Fekety FR, Cluff LE: Studies of the epidemiology of staphylococcal infection: Seasonal variation. N Engl J Med 1964; 271: 1333–1337.
106. Savitz MH, Mails LI: Prophylactic clindamycin for neurosurgical patients. NY State J Med 1976; 76: 64–67.
107. Buckwold FJ, Hand R, Hansebour RR: Hospital-acquired bacterial meningitis in neurosurgical patients. J Neurosurg 1977; 46: 494–500.
108. Malis LI: Prevention of neurosurgical infection by intraoperative antibiotics. Neurosurg 1979; 5: 339–343.
109. Savitz MH, Katz SS: Prevention of primary wound infection in neurosurgical patients: A 10-year study. Neurosurg 1986; 18: 685–688.
110. Geraghty J, Feely M: Antibiotic prophylaxis in neurosurgery: A randomized, controlled trial. J Neurosurg 1984; 60: 724–726.
111. Kartush JM, Cannon SC, Bojrab DI, et al.: Use of bacitracin for neurotologic surgery. Laryngoscope 1988; 98: 1050–1054.

Martha E. Corcoran
John Y. Lim
Richard A. Chole

CHAPTER SEVENTY-ONE

Prophylaxis for Oral Surgery and Fractures of the Facial Skeleton

▼

Oral and maxillofacial surgical procedures may involve any class of wound. Procedures not involving an intraoral approach or violation of the upper respiratory tract fall into the class I category and should have correspondingly low postoperative infection rates. Transoral oral surgical procedures, transoral orthognathic procedures, and open facial fracture repair fall into class II and class III categories with correspondingly increased risks of postoperative wound complications. It is for these procedures and wound classifications that prophylactic antibiotics may be of benefit. Antibiotic therapy for class IV wounds (infected wounds) falls into the category of therapeutic rather than prophylactic treatment.

In transoral oral and maxillofacial surgery, microorganisms belonging to the endogenous oral microflora are the most frequent pathogens. The most likely contaminating organisms are streptococci, anaerobic gram-positive cocci, and anaerobic gram-negative rods.[1-3] According to Peterson,[4] it is unlikely that many postoperative infections following transoral procedures are the result of anaerobic bacteria; rather, the infections are more likely due to aerobic streptococci. And if the surgical procedure is to be done transcutaneously, the most likely organisms that would cause infection are colonizing staphylococci from the skin.

Midface fractures usually involve one or more sinuses. A healthy sinus is relatively sterile, but an infected sinus differs from the oral cavity with the addition of pathogenic *Streptococcus pneumoniae* and *Haemophilus influenzae*.[5]

When considering dental work and tooth extractions, including root canal work, microbes include the potentially dangerous obligate anaerobes. These are found in pulps of teeth with pulpal necrosis and periapical lucencies.[6]

The primary benefit of prophylactic antibiotics is reduction of the inoculum of viable bacteria in the wound at the time of surgery. Important factors in the selection of an antibiotic include the pharmacokinetics, the route, and the timing of administration. Two basic principles regarding antibiotic prophylaxis have been supported in the literature. First, to be effective, an antibiotic that is active against potential pathogens should be present in the tissue at the time of bacterial inoculation.[7] This is impossible to achieve in traumatic wounds. However, because bacteremia and reinoculation of potential pathogens may occur at the time of manipulation and fracture repair, perioperative antibiotic prophylaxis may be warranted. Second, a tissue concentration of antibiotic that is adequate to inhibit bacterial growth should be maintained for a sufficient period of time following the inoculation, generally not exceeding 24 hours.[7, 8]

CURRENT RECOMMENDATIONS

Fractures of the Facial Skeleton

Mandibular Fractures. Much has been written regarding the use of antibiotics with mandible fractures. Reported rates of infection following mandibular fractures vary 6%–50%.[9-11] In a nonrandomized prospective study James and colleagues[10] evaluated 422 mandible fractures. They found a postoperative infection rate of approximately 7% when antibiotics were used routinely for all patients with open fractures. In another nonrandomized study Zallen and Curry[11] treated 64 patients with open mandible fractures. They found a 6% rate of infection in patients treated with antibiotics and a 50% rate of infection without antibiotic treatment. There were no control groups in either of these reports. In a prospective randomized clinical trial Chole and Yee[9] examined the effectiveness of cefazolin administration during the perioperative period in preventing postoperative infections in a variety of facial fractures. When all patients were considered there was an overall prevalence of postoperative infections of 42% in the non–antibiotic-treated group and a 9% infection rate in the antibiotic-treated group. Antibiotic treatment resulted in a significantly reduced incidence of infection over controls (p = .0001). All infections in patients with facial fractures occurred at the site of the parasymphyseal body or angle jaw fractures with one exception. There were no infections in patients with subcondylar (closed) mandibular fractures.

Potential sources of bacterial contamination following open mandibular fractures include mucous membrane tears, lacerations of skin, and teeth. If teeth are carious or nonvital they may pose an even greater risk of infection secondary to the greater bacterial inoculum or the potential foreign body reaction caused by a nonvital tooth.

All mandibular fractures involving teeth must be considered open (compound) fractures and at higher risk for infection. In a large series of patients undergoing open reduction and internal fixation of mandibular fractures, 50% of the patients who acquired postoperative infections had angle fractures with a tooth in the fracture line. Extraction of the tooth in the fracture line had no bearing on the postoperative infection rate.[10] In the study by Zallen and Curry,[11] there was no correlation between removal or retention of teeth and an increased complication rate. Chuong and colleagues,[12] in a retrospective analysis of 327 fractures of the mandible, found no significant difference in complication rates when cases with teeth in the line of injury treated by extraction were compared with those cases treated with retention of teeth. Their indications for extractions include teeth in the line of injury that are significantly mobile, teeth that have root exposure in distracted fractures, or teeth that interfere with either reduction or fixation of fractures.

The evidence supports the use of perioperative antibiotics for all open mandible fractures, and there is little evidence to support the use of perioperative antibiotics for closed fractures. With appropriate case selection and antibiotic treatment, healthy teeth can be retained in a fracture line. Because of the high bacterial inoculum in infected teeth (i.e., gross caries, pulpal necrosis, and periapical lucencies), therapeutic rather than prophylactic doses of antibiotics should be considered. Cefazolin, penicillin, and erythromycin have been used successfully as prophylaxis in mandibular fracture repair.[9, 11]

- Antibiotic prophylaxis is effective for open mandibular fractures, and there is no evidence to support its use in closed fractures.

Midface Fractures: Le Fort and Zygomatic Complex. Midface fractures may be open or closed. Open fractures potentially communicate with the sinuses, the nasal cavity, the nasopharynx, or the oral cavity including upper dentition. The sinuses are usually considered sterile, but they may become infected when blood and secretions within sinuses act as culture media. They also have potential for skull base involvement including cerebrospinal fluid leak and orbital penetration. Open fractures are considered class II wounds, and significant postoperative infection rates may be expected. Closed fractures, such as an isolated zygomatic arch fracture, are considered clean or class I wounds with correspondingly low infection rates.

Infection rates following maxillary fractures or fracture repair are low.[9, 13, 14] Ellis[14] states that the rate of infection following either a zygomatic fracture or fracture reduction is extremely low; however it is difficult to discern because many surgeons use prophylaxis as a matter of routine. In a prospective randomized clinical trial, Chole and Yee[9] found no infections in patients treated for maxillary fractures or zygomatic fractures. Of 101 patients evaluated there were 24 zygomatic fractures and 6 Le Fort fractures with no postoperative infections regardless of therapy. In a double-blind, randomized study evaluating the efficacy of perioperative antibiotic therapy in head and neck surgery, Eschelman and colleagues[13] found no infections in patients with maxillary and zygomatic fractures treated by open reduction and internal fixation (nine patients received antibiotics perioperatively, and six patients received placebo).

Infectious orbital complications including cellulitis, abscess, cavernous sinus thrombophlebitis, brain abscess, and meningitis may follow a traumatic orbital injury; therefore, some authors recommend antibiotic coverage during orbital repair.[15]

Because the sinuses, nasal cavity, nasopharynx, or oral cavity may be involved in these fractures, prophylactic antibiotics are appropriate on a theoretical basis. However, in the absence of infection there are 10 data to support the routine use of antibiotic prophylaxis for these fractures.

- There is no support for the routine use of antibiotics in the treatment of midface fractures.

Frontal Sinus Fractures. Complications following repair of frontal sinus fractures include wound infections, cerebrospinal fluid (CSF) leak, meningitis, and mucocele formation. The overall rate of wound complications after fracture repair is approximately 10%.[16–18]

Two retrospective reviews reported 10% and 11% infection rates following surgery.[16, 17] These reviews did not clarify whether antibiotics were used in the perioperative period. Duvall and colleagues[19] reported very few postoperative wound infections in their retrospective review of 112 patients treated for frontal sinus fractures. Antibiotics were used in all cases of displaced anterior and posterior wall fractures. Two thirds of the patients with nondisplaced anterior wall fractures received antibiotics. A variety of antibiotic regimens were used in therapeutic rather than prophylactic doses (10- to 15-day therapy). These data suggest that antibiotic therapy for most frontal sinus fractures results in a low rate of postoperative infection. However, it is not clear from the available data whether antibiotic therapy is indicated for anterior wall fractures, nor is it clear whether antibiotic administration in prophylactic rather than therapeutic doses is beneficial.

Antibiotic prophylaxis to prevent meningitis with traumatic CSF leak is controversial because studies have not shown a reduction in the incidence of meningitis in patients who have received prophylaxis. In fact, after 5 days of systemic antibiotics the nasopharynx usually becomes colonized with more resistant organisms, usually acquired in the hospital setting, making ultimate therapy for meningitis more complicated.[20]

- Antibiotics are probably indicated for displaced anterior and posterior wall fractures and probably not indicated for isolated anterior wall fractures (Table 71–1).

Oral Surgical and Dental Procedures

The incidence of postoperative infections for oral surgical procedures varies depending on the procedure. Dentoalveolar surgery, including extraction of erupted and impacted teeth,

Table 71–1. ROUTINE ANTIBIOTIC PROPHYLAXIS AND MAXILLOFACIAL SURGERY

Operation Type		Antibiotic	Special Notes
Mandibular Fractures	Open	Cefazolin	Antibiotics not needed for closed fractures
Maxillary Fractures	Zygomatic	None	
	Le Fort	None	
Frontal Sinus Fractures		Unclear	Not needed for isolated anterior wall
Oral Surgery		Penicillin or erythromycin	
Orthognathic Surgery		None	

cystectomies, apical surgery, periodontal surgery, and other minor surgical procedures on soft and hard oral tissues, has an overall postoperative infection rate of approximately 4%. Infection rates with other procedures range 2%–37%.[1, 21–26]

Many patients with periapical lucencies and pulpal necrosis may require extensive dental intervention, including root canal procedures and periapical instrumentation. It has been shown that pulpal tissue in patients with pulpal necrosis and periapical lucencies is invariably infected.[6] With root canal and periapical work, postoperative infections may be indicated by flare-ups. Flare-ups are considered by most authors to be related to infection.[4] Postoperative flare-ups may be reduced by treatment with antibiotics perioperatively as shown by several authors.

In a series of studies by Morse and colleagues[21–24, 26] antibiotic administration in patients with asymptomatic pulpal necrosis and periapical radiographic lucencies was evaluated. A 20% flare-up prevalence was found in the nontreatment group, whereas the flare-up prevalence fell to 1% in the patient group treated with perioperative penicillin. Their overall flare-up prevalence was 2%. In a double-blind, randomized trial of 100 patients treated for pulpal necrosis and periapical lucencies, Mata and colleagues[25] also found a significant difference between placebo and penicillin groups with respect to flare-ups. The postoperative flare-up prevalence for the placebo group was 18% and only 2% for the group treated with penicillin (p<.05). Similar postoperative flare-up rates (2%) have occurred with high-dose, 1-day regimens of erythromycin as well.[21, 22, 26]

The reduction in prevalence of postoperative flare-ups is important; serious complications may occur after therapy from originally asymptomatic pulpal necrosis and periapical lucencies as evidenced by septicemias and early Ludwig's angina as seen in other studies.[24] In overview, the evidence is substantial that the use of perioperative (prophylactic) antibiotic therapy with either penicillin or erythromycin significantly reduced the incidence of flare-ups than when antibiotics were not used.

Josefsson and colleagues[27] looked at the effect of antibiotic prophylaxis on bacteremia in 60 oral surgical procedures, consisting mainly of noninfected mandibular third-molar extractions. They found that during the operation, the total number of bacteria in blood was lower in the antibiotic treatment groups than in the nonantibiotic treatment groups. In Josefsson's study, the number of patients with anaerobic bacteremias during surgery was similar in all groups. But 10 minutes after surgery, levels of anaerobic bacteria were significantly lower in the groups administered antibiotics. This study demonstrates the value of perioperative antibiotics in reducing bacteremias during and following surgery. These findings support the use of antibiotics for third-molar extraction procedures in situations where minimization of bacteremias is desirable (i.e., endocarditis prophylaxis).

- Antibiotics are indicated in patients undergoing treatment for periapical lucencies and pulpal necrosis.
- Perioperative antibiotics are indicated for selected patients undergoing third-molar extractions.

Orthognathic Surgery

Infection rates following orthognathic surgery are relatively low. Reported infection rates vary 1%–11%.[28–30] Extraoral

procedures performed with sterile technique without communication with the oral cavity should have a very low risk of postoperative infection and therefore require no antibiotic coverage.[31] The role of prophylactic antibiotic therapy in intraoral orthognathic surgery remains controversial.

A survey of 114 oral and maxillofacial surgery residency programs demonstrated that most used antibiotics routinely with intraoral orthognathic procedures. However, no consistent protocol for the type, method, or duration of antibiotic administration was found.[32]

Martis and Karabouta[30] reviewed a large series of orthognathic procedures. Multiple procedures were performed through the intraoral approach. These included sagittal splitting osteotomy, anterior maxillary osteotomy, subapical osteotomy, sliding genioplasty, corticotomy, and vertical ramus osteotomy. Of 76 procedures undertaken without antibiotic prophylaxis, none caused acute perioperative infections. The authors also found a very low rate of infection (0.26%) in the antibiotic-treated group. Their results confirm that infections after orthognathic surgery are rare even in the absence of prophylactic antibiotics.

Peterson and Booth[29] looked at the effect of prophylactic antibiotics on the prevalence of postoperative wound infections in intraoral orthognathic surgery. The types of intraoral surgery examined included alveolar segmental osteotomies of the maxilla and mandible and subcondylar and sagittal osteotomies of the ramus of the mandible. Antibiotic prophylaxis was used in 35 cases, and no prophylaxis was used in 65. The overall prevalence of infection was 11.4% and 11.1%, respectively. On the basis of the data gathered, they concluded that antibiotics should not be used routinely in intraoral orthognathic surgery.

Yratstorza[28] reviewed 148 orthognathic surgery patients during an 11-year span. Fifty-eight received antibiotic prophylaxis, with infections developing in three of these patients. No infections occurred in the patients who did not receive antibiotic prophylaxis. He concluded that this study disproves the necessity for routine prophylactic use of antibiotics in maxillomandibular osteotomies by either intraoral or extraoral approaches.

It appears that the routine use of prophylactic antibiotics for orthognathic surgery is not justified. Their use should be considered in patients with systemic problems or for those patients undergoing procedures requiring sizable bone grafts or alloplastic material implants.

- The routine use of prophylactic antibiotics for orthognathic surgery is not justified. Their use should be considered in patients with systemic problems or for those patients undergoing procedures requiring sizable bone grafts or alloplastic material implants.

Special Considerations

Dental Hygiene. Chole and Yee[9] suggested factors likely to contribute to an increased risk of infection following mandibular fracture repair. These include poor dental hygiene, lack of dental care, and complex injuries in some patients. A logistic regression in their study showed no significant effect of delay of therapy on infection rate in either the antibiotic or the control groups. Other investigators have also shown no increase in postoperative infection rates when mandibular fracture repair was delayed beyond 24 hours.

References

1. Heimdahl A, Nord CE: Antimicrobial prophylaxis in oral surgery. Scan J Infect Dis (Suppl) 1990; 70: 91–101.
2. Matsen JM: The frequency of bacterial pathogens in infections potentially preventable by antimicrobial prophylaxis. Scan J Infect Dis (Suppl) 1990; 70: 9–17.
3. Olson M, O'Connor M, Schwartz ML: Surgical wound infections: A 5-year prospective study of 20,193 wounds at the Minneapolis VA Medical Center. Ann Surg 1984; 199: 253–259.
4. Peterson LJ: Antibiotic prophylaxis against wound infections in oral and maxillofacial surgery. J Oral Maxillofac Surg 1990; 48: 617.
5. Cook HE, Haber J: Bacteriology of the maxillary sinus. J Oral Maxillofac Surg 1987; 45: 1011.
6. Finegold SM, Sutter VL: Anaerobic Infections. Kalamazoo: The Upjohn Co., 1983, p 58.
7. Burke JF: The effective period of preventive antibiotic action in experimental incisions and dermal lesions. Surg 1961; 50: 161–168.
8. Stone HH, Haney BB, Kolb LD, et al.: Prophylactic and preventive antibiotic therapy. Ann Surg 1979; 189: 691–699.
9. Chole RA, Yee J: Antibiotic prophylaxis for facial fractures. Arch Otolaryngol 1987; 113: 1055.
10. James RB, Fredrickson C, Kent JN: Prospective study of mandibular fractures. J Oral Surg 1981; 39: 275–281.
11. Zallen RD, Curry JT: A study of antibiotic usage in compound mandibular fractures. J Oral Surg 1975; 3: 431–434.
12. Chuong R, Donoff RB, Guralnick WC: A retrospective analysis of 327 mandibular fractures. J Oral Maxillofac Surg 1983; 41: 305–309.
13. Eschelman LT, Schleuning AJ, Frummett RE: Prophylactic antibiotics in otolaryngologic surgery: A double-blind study. Trans Am Acad Ophthamol Otolaryngol 1971; 75: 387–394.
14. Ellis E: Fractures of the zygomatic complex and arch. In: Finseca RJ, and Walker RW (eds): Oral and Maxillofacial Trauma, vol. 1. Philadelphia: WB Saunders Co., 1991, p 435.
15. Mathog RH, Crane LR, Nowak GS: Antimicrobial therapy following head and neck trauma. In: Johnson JT (ed): Antibiotic Therapy in Head and Neck Surgery. New York: Marcel Dekker, 1987, pp 31–49.
16. Wallis A, Donald PJ: Frontal sinus fractures: A review of 72 cases. Laryngoscope 1988; 98: 593–598.
17. Wilson BC, Davidson B, Corey JP, Haydon RC: Comparison of complications following frontal sinus fractures managed with exploration with or without obliteration over 10 years. Laryngoscope 1988; 98: 516–520.
18. Larabee WF, Travis LW, Tabb HG: Frontal sinus fractures: Their suppurative complications and surgical management. Laryngoscope 1980; 90: 1810–1813.
19. Duvall AJ, Porto DP, Lyons D, Boies LR: Frontal sinus fractures: Arch Otolaryngol Head Neck Surg 1987; 113: 933–935.
20. Neely JG, Fine DP, Reynolds AF: The use of prophylactic antibiotics in patients with cerebrospinal fluid otorrhea and rhinorrhea. In: Johnson JT (ed): Antibiotic Treatment in Head and Neck Surgery. New York: Marcel Dekker, 1987, pp 103–111.
21. Morse DR, Koran LZ, Esposito JV, et al.: Asymptomatic teeth with necrotic pulps and associated periapical radiolucencies: Relationship of flare-ups to endodontic instrumentation, antibiotic usage, and stress in three separate practices at three different time periods. Part 1: 1963–1970. Int J Psychosom 1986; 33: 5–17.
22. Morse DR, Koran LZ, Esposito JV, et al.: Asymptomatic teeth with necrotic pulps and associated periapical radiolucencies: Relationship of flare-ups to endodontic instrumentation, antibiotic usage, and stress in three separate practices at three different time periods. Part 2: 1978–1983. Int J Psychosom 1986; 33: 18–30.
23. Morse DR, Koran LZ, Esposito JV, et al.: Asymptomatic teeth with necrotic pulps and associated periapical radiolucencies: Relationship of flare-ups to endodontic instrumentation, antibiotic usage, and stress in three separate practices at three different time periods. Part 3: 1983–1985. In J Psychosom 1986; 33: 31–37.
24. Morse DR, Furst ML, Belott RM, et al.: Infectious flare-ups and serious sequelae following endodontic treatment: A prospective randomized trial on efficacy of antibiotic prophylaxis in cases of asymptomatic pulpal-periapical lesions. Oral Surg Oral Med Oral Pathol 1987; 64: 96–109.
25. Mata E, Koren LZ, Morse DR, Sinai IH: Prophylactic use of penicillin V in teeth with necrotic pulps and asymptomatic periapical radiolucencies. Oral Surg Oral Med Oral Pathol 1985; 60: 201–207.
26. Abbott AA, Koren LZ, Morse DR, et al.: A prospective randomized trial on efficacy of antibiotic prophylaxis in asymptomatic teeth with pulpal necrosis and associated periapical pathosis. Oral Surg Oral Med Oral Path 1988; 66: 722–733.
27. Josefsson K, Heimdahl A, von Konow L, Nord CE: Effect of phenoxymethylpenicillin and erythromycin prophylaxis on anaerobic bacteremia after oral surgery. J Antimicrob Chemother 1985; 16: 243–251.
28. Yratstorza JA: Indications for antibiotics in orthognathic surgery. J Oral Surg 1976; 34: 514–516.
29. Peterson LJ, Booth DF: Efficacy of antibiotic prophylaxis in intraoral orthognathic surgery. J Oral Surg 1976; 34: 1088–1091.
30. Martis C, Karabouta I: Infection after orthognathic surgery, with and without preventive antibiotics. Int J Oral Surg 1984; 13: 490–494.
31. Zallen RD, Strader RJ: The use of prophylactic antibiotics in extraoral procedures for mandibular prognathism. J Oral Surg 1971; 29: 178–179.
32. Heit JM, Farhood VW, Edwards RC: Survey of antibiotic prophylaxis for intraoral orthognathic surgery. J Oral Maxillofac Surg 1991; 49: 340–342.

Index

▼